EDITION

10

Lippincott Review for
NCLEX-PN®

Barbara Kuhn Timby, RN, BC, BSN, MA
Professor Emeritus
Glen Oaks Community College
Centreville, Michigan

Diana L. Rupert, RN, CNE, MSN, PhD
Administrator
Indiana County Technology Center
School of Practical Nursing
Assistant Professor,
Nursing and Allied Health Professions
Indiana University of Pennsylvania
Indiana, Pennsylvania

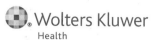
Wolters Kluwer
Health

Philadelphia • Baltimore • New York • London
Buenos Aires • Hong Kong • Sydney • Tokyo

Acquisitions Editor: Renee Gagliardi
Product Development Editor: Bernadette Enneg
Design Coordinator: Joan Wendt
Production Project Manager: Cynthia Rudy
Manufacturing Coordinator: Kathleen Brown
Production Service: SPi Global

10th edition

9 8 7 6 5 4 3 2 1

Printed in China

Library of Congress Cataloging-in-Publication Data
Timby, Barbara Kuhn, author.
  Lippincott's review for NCLEX-PN®. — Tenth edition / Barbara Kuhn Timby, Diana L. Rupert.
      p. ; cm.
  Includes bibliographical references and index.
  ISBN 978-1-4698-4534-0 (alk. paper)
  I. Rupert, Diana L., author. II. Title.
  [DNLM: 1. Nursing, Practical—Examination Questions. WY 18.2]
  RT62
  610.7306'93076—dc23
                                                                                      2013049592

LWW.com

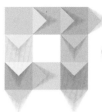 **Contributors**

Coauthors of Previous Editions

Ann Carmack, RN, MSN
Director of Nursing
Brown Mackie College
Lenexa, Kansas

Jeanne C. Scherer, RN, BSN, MS
*Formerly Assistant Director and Medical-Surgical
  Coordinator*
Sisters School of Nursing
Buffalo, New York

Contributor to Previous Editions

Bennita W. Vaughans, RN, MSN
Instructor
Practical Nursing Program
Councill Trenholm State Technical College
Montgomery, Alabama

Reviewers for Current and Previous Editions

Barbara Avent, BSN, RN
Program Coordinator
Tennessee Technology Center at Jackson
Jackson, Tennessee

Holli Benge, MSN, RN
Department Chair, Vocational Nursing
Tyler Junior College
Tyler, Texas

Robin Brown, RN, MS
Practical Nursing Department Head
Lake Area Technical Institute
Watertown, South Dakota

Maureen Heaton, RN, MSN
Associate Professor
Northern Michigan University
School of Nursing
Marquette, Michigan

Frances Leibfreid, RN, BSN, MEd
Professor and Director of Nursing Education
Allegany College of Maryland
Cumberland, Maryland

Paula Molina-Shaver, RN-BS, BSN
Program Head, Practical Nursing
Boise State University
College of Applied Technology
Nampa, Idaho

Nancy Strassner, BS, MPA
PN Coordinator
Wayne-Finger Lakes Board of Cooperative
  Educational Services
Newark, New Jersey

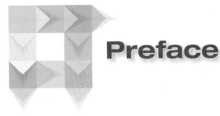

Preface

Lippincott Review for NCLEX-PN®, Tenth Edition, has been written to help the candidate prepare for the National Council Licensure Examination for Practical/Vocational Nurses (NCLEX-PN®). Several features make this review book especially helpful.

First and foremost, the most recent NCLEX-PN® Test Plan approved by the National Council of State Boards of Nursing (effective April 2014) was used as a guide for preparing this book. Consequently, the review questions presented here reflect the components in the Test Plan as well as current nursing practice. In addition, the substance of the questions is based entirely on information contained in textbooks that are widely used in practical nursing programs throughout the United States.

An effort has also been made to divide the book content into comprehensive yet manageable sections. To accomplish this goal, the topics for review are organized into four major units according to specialty areas of nursing practice:

- Unit 1: The Nursing Care of Adults with Medical-Surgical Disorders
- Unit 2: The Nursing Care of the Childbearing Family
- Unit 3: The Nursing Care of Children
- Unit 4: The Nursing Care of Clients with Mental Health Needs.

The decision to arrange the content according to specific subject areas was made for several reasons. First, it helps correlate the review with courses commonly taught in most practical nursing programs. Second, it allows energy to be focused on reviewing a limited amount of information at any one time.

The four major units are further subdivided into a total of 16 separate review tests. The first unit, which pertains to the nursing care of clients with medical-surgical disorders, contains 10 review tests. The remaining three units each contain 2 review tests. This distribution is appropriate because medical-surgical nursing is the most common clinical area where new practical nurses are employed. In addition, the Test Plan is based on a job survey of newly employed practical nurses 6 months after

their graduation; therefore, it is logical to assume that most of the licensing examination questions will reflect items of a medical-surgical nature.

All of the questions in the review tests are integrated in the same manner as in the licensing examination. This means that each test question—whether it concerns a medical-surgical, obstetric, pediatric, or mental health situation—reflects a specific category and subcategory of client need. Both of these test components are discussed further in *Frequently Asked Questions*, page vii.

Another helpful feature of this review book is the fifth unit, which consists of a two-part Comprehensive Examination that follows the 16 review tests. The examination, beginning on page 619, is as much like the national licensing examination as possible. Like the NCLEX-PN®, the questions in the Comprehensive Examination are a mix of all nursing content areas and the Test Plan components.

The two Comprehensive Examinations contain a total of 261 items. The number of questions in each test is slightly higher than the average number of items answered by candidates on the NCLEX-PN®—112 items in an average of 2 hours, 14 minutes in 2011 (National Council of State Boards of Nursing, 2013). Taken in total, the Comprehensive Examination provides practice with more than the maximum of 205 questions asked on the NCLEX-PN®, and it offers a rough estimate of how long it might take to answer all the potential NCLEX-PN® items, should that possibility occur.

In addition to the review tests and two-part Comprehensive Examination in the text, the accompanying Web site (http://thepoint.lww.com/TimbyNCLEX10e) provides a way to realistically simulate the computerized method for taking the NCLEX-PN®. You can use the questions on the Web site to test yourself in several ways: by general content area, by number of questions, or by time. This functionality allows you to tailor your studying to the specific areas in which you need practice or to the time you have available in a study session, while simulating the NCLEX-PN® as closely as possible.

Other advantages to using this book include the sections containing the *Correct Answers, Rationales, and*

Test Taking Strategies, which follow each review test and comprehensive examination. These sections provide the best answer to each test question; the rationale for the correct answer, and reasons why the other answer choices are incorrect; a test taking strategy to guide the selection of the answer to the question; the Cognitive Level of the question; and the Test Plan Category and Subcategory. These are discussed later in the *Frequently Asked Questions* section. Reading the rationales and information included in the test-taking strategies is an excellent technique for reviewing the domain of practical nursing.

In summary, there are more than 1,800 items in the 16 review tests and 261 items in the two-part comprehensive examination, for a total of more than 2,000 items. The items that compose the 16 review tests and comprehensive exams are found on the Web site (http://thepoint.lww.com/ TimbyNCLEX10e), along with additional alternative-format items with audio clips. Although it is unreasonable to believe that any item in this book will be identical to one in the national examination, it is reasonable to expect that the NCLEX-PN® will test similar content, knowledge, and skills. Although no review book or licensing examination can cover all aspects of nursing, this book serves as a resource for a comprehensive review and realistic simulation of the NCLEX-PN® process.

As a candidate for the NCLEX-PN®, you will benefit by reading the section titled *Frequently Asked Questions,* which begins on page vii. This section provides information about the NCLEX-PN® testing process, how the test is designed, and suggestions on how to prepare for the examination. The National Council of State Boards of Nursing Web site (www.ncsbn.org) provides the most up-to-date information on the Test Plan and the testing process. The *How to Use This Book* section, which begins on page xv, introduces you to the testing format used in this review book.

Although this book's primary purpose is to help practical nurses prepare for the national licensing examination, it can serve other purposes as well. For example, it can be used to study for various types of achievement tests in nursing. Inactive practical nurses who wish to return to nursing will also find the book useful for review and self-appraisal, as will others who seek course credit by taking challenge examinations for advanced placement. And, finally, faculty may find the book helpful for developing expertise in test construction. However, regardless of the many purposes for which this book may be used, its ultimate goal is to help candidates prepare for the national licensing examination (NCLEX-PN®), demonstrating their ability to provide safe, effective nursing care.

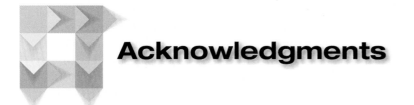

Acknowledgments

Many thanks to Diana Rupert, coauthor of this edition, for updating and revising test items as well as generating new material. The authors express sincere thanks for the contributions of Ann Carmack, RN, MSN, coauthor of the ninth edition, Bennita Vaughans, RN, MSN, contributor to the sixth edition, and Jeanne C. Scherer, RN, BSN, MS, coauthor of the fourth edition, whose previous work made this revision easier.

Finally, recognition is due for the conscientious assistance from the editors and staff who have helped develop this book through its various stages of production. Among that legion, the authors wish to thank Renee Gagliardi, Digital Product Manager, Bernadette Enneg, Associate Digital Product Manager, and Cynthia Rudy, Production Manager.

Barbara Kuhn Timby, RN, BC, BSN, MA

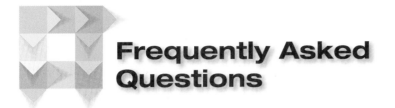

Frequently Asked Questions

The following are frequently asked questions concerning the NCLEX-PN® and the most current information that is available about the testing process.

What is the NCLEX-PN®?

The abbreviation *NCLEX-PN*® stands for the National Council Licensure Examination for Practical/Vocational Nurses. In short, the NCLEX-PN® is a computerized test developed by the National Council of State Boards of Nursing. The test is used to regulate the licensing of practical and vocational nurses in each of its member states.

> **MEMBERS OF THE NATIONAL COUNCIL OF STATE BOARDS OF NURSING**
>
> Members include representatives from:
>
> - All 50 United States
> - District of Columbia
> - Guam
> - American Samoa
> - Virgin Islands
> - Northern Mariana Islands

What is the purpose of the NCLEX-PN®?

All National Council member states and territories currently use the NCLEX-PN® as the standard for licensing practical and vocational nurses. *Practical nurse* and *vocational nurse* are regional terms; they differ in name only. Whether referred to as practical or vocational, each nurse completes similar educational programs, and graduates from both take the NCLEX-PN®. The terms *practical nurse* and *practical nursing* are used in this book to refer to both.

Licensing serves to assure the public that a graduate practical nurse is a competent practitioner. Passing the NCLEX-PN® demonstrates that a graduate of a practical nursing program can perform entry-level nursing skills that meet the needs of clients who have common health problems with predictable outcomes and demonstrate at least a minimum level of competency.

Can foreign-educated nurses take the NCLEX-PN®?

Foreign-educated nurses can take the NCLEX-PN®. However, before taking the test, they must first meet eligibility requirements in the state where they wish to practice. In most states, foreign-educated nurses are asked to present credentials describing their course of study in the country where they were schooled.

How is the NCLEX-PN® developed?

Before the examination is administered, it goes through several stages of development.

> **STEPS IN THE NCLEX-PN® TEST DEVELOPMENT**
>
> - Survey newly licensed practical nurses every 3 years
> - Analyze practical nurse job responsibilities
> - Formulate a test plan based on the data
> - Select and approve item writers
> - Submit questions to item reviewers
> - Implement trial testing of items
> - Give state boards of nursing an opportunity to review items
> - Obtain approval of NCLEX-PN® test items
> - Maintain two alternating NCLEX-PN® test pools

What is the NCLEX-PN® Test Plan?

The Test Plan, which changes from time to time, serves as the framework for the content that is included in the NCLEX-PN®. The current Test Plan, implemented in April 2014, is based on the results of a study called the *Report of Findings from the 2012 LPN/LVN Practical Analysis: Linking the NCLEX-PN® Examination to Practice*. This study sampled data from newly licensed practical nurses who provided information on how often they performed each of the studied nursing activities, the impact of the nursing activities on their clients' well-being, and the settings in which the activities were performed.

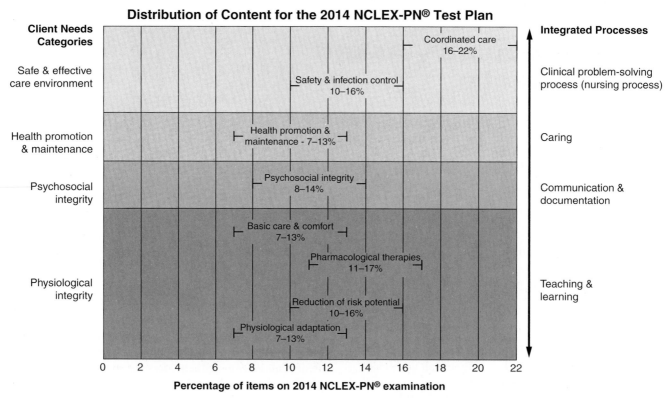

Distribution of Content for the 2014 NCLEX-PN® Test Plan

(From National Council of State Boards of Nursing, Inc. [NCSBN]. *NCLEX-PN® Examination: Test Plan for the National Council Licensure Examination for Licensed Practical/Vocational Nurses.* Chicago, IL: National Council of State Boards of Nursing, Inc. [NCSBN]. Copyright by the National Council of State Boards of Nursing, Inc. All rights reserved.)

The tabulated results of the job analysis study influence the subject matter tested and the percentage of questions asked in particular NCLEX-PN® test categories. The test categories on the current NCLEX-PN® Test Plan follow the framework of Client Needs Categories and Client Needs Subcategories. (See Structure of the Test Plan below.)

The distribution of 2014 NCLEX-PN® test items in the Client Needs Categories and Subcategories is as follows:

- Physiological integrity
  – Basic care and comfort, 7% to 13%
  – Pharmacological therapies, 11% to 17%
  – Reduction of risk potential, 10% to 16%
  – Physiological adaptation, 7% to 13%
- Safe and effective care environment
  – Coordinated care, 16% to 22%
  – Safety and infection control, 10% to 16%
- Health promotion and maintenance, 7% to 13%
- Psychosocial integrity, 8% to 14%

Client Needs Categories and Subcategories

Of the four Client Needs Categories, the emphasis is on physiological integrity. Safe and effective care environment is the next most important; health promotion and maintenance and psychosocial integrity are equally rated.

Physiological Integrity

This category tests the candidates' knowledge in the following areas:

- Basic care and comfort—providing comfort and assistance in performance of activities of daily living
- Pharmacologic therapies—providing care related to administration of medications and monitoring clients receiving parenteral therapies
- Reduction of risk potential—reducing the possibility of developing complications or additional health problems related to treatments, procedures, or existing conditions
- Physiological adaptation—providing care during acute and chronic phases of health disorders, including emergency situations.

Safe, Effective Care Environment

This category covers questions concerning:

- Coordinated care—providing care and collaborating with health team members to coordinate client care, including legal and ethical issues
- Safety and infection control—protecting clients and health care personnel from injury.

Health Promotion and Maintenance

This category tests the candidate's ability to answer questions about the expected stages of growth and development and the prevention or early detection of health problems.

Psychosocial Integrity

This category covers questions concerning the promotion and support of the emotional, mental, and social well-being of clients.

Integrated processes

Clinical problem solving process (nursing process) is integrated throughout the Client Needs Categories and Subcategories. This review book codes all questions according to the Client Needs Categories and Subcategories. Other integrated processes—caring, communication and documentation, teaching, and learning—are represented as well.

What is the style of questions asked on the NCLEX-PN®?

The NCLEX-PN® is composed primarily of multiple-choice questions. A multiple-choice question, also called an *item,* has two main parts: the *stem* and the *options.*

The stem

The *stem* presents the problem or situation that requires a solution. The stem of an NCLEX-PN® multiple-choice item is stated as a question in a complete sentence. If all the essential information for answering the question is contained in the stem, it is called a *stand-alone item.* Sometimes in this book the stem is preceded by a *case scenario,* which gives background information that is pertinent to the item or to a group of items that follow the case scenario.

The options

The *options* are the choices from which an answer is selected. There are four options in multiple-choice questions. The options on the NCLEX-PN® are labeled *1, 2, 3,* and *4.* In this type of question, there is one correct answer among the choices given. The three incorrect options, called *distractors,* are intended to appear as good answers; they may even be partially correct. But an option is incorrect if it is not the best answer to the question.

Alternative-format questions

In addition to the traditional four-option multiple-choice questions, the NCLEX-PN® also includes alternative-format questions. These are as follows:

- Multiple-response multiple-choice questions that provide four to six options from which the candidate must select all applicable answers, of which a minimum of two options are correct; at least one option is incorrect; and all options will never be correct
- Fill-in-the-blank questions, which require the candidate to use an on-screen calculator to solve dosage problems or make conversions; instructions for rounding are provided in the stem
- Hot-spot questions, which require the candidate to use the computer mouse to click onto an appropriate area on a graphic image appearing on the computer screen
- Ordered-response questions, which require the candidate to arrange all the options sequentially or chronologically by clicking and dragging the items using the computer mouse

- Multimedia-response questions, which require the candidate to arrive at the correct answer by reviewing information presented in a chart, table, graph, sound, or video clip.

Most of the questions on the NCLEX-PN®, however, are of the traditional variety—multiple-choice questions with four options—and these standard questions make up the bulk of this review book.

STANDARD MULTIPLE-CHOICE STEM AND OPTIONS

Which nursing assessment finding best justifies withholding the continued I.M. administration of penicillin (Bicillin) until consulting with the prescribing physician?

[ ]   1. The client states that the injection sites are painful.
[ ]   2. The client shows the nurse a red, itchy rash.*
[ ]   3. The client's oral body temperature is 100° F (37.8° C).
[ ]   4. The client has been having two stools a day.

*Correct answer

How is the NCLEX-PN® administered?

The NCLEX-PN® is a computerized adaptive test. The term *adaptive* means that the computer creates a unique test for each candidate. (See "How does the computer select test questions?" for more information.)

The computerized method of testing offers several advantages over the earlier pencil and paper method of taking the NCLEX-PN® that was offered only twice a year. For example, it:

- Facilitates year-round testing
- Offers convenient scheduling choices
- Personalizes the test for each candidate
- Shortens the length of the examination
- Expedites notification of test results.

A candidate may request any testing site regardless of the state in which he or she wishes to be licensed. Because the test is adapted to each candidate, it can be completed in 5 hours or less; the average time is just over 2 hours (National Council of State Boards of Nursing, 2013). Also, because scoring is computerized, examination results are available more rapidly than in the past.

What is the testing site like?

Each of more than 4,400 Pearson VUE testing sites, the world's largest network of test centers in 175 countries around the world, is able to accommodate multiple candidates at the same time. Each candidate is assigned to a separate testing cubicle that contains a computer with an on-screen calculator and other functional keys, note board, and marker. Personal articles can be placed in secured storage or lockers outside the test room.

Persons with special physical needs, or those requesting modifications in the testing process or environment, must make that information known to the board of nursing at the time of application. A letter from a professional (usually the director of the nursing program) confirming the candidate's disability is also required. If the board of nursing approves the applicant's request, special accommodations are made if they do not jeopardize the security of the test or give the candidate an unfair advantage.

Precautions are taken to ensure that the candidate who is registered for the NCLEX-PN® and the person about to take the test are one and the same.

Once the examination commences, test security is maintained in two ways. All candidates are observed directly and continuously by a proctor who can view the testing cubicles without entering the room. In addition, candidates are monitored by video and audio equipment that has taping capability.

TEST SITE SECURITY POLICIES

Before the test, each person must:

- Possess an Authorization to Test (ATT) affidavit.*
- Present two forms of signature identification.
  - One must contain a recent photograph.
  - The name on the photograph identification must match exactly the name on the ATT.
- Be photographed, fingerprinted, and provide a signature at the test site. A fingerprint is required each time a candidate exits and reenters the testing area.
- No hats, scarves, coats, papers, books, food, drinks, lip balm, medical aids or devices, pens, wallets, watches, cameras, beepers, cell phones, or other electronic devices like pagers or hand-held computers are allowed in the testing room, and in the case of weapons they are not allowed in the testing center itself. Personal items must be stored in a locker; certain items such as medical aids or devices, food and beverages may be accessed during a break.

*See "How do I register for the NCLEX-PN®?" on page xii.

Will I be given a chance to practice using the computer?

Regardless of the candidates' computer skills, each is given an opportunity to practice before the actual test begins. If necessary, computer assistance is also available during the examination. Thus far, candidates with computer experience have not demonstrated any advantage in test performance.

How does the computer select test questions?

The NCLEX-PN® questions vary in their level of difficulty. When the test begins, the first questions are generally at a moderately difficult level. If the candidate answers such a question incorrectly, the computer selects an easier question next. Conversely, if the candidate answers a moderately difficult item correctly, the next question is more difficult. Passing the examination depends on both the number of correctly answered questions and their level of difficulty.

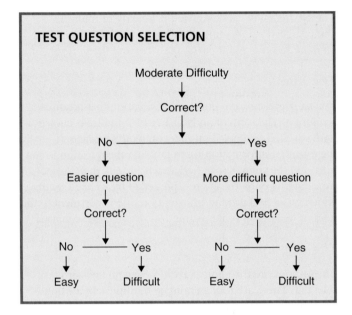

The difficulty of each item is based on *Bloom's Taxonomy* (1956), a classification of six cognitive learning levels that range from basic to advanced. The taxonomy was more recently revised in 2011 by a former student of Bloom's, replacing nouns that were originally used with verbs. The six cognitive levels include (in order of increasing difficulty): remembering, understanding, applying, analyzing, evaluating, and creating.

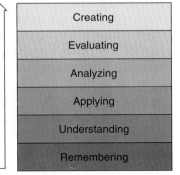

Remembering, the lowest level of cognition, requires recalling information from prior memorization.

Understanding, the next level, requires explaining ideas or concepts, with skills such as locating, selecting, reporting, and paraphrasing information. *Applying,* the cognitive level (or higher) at which the majority of NCLEX-PN® items are written, requires using principles to solve or interpret information related to a client's health and its deviations. *Analyzing,* a cognitive level of further increasing difficulty, requires using abstract and logical thought processes that form the basis for a nursing action. This level of thinking necessitates, for example, that a person compare or contrast information, distinguish cause and effect, identify fine differences, and question actions. *Evaluating,* the next to highest cognitive level, involves, for example, an ability to appraise a situation or information and to defend or support a selected action. *Creating,* the level that ranks as the highest and most challenging degree of thinking, requires such activities as inventing, modifying, substituting, and reorganizing information to fashion new ideas.

How do I indicate my answers to the NCLEX-PN® questions?

Answers are selected by using the keyboard or mouse. The most used keys are the *space bar* and the *enter key.* The space bar moves the cursor to highlight a choice. The enter key is pressed to record the highlighted choice. Exhibit items are accessed by selecting the "exhibit item" button on the screen. Ordered-response items, which require sequencing, are answered by clicking on a choice with the computer mouse and dragging the choice to the order within the sequence. Hot-spot items are answered by clicking an area that you want to represent as the answer. A description of the functional keys, along with a written explanation on how to use them, is included at each computer terminal. A mouse interface and on-screen calculator can be accessed by clicking on the "calculator" button. The item indicates how many decimal places should be in the answer. The unit of measure will be provided. The question bank on the Web site included with this book also features an on-screen calculator. Noteboards and markers are provided by the test center but may not be removed.

How long do the questions remain on the screen?

Each question remains on the screen until an answer is recorded. Candidates are *not* able to:

• Skip a question
• Review previous questions
• Change answers after moving on to the next item.

The underlying reason is that the difficulty of each test question is based on the candidate's answer to preceding test questions.

How many questions are asked on the NCLEX-PN®?

Each candidate's test is unique. The test is made up of a comparatively small number of items from among the vast quantity stored in the memory of the computerized test pool. However, each candidate must answer a minimum of 85 questions. Of these questions, 60 are scored questions and 25 are tryout items that may be used in subsequent test pools. The maximum number of questions given to any candidate is 205—180 of which are scored, the remainder being tryout items.

There is no way for a candidate to determine which questions are tryout items. The tryout items are *not* calculated in the final NCLEX-PN® score, regardless of whether the candidate answers the questions correctly.

In 2011, approximately 57% of NCLEX-PN® candidates answered the minimum number of test items (National Council of State Boards of Nursing, 2013). Approximately 14%, of NCLEX-PN® candidates answered the maximum number of questions (National Council of State Boards of Nursing, 2013). The latter group usually consists of those whose test performances are on the borderline between passing and failing. The remaining test candidates answered between 86 and 112 items.

NCLEX-PN® TESTING PARAMETERS	
Minimum number of questions	85
Maximum number of questions	205
Minimum testing time	None
Maximum testing time	5 hours
Scheduled breaks	
Personal break, anytime by raising hand	After 2 hours
All breaks count against testing time	After 3½ hours

How long does the NCLEX-PN® take?

Because each test is tailor-made for the candidate, there is no minimum amount of time for the test. The maximum length of time allowed for the NCLEX-PN® is 5 hours; however, most candidates finish in less than half that time. The examination time varies, depending on how speedily the candidate reads and answers each test item and how well or poorly the questions are answered.

The test is terminated when the computer has sufficient data to determine with 95% confidence whether the candidate has demonstrated sufficient knowledge to pass the examination. The test ends automatically when the candidate:

• Answers at least a minimum number of 85 questions correctly
• Answers 85 to 205 questions at or below the passing standard

- Answers 205 questions without enough certainty to determine a passing or failing score
- Is still testing when the 5-hour time limit expires.

Who decides the pass/fail score for the NCLEX-PN®?

The National Council's Board of Directors ultimately establishes the official minimum passing standard for the NCLEX-PN®. The Board of Directors' decision is made after receiving recommendations from a panel of nine judges. The panel, which represents diverse geographic regions and areas of clinical practice, determines what portion of minimally competent practical nurses would correctly answer each test question in a sample test.

The passing standard for the NCLEX-PN® is reevaluated whenever the Test Plan changes or at 3-year intervals, whichever comes first. Each state has the authority to set the minimum passing score in its own jurisdiction. However, most states use the same minimum passing score proposed by the National Council of State Boards of Nursing.

How do I register for the NCLEX-PN®?

There are several basic steps that all candidates must complete before taking the NCLEX-PN®.

NCLEX-PN® applications may be obtained on request from the state board of nursing, or they may be available from the candidate's school of nursing. After receiving an application, the state board of nursing determines if the applicant meets licensure eligibility requirements.

Once the candidate's eligibility is confirmed, NCLEX-PN® registration with Pearson VUE, an electronic testing service, can go forward. Pearson VUE offers three different methods of registration: through its Web site (www.pearsonvue.com), by contacting a Pearson VUE agent, or by contacting the test center directly. Forms and information on registering for the NCLEX-PN® can be obtained by requesting the *NCLEX Candidate Bulletin* from the National Council of State Boards of Nursing (available at www.ncsbn.org). Fee payment of $200 is required at the time of registration.

Anyone who schedules a test outside the U.S., must pay an additional $150 fee and a Value Added Tax (VAT) where applicable. There is a $50 fee to change the location where licensure is requested.

After registration with Pearson VUE has been processed, the candidate is sent a publication titled *Scheduling and Taking Your NCLEX*, along with a printed form called an *Authorization to Test* (ATT). There are three pieces of important information on the ATT: a candidate examination number, an authorization number, and an expiration date.

STEPS FOR NCLEX-PN® REGISTRATION

1. Apply to the board of nursing in the state from which licensure is sought.
2. Request that the nursing program provide the board with proof of eligibility to take the NCLEX-PN®.
3. Register with Pearson VUE.
4. Pay a fee of $200 if testing in the U.S.

When and how do I arrange to take the NCLEX-PN®?

After receiving an ATT, candidates can schedule a test date by phone with the test site of their choice or online at Pearson VUE's Web site before the expiration date that appears on the ATT. The locations and phone numbers of all available test sites are provided in the scheduling brochure and can also be found online by using the Test Center Locator function of the Pearson VUE Web site.

After contacting the test site, first-time candidates are offered a test date within 30 days; repeating candidates may be scheduled within a 45-day period. Either type of candidate can request a date beyond the 30 or 45 days as long as the date occurs before the expiration date on the ATT.

If the candidate wishes to cancel or reschedule a testing date, it must be done within 3 business days of the original appointment; otherwise, all fees are forfeited and the ATT is revoked. The same policy applies if a candidate is more than 30 minutes late on the date of the test.

How will I be informed of my NCLEX-PN® results?

Test results, either Pass or Fail, are reported by mail from the state board of nursing where the candidate desires licensure. Although each candidate's score is electronically transmitted from the testing service to the respective board of nursing within 48 hours after an examination, the interim for informing the candidate varies from state to state. Generally, most candidates receive their test results one month after taking the examination.

A candidate who fails the NCLEX-PN® is provided with a testing analysis in the form of a printed diagnostic profile. The profile gives data on how close the candidate came to the minimum passing score, how many items were answered, and performance achieved in each of the Test Plan categories. The statistical data are offered to assist failing candidates to improve their potential for success when retaking the NCLEX-PN®. Weak areas suggest where an unsuccessful candidate might concentrate his or her review.

What if I feel my test result is incorrect?

Some (but not all) states provide a process for reviewing and challenging NCLEX-PN® results. If a failed candidate feels that his or her test performance measurement is invalid, or wants the opportunity to dispute the answer to missed items, arrangements can be made to examine the questions that were answered in error. The review and challenge involves a fee and is limited to no more than 2½ hours.

When can I retake the NCLEX-PN® if I fail?

Presently, a repeating candidate can retake the examination eight times a year but no more than once in any 45-day period. This allows for a variation in items within the existing test pool. When, and if, the test pool of items increases, the frequency for retesting may be amended by the board of nursing in the jurisdiction where licensure is desired.

What are some strategies for NCLEX-PN® success?

There are certain strategies that promote success on the NCLEX-PN®. Some are more appropriate for long-term planning; others are more pertinent as the test date nears.

STRATEGIC PLAN FOR NCLEX-PN® PREPARATION

- Develop a time schedule for a comprehensive review.
- Divide the review topics into manageable amounts.
- Refresh your knowledge of topics in nursing courses.
- Reread sections in nursing textbooks, classroom notes, and written assignments.
- Reexamine tests from previous nursing courses.
- Use this review book to assess your areas of competence.
- Identify weak areas, and restudy or clarify information.

Long-term strategies

Long-term strategies are best implemented as early as possible after completion of a nursing program. In fact, some nursing programs include standardized comprehensive examinations for graduating nurses to help predict how well the potential graduate will perform on the NCLEX-PN®. But most new graduates are left to their own initiative when it comes to preparing for the licensing examination. Whatever approaches are used, it is best to begin preparing for the NCLEX-PN® well in advance.

A systematic and comprehensive review is more effective than last-minute cramming. Cramming contributes to disorganized thinking; facts and concepts are likely to be confused. Also, with cramming there is always an underlying fear of being unprepared, which only heightens test anxiety.

One method of continued learning and retention of learned material is to focus on the review of subjects recently covered in the classroom. For example, after a focused review of the nursing care of clients with disorders of the cardiovascular system, it is advantageous to take the corresponding review test in this book. This is considered a practical approach because, although the NCLEX-PN® basically tests the four categories in the Test Plan, the test questions are asked from a medical, surgical, obstetric, pediatric, or mental health perspective.

LONG-TERM REVIEW STRATEGIES

- Give priority attention to your weaker subjects first.
- Review key concepts in nursing textbooks.
- Summarize information identified in chapter objectives.
- Process critical-thinking questions in nursing books.
- Concentrate on how each Client Needs Category and Subcategory applies to the specific review topic.
- Organize or join a study group preparing for the NCLEX-PN®.
- Select an environment that is conducive to concentration.
- Choose to review when you are the most energetic and focused.
- Keep review periods short, regular, and on task.
- Take an NCLEX-PN® review course if your motivation weakens.
- Invest in NCLEX-PN® computerized testing programs.

Above all, it is best to include review strategies that have been successful in the past.

Short-term strategies

Some strategies are more appropriate as the testing date draws near.

SHORT-TERM STRATEGIES FOR ENSURING SUCCESS

- Correct vision or hearing problems before the test date.
- Make a trial run to the test site location.
- Obtain hotel or motel reservations if the test site is distant.
- Plan some leisure activity the day before the test.
- Get an adequate amount of sleep the night before the test.
- Awaken early.
- Eat sensibly.
- Avoid taking any mind- or mood-altering drugs.
- Take required admission papers and identification.
- Bring a snack or beverage for scheduled breaks.
- Distance yourself from anyone who looks frantic; anxiety is contagious.
- Locate the restroom, and use it shortly before the test.
- Use relaxation techniques.
- Make positive statements to yourself about your ability.

If you use several of the suggested long- and short-term strategies, you can approach the NCLEX-PN® with a feeling of confidence and a positive mental attitude. You will be off to a good start by continuing to work your way through this review book.

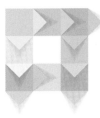

How to Use This Book

Lippincott Review for NCLEX-PN®, Tenth Edition, contains a series of tests covering a wide variety of health-related problems that can be used as a helpful adjunct for preparing for the NCLEX-PN®. Although one of its objectives is to simulate the NCLEX-PN® as much as possible, this book's primary purpose is to provide graduate nurses with an effective resource for reviewing nursing content. By answering most questions correctly, you will have a solid foundation for taking the national licensure examination, as well as a keen understanding of how to manage client situations in real-life clinical settings.

Reading the book's *Preface* and the section on *Frequently Asked Questions* will provide you with a thorough overview of the latest NCLEX Test Plan and address your concerns about the number and types of questions you may be asked on the actual examination. A copy of the detailed NCLEX-PN® Test Plan for 2014 can be obtained at https://www.ncsbn.org/2014_PN_TestPlan.pdf. You will also learn valuable information about how to register for testing, what to expect at the test site facility, and helpful review strategies to ensure a successful test-taking experience.

In the sections below, you will learn how this book is organized, practical tips for choosing correct responses to test questions, and important information about the book's answers and rationales, classification of test items, and comprehensive examinations.

How the book is organized

This review book is divided into five units. The first four units are devoted to specific specialty areas of clinical practice—including adult medical-surgical disorders, care of the childbearing family, care of children, and care of clients with mental health needs. These units are further subdivided into two or more review tests that concentrate on particular types of clients, health problems, and nursing care.

The last unit—a two-part printed Comprehensive Examination—and the Web site containing all the questions in the book serve as the final resources for your NCLEX-PN® review.

DIVISIONS FOR REVIEW

- Unit 1: The Nursing Care of Adults with Medical-Surgical Disorders
- Unit 2: The Nursing Care of the Childbearing Family
- Unit 3: The Nursing Care of Children
- Unit 4: The Nursing Care of Clients with Mental Health Needs
- Unit 5: Postreview Tests

Editorial policies

Throughout the book, the word *client* is used when referring to the person receiving nursing services. Although the word *patient* is more familiar to some, *client* is the term that is used throughout the NCLEX-PN®.

Clients are identified generically by age, medical information, and gender when it is germane to the question. The same principle is followed on the NCLEX-PN®.

An effort has also been made to avoid using feminine pronouns when referring to the nurse because more and more men are joining their female colleagues in nursing practice. A similar decision was made regarding the use of only masculine pronouns when referring to physicians. In most cases, they are identified as the *nurse* or the *physician*. You can assume that the nurse to which the question refers is a practical nurse; if not, that information is identified.

Last, in multiple-choice questions involving drugs, both the generic name and a brand name are provided wherever possible. The generic name is given first; a common brand or trade name follows in parentheses.

Testing format

Just like the latest NCLEX-PN® examination, this review book primarily includes traditional multiple-choice questions consisting of a stem and four answer choices (options). However, a small percentage of alternative-format questions—such as multiple-response multiple-choice (typically, six-option questions), fill-in-the-blank (a calculation), hot-spot (graphically illustrated), and ordered-response (including options which the test-taker must place in chronologic order)—are also included in each test, reflecting the most recent changes to the NCLEX Test Plan. These alternative-format questions are highlighted in color in the book. Audio items are also included on the Web site that accompanies this book.

In some cases, test questions are preceded by a case scenario that contains descriptive information about a client's condition or circumstances that are pertinent to answering the question. Such descriptions are italicized and appear above the stem, as shown below.

Sample case scenario

The nurse is caring for a 49-year-old client who is short of breath, has a heart rate of 110 beats/minute, and has moist breath sounds.

       1. Which position is best for promoting ventilation in this client?   **<stem**

    [ ] **1.** Supine   **<distractor**
    [ ] **2.** Fowler's   **<correct answer**
    [ ] **3.** Prone   **<distractor**
    [ ] **4.** Sims'   **<distractor**

Choosing answers

There are several necessary steps in choosing an answer. They include analyzing the information, looking for key words or terms, using a process of elimination or other test-taking strategy, selecting an option, and making your choice.

Additional methods that are helpful in selecting an option for an answer include:

- Using the steps in the nursing process when a question asks what to do next; in other words, gathering data before intervening, and so on
- Using Maslow's hierarchy to determine which health-related problem needs to be addressed first, following the sequence of managing *physiological needs*, such as breathing, followed by *needs for safety and security*, *needs for love and belonging*, *needs for esteem and self-esteem*, and a *need for self-actualization,* in that order
- Considering safety issues when a client requires care, but is physiologically stable
- Responding to communication questions by selecting an option that supports principles of therapeutic communication, especially those that promote verbalization by the client (Some examples include asking open-ended questions, reflecting, offering general leads, clarifying, and sharing perceptions. Nontherapeutic communication techniques that should be avoided include giving false reassurance, giving advice, changing the subject, demanding an explanation, using clichés, and showing disapproval.)

- Applying knowledge of common laboratory test results, such as normal blood counts, blood chemistry values, and blood gases
- Recognizing and identifying basic ECG waveforms
- Applying knowledge of normal nutrition and therapeutic diets

Analyzing the information

It is always best to read each case scenario and stem carefully. Focus on the subject or content in the information that makes the situation unique. Arriving at a correct answer involves integrating the pertinent facts within the context of the question. For example, if you are informed that a client is 3 years old, the answer to the question might be different than if the client is 65 years old, based on variations in the life cycle.

Looking for key terms

Key terms are words and their modifiers that help call attention to the critical information in the question. Identifying key terms can help you select the answer that fits the intent of the question.

EXAMPLES OF KEY WORDS AND MODIFIERS

Key words

Best	Least
Most	Except
Next	Earliest
At this time	Essential
Immediately	Initially

Key words and modifiers

Best response	Most important
Best evidence	Most appropriate
Best measure	Most accurate
Best answer	Most indicative
Best explanation	Most suggestive

Selecting an option

When selecting an option, make sure you have read each one carefully because there may only be subtle differences between them. It is always helpful to narrow your options by using the process of elimination, being aware of distractor choices. Remember, the process of selecting an option may be different when answering alternative-format questions. For example, with multiple-response multiple-choice questions, more than one option is correct.

Making your choice

Once you have decided which option is best, you can record your answer in the printed book by blackening the box in front of that option in the review test. If you are answering alternative-format questions: blacken the boxes in front of all of the options you think are correct for multiple-response multiple-choice questions; write your answer on the blank line provided for fill-in-the-blank questions; draw an *X* over the appropriate place on the illustration for hot-spot questions; and place the options in the correct order by writing the desired sequence for the ordered-response questions.

A word of warning: As in the actual NCLEX-PN®, the correct answers are *randomized;* that is, they do not follow any particular pattern. It is therefore foolhardy to choose an answer by trying to predict some planned sequence in the numbered choices.

Correct answers and rationales

See the sections in each test titled Correct Answers, Rationales, and Test Taking Strategies after completing each test and the Comprehensive Examinations. Compare your answers with those identified as the correct answers. Remember to place a check mark next to any items you answered incorrectly.

Study the rationale and discussion of the test-taking strategy for each item regardless of whether you answered it correctly or incorrectly. The rationales often contain additional information that will enhance your NCLEX-PN® review.

Next, analyze the reason you chose an incorrect answer. If you answered incorrectly because you did not read the item carefully or because you blackened the wrong box, plan to concentrate more on reading and marking the answers more accurately. If you made an error because you lacked the knowledge required to answer the question correctly, make a point of restudying that specific health-related problem.

Comprehensive Examinations

Once you have taken all the individual tests and completed your review, you will be ready to take the two-part Comprehensive Examination in the book or the examination on the Web site, or both. Whatever your decision, take these examinations as seriously as if you were taking the actual licensing examination.

Both of these practice examinations are intended to simulate the NCLEX-PN®. The printed version contains more items than the maximum number asked on the NCLEX-PN®. Because of its length, it provides the greatest opportunity for practice in answering a mix of questions from all of the review test material.

The Web site can generate mixes of questions that relate to topics in each of the four review test units. You can use the Web site to practice by time or by number of questions and compare your results with those of previous NCLEX-PN® candidates identified in this book. In addition, the computerized version simulates the same testing process candidates are required to use when taking the NCLEX-PN®.

When all the components of this book and Web site are utilized, along with recommended areas for further review, most candidates can acquire the self-confidence that will make passing the NCLEX-PN® that much easier.

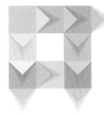

Contents

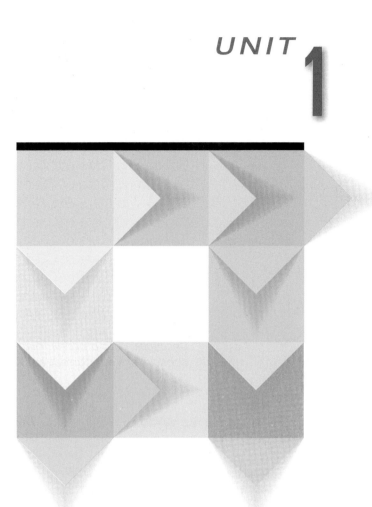

The Nursing Care of Adults with Medical-Surgical Disorders

The Nursing Care of Clients with Musculoskeletal Disorders

■ Nursing Care of Clients with Musculoskeletal Injuries
■ Nursing Care of Clients with Fractures
■ Nursing Care of Clients with Casts
■ Nursing Care of Clients in Traction
■ Nursing Care of Clients with Inflammatory Joint Disorders
■ Nursing Care of Clients with Degenerative Bone Disorders
■ Nursing Care of Clients with Amputations
■ Nursing Care of Clients with Skeletal Tumors
■ Nursing Care of Clients with Herniated Intervertebral Disks
■ Correct Answers, Rationales, and Test Taking Strategies

Directions: *With a pencil, blacken the space in front of the option you have chosen for your correct answer.*

Nursing Care of Clients with Musculoskeletal Injuries

A client who golfs at least three times a week has been experiencing wrist pain aggravated by movement. The physician diagnoses the condition as tenosynovitis and recommends temporarily avoiding repetitive wrist motion.

1. Which statement made by the client to the nurse provides the best evidence that the client understands the therapeutic plan?
[ ] **1.** "I should keep my hand as still as possible."
[ ] **2.** "I should stop playing golf for the time being."
[ ] **3.** "I can substitute playing miniature golf."
[ ] **4.** "I can wear a tight leather glove when golfing."

The nurse examines a client who slipped and fell while climbing stairs and now has ankle swelling and pain on movement.

2. While the client is waiting for the ankle to be X-rayed, which nursing measure is most helpful for relieving the soft-tissue swelling?
[ ] **1.** Place a heating pad on the ankle.
[ ] **2.** Apply ice to the ankle.
[ ] **3.** Exercise the client's foot.
[ ] **4.** Immobilize the client's foot.

The ankle X-ray reveals that the bones are not fractured. The physician tells the client that the ankle is severely sprained.

3. The physician directs the nurse to wrap the client's lower extremity with an elastic bandage. Where should the nurse begin applying the bandage?
[ ] **1.** Below the knee
[ ] **2.** Above the ankle
[ ] **3.** Across the phalanges
[ ] **4.** At the metatarsals

4. Which is the best technique for the nurse to use when applying the elastic bandage to the client's lower extremity?
[ ] **1.** Making figure-eight turns with the bandage
[ ] **2.** Making spiral-reverse turns with the bandage
[ ] **3.** Making recurrent turns with the bandage
[ ] **4.** Making spica turns with the bandage

Before the client is discharged from the emergency department, the nurse provides instructions on how to care for the sprained ankle at home.

5. The nurse advises the client on the need for maintenance of the bandage. When should the nurse advise the client with a sprained ankle to rewrap the elastic bandage?
[ ] **1.** When the toes appear pink
[ ] **2.** When the ankle feels painful
[ ] **3.** When the toes look swollen
[ ] **4.** When the joint feels stiff

A client arrives in the emergency department with a shoulder injury after falling from a stepladder.

6. When the nurse assesses the client, which finding is the best indication that the shoulder has been dislocated?
[ ] **1.** The client is experiencing intense pain.
[ ] **2.** There is obvious swelling about the joint.
[ ] **3.** The client is hesitant to move the arm.
[ ] **4.** The affected arm is longer than the other.

The physician informs the client of plans to correct the shoulder dislocation by manipulation.

7. When the client asks the nurse what is meant by the term *manipulation*, which explanation is most accurate?
[ ] **1.** Manipulation involves making an incision to realign the bones.
[ ] **2.** Manipulation involves the insertion of a pin or wire into the joint.
[ ] **3.** Manipulation repositions the bone ends manually.
[ ] **4.** Manipulation strengthens the joint with exercise.

Before discharge, the nurse informs the client that a sling needs to be worn to immobilize the injured shoulder. The client tells the nurse that there is no insurance to pay for the hospital bill or a sling. The nurse teaches a family member how to apply a triangular sling made from muslin.

8. Which statement made by the family member indicates the need for further teaching?
[ ] **1.** "The hand should be elevated higher than the elbow."
[ ] **2.** "The knot should be tied at the back of the neck."
[ ] **3.** "The elbow should be flexed within the sling."
[ ] **4.** "The sling is used to elevate and support the arm."

Nursing Care of Clients with Fractures

While backpacking with a youth group, a 17-year-old falls and sustains an injury to the lower leg. A nurse who is accompanying the group suspects a fracture of the tibia.

9. To immobilize the suspected fracture, how should the nurse apply a splint?
[ ] **1.** Below the knee to above the hip
[ ] **2.** Above the knee to below the hip
[ ] **3.** Above the ankle to below the knee
[ ] **4.** Below the ankle to above the knee

An X-ray of the injured teenager's leg reveals a comminuted fracture of the distal tibia.

10. Which explanation by the nurse can best help this client understand the injury that has occurred?
[ ] **1.** One bone end is driven into the other.
[ ] **2.** The bone is splintered into pieces.
[ ] **3.** There is no open break in the skin.
[ ] **4.** A portion of the bone is split away.

After consulting the attending physician, the nurse learns that the teenager will require surgery to realign the bones in the fractured tibia.

11. In this case, from whom is it most appropriate for the physician, with the nurse as a witness, to obtain consent to perform the surgical procedure?
[ ] **1.** The injured client
[ ] **2.** The client's physician
[ ] **3.** The client's youth leader
[ ] **4.** The client's parent

12. The client is about to go to surgery but is still wearing a class ring. Which nursing action is most appropriate regarding care of the client's valuables?
[ ] **1.** Put the ring in the bedside stand.
[ ] **2.** Tape the ring to the client's finger.
[ ] **3.** Give the ring to a security guard.
[ ] **4.** Take the ring to the hospital safe.

The client has returned from surgery with a leg cast, and the nurse is assisting the client back to bed.

13. Which of the following would the nurse identify as the highest priority when documenting the postoperative circulation status of the recently casted extremity?
[ ] **1.** Adequate neurovascular functioning
[ ] **2.** Minimal pain on movement
[ ] **3.** Vital signs within normal limits
[ ] **4.** No drainage noted on the cast

14. The nurse knows that a client who sustains multiple fractures of long bones is at risk for developing fat embolism syndrome. Which findings suggest that the client is developing this complication? Select all that apply.
[ ] **1.** Bradycardia
[ ] **2.** Petechiae
[ ] **3.** Dyspnea
[ ] **4.** Mental status changes
[ ] **5.** Hypertension
[ ] **6.** Hematuria

A nurse stops to assist an individual who was involved in a motor vehicle accident. The victim was not wearing a seat belt and was thrown from the car.

15. Of the following emergency measures, which one should the nurse perform first?
[ ] **1.** Check the victim's breathing.
[ ] **2.** Cover the victim with a blanket.
[ ] **3.** Move the victim to the curb.
[ ] **4.** Assess the victim for injuries.

The nurse suspects that the victim has sustained rib fractures.

16. Which assessment finding is the best indication that the client is experiencing secondary complications from the fractured ribs?
[ ] **1.** Irregular pulse rate
[ ] **2.** Asymmetrical chest expansion
[ ] **3.** Expiratory wheezing on auscultation
[ ] **4.** Coughing up pink, frothy sputum

Aside from the suspected rib fractures, the nurse sees a bone fragment protruding from the client's thigh as well as profuse bleeding from the wound.

17. Which technique is most appropriate to control the bleeding?
[ ] **1.** Place a tourniquet around the leg.
[ ] **2.** Apply direct pressure on the wound.
[ ] **3.** Compress the femoral artery.
[ ] **4.** Elevate the injured extremity.

The nurse suspects that the accident victim might also have a broken back.

18. Which is the most preferred position when transporting a victim with a possible back injury?
[ ] **1.** Side-lying
[ ] **2.** Prone
[ ] **3.** Supine
[ ] **4.** Semi-Fowler's

An 80-year-old client who sustained a fall at a long-term care facility is suspected of having a fractured right hip.

19. Which statements support the nurse's belief that the client has a fractured hip? Select all that apply.
[ ] **1.** The client has pain near the distal femur.
[ ] **2.** The client cannot bear weight on the affected leg.
[ ] **3.** The client's affected leg is shorter.
[ ] **4.** The client's affected leg is adducted.
[ ] **5.** The client's affected leg is externally rotated.
[ ] **6.** The client prefers to sit rather than lie flat.

20. Which risk factor found in the client's medical record does the nurse identify as most significant for sustaining a hip fracture?
[ ] **1.** The client is postmenopausal.
[ ] **2.** The client is somewhat obese.
[ ] **3.** The client has type 2 diabetes.
[ ] **4.** The client is lactose intolerant.

21. Which of the following evening snacks would the nurse encourage for the client with immobility due to the fractured hip?
[ ] **1.** An orange
[ ] **2.** Rice cakes
[ ] **3.** Cheese sticks
[ ] **4.** Potato chips

22. The nurse uses a diagram of the hip to explain to the client and the family where an intertrochanteric fracture of the femur has occurred. Identify with an *X* the anatomic location of the injury.

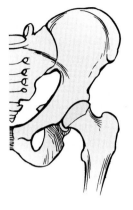

After the client's fractured hip is stabilized with an open reduction and internal fixation (ORIF), the nurse teaches the client to perform isometric quadriceps-setting exercises.

23. Which instruction should the nurse reinforce to ensure that the exercises are done correctly?
[ ] **1.** Move your toes toward and away from your head.
[ ] **2.** Contract and relax your thigh muscles.
[ ] **3.** Lift your lower leg up and down from the bed.
[ ] **4.** Bend your knee and pull your lower leg upward.

After surgery, the client is instructed to wear thigh-high antiembolism stockings.

24. Which statement by the nurse provides the best explanation about the purpose of antiembolism stockings?
[ ] **1.** Antiembolism stockings prevent blood from pooling in the legs.
[ ] **2.** Antiembolism stockings reduce blood flow to the extremities.
[ ] **3.** Antiembolism stockings keep the blood pressure lower in the legs.
[ ] **4.** Antiembolism stockings keep the blood vessels constricted.

25. The nurse supervises a nursing assistant who is applying the client's antiembolism stockings. What is the correct technique for applying these stockings?
[ ] **1.** The nursing assistant applies the stockings before getting the client out of bed.
[ ] **2.** The nursing assistant applies the stockings just before helping the client do leg exercises.
[ ] **3.** The nursing assistant applies the stockings after noting that the client's legs are cool.
[ ] **4.** The nursing assistant applies the stockings at night before the client's bedtime.

26. Postoperatively, which intervention should be completed before turning the client onto the nonoperative side?
[ ] **1.** Placing pillows between the client's legs
[ ] **2.** Having the client point the toes downward
[ ] **3.** Flexing the client's knee on the affected side
[ ] **4.** Elevating the head of the client's bed

27. The physician orders that the client may be out of bed to sit in a chair. How should the nurse position the chair to facilitate transferring the client from the bed?
[ ] **1.** At the end of the bed
[ ] **2.** Perpendicular to the bed
[ ] **3.** Parallel with the bed
[ ] **4.** Against a side wall

A client with a hip prosthesis is allowed to ambulate with a walker using a three-point partial weight-bearing gait.

28. Which return demonstration indicates that the client has understood the correct way to ambulate with the walker?
[ ] **1.** The client advances the walker and operative leg while putting most of the weight on the walker's handgrips.
[ ] **2.** The client advances the walker and operative leg while putting most of the weight on the back legs of the walker.
[ ] **3.** The client advances the walker and operative leg while putting most of the weight on the toes of the operative leg.
[ ] **4.** The client advances the walker and operative leg while putting most of the weight on the heel of the nonoperative leg.

A client who has degenerative arthritis involving the hips undergoes a total hip replacement.

29. After the client's total hip replacement surgery, which nursing actions are essential? Select all that apply.
[ ] **1.** Keeping the client's knees apart at all times
[ ] **2.** Avoiding more than 90 degrees of hip flexion
[ ] **3.** Having the client use a raised toilet seat
[ ] **4.** Raising the head of the client's bed 90 degrees
[ ] **5.** Placing two pillows beneath the client's knees
[ ] **6.** Keeping the client's legs internally rotated

Nursing Care of Clients with Casts

A plaster arm cast will be applied to an adult client with a compound fracture of the radius.

30. When preparing the client for cast application, which statement by the nurse is most accurate?
[ ] **1.** "The cast will feel tight as it's applied."
[ ] **2.** "Your arm will feel warm as the wet plaster sets."
[ ] **3.** "You can expect a foul odor until the cast is dry."
[ ] **4.** "You may feel itchy while the cast is wet."

31. How can the nurse best support the wet cast while the physician wraps the arm with rolls of wet plaster?
[ ] **1.** By using a soft mattress
[ ] **2.** By resting it on a firm surface
[ ] **3.** By using the tips of the fingers
[ ] **4.** By using the palms of the hands

32. After the arm cast has been applied, which nursing observation is the best indication that the client may be developing compartment syndrome?
[ ] **1.** The client experiences severe pain.
[ ] **2.** The client's hand becomes reddened.
[ ] **3.** The fingers develop muscle spasms.
[ ] **4.** The radial pulse feels bounding.

33. Which is the best material for the nurse to place under a wet plaster cast immediately after application?
[ ] **1.** Synthetic sheepskin
[ ] **2.** A vinyl sheet
[ ] **3.** An absorbent pad
[ ] **4.** Several pillows

34. What is the best technique a nurse can use for drying the wet plaster arm cast?
[ ] **1.** Leave the casted arm uncovered.
[ ] **2.** Apply a heating blanket to the cast.
[ ] **3.** Use a hair dryer to blow hot air onto the cast.
[ ] **4.** Place a heat lamp directly above the cast.

35. Which is the best method to assess circulation in the casted extremity?
[ ] **1.** Ask the client to wiggle the fingers.
[ ] **2.** Feel the cast to determine if it is unusually hot or cold.
[ ] **3.** Depress the client's nail beds, and document the time it takes for the color to return.
[ ] **4.** See if there is enough room to insert a finger between the cast and the extremity.

While waiting for the cast to dry, the client asks the nurse about the differences between plaster casts and those made of synthetic materials such as fiberglass.

36. Which statement by the nurse about fiberglass casts is most accurate?
[ ] **1.** Fiberglass casts are less expensive.
[ ] **2.** Fiberglass casts are lighter weight.
[ ] **3.** Fiberglass casts are easier to apply.
[ ] **4.** Fiberglass casts are less restrictive.

Before discharging the client, the nurse provides the client with plaster cast care instructions and information about signs and symptoms of complications. The client returns to the clinic several hours later with bloody drainage seeping through the cast.

37. After assessing the client's cast, what action should the nurse take next?
[ ] **1.** Document the finding in the medical record.
[ ] **2.** Call the physician and report the finding.
[ ] **3.** Circle the area, then record the time.
[ ] **4.** Apply an ice bag over the drainage area.

A hip-spica cast is applied to a 16-year-old who sustained a fractured femur in a motorcycle accident.

38. The client tells the nurse, "My father is furious with me. He does not want me to ride a motorcycle." Which response by the nurse is most appropriate?
[ ] **1.** "As they say, 'Father knows best.'"
[ ] **2.** "All parents want their children to be safe."
[ ] **3.** "It can be frustrating when you disagree with your father."
[ ] **4.** "I think you should comply, but the decision is yours."

39. Which developmental task should the nurse keep in mind while planning the client's care?
[ ] **1.** The client is searching for sexual identity.
[ ] **2.** The client is testing physical abilities.
[ ] **3.** The client is acquiring independence.
[ ] **4.** The client is learning to control emotions.

40. Which equipment should the nurse anticipate needing to facilitate the client's bowel elimination?
[ ] **1.** Bedside commode
[ ] **2.** Fracture bedpan
[ ] **3.** Mechanical lift
[ ] **4.** Raised toilet seat

The client asks the nurse to explain the purpose of the bar running between the thighs on the hip-spica cast.

41. Which statement by the nurse about the cast's bar is most accurate?
[ ] **1.** The bar facilitates lifting and turning clients.
[ ] **2.** The bar enhances physical exercise.
[ ] **3.** The bar strengthens the cast.
[ ] **4.** The bar maintains the proper position.

After several days, the client tells the nurse that the skin itches terribly beneath the cast.

42. Which nursing action is most appropriate at this time?
[ ] **1.** Collaborate with the physician on prescribing an antipruritic medication.
[ ] **2.** Provide powder for the client to sprinkle in the cast.
[ ] **3.** Obtain a flat ruler so the client can scratch inside the cast.
[ ] **4.** Apply a commercially prepared ice bag to the outside of the cast.

After the client has had the hip-spica cast for nearly 3 weeks, the nurse detects a foul odor coming from the cast.

43. Which statement is most accurate regarding the cause of the cast's unpleasant odor?
[ ] **1.** The plaster has dried improperly.
[ ] **2.** There is bleeding under the cast.
[ ] **3.** The cast is disintegrating.
[ ] **4.** There is an infected wound.

The physician cuts a small window in the hip-spica cast to inspect the underlying tissue.

44. Which nursing action is most appropriate after the piece of plaster is removed to create a window in the cast?
[ ] **1.** Dispose of the piece of plaster in a plastic biohazard bag.
[ ] **2.** Replace the piece of plaster in the cast hole with tape.
[ ] **3.** Put the piece of plaster in the client's bedside drawer.
[ ] **4.** Send the piece of plaster to the laboratory for culturing.

45. Which nursing action is most correct when the rough edges on the client's hip-spica cast begin to threaten the integrity of the skin?
[ ] **1.** Line the cast edge with adhesive petals of moleskin.
[ ] **2.** Apply a fresh strip of plaster to the cast edge.
[ ] **3.** Trim the rough cast edge with a cast cutter.
[ ] **4.** Cover the cast edge with a gauze dressing.

46. Which assessment finding suggests that the client in the hip-spica cast may be developing a response to room confinement known as *cast syndrome*?
[ ] **1.** The client becomes nauseated and vomits.
[ ] **2.** The client becomes disoriented and confused.
[ ] **3.** The client becomes feverish and hypotensive.
[ ] **4.** The client becomes dyspneic and hyperventilates.

Nursing Care of Clients in Traction

Before undergoing surgery for a fractured hip, an older client is placed in Buck's traction.

47. Which nursing technique is best when planning to change the client's bed linens?
[ ] **1.** Roll the client from one side of the bed to the other.
[ ] **2.** Apply the linens from the foot to the top of the bed.
[ ] **3.** Leave the bottom sheets in place until after surgery.
[ ] **4.** Raise the client from the bed with a mechanical lift.

48. Which assessment finding warrants immediate action by the nurse when a client is in Buck's traction?
[ ] **1.** The traction weights are hanging above the floor.
[ ] **2.** The leg is in line with the pull of the traction.
[ ] **3.** The client's foot is touching the end of the bed.
[ ] **4.** The rope is in the groove of the traction pulley.

49. Which technique is the best strategy for assessing circulation in the leg in Buck's traction?
[ ] **1.** Observe whether the client can wiggle or move the toes.
[ ] **2.** Palpate for pulsation of the dorsalis pedis artery.
[ ] **3.** Take the client's blood pressure with a thigh cuff positioned on the affected leg.
[ ] **4.** Determine whether the client can feel sharp and dull sensations.

An older client is placed in Russell's traction while awaiting surgery.

50. To prevent skin breakdown while the client is in traction, the nurse must frequently inspect the skin in which area?
[ ] **1.** Over the ischial spines
[ ] **2.** In the popliteal space
[ ] **3.** Near the iliac crests
[ ] **4.** At the zygomatic arch

The nurse enters the client's room to assess the traction apparatus.

51. Which of the following might interfere with the effectiveness of Russell's traction?
[ ] **1.** The rope is strung tautly from pulley to pulley.
[ ] **2.** The trapeze is hanging above the client's chest.
[ ] **3.** The rope is knotted at the location of a pulley.
[ ] **4.** The weight is about 24″ (61 cm) from the floor.

On the day of surgery, the client in Russell's traction is transported to the operating room in the bed.

52. Which nursing action is appropriate while the client is being transported?
[ ] **1.** The nurse maintains the traction as applied.
[ ] **2.** The nurse removes the weights during the transport.
[ ] **3.** The nurse rests the weights on the end of the bed.
[ ] **4.** The nurse takes the client's leg out of the traction.

A cervical halter type of skin traction is applied to a client who has experienced a whiplash injury in a motor vehicle accident.

53. When the nurse makes rounds at the beginning of the shift, which observation requires the nurse's immediate attention?
[ ] **1.** The halter rests under the client's chin and occiput.
[ ] **2.** The client's ears are clear of the traction ropes.
[ ] **3.** The weight hangs between the headboard and wall.
[ ] **4.** There is a soft pillow beneath the client's head.

A client with a fractured femur is in skeletal traction with a pin through the distal femur. The affected leg is supported by balanced suspension.

54. Which material added by the nurse is best for covering the tips of the pin to prevent injuries while the client is in skeletal leg traction?
[ ] **1.** Gauze squares
[ ] **2.** Cotton balls
[ ] **3.** Cork blocks
[ ] **4.** Rubber tubes

55. The nurse is evaluating the status of the pin sites for signs of infection. Which finding is most important to bring to the physician's attention?
[ ] **1.** Serous drainage at the pin site
[ ] **2.** Bloody drainage at the pin site
[ ] **3.** Mucoid drainage at the pin site
[ ] **4.** Purulent drainage at the pin site

The physician orders antibiotic therapy for the client's infection.

56. If the client is allergic to penicillin, the nurse must question a medical order for which type of antibiotic?
[ ] **1.** An aminoglycoside such as gentamicin sulfate (Garamycin)
[ ] **2.** A cephalosporin such as cefaclor (Ceclor)
[ ] **3.** A tetracycline such as doxycycline (Vibramycin)
[ ] **4.** A sulfonamide such as trimethoprim/sulfamethoxazole (Bactrim)

A client with a fractured cervical vertebra is placed in halo-cervical traction, a type of skeletal traction consisting of pins inserted into the skull that are incorporated into a vest of plaster.

57. Which description by the nurse most accurately states the purpose of halo-cervical traction?
[ ] **1.** "It restricts neck movement but enables physical activity."
[ ] **2.** "It allows head movement while immobilizing the spine."
[ ] **3.** "It accelerates healing by facilitating physical therapy."
[ ] **4.** "It promotes faster bone repair within a shorter time span."

58. Which nursing observation provides the best indication that the halo-cervical traction device is applied appropriately?
[ ] **1.** The client has full range of motion in the neck.
[ ] **2.** The client's neck pain is within a tolerable level.
[ ] **3.** The client can speak and hear at preinjury levels.
[ ] **4.** The client reports the ability to see straight ahead.

59. Which assessment finding is the best indication that the client in halo traction is developing a serious complication?
[ ] **1.** The client experiences orthostatic hypotension.
[ ] **2.** The client needs assistance with shaving.
[ ] **3.** The client cannot open the mouth widely.
[ ] **4.** The client complains about irritation under the axillae.

Nursing Care of Clients with Inflammatory Joint Disorders

An adult consults a physician about persistent joint pain and stiffness.

60. Which laboratory test value, if elevated, is the best diagnostic indicator of rheumatoid arthritis?
[ ] **1.** Erythrocyte sedimentation rate (ESR)
[ ] **2.** Partial thromboplastin time (PTT)
[ ] **3.** Fasting blood sugar (FBS)
[ ] **4.** Blood urea nitrogen (BUN)

61. The nurse is reviewing the history and physical of the client with possible rheumatoid arthritis. If the diagnosis is confirmed, during which period would the nurse anticipate documentation of symptoms?
[ ] **1.** In very early childhood
[ ] **2.** At the onset of puberty
[ ] **3.** During young adulthood
[ ] **4.** Within older adulthood

The physician diagnoses rheumatoid arthritis and prescribes a total of 5 g of aspirin per day. The client is surprised the physician prescribed a common drug such as aspirin to treat the condition.

62. The nurse should plan to include which information related to the therapeutic benefits of aspirin in the teaching plan for this client?
[ ] **1.** Aspirin stimulates the immune system.
[ ] **2.** Aspirin relaxes skeletal muscles.
[ ] **3.** Aspirin reduces joint inflammation.
[ ] **4.** Aspirin interrupts nerve synapses.

The client tells the nurse about experiencing an upset stomach when taking aspirin.

63. Which modification in the client's care plan is most appropriate to relieve the client's stomach discomfort?
[ ] **1.** Give aspirin before meals only.
[ ] **2.** Give aspirin with cold water.
[ ] **3.** Give aspirin with hot tea.
[ ] **4.** Give aspirin with food or meals.

64. Because the client takes large amounts of aspirin daily, the nurse monitors for signs and symptoms of aspirin toxicity. Which assessment finding is the best indication of aspirin toxicity?
[ ] **1.** Ringing in the ears
[ ] **2.** Dizziness
[ ] **3.** Metallic taste in the mouth
[ ] **4.** Proteinuria

65. When the client experiences an exacerbation of symptoms of rheumatoid arthritis, which adjunct medication, in addition to aspirin, is anticipated?
[ ] **1.** Ibuprofen (Advil)
[ ] **2.** Prednisone (Deltasone)
[ ] **3.** Etanercept (Enbrel)
[ ] **4.** Levofloxacin (Levaquin)

66. Which statement made by the client indicates that further instruction regarding corticosteroid therapy is necessary?
[ ] **1.** "I'm susceptible to getting infections."
[ ] **2.** "I should never stop taking my medication abruptly."
[ ] **3.** "I may become very depressed and perhaps suicidal."
[ ] **4.** "I may develop low blood sugar and need glucose."

The client tells the nurse that watching television helps decrease the discomfort.

67. Which conclusion made by the nurse is most accurate given the above information?
[ ] **1.** The client's condition is improving due to electronic signals.
[ ] **2.** The client is having less pain transmission.
[ ] **3.** The client is experiencing a slight case of arthritis.
[ ] **4.** The client is being distracted from the pain.

68. Which finger joints would the nurse expect to be most affected by the client's rheumatoid arthritis?
[ ] **1.** Proximal finger joints
[ ] **2.** Medial finger joints
[ ] **3.** Distal finger joints
[ ] **4.** Lateral finger joints

The physician recommends applying heat to the client's hands to relieve discomfort.

69. When determining client-specific nursing interventions to add to the plan of care, which heat application method is best?
[ ] **1.** Hot wax treatment
[ ] **2.** Warm moist compresses
[ ] **3.** Electric heating pad
[ ] **4.** Infrared heat lamp

70. While planning care for the client, when would the nurse expect a need for more time and assistance with activities of daily living?
[ ] **1.** In the early morning
[ ] **2.** At noon
[ ] **3.** In the late afternoon
[ ] **4.** Before bed

71. Which nursing recommendation has the greatest potential for helping the client maintain the ability to perform self-care?
[ ] 1. Move to a warm climate like Arizona.
[ ] 2. Buy clothes that are easy to pull up or slip on.
[ ] 3. Enroll in an aerobics exercise class.
[ ] 4. Sleep on a warm waterbed or heating pad.

During an acute episode of rheumatoid arthritis, the physician asks the nurse to apply a splint to each of the client's hands.

72. Which explanation most accurately explains to the client the primary purpose of the splints?
[ ] 1. Splints are used to rest affected joints.
[ ] 2. Splints are used to slow joint deterioration.
[ ] 3. Splints are used to improve hand strength.
[ ] 4. Splints are used to increase range of motion.

The client has not responded to the current drug therapy and the physician has added methotrexate (Rheumatrex) and cyclosporine (Sandimmune) to the medication regimen.

73. Which statement to the nurse indicates a good understanding by the client of the use of methotrexate and cyclosporine together?
[ ] 1. "I am having an exacerbation of symptoms so two medications are needed."
[ ] 2. "Cyclosporine is given to enhance the effect of the methotrexate."
[ ] 3. "Methotrexate and cyclosporine together decrease unwanted side effects."
[ ] 4. "My symptoms are severe enough to indicate the use of two strong medications."

74. Which assessment finding would the nurse consider a likely adverse effect of the client's methotrexate (Rheumatrex) therapy?
[ ] 1. Constipation
[ ] 2. Polyuria
[ ] 3. Mouth sores
[ ] 4. Chest pain

A 75-year-old client with osteoarthritis in the left hip has been told by the physician to apply a heating pad to the area several times a day.

75. Which nursing instruction about heating pads is essential to include in the client's teaching plan?
[ ] 1. Keep the heating pad on the low setting.
[ ] 2. Place the heating pad directly on the skin.
[ ] 3. Cover the heating pad with plastic during use.
[ ] 4. Apply the heating pad for 2 hours at a time.

76. Which nursing instruction is most beneficial to minimize stress on the client's painful joints?
[ ] 1. Maintain a normal weight.
[ ] 2. Apply a topical analgesic cream.
[ ] 3. Take a calcium supplement.
[ ] 4. Become more physically active.

77. The client uses a cane when ambulating. When the nurse observes the client walking, which assessment finding indicates the need for more instruction regarding the use of the cane?
[ ] 1. The tip of the cane is covered with a rubber cap.
[ ] 2. The client wears athletic shoes with nonskid soles.
[ ] 3. The client uses the cane on the painful side.
[ ] 4. The client looks straight ahead when walking.

The client reports taking 400 mg of ibuprofen (Motrin) four times a day at home.

78. Which question best helps the nurse determine whether the client is experiencing an adverse effect from taking nonsteroidal anti-inflammatory drugs (NSAIDs) such as ibuprofen (Motrin)?
[ ] 1. "Have you noticed any hand tremors?"
[ ] 2. "Are you urinating more frequently?"
[ ] 3. "Has your interest in food changed?"
[ ] 4. "What color are your stools?"

A total hip replacement (hip arthroplasty) is planned for a 70-year-old client with osteoarthritis. The physician instructs the client to stop taking enteric-coated aspirin (Ecotrin) 1 week before surgery.

79. Which statement by the nurse best explains the rationale for the physician's instructions?
[ ] 1. "Aspirin can increase your risk of wound infection."
[ ] 2. "Aspirin impairs your ability to control bleeding."
[ ] 3. "Aspirin can make it difficult to assess your pain."
[ ] 4. "Aspirin interferes with your ability to heal."

Before the total hip replacement, the nurse teaches the client how to use an incentive spirometer.

80. Which statement indicates that the client understands how to use the incentive spirometer correctly?
[ ] 1. "I should position the mouthpiece and inhale deeply."
[ ] 2. "I should position the mouthpiece and exhale forcefully."
[ ] 3. "I should position the mouthpiece and cough effectively."
[ ] 4. "I should position the mouthpiece and breathe naturally."

Just before the total hip replacement, the nurse prepares a large area of the client's skin for surgery.

81. Which technique is most appropriate for the nurse to use when preparing the operative site?
[ ] 1. Washing the area with soap and water
[ ] 2. Pressing the razor deeply into the skin while shaving
[ ] 3. Clipping the hair around the intended incisional area
[ ] 4. Shaving in the direction of hair growth

82. After the client undergoes a total hip replacement, how should the nurse position the affected hip?

[ ] **1.** Adduct the hip
[ ] **2.** Abduct the hip
[ ] **3.** Flex the hip
[ ] **4.** Extend the hip

83. The nurse and nursing assistant are caring for the client postoperatively. Which piece of equipment would the nurse instruct the nursing assistant to obtain?

[ ] **1.** A bed cradle
[ ] **2.** A bed board
[ ] **3.** An overhead trapeze
[ ] **4.** Lower side rails

84. What equipment is best for preventing external rotation of the operative leg when caring for a client with a total hip replacement?

[ ] **1.** A footboard
[ ] **2.** A trochanter roll
[ ] **3.** A turning sheet
[ ] **4.** A foam mattress

After the client's total hip replacement, the nurse provides discharge instructions regarding positions to be temporarily avoided.

85. Which statement indicates that the client understands the restrictions to be followed?

[ ] **1.** "I shouldn't cross my legs."
[ ] **2.** "I should avoid pointing my toes."
[ ] **3.** "I shouldn't lie flat in bed."
[ ] **4.** "I shouldn't stand upright."

86. When coordinating discharge care with a home health nurse, which piece of equipment is essential for home care?

[ ] **1.** A wheelchair
[ ] **2.** A hospital bed
[ ] **3.** A raised toilet seat
[ ] **4.** A mechanical lift

87. Which area of health teaching is essential to include in the discharge instructions for a client who has undergone a total hip replacement?

[ ] **1.** Modifying ways of donning clothing
[ ] **2.** Using special equipment for bathing
[ ] **3.** Taking vigorous daily walks
[ ] **4.** Receiving a daily stool softener

A 36-year-old client undergoes an arthroscopy of the right knee for diagnosing and treating chronic joint pain.

88. When assessing the preoperative teaching, which information is considered a priority?

[ ] **1.** Signs and symptoms of arthritis
[ ] **2.** Technique for using crutches
[ ] **3.** Adverse effects of drug therapy
[ ] **4.** The need to balance rest and exercise

A 60-year-old client with osteoarthritis is scheduled to undergo knee arthroplasty in which an artificial joint will replace the natural knee joint. A continuous passive motion (CPM) machine will be used postoperatively.

89. To obtain client compliance with medical regimen, which information regarding continuous passive motion (CPM) machine use is essential?

[ ] **1.** A CPM machine strengthens the leg muscles.
[ ] **2.** A CPM machine relieves foot swelling.
[ ] **3.** A CPM machine reduces surgical pain.
[ ] **4.** A CPM machine restores joint function.

90. When the nurse is documenting the client's progress while using a continuous passive motion (CPM) machine, which assessment data are essential to include?

[ ] **1.** Degree of flexion, number of cycles, and condition of the sutures around the incision
[ ] **2.** Degree of flexion, number of cycles, and amount of time the client used the machine
[ ] **3.** Degree of flexion, number of cycles, and characteristics of drainage from the wound
[ ] **4.** Degree of flexion, number of cycles, and presence and quality of arterial pulses

91. Which evidence is the best indication that the client who had a knee arthroplasty is recovering according to expected outcomes and no longer needs the continuous passive motion (CPM) machine?

[ ] **1.** The client has minimal pain when ambulating.
[ ] **2.** The client can flex the operative knee 90 degrees.
[ ] **3.** The client can perform straight-leg raising.
[ ] **4.** The client's surgical wound is approximated.

A 54-year-old client is being treated for gout.

92. When the nurse examines the client, which body part is usually affected by gout?

[ ] **1.** Great toe
[ ] **2.** Index finger
[ ] **3.** Sacrococcygeal vertebrae
[ ] **4.** Temporomandibular joint

93. When the nurse is providing shift report for the client diagnosed with gout, which lab result is essential to communicate with the next shift?

[ ] **1.** Creatinine clearance
[ ] **2.** Blood urea nitrogen
[ ] **3.** Serum uric acid
[ ] **4.** Serum calcium

After the physician orders a low-purine diet for the client, the nurse assesses the client's dietary needs and knowledge of appropriate foods.

94. The nurse would be correct to request a consultation with a dietitian if the client chooses a meal that includes which food?
[ ] **1.** Beets
[ ] **2.** Milk
[ ] **3.** Eggs
[ ] **4.** Liver

The client suffers an acute attack of gout. The physician prescribes colchicine to be given every hour until the client's pain is relieved.

95. Which client symptom indicates that the nurse should discontinue the medication and notify the physician even if the client's pain is unrelieved?
[ ] **1.** Vomiting
[ ] **2.** Dizziness
[ ] **3.** Drowsiness
[ ] **4.** Headache

The client with gout is at risk for forming kidney stones and has been instructed by the nurse to drink 3,000 mL of fluid daily.

96. When implementing the care plan, the nurse should encourage the major intake of fluids at which time of the day?
[ ] **1.** Before bedtime
[ ] **2.** Early evening
[ ] **3.** In the morning
[ ] **4.** Midafternoon

The nurse advises the client to continue consuming a high intake of fluid after discharge.

97. When the client describes usual fluids in the diet, which would the nurse instruct the client to avoid?
[ ] **1.** Coffee
[ ] **2.** Alcohol
[ ] **3.** Cranberry juice
[ ] **4.** Carbonated drinks

Nursing Care of Clients with Degenerative Bone Disorders

98. The physician orders passive range-of-motion (ROM) exercises for an elderly client on bed rest. Which statement regarding the performance of ROM exercises is correct?
[ ] **1.** ROM exercises should be completed independently with verbal cues from the nurse.
[ ] **2.** Force may be needed during ROM exercises to achieve maximum benefit.
[ ] **3.** Support should be maintained to the proximal and distal areas of the joint during ROM exercise.
[ ] **4.** ROM exercises should be performed until the client verbalizes discomfort.

A middle-aged client asks the nurse about methods for preventing or delaying the onset of osteoporosis.

99. Which assessment finding most likely indicates that a client has osteoporosis?
[ ] **1.** Swollen joints
[ ] **2.** Discomfort when sitting
[ ] **3.** Spinal deformity
[ ] **4.** Diminished energy level

100. A client diagnosed with osteoporosis receives nursing instructions on methods to reduce disease progression. Which substances should the nurse advise the client to avoid?
[ ] **1.** Aspirin and fiber-containing laxatives
[ ] **2.** Tobacco products and carbonated beverages
[ ] **3.** Orange juice and caffeinated drinks
[ ] **4.** Calcium-enriched dairy products

101. The nurse is caring for a client who was just diagnosed with osteoporosis. In this lateral view of the spine, identify with an *X* the area where an abnormality will most likely be observed.

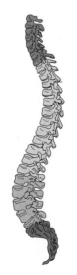

A 55-year-old client has developed bone necrosis as a result of chronic osteomyelitis in the tibia of the left leg.

102. Which nursing intervention is most appropriate for preventing a pathological fracture?
[ ] **1.** Encouraging a high fluid intake
[ ] **2.** Providing a nutritional diet
[ ] **3.** Supporting the limb during movement
[ ] **4.** Relieving pressure on bony prominences

A 68-year-old Hispanic client immigrated to the United States 3 months ago. The client comes to the emergency department with complaints of severe pain in the shoulder, elbow, and knee. The physician diagnoses bursitis.

103. On the basis of the nurse's knowledge of the client's culture and beliefs, which statement regarding the health-seeking behavior is probably most accurate?
[ ] **1.** Home remedies have been unsuccessful, and the condition threatens the client's self-image.
[ ] **2.** The power to cure comes from physicians and is based on advances in medical technology.
[ ] **3.** The client has lost faith in prayer, supernatural forces, and the *curandero*.
[ ] **4.** The client's condition is the result of the *mal de ojo* (evil eye).

A client diagnosed with osteomalacia has been told that the condition may improve with the addition of vitamin D.

104. Aside from recommending the consumption of foods fortified with vitamin D, which suggestion by the nurse is most appropriate?
[ ] **1.** Obtain more direct exposure to sunlight.
[ ] **2.** Eat meat from growth-stimulated cattle.
[ ] **3.** Consume bright orange vegetables.
[ ] **4.** Purchase organically grown produce.

Nursing Care of Clients with Amputations

During a farming accident, the arm of a 50-year-old person was caught in a grain elevator. The lower left arm and hand were crushed.

105. If the client is in shock, how should the nurse position the accident victim's body while continuing to assess and provide care?
[ ] **1.** Prone with the arm supported
[ ] **2.** In Fowler's position with the knees flexed
[ ] **3.** Supine with the legs elevated
[ ] **4.** Lateral with the back extended

The client is rushed to surgery where the injured arm is amputated above the elbow.

106. Postoperatively, the client screams obscenities at the nurse after realizing that the injured forearm is missing. Which nursing action is most appropriate at this time?
[ ] **1.** Leave until the client works through the anger.
[ ] **2.** Stay quietly with the client at the bedside.
[ ] **3.** Tell the client to gain emotional control.
[ ] **4.** Call the physician and request a sedative.

Later the client says, "I know my arm isn't there, but I feel it throbbing."

107. Which response by the nurse would be most accurate?
[ ] **1.** "You may be experiencing referred pain from an adjacent muscle."
[ ] **2.** "You may be experiencing phantom pain from the amputated site."
[ ] **3.** "You may be experiencing psychogenic pain from emotional distress."
[ ] **4.** "You may be experiencing intractable pain that can best be treated with opioids."

An older diabetic client is admitted with vascular problems. The nurse notes that some toes on the left foot are black. The client is scheduled for a below-the-knee amputation (BKA).

108. When planning the client's postoperative care, which position is least desirable as it could lead to long-term complications?
[ ] **1.** Lying prone
[ ] **2.** Lying supine
[ ] **3.** Sitting in a chair
[ ] **4.** Standing to shower

The nursing team meets to develop a plan for strengthening the client's muscles to prepare for ambulating with crutches after surgery.

109. Which activity is best to begin implementing immediately after the client's surgery?
[ ] **1.** Standing at the side of the bed
[ ] **2.** Balancing between parallel bars
[ ] **3.** Lifting oneself with the trapeze
[ ] **4.** Transferring from the bed to a chair

The client asks the nurse why the stump is rewrapped with elastic bandages several times a day.

110. While teaching the client, what can the nurse explain about the purpose of stump bandaging?
[ ] **1.** It lengthens and tones the muscles.
[ ] **2.** It shrinks and shapes the stump.
[ ] **3.** It maintains joint flexibility.
[ ] **4.** It absorbs blood and drainage.

111. When caring for a client with a below-the-knee amputation, the nurse promotes the client's potential use of a prosthesis. To ensure optimum rehabilitation, what nursing actions are appropriate? Select all that apply.
[ ] 1. Encourage the client to dangle at the bedside during personal care and for meals.
[ ] 2. Instruct the client to place a pillow under the thigh of the amputated limb while in bed.
[ ] 3. Teach the client to wrap the stump distally to proximally with an elastic bandage.
[ ] 4. Have the client tighten the thigh muscles and press the knee into the bed several times a day.
[ ] 5. Have the client remove and replace the stump bandage every other day.

Nursing Care of Clients with Skeletal Tumors

An 18-year-old client is diagnosed with a cancerous bone tumor (osteogenic sarcoma) in the femur. An above-the-knee amputation (AKA) is performed.

112. What equipment should be kept at the client's bedside during the immediate postoperative period?
[ ] 1. Gauze dressings
[ ] 2. Rubber tourniquet
[ ] 3. Oropharyngeal airway
[ ] 4. Oxygen equipment

A rigid plaster shell surrounds the client's stump. A pylon, or temporary prosthesis, allows the client to ambulate with crutches soon after surgery.

113. Which observation by the nurse best suggests that the client's crutches need further adjustment?
[ ] 1. The client stands straight without bending forward.
[ ] 2. The client's elbows are slightly flexed when standing in place.
[ ] 3. The top bars of the crutches fit snugly into the axillae.
[ ] 4. The client's wrists are hyperextended when grasping the handgrips.

114. Because of the location of a malignant bone tumor like osteogenic sarcoma, the nurse knows to assess for which possible complication?
[ ] 1. Bowel obstruction
[ ] 2. Liver dysfunction
[ ] 3. Mental status changes
[ ] 4. Anemia

115. The nurse is completing duties on a busy orthopedic unit. Which task is most appropriate to delegate to a skilled nursing assistant?
[ ] 1. Adjusting the client's prosthesis for ambulation
[ ] 2. Instructing the client on the use of a shower chair
[ ] 3. Retrieving requested labwork results
[ ] 4. Completing assessment of stump drainage

Nursing Care of Clients with Herniated Intervertebral Disks

A construction worker has an acute onset of severe low back pain. The physician suspects that the client has a herniated intervertebral disk in the lumbar spine.

116. When assessing the characteristics of pain in a client with a herniated disk, the nurse would expect to document increased intensity of pain during which activity?
[ ] 1. Eating
[ ] 2. Sneezing
[ ] 3. Sleeping
[ ] 4. Urinating

117. If the client is typical of others with a herniated disk, the nurse would expect the client to report which additional symptom?
[ ] 1. Pain radiating into the buttocks and leg
[ ] 2. Tenderness over one or both iliac crests
[ ] 3. Diminished sensation in one or both knees
[ ] 4. Brief periods when the toes feel quite cold

The physician makes a tentative diagnosis of herniated intervertebral disk and prescribes 30 mg of cyclobenzaprine hydrochloride (Flexeril) orally b.i.d.

118. While teaching the client, what can the nurse explain is the purpose for prescribing this medication?
[ ] 1. To reduce emotional depression
[ ] 2. To relax skeletal muscles
[ ] 3. To promote restful sleep
[ ] 4. To relieve inflammation

The physician orders a transcutaneous electric nerve stimulation (TENS) unit for the client with lower back pain.

119. Which statement reflects the most widely recognized theory for the use of transcutaneous electric nerve stimulation (TENS)?
[ ] 1. The sensation created by the TENS unit blocks the brain's perception of pain impulses.
[ ] 2. The sensation created by the TENS unit travels to the nerve root of the injury.
[ ] 3. The sensation created by the TENS unit destroys the brain's pain center.
[ ] 4. The sensation created by the TENS unit weakens nociceptor sensory nerves.

The physician orders a myelogram with a water-soluble contrast dye to confirm the diagnosis of a herniated intervertebral disk.

120. Which nursing intervention is most important after the client returns from the myelogram?
[ ] 1. Reducing glare from bright lights
[ ] 2. Withholding food and fluids for 12 hours
[ ] 3. Administering sedatives every 6 hours
[ ] 4. Encouraging a high fluid intake

Conservative treatment does not relieve the client's symptoms and physical disability. The client consents to have a laminectomy and spinal fusion in the lumbar area of the spine.

121. Before turning the client postoperatively, which nursing instruction is especially important to prevent postoperative complications?
[ ] **1.** "Hold your breath as you are turning."
[ ] **2.** "Move your lower body first, then your chest."
[ ] **3.** "As you hold onto the trapeze, lift your hips off the bed."
[ ] **4.** "Let me roll you as if you were a log."

The nurse includes principles of good body mechanics in the discharge teaching for a client who has undergone spinal surgery. The client is from a foreign country and speaks English as a second language.

122. Until a translator is available, which nursing action is best when teaching the client who speaks English as a second language about body mechanics?
[ ] **1.** Speak slowly while looking at the client.
[ ] **2.** Write the instructions on paper.
[ ] **3.** Use colorful pictures or diagrams.
[ ] **4.** Have the client watch a video.

123. With the assistance of the translator, the nurse correctly instructs the client to use which technique when picking something up?
[ ] **1.** Flex both knees.
[ ] **2.** Keep both feet together.
[ ] **3.** Lift with the arms extended.
[ ] **4.** Bend from the waist.

 # Correct Answers, Rationales, and Test Taking Strategies

Nursing Care of Clients with Musculoskeletal Injuries

1. 2. Tenosynovitis is an inflammation of the sheath that surrounds the tendons. Tendons connect muscle to bone. Typically tenosynovitis is found in the wrist and ankle and is caused by similar repeated movements (pinching, grasping, rotating). Temporarily eliminating the activity that has injured the tendons, in this case playing golf, is the best action to take at this time. Keeping the hand and wrist immobile is unnecessary. Playing miniature golf would continue to injure the tendon. Golfers wear gloves for a variety of reasons, such as preventing blisters. Although wearing a tight glove may give the wrist support, it does not protect the joint from injury.
> *Test Taking Strategy—Use the process of elimination to identify the option that provides the best evidence that the client understands how to implement the therapeutic measure for promoting symptom relief. Recall that this condition is related to repeated movements of the same kind; therefore, discontinuing playing golf temporarily (option 2) will facilitate relief of the client's symptoms. Review how tenosynovitis is managed if you had difficulty answering this question.*
> *Cognitive Level—Analyzing*
> *Client Needs Category—Health promotion and maintenance*
> *Client Needs Subcategory—None*

2. 2. Applying ice and elevating a swollen extremity relieves swelling. Heat is not used immediately after injury because it increases circulation to the injured part, causing more swelling. Exercise causes pain and further swelling in the early stage of an injury. Immobilization can help relieve pain and promote healing.
> *Test Taking Strategy—Look for the key words "most helpful" in reference to a method for reducing soft-tissue swelling. Recall that the acronym RICE—Rest, Ice, Compression, Elevation—is used to manage early symptoms caused by soft-tissue injuries, making option 2 the best answer. Review methods for treating sprains if you had difficulty answering this question.*
> *Cognitive Level—Applying*
> *Client Needs Category—Physiological integrity*
> *Client Needs Subcategory—Basic care and comfort*

3. 4. When wrapping the lower extremity with an elastic bandage, bandaging starts at the metatarsal bones, which form the ball of the foot and instep. The toes, or phalanges, are left uncovered to assess circulation. To relieve swelling, the injured area is wrapped distally (from the metatarsals) to proximally (the calf). Wrapping from below the knee toward the foot would not relieve swelling.

> *Test Taking Strategy*—*Analyze to determine what information the question asks for, which is the location where an elastic bandage should be started when wrapping the ankle area. Recall that to correctly apply an elastic bandage to an ankle, wrapping begins at the foot (option 4), moving upward above the ankle. Review the techniques for applying elastic bandages if you had difficulty answering this question.*
> *Cognitive Level*—*Understanding*
> *Client Needs Category*—*Physiological integrity*
> *Client Needs Subcategory*—*Basic care and comfort*

4. 1. By overlapping the elastic bandage in an alternately ascending and descending oblique pattern around a joint, the figure-eight turn is made. Each turn crosses the one preceding it so that it resembles the number eight. This method is used frequently for sprained ankles. A spiral-reverse turn is used to bandage a cone-shaped body part, such as the thigh or leg. The recurrent turn is used to cover the tip of a body part, such as the stump of an amputated limb. A spica turn is an adaptation of the figure-eight wrap; it is used when the wrap goes around an adjacent body part such as the thumb and hand or the thigh and hip.

> *Test Taking Strategy*—*Use the process of elimination to help select the option that identifies the best technique for wrapping the client's area of injury. Recall that using a figure-eight turn (option 1) is best when wrapping an ankle. Review techniques for wrapping parts of the body using an elastic bandage if you had difficulty answering this question.*
> *Cognitive Level*—*Understanding*
> *Client Needs Category*—*Physiological integrity*
> *Client Needs Subcategory*—*Basic care and comfort*

5. 3. The purpose of wrapping the injured area with an elastic bandage is to reduce pain and decrease swelling without interfering with circulation. If the bandage is applied too tightly, venous blood and lymph may become trapped in the toes, producing a swollen appearance. Some swelling of the toes may be the result of the initial injury. The toes may also feel numb or look blue. It is good to conduct a baseline assessment of color and swelling in the toes before applying the elastic bandage. Rewrapping the extremity may restore or improve circulation. The injured area will not be pain-free until the swelling subsides and injured tissue heals. Typically, there is some stiffness when maintaining a joint in a position.

> *Test Taking Strategy*—*Analyze to determine what information the question asks for, which is when it is essential to remove and rewrap a elastic bandage. Impaired circulation is characterized by cold, pale, or blue swollen toes (option 3). Review the potential for a tourniquet effect if an elastic bandage*

is applied too tightly or the wrapped tissue continues to swell after the bandage has been applied if you had difficulty answering this question.
> *Cognitive Level*—*Applying*
> *Client Needs Category*—*Health promotion and maintenance*
> *Client Needs Subcategory*—*None*

6. 4. A dislocation is caused by the tearing of the ligaments that connect and hold two bone ends within a joint, resulting in temporary displacement of the bone from its normal position. When the nurse assesses the client's injury, the affected arm will look longer than the other arm. Most traumatic musculoskeletal injuries, including sprains, strains, and fractures, are accompanied by pain, swelling, and compromised mobility. Consequently, these symptoms do not provide the best evidence of a dislocation.

> *Test Taking Strategy*—*Use the process of elimination to help select the option that identifies the best indication that the client has experienced a shoulder dislocation. Options 1, 2, and 3 can be eliminated because they are too nonspecific for a dislocation involving the shoulder. Option 4 is the best answer because a classic sign of a shoulder dislocation is that the arm with the injury is longer than the other. Review the signs and symptoms of a shoulder dislocation if you had difficulty answering this question.*
> *Cognitive Level*—*Applying*
> *Client Needs Category*—*Physiological integrity*
> *Client Needs Subcategory*—*Physiological adaptation*

7. 3. Restoring function for a dislocation involves repositioning two adjacent bones so that they are again in contact with one another. The physician does the repositioning manually, with or without anesthesia. A surgical incision is necessary when doing a procedure called an *open reduction*. Inserting a pin or wire is a type of internal fixation. To allow time for healing, exercise is prescribed only after a period of stabilization.

> *Test Taking Strategy*—*Look at the key words "most accurate" used in reference to the meaning for the term manipulation. Recall that manipulation is a procedure in which an area of an orthopedic injury is repositioned by the physician without creating a surgical incision. Review the definition of the word manipulation and a description for how it is performed if you had difficulty answering this question.*
> *Cognitive Level*—*Understanding*
> *Client Needs Category*—*Physiological integrity*
> *Client Needs Subcategory*—*Physiological adaptation*

8. 2. When a triangular sling is used, the knot is tied at the side of the neck to avoid pressure on the cervical vertebrae. All the other statements made by the family member indicate correct information concerning the application and use of a triangular sling.

Test Taking Strategy—Analyze to determine what information the question asks for, which is evidence that more teaching is required about the method for applying a triangular arm sling. Recall that there is a bony cervical vertebral prominence at the back of the neck. Therefore, the knot on the sling should be located on either side of the neck rather than in the posterior center area (option 2). Review how to apply a triangular sling to an injured arm if you had difficulty answering this question.
Cognitive Level—*Analyzing*
Client Needs Category—*Health promotion and maintenance*
Client Needs Subcategory—*None*

Nursing Care of Clients with Fractures

9. 4. To immobilize a broken bone, a splint is applied to prevent movement of the joints above and below the injury. The tibia is located between the knee and the ankle. Therefore, it is correct to apply the splint from below the ankle to above the knee. All other areas mentioned would not stabilize the injury correctly.
   Test Taking Strategy—Analyze to determine what information the question asks for, which is how to immobilize a lower extremity using a splint. Recall that a fracture causes instability in a bone that ordinarily is continuous between its proximal and distal attachments. To limit further injury and reduce the discomfort associated with the injury, joints above and below the injured bone (option 4) must be stabilized. Review the principles involved in applying an immobilizing splint if you had difficulty answering this question.
   Cognitive Level—*Applying*
   Client Needs Category—*Physiological integrity*
   Client Needs Subcategory—*Basic care and comfort*

10. 2. A comminuted fracture means that there are pieces, fragments, or splinters of bone in the area where the bone was broken. An impacted fracture is one in which the bone ends are driven together. A simple or closed fracture is one in which there is no break in the skin. A green-stick fracture involves a longitudinal split that extends partially through one side of the bone.
   Test Taking Strategy—Analyze to determine what information the question asks for, which is a description of a comminuted fracture. Recall that when a bone is broken into more than two pieces (option 2), the term comminuted is used to describe it. Review the words used to describe various types of fractures, with a focus on the description of a comminuted fracture, if you had difficulty answering this question.
   Cognitive Level—*Applying*
   Client Needs Category—*Physiological integrity*
   Client Needs Subcategory—*Physiological adaptation*

11. 4. The physician or hospital personnel should first attempt to obtain permission from a minor client's parent or guardian. Minors cannot give permission under most circumstances. If permission is obtained over the telephone, at least two people must hear the verbal consent and cosign as witnesses to what they heard. The physician's role is to explain the procedure and the risk factors associated with the surgery. The nurse's responsibility is to witness the signing of the consent. The youth leader is not an appropriate person to give consent unless previous arrangements were made in case of emergency. The best choice is the parent or guardian.
   Test Taking Strategy—Look at the key words "most appropriate," which are used when asking who can legally give consent for treatment when the client is a minor child. Recall that unless a minor is emancipated (i.e., living independently from his or her parents), consent for treatment must be obtained from a parent (option 4) or legal guardian. Review legal implications regarding obtaining consents for treatment if you had difficulty answering this question.
   Cognitive Level—*Applying*
   Client Needs Category—*Safe and effective care environment*
   Client Needs Subcategory—*Coordinated care*

12. 4. Jewelry is removed preoperatively, then itemized, identified, and locked in a secure area such as the hospital safe. The nurse is responsible for documenting in the client's record the items that were taken and how they are being kept secure. In some health care facilities, the client is given a receipt for this property. If a client asks that a wedding ring be left on, the nurse can secure it to the finger or hand with tape or a strip of gauze. Class rings, however, generally contain multiple grooves or crevices that can trap and hold microorganisms. Therefore, to reduce the risk of infection, it is best to remove and safeguard the ring. The ring is subject to theft if left in the bedside stand. Security guards usually are not responsible for the safekeeping of personal valuables. Another alternative is to give the client's valuables to a family member.
   Test Taking Strategy—Look at the key words "most appropriate," which are used when asking how a client's class ring as well as other valuables should be cared for before the client has surgery. Recall that the nurse is responsible for keeping valuables safe if they cannot be given to a responsible family member. Hospitals can retain clients' identified valuables temporarily in their safe (option 4). Review policies for safeguarding items of value when a client does not have the capacity to personally do so if you had difficulty answering this question.
   Cognitive Level—*Applying*
   Client Needs Category—*Safe and effective care environment*
   Client Needs Subcategory—*Coordinated care*

13. 1. In documenting the client's postoperative circulation status to the affected extremity, a detailed neurovascular assessment, including a circulation check ensuring adequate capillary refill and warm and pink toes, a sensation check requiring the client to identify touch, and a motion check requiring the client to move the toes, is a priority. Pain on movement is to be expected. An assessment of vital signs and inspection of the cast for drainage are important for documentation but are not of the highest priority regarding the circulatory status.

> *Test Taking Strategy—Use the process of elimination to help select the option identifying the highest priority to document when assessing circulatory status. Although options 2, 3, and 4 are valid assessment findings that indicate the absence of complications, option 1 represents a priority assessment in relation to this client's surgical procedure. Review the importance of assessing a client's neurovascular status after orthopedic surgery and a method for doing so if you had difficulty answering this question.*

Cognitive Level—*Analyzing*
Client Needs Category—*Physiological integrity*
Client Needs Subcategory—*Reduction of risk potential*

14. 2, 3, 4. During the first 72 hours after a traumatic injury, especially to long bones, the nurse should suspect fat embolism syndrome if the client manifests the following cluster of signs and symptoms: chest pain, dyspnea, tachycardia, tachypnea, fever, disorientation, restlessness, and petechiae over the chest, axillary folds, conjunctiva, buccal membrane, and hard palate.

> *Test Taking Strategy—Analyze to determine what information the question asks for, which is the signs and symptoms of fat embolism. Alternative-format "select all that apply" questions require considering each option independently to decide its merit in answering the question. Choose the options that best correlate with the signs and symptoms caused by a fat embolism. Review references for clinical manifestations experienced by a client who develops a fat embolism if you had difficulty answering this question.*

Cognitive Level—*Applying*
Client Needs Category—*Physiological integrity*
Client Needs Subcategory—*Reduction of risk potential*

15. 1. The first step a rescuer should take is to see that the victim is breathing, because maintaining ventilation is essential for sustaining life—assessing airway and breathing are a nurse's highest priority. The nurse should be careful about moving the client until spinal cord injuries are confirmed or ruled out. Observing for injuries and covering the client with a blanket are important, but only after breathing has been assessed.

> *Test Taking Strategy—Look at the key word "first" in relation to the action that is the highest priority when assisting a person involved in a motor vehicle accident. Recall Maslow's hierarchy of needs, which*

indicates life-sustaining physical needs (option 1) demand the priority for attention and care. Review how a patent airway and breathing supersede subsequent emergency actions, other than those in which a cardiac arrest has occurred, if you had difficulty answering this question.

Cognitive Level—*Analyzing*
Client Needs Category—*Physiological integrity*
Client Needs Subcategory—*Physiological adaptation*

16. 2. The ribs enclose the lungs. This makes injuries to the pulmonary system the primary complication associated with fractured ribs. Broken ribs may puncture the pleura and collapse a lung. One classic sign of a flail chest injury is asymmetrical or paradoxical chest expansion, which results in dyspnea. Although the heart is also in the thorax, it is somewhat better protected in the center of the chest. Tachycardia and a weak, thready pulse (rather than an irregular pulse rate) are more likely to indicate damage to major blood vessels. Expiratory wheezing is generally associated with asthma; pink, frothy sputum is commonly found with heart failure.

> *Test Taking Strategy—Use the process of elimination to help select the option that identifies the best indication of a complication associated with fractured ribs. Although options 1, 3, and 4 are abnormal findings, option 2 correlates most with a complication known as flail chest. Flail chest occurs when a segment of the ribs is broken in two or more places, resulting in paradoxical chest movement due to the loss of rib continuity. Review the signs and symptoms of a flail chest if you had difficulty answering this question.*

Cognitive Level—*Applying*
Client Needs Category—*Physiological integrity*
Client Needs Subcategory—*Reduction of risk potential*

17. 3. The best method to control bleeding in the case of a compound fracture is to compress the major artery above the injury site. Direct pressure on the wound may cause additional injuries to the soft tissue surrounding the fracture. A tourniquet is only used if all other efforts to control bleeding are unsuccessful. When used, a tourniquet is periodically released to allow oxygenated blood to the distal tissue. Elevating the extremity is helpful after applying pressure on the artery, but should be done with caution to prevent further damage to the bone and soft tissue.

> *Test Taking Strategy—Look at the key words "most appropriate," which are used when asking for a method to control bleeding that involves an open fracture. Recall that ordinarily pressure is used to control bleeding, but in the case of an open fracture, direct pressure may contribute to further injury. Therefore, pressure on the artery above the injury (option 3) is most appropriate. Review techniques for controlling bleeding and hemorrhage from a wound, especially one associated with an open fracture, if you had difficulty answering this question.*

Cognitive Level—Applying
Client Needs Category—Physiological integrity
Client Needs Subcategory—Physiological adaptation

18. 3. The neck and back of any accident victim with a suspected spinal injury should be immobilized before transport. The victim is typically positioned flat on the back (supine) and secured to a rigid stretcher before being moved and transported. Rescuers need to keep the head and spine extended and straight. Emergency medical personnel use a back board in such instances. Placing the client in a side-lying, face-lying (prone), or semisitting (semi-Fowler's) position may cause more injury to the vertebrae or the spinal cord because of the flexion and extra movement.

> *Test Taking Strategy—Look at the key words "most preferred," which are used when asking about the position for transporting a person with a possible back injury. Recall that it is imperative that the vertebrae be immobilized through positioning (option 3) and mechanical devices to prevent spinal cord injuries. Review the positions listed, focusing on which position is most useful for protecting the spinal cord, if you had difficulty answering this question.*
> *Cognitive Level—Applying*
> *Client Needs Category—Physiological integrity*
> *Client Needs Subcategory—Physiological adaptation*

19. 2, 3, 5. A client with a fractured hip develops pain in the injured area—the joint between the proximal end of the femur and the acetabulum of the pelvis—and weight bearing on the affected leg is impossible or difficult. The fracture results in shortening and external rotation of the affected leg because of discontinuity of the femur. Also, the client typically has muscle spasms involving the iliopsoas muscle attached to the lesser trochanter of the femur, and the abductor and rotator muscles that are inserted on the greater trochanter of the femur. Therefore, the client's affected leg is not drawn toward the midline in an adducted position. The client would probably be too uncomfortable in an adducted position or when sitting or lying.

> *Test Taking Strategy—Analyze to determine what information the question asks for, which is the signs and symptoms of a fractured hip. Alternative-format "select all that apply" questions require considering each option independently to decide its merit in answering the question. Choose the options that best correlate with the signs and symptoms experienced by a client who has a fractured hip. Review the signs and symptoms of a fractured hip if you had difficulty answering this question.*
> *Cognitive Level—Applying*
> *Client Needs Category—Physiological integrity*
> *Client Needs Subcategory—Physiological adaptation*

20. 1. Estrogen deficiency, which occurs postmenopausally, is linked to loss of calcium from the bones. Decreased bone mass weakens the skeletal system, increasing a person's susceptibility for fractures. Being overweight exerts more stress on the skeletal system; however, as long as bone integrity remains intact, the risk of fractures is the same as that for the general population. Individuals with type 2 diabetes have the same risk for fractures as the general population. Lactose intolerance is not necessarily a risk factor as long as the client gets calcium from other sources such as vegetables or a calcium supplement.

> *Test Taking Strategy—Look at the key words "most significant," which direct the selection of a risk factor from among the four options that predisposes an 80-year-old female to fracturing a hip. Note that the client is beyond childbearing years, indicating a reduced level of estrogen (option 1). Review the relationship between estrogen and its effect on bone density if you had difficulty answering this question.*
> *Cognitive Level—Understanding*
> *Client Needs Category—Physiological integrity*
> *Client Needs Subcategory—Reduction of risk potential*

21. 3. Protein requirements increase during prolonged immobility, such as when a client has a fractured hip. Protein is the only nutrient that can build and repair tissue. To promote healing and prevent skin breakdown and infection, increasing protein in the diet by adding protein-rich snacks such as cheese sticks celery with peanut butter is important. An orange provides vitamin C. A rice cake is a good snack when dieting. Potato chips have limited nutritional value.

> *Test Taking Strategy—Analyze to determine what information the question asks for, which is the snack that would be best for a client who has sustained a fractured hip. Recall that a primary function of dietary protein is the growth and repair of tissue, making a snack of sticks of cheese or (option 3) the best answer. Review the nutrient content of each snack, eliminating those that do not include protein, if you had difficulty answering this question.*
> *Cognitive Level—Applying*
> *Client Needs Category—Health promotion and maintenance*
> *Client Needs Subcategory—None*

22.

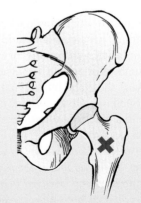

An intertrochanteric fracture refers to a break in the continuity of the femur between the greater and lesser trochanters, the bony prominences that lie outside the joint capsule. An intertrochanteric fracture is also referred to as an extracapsular fracture. The head and neck of the proximal femur are within the acetabulum. A fracture below the head of the femur (subcapital) or across the neck of the femur (transcervical) is referred to as an intracapsular fracture.

Test Taking Strategy—Analyze to determine what information the question asks for, which is the location of an intertrochanteric fracture of the femur. Refer to the anatomy of the femur if you had difficulty answering this question.
Cognitive Level—Understanding
Client Needs Category—Physiological integrity
Client Needs Subcategory—Physiological adaptation

23. 2. Isometric exercises are used to strengthen muscles and provide stamina. To perform isometric exercises, a client tenses and releases certain groups of muscles. These exercises do not involve any appreciable movement of a joint. The quadriceps muscles are on the anterior aspect of the thigh. All other options describe isotonic exercises, which involve joint movement.

Test Taking Strategy—Analyze to determine what information the question asks for, which is an isometric exercise involving the quadriceps group of muscles. Recall that isometric exercises are done "in place"; in other words, without moving about, which corresponds to the description in option 2. Review the differences between isotonic and isometric exercises, focusing on how the quadriceps muscles are exercised isometrically, if you had difficulty answering this question.
Cognitive Level—Applying
Client Needs Category—Health promotion and maintenance
Client Needs Subcategory—None

24. 1. Muscle contraction helps to move venous blood toward the heart. Clients who are inactive or immobile have reduced muscle activity in the lower extremities, predisposing to pooling of venous blood. The stagnation of blood places the client at risk for clot (thrombus) formation. Elastic stockings, known as *antiembolism stockings* or *thromboembolic disease hose*, support the valves within veins. The supported valves keep the blood flowing forward toward the heart. When blood moves, rather than pools in the lower extremities, it is less likely to form a clot (thrombus). Properly fitted antiembolism stockings should neither restrict arterial blood from flowing into the lower extremities nor affect blood pressure. Even though they are tight-fitting, antiembolism stockings do not constrict the blood vessels. Sequential compression devices (SCDs) are another commonly used method designed to limit the development of deep vein thrombosis (DVT) and peripheral edema in immobile clients or those recovering from vascular or orthopedic surgery.

Test Taking Strategy—Use the process of elimination to help select the option that provides the best explanation for the purpose of antiembolism stockings. Recall that valves within the veins promote the forward motion of venous blood to the heart. Keeping the valves supported with elastic antiembolism stockings prevents stagnation of venous blood (option 1), which predisposes to forming blood clots. Review factors that predispose clients to forming venous blood clots if you had difficulty answering this question.
Cognitive Level—Understanding
Client Needs Category—Physiological adaptation
Client Needs Subcategory—Reduction of risk potential

25. 1. To prevent trapping venous blood in the lower extremities, antiembolism stockings are applied while the legs are in a nondependent position. The best time to apply these stockings is in the morning, before the client gets out of bed, or after elevating the legs a short time. Antiembolism stockings are worn almost continuously. They are removed once per shift or once per day to assess the skin.

Test Taking Strategy—Analyze to determine what information the question asks for, which is the correct technique for applying antiembolism stockings. Recall that gravity causes venous blood to pool in the lower legs. To minimize pooling, antiembolism stockings are applied before the client gets out of bed before pooling can occur. Review the guidelines for applying antiembolism stockings to provide the most therapeutic benefit if you had difficulty answering this question.
Cognitive Level—Understanding
Client Needs Category—Safe and effective care environment
Client Needs Subcategory—Coordinated care

26. 1. A client who has had a repair of a fractured hip is turned using sufficient pillows so that the operative leg remains slightly abducted. Hip abduction prevents displacement of the fixation device. Pointing the toes, flexing the knee, or elevating the head will not promote hip abduction.

Test Taking Strategy—Analyze to determine what information the question asks for, which is the correct manner in which clients with a hip repair should be turned postoperatively. Recall that abduction of the hip (option 1) using pillows between the client's legs helps to maintain the hip within the hip joint. Review precautions to take when turning a postoperative client who has had a fractured hip repaired if you had difficulty answering this question.
Cognitive Level—Applying
Client Needs Category—Physiological integrity
Client Needs Subcategory—Reduction of risk potential

27. 3. When helping the client transfer from the bed to a chair, it is best to place the chair parallel to and near the head of the bed on the client's stronger side. The distance between the bed and chair should be as short as possible because the client is weak and at risk for losing balance. Transferring to a chair at the end of the bed or against a side wall requires much more physical effort and poses safety hazards. Placing the chair perpendicularly interferes with assisting the client.

> *Test Taking Strategy—Analyze to determine what information the question asks for, which is the best placement of a chair to allow transferring the client with a hip prosthesis from bed. Recall that the primary concern is to prevent the client from falling and reinjuring the repaired hip as well as reducing the work of the nurse. If the chair is placed parallel with the client's stronger side and near the head of the bed (option 3), the client can support weight on the unaffected left leg during the transfer. Review the technique for transferring clients from bed to a chair if you had difficulty answering this question.*
> *Cognitive Level—Applying*
> *Client Needs Category—Safe and effective care environment*
> *Client Needs Subcategory—Safety and infection control*

28. 1. In a three-point partial weight-bearing gait, the weaker leg and walker are advanced together. The hands support most of the weight while the stronger leg is lifted and advanced. This distributes the client's weight correctly.

> *Test Taking Strategy—Analyze to determine what information the question asks for, which is a correct description of a three-point partial weight-bearing gait. When using a walker to perform a three-point partial weight-bearing gait, the body weight is supported with both hands on the handgrips while placing some weight on the affected leg to move forward (i.e., 2 hands + 1 leg = 3 points), which is option 1. Review the various ambulatory gaits that may be used when using a walker or crutches and the manner in which they are performed if you had difficulty answering this question.*
> *Cognitive Level—Analyzing*
> *Client Needs Category—Health promotion and maintenance*
> *Client Needs Subcategory—None*

29. 1, 2, 3. Until healing occurs, the client's legs must be spread outward (abducted) from the body. Adduction of the hip or flexion greater than 90 degrees may dislocate the prosthesis from the joint. Postoperative nursing care also requires using a foam wedge splint between the legs while the client is in bed, using a raised toilet seat for elimination, keeping the knees lower than the hips when sitting, and reminding the client to avoid bending forward when dressing. Raising the head of the bed 90 degrees creates excessive hip flexion and can dislocate the hip. The leg should be in neutral position after hip replacement surgery.

> *Test Taking Strategy—Analyze to determine what information the question asks for, which is proper positioning of a client who has undergone total hip replacement. Alternative-format "select all that apply" questions require considering each option independently to decide its merit in answering the question. Choose the options that best correlate with the postoperative nursing care of a client with a total hip replacement. Review the postoperative care of clients undergoing a total hip replacement if you had difficulty answering this question.*
> *Cognitive Level—Applying*
> *Client Needs Category—Physiological integrity*
> *Client Needs Subcategory—Reduction of risk potential*

Nursing Care of Clients with Casts

30. 2. Casts are used to immobilize a body part until a bone can heal. When plaster combines with water, a chemical reaction takes place. Energy is given off in the form of heat. Therefore, it is appropriate to warn the client that the arm may feel quite warm temporarily. Steam or heat waves may even be seen rising from the surface of the wet cast. The cast supports the broken bone, but it should not constrict the underlying tissue or feel tight. Wet plaster does not produce a disagreeable odor. The client should not feel itchy when the cast is applied.

> *Test Taking Strategy—Look at the key words "most accurate" as they relate to information provided by the nurse to a client who will have a cast applied. Recall that heat (option 2) is a by-product of the chemical reaction that occurs when plaster is mixed with water. Review the teaching that is appropriate to provide a client on whom a cast will be applied if you had difficulty answering this question.*
> *Cognitive Level—Applying*
> *Client Needs Category—Physiological integrity*
> *Client Needs Subcategory—Reduction of risk potential*

31. 4. A wet cast is held and supported with the palms of the hands. Using the fingers is likely to cause indentations in the cast, which may create pressure areas on the underlying tissue. After the cast is applied, it is dried while supported on a soft surface like pillows. A wet cast on a hard surface can become flattened.

> *Test Taking Strategy—Use the process of elimination to select the option that identifies the best method for supporting a plaster cast as it is being applied. Options 2 and 3 can be eliminated immediately because the methods they describe will cause changes in the cast contour and internal dents that can cause pressure ulcers. Option 1 has some merit, but not until later; supporting the cast on pillows*

interferes with the application of the cast. Option 4 remains the best answer because it will not cause changes in the external or internal surfaces of the cast. Review how to assist with a cast application if you had difficulty answering this question.
***Cognitive Level**—Applying*
***Client Needs Category**—Physiological integrity*
***Client Needs Subcategory**—Reduction of risk potential*

32. 1. Compartment syndrome occurs when the muscle swells but the muscle tissue, blood vessels, and nerves are constricted by surrounding nonexpansive fascia or a rigid cast. Unrelenting sharp pain that is not relieved using standard measures is the first symptom of compartment syndrome. Ischemia, the impairment of arterial blood flow that is caused by swelling of the surrounding muscle within the inelastic fascia, causes pain. Paralysis and sensory loss follow as nerves become damaged by compression and lack of blood supply. Muscle spasms do not typically occur. The hand may appear pale or white, not reddened, and may feel cold because of inadequate arterial blood. If the radial artery is assessed, the nurse typically finds that the pulse is weak or absent.

> *Test Taking Strategy—Use the process of elimination to select the option that identifies the best indication that compartment syndrome is developing. Refer to the rationale for why options 2 and 4 can be eliminated because they describe findings unrelated to compartment syndrome. Option 3 can be eliminated because muscle spasms do not occur. Option 1 remains the correct answer because pain is the classic symptom of ischemia. Review the etiology of compartment syndrome and the signs and symptoms related to it if you had difficulty answering this question.*

***Cognitive Level**—Applying*
***Client Needs Category**—Physiological integrity*
***Client Needs Subcategory**—Reduction of risk potential*

33. 4. A wet cast is supported along its entire length with soft pillows as it dries. This soft support distributes the weight of the cast over a greater surface and prevents flattening of the underlying portion. Using pillows also elevates the extremity, which relieves temporary swelling. A synthetic sheepskin or vinyl sheet would interfere with water evaporation from the wet plaster. An absorbent pad would not sufficiently cushion the weight of the cast.

> *Test Taking Strategy—Use the process of elimination to help select the option that identifies the best material to place beneath a wet cast. Options 2 and 3 can be eliminated immediately because they cause the cast to retain water. Option 1 looks like an attractive answer because of the word "absorbent"; however, this type of pad is thin and will increase the risk for flattening the contour of the cast. Option 4 remains the best answer because it conforms to the round shape of the cast. Review the care of a client with*

a freshly applied plaster cast if you had difficulty answering this question.
***Cognitive Level**—Applying*
***Client Needs Category**—Physiological integrity*
***Client Needs Subcategory**—Physiological adaptation*

34. 1. Natural evaporation is the best way to dry a plaster cast. This process takes 24 to 48 hours. It involves leaving the casted area uncovered and turning the client at frequent intervals so that the entire cast circumference is exposed to the air. Intense heat, such as with a heating blanket, hair dryer, or heat lamp, may burn the client or just dry the superficial surface of the cast.

> *Test Taking Strategy—Use the process of elimination to help select the option that identifies the best method for drying a wet cast. Although the surface of the cast will feel dry using options 2, 3, and 4, they can be eliminated because the inside of the cast will remain wet. Therefore, option 1 is the best answer because over time the entire cast will become thoroughly dry. Review how to facilitate drying a wet plaster cast if you had difficulty answering this question.*

***Cognitive Level**—Applying*
***Client Needs Category**—Physiological integrity*
***Client Needs Subcategory**—Basic care and comfort*

35. 3. There is a difference between a circulatory assessment and a neurovascular assessment. Circulation is assessed by compressing nail beds to observe capillary refill. After pressure on a nail bed is released, the color returns to normal within 2 to 3 seconds. This assessment is also performed on the opposite extremity. If the capillary refill time is normal and similar in the nail beds of both extremities, circulation can be considered adequate. Determining that there is space between the cast and the skin is not totally reliable. If circulation is impaired due to compartment syndrome, there may still be room to insert a finger at the cast margins. Moving the fingers reflects nerve function.

> *Test Taking Strategy—Use the process of elimination to select the option that describes the best method for assessing circulation in the casted extremity. Option 3 is the best answer because it describes a standard of care for assessing circulatory status referred to as the blanching test. Review the purpose for the blanching test and the method for performing it if you had difficulty answering this question.*

***Cognitive Level**—Applying*
***Client Needs Category**—Physiological integrity*
***Client Needs Subcategory**—Reduction of risk potential*

36. 2. Casts made of fiberglass, a molded plastic material, have several advantages, one of which is that they are lighter than plaster casts. A synthetic cast dries more quickly, is more durable, and is unlikely to soften if it becomes wet; that is not to say that the padding beneath the fiberglass cast will be water-resistant. Fiberglass casts are more difficult to mold around an extremity when being applied. Because of their rigidity, they are more likely to impair skin where rough edges may develop.

> *Test Taking Strategy—Look at the key words "most accurate," which requires analyzing the options to identify one that correlates with a characteristic of fiberglass casts. Recall that this type of synthetic cast is made of cotton-polyester knit that is impregnated with fiberglass, making it much lighter (option 2) than plaster of paris. Fiberglass casts are no less flexible (option 3) or less restrictive (option 4) than plaster ones. The major disadvantage is that they are more expensive (option 1) than traditional plaster casts. Review the advantages and disadvantages of fiberglass casts if you had difficulty answering this question.*
> *Cognitive Level—Applying*
> *Client Needs Category—Physiological integrity*
> *Client Needs Subcategory—Physiological adaptation*

37. **3.** Marking the outer margin of the drainage on the cast helps the nurse evaluate the status of the bleeding. The nurse should reassess the client's cast for drainage every few minutes thereafter. By comparing the subsequent size of the bloody spot, the nurse evaluates the seriousness of the bleeding. It is important to monitor vital signs each time the drainage is assessed. All information is documented. If the bleeding is not controlled and vital signs indicate that the client's condition is changing, the physician must be notified immediately. An ice bag is generally used to control swelling postoperatively; it may also help decrease bleeding.

> *Test Taking Strategy—Analyze to determine what information the question asks for, which is the nursing action that should be performed after observing a bloody discoloration on the surface of a cast. Recall that assessment is the first step in the nursing process. Observing whether the circled drainage (option 3) increases helps the nurse determine if the bleeding is significant. Review references that describe care of a client with a cast if you had difficulty answering this question.*
> *Cognitive Level—Applying*
> *Client Needs Category—Physiological integrity*
> *Client Needs Subcategory—Physiological adaptation*

38. **3.** When a client expresses a concern, it is best for the nurse to verbalize the feeling or message that the sender conveyed. This response shows understanding and a willingness to listen. Using cliches, agreeing with the client, stereotyping the family, or offering opinions are all nontherapeutic. They are of little help to a client who is struggling with a personal problem.

> *Test Taking Strategy—Look at the key words "most appropriate." Apply the key words to identify the*

option that is an example of a therapeutic response. Recall that by sharing perceptions (option 3), the nurse shows empathy for the client's feelings. Review types and examples of therapeutic and nontherapeutic communication techniques if you had difficulty answering this question.
> *Cognitive Level—Applying*
> *Client Needs Category—Psychosocial integrity*
> *Client Needs Subcategory—None*

39. **3.** Most adolescents seek to become independent of their parents and develop relationships with nonrelatives. Developmental tasks concerned with self-identity, sexuality, testing the body's abilities, and learning to control emotional behavior occur more commonly just before young adulthood.

> *Test Taking Strategy—Analyze to determine what information the question asks for, which is the developmental task of an adolescent. Recall that adolescence is a time during which teenagers are learning and testing behaviors that promote independence. Review references that discuss the developmental tasks of adolescence if you had difficulty answering this question.*
> *Cognitive Level—Applying*
> *Client Needs Category—Health promotion and maintenance*
> *Client Needs Subcategory—None*

40. **2.** A hip-spica cast is used to immobilize and promote healing of a hip joint or fractured femur. This type of cast covers the trunk of the body and includes one or both legs to the knee or ankle, depending on the injury. The cast interferes with hip flexion and assuming a sitting position. A fracture bedpan elevates the buttocks just slightly enough for bowel elimination.

> *Test Taking Strategy—Analyze to determine what information the question asks for, which is identifying an item that can be used to facilitate the client's bowel elimination. Recall that the rigidity of the cast will not allow flexion of the hip, making a fracture bedpan (option 2) the best answer. Because this client cannot sit, a bedside commode (option 1), mechanical lift (option 3), and raised toilet seat (option 4) are inappropriate. Refer to illustrations of a hip-spica cast and discussions of nursing measures when caring for a client with this type of cast if you had difficulty answering this question.*
> *Cognitive Level—Applying*
> *Client Needs Category—Physiological integrity*
> *Client Needs Subcategory—Basic care and comfort*

41. **3.** One of the weakest areas of a hip-spica cast is at the groin. This area tends to crack because it is stressed when the client is turned and repositioned. The bar helps to strengthen the cast. The bar is never used for lifting, turning, or performing physical exercise. The bar will maintain proper alignment, but this is not its primary purpose.

> *Test Taking Strategy—Look at the key words "most accurate" and apply them to identify the option that correlates with a correct statement regarding the purpose of the bar within a hip-spica cast. Recall that the hips and legs are generally abducted when this type of cast is used, making the cast subject to damage during position changes. The bar helps to provide more stability (option 3) to avoid cracking or breaking. Review the construction of a hip-spica cast and areas that are subject to damage if you had difficulty answering this question.*
> *Cognitive Level—Understanding*
> *Client Needs Category—Health promotion and maintenance*
> *Client Needs Subcategory—None*

42. 1. Obtaining a medical order for administering an antihistamine/antipruritic drug such as cyproheptadine (Periactin) can chemically relieve the client's itching. Distraction may also be an alternative technique for relieving discomfort, but it takes commitment and repeated practice to be effective. The client should be cautioned against using a flat ruler or any method that scratches the skin under the cast. If the integrity of the skin is impaired, organisms may begin to grow in the warm, dark, moist environment. Powder is inappropriate because it can cake under the cast, causing potential skin breakdown. Ice bags to the outside of the cast are ineffective in preventing itching.

> *Test Taking Strategy—Look at the key words "most appropriate" and select the best method for relieving itching beneath a cast. Recall that the primary goal is to prevent the client from scratching and impairing the skin. One method is to administer a medication (option 1) that relieves itching. Review interventions that can assist with safely relieving itching while preventing impairment of skin integrity if you had difficulty answering this question.*
> *Cognitive Level—Applying*
> *Client Needs Category—Physiological integrity*
> *Client Needs Subcategory—Pharmacological therapies*

43. 4. The most common cause of an odor from a cast is an infected wound. Infected wounds produce purulent drainage, causing unpleasant odors as the pus accumulates. To confirm the suspicion that an infection exists, the nurse should monitor the client for a cluster of additional signs and symptoms, including elevated temperature, tachycardia, anorexia, and malaise.

> *Test Taking Strategy—Look at the key words "most accurate" and select the option that explains a cause for a foul odor coming from the cast. Recall that infected exudate (option 4) can create an odor, especially when it is confined beneath a cast*

for an extended time. Review characteristics that accompany purulent drainage if you had difficulty answering this question.
> *Cognitive Level—Understanding*
> *Client Needs Category—Physiological integrity*
> *Client Needs Subcategory—Physiological adaptation*

44. 2. The piece of plaster that is removed to make a window should be replaced in the opening and secured with tape or an elastic bandage. Allowing the window to remain unplugged may cause the tissue to bulge into the opening. This uneven pressure on the skin can cause it to break down. There is no need to store the plaster piece, dispose of it, or send it to the laboratory.

> *Test Taking Strategy—Look at the key words "most appropriate" and select the option that correlates with the best action to take when a window has been created in a cast. Recall that a "window" facilitates assessing and treating impaired skin or the site of an infection beneath the cast. The tissue, however, will bulge through the open space unless the piece of plaster is replaced (option 2). Review the care that is required for a cast with a window if you had difficulty answering this question.*
> *Cognitive Level—Applying*
> *Client Needs Category—Physiological integrity*
> *Client Needs Subcategory—Physiological adaptation*

45. 1. Rough or crumbling edges of a plaster cast are smoothed or repaired by applying petals made from moleskin or adhesive tape. Petals, formed in rectangular or oval pieces, are inserted on the inside of the cast edge and then folded over the outside edge of the cast. The strips are made to overlap, resembling the appearance of flower petals. The physician usually applies more plaster strips or uses a cast cutter if needed. Trimming a cast does not usually stop it from crumbling. Fragments of plaster are likely to continue breaking off if the nurse uses gauze to cover the cast edge.

> *Test Taking Strategy—Look at the key words "most correct" in reference to the best action to take when rough cast edges threaten the integrity of the skin. Recall that rather than remove and replace the cast, the rough edges can be smoothed by applying petals made from tape or moleskin (option 1). Review how to manage the care of a client in a cast, focusing on methods to prevent impaired skin, if you had difficulty answering this question.*
> *Cognitive Level—Applying*
> *Client Needs Category—Physiological integrity*
> *Client Needs Subcategory—Physiological adaptation*

46. 1. Cast syndrome, also known as *superior mesenteric syndrome,* causes GI symptoms, such as abdominal distention, bloating, nausea, vomiting, and abdominal pain. The symptoms are caused by a partial or total intestinal obstruction. Symptoms related to anxiety may also be present.

> *Test Taking Strategy—Analyze to determine what information the question asks for, which is the signs and symptoms of cast syndrome. Recall that a hip-spica cast encircles the trunk of the body; its rigidity interferes with expansion if intestinal gas accumulates or other digestive symptoms develop (option 1). The other options, if they develop, are more likely to be caused by complications other than cast syndrome. Review cast syndrome, also known as superior mesenteric syndrome, if you had difficulty answering this question.*
> **Cognitive Level**—*Applying*
> **Client Needs Category**—*Physiological integrity*
> **Client Needs Subcategory**—*Physiological adaptation*

Nursing Care of Clients with Traction

47. 2. Buck's traction is a type of skin traction used to immobilize, position, and align one or more lower extremities. The leg of the client in Buck's traction must remain in alignment with the pull of the traction. This means, rather than making the bed as usual from side to side, the nurse removes and applies the linens at the top or bottom of the bed and pulls them underneath the client. A person in Buck's traction is not turned from side to side or raised with a mechanical lift. A client in traction, as any other hospitalized client, has bed linens changed whenever they are soiled, wet, or need replacement.

> *Test Taking Strategy—Use the process of elimination to help select the option that identifies the best nursing technique when changing the linen on the bed of a client in Buck's traction. Options 1 and 4 can be eliminated immediately because the extremity or extremities must be kept in alignment with the pull of traction. Option 3 can be eliminated because it is not appropriate to delay changing the linen. This leaves option 2 as the correct answer because the linens can be pulled beneath the client's posterior without disturbing the pull of traction. Review nursing care of a client in Buck's traction if you had difficulty answering this question.*
> **Cognitive Level**—*Applying*
> **Client Needs Category**—*Physiological integrity*
> **Client Needs Subcategory**—*Basic care and comfort*

48. 3. To maintain countertraction, the client's foot must never press against the foot of the bed. If this occurs, the nurse should help pull the client toward the head of the bed. The weights must always hang free, rather than rest on the floor or the bed. The body must be in alignment with the pull of the traction. The traction rope must move freely within the groove of the pulley.

> *Test Taking Strategy—Analyze to determine what information the question asks for, which is an assessment*

finding that requires immediate action. Finding the client's foot at the end of the bed (option 3) is a cause for immediate action because it indicates that the traction is ineffective. Review the care of a client in traction if you had difficulty answering this question.*
> **Cognitive Level**—*Applying*
> **Client Needs Category**—*Physiological integrity*
> **Client Needs Subcategory**—*Reduction of risk potential*

49. 2. The best technique for assessing circulation among the options provided is to palpate the distal peripheral pulse, such as the dorsalis pedis artery, which is on the top of the foot. Other pertinent circulatory assessments include checking the client's skin color, temperature, capillary refill time, and subjective complaints concerning pain. Checking movement and sensation are neurologic assessment techniques. Taking the blood pressure on the thigh rather than the arm is unnecessary.

> *Test Taking Strategy—Use the process of elimination to help select the option that describes the best technique for assessing the quality of circulation in an extremity in Buck's traction. Options 1 and 4 can be eliminated immediately because they describe neurologic assessment techniques. Option 3 can be eliminated, because assessing a blood pressure in the thigh does not provide information about distal blood flow. Option 2 remains as the best answer because arterial blood flow is best assessed by palpating distal pulses and comparing them on both feet. Review how to perform a vascular assessment if you had difficulty answering this question.*
> **Cognitive Level**—*Applying*
> **Client Needs Category**—*Physiological integrity*
> **Client Needs Subcategory**—*Reduction of risk potential*

50. 2. Russell's traction is used to align a fractured femur. The affected leg is supported in a sling just below the knee and pulling forces are exerted upward and longitudinally by means of pulleys and weights. The popliteal space behind the knee is especially prone to pressure and irritation when Russell's traction is used. This area is suspended in a sling, which can become wrinkled. A piece of thick felt is sometimes used to line the sling to keep the surface smooth. The ischial spines are part of the inferior portion of the pelvic bones. The iliac crests are the upper flared portions of the bony pelvis. Neither of these areas is included in Russell's traction. The zygomatic arches are in the cheek.

> *Test Taking Strategy—Analyze to determine what information the question asks for, which is the location where the skin is most likely to become impaired when a client is in Russell's traction. Recall the description of Russell's traction, which indicates that the skin in the popliteal space is vulnerable to skin*

breakdown. Refer to images of this type of traction if you had difficulty answering this question.
Cognitive Level—Applying
Client Needs Category—Physiological integrity
Client Needs Subcategory—Reduction of risk potential

51. 3. Two pieces of rope are sometimes spliced together with a knot to provide sufficient length for traction. However, if the knot prevents free movement over and within a pulley, it interferes with the traction's effectiveness. Traction ropes are taut. Locating the trapeze above the client's chest facilitates its use. Traction weights must hang freely above the floor for effective use.
Test Taking Strategy—Analyze to determine what information the question asks for, which is identifying something that is interfering with the function of the traction. Recall that the ropes in any type of traction must move freely through the series of pulleys, making option 3 the correct answer. Review principles that apply to using traction for orthopedic injuries or disorders if you had difficulty answering this question.
Cognitive Level—Applying
Client Needs Category—Physiological integrity
Client Needs Subcategory—Reduction of risk potential

52. 1. Preoperatively, the traction remains applied to the client at all times, even during transport to the operating room. Its purpose is to relieve muscle spasms and immobilize the fractured bone. If the nurse removes the traction or releases the weights, muscle spasms can recur. Any realignment that may have been achieved with the use of traction is jeopardized.
Test Taking Strategy—Analyze to determine what information the question asks for, which is the appropriate action the nurse should take when transporting a client in traction to the operating room. Recall that traction must be maintained at all times, even during transport to surgery, making option 1 the correct answer. Review how to manage the care of a client in traction if you had difficulty answering this question.
Cognitive Level—Applying
Client Needs Category—Physiological integrity
Client Needs Subcategory—Reduction of risk potential

53. 4. A pillow is usually contraindicated when a client is in cervical skin traction because it alters the direction of pull. If any kind of head support is necessary, it is usually provided with a cervical or neck pillow that fits under the nape of the neck. The other options are correct and do not require the nurse's attention.
Test Taking Strategy—Analyze to determine what information the question asks for, which is a situation that requires immediate attention upon being observed by the nurse. Recall that the cervical vertebrae must

be aligned with the pull of the traction; because a pillow alters the alignment, option 4 is the correct answer. Review how to care for a client in cervical skin traction if you had difficulty answering this question.
Cognitive Level—Applying
Client Needs Category—Physiological integrity
Client Needs Subcategory—Reduction of risk potential

54. 3. The tips of the pin used for skeletal traction are skewered into a block of cork or a rubber ball similar to one used for playing jacks. Gauze and cotton are inadequate for preventing punctures and abrasions. The pin may also pierce rubber tubes, thereby exposing the sharp tip.
Test Taking Strategy—Use the process of elimination to identify the option that describes the best material for covering the pin used in skeletal traction. Recall that the choice of material must be sturdy enough to cover the tips of the pins, but safe enough that it will not injure the nurse or other caregivers. Option 3 meets those qualifications. Gauze squares and cotton balls (options 1 and 2) are too soft to prevent punctures. Pins can also pierce rubber tubes (option 4). Review nursing measures when caring for a client with skeletal traction if you had difficulty answering this question.
Cognitive Level—Applying
Client Needs Category—Safe and effective care environment
Client Needs Subcategory—Safety and infection control

55. 4. Purulent drainage, sometimes referred to as *pus*, indicates an infection. Purulent drainage is a collection of fluid containing white blood cells and pathogens. The presence of white blood cells indicates that the body is attempting to destroy and remove infecting organisms. Serous drainage, which is clear, is made up of plasma or serum. Bloody drainage indicates trauma. Mucoid drainage, which is released from mucous membranes, is sticky and transparent.
Test Taking Strategy—Use the process of elimination to identify the best indication that there is an infection at the pin site. Recall that the term purulent (option 4) refers to pus, which corresponds to an infectious exudate. Review a description of purulent drainage and the conditions under which it may be noted if you had difficulty answering this question.
Cognitive Level—Evaluating
Client Needs Category—Physiological integrity
Client Needs Subcategory—Physiological adaptation

56. 2. There is a high probability that individuals who are allergic to penicillin will also exhibit a cross-sensitivity to cephalosporins. Both types of drugs are similar in their structure. All clients with known drug sensitivity are closely observed when a new medication, especially an antibiotic, is administered. Individuals with a penicillin allergy seem to react more frequently to cephalosporins than to the other types of antibiotics mentioned.

> *Test Taking Strategy*—*Analyze to determine what information the question asks for, which involves a class of antibiotics that should be questioned if written in the medical orders of a client who is allergic to penicillin. Recall that some clients who are allergic to penicillin may have a cross-sensitivity to cephalosporin antibiotics as well. Review these classes of antibiotics, looking for a group that should be used with caution in clients who are allergic to penicillin, if you had difficulty answering this question.*
> *Cognitive Level*—*Applying*
> *Client Needs Category*—*Physiological integrity*
> *Client Needs Subcategory*—*Pharmacological therapies*

57. 1. Halo-cervical traction immobilizes the vertebrae in the neck while allowing clients to assume physical activity, such as standing, sitting, and walking. Halo-cervical traction restricts head movement. Vertebral fractures proceed to heal at a standard rate regardless of whether halo traction or some other medical or surgical management is instituted. Physical therapy is not prescribed until the vertebral fracture is stabilized and the halo traction is removed.

> *Test Taking Strategy*—*Look at the key words "most accurately," which are used to describe statements about the purpose for applying halo-cervical traction. Recall that this type of traction may be used in preference to keeping a client confined to bed with some other type of immobilizing traction. Option 2 can be eliminated because this type of traction restricts head movement. Options 3 and 4 can be eliminated because the type of traction does not affect the rate of healing, and physical therapy cannot be instituted until the vertebral fracture is stabilized. Refer to illustrations of halo-cervical traction and the reasons for its use if you had difficulty answering this question.*
> *Cognitive Level*—*Applying*
> *Client Needs Category*—*Physiological integrity*
> *Client Needs Subcategory*—*Physiological adaptation*

58. 4. A client's ability to see straight ahead is the best sign that halo-cervical traction is keeping the neck immobilized in a neutral position. Clients should not be able to move the neck at will while in halo-cervical traction. Clients may experience mild neck discomfort even though the traction is applied appropriately. The ability to speak and to hear are unrelated to the use of traction.

> *Test Taking Strategy*—*Use the process of elimination to help select the option that correlates with the best indication that halo-cervical traction is appropriately applied. Option 1 can be eliminated immediately because the client's head should be fixated in neutral position. Option 2 can be eliminated because the*

pain level experienced by a client can be variable. Option 3 can be eliminated because sensory functions are not a consequence of appropriately applied traction. Recall that the purpose of this type of traction is immobilization of the vertebrae; therefore, keeping the head in a straight anatomical position (option 4) is the best answer. Review how to assess if halo-cervical traction has been applied appropriately if you had difficulty answering this question.*
> *Cognitive Level*—*Applying*
> *Client Needs Category*—*Physiological integrity*
> *Client Needs Subcategory*—*Physiological adaptation*

59. 3. Signs of a developing complication related to halo traction include an inability to fully open the mouth and difficulty swallowing. Orthostatic hypotension, if it occurs, is not because of the malfunction of the halo traction. Men in halo traction typically need help with shaving because they cannot change their head position to see where to shave. Women in halo traction typically need help with shaving their axillae or legs; the nurse should anticipate offering assistance. Irritation in the axillae is usually related to the plaster vest and does not indicate a need for readjustment. Nursing intervention, however, is needed to prevent further skin breakdown.

> *Test Taking Strategy*—*Use the process of elimination to help select the option that identifies the best indication of a developing complication in a client in halo traction. Option 1 can be eliminated because it is not related to the traction. Options 2 and 4 can be eliminated because these are common discomforts but do not indicate complications of halo traction. Recall that halo traction is generally used to immobilize an injury of the cervical spine. Neurologic complications may be suspected if the client has impaired jaw movements, such as an inability to open the mouth (option 3), bite down, extend the tongue, or weakness swallowing. Review pertinent assessments of the client in halo traction if you had difficulty answering this question.*
> *Cognitive Level*—*Analyzing*
> *Client Needs Category*—*Physiological integrity*
> *Client Needs Subcategory*—*Reduction of risk potential*

Nursing Care of Clients with Inflammatory Joint Disorders

60. 1. Rheumatoid arthritis (RA) is a chronic, autoimmune, systemic inflammatory disorder affecting the joints. The erythrocyte sedimentation rate (ESR) test is a nonspecific test that indicates the presence and progress of an inflammatory disease. It is elevated in a number of inflammatory conditions, including RA. A partial thromboplastin time (PTT) helps determine a person's ability to clot blood; it is commonly ordered for clients receiving heparin therapy. A fasting blood sugar (FBS) test is performed to diagnose and evaluate the treatment of diabetes mellitus. Blood urea nitrogen (BUN) levels are commonly checked to assess renal function.

> *Test Taking Strategy*—*Use the process of elimination to help select the option that identifies the best test for diagnosing RA. Recall that an ESR is used to detect the presence of an inflammatory process. RA causes not only inflammation of joints, but also systemic inflammation. The severity of RA is indicated by the degree of ESR elevation (option 1); the client's response to treatment also can be determined by a decrease in the ESR. PTT (option 1) tests clotting ability, FBS (option 3) is a test for diabetes, and BUN (option 4) is used to assess renal function. Review signs and symptoms of RA if you had difficulty answering this question.*
> *Cognitive Level*—*Understanding*
> *Client Needs Category*—*Physiological integrity*
> *Client Needs Subcategory*—*Reduction of risk potential*

61. 3. Although some people acquire juvenile rheumatoid arthritis, most experience the onset of rheumatoid arthritis (RA) early in adult life. The disease profoundly affects the ability to maintain employment during the productive years of life.

> *Test Taking Strategy*—*Analyze to determine what information the question asks for, which is the usual time at which there is an onset of symptoms among those who develop RA. Recall that unlike osteoarthritis, which affects older adults, clients with RA typically present with signs and symptoms in early adulthood (in their twenties), which corresponds with option 3. Review the disease process, focusing on when signs and symptoms of RA are generally first manifested if you had difficulty answering this question.*
> *Cognitive Level*—*Applying*
> *Client Needs Category*—*Physiological integrity*
> *Client Needs Subcategory*—*Physiological adaptation*

62. 3. Aspirin produces analgesic, anti-inflammatory, and antipyretic effects. Its analgesic and anti-inflammatory effects are probably achieved by inhibiting chemicals called *prostaglandins*, not by interrupting nerve synapses. Prostaglandins increase sensitivity of peripheral pain receptors. Aspirin does not relax skeletal muscles or stimulate the immune system.

> *Test Taking Strategy*—*Analyze to determine what information the question asks for, which is the rationale for prescribing aspirin for a client with rheumatoid arthritis. Recall that aspirin is a salicylate, and its therapeutic effects include relief of the client's pain as well as inflammatory symptoms (option 3). Review the mechanism by which aspirin has an effect and*

the conditions for which it is prescribed if you had difficulty answering this question.
> *Cognitive Level*—*Understanding*
> *Client Needs Category*—*Physiological integrity*
> *Client Needs Subcategory*—*Pharmacological therapies*

63. 4. Taking irritating drugs with food or at mealtimes helps to decrease gastric distress. Aspirin, especially in large doses, tends to irritate the stomach mucosa, resulting in bleeding. Giving aspirin on an empty stomach increases discomfort because of the combination of gastric acidity and the acidity of aspirin (acetylsalicylic acid). Cold water and hot tea do not protect the stomach or alter aspirin's acidity. The caffeine in tea actually stimulates an increase in the production of stomach acid. Enteric-coated aspirin is needed for clients who take large doses of aspirin because the enteric coating protects the stomach.

> *Test Taking Strategy*—*Look at the key words "most appropriate" in reference to a nursing measure for relieving stomach discomfort caused by the prescribed aspirin. Recall that if food is consumed when gastric-irritating medications are administered, it may prevent or reduce gastric burning and nausea (option 4). Review nursing interventions related to the administration of aspirin if you had difficulty answering this question.*
> *Cognitive Level*—*Applying*
> *Client Needs Category*—*Physiological integrity*
> *Client Needs Subcategory*—*Pharmacological therapies*

64. 1. Ringing in the ears, called *tinnitus*, is a sign of aspirin toxicity and is seen when clients take large amounts of salicylates on a daily basis. Clients may also report a buzzing, tinkling, or hissing sound. Diseases or conditions affecting the ear can also cause tinnitus. Dizziness, metallic tastes in the mouth, and proteinuria are not typically associated with aspirin toxicity.

> *Test Taking Strategy*—*Use the process of elimination to help select the option that correlates with a symptom of aspirin toxicity. Many medications may cause side effects like those identified in options 2, 3, and 4, but tinnitus (option 1) is a classic sign of aspirin toxicity. Review aspirin toxicity and factors that contribute to it if you had difficulty answering this question.*
> *Cognitive Level*—*Applying*
> *Client Needs Category*—*Physiological integrity*
> *Client Needs Subcategory*—*Pharmacological therapies*

65. 2. A glucocorticord such as prednisone is used at low doses for short-term relief of pain and inflammation frequently brought on by periods of disease exacerbation in rheumatoid arthritis. A nonsteroidal anti-inflammatory drug (NSAID) such as ibuprofen is used in the early stages of the disease process. Etanercept (Enbrel) is a biological response modifier used when other treatments have failed.

Levofloxacin (Levaquin) is an antibiotic and will not improve the disease process.

> *Test Taking Strategy*—*Analyze to determine what information the question asks for, which is a medication that may be temporarily prescribed in addition to aspirin to control a recurrence of severe arthritis symptoms. Determine which of the medications in the four options may be used short-term to produce an anti-inflammatory effect. Although ibuprofen and etanercept are both used to manage symptoms of arthritis, they are more often given on an ongoing long-term basis. When symptoms of arthritis exacerbate, prednisone (option 2), which is a steroid, may be prescribed and then tapered before being discontinued. Review the actions and uses for each drug in the four options if you had difficulty answering this question.*
> *Cognitive Level*—*Analyzing*
> *Client Needs Category*—*Physiological integrity*
> *Client Needs Subcategory*—*Pharmacological therapies*

66. 4. Individuals receiving corticosteroids tend to have elevated blood glucose levels. Diabetic clients may need to increase their dosage of insulin or oral hypoglycemic agents. Nondiabetic clients should also be monitored for hyperglycemia and glycosuria. Because steroids depress the inflammatory response, they place the client at high risk for acquiring infections. To prevent acute adrenal insufficiency, steroids are tapered and withdrawn gradually if therapy is discontinued. Depression is common among individuals receiving corticosteroids.

> *Test Taking Strategy*—*Analyze to determine what information the question asks for, which is an incorrect statement that requires further teaching or clarification. Read the options carefully because you are looking for a statement that is wrong. Option 4 requires correction because a common side effect of steroids is an elevation of blood glucose, not a decrease. This becomes particularly problematic for diabetic clients who require steroids for an anti-inflammatory response. Review information on corticosteroid therapy if you had difficulty answering this question.*
> *Cognitive Level*—*Analyzing*
> *Client Needs Category*—*Physiological integrity*
> *Client Needs Subcategory*—*Pharmacological therapies*

67. 4. Distraction is a legitimate and often very effective method for relieving discomfort. Watching television is one method of distraction. There are no reports that electronic television signals are an effective treatment for arthritis. The client who has only a slight case of arthritis would be likely to feel pain relief at times other than when watching television.

> *Test Taking Strategy*—*Look at the key words "most accurate" when used to identify the conclusion*

the nurse can draw from the client's observation that watching television is associated with relief of discomfort. Recall that diversionary activities can decrease pain because the mind is focused on something other than discomfort (option 4). Review nonpharmacological methods for reducing pain if you had difficulty answering this question.
> *Cognitive Level*—*Applying*
> *Client Needs Category*—*Physiological integrity*
> *Client Needs Subcategory*—*Physiological adaptation*

68. 1. The proximal finger joints are most commonly affected in clients with rheumatoid arthritis. In some cases, the joints are so affected that the fingers actually turn laterally. In osteoarthritis, the distal finger joints are more commonly deformed. Traumatic arthritis, which is associated with a specific injury, can affect any joint.

> *Test Taking Strategy*—*Analyze to determine what information the question asks for, which is the finger joints most affected by rheumatoid arthritis. Recall that the joints at the bases of the fingers are affected by rheumatoid arthritis and ultimately destroyed by the inflammatory process. Review the signs and symptoms of rheumatoid arthritis, focusing on the locations where joints are most affected, if you had difficulty answering this question.*
> *Cognitive Level*—*Applying*
> *Client Needs Category*—*Physiological integrity*
> *Client Needs Subcategory*—*Physiological adaptation*

69. 2. Moist heat is more effective than forms of dry heat, such as hot wax treatments, an electric heating pad, or an infrared heat lamp. This phenomenon is attributed to the fact that water is a better conductor of heat than air. Whenever any form of heat is used, the nurse must take care to ensure that the client is not accidentally burned.

> *Test Taking Strategy*—*Use the process of elimination to help select the option that identifies the best method for applying heat to the client's joints that are affected by rheumatoid arthritis. Options 3 and 4 can be eliminated immediately because they are examples of devices that utilize dry heat. Melted wax (option 1) has some merit, but the modifying word "hot" disqualifies it because it suggests a potential for burning the skin. Option 2 is the best answer because it describes using "warm, moist" heat, which is more effective. Review the principles that apply to the therapeutic use of heat if you had difficulty answering this question.*
> *Cognitive Level*—*Applying*
> *Client Needs Category*—*Physiological integrity*
> *Client Needs Subcategory*—*Basic care and comfort*

70. 1. People with rheumatoid arthritis (RA) are stiffer and more uncomfortable in the early morning hours after being inactive during the hours of sleep. Therefore, it is best to allow extra time and to distribute self-care activities over later hours of the day.

> *Test Taking Strategy—Analyze to determine what information the question asks for, which is the time of day during which a client with RA has the greatest need for additional time and assistance with activities of daily living. Recall that clients with RA experience greater stiffness and impaired movement after being inactive during the night. Consequently, option 1 is the best answer. Review the effects the disease process has on joints and the time of day the client's activities are most affected if you had difficulty answering this question.*
> *Cognitive Level—Applying*
> *Client Needs Category—Physiological integrity*
> *Client Needs Subcategory—Basic care and comfort*

71. 2. Hand deformities and muscle atrophy make it difficult for the client with rheumatoid arthritis to perform fine motor movement with the fingers. Purchasing clothes that can be easily pulled or slipped on enables the client to maintain a degree of independence. Although exercise is important to help maintain the client's joint mobility, aerobic exercise is unrealistic because it is likely to be too strenuous and tiring (clients with rheumatoid arthritis are often anemic and tire easily). Sleeping on a waterbed or moving to a warm climate will have little, if any, effect on the disease process.

> *Test Taking Strategy—Look at the key words "greatest potential." Analyze the options for one that suggests a method for helping the client gain or maintain independence. Exercise, if it is low-impact rather than aerobic, would be beneficial. But option 2, selecting garments that can be easily donned or removed, is the best answer from among the options. Review methods for reducing the client's need for assistance with self-care activities if you had difficulty answering this question.*
> *Cognitive Level—Analyzing*
> *Client Needs Category—Physiological integrity*
> *Client Needs Subcategory—Basic care and comfort*

72. 1. During an acute attack, splints are used primarily to keep the inflamed joints somewhat inactive. Resting the affected joint in a splint limits the movement and alleviates additional stress on the diseased joints. The acute inflammation subsides with a combination of drug therapy and the body's natural healing processes. By limiting the damage during the acute attack, a certain amount of strength and joint flexibility is preserved, but these are not the primary purpose of splints. Splinting the affected fingers will not slow joint deterioration.

> *Test Taking Strategy—Analyze to determine what information the question asks for, which is the primary purpose for applying splints to the client's hands during an episode of acute symptoms. Recall that*

movement increases pain intensity, which leads to selecting option 1 as the best answer. Review symptoms experienced by a client with rheumatoid arthritis and the measures used to manage the symptoms if you had difficulty answering this question.
> *Cognitive Level—Applying*
> *Client Needs Category—Physiological integrity*
> *Client Needs Subcategory—Reduction of risk potential*

73. 2. Methotrexate (Rheumatrex) and cyclosporine, an immunomodulator, are two of several disease-modifying antirheumatic drugs (DMARDs). When used in combination, there is a greater reduction of rheumatoid arthritis (RA) symptoms than when monotherapy (one drug) is used. Dual therapy enhances the effects of the methotrexate—possibly because, as some clinicians believe, the combination provides additional suppression of the immune system. Combining the medications is not used for diminishing an exacerbation or for decreasing unwanted side effects associated with drug therapy. It is also not prescribed because the client's status is declining, thereby having severe symptoms.

> *Test Taking Strategy—Analyze to determine what information the question asks for, which is the reason for prescribing combination drug therapy. Because RA is associated with destruction of joints and is believed to have an autoimmune etiology, combination drug therapy potentiates greater effectiveness (option 2). Review references that discuss combining DMARDs such as methotrexate and cyclosporine if you had difficulty answering this question.*
> *Cognitive Level—Applying*
> *Client Needs Category—Physiological integrity*
> *Client Needs Subcategory—Pharmacological therapies*

74. 3. The mucosa of the mouth and entire GI tract may become ulcerated as a consequence of taking methotrexate (Rheumatrex). Therefore, it is especially important to inspect the oral cavity. This drug also causes many other side and adverse effects, including diarrhea and renal failure. Chest pain is not a usual adverse effect of methotrexate.

> *Test Taking Strategy—Analyze to determine what information the question asks for, which is an adverse effect of methotrexate. Recall that this drug is also classified as a cancer chemotherapeutic agent and, as such, destroys rapidly proliferating cells like those in the mucosa of the GI tract. Ulcerative stomatitis (mouth sores), option 3, requires an interruption of drug therapy. Review adverse effects associated with methotrexate if you had difficulty answering this question.*
> *Cognitive Level—Applying*
> *Client Needs Category—Physiological integrity*
> *Client Needs Subcategory—Pharmacological therapies*

75. 1. To avoid burning the skin, a heating pad is always kept on a low setting. The client is cautioned to avoid turning the heat setting higher when becoming adapted to the sensation of warmth. Because of the client's age and changes in skin and sensory functioning, the risk of burns is high if the heating pad is placed directly next to the skin. A heating pad is covered with fabric such as flannel. Heat is not applied for longer than 20 to 30 minutes at a time.

Test Taking Strategy—Analyze to determine what information the question asks for, which is an essential instruction that the nurse should include when teaching a client about using a heating pad. Instructions that promote the client's safety are always a priority, making option 1 the best answer. Review principles of heat application if you had difficulty answering this question.

Cognitive Level—*Remembering*
Client Needs Category—*Safe and effective care environment*
Client Needs Subcategory—*Safety and infection control*

76. 1. Because obesity puts additional stress on weight-bearing joints and contributes to the discomfort of osteoarthritis, maintaining a desired weight will help to minimize stress and decrease pain. Applying a topical analgesic cream may improve joint mobility and help with sore muscles, but it does not directly relieve the joint stress related to arthritis. Taking a calcium supplement may help to maintain bone density, but it will not reduce stress on arthritic joints. Physical activity is likely to cause more discomfort to a person whose hips are affected by osteoarthritis.

Test Taking Strategy—Look at the key words "most beneficial." Read the options, looking for one that correlates with client teaching that will reduce stress on painful weight-bearing joints. Recall that stress on joints is increased by excessive body weight. Therefore, achieving an appropriate weight (option 1) in relation to height will reduce the weight-bearing load on diseased joints. Review methods that preserve or promote joint function, especially in clients with osteoarthritis, if you had difficulty answering this question.

Cognitive Level—*Applying*
Client Needs Category—*Health promotion and maintenance*
Client Needs Subcategory—*None*

77. 3. A cane should always be held on the unaffected side. This allows the client to transfer or redistribute body weight from the painful joint to the hand with the cane when taking a step. Covering the tip with a rubber cap, wearing supportive shoes, and maintaining good posture are all appropriate techniques for using a cane.

Test Taking Strategy—Analyze to determine what information the question asks for, which is an option that indicates the client is using a cane incorrectly (option 3). Review how to correctly instruct a client on the use of a cane if you had difficulty answering this question.

Cognitive Level—*Applying*
Client Needs Category—*Physiological integrity*
Client Needs Subcategory—*Basic care and comfort*

78. 4. Gastrointestinal adverse effects and the potential for bleeding are common among clients who take non-steroidal anti-inflammatory drugs (NSAIDs). By asking the client to identify the color of the stools, the nurse is assessing if the drug is causing GI bleeding. NSAIDs are not known to cause increased urination or hand tremors. NSAIDs may or may not affect appetite, depending on the amount of GI upset.

Test Taking Strategy—Use the process of elimination to help select the option that allows the nurse to assess the possibility that the client is experiencing a side effect of NSAID therapy. Options 1 and 2 can be eliminated, because NSAIDs are not known to cause increased urination or hand tremors. Loss of appetite (option 3) may occur, depending on the amount of GI upset, but option 4 remains as the best answer because a change of stool color from brown to black suggests the client is experiencing bleeding in the upper GI tract from NSAID therapy. Review the side effects of drugs that are classified as NSAIDs if you had difficulty answering this question.

Cognitive Level—*Applying*
Client Needs Category—*Physiological integrity*
Client Needs Subcategory—*Pharmacological therapies*

79. 2. Aspirin increases the possibility of postoperative bleeding. It interferes with the ability of platelets to clump together, one of the first mechanisms in clot formation. Aspirin does not increase the risk of wound infection or affect the body's ability to heal. Aspirin is not discontinued to facilitate assessing the client's pain. However, if the client takes aspirin for arthritis and is asked to discontinue it for a week, signs of joint stiffness, tenderness, swelling, and immobility may occur.

Test Taking Strategy—Use the process of elimination to select the option that provides the best rationale for discontinuing the self-administration of enteric-coated aspirin preoperatively. Recall that the antiplatelet properties of aspirin may contribute to or prolong bleeding (option 2) during and immediately after surgery. Review the actions of aspirin and its side effects if you had difficulty answering this question.

Cognitive Level—*Understanding*
Client Needs Category—*Physiological integrity*
Client Needs Subcategory—*Pharmacological therapies*

80. 1. An incentive spirometer helps a client measure the effectiveness of deep inhalation. Postoperatively, it is important for the client to breathe deeply to open the airways and alveoli. This helps improve the oxygenation of blood, eliminate carbon dioxide, and prevent atelectasis and pneumonia. None of the other options indicates the correct use of an incentive spirometer.

> *Test Taking Strategy—Analyze to determine what information the question asks for, which is a correct description on how an incentive spirometer is used. Recall that inhaling deeply (option 1) increases the volume of inspired air and inflates alveoli, which helps improve external and internal respiration. Review the technique for using an incentive spirometer if you had difficulty answering this question.*
> **Cognitive Level**—*Understanding*
> **Client Needs Category**—*Health promotion and maintenance*
> **Client Needs Subcategory**—*None*

81. 3. Clipping the hair around the intended incisional area is preferred over shaving to avoid microabrasions that support bacterial growth. Pressing the razor firmly or deeply onto the skin can cause cuts. Altering the integrity of the skin because of cuts and bleeding increases the risk of postoperative wound infections. Soap is used to decrease the number of transient skin organisms. For surgery, a stronger antiseptic is usually used.

> *Test Taking Strategy—Apply the key words "most appropriate" when evaluating the descriptions in the options regarding preoperative skin preparation. Recall that the Joint Commission's National Patient Safety Goals require clipping (option 3) not shaving hair before surgery to reduce the risk of surgical infections. Review the preoperative care of clients, focusing on practices involved in skin preparation, if you had difficulty answering this question.*
> **Cognitive Level**—*Applying*
> **Client Needs Category**—*Safe and effective care environment*
> **Client Needs Subcategory**—*Safety and infection control*

82. 2. The hip of a client who has undergone a total hip replacement (arthroplasty) is maintained in a position of abduction, or away from the midline. Adduction is positioned toward the midline, and flexion is a bent position. Extension is keeping the body part straight. If the client flexes the hip more than 90 degrees or adducts the hip, the prosthetic femoral head may become dislocated. A triangular foam wedge is generally kept between the client's legs while the client is in bed.

> *Test Taking Strategy—Analyze to determine what information the question asks for, which is the position that must be maintained after a total hip replacement. Recall that to maintain the prosthetic device within its appropriate joint location, the leg must be abducted (option 2). Adduction may lead to displacement of the prosthetic device. Review the postoperative care of a client who has had a total hip replacement if you had difficulty answering this question.*

> **Cognitive Level**—*Applying*
> **Client Needs Category**—*Physiological integrity*
> **Client Needs Subcategory**—*Physiological adaptation*

83. 3. A trapeze helps the client move and lift his or her body. Encouraging the client to participate actively helps maintain muscular strength and reduces the nurse's effort when moving and positioning a client. A bed cradle is used to keep bed linens off lower extremities. A bed board is used to support the client's spine. Lower side rails are appropriate when maintaining the safety of a confused client or one with a perceptual disorder.

> *Test Taking Strategy—Look at the key words "most helpful," and apply them to the listed items. Select the one that would assist most in the client's postoperative care. Recall that the client has unrestricted upper body function despite compromised movement of the operative leg. A trapeze (option 3) reduces the work-related effort required of the nurse and strengthens the client's arm muscles needed to eventually ambulate with a walker. If you had difficulty answering this question, review equipment that will help manage the care of a client after a total hip replacement.*
> **Cognitive Level**—*Applying*
> **Client Needs Category**—*Physiological integrity*
> **Client Needs Subcategory**—*Physiological adaptation*

84. 2. A trochanter roll is used to maintain the hip in a position of extension. Placing this positioning device at the trochanter helps keep the hip from rotating outward. A footboard is used to prevent plantar flexion and footdrop deformity. A turning sheet is used to reposition a client. A foam mattress helps relieve pressure over bony prominences.

> *Test Taking Strategy—Use the process of elimination to help select the option that identifies the best item for preventing external rotation of the postoperative client's leg. Options 1, 3, and 4 can be eliminated because they describe devices that serve other functions; the footboard (option 1) prevents plantar flexion, the foam mattress (option 4) relieves pressure on bony prominences, and the turning sheet (option 3) is used for repositioning. Option 2 remains as the best answer because if the trochanter roll is positioned correctly, it reduces the potential for external rotation. Review the purpose and technique for using a trochanter roll if you had difficulty answering this question.*
> **Cognitive Level**—*Applying*
> **Client Needs Category**—*Physiological integrity*
> **Client Needs Subcategory**—*Reduction of risk potential*

85. 1. A client with a total hip replacement is instructed to avoid crossing the legs because this places the hip in a position of adduction and flexion. These two positions can displace the prosthetic device. Pointing the toes, as in plantar flexion or dorsiflexion, will not displace the device. Lying flat and standing upright are not harmful.

> *Test Taking Strategy*—*Analyze to determine what information the question asks for, which is accurate information about a position that must be avoided to prevent displacing the hip prosthesis. Recall that hip adduction and flexion, which would occur if the legs are crossed (option 1), must be avoided. Review discharge teaching after a total hip prosthesis, especially as it relates to preventing hip adduction, if you had difficulty answering this question.*
> *Cognitive Level*—*Analyzing*
> *Client Needs Category*—*Physiological integrity*
> *Client Needs Subcategory*—*Reduction of risk potential*

86. 3. Postoperatively and for an extended time afterward, a client with a total hip replacement must avoid flexing the hip more than 90 degrees. This necessitates using a raised toilet seat. The client does not need a wheelchair and can ambulate using a walker. The client can continue to use the bed at home. The nurse teaches the client the proper techniques for transferring from bed to a chair; therefore, a mechanical lift is unnecessary.

> *Test Taking Strategy*—*Analyze to determine what information the question asks for, which is a home-care item that is essential after being discharged from the hospital. Recall that bending (flexing) the hips severely is contraindicated because it may displace the hip prosthesis. Using a raised toilet seat facilitates elimination, but reduces the degree of hip flexion. Review the purpose of using a raised toilet seat after a total hip replacement if you had difficulty answering this question.*
> *Cognitive Level*—*Understanding*
> *Client Needs Category*—*Safe and effective care environment*
> *Client Needs Subcategory*—*Coordinated care*

87. 1. The client with a total hip replacement must avoid bending over to put on or take off socks, pants, underwear, and shoes. Someone should help with these items of clothing, or assistive devices may be used. Another approach is to modify the clothing so that the client can slip items on without flexing the hip more than 90 degrees. No special equipment is needed for bathing; however, the client must be cautious when getting in and out of the shower and with the water temperature. Instructing the client about home safety is also important. Additional areas to cover include water and environmental temperatures, furniture placement, lighting, medication administration, and fire safety. Taking vigorous walks is inappropriate immediately after discharge because the client's activity level should be increased gradually. Stool softeners are not usually included in the client's discharge instructions.

> *Test Taking Strategy*—*Analyze to determine what information the question asks for, which is essential*

discharge instructions for a client who has had a total hip replacement. Recall that dressing and removing clothing often involves flexing the hip. Therefore, the nurse must include information about dressing techniques that can be substituted to avoid these positions. Review modifications in self-care that are necessary when recovering from a total hip replacement if you had difficulty answering this question.*
> *Cognitive Level*—*Applying*
> *Client Needs Category*—*Safe and effective care environment*
> *Client Needs Subcategory*—*Coordinated care*

88. 2. Arthroscopy is a minimally invasive surgery used most often to diagnose problems with the knee, but it also may be used to examine other joints. The arthroscope contains a lens that is inserted into the joint to visually inspect the internal structure and repair gross damage if necessary. Most clients who undergo arthroscopy of the knee use crutches for some time after the procedure. Because postprocedural discomfort and recovery from anesthesia or light conscious sedation interfere with learning and practice, it is best to teach clients how to use crutches during their preoperative preparation. Most clients who undergo arthroscopy have already personally experienced the signs and symptoms of arthritis. Drug teaching is postponed until the physician writes postoperative orders. Balancing rest with exercise is important, but the physician indicates those specific orders after the procedure.

> *Test Taking Strategy*—*Look at the key words "most appropriate," and apply them to the information in each of the four options. Determine which option correlates with teaching that should be included when a client undergoes an arthroscopy of the knee. Recall that the client's mobility will be temporarily impaired, which leads to selecting option 2 as the best answer. Review teaching that is provided when a client undergoes arthroscopic knee surgery if you had difficulty answering this question.*
> *Cognitive Level*—*Applying*
> *Client Needs Category*—*Physiological integrity*
> *Client Needs Subcategory*—*Reduction of risk potential*

89. 4. A continuous passive motion (CPM) machine is used primarily to restore full range of joint motion to the affected knee postoperatively. Clients with knee joint replacement are often reluctant to exercise the operative knee actively because of pain. Discomfort usually accompanies use of the CPM machine. Exercise tones and strengthens muscles and relieves dependent swelling by promoting venous circulation; however, these are considered secondary benefits. It is appropriate for the nurse to administer a prescribed analgesic before the client uses a CPM machine.

> *Test Taking Strategy*—*Analyze to determine what information the question asks for, which is the purpose*

for using a CPM machine. Recall that exercise is important for maintaining joint mobility (option 4). To compensate for a client's reluctance to exercise actively to maintain restored function, the machine exercises the operative joint mechanically. Review the purpose for using a CPM machine if you had difficulty answering this question.
Cognitive Level—Applying
Client Needs Category—Health promotion and maintenance
Client Needs Subcategory—None

90. 2. The length of time the client spends on the continuous passive motion (CPM) machine helps determine a response to treatment after arthroplasty. Inspecting and documenting the wound's appearance and the drainage on the dressing, and checking the presence and quality of arterial pulses, are important data to record. However, this information is more pertinent to the client's general physical health, not the progress of treatment.
Test Taking Strategy—Analyze to determine what information the question asks for, which is data that is essential to document in relation to the client's use of a CPM machine. Recall that the surgeon will be interested in knowing information about the degree of joint flexion, the number of cycles provided by the machine, and the client's compliance with its use (option 2). Review pertinent information to document when a client's nursing care involves a CPM machine if you had difficulty answering this question.
Cognitive Level—Applying
Client Needs Category—Physiological integrity
Client Needs Subcategory—Reduction of risk potential

91. 2. The ability to flex the operative knee 90 degrees is an expected outcome before discharge. It is a criterion that supports discharging the client after surgery. The ability to perform straight-leg raises demonstrates sufficient quadriceps strength to discontinue the use of a resting knee extension splint (immobilizer), which may be used to prevent dislocation of the knee prosthesis. A decrease in pain and wound approximation are positive signs of healing and rehabilitation, but they are not criteria for discontinuing the use of a continuous positive motion (CPM) machine.
Test Taking Strategy—Use the process of elimination to help select the option that identifies the best indication that a CPM machine is no longer needed after a knee arthroplasty. Options 1 and 4 can be immediately eliminated because they are unrelated to achieving the desired range of motion. Option 3 looks appealing, but performing straight-leg raises is a criterion for discontinuing the use of a leg immobilizer, not a CPM machine. Option 2 remains as the best answer because it correlates with the joint mobility necessary for gait and function of the

operative knee. Review criteria used to discontinue use of a CPM after knee replacement surgery if you had difficulty answering this question.
Cognitive Level—Analyzing
Client Needs Category—Physiological integrity
Client Needs Subcategory—Physiological adaptation

92. 1. Gout is a metabolic disease caused by hyperuricemia as well as a form of acute arthritis. Marked by acute inflammation, gout can affect any joint; however, approximately 80% of those with the disease experience symptoms in their great toe, which makes ambulation painful.
Test Taking Strategy—Analyze to determine what information the question asks for, which is the joint that is characteristically affected by gout. Recall that the majority of individuals with gout have pain and swelling of the joint in one or both great toes. Review the signs and symptoms of gout focusing on the joints that are typically affected if you had difficulty answering this question.
Cognitive Level—Understanding
Client Needs Category—Physiological integrity
Client Needs Subcategory—Physiological adaptation

93. 3. An elevated serum uric acid level is diagnostic among clients with gout. An elevated serum creatinine clearance and blood urea nitrogen level are indicative of renal failure. Serum calcium is elevated in hyperparathyroidism, primary cancers such as Hodgkin's disease or multiple myeloma, and bone metastasis.
Test Taking Strategy—Analyze to determine what information the question asks for, which is the test result that is used to support a diagnosis of gout. Remember that gout is associated with an excess of uric acid (option 3). Review diagnostic laboratory tests performed on clients with symptoms of gout if you had difficulty answering this question.
Cognitive Level—Applying
Client Needs Category—Physiological integrity
Client Needs Subcategory—Reduction of risk potential

94. 4. Purines are chemicals in the body that eventually break down into uric acid. The accumulation of uric acid causes the signs and symptoms related to gout. Organ meats, such as liver, kidney, brain, and sweetbreads, are high in purines. Other food sources high in purines include fish roe (eggs), sardines, and anchovies. Foods that are moderately high in purines are meats, seafood, dried beans, lentils, spinach, and peas. The other choices are not high in purines and may be included in the client's diet.
Test Taking Strategy—Analyze to determine what information the question asks for, which is a food or beverage that increases uric acid levels. Read the food items listed, and select the one that should be avoided by a person who has gout. Recall that the client must avoid food and beverages that increase

uric acid levels. *Review food items, such as liver (option 4) and other organ meats that are high in purines, if you had difficulty answering this question.*
Cognitive Level—*Analyzing*
Client Needs Category—*Safe and effective care environment*
Client Needs Subcategory—*Coordinated care*

95. 1. Colchicine is an antigout agent used to treat acute attacks and to prevent recurrences of gout. The nurse would withhold this drug if the client manifests GI disturbances such as nausea and vomiting, abdominal pain, and diarrhea. While the client is receiving the drug, the nurse should frequently assess the joints for pain, mobility, and edema. Dizziness, drowsiness, and headache are not signs of an adverse reaction to this drug.
Test Taking Strategy—Analyze to determine what information the question asks for, which is a symptom of an adverse reaction to colchicines. Review the symptoms and select the criterion that is used as the basis for withholding further doses of colchicine. Recall that vomiting is evidence that the accumulating colchicine dosage is having a negative effect on the client. Review the administration of colchicines if you had difficulty answering this question.
Cognitive Level—*Applying*
Client Needs Category—*Physiological integrity*
Client Needs Subcategory—*Pharmacological therapies*

96. 3. It is best to provide the greater share of fluid in the morning to compensate for the long period without oral fluids while sleeping. Frequent urination related to increased intake will most likely occur during the day. Providing a large volume of fluid after a meal contributes to GI fullness or upset. Consuming large amounts of fluid during evening hours or before bedtime usually results in nocturia and interferes with sleep.
Test Taking Strategy—Analyze to determine what information the question asks for, which is the time when most oral fluid intake should occur. Recall that to avoid disturbing the client's sleep for the purpose of urination, the majority of fluid should be consumed in the morning (option 3). Review how the volume of oral fluid intake should be distributed in a 24-hour period if you had difficulty answering this question.
Cognitive Level—*Applying*
Client Needs Category—*Physiological integrity*
Client Needs Subcategory—*Basic care and comfort*

97. 2. There is a correlation between the consumption of alcohol and the recurrence of gout symptoms. Therefore, it is best to instruct clients with gout to abstain from drinking alcohol. Coffee, cranberry juice, and carbonated beverages are safe to consume.

Test Taking Strategy—Analyze to determine what information the question asks for, which is a beverage that should be avoided by a client with gout. Recall that drinking alcohol (option 2), straight or in mixed drinks, increases the risk for exacerbating the symptoms of gout. Review foods and beverages that are most likely to aggravate gouty symptoms if you had difficulty answering this question.
Cognitive Level—*Applying*
Client Needs Category—*Health promotion and maintenance*
Client Needs Subcategory—*None*

Nursing Care of Clients with Degenerative Bone Disorders

98. 3. The nurse is correct to support the joint being exercised by holding areas proximal and distal to the joint. Range-of-motion (ROM) exercises do not necessarily need to be completed independently. Force on a joint is not needed and can have serious consequences. Exercise should be stopped when discomfort occurs.
Test Taking Strategy—Analyze to determine what information the question asks for, which is a correct statement about performing ROM exercises. Recall that when moving the joint through its range of motion, the area above and below the joint should be supported (option 3). Review the technique for performing passive ROM exercises if you had difficulty answering this question.
Cognitive Level—*Applying*
Client Needs Category—*Health promotion and maintenance*
Client Needs Subcategory—*None*

99. 3. Osteoporosis is a gradually progressive disease, usually seen more frequently in women, in which the density of bone tissue decreases over time. The thinning of the bone places the client at risk for fractures. Clients with osteoporosis tend to present with spinal deformities such as kyphosis (dowager's hump) or an inability to assume an erect posture. Although clients with osteoporosis may experience swollen joints, discomfort in sitting, and diminished energy, these conditions are not uniquely associated with this disorder.
Test Taking Strategy—Look at the key words "most likely" when asking for the evidence that suggests a client has osteoporosis. Recall that as the bones in the spine become less dense, the client's height decreases and there is a distortion in the normal curvature of the spine (option 3). Review the clinical manifestations of osteoporosis if you had difficulty answering this question.
Cognitive Level—*Remembering*
Client Needs Category—*Physiological integrity*
Client Needs Subcategory—*Physiological adaptation*

100. 2. Smoking and consuming carbonated beverages contribute to the severity of osteoporosis. Smoking tobacco products inhibits the action of osteoblasts, cells that help form and replace bone cells. The phosphoric acid in carbonated beverages may interfere with bone density; also, substituting carbonated soft drinks for milk decreases the amount of calcium in a person's diet. Although caffeine has been contraindicated in the past, recent studies show no strong evidence linking it with osteoporosis. Aspirin, fiber-containing laxatives, and orange juice are safe to consume unless there are other reasons for which they are contraindicated. Supplemental calcium and consumption of dairy products are therapeutic measures for individuals who are at risk for or who have acquired osteoporosis.

> *Test Taking Strategy—Analyze to determine what information the question asks for, which is substances that should be avoided to slow the progression of bone demineralization. Tobacco products and carbonated beverages have adverse effects on bone growth and mineralization, and should be avoided. Review lifestyle changes that reduce the severity of osteoporosis if you had difficulty answering this question.*
> **Cognitive Level**—*Understanding*
> **Client Needs Category**—*Health promotion and maintenance*
> **Client Needs Subcategory**—*None*

101.

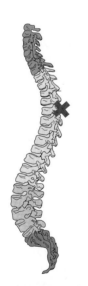

The client with osteoporosis typically develops progressive kyphosis, an exaggerated curvature of the thoracic spinal vertebrae. Kyphosis accompanies a loss of height. Osteoporosis of the spine can also cause back pain from spinal compression fractures.

> *Test Taking Strategy—Look at the key words "most likely," which are used when asking for the spinal location typically affected by osteoporosis. Recall that kyphosis is common among individuals with advanced osteoporosis. Kyphosis describes*

an abnormality in the thoracic vertebrae. Review illustrations and descriptions of the spinal deformity associated with osteoporosis if you had difficulty answering this question.
> **Cognitive Level**—*Understanding*
> **Client Needs Category**—*Physiological integrity*
> **Client Needs Subcategory**—*Physiological adaptation*

102. 3. Osteomyelitis is an infection in the bone and can be either acute or chronic. Bone infection typically occurs because of trauma, orthopedic surgery, or generalized sepsis. Fractures are possible with this condition; therefore, supporting the limb affected by osteomyelitis and handling it gently help reduce the risk of a pathologic fracture. Meeting the client's needs for nutrition and fluids addresses the metabolic problems (such as fever) that accompany an infection. Because the activity of a client with osteomyelitis is often limited, using pressure-relieving devices becomes imperative in maintaining skin integrity.

> *Test Taking Strategy—Look at the key words "most appropriate," which are used to ask about a nursing intervention that will help prevent a pathological fracture. Recall that to prevent a fracture of a bone weakened by disease, it must be supported (option 3) and handled with care during movement. Review the methods for preventing secondary complications associated with osteomyelitis if you had difficulty answering this question.*
> **Cognitive Level**—*Applying*
> **Client Needs Category**—*Physiological integrity*
> **Client Needs Subcategory**—*Basic care and comfort*

103. 1. Health-seeking behaviors and illness beliefs vary among Hispanic Americans. These behaviors and beliefs are influenced by geography, length of time spent in the United States, financial issues, age, and social standing. Because this client is an older adult and has just immigrated to the United States, the nurse may assume that health-seeking behaviors are deeply rooted in traditional Hispanic culture and health care practices. In a traditional Hispanic home, female members of the household provide medical care. Many clients will not go to a hospital or physician until all attempts at treating the illness with home remedies have been exhausted. Traditionally, Hispanic American men are expected to be *macho,* or strong; having an illness may be perceived as being weak. Some Hispanic Americans who have established themselves within the United States believe that medical technology assists the physician in curing illnesses; however, because the client in the scenario has been in the United States for a short time, the client's long-standing cultural health beliefs most likely take precedence. A *curandero* is a faith healer. There is no evidence in this question to validate that the client no longer believes in *curanderos.* Some Hispanic Americans believe that illness is caused by the "evil eye," which would be treated by spiritual ceremonies, candles, and prayer.

> *Test Taking Strategy—Analyze to determine what information the question asks for, which is Hispanic culture and health care beliefs that combine spiritualistic approaches and safe, simple home remedies. Recall that when an illness or injury occurs, Hispanics traditionally turn first to family members, especially those who are older, or a curandero for advice and care. Review Hispanic cultural beliefs as they relate to health care if you had difficulty answering this question.*
> **Cognitive Level**—*Analyzing*
> **Client Needs Category**—*Psychosocial integrity*
> **Client Needs Subcategory**—*None*

104. 1. Osteomalacia is a disease characterized by soft, brittle, easily fractured, or deformed bones. In adults the disease is called *osteomalacia*, but in children it is known as *rickets*. It is commonly caused by a lack of vitamin D. Vitamin D is necessary for calcium absorption. Exposure to sunlight helps to convert dehydrocholesterol in the skin and ergosterol, a plant precursor, to provitamins that eventually become vitamin D. The beneficial and harmful effects of eating cattle injected with bovine growth hormone have not been conclusively determined. Orange vegetables are good sources of beta carotene, a precursor of vitamin A. Organically grown produce does not provide any additional nutritional benefit over other produce; however, eliminating the ingestion of chemical fertilizers, herbicides, and pesticides may be beneficial.

> *Test Taking Strategy—Look at the key words "most appropriate." Review the options to determine which additional nursing suggestion from those listed will contribute to improving the client's condition. Recall that vitamin D is synthesized when the skin is exposed to ultraviolet rays from natural sunlight (option 1). Review the contributions of vitamin D, sunlight, and calcium to healthy bone structure if you had difficulty answering this question.*
> **Cognitive Level**—*Applying*
> **Client Needs Category**—*Health promotion and maintenance*
> **Client Needs Subcategory**—*None*

Nursing Care of Clients with Amputations

105. 3. With very few exceptions, a person in shock is kept flat (supine) with the lower extremities slightly elevated (modified Trendelenburg position). Gravity helps to maintain blood in the area of the vital organs. Keeping the client prone (in a face-down position), in a side-lying position (lateral), or sitting up (Fowler's position) would not help circulate blood where it is critically needed. In fact, some of the described positions would interfere with emergency assessment and care.

> *Test Taking Strategy—Analyze to determine what information the question asks for, which is a standard position when managing the care of a client in shock. There are many types of shock, but in this scenario the client is experiencing hypovolemic shock. Raising the feet and legs about 12″ (option 3) helps promote circulation. Review nursing care of a client in shock if you had difficulty answering this question.*
> **Cognitive Level**—*Applying*
> **Client Needs Category**—*Physiological integrity*
> **Client Needs Subcategory**—*Physiological adaptation*

106. 2. Staying with a grief-stricken client provides emotional support and may help the client feel the nurse will be available to respond during future needs. Leaving an uncomfortable situation is one method health professionals use to cope with their own feelings of inadequacy; however, the client would probably interpret the desertion as a sign that the nurse is not a caring individual. Allowing the client to release the rage can be therapeutic as long as it does not endanger the client or others. Feeling angry is one of the early steps in the grieving process. Calling the physician is inappropriate because it does not address the real problem of anger related to the missing limb.

> *Test Taking Strategy—Look at the key words "most appropriate," and apply them to each of the options to select the one that is best for responding to a client who is distraught and screaming obscenities. Recall that it is not therapeutic to abandon, sedate, or be critical with a client who is overcome with emotion. The most therapeutic action is option 1. The nurse's very presence, despite being a verbal target, is a form of support. Review the stages of loss and grieving and therapeutic communication skills if you had difficulty correctly answering this question.*
> **Cognitive Level**—*Applying*
> **Client Needs Category**—*Psychosocial integrity*
> **Client Needs Subcategory**—*None*

107. 2. Phantom pain or sensation is a phenomenon experienced by some people who have had a limb amputated. The person typically feels a physical sensation in the location of the missing limb. The feelings range from a sense that the amputated part is still there to other sensations that cause discomfort, such as pain, cramping, burning, and itching. Referred pain is discomfort experienced in a location that is distant from the actual area of pathology. Psychogenic pain, which the nurse should explain to the client in lay terms, is discomfort that is emotional in origin. Intractable pain is severe and unrelenting and may require a combination of therapies.

> *Test Taking Strategy—Look at the key words, "most accurate" when evaluating the type of pain that the client is experiencing. Recall that phantom limb pain (option 2) is very real to the client, who may be unfamiliar with its manifestation. Review the definition*

and cause of phantom limb pain if you had difficulty correctly answering this question.
Cognitive Level—*Applying*
Client Needs Category—*Physiological integrity*
Client Needs Subcategory—*Physiological adaptation*

108. **3.** Sitting in a chair, especially frequently or for long periods, is undesirable because below-the-knee amputees are prone to knee flexion contractures. A knee flexion contracture interferes with wearing a prosthesis and being able to walk again. For this reason, the stump is kept in an extended or neutral position as much as possible. The prone, supine, and standing positions all allow for extension of the stump.

> *Test Taking Strategy—Look at the key words "least desirable," and apply them to select the option that would be detrimental to the client who has undergone a below-the-knee amputation (BKA). Recall that the best rehabilitation outcome after an amputation requires functional use of the remaining joints. A sitting position (option 3) jeopardizes the use of a prosthesis if a knee flexion contracture develops. Review the nursing care of a client undergoing a BKA, focusing on the prevention of contractures, if you had difficulty answering this question.*
> **Cognitive Level**—*Applying*
> **Client Needs Category**—*Physiological integrity*
> **Client Needs Subcategory**—*Basic care and comfort*

109. **3.** Almost immediately after surgery, the client should begin to use the trapeze to build up muscle strength in preparation for using crutches. The muscles that need the most strengthening are those in the arms, neck, shoulders, chest, and back. The client may also squeeze rubber balls and perform arm push-ups. Doing arm push-ups involves placing the palms flat on the bed and raising the buttocks. Some health care professionals provide the client with sawed-off crutches to use in bed to condition the same muscles needed during ambulation. Standing at the side of the bed and transferring from the bed to a chair should not be attempted without assistance because of the risk of falling. The client needs to get used to balancing with one leg; therefore, parallel bars are contraindicated at this time.

> *Test Taking Strategy—Use the process of elimination to help select the option that identifies the best activity for the client to perform immediately after surgery to prepare for using crutches. Option 2 can be eliminated because using parallel bars would occur later in the client's rehabilitation. Options 1 and 4 involve leg muscles, but they can be eliminated because leg strength is secondary to conditioning the arm muscles (option 3) for support and ambulation with crutches. Review methods for preparing a client for using crutches if you had difficulty answering this question.*

Cognitive Level—*Applying*
Client Needs Category—*Health promotion and maintenance*
Client Needs Subcategory—*None*

110. **2.** Wrapping the stump decreases stump edema, thereby shrinking and shaping the stump. A permanent prosthesis is not constructed until the stump is cone shaped and no longer undergoing changes in size. An equal amount of compression is applied with each turn of the elastic bandage. Isotonic and isometric exercises are used to tone muscles. Range-of-motion exercises help maintain joint flexibility. Gauze dressings absorb blood and drainage.

> *Test Taking Strategy—Analyze to determine what information the question asks for, which is the purpose for wrapping the stump with elastic bandages. Recall that the stump cannot be fitted with a permanent prosthesis until it has achieved a final size and shape (option 2). Review the purpose for frequently wrapping the stump if you had difficulty answering this question.*
> **Cognitive Level**—*Applying*
> **Client Needs Category**—*Physiological integrity*
> **Client Needs Subcategory**—*Physiological adaptation*

111. **3, 4.** To ensure optimal rehabilitation, the client needs to wrap the stump to control edema and shrink it to its final shape and size before a permanent prosthesis can be made. Active isometric exercises, such as quadriceps and gluteal setting exercises, help strengthen the muscles required for ambulation. The client should be taught to tighten the thigh muscles and to press the knee into the bed several times a day. Flexion, abduction, and external rotation should be avoided. Therefore, the client must avoid sitting for long periods, dangling the stump over the bedside, or putting a pillow under the thigh. The client is encouraged to keep the knee and leg in a neutral position. The stump bandage should be removed and reapplied at least two or three times a day, or whenever it becomes soiled or loose.

> *Test Taking Strategy—Analyze to determine what information the question asks for, which is nursing actions that aid rehabilitation after a below-the-knee amputation (BKA). Alternative-format "select all that apply" questions require considering each option independently to decide its merit in answering the question. Choose the options that best correlate with nursing actions that facilitate rehabilitation after a BKA. Review nursing measures that help prepare a client for using a prosthesis if you had difficulty answering this question.*

Cognitive Level—*Applying*
Client Needs Category—*Physiological integrity*
Client Needs Subcategory—*Reduction of risk potential*

Nursing Care of Clients with Skeletal Tumors

112. 2. A rubber tourniquet is usually kept at the bedside in case the client begins to hemorrhage when elevating the stump and applying direct pressure cannot control bleeding. An emergency supply of gauze dressings should not be necessary. If the airway becomes compromised, the nurse would maintain temporary patency by using the chin-lift/head-tilt maneuver. Most clients are transferred to the nursing unit from the recovery room with oxygen already in place.

Test Taking Strategy—Analyze to determine what information the question asks for, which is an item important to have available when providing care of a client with an above-the-knee amputation (AKA) in the immediate postoperative period. Recall that hemorrhage is always a potential postoperative complication, especially in this case when arteries and veins have been severed. This leads to selecting option 2 because the use of a tourniquet to control hemorrhage would be an alternative life-saving measure. Review the nursing care of a client immediately after an AKA, focusing especially on how hemorrhage would be controlled, if you had difficulty answering this question.
Cognitive Level—Applying
Client Needs Category—Physiological integrity
Client Needs Subcategory—Physiological adaptation

113. 3. If crutches are measured and fitted appropriately, there should be enough room to fit at least two fingers between the axilla and the axillary bar of the crutch. Prolonged pressure under the arm can affect circulation or impair nerve function, resulting in permanent paralysis. All of the other options indicate that the crutch length and the handgrip position are correct.

Test Taking Strategy—Use the process of elimination to help select the option that identifies an indication that the client's crutches require adjustment. Options 1, 2, and 4 can be eliminated because they describe well-fitting crutches. Option 3 remains as the best answer because pressure on nerves and blood vessels in the axillae from crutches that are too long can cause neurovascular damage. Review the assessments that indicate that the length of the crutches and position of the hand grips are appropriate for a client if you had difficulty answering this question.
Cognitive Level—Applying
Client Needs Category—Physiological integrity
Client Needs Subcategory—Physiological adaptation

114. 4. Malignant bone tumors cause secondary anemia if bone marrow function is disrupted. Although primary bone tumors can spread to any organ, the bowel and liver are not common metastatic sites. Mental status changes may occur, but they are not related to the location of a bone tumor.

Test Taking Strategy—Analyze to determine what information the question asks for, which is a potential complication of osteogenic sarcoma. Recall that blood cells (option 4) are manufactured in bone marrow, which, in this case, may be affected by the tumor. Review the pathophysiology associated with osteogenic sarcoma if you had difficulty answering this question.
Cognitive Level—Applying
Client Needs Category—Physiological integrity
Client Needs Subcategory—Physiological adaptation

115. 2. A skilled nursing assistant on an orthopedic floor is able to provide complete instructions on how to use a shower chair. It is in the scope of nursing practice to position a prosthesis in the appropriate manner for ambulation, discuss lab work, and assess drainage.

Test Taking Strategy—Analyze to determine what information the question asks for, which is the most appropriate task to delegate to a skilled nursing assistant. Recall that nursing assistants help clients with basic tasks such as personal hygiene, which may involve the use of a shower chair and assistance with toileting, eating, and ambulating safely. Review the job description of a person who is hired as a skilled nursing assistant if you had difficulty answering this question.
Cognitive Level—Analyzing
Client Needs Category—Safe and effective care environment
Client Needs Subcategory—Coordinated care

Nursing Care of Clients with a Herniated Intervertebral Disk

116. 2. Any activity that increases intraspinal pressure, such as sneezing, causes lower back pain to intensify. Other activities that can worsen back pain include coughing, lifting an object, and straining to have a bowel movement. Eating and urinating do not normally affect the intensity of pain. Resting and inactivity help relieve pain caused by a herniated intervertebral disk.

Test Taking Strategy—Analyze to determine what information the question asks for, which is an activity that is accompanied by an increase in the intensity of the client's pain. Recall that when intraspinal pressure is increased, such as when sneezing (option 2), coughing, or bearing down during bowel elimination, pain is increased. Review the factors that intensify the pain experienced by someone with a herniated intervertebral disk if you had difficulty answering this question.
Cognitive Level—Applying
Client Needs Category—Physiological integrity
Client Needs Subcategory—Basic care and comfort

117. 1. Many clients feel pain radiate into their buttocks and down the leg where the herniating disk protrudes on the spinal nerve root. The sciatic nerve is commonly affected when the herniated disk occurs between lumbar vertebrae. The iliac crests, knees, and toes are not generally symptomatic.
> *Test Taking Strategy—Analyze to determine what information the question asks for, which is a typical symptom experienced by a client with a herniated intervertebral disk. Recall that when a portion of the disk protrudes and presses on a spinal nerve, the client experiences pain along its length. Disks in the lumbar spine are most affected, causing sciatic nerve involvement. Consequently, option 1 is the best answer. Review the signs and symptoms associated with a herniated intervertebral disk, especially one in the lumbar area, if you had difficulty answering this question.*
> *Cognitive Level—Applying*
> *Client Needs Category—Physiological integrity*
> *Client Needs Subcategory—Physiological adaptation*

118. 2. Cyclobenzaprine hydrochloride (Flexeril) is a central-acting skeletal muscle relaxant. Clients with low back pain often maintain tensed muscles to reduce movement that aggravates the pain. After being contracted for a substantial amount of time, the muscles may spasm, which contributes to the pain instead of providing relief. Cyclobenzaprine does not reduce depression and should not be given with alcohol or other central nervous system depressants. Nonsteroidal anti-inflammatory drugs (NSAIDs) are given to decrease inflammation; sedatives and hypnotics are used to promote rest and sleep.
> *Test Taking Strategy—Analyze to determine what information the question asks for, which is the purpose for prescribing cyclobenzaprine hydrochloride (Flexeril). Recall that this drug is categorized as a skeletal muscle relaxant (option 2). Review the action and uses for cyclobenzaprine hydrochloride (Flexeril) if you had difficulty answering this question.*
> *Cognitive Level—Applying*
> *Client Needs Category—Physiological integrity*
> *Client Needs Subcategory—Pharmacological therapies*

119. 1. Most clinicians believe the transcutaneous electric nerve stimulation (TENS) unit generates sensations that the brain perceives rather than the pain that is being transmitted from the location where it originates. The process is compared to a car waiting while a train crosses the highway. The impulses from the TENS unit are like the train. As long as the TENS impulses flood the brain, the pain impulses are blocked. Thus, the TENS unit does not travel to a nerve root, weaken nociceptor sensory muscles, or destroy the brain's pain center.
> *Test Taking Strategy—Use the process of elimination to help select the option that describes the most widely held theory about the method by which a TENS unit achieves its pain-relieving effect. Recall that pain is transmitted over nociceptors in the peripheral nervous system to the brain. Because the brain responds to only one sensation at a time, providing a stimulus other than pain will reduce pain perception. Review the hypothesis that explains the effect produced by a TENS unit if you had difficulty answering this question.*
> *Cognitive Level—Understanding*
> *Client Needs Category—Physiological integrity*
> *Client Needs Subcategory—Physiological adaptation*

120. 4. Encouraging extra fluids and maintaining a quiet environment can help prevent headaches after a myelogram. Drinking fluid dilutes and hastens excretion of the contrast medium used during the procedure. Increasing oral fluid intake also helps replace cerebrospinal fluid withdrawn before or after the procedure. Keeping the room dim can help relieve a spinal headache once it manifests; however, this is not generally done as a standard of care after a myelogram. Food may be withheld if the client becomes nauseated, but this is not routinely done. Administering sedatives at scheduled intervals after a myelogram can mask early signs of central nervous system complications.
> *Test Taking Strategy—Look at the key words "most important." Review the nursing interventions described and select the one that should be performed after a client has a myelogram. Recall that during this procedure cerebrospinal fluid is withdrawn and contrast media is instilled. Increasing a client's oral fluid intake (option 4) replaces the volume of withdrawn fluid and dilutes the dye, which promotes its excretion. Review nursing care of a client after a myelogram if you had difficulty answering this question.*
> *Cognitive Level—Applying*
> *Client Needs Category—Physiological integrity*
> *Client Needs Subcategory—Physiological adaptation*

121. 4. A laminectomy is performed to relieve pressure on the nerves that are causing pain that radiates down the leg. Spinal fusion stabilizes the portion of the vertebrae in which the laminae were removed. The client with a laminectomy and spinal fusion should be rolled from side to side without twisting the spine. This type of movement, called *logrolling*, prevents displacing bone grafts until they have become solidly fused. Holding one's breath increases discomfort when accompanied by bearing down. Because the client cannot twist the spine, moving the lower body and then the upper body would be harmful. Likewise, raising the upper body and hips off the bed would be contraindicated.
> *Test Taking Strategy—Analyze to determine what information the question asks for, which is an instruction from the nurse that will prevent a complication after a laminectomy and spinal fusion. Recall that the site*

where the surgery was performed has not permanently fused at this time. To prevent displacing the unstable area in the spine as a result of flexing or rotating the vertebrae, a client is logrolled (option 4). Review how to change a postoperative client's position after a laminectomy and spinal fusion if you had difficulty answering this question.

Cognitive Level—*Applying*
Client Needs Category—*Physiological integrity*
Client Needs Subcategory—*Reduction of risk potential*

122. 3. Ideally, it is best to have a translator assist with interpreting health teaching provided to a client who does not speak English well. Providing printed instructions in the client's primary language is another alternative. If those options are not available, showing the client pictures and diagrams is the most appropriate action to supplement what the client may somewhat understand verbally. Demonstrating may also help to get the point across. Speaking slowly and looking at the client may or may not facilitate the understanding of the verbal instructions. In some cultures, looking directly at a person is considered offensive. Similarly, writing the instructions on paper or watching a video in English does not address the client's inability to understand or speak English.

> **Test Taking Strategy**—*Use the process of elimination to help select the best nursing action in the absence of a translator for teaching a client who speaks English as a second language about body mechanics. Recall that pictures and diagrams (option 3) can*

be universally understood regardless of a person's preferred language. Review techniques for communicating with non-English-speaking clients or those who do not speak English well if you had difficulty answering this question.

Cognitive Level—*Applying*
Client Needs Category—*Health promotion and maintenance*
Client Needs Subcategory—*None*

123. 1. Bending both knees and keeping the back straight makes best use of the longest and strongest muscles in the body. The feet are spread apart for a broad base of support. Extending the arms strains the weaker muscles by placing the weight of the lifted object outside the body's center of gravity.

> **Test Taking Strategy**—*Analyze to determine what information the question asks for, which is how to pick up objects using good body mechanics. Recall that principles of body mechanics stress bending the knees (option 1) while keeping the back straight to reduce strain on the lower back. Review principles of body mechanics if you had difficulty answering this question.*

Cognitive Level—*Applying*
Client Needs Category—*Health promotion and maintenance*
Client Needs Subcategory—*None*

The Nursing Care of Clients with Neurologic System Disorders

- Nursing Care of Clients with Infectious and Inflammatory Conditions
- Nursing Care of Clients with Seizure Disorders
- Nursing Care of Clients with Neurologic Trauma
- Nursing Care of Clients with Degenerative Disorders
- Nursing Care of Clients with Cerebrovascular Disorders
- Nursing Care of Clients with Tumors of the Neurologic System
- Nursing Care of Clients with Nerve Disorders
- Correct Answers, Rationales, and Test Taking Strategies

Directions: With a pencil, blacken the space in front of the option you have chosen for your correct answer.

Nursing Care of Clients with Infectious and Inflammatory Conditions

A 23-year-old is brought to the hospital after efforts to relieve a fever are unsuccessful. The tentative diagnosis is meningitis.

1. If the diagnosis is accurate, which nursing assessment findings support the diagnosis? Select all that apply.
[ ] **1.** Photophobia
[ ] **2.** A stiff neck
[ ] **3.** Muscle weakness
[ ] **4.** Diarrhea
[ ] **5.** Vertigo
[ ] **6.** Fever

The physician plans to perform a lumbar puncture (spinal tap) to confirm the diagnosis of meningitis.

2. When assisting the client on the examination table, the nurse should place the client in which position?
[ ] **1.** Knee–chest (genupectoral) position
[ ] **2.** Sitting in an orthopneic position
[ ] **3.** Side-lying position with his neck flexed
[ ] **4.** Prone position with the head turned to the left side

3. Which nursing intervention is most appropriate after the lumbar puncture has been performed?
[ ] **1.** Keep the client in a side-lying position.
[ ] **2.** Assist the client into a sitting position.
[ ] **3.** Withhold food and fluids for 1 hour.
[ ] **4.** Keep the client flat for several hours.

4. While awaiting the diagnostic test results for a client with possible meningitis, which transmission-based precautions are best to implement?
[ ] **1.** Droplet precautions
[ ] **2.** Airborne precautions
[ ] **3.** Contact precautions
[ ] **4.** Standard precautions

The physician orders a cooling blanket to reduce the fever of a client with meningitis.

5. When implementing this medical order, which nursing action is most appropriate?
[ ] **1.** Place the cooling blanket on top of the client.
[ ] **2.** Wrap the cooling blanket in a light cloth cover.
[ ] **3.** Add normal saline solution to the fluid chamber.
[ ] **4.** Replace crushed ice periodically as it melts.

The care plan for a client with viral encephalitis indicates that the nurse should perform neurologic checks every 2 hours.

6. If the client had been unresponsive except to painful stimuli, which new assessment finding indicates that the client is improving?
[ ] **1.** Pupils are fixed when stimulated with light.
[ ] **2.** Pupils are unequal when stimulated with light.
[ ] **3.** Client's Glasgow Coma Scale score is 12.
[ ] **4.** Stroking the cheek with a swab causes swallowing.

The nursing team discusses the care of a new client who has Guillain-Barré syndrome.

7. When the medical history is reviewed, which finding is most likely related to the client's diagnosis?
[ ] **1.** The client had an influenza immunization in the past week.
[ ] **2.** The client was bitten by a spider several days ago.
[ ] **3.** The client drinks fresh, unpasteurized milk daily.
[ ] **4.** The client sprayed the garden with insecticide yesterday.

8. When the nursing team plans the care of a client with Guillain-Barré syndrome, which assessment finding most accurately determines whether the client is developing ineffective breathing?
[ ] **1.** Respiratory rate is 24.
[ ] **2.** Skin is flushed.
[ ] **3.** Activity is decreased.
[ ] **4.** Pulse oximetry reading is 82%.

The client with Guillain-Barré syndrome begins to have difficulty swallowing food.

9. Which method is most appropriate to provide adequate nutrition for the client at this time?
[ ] **1.** Crystalloid I.V. fluid
[ ] **2.** Nasogastric tube feedings
[ ] **3.** Total parenteral nutrition
[ ] **4.** Gastrostomy tube feedings

A hospice nurse makes a visit to the home of a client with acquired immunodeficiency syndrome (AIDS) dementia complex.

10. Which nursing approach for communication would be best if the client becomes confused?
[ ] **1.** Turn the television on so the client can hear human voices.
[ ] **2.** Play some music when the client is aggressive.
[ ] **3.** Orient the client to the surroundings and current situations.
[ ] **4.** Look at and talk about pictures in a photo album of the client's life.

Nursing Care of Clients with Seizure Disorders

A 23-year-old who experienced a generalized seizure while at work is admitted to the hospital and is undergoing diagnostic tests.

11. Which of the following indicates an autonomic nervous system manifestation of a seizure?
[ ] **1.** Numbness and tingling of the hands
[ ] **2.** Changes in taste and speech
[ ] **3.** Flushing and increased sweating
[ ] **4.** A subjective aura or sensation

The nurse enters seizure precautions into the client's care plan.

12. Which environmental modifications should the nurse implement? Select all that apply.
[ ] **1.** Keep the room dark and quiet.
[ ] **2.** Lower the bed to the lowest position.
[ ] **3.** Keep the side rails up and padded.
[ ] **4.** Provide soft, soothing music.
[ ] **5.** Ensure a warm, well-lit room.
[ ] **6.** Make sure suction equipment is available.

13. When implementing seizure precautions, which nursing action is most appropriate?
[ ] **1.** Move the client to a room close to the nurses' station.
[ ] **2.** Serve the client's food in paper and plastic containers.
[ ] **3.** Maintain the client's bed in the lowest position.
[ ] **4.** Ensure that soft wrist restraints are applied.

14. When preparing the client for an EEG, which nursing action is most appropriate?
[ ] **1.** Administer a sedative 1 hour before the test.
[ ] **2.** Withhold food and water after midnight on the day of the test.
[ ] **3.** Assist with shampooing the client's hair.
[ ] **4.** Take the client's blood pressure while lying and sitting.

15. If the client begins to have a seizure after the EEG, which action should the nurse take first?
[ ] **1.** Administer oxygen by nasal cannula.
[ ] **2.** Measure the blood pressure and pulse.
[ ] **3.** Check the client's pupils.
[ ] **4.** Place the client in a side-lying position.

16. When documenting a seizure, which information is most important to include initially?
[ ] **1.** The time the seizure started
[ ] **2.** The duration of the seizure
[ ] **3.** The client's mood just before the seizure
[ ] **4.** The client's comments after the seizure

17. Which nursing actions are essential when finding a client experiencing a tonic-clonic seizure? Select all that apply.
[ ] **1.** Calling out the client's name
[ ] **2.** Holding the client's body during the seizure activity
[ ] **3.** Placing an emesis basin close to the client's mouth
[ ] **4.** Rolling the client's body to the side
[ ] **5.** Removing environmental hazards to protect the client
[ ] **6.** Calling the respiratory therapy department

18. When a client is injured during a seizure, which fact is most important to document on the incident (accident) report to reduce the risk of liability?
[ ] **1.** The client was assigned to a licensed nurse.
[ ] **2.** The signal cord was within the client's reach.
[ ] **3.** The client's vital signs had been stable.
[ ] **4.** The client was last observed reading.

After a tonic–clonic (grand mal) seizure, the client progresses to the postictal phase.

19. Which clinical manifestation will the nurse most likely observe first?
[ ] **1.** Excessive jerking of the entire body
[ ] **2.** Staring with a brief loss of consciousness
[ ] **3.** Fluttering of the eyelids and movement of the lips
[ ] **4.** Confusion followed by deep sleep

20. What is the priority nursing intervention in the postictal phase of a seizure?
[ ] **1.** Assess the client's level of arousal.
[ ] **2.** Assess the client's breathing pattern.
[ ] **3.** Reorient the client to the surroundings.
[ ] **4.** Change the client's clothing.

The medical record of a client with epilepsy indicates two previous episodes of status epilepticus.

21. Which emergency drug should the nurse plan to have available in case the client has a similar episode?
[ ] **1.** Diazepam (Valium)
[ ] **2.** Phenytoin (Dilantin)
[ ] **3.** Carbamazepine (Tegretol)
[ ] **4.** Phenobarbital sodium (Luminal)

22. Before discharge, the nurse instructs the client who will take phenytoin sodium (Dilantin) at home to perform which hygiene measure?
[ ] **1.** Frequent shampooing of the hair
[ ] **2.** Weekly trimming of fingernails
[ ] **3.** Brushing teeth at least twice daily
[ ] **4.** Daily bathing using mild soap

Nursing Care of Clients with Neurologic Trauma

A nurse who witnesses a motor vehicle accident stops to provide emergency assistance to the injured motorists.

23. When the nurse assesses a victim who has been thrown from the vehicle, which assessment finding is most suggestive of a serious head injury?
[ ] **1.** The victim has a bad headache.
[ ] **2.** The victim asks the nurse, "What happened?"
[ ] **3.** The victim is hesitant to move.
[ ] **4.** The victim has clear fluid draining from the ears.

24. Which nursing action is most important to do next?
[ ] **1.** Maintain the victim's present position.
[ ] **2.** Assist in obtaining the victim's insurance card.
[ ] **3.** Cover the victim with a light blanket.
[ ] **4.** Give the victim some water to drink.

25. To reduce the risk of liability, which is the most appropriate action for the nurse to take?
[ ] **1.** Avoid giving the accident victim any personal identification.
[ ] **2.** Remain with the accident victim until paramedics arrive.
[ ] **3.** Provide a report of who caused the accident to law enforcement officials.
[ ] **4.** Let others at the scene provide direct care.

The accident victim is taken to the emergency department for evaluation.

26. While waiting for the physician to examine the client, how should the nurse position the client?
[ ] **1.** Dorsal recumbent with the legs elevated
[ ] **2.** Supine with the head slightly elevated
[ ] **3.** Flat with a neck immobilizer in place
[ ] **4.** Right lateral with the neck flexed

After X-rays are taken of the head, neck, and spine, the client is diagnosed with a head injury and admitted for inpatient care.

27. When assessing the client with a head injury, which assessment finding should receive priority attention?
[ ] **1.** Lung sounds
[ ] **2.** Clarity of speech
[ ] **3.** Mobility of fingers
[ ] **4.** Pupillary responses

28. If the nurse obtains the following data, which finding should be reported to the physician immediately?
[ ] **1.** The client rates a headache as 5 on a scale of 0 to 10.
[ ] **2.** The client leaves most of the food on the dietary tray.
[ ] **3.** The client is difficult to arouse with stimulation.
[ ] **4.** The client complains of feeling cold.

29. When assessing the client's head injury, the nurse observes a worsening in the client's condition. Which finding is most likely contributing to the change?
[ ] **1.** The client has been disturbed every hour.
[ ] **2.** The client has had very little fluid intake.
[ ] **3.** The client's neck is flexed toward the chest.
[ ] **4.** The client's bladder is becoming quite full.

The client is treated with mannitol (Osmitrol).

30. When providing an update of client status to the physician via a phone report, which assessment finding relates directly to the administration of mannitol (Osmitrol)?
[ ] **1.** Urine output
[ ] **2.** Respiratory rate
[ ] **3.** Level of pain
[ ] **4.** Blood pressure

After a diving accident, a 22-year-old suffers a complete transection of the spinal cord at the level of the fifth thoracic (T5) vertebra.

31. Which statement indicates that the client has an accurate understanding of the prognosis?
[ ] 1. "After surgery, I can expect full function."
[ ] 2. "I will have to have someone feed and bathe me."
[ ] 3. "I will retain functions above my chest."
[ ] 4. "No one can predict my potential outcome."

32. The nurse is providing instruction to the family on the location of the client's injury. In this lateral view of the spine, identify with an X the area on the thoracic vertebrae where the injury to the spinal cord has occurred.

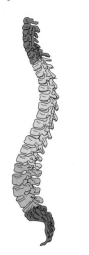

After medical stabilization, the client is transferred to a rehabilitation unit.

33. When the nursing team discusses the client's plan of care, which has the highest priority?
[ ] 1. Teaching the client about prevention of skin breakdown
[ ] 2. Strengthening the client's upper body muscles
[ ] 3. Confronting the client's denial of the prognosis
[ ] 4. Letting the client verbalize about the accident

34. The client with a spinal cord injury presents with characteristics related to autonomic dysreflexia. Which signs and symptoms will the nurse detect with this disorder? Select all that apply.
[ ] 1. Severe hypertension
[ ] 2. Rapid heart rate
[ ] 3. Pounding headache
[ ] 4. Pale skin
[ ] 5. Blurred vision
[ ] 6. Nasal stuffiness

35. When planning a bowel retraining program for a client with a spinal cord injury, which nursing intervention is most appropriate?
[ ] 1. Administering a stool softener twice per week
[ ] 2. Encouraging the client to consume a high-fiber diet
[ ] 3. Having the client drink two glasses of water every morning
[ ] 4. Teaching the client to self-administer daily enemas

36. The nurse plans for the client's discharge and discusses the home environment with the client. Which home care suggestion is best for promoting the mobility of the client with a spinal cord injury?
[ ] 1. Rent or buy a conventional hospital bed.
[ ] 2. Build a wheelchair ramp to the door.
[ ] 3. Apply for a handicapped parking sticker.
[ ] 4. Provide a raised toilet seat with grab bars.

Nursing Care of Clients with Degenerative Disorders

An older adult diagnosed with Parkinson's disease is admitted to a nursing home for basic nursing care.

37. Which assessment finding is most important to consider before developing the client's care plan?
[ ] 1. The client's ability to perform activities of daily living
[ ] 2. The client's preferences for and dislikes of various foods
[ ] 3. The family members' views about nursing home placement
[ ] 4. The client's feelings about giving up independent living

38. The nurse educator provides an inservice program about Parkinson's disease. Which clinical manifestation is the educator most likely to include as the initial sign of Parkinson's disease?
[ ] 1. Muscle rigidity
[ ] 2. Muscle tremors
[ ] 3. Muscle weakness
[ ] 4. Muscle deterioration

The client with Parkinson's disease takes levodopa/carbidopa (Sinemet) three times a day.

39. When the nurse observes that the client has difficulty swallowing the capsule of medication, which action is best to take?
[ ] 1. Soak the capsule in water until soft.
[ ] 2. Tell the client to chew the capsule.
[ ] 3. Empty the capsule in the client's mouth.
[ ] 4. Offer water before giving the capsule.

The nurse initiates a teaching plan for the client with Parkinson's disease.

40. Which instruction should be the nurse's priority in this situation?
[ ] 1. Steps to enhance the client's immune system
[ ] 2. Importance of maintaining a balanced diet
[ ] 3. Need to remove all safety hazards
[ ] 4. Importance of social interactions

41. Which goal is most realistic for a client diagnosed with Parkinson's disease?
[ ] 1. To reverse the symptoms and cure the disease
[ ] 2. To stop the progression of the disease process
[ ] 3. To maintain optimal muscle and motor function
[ ] 4. To prepare for a progressive terminal disease

42. Because the client with Parkinson's disease is prone to constipation, the nurse should encourage increased consumption of which food?
[ ] 1. Fresh fruits
[ ] 2. Wheat pasta
[ ] 3. Low-fat cheese
[ ] 4. Canned vegetables

An older client with dementia is admitted to the Alzheimer's unit of an extended care facility.

43. The nurse discusses the client's condition with the family. Based on the nurse's knowledge, which characteristic is found in Alzheimer's disease that distinguishes it from other dementias?
[ ] 1. Destruction of brain cells from hypoxia
[ ] 2. Destruction of brain cells from a stroke
[ ] 3. Neurofibrillary tangles and plaques in the brain
[ ] 4. A superficial infection in the meninges of the brain

44. When the client is observed wandering about the facility, the nurse modifies the client's care plan to provide for safety. Which nursing intervention is most appropriate at this time?
[ ] 1. Keep the client confined to the room.
[ ] 2. Attach an identity tag to the client's clothes.
[ ] 3. Lock all the outside doors in the facility.
[ ] 4. Make sure the client knows the location of the facility.

45. What nursing approach is best when managing the care of a client with dementia who insists on carrying a purse at all times?
[ ] 1. Ask the client where the purse can be stored.
[ ] 2. Ensure that the client is never without the purse.
[ ] 3. Inform the client that the purse may become lost.
[ ] 4. Find out why the client feels the need for a purse.

46. The client repeatedly asks, "Where is my mother?" Which response by the nurse would be best to prevent client frustration and agitation?
[ ] 1. Explain to the client, "Your mother died several years ago."
[ ] 2. Tell the client, "Your mother will visit later."
[ ] 3. State, "You miss your mother. What was she like?"
[ ] 4. Ask the client, "When did you last see your mother?"

A 48-year-old client experiences an exacerbation of multiple sclerosis after being asymptomatic for the past 6 months.

47. How can the nurse best help the client deal with personal fears at this time?
[ ] 1. Encourage the client to verbalize feelings.
[ ] 2. Provide a detailed explanation of the disease progression.
[ ] 3. Tell the client about physical assessment findings.
[ ] 4. Explain that the disease may become periodically acute.

48. When assisting the client with activities of daily living (ADLs), which approach is best?
[ ] 1. Limit the time for performing ADLs to 30 minutes.
[ ] 2. Eliminate whatever tasks the client cannot perform.
[ ] 3. Let the client rest between activities.
[ ] 4. Perform all of the client's ADLs at this time.

49. The nurse is providing suggestions to the family of a client with multiple sclerosis on vacationing areas to avoid. Which areas would the nurse stress?
[ ] 1. Areas with predominantly hot weather
[ ] 2. Areas where the climate is generally wet
[ ] 3. Places with dry arid environments
[ ] 4. Locations that are usually cold

The physician prescribes interferon beta-1a (Avonex) by the subcutaneous route for a client with multiple sclerosis.

50. When the nurse alternates injection sites on the client's upper arms, how far apart should the injections be spaced?
[ ] 1. ¼" (0.6 cm)
[ ] 2. ½" (1.3 cm)
[ ] 3. 1" (2.5 cm)
[ ] 4. 2" (5 cm)

51. Before discharge, the nurse instructs the client about administering subcutaneous injections and correctly explains that the client should rotate injections between which two areas?
[ ] 1. Thighs and hips
[ ] 2. Forearms and hips
[ ] 3. Thighs and abdomen
[ ] 4. Abdomen and buttocks

52. Which nursing action would be most appropriate if the client develops anorexia and nausea while taking interferon beta-1a (Avonex)?
[ ] 1. Withhold the medication.
[ ] 2. Offer frequent mouth care.
[ ] 3. Administer the drug after meals.
[ ] 4. Provide small, easy to digest meals.

During a physical assessment, the nurse notes that the client experiences weakness and numbness in various parts of the body.

53. Which measure for preventing impaired skin integrity is appropriate to add to the care plan at this time?
[ ] **1.** Use an air-fluidized (Clinitron) bed.
[ ] **2.** Change the client's position every 2 hours.
[ ] **3.** Rub any reddened areas every 2 hours.
[ ] **4.** Provide daily treatment in a hyperbaric oxygen chamber.

The nurse is caring for an older client who has been diagnosed with myasthenia gravis.

54. Which sign or symptom in the client's medical history would most likely indicate a manifestation of the client's disease?
[ ] **1.** Sudden hearing loss
[ ] **2.** Sensitivity to light
[ ] **3.** Drooping eyelids
[ ] **4.** Protruding tongue

55. Which assessment finding is especially important to monitor when caring for a client with myasthenia gravis who is in crisis?
[ ] **1.** Breathing
[ ] **2.** Temperature
[ ] **3.** Blood pressure
[ ] **4.** Mental status

56. When planning care for this client, which equipment is most important for the nurse to keep at the bedside?
[ ] **1.** A bite block in case of seizures
[ ] **2.** A cardiac defibrillator in case of cardiac arrest
[ ] **3.** A suction machine in case of compromised swallowing
[ ] **4.** A cooling blanket in case of hyperthermia

The physician orders pyridostigmine bromide (Mestinon) for the client. The dosage will be adjusted according to the client's response.

57. Which nursing action is best for controlling the symptoms of the client diagnosed with myasthenia gravis?
[ ] **1.** Ensure that the client has regular bowel and bladder elimination.
[ ] **2.** Administer each dose of medication at the precise scheduled time.
[ ] **3.** Encourage the client to exercise twice daily for 30 minutes.
[ ] **4.** Provide nutritional supplements between each meal and at bedtime.

The client's care plan indicates to use Crede's maneuver to promote urination.

58. Which action by the client demonstrates that Crede's manuever is performed correctly?
[ ] **1.** Contracting and relaxing the urinary sphincter 10 to 25 times daily
[ ] **2.** Squeezing the urinary sphincter and holding for 3 seconds, then repeating
[ ] **3.** Bearing down, taking a deep breath, and slowly releasing it
[ ] **4.** Applying downward hand pressure at the umbilicus toward the symphysis pubis

A 60-year-old client in the late stage of amyotrophic lateral sclerosis (Lou Gehrig disease) is admitted to the hospital.

59. On the basis of the usual course of this disease, which nursing diagnosis is most likely included in the client's care plan?
[ ] **1.** Sexual dysfunction
[ ] **2.** Disturbed body image
[ ] **3.** Impaired memory
[ ] **4.** Self-care deficit

Nursing Care of Clients with Cerebrovascular Disorders

The nurse makes a home health visit to evaluate a 79-year-old client.

60. The nurse notes that the client has had a change in baseline neurologic functioning. Which symptom suggests that the client may be having transient ischemic attacks (TIAs)?
[ ] **1.** Brief periods of unilateral weakness
[ ] **2.** Brief periods of hand numbness
[ ] **3.** Brief periods of photosensitivity
[ ] **4.** Brief periods of stabbing head pain

61. After the nurse gathers more data concerning the client's signs and symptoms, which action is most appropriate?
[ ] **1.** Explain the event in understandable language.
[ ] **2.** Refer the client for immediate medical evaluation.
[ ] **3.** Recommend taking a low-dose aspirin once daily.
[ ] **4.** Advise the client to call 911 if symptoms persist.

Later in the day, the client is admitted to the hospital after emergency medical personnel respond to a call that the client has been found unconscious. The physician orders frequent neurologic checks.

62. The nurse in the emergency department assesses the client's neurologic function. When checking the client's pupils, which technique is correct?
[ ] **1.** Shine the penlight from the temple into each pupil.
[ ] **2.** Cover one of the client's eyes, then the other eye.
[ ] **3.** Brighten the lights in the examination area.
[ ] **4.** Observe for extraocular eye movement.

The physician orders a computed tomography scan of the client's brain with contrast dye.

63. The nurse describes the purpose of the computed tomography (CT) scan to the client and spouse and asks about the client's allergy history. The client's spouse reports that the client has several allergies. Which one must be reported to the physician before the CT scan?
[ ] **1.** Penicillin
[ ] **2.** Shellfish
[ ] **3.** Latex
[ ] **4.** Metal

It is determined that the client has had a stroke, and the client is admitted to the medical unit. A member of the client's church comes to the hospital to visit the client and asks the nurse, "What is my friend's condition?"

64. On the basis of Health Insurance Portability and Accountability Act (HIPAA) regulations, what client information is protected and should not be disclosed? Select all that apply.
[ ] **1.** Client's date of birth
[ ] **2.** Client's Social Security number
[ ] **3.** Client's insurance information
[ ] **4.** Client's address
[ ] **5.** Client's occupation
[ ] **6.** Client's diagnosis

The nursing team begins developing a care plan for the stroke victim.

65. When the nurse monitors the client's neurologic status, which finding is most suggestive that the client's intracranial pressure is increasing?
[ ] **1.** Systolic pressure increases and diastolic pressure decreases.
[ ] **2.** Systolic pressure decreases and diastolic pressure increases.
[ ] **3.** Apical heart rate is greater than the radial rate.
[ ] **4.** Radial pulse rate is greater than the apical rate.

The charge nurse enters the nursing diagnosis "Risk for ineffective airway clearance related to an inability to swallow" on the client's care plan.

66. Which nursing intervention is most appropriate for managing the identified problem?
[ ] **1.** Keeping the client supine
[ ] **2.** Removing all head pillows
[ ] **3.** Performing oral suctioning
[ ] **4.** Providing frequent oral hygiene

The neurologist determines that the stroke victim has right-sided hemiplegia.

67. The nurse documents that the client is at risk for falls. Which risk factors increase any client's risk for falls? Select all that apply.
[ ] **1.** The client is male.
[ ] **2.** The client is taking antibiotics.
[ ] **3.** The client is confused.
[ ] **4.** The client has vertigo.
[ ] **5.** The client has impaired vision.
[ ] **6.** The client needs help with toileting.

The nurse evaluates the stroke victim's medication profile because of the increased risk for falls.

68. Which classifications of drugs are most likely to result in falls? Select all that apply.
[ ] **1.** Antihyperlipidemics
[ ] **2.** Benzodiazepines
[ ] **3.** Sedatives
[ ] **4.** Opioids
[ ] **5.** Anticonvulsants
[ ] **6.** Antihypertensives

69. On the basis of the client's fall risk assessment, which interventions should the nurse implement? Select all that apply.
[ ] **1.** Instruct the client to ask for help before getting up.
[ ] **2.** Turn on the bed alarm.
[ ] **3.** Apply restraints to the upper extremities.
[ ] **4.** Advise the client's family to inform the staff when leaving.
[ ] **5.** Place the bed in the lowest position.
[ ] **6.** Obtain an order for a physical therapy consult.

70. When the client is stable enough to transfer from the bed to a wheelchair, which nursing action is correct?
[ ] **1.** Instruct the client about how to balance with a walker.
[ ] **2.** Position the wheelchair perpendicular to the bed.
[ ] **3.** Ask the client if a gait belt is preferred.
[ ] **4.** Brace the paralyzed foot and knee.

Because of the client's diagnosis of right-sided hemiplegia, the nurse instructs the client's spouse how to perform passive range-of-motion (ROM) exercises.

71. When teaching the client's spouse about these exercises, which instructions are most accurate? Select all that apply.
[ ] **1.** Move the paralyzed limbs in as many directions as possible.
[ ] **2.** Perform the exercises every hour while awake.
[ ] **3.** Repeat each exercise three times.
[ ] **4.** Take the pulse before exercising.
[ ] **5.** Allow rest periods between exercises.
[ ] **6.** Begin the exercises starting with the affected leg.

The nurse attaches a footboard to the client's bed.

72. Which statement best describes how the nurse positions the client's feet when a footboard is used?
[ ] **1.** The soles are perpendicular to the board.
[ ] **2.** The soles are parallel to the board.
[ ] **3.** The knees are flexed less than 90 degrees.
[ ] **4.** The ankles are extended more than 90 degrees.

The speech therapist reports to the nurse that the client has expressive aphasia.

73. Which nursing intervention is best for communicating with the client at this time?
[ ] **1.** Speak using a low tone of voice.
[ ] **2.** Have the client point to key phrases printed on a clipboard.
[ ] **3.** Complete the sentence if the client becomes frustrated.
[ ] **4.** Encourage the client to practice verbalizing key words.

74. Which nursing goal is most important to the client's rehabilitation?
[ ] **1.** To regulate bowel and bladder elimination
[ ] **2.** To prevent contractures and joint deformities
[ ] **3.** To deal with problems of altered body image
[ ] **4.** To foster positive outcomes from depression

75. The client's spouse notices situations during which the client laughs or cries inappropriately. The spouse asks the nurse, "Why are these mood swings occurring?" Which is the best response by the nurse?
[ ] **1.** Your spouse is trying to gain control over the situation by these mood swings.
[ ] **2.** Emotional fluctuations are common for many after experiencing a stroke.
[ ] **3.** The stroke has destroyed the part of the brain dealing with emotions.
[ ] **4.** It is common to be very emotional after a major life event.

76. The client's spouse will be the primary caretaker upon discharge. The physician has written a new prescription for warfarin (Coumadin). Which teaching topics should the nurse cover before discharge? Select all that apply.
[ ] **1.** Dietary restrictions
[ ] **2.** Avoiding heavy lifting
[ ] **3.** Staying out of bright sunlight
[ ] **4.** Missed doses
[ ] **5.** Bruising or blood in urine
[ ] **6.** Need for frequent laboratory work

Assessment reveals that the stroke victim has hemianopia.

77. Which intervention should be added to the client's care plan in relation to this latest finding?
[ ] **1.** Have the client wear dark glasses when in bright light.
[ ] **2.** Cover the client's affected eye with an eye patch.
[ ] **3.** Approach the client from the unaffected side.
[ ] **4.** Position food on the tray resembling the face of a clock.

A client with a leaking cerebral aneurysm is being treated conservatively with complete bed rest, anticonvulsants, and sedatives.

78. Of the following nursing observations, which is most important to address in view of the client's condition?
[ ] **1.** The client has a chronic cough.
[ ] **2.** The client is becoming jittery.
[ ] **3.** The client's skin is warm and clammy.
[ ] **4.** The client develops diarrhea.

79. The nurse is preparing to examine a client with a cerebral aneurysm. Place all of the following assessment areas in order of priority, listing the top priority first. Use all the options.

1. Bowel elimination	
2. Motor strength	
3. Vital signs	
4. Skin integrity	
5. Urine output	
6. Level of consciousness (LOC)	

The client with a cerebral aneurysm tells the nurse that the nonopioid analgesic administered 2 hours ago has not adequately relieved a headache.

80. If the drug is administered every 3 to 4 hours, which nursing action is most appropriate at this time in response to the client's statement?
[ ] **1.** Administer another dose of the nonopioid analgesic immediately.
[ ] **2.** Rearrange medication times so that the client receives pain medication hourly.
[ ] **3.** Consult the physician about ordering an opioid analgesic.
[ ] **4.** Use a nondrug intervention such as listening to a guided imagery tape.

Nursing Care of Clients with Tumors of the Neurologic System

A client with a suspected brain tumor is scheduled for a positron emission tomography scan.

81. When preparing the client for the upcoming positron emission tomography (PET) scan, the nurse instructs the client to avoid which substances the day before the test? Select all that apply.
[ ] **1.** Caffeine
[ ] **2.** Shampoo
[ ] **3.** Diuretics
[ ] **4.** Shellfish
[ ] **5.** Alcohol
[ ] **6.** Tobacco

82. Which discharge instruction is most appropriate following the positron emission tomography scan?
[ ] **1.** Take a mild sedative tonight.
[ ] **2.** Increase your fluid intake.
[ ] **3.** Avoid excessive sitting.
[ ] **4.** Report signs of a fever.

Positron emission tomography confirms a brain tumor, and the client is scheduled for a craniotomy.

83. Which preoperative assessment is most important to document as a basis for postoperative comparison?
[ ] **1.** Motor strength in all extremities
[ ] **2.** Sodium and potassium laboratory values
[ ] **3.** Pulses in lower extremities
[ ] **4.** Glucometer blood glucose levels

84. Before the client undergoes the craniotomy, the nurse inserts a urinary catheter. How far should the catheter be inserted if the client is a male?
[ ] **1.** 2″ to 4″ (5 to 10 cm)
[ ] **2.** 4″ to 6″ (10 to 15 cm)
[ ] **3.** 6″ to 8″ (15 to 20 cm)
[ ] **4.** 8″ to 10″ (20 to 25.5 cm)

Before surgery, the nurse explains to the client about the need for skin preparation involving hair removal from the scalp.

85. When is the best time to clip the client's hair?
[ ] **1.** The night before surgery
[ ] **2.** In the morning, after a shower
[ ] **3.** Before administering preoperative sedation
[ ] **4.** Before surgery, in the operating room area

86. The client asks the nurse why the hair is being clipped and not shaved. Which response by the nurse is most appropriate?
[ ] **1.** "Clipping the hair is hospital policy."
[ ] **2.** "This method is safer for you."
[ ] **3.** "Shaving the head causes microscopic cuts, resulting in risk for infection."
[ ] **4.** "Surgery could be postponed if bleeding from the scalp occurs."

The client is returned to the nursing unit after 6 hours of surgery.

87. During the immediate postoperative assessment, the nurse notes that the client's dressing is moist. Which action is most appropriate to take first?
[ ] **1.** Change the dressing.
[ ] **2.** Reinforce the dressing.
[ ] **3.** Remove the dressing.
[ ] **4.** Document the findings.

After the craniotomy, the client has periods of confusion.

88. Which nursing intervention is best during the confused episodes?
[ ] **1.** Reading a newspaper or magazine to the client
[ ] **2.** Informing the client that confusion is temporary
[ ] **3.** Withholding verbal communication temporarily
[ ] **4.** Reorienting the client to place and situation

The physician orders a clear liquid diet for the client and restricts oral intake to no more than 1,000 mL.

89. Before requesting the clear liquids prescribed by the physician, which assessment information is essential for the nurse to know?
[ ] **1.** The client's ability to raise the head
[ ] **2.** The client's preferences of clear liquids
[ ] **3.** Whether the client's bowel sounds have returned
[ ] **4.** The client's ability to swallow effectively

90. The nurse is managing care in the postoperative period. In which situation does the nurse practice beneficence?
[ ] **1.** When the nurse practices good handwashing
[ ] **2.** When the nurse reports a breech in client confidentiality
[ ] **3.** When the nurse refers the client to a support group
[ ] **4.** When the nurse advocates for the wishes of the client

Nursing Care of Clients with Nerve Disorders

A nurse is assessing the neurologic status of a client exhibiting neurologic difficulties.

91. Which client response depicts normal function of cranial nerve XI?
[ ] **1.** A client wrinkling the forehead
[ ] **2.** A client puffing out the cheeks
[ ] **3.** A client sticking out the tongue
[ ] **4.** A client shrugging the shoulders

A client is diagnosed with trigeminal neuralgia (tic douloureux).

92. On the basis of the factors that cause the client to experience paroxysmal pain, which intervention is most appropriate to include in this client's care plan?
[ ] **1.** Direct a fan toward the client's face.
[ ] **2.** Avoid care that involves touching the client's face.
[ ] **3.** Keep ice chips available at the client's bedside.
[ ] **4.** Apply warm facial compresses for pain.

The physician treats the client with carbamazepine (Tegretol).

93. Because carbamazepine (Tegretol) can cause liver dysfunction, the client's discharge plan should include instructions to report which symptom?
[ ] **1.** Unusual bleeding
[ ] **2.** Black stools
[ ] **3.** Cloudy urine
[ ] **4.** Mottled skin

Drug therapy is unsuccessful for a client with trigeminal neuralgia. The physician severs one of the branches of the trigeminal nerve and orders eye irrigations postoperatively.

94. To correctly perform the eye irrigation, the nurse instills the eye irrigant in which direction?
[ ] **1.** From the lower conjunctiva toward the corneal surface
[ ] **2.** From the outer canthus of the eye to the inner canthus
[ ] **3.** From the nasal corner of the eye toward the temple
[ ] **4.** From the margins of the eyelashes to the folds of the lids

A client develops Bell's palsy due to inflammation around cranial nerve VII.

95. When the nurse performs a physical assessment, which finding is most indicative of the client's disorder?
[ ] **1.** Quivering eye movement
[ ] **2.** Muscle spasms in the lower extremities
[ ] **3.** Loss of motor function on the affected side
[ ] **4.** Unilateral facial paralysis

96. Which intervention is most appropriate for a client diagnosed with Bell's palsy?
[ ] **1.** Reduce the amount of light in the room.
[ ] **2.** Advise the client to drink liquids from a straw.
[ ] **3.** Inspect the buccal pouch for food after eating.
[ ] **4.** Instruct the client on how to walk with a cane.

The nurse is completing a history on a client who has been having right sciatic pain.

97. On this view of the pelvis, identify with an *X* the area where right sciatic pain occurs.

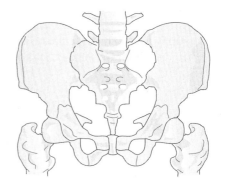

A client who experiences recurrent pain along the sciatic nerve is scheduled for a myelogram.

98. When the nurse describes the myelogram procedure to the client, which statement is most accurate?
[ ] **1.** "Part of the test involves a lumbar puncture."
[ ] **2.** "You will be asked to change positions frequently."
[ ] **3.** "Dye is instilled into a vein in your arm."
[ ] **4.** "Light anesthesia is administered during the test."

The myelogram shows that the client has a herniated intervertebral lumbar disk.

99. The nurse begins developing a teaching plan for the client. Which instruction is most applicable after symptoms are relieved?
[ ] **1.** Carry heavy objects away from your center of gravity.
[ ] **2.** Lift with your knees bent and your back straight.
[ ] **3.** Create a base of support by keeping your feet together.
[ ] **4.** Select a soft, spongy mattress for your bed.

The client eventually undergoes diskectomy with spinal fusion for the herniated disk.

100. When changing the client's position postoperatively, which nursing action is best?
[ ] **1.** Raise the client with a mechanical lift.
[ ] **2.** Logroll the client from side to side.
[ ] **3.** Have the client flex the knees and lift.
[ ] **4.** Pull the client's arms and then the legs.

101. When planning for the client's discharge after the diskectomy and spinal fusion, the nurse should include which instructions? Select all that apply.
[ ] 1. Avoid twisting or jerking the back.
[ ] 2. Sit in a chair with a soft back.
[ ] 3. Avoid sitting for long periods during the first week.
[ ] 4. Bend from the waist when picking up items from the floor.
[ ] 5. Monitor urine output for the first week.
[ ] 6. Report lower extremity color changes to the physician.

A client has been pronounced brain dead.

102. Which clinical findings would the nurse find on assessment in the brain-dead client? Select all that apply.
[ ] 1. Poor skin turgor
[ ] 2. Decerebrate posturing
[ ] 3. Deep tendon reflexes
[ ] 4. Absent corneal reflex
[ ] 5. Dilated nonreactive pupils
[ ] 6. Dry mucous membranes

103. The nurse is preparing the deceased client's body prior to the family's arrival. Which action provides a more aesthetic appearance to the body?
[ ] 1. Place the arms at the side and cover with a sheet.
[ ] 2. Place a rolled towel under the chin until the family arrives.
[ ] 3. Bathe the body and place a perineal pad between the legs.
[ ] 4. Remove all tubes and dressings allowing family access.

Correct Answers, Rationales, and Test Taking Strategies

Nursing Care of Clients with Infectious and Inflammatory Conditions

1. 1, 2, 6. Meningitis is an inflammation of the meninges and can be caused by bacteria, viruses, fungi, or parasites. Bacterial meningitis is the most serious form and is contagious. Neck stiffness, also called *nuchal rigidity*, is a common symptom among those who contract meningitis. Other common signs and symptoms include photophobia, nausea, vomiting, restlessness, irritability, seizures, headache, and fever. Muscle weakness, diarrhea, and vertigo are not typical signs and symptoms of meningitis.
> *Test Taking Strategy—Analyze the information about which the question asks, which involves the symptoms of meningitis. Alternative-format "select all that apply" questions require considering each option independently to decide its merit in answering the question. Select all of the symptoms of meningitis. Review the symptoms of meningitis in the neurologic chapter of a textbook if you had difficulty answering this question.*
> **Cognitive Level**—*Understanding*
> **Client Needs Category**—*Physiological integrity*
> **Client Needs Subcategory**—*Physiological adaptation*

2. 3. A lumbar puncture is performed by placing an aspiration needle into the subarachnoid space of the spinal cord, usually in the lumbar area at the level of the fourth intervertebral space, and obtaining cerebrospinal fluid, which is then sent for analysis. The client is typically positioned on his or her side, with the neck and knees flexed to increase the space between the vertebrae. It is anatomically difficult for the physician to perform this test with the client placed in a knee-chest position or in an orthopneic or prone position.
> *Test Taking Strategy—Use the process of elimination to identify the position that best flexes the vertebrae for ease and accuracy of needle placement. Review the procedure, recalling that the position of the client must give access to the subarachnoid space, if you had difficulty with this question.*
> **Cognitive Level**—*Applying*
> **Client Needs Category**—*Physiological integrity*
> **Client Needs Subcategory**—*Reduction of risk potential*

3. 4. To prevent complications and allow time for more cerebrospinal fluid (CSF) to form, clients are kept flat in bed for several hours after undergoing lumbar puncture. Increasing fluids helps re-form CSF at a faster rate. To apply pressure on the puncture site, a supine position rather than a side-lying position is preferred. Assisting the client into a sitting position is unsafe; it can lead to a severe headache or neurologic complications.

Test Taking Strategy—Note the strategic key term "most appropriate." Understanding that lumbar puncture lowers CSF pressure leads to the answer. Review the lumbar puncture procedure and nursing actions if you had difficulty answering this question.
Cognitive Level—*Applying*
Client Needs Category—*Physiological integrity*
Client Needs Subcategory—*Physiological adaptation*

4. 1. The three categories of transmission-based precautions include airborne, droplet, and contact precautions. Most forms of meningitis are spread within a 3-foot radius from an infected person to an uninfected person via moist oral and respiratory secretions released during coughing, sneezing, or talking. The Centers for Disease Control and Prevention, therefore, advises that droplet precautions are most appropriate in a client with possible meningitis. Airborne precautions are implemented to prevent the transmission of pathogens such as those from tuberculosis, for example, within the residue of evaporated droplets that remain suspended in the air or attached to dust particles. Contact precautions are used for pathogens that may be transmitted from skin-to-skin contact or from contact with contaminated objects in the client's environment. Standard precautions are followed when caring for all clients, regardless of their infectious status.

Test Taking Strategy—Use the process of elimination to select the option that identifies the transmission-based precautions for controlling the spread of meningitis. Review transmission-based precautions if you had difficulty answering this question.
Cognitive Level—*Applying*
Client Needs Category—*Safe and effective care environment*
Client Needs Subcategory—*Safety and infection control*

5. 2. To protect the client's skin, there should be a layer of light cloth between the client and the cooling blanket. The cooling blanket is placed beneath the client, not on top. Distilled water is used to fill the fluid chamber, not normal saline. Ice is not used; the distilled water is chilled electronically.

Test Taking Strategy—Use the process of elimination to select the intervention that is most appropriate for reducing a fever. To answer this question correctly, recall that the cooling process can cause significant vasoconstriction in unprotected skin, thus reducing the distribution of oxygen and nutrients to cells and causing local thermal injury. To reduce the risk of damage to the client's skin, a protective surface must be placed between the cooling blanket and the client. Option 1 is not the most efficient method for the transfer of body heat via conduction. Options 3 and 4 represent incorrect actions. Review the procedure

for implementing a cooling blanket if you had difficulty answering this question.
Cognitive Level—*Applying*
Client Needs Category—*Safe and effective care environment*
Client Needs Subcategory—*Safety and infection control*

6. 3. The best sign of improvement is when a previously unresponsive client now has an improvement in the Glasgow Coma Scale score. The Glasgow Coma Scale is a tool that assesses a client's response to stimuli. The scores range from 3 to 15. A score of 7 or less is interpreted as comatose; a score of 15 indicates normal functioning. When checking the pupils, a normal finding is that both pupils constrict when stimulated with light. Fixed, dilated pupils indicate brain dysfunction. Swallowing is a reflex and is not a measure of cognitive improvement.

Test Taking Strategy—Look for the key words "new assessment finding," indicating a change, and "improving." Evaluating the difference between the past status of being unresponsive and a condition that would include the improved status as noted in a nursing assessment is key. Review neurologic assessments and significant findings, including the Glasgow Coma Scale, if you had difficulty answering this question.
Cognitive Level—*Evaluating*
Client Needs Category—*Physiological integrity*
Client Needs Subcategory—*Physiological adaptation*

7. 1. Guillain-Barré syndrome is characterized by an acute autoimmune inflammatory destruction of the myelin sheath covering the peripheral nerves, which causes rapid, progressive symmetrical loss of motor function; however, the sensory nerves remain intact. Most clients show signs of recovery several weeks after symptoms cease. The exact cause of Guillain-Barré syndrome is unknown, but there seems to be a relationship to prior exposure to infectious agents, either by an actual infection or their attenuated form in an immunization (e.g., flu shot). This condition is not associated with spider bites, unpasteurized milk, or insecticides.

Test Taking Strategy—Analyze to determine what information the question asks for, which is the relationship between an occurrence in the client's history and the disease process. Understanding the potential causes for Guillain-Barré syndrome or relationships of events in the history with the syndrome allows for successfully answering the question. Recalling that Guillain-Barré is linked to a postinfectious inflammatory process, option 1 has the highest possibility of a connection. Review Guillain-Barré syndrome if you had difficulty answering this question.
Cognitive Level—*Understanding*
Client Needs Category—*Physiological integrity*
Client Needs Subcategory—*Physiological adaptation*

8. 4. When planning client care, it is important to know that in clients diagnosed with Guillain-Barré syndrome, weakness often begins in the extremities and progresses to the upper areas, including the chest. The diaphragm may become paralyzed, resulting in apnea with no respiratory effort. The pulse oximetry reading, which can be monitored continuously, is the most accurate technique for assessing whether a client is breathing effectively. Normal pulse oximetry readings are between 92% and 100%, so a reading of 82% indicates major respiratory compromise. Cyanosis is a result of respiratory distress; therefore, flushed skin is an inaccurate finding. Chest tightness is also not a typical finding.

> *Test Taking Strategy—Look for the key words "developing ineffective breathing," which suggests choosing an option that requires knowledge of respiratory compromise. A respiratory rate of 24 (option 1), although somewhat above normal, is not significantly elevated. Similarly, option 2 could be suggestive of compromised breathing, but the best evidence is provided by using a pulse oximeter to document oxygen saturation of the blood. Option 4 provides a significant indication of respiratory distress. Review signs of hypoxia to determine evidence of respiratory compromise if you had difficulty answering this question.*
> **Cognitive Level**—*Analyzing*
> **Client Needs Category**—*Physiological integrity*
> **Client Needs Subcategory**—*Physiological adaptation*

9. 2. Tube feedings utilize the normal route for digestion, absorption, and elimination of nutrients. Nasogastric (NG) tube feedings are less invasive than gastrostomy tube feedings. Crystalloid I.V. fluid does not supply all the nutrients that a person needs to maintain a healthy state. Total parenteral nutrition (TPN) requires a more invasive administration technique for administration than NG tube feedings.

> *Test Taking Strategy—Use the process of elimination to select the option that identifies the best temporary nutritional method to use in place of the oral route while still utilizing normal digestive processes. Understanding other nutritional routes allows the student to assess which route is best for this disease process. Options 3 and 4 can be eliminated because they are routes needing invasive techniques that are more appropriate for clients requiring nutritional support over a prolonged period of time. Option 1 can be eliminated due to the inadequacy of the nutrition provided. Review enteral and parenteral methods for meeting the nutritional needs of clients if you had difficulty answering this question.*
> **Cognitive Level**—*Applying*
> **Client Needs Category**—*Physiological integrity*
> **Client Needs Subcategory**—*Physiological adaptation*

10. 3. Human immunodeficiency virus encephalopathy, also known as *acquired immunodeficiency syndrome (AIDS) dementia complex,* occurs in at least two-thirds of clients with AIDS. It is characterized by a progressive decline in cognitive, behavioral, and motor function. The best technique to reduce the client's confusion is reorientation to person, place, and circumstances. Reorientation may have to be repeated frequently. Encouraging the family to turn on the television, play the client's favorite music, or look at a photo album with the client are techniques for providing sensory stimulation and do not help with confusion.

> *Test Taking Strategy—Use the process of elimination to select the option that identifies a key principle for reorienting a confused client. Option 3 specifically addresses a technique for reorientation. All other options can be eliminated because they do not address reorientation. Review how to reorient a confused client if you have difficulty answering this question.*
> **Cognitive Level**—*Applying*
> **Client Needs Category**—*Physiological integrity*
> **Client Needs Subcategory**—*Basic care and comfort*

Nursing Care of Clients with Seizure Disorders

11. 3. Autonomic nervous system manifestations of a seizure include an increase in epigastric secretions, pallor, sweating, flushing, piloerection, pupillary dilation, and tachycardia. Numbness and tingling and changes in taste and speech are somatosensory changes. Psychic changes include an aura that may be associated with a smell, noise, or sensation.

> *Test Taking Strategy—Analyze to determine what information the question asks for, which is an assessment that correlates with autonomic nervous system manifestations. Options 1, 2, and 4 are associated with the central nervous system. Review the function of the autonomic nervous system if you had difficulty answering this question.*
> **Cognitive Level**—*Understanding*
> **Client Needs Category**—*Physiological integrity*
> **Client Needs Subcategory**—*Physiological adaptation*

12. 1, 2, 3, 6. Safety is a priority for a client diagnosed with a seizure disorder. Should a seizure occur, modifying the environment helps reduce the potential for injuries. The nurse should keep the room dark and quiet, lower the bed to its lowest position, and keep the side rails up and padded. Suction and oxygen equipment should also be available. Lights, noise, and warm temperatures have been known to cause seizures. Providing soft, soothing music can cause relaxation but does not decrease the potential for injuries.

> *Test Taking Strategy—Analyze to determine what information the question asks for, which is environmental*

modifications associated with seizure precautions. Include those options that protect the client from injury. Alternative-format "select all that apply" questions require considering each option independently to decide its merit in answering the question. Eliminate options 1 and 4, which promote comfort, but do not affect the safety of the client. Review seizure precautions if you had difficulty answering this question.
Cognitive Level—*Applying*
Client Needs Category—*Safe and effective care environment*
Client Needs Subcategory—*Safety and infection control*

13. 3. To protect a client with a known or suspected seizure disorder, the bed should be kept in the lowest position, decreasing the chance of injury from falling to the floor during seizure activity. Although glass or metal utensils on a tray may injure a client, they are not usually restricted. The nurse may be able to observe the client more closely if the client is in a room close to the nurses' station, but such room arrangements are not always available. Restraining a client is not warranted.
Test Taking Strategy—*The key words are "most appropriate," indicating that one option is best. Use the process of elimination to identify the seizure precaution and specific nursing action that would best limit injury. Option 3 limits injuries from a fall. Options 2 and 4 are not standards of care for seizure precautions. Option 1 has merit, but it is not the "most appropriate" action from among the options provided. Review seizure precautions if you had difficulty answering this question.*
Cognitive Level—*Applying*
Client Needs Category—*Safe and effective care environment*
Client Needs Subcategory—*Safety and infection control*

14. 3. An EEG is a record of the brain's electrical activity. To ensure that the electrodes of the EEG remain attached to the skull during the test, hair should be clean and dry. Therefore, assisting the client in shampooing the hair is the most appropriate intervention at this time. Fasting is not required, although beverages containing caffeine are restricted 8 hours before an EEG. The blood pressure is assessed before the test; however, it is unnecessary to have the client lie down and then sit during the assessment. Drugs that affect brain activity, such as sedatives, are withheld for 24 to 48 hours because they can affect the test outcome. To increase the chances of recording seizure activity, it is sometimes recommended that the client be deprived of sleep.
Test Taking Strategy—*Analyze to determine what information the question asks for, which is the preparation of the client for an EEG. With the goal of obtaining an accurate EEG for diagnostic purposes, recall that contact between the electrode and*

the scalp throughout the test is crucial to obtaining accurate results. Removing oil from the hair and scalp with shampoo before the test promotes electrode and scalp contact, making option 3 most appropriate. Review the procedure to prepare a client for an EEG if you had difficulty answering this question.
Cognitive Level—*Applying*
Client Needs Category—*Physiological integrity*
Client Needs Subcategory—*Reduction of risk potential*

15. 4. When a client begins to convulse, the highest priority is maintaining a patent airway. Turning the client on his or her side, which allows saliva and vomitus (if present) to drain from the mouth, is the most immediate method of doing so. Turning the client also prevents the tongue from blocking the airway. Oxygen is administered after the airway is open and clear. Vital signs are taken after the seizure is completed. Checking a client's pupils would be a very difficult task to perform while the client is having a seizure.
Test Taking Strategy—*Look for the key words "first action," indicating a priority. Maslow's hierarchy addresses physiologic needs, which include maintaining the airway and breathing as a priority; thus, maintaining a patent airway (option 4) is the best answer. Although option 1 helps to improve oxygenation, it would be ineffective if the airway is not patent. Options 2 and 3 only provide assessment data. Review nursing care during the ictal phase of a seizure if you had difficulty answering this question.*
Cognitive Level—*Analyzing*
Client Needs Category—*Physiological integrity*
Client Needs Subcategory—*Reduction of risk potential*

16. 2. Although the time that the seizure started is important information to document, it is not as valuable to the diagnostic process as identifying the seizure's duration. The client's mood before the seizure and comments afterward may be diagnostic, but they are not higher priorities than documenting the duration of the seizure.
Test Taking Strategies—*Look for the key words "initially" and "most important." Recalling the crucial information to relay to the physician (option 2) is the priority. Options 1, 3, and 4 provide secondary or inconsequential information. Review nursing assessment findings that are pertinent to document during the ictal phase of a seizure if you had difficulty answering this question.*
Cognitive Level—*Analyzing*
Client Needs Category—*Physiological integrity*
Client Needs Subcategory—*Physiological adaptation*

17. 4, 5, 6. When responding to the client who is experiencing a tonic–clonic seizure, safety and maintenance of the airway are the priority concerns. Rolling the client's whole body to the side facilitates any drainage that may occur from the mouth and keeps the airway open. Objects or situations that could harm the client should be removed from the environment. The respiratory therapy department (or the rapid response team) should be activated for additional support, such as oxygen therapy.

The jaw is typically clenched during a seizure; therefore, placing an emesis basin close to the mouth is not an effective action. Furthermore, it may cause the client harm. Calling out the client's name is not essential because the client may lose consciousness for up to several minutes during a seizure. Holding the client down during the seizure activity can harm the client and does nothing to stop the seizure.

> *Test Taking Strategy—Analyze to determine what information the question asks for, which are essential actions to take when finding a client experiencing a tonic–clonic seizure. Essential actions are those for maintaining physiologic needs and protecting the client from harm until the seizure concludes. Alternative-format "select all that apply" questions require considering each option independently to decide its merit in answering the question. Options 4, 5, and 6 focus on maintaining an airway, protecting the client from harm, and improving oxygenation. Review nursing actions when managing the care of a client experiencing a tonic–clonic seizure if you had difficulty answering this question.*

Cognitive Level—Applying
Client Needs Category—Safe and effective care environment
Client Needs Subcategory—Safety and infection control

18. 2. In the event of a lawsuit, it is important to prove that safety standards were being followed. The best evidence is noting that the signal cord was within the client's reach. This information may relieve the nurse from liability. It is important to document the vital signs at the time that the client was found. The time that the client was last observed is more pertinent legally than what the client was doing when observed. Having a client assigned to a licensed nurse does not relieve the nurse from liability. Safety precautions must always be followed.

> *Test Taking Strategy—Analyze to determine what information the question asks for, which involves legal requirements when completing an incident report. Remember that nurses are required to follow safety standards and policies within their health care institution. Documenting actions from specific nursing standards of care, such as those that require the client's access to a device for summoning help, protects the nurse and facility from litigation. Option 2 is the only option that upholds a safety standard of care. Review the purposes of an incident report and the information included in an incident report if you had difficulty answering this question.*

Cognitive Level—Applying
Client Needs Category—Safe and effective care environment
Client Needs Subcategory—Safety and infection control

19. 4. A tonic–clonic (generalized) seizure involves both a tonic phase and a clonic phase. Within the tonic phase, loss of consciousness, dilated pupils, and muscular stiffening are common clinical manifestations. This period lasts approximately 20 to 30 seconds. The clonic phase of a generalized seizure results in repetitive movements of muscle contraction. The generalized seizure ends with confusion, drowsiness, deep sleep, and resumption of regular respirations. Jerking in one extremity is a clinical manifestation of a partial seizure. An absence seizure, which frequently goes unnoticed, involves staring with brief loss of consciousness and fluttering of the eyelids and lip movement. Excessive jerking of the entire body is a manifestation of myoclonic seizures.

> *Test Taking Strategy—Note the key word "first" in the question. Knowledge of the postictal stage is essential. Elimination of signs of other types of seizures (myoclonic, partial and absence) leaves option 4 as the correct answer. Review the sequence of events that accompany tonic-clonic seizures if you had difficulty answering this question.*

Cognitive Level—Analyzing
Client Needs Category—Physiological integrity
Client Needs Subcategory—Physiological adaptation

20. 2. A priority nursing measure during the postictal phase of a seizure is to maintain the client's airway and assess the client's breathing pattern for an effective rate, rhythm, and depth. Oxygen administration may be necessary. Assessing the levels of consciousness and arousability as well as reorientation to person, place, and time is important to complete but only after a patent airway and regular respiratory pattern have been established. Incontinence of bowel and bladder is common during a seizure, and providing hygiene is important to provide dignity for the client, but not as important as maintaining an airway and assessing breathing.

> *Test Taking Strategy—Look for the key word "priority." It can be anticipated that more than one option is correct, but choosing the option that is most important or holds the most significance is the best strategy. Remember to use airway and breathing to identify the priority nursing intervention. According to this strategy, airway and breathing pattern (option 2) takes priority over the other options. Review the nursing management of a client during the postictal phase of a seizure if you had difficulty answering this question.*

Cognitive Level—Applying
Client Needs Category—Physiological integrity
Client Needs Subcategory—Physiological adaptation

21. 1. Carbamazepine (Tegretol), phenytoin (Dilantin), and phenobarbital sodium (Luminal) are used as anticonvulsants to treat various seizure disorders. Diazepam (Valium) is classified as a benzodiazepine. It and lorazepam (Ativan) are the drugs of choice for treating status epilepticus by the I.V. route.

Test Taking Strategy—Use the process of elimination to select an option identifying an emergency drug for managing a seizure. Carbamazepine (Tegretol), phenytoin (Dilantin), and phenobarbital sodium (Luminal) are all anticonvulsants that are used on a scheduled daily basis for managing seizure disorders. Diazepam (option 1) is a benzodiazepine that is administered intravenously in an emergency to abort episodes of status epilepticus. Therefore, option 1 emerges as the best choice. Review seizure medications if you had difficulty answering this question.
Cognitive Level—Understanding
Client Needs Category—Physiological integrity
Client Needs Subcategory—Pharmacological therapies

22. 3. Phenytoin sodium (Dilantin) causes gingival hyperplasia. Thorough oral hygiene, gum massage, daily flossing, and regular dental care are essential. Therefore, brushing the teeth becomes especially important for preventing oral complications. Shampooing the hair, trimming the fingernails, and bathing the skin are important components of good hygiene for all clients.

Test Taking Strategy—Analyze to determine what information the question asks for, which is a hygiene measure to reduce the side effects of phenytoin (Dilantin). A helpful hint is that phenytoin causes oral problems, so routine oral and dental care is a priority and an essential teaching point. Review side effects of phenytoin if you had difficulty answering this question.
Cognitive Level—Applying
Client Needs Category—Physiological integrity
Client Needs Subcategory—Pharmacological therapies

Nursing Care of Clients with Neurologic Trauma

23. 4. All the identified assessment findings are possible with a head injury, but the most serious is observing serous drainage from the ears. Serous drainage from the ears or nose suggests that the meninges have been lacerated and the drainage is cerebrospinal fluid.

Test Taking Strategies—Look at the key words "most suggestive" and "serious head injury." Options 1, 2, and 3 are significant, but option 4 is a definite indication of a serious head injury. Review signs and symptoms of head trauma if you had difficulty answering this question.
Cognitive Level—Analyzing
Client Needs Category—Physiological integrity
Client Needs Subcategory—Physiological adaptation

24. 1. As long as the accident victim is breathing and alert, it is best to keep the head and neck from moving. Movement may further damage the neck and spinal cord. Therefore, ambulating or moving the victim before the neck is immobilized is potentially unsafe. Covering the victim with a light blanket is appropriate if the environmental temperature is cold or the client is manifesting signs of shock. Water is generally withheld until the need for surgery is ruled out. Providing care and support for the client until help arrives is more important than finding the client's insurance card.

Test Taking Strategy—Look at the key word is "next," a follow-up on the previous scenario, which identifies that the client has experienced a head injury during a motor vehicle accident. The "next" priority would be preventing further injury. Of the choices, option 1 prevents further injury. Review measures for preventing spinal cord injuries if you had difficulty answering this question.
Cognitive Level—Analyzing
Client Needs Category—Physiological integrity
Client Needs Subcategory—Physiological adaptation

25. 2. According to most Good Samaritan laws, after stopping to provide aid, nurses have an obligation to remain with the victim until someone else with comparable knowledge and skills arrives. The other options describe actions that are legal but unethical.

Test Taking Strategy—Analyze to determine what information the question asks for, which is an option that identifies how to limit legal liability. When there is a liability question, follow policies, regulations, and practice acts. Option 2 is the only option that follows a legal standard. Review legal aspects that relate to a professional who provides care under a Good Samaritan law if you had difficulty answering this question.
Cognitive Level—Applying
Client Needs Category—Safe and effective care environment
Client Needs Subcategory—Coordinated care

26. 3. Until spinal cord injury is ruled out, the client should be kept flat with the head immobile. Keeping the head elevated 30 to 45 degrees aids in promoting venous return, which helps to reduce intracranial pressure. This choice is appropriate but only after spinal cord injury has been ruled out. None of the other positions allows for elevation of the victim's head and, therefore, will not help to reduce or stabilize the intracranial pressure.

Test Taking Strategy—Analyze to determine what information the question asks for, which is a position that increases the potential for a positive outcome after head injury. When the diagnosis is a head injury, maintaining a neutral anatomic position is essential to avoid possible or further damage to the spinal

cord before the client is seen by a physician. Option 3 keeps the client flat and, combined with the neck immobilizer, prevents flexion of the neck or other potentially injurious positions. Review nursing care that is appropriate for clients experiencing trauma to the head and neck if you had difficulty answering this question.
Cognitive Level—*Applying*
Client Needs Category—*Physiological integrity*
Client Needs Subcategory—*Physiological adaptation*

27. 4. Changes in pupil response indicate increasing intracranial pressure and provide vital information regarding the client's neurologic status. Preventing and stabilizing intracranial pressure is a priority because elevated intracranial pressure could lead to brain damage. The other assessments are appropriate when caring for any client, but they do not provide information about the client's neurologic status.
> *Test Taking Strategy*—*Use the process of elimination to identify the option that has the greatest significance in relation to the diagnosis. Option 4 directly relates to a pathologic change affecting the status of the neurologic system and a need for immediate medical intervention. Review nursing assessments that are pertinent to head injuries if you had difficulty answering this question.*
> **Cognitive Level**—*Analyzing*
> **Client Needs Category**—*Physiological integrity*
> **Client Needs Subcategory**—*Physiological adaptation*

28. 3. A change in the client's level of consciousness is the most significant indication that intracranial pressure is increasing and possible secondary brain damage is imminent. The information in the other options is important to document but not serious enough to notify the physician.
> *Test Taking Strategy*—*Look for the key word "immediately" in relation to an assessment finding that indicates a significant problem. Look for an option in which the client's condition could be in jeopardy. Option 3 directly relates to a change in neurologic status with a potential for progressing deterioration. Review the symptoms of head injuries and increased intracranial pressure if you had difficulty answering this question.*
> **Cognitive Level**—*Analyzing*
> **Client Needs Category**—*Physiological integrity*
> **Client Needs Subcategory**—*Physiological adaptation*

29. 3. Flexing the neck interferes with venous outflow from the brain. Venous congestion raises intracranial pressure. Fluids are generally restricted for a client with a head injury to reduce the potential for raising intracranial pressure. Being frequently disturbed interferes with the client's

sleep pattern, but that is not as significant a consequence as identifying the relationship between neck flexion and increased intracranial pressure. A full bladder causes autonomic dysreflexia in a client with a spinal cord injury.
> *Test Taking Strategy*—*Analyze to determine what information the question asks for, which involves correlating the client's changing neurologic status and identifying a contributing factor for that change. Begin by evaluating each option and ask if this finding would cause the change in neurologic status. Option 3 relates directly to the spinal cord and altered neurologic status, making it the best option. Options 1, 2, and 4 relate to potential problem situations, but these do not affect the neurologic status in this case. Review nursing assessments that are pertinent to head injuries if you had difficulty answering this question.*
> **Cognitive Level**—*Evaluating*
> **Client Needs Category**—*Physiological integrity*
> **Client Needs Subcategory**—*Physiological adaptation*

30. 1. Mannitol (Osmitrol) is a potent osmotic diuretic used to reduce cerebrospinal pressure. Urine output is one of the data that indicates the client's response to drug therapy. Adverse effects associated with mannitol therapy include dehydration, electrolyte loss, vomiting, and diarrhea. The other options are not related to mannitol.
> *Test Taking Strategy*—*Analyze to determine what information the question asks for, which is the therapeutic action of mannitol. If you have no idea, you may deduce its action by analyzing the trade name or by critically thinking what the desired therapeutic response may be. Identify the assessment finding that would document this occurrence. Option 1 is best because it documents the diuretic effect the medication has on reducing cerebrospinal fluid. Review the actions of mannitol and nursing considerations in administering the drug if you had difficulty answering this question.*
> **Cognitive Level**—*Analyzing*
> **Client Needs Category**—*Physiological integrity*
> **Client Needs Subcategory**—*Pharmacological therapies*

31. 3. The client is correct in stating that function will be retained above the chest and including function of the upper extremities; however, with a complete transection of the spinal cord at the T5 level, the client will have permanent paraplegia. The client will be able to eat independently.
> *Test Taking Strategy*—*Use the process of elimination to select the option that best describes the structure and function of spinal nerves. Option 1 can be eliminated because it is known that the client has a complete transection of the spinal cord at the thoracic level. Thus, one can expect that there will not be full neuromuscular function. Option 4 can also be*

eliminated because with a complete transection of the spinal cord, there is a definite disruption of nerve transmission that nullifies any improved outcome in the future. Option 2 can be eliminated because the injury is at the thoracic, not cervical, level. Review the significance of an injury that involves transection of the spinal cord and function at the thoracic level of spinal nerves if you had difficulty answering this question.
Cognitive Level—*Analyzing*
Client Needs Category—*Physiological integrity*
Client Needs Subcategory—*Physiological adaptation*

32.

Understanding the area of injury and the neurologic deficits that accompany it are important aspects of nursing care. At the top of the vertebral column are the cervical vertebrae (C1–8), followed by the thoracic vertebrae (T1–12), then the lumbar vertebrae (L1–5), and the sacral vertebrae (S1–5). The correct placement of the X is at the level of T5 where the injury occurred.

> *Test Taking Strategy—Analyze to determine what information the question asks for, which involves the various anatomic groups of vertebrae and the location of the injury. Focus on the location of the thoracic region and then mark the site of the fifth thoracic vertebrae. Refer to pictorial depictions of the spine if you had difficulty answering this question.*
> **Cognitive Level**—*Understanding*
> **Client Needs Category**—*Physiological integrity*
> **Client Needs Subcategory**—*Physiological adaptation*

33. 2. All of the goals listed are appropriate, but the highest priority for maintaining the client's physical abilities is to strengthen and retain as much upper body function as possible. Upper body strength is the key to ensuring the client's mobility, self-care, and self-worth. Preventing skin breakdown, addressing the client's denial of his condition, and allowing the client to verbalize feelings are important, but are not the priority at this time.

> *Test Taking Strategy—Use the process of elimination to identify the option that identifies the highest priority in the rehabilitation setting. Strengthening the upper body muscles (option 2) is an appropriate priority goal for the rehabilitation setting. Review the consequences of spinal cord injuries and how they are managed to maintain the greatest potential for function if you had difficulty answering this question.*
> **Cognitive Level**—*Analyzing*
> **Client Needs Category**—*Health promotion and maintenance*
> **Client Needs Subcategory**—*None*

34. 1, 3, 5, 6. Autonomic dysreflexia is an acute emergency that occurs as a result of exaggerated autonomic responses to stimuli. Signs and symptoms include severe hypertension, slow heart rate, pounding headache, nausea, blurry vision, flushed skin, sweating, nasal stuffiness, and goose bumps. Clinical manifestations occur after spinal shock has been resolved and are often triggered by a full bladder or fecal impaction. Therefore, checking the client's catheter for patency is an appropriate action to take. Autonomic dysreflexia can have life-threatening consequences if unrelieved.

> *Test Taking Strategy—Analyze to determine what information the question asks for, which are signs and symptoms of autonomic dysreflexia. Review common manifestations of autonomic dysreflexia if you had difficulty answering this question.*
> **Cognitive Level**—*Applying*
> **Client Needs Category**—*Physiological integrity*
> **Client Needs Subcategory**—*Physiological adaptation*

35. 2. Adding fiber increases bulk to the stool, promoting regular bowel elimination. Fiber attracts fluid to moisten stool, which reduces or prevents fecal impaction. The presence of fecal impaction may also cause autonomic dysreflexia. Some paraplegics perform manual disimpaction on a regular basis to promote bowel elimination. Daily enemas are excessive; however, if an enema is necessary, it is more effective if administered after a meal, when the gastrocolic reflex is more active. Stool softeners twice per week will not promote daily bowel function. Water is necessary for both bowel and bladder function, but the recommended daily requirement for water is eight glasses, not two.

> *Test Taking Strategy—Use the process of elimination to identify an option that identifies a nursing action for establishing independent bowel elimination with the least harsh and invasive measures. Options 1 and 4 require medication administration, so they can be eliminated. Option 3 does not meet the daily requirements; thus, it will not improve bowel function. Option 2 is not invasive and promotes regular bowel elimination, so it is the best choice. Review nursing management of elimination during bowel retraining if you had difficulty answering this question.*

Cognitive Level—Applying
Client Needs Category—Physiological integrity
Client Needs Subcategory—Physiological adaptation

36. **2.** A wheelchair ramp will promote mobility by enabling the client to get in and out of the house easily. A hospital bed will assist with positioning the client. A handicapped parking sticker ensures that the client will not have to travel long distances to get in and out of public facilities, but it does not ultimately promote mobility. A raised toilet seat is an inappropriate choice, especially if it is higher than the level of the wheelchair. This would promote inconvenience rather than mobility.

> *Test Taking Strategies—Use the process of elimination to select the option that best fulfills the goal of promoting client mobility after discharge. Options 1, 3, and 4 are all good suggestions, but option 2 is the only choice that promotes mobility. Review approaches for promoting mobility for a client who has compromised neuromuscular function if you had difficulty answering this question.*
> *Cognitive Level—Applying*
> *Client Needs Category—Safe and effective care environment*
> *Client Needs Subcategory—Coordinated care*

Nursing Care of Clients with Degenerative Disorders

37. **1.** Parkinson's disease is the result of a deficiency in dopamine, a neurotransmitter. It is usually seen in clients older than age 50; early signs and symptoms include stiffness, tremors of the hands, and pill rolling (rhythmic motions of thumb against the fingers). Later signs and symptoms include stooped posture, slow shuffling gait, and drooling. Assessing the client's ability to carry out various activities of daily living (ADLs) is the most appropriate nursing intervention at this time. It also allows for proper planning with the various disciplines that will be involved in the client's care. All the other data are important to the care of the client, but physiologic needs are a higher priority.

> *Test Taking Strategies—Use the process of elimination to identify the option that describes an assessment finding that is "most important" from among all the others. According to Maslow, physiologic needs are of highest priority. Option 1 is the only assessment that relates to physical ability. All other options, which address preferences and feelings, are less important than determining the client's ability for self-care, leaving option 1 as the best answer. Review Maslow's hierarchy of needs if you had difficulty answering this question.*
> *Cognitive Level—Applying*
> *Client Needs Category—Safe and effective care environment*
> *Client Needs Subcategory—Coordinated care*

38. **2.** The first sign of Parkinson's disease is usually fine motor tremors. The client is often the first person to notice this sign. Muscle rigidity is the second sign. Owing to the tremors and muscle rigidity, muscle deterioration and muscle weakness may occur if the muscles are not regularly used.

> *Test Taking Strategy—Use the process of elimination to identify an option that describes an initial sign of Parkinson's disease. Apply knowledge of the disease process and progression of symptoms to select from among the options. Option 2 is one of the first signs of Parkinson's disease. Review the signs and symptoms of Parkinson's disease and its progression of symptoms if you had difficulty with this question.*
> *Cognitive Level—Understanding*
> *Client Needs Category—Safe and effective care environment*
> *Client Needs Subcategory—Coordinated care*

39. **4.** Offering a few sips of water before placing the capsule in the client's mouth should help moisten the oral cavity and help the client swallow the medication. Capsules are never softened by placing them in water before administration nor should clients be instructed to chew capsules. Emptying the contents of the capsule into the client's mouth will produce an unpleasant taste. At the worst, an opened capsule may be absorbed at an undesirable rate.

> *Test Taking Strategy—Use the process of elimination to identify the best nursing action to use when a client has difficulty swallowing oral medication. Eliminate options 1 and 2 because capsules decompose in water and option 3 because it does not address the question. Option 4 provides an appropriate nursing strategy. Refer to medication administration guidelines if you had difficulty with this question.*
> *Cognitive Level—Applying*
> *Client Needs Category—Safe and effective care environment*
> *Client Needs Subcategory—Safety and infection control*

40. **3.** The primary focus for the client with Parkinson's disease is safety because much of the disease progression renders the client at risk for falling. The client typically has a propulsive unsteady gait, characterized by a tendency to take increasingly quicker steps while walking. The client may have difficulty beginning to walk, then difficulty returning to a seated position.

> *Test Taking Strategy—Look at the key words "nursing priority." Safety is always a priority. Always consider an action that avoids injury in options when the word "safety" is used. Review Parkinson's disease and its effects if you had difficulty answering this question.*
> *Cognitive Level—Applying*
> *Client Needs Category—Safe and effective care environment*
> *Client Needs Subcategory—None*

41. 3. The most realistic goal is to slow further deterioration, including that of muscle and motor activity. Intensity and duration of symptoms may vary based on the client's status from day to day or between medication doses. There is no known cure for Parkinson's disease and no way to stop its progression. However, many clients live with the disease for years.

> *Test Taking Strategy—Use the process of elimination to identify the option that identifies the most realistic goal for a client with Parkinson's disease. Eliminate options 1 and 2 because Parkinson's disease cannot be cured nor can the inevitable progression be stopped. Option 4 is inaccurate because Parkinson's disease is not in itself a terminal disease; most clients with Parkinson's disease die from complications such as aspiration or pneumonia. Option 3 is the most realistic choice and falls within the realm of nursing. Review Parkinson's disease, its management, and complications if you had difficulty answering this question.*
> **Cognitive Level**—*Evaluating*
> **Client Needs Category**—*Health promotion and maintenance*
> **Client Needs Subcategory**—*None*

42. 1. Fresh fruits and vegetables are good sources of fiber, which increases the bulk and water content of the stool. Most pasta is made from some type of refined wheat flour. Whole grains are a better source of fiber. Canned vegetables contain fiber but also a great deal of sodium. Cooking softens the fiber in vegetables and fruit; consequently, the cooking process reduces the indigestible bulk. Cheese is known to cause constipation, not help control it.

> *Test Taking Strategies—Analyze to determine what information the question asks for, which involves the application of nutritional strategies for managing constipation. Recall the foods that can decrease constipation. Fresh fruits (option 1) are an excellent source of fiber and contain fructose, a natural sweetener with laxative effects, making it the best choice. Refer to texts on nutrition if you had difficulty answering this question.*
> **Cognitive Level**—*Applying*
> **Client Needs Category**—*Physiological integrity*
> **Client Needs Subcategory**—*Basic care and comfort*

43. 3. Neurofibrillary tangles and plaques are found in postmortem examinations of clients with Alzheimer's disease. This clinical manifestation makes Alzheimer's disease different from other types of dementias. Hypoxia of the brain cells may result from a cerebrovascular accident or stroke or any type of ischemic insult. Evidence of infection of the meninges is common in meningitis but not in Alzheimer's disease.

> *Test Taking Strategy—Analyze to determine what information the question asks for, which requires knowledge of the pathophysiology that contributes to the unique feature or special "characteristic" of Alzheimer's disease. Options 1 and 2 relate to a stroke and cerebral hypoxia. Option 4 relates to an infection, which is incorrect, because an infection could be treated and reversed. Option 3 remains as the correct specific characteristic. Review the etiology of Alzheimer's disease if you had difficulty answering this question.*
> **Cognitive Level**—*Understanding*
> **Client Needs Category**—*Physiological integrity*
> **Client Needs Subcategory**—*Physiological adaptation*

44. 2. Make sure the client can be identified and returned to the care-providing agency. The Alzheimer's Association distributes identification tags and keeps a registry of client names as well. Confining the client to the room is inappropriate. Locking the outside doors is a fire and safety hazard. It is better to install doors that sound an alarm when opened. Memory loss is a classic sign of Alzheimer's disease. The client will most likely have to be redirected several times during the day.

> *Test Taking Strategy—Use the process of elimination to identify an option that is appropriate for maintaining mobility yet protects a confused client's safety and the safety of others. Safety is always a priority. Memory loss makes the individual unsafe because he or she could wander away and become lost. Option 2 provides the most appropriate means of client identification and safety. Option 1 interferes with the client's freedom to move about. Option 3 can be eliminated because it jeopardizes the safety of all of the clients and personnel in the case of a fire; therefore, it is an inappropriate nursing action. Option 4 is not reasonable due to the effects caused by the disease process. Review measures for maintaining safety in a long-term care facility for clients who are experiencing confusion if you had difficulty answering this question.*
> **Cognitive Level**—*Applying*
> **Client Needs Category**—*Safe and effective care environment*
> **Client Needs Subcategory**—*Safety and infection control*

45. 2. The purse may be a symbol of security for the client. Therefore, it is best to accommodate the client's idiosyncrasy. Trying to alter the client's behavior may increase the client's confusion and lead to aggressive behavior. The client may not have the cognitive ability to offer a reason, choose a storage place, or understand the concept of loss.

> *Test Taking Strategy—Use the process of elimination to identify a nursing intervention that supports the client's psychological need for security. If ensuring that the client has the purse at all times does not endanger the safety of the client or others, it is*

appropriate. Eliminate options 1 and 3 because they are similar and suggest that the purse should be put away. Eliminate option 4; the client has a disease process affecting the ability to logically communicate. Review methods for avoiding agitation among clients who have deteriorating cognitive function if you had difficulty answering this question.
Cognitive Level—*Applying*
Client Needs Category—*Psychosocial integrity*
Client Needs Subcategory—*None*

46. 3. Clients with dementia can sometimes be distracted from their original thoughts; therefore, stating that the client misses the mother and asking questions that foster long-term memory are most appropriate. In many cases, the short-term memory of a client with dementia has deteriorated; however, long-term memory may be intact. Reminding the client about the mother's death may cause distress. Lying by saying the client's mother will visit later is unethical. Frustration may develop when asking the client to identify the mother's last visit.
Test Taking Strategy—*Use the process of elimination to identify the most therapeutic response. The goal is to prevent client frustration by using a therapeutic communication technique in relation to a client's cognitive deficits. Eliminate option 2 because it is misleading and untrue. Eliminate option 4 because it may be beyond the capacity of a client with dementia. Option 1, though honest, is harsh, and therefore can be eliminated. Review the process of communication with dementia clients if you had difficulty answering this question.*
Cognitive Level—*Applying*
Client Needs Category—*Psychosocial integrity*
Client Needs Subcategory—*None*

47. 1. Multiple sclerosis is a progressive, debilitating disease affecting the myelin sheath of the peripheral nerves. The cause is unknown and onset affects clients usually between ages 20 and 40. Myelin is necessary for the transmission of nerve impulses to and from the brain. Being able to verbalize feelings of fear and frustration about a debilitating disease can be extremely therapeutic for the client. Sharing possibly irrational fears with a caring individual may help put them in a more realistic light. Giving accurate information, identifying assessment findings, and validating that the present health experience is common are appropriate nursing measures once the client verbalizes fears.
Test Taking Strategy—*Use the process of elimination to identify a principle of therapeutic communication that allows the client to discuss his or her personal basis for fears. The client's fears may or may not be due to a lack of understanding about the diagnosis and its effects. Options 2, 3, and 4 are similar because the nurse assumes the client is fearful from a lack of general information without confirming that as the cause; therefore, all three options may be eliminated. Option 1 is the only option in which the client*

is allowed to verbalize feelings; thus it is the best choice. Review techniques of therapeutic communication if you had difficulty answering this question.
Cognitive Level—*Applying*
Client Needs Category—*Psychosocial integrity*
Client Needs Subcategory—*None*

48. 3. A client with multiple sclerosis is typically weak and tires easily. Scheduling rest periods between activities will help manage these symptoms; it may also facilitate more self-care measures and elevate the client's self-esteem. The client is entitled to have basic needs met; if unable to do so independently, staff must carry out the responsibility. Hurrying through tasks would probably tire the client. Doing tasks that the client is capable of performing is demeaning.
Test Taking Strategy—*Use the process of elimination to identify the best approach that promotes completion of activities of daily living (ADLs) while maintaining the client's dignity. Weakness and fatigue most often interfere with successful completion of ADLs; thus, option 3 enables the client to better tolerate activity, which enables care to be completed. Options 1, 2, and 4 propose inappropriate nursing care. Review nursing approaches that promote completion of ADLs by distributing them over a longer period of time if you had difficulty answering this question.*
Cognitive Level—*Applying*
Client Needs Category—*Physiological integrity*
Client Needs Subcategory—*Basic care and comfort*

49. 1. Hot weather, even hot baths, increases the weakness common among clients with multiple sclerosis. Clients are not usually as adversely affected by rainy, dry, or cold environments.
Test Taking Strategy—*Analyze to determine what information the question asks for, which involves knowledge of the disease process and information that promotes safety. Warning a client implies that there is a safety issue. Look for the option that may place the client at risk for an exacerbation of the illness. Review information about clients with multiple sclerosis and information the nurse should provide if you have difficulty with this question.*
Cognitive Level—*Applying*
Client Needs Category—*Health promotion and maintenance*
Client Needs Subcategory—*None*

50. 3. Subcutaneous injections are placed no closer than 1″ in all directions from another recent injection. Use the size of a small dot adhesive bandage to estimate this distance. Injecting medications too close to another site can affect the absorption of the medication. In addition, subcutaneous injections should be avoided when the site is bruised, tender, hard, swollen, inflamed, or scarred.

Test Taking Strategy—*Analyze to determine what information the question asks for, which involves the principles for administering medications subcutaneously. Understanding the rationale for the distance between sites can narrow your choice. Review subcutaneous injection procedures if you had difficulty with this question.*
Cognitive Level—*Applying*
Client Needs Category—*Safe and effective care environment*
Client Needs Subcategory—*Safety and infection control*

51. 3. The thighs and abdomen are commonly used for administering subcutaneous interferon injections because they are more accessible for self-administration than the arms. The abdominal site provides the fastest rate of drug absorption. Activity, such as walking, will speed the rate of absorption of medications injected in the thighs.

Test Taking Strategy—*Use the process of elimination to select an option that identifies subcutaneous injection sites most appropriate for self-administration. Because the client is administering the medication, consider the sites more easily accessible for the client. Eliminate options 1, 2, and 4 because they contain sites that are difficult or inaccessible for self-administration. Review recommended sites for subcutaneous injections if you had difficulty answering this question.*
Cognitive Level—*Applying*
Client Needs Category—*Health promotion and maintenance*
Client Needs Subcategory—*None*

52. 4. Interferon beta-1a (Avonex) is essential for reducing the frequency of exacerbations in relapsing forms of multiple sclerosis. The drug slows the progression of physical disability. Therefore, withholding the drug because of anorexia and nausea is not an option. Mouth care improves the client's appetite, but it will not relieve the client's nausea. Administering the drug after meals will neither improve the client's appetite nor will it relieve nausea. Therefore, the best approach is to meet the client's nutritional needs by providing small, frequent meals that are easy to digest.

Test Taking Strategy—*Use the process of elimination to identify a nursing measure for managing medication side effects of anorexia and nausea. Eliminate option 1; a nurse would not withhold a medication without consulting the physician. Eliminate options 2 and 3 because frequent mouth care and administering the drug after meals will not reduce the side effects. Recalling that this medication is injected, the medication is not causing gastric distress. Option 4 is the option that directly affects the GI system to help cope with anorexia and diminish symptoms of nausea. Review interventions that prevent or reduce nausea and vomiting associated with the side effects of medications if you had difficulty answering this question.*

Cognitive Level—*Applying*
Client Needs Category—*Physiological integrity*
Client Needs Subcategory—*Pharmacological therapies*

53. 2. Clients with multiple sclerosis may experience numbness or decreased sensations; consequently, they may be unable to tell when an area of pressure is developing. Changing the client's position every 2 hours is sufficient in most circumstances to maintain skin that is still intact. An air-fluidized bed is appropriate for clients who are totally immobile or who have already developed stage 3 or 4 pressure ulcers. Rubbing a reddened skin area is inappropriate because this further damages the skin. Hyperbaric oxygen chambers promote healing by administering 100% oxygen at pressure three times greater than atmospheric pressure and are used when skin breakdown does not heal. Hyperbaric therapy is not used to prevent skin breakdown. Daily treatments can be costly and inconvenient because few hospitals have this type of therapy available.

Test Taking Strategy—*Analyze to determine what information the question asks for, which is preventive nursing measures for promoting skin integrity. Eliminate options 1 and 4 because they address issues of preventing further deterioration of pressure ulcers that already exist. Option 3 is inaccurate. Option 2 specifically addresses and provides the best intervention for preventing skin breakdown. Review the etiology, prevention, and management of pressure ulcers if you had difficulty with this question.*
Cognitive Level—*Applying*
Client Needs Category—*Physiological integrity*
Client Needs Subcategory—*Basic care and comfort*

54. 3. Myasthenia gravis is a neuromuscular disorder characterized by severe weakness of one or more skeletal muscles. Ptosis, which is drooping of the eyelids, is one of the more common signs of this disease and probably would be noticed by the client. Other common signs of generalized weakness include difficulty chewing and swallowing, masklike facial expressions, and inarticulate speech. The client's hearing and pupillary reflex would be unaffected by the disease. The client may have some problems moving the tongue during speech, but the tongue does not generally protrude.

Test Taking Strategy—*Use the process of elimination to select a sign or symptom most associated with myasthenia gravis. Recalling that muscular weakness is a classic symptom, option 3 is the only option that correlates with this symptom. Options 1, 2, and 4 can be eliminated because they are not evidence of skeletal muscle weakness. Review the signs and symptoms of myasthenia gravis if you had difficulty answering this question.*
Cognitive Level—*Understanding*
Client Needs Category—*Physiological integrity*
Client Needs Subcategory—*Physiological adaptation*

55. 1. Clients with myasthenia gravis are prone to upper body muscular weakness that can compromise the ability to breathe. Because ventilation is critical to life, this assessment is the most appropriate and critical to make. During a myasthenic crisis, the client experiences respiratory difficulty, increased weakness, and problems talking and swallowing. Confusion, hypertension, and elevated temperature are not associated with this disorder.

    Test Taking Strategy—Look at the key words "in crisis." Eliminate options that do not have a connection with muscle weakness and then prioritize to choose the option with the greatest health risk. Recall that muscle weakness can cause respiratory compromise, leading to an emergency situation. Breathing (option 1) utilizes muscle activity and is the highest priority. Options 2, 3, and 4 are not associated with muscle weakness. Review the nursing care of a client with myasthenia gravis if you had difficulty answering this question.
    Cognitive Level—Applying
    Client Needs Category—Physiological integrity
    Client Needs Subcategory—Physiological adaptation

56. 3. Because swallowing, which requires muscular strength, is compromised, an oral suction machine is best kept at the bedside of a client with myasthenia gravis. Suctioning may be needed quickly if the client cannot clear his or her airway. A cardiac defibrillator should remain centrally located near the nurses' station when not in use. Typically, clients with myasthenia gravis do not have seizures nor do they develop hyperthermia, so a bite block and cooling blanket are not necessary.

    Test Taking Strategy—Use the process of elimination to identify the equipment that is most important to maintaining the safety of a client with respiratory muscle weakness. Options 1, 2, and 4 can be eliminated as not having a correlation with muscle weakness or other symptoms of myasthenia gravis. Having a suction machine at the bedside is the best choice for keeping the airway open when swallowing becomes compromised; thus, option 3 is the best choice. Review the nursing management of clients with myasthenia gravis if you had difficulty with this question.
    Cognitive Level—Applying
    Client Needs Category—Physiological integrity
    Client Needs Subcategory—Reduction of risk potential

57. 2. Administering medications for myasthenia gravis at precise times prevents the worsening of symptoms as the medication wears off. Getting adequate nourishment is a healthy behavior, but dietary measures do not affect the symptoms of myasthenia gravis. Exercise may actually precipitate muscular weakness. Ensuring elimination is an appropriate nursing measure for managing the consequences of myasthenia gravis, but not for controlling the muscular weakness that causes elimination problems.

    Test Taking Strategy—Use the process of elimination to identify a medication administration technique that would best control symptoms associated with myasthenia gravis. Option 2 maintains muscle strength, which directly relates to the disease symptoms. All other options do not address the primary symptom. Review drug therapy as it relates to relieving the symptoms of myasthenia gravis if you had difficulty answering this question.
    Cognitive Level—Applying
    Client Needs Category—Physiological integrity
    Client Needs Subcategory—Pharmacological therapies

58. 4. Applying gentle downward pressure to the bladder while voiding is the correct way to perform a Crede maneuver to help empty the bladder. Kegel exercises are used to restore muscle function to the pelvic floor; they are used after childbirth and to help with urinary incontinence, and involve contracting of the urinary sphincter. The Valsalva maneuver is used to aid in defecation.

    Test Taking Strategy—Use the process of elimination to select the option that may initiate and promote complete emptying of the bladder. Options 1, 2, and 3 describe physical activities that address other problems of elimination. Option 4 then emerges as the best choice. Review the Crede manuever for promoting urinary elimination if you had difficulty with this question.
    Cognitive Level—Applying
    Client Needs Category—Health promotion and maintenance
    Client Needs Subcategory—None

59. 4. Amyotrophic lateral sclerosis (ALS) also known as *Lou Gehrig disease*, is a progressive, fatal neurologic disorder that affects men more than women. The cause of ALS is unknown, but it is characterized by degeneration of the motor neurons of the spinal cord and brain stem. As ALS progresses, clients generally become totally dependent on family or health care workers for all of their basic needs; therefore, the nursing diagnosis *Self-care deficit* is likely to be included in the client's care plan. Death is usually a consequence of respiratory failure or pneumonia. *Sexual dysfunction, Disturbed body image*, and *Impaired memory* may also be in the care plan, depending on the client's circumstances.

    Test Taking Strategy—Analyze to determine what information the question asks for, which involves the identification of a nursing diagnosis for a client with progressive loss of motor function. A diagnosis that corresponds to a physiologic need is of highest priority, according to Maslow. Because this is a progressive neurologic disorder, the client will have an inability to care for himself or herself. The nurse may develop a care plan for options 1, 2, and 3 at some point in the client's care, but it is essential that the care plan include nursing measures for managing a self-care deficit. Review principles for identifying a priority nursing diagnosis if you had difficulty answering this question.

Cognitive Level—Analyzing
Client Needs Category—Physiological integrity
Client Needs Subcategory—Physiological
adaptation

Nursing Care of Clients with Cerebrovascular Disorders

60. 1. A client who is experiencing a transient ischemic attack (TIA) may have weakness, dizziness, speech disturbances, visual loss, or double vision. Although the client may report visual changes, photosensitivity is not one of them. Stabbing head pain is more characteristic of a cerebral hemorrhage. Numbness and tingling in the hand is associated with nerve damage such as a pinched nerve in the neck is not associated with TIAs.

> *Test Taking Strategy—Analyze to determine what information the question asks for, which is a symptom that could indicate a transient ischemic attack (TIA). Eliminate options 2, 3, and 4 because they are not usually common among clients who experience a TIA. Review the symptoms of TIAs in a textbook if you had difficulty with this question.*
> *Cognitive Level—Evaluating*
> *Client Needs Category—Physiological integrity*
> *Client Needs Subcategory—Physiological adaptation*

61. 2. A transient ischemic attack (TIA) signals that a stroke may occur in the very near future; it is therefore inappropriate to ignore the symptoms or see if the symptoms persist. Providing an explanation is appropriate, but referring the client for immediate medical evaluation is the nurse's priority. Taking a low-dose aspirin daily may prevent vascular thrombosis; however, it does not supersede seeking evaluation and treatment of the underlying cause of symptoms.

> *Test Taking Strategy—Use the process of elimination to select the option describing the most appropriate action to take if a TIA is suspected. Recognize that client safety is always a first priority, and so referring the client for immediate medical attention (option 2) provides the most appropriate action to ensure client safety. Providing an explanation (option 1) does not address the potential seriousness of the event. Taking a daily aspirin (option 3) may be beneficial eventually, but it does not address the current danger for this client. Waiting to call 911 delays adequate treatment to prevent potential complications. Review the significance of and potential complications associated with a TIA if you had difficulty answering this question.*
> *Cognitive Level—Analyzing*
> *Client Needs Category—Physiological integrity*
> *Client Needs Subcategory—Physiological adaptation*

62. 1. To obtain valid assessment data, the nurse should dim the lights in the examination area and shine the penlight from the side of the temple into each pupil. If

conscious, the client is typically instructed to stare into the distance, not directly at the light. Both eyes are open, and the response of each pupil is observed separately before the opposite eye is directly stimulated. The nurse is primarily observing for constriction of the stimulated pupil, not extraocular eye movement.

> *Test Taking Strategy—Use the process of elimination to select the option that identifies the correct procedure for checking the client's pupillary response, which is a component of the neurologic exam. Recalling the procedure, options 2 and 3 can be eliminated as incorrect. Option 4 does not relate to assessing the pupils. Option 1 describes the correct assessment technique. Review the neurologic assessment procedure and manner for checking pupillary responses if you had difficulty answering this question.*
> *Cognitive Level—Applying*
> *Client Needs Category—Physiological integrity*
> *Client Needs Subcategory—Physiological adaptation*

63. 2. An allergy to shellfish indicates sensitivity to iodine, which is a component in many contrast dyes. To avoid a reaction, an allergy to shellfish must be reported. Allergy to any of the other substances does not affect the computed tomography (CT) scan.

> *Test Taking Strategy—Analyze to determine what information the question asks for, which is identifying a substance that correlates with a cross-sensitivity to contrast dye. An allergy to that substance must be reported to the physician before the CT scan. Recall that an allergy to shellfish could indicate that the client has an allergy to iodine, which is a component in many contrast dyes. Refer to CT procedures if you had difficulty with this question.*
> *Cognitive Level—Understanding*
> *Client Needs Category—Physiological integrity*
> *Client Needs Subcategory—Reduction of risk potential*

64. 1, 2, 3, 4, 6. The Health Insurance Portability and Accountability Act (HIPAA) of 1996 was passed by the federal government to protect clients' health information. It maintains confidentiality and regulates those who can access client records. It also has strict standards for storage and release of medical records. Unless the client has authorized that his or her health information may be given out, it is illegal for the nurse to do so. Protected information includes the client's diagnosis, date of birth, Social Security number, insurance information, address, phone numbers, past and present medical history, and future plans for treatment. HIPAA regulations do not include the client's occupation.

> *Test Taking Strategy—Analyze to determine what information the question asks for, which is client information that is protected by the Health Insurance Portability and Accountability Act (HIPAA). Alternative-format "select all that apply" questions require considering each option independently to*

decide its merit in answering the question. Options 1 through 4 and 6 are all protected information. Option 5 is not protected information. Review HIPPA and its implications if you had difficulty answering this question.
Cognitive Level—*Applying*
Client Needs Category—*Safe and effective care environment*
Client Needs Subcategory—*Coordinated care*

65. 1. A widened pulse pressure is an ominous sign that accompanies increased intracranial pressure. Pulse pressure is the difference between systolic and diastolic blood pressures. A pulse pressure between 30 and 50 mm Hg is considered normal. A widened pulse pressure is one that exceeds 50 mm Hg. If a trend is developing, however, it should be reported early rather than waiting until the pulse pressure equals or exceeds 50 mm Hg. The remaining choices are not indicators that intracranial pressure is increasing.

> **Test Taking Strategy**—*Use the process of elimination to select an answer that identifies an increase in intracranial pressure. Notice that is options 1 and 2 are opposites and options 3 and 4 are opposites. By eliminating either changes in blood pressure or heart rate as indications associated with increased intracranial pressure, the choice for an answer is narrowed to the remaining two options. Recalling that widened pulse pressure is the difference in blood pressures eliminates options 3 and 4. Review symptoms that suggest increased intracranial pressure if you had difficulty with this question.*
> **Cognitive Level**—*Analyzing*
> **Client Needs Category**—*Physiological integrity*
> **Client Needs Subcategory**—*Physiological adaptation*

66. 3. Suctioning is required whenever a client cannot clear his or her own airway. An unconscious client should be positioned on the side rather than supine. Removing pillows is inconsequential to maintaining a clear airway. Oral hygiene is an appropriate nursing measure for meeting the client's basic needs, but it does not clear the airway.

> **Test Taking Strategy**—*Use the process of elimination to identify the most appropriate measure for managing the etiology of the nursing diagnosis. Consider the nursing intervention that specifically helps to maintain a clear airway, which is option 3. Option 1 is incorrect because a side-lying position helps to prevent aspiration of secretions. Options 2 and 4 are not useful in keeping the airway clear. Review nursing measures for preventing aspiration experienced by a client who has neuromuscular deficits if you had difficulty answering this question.*
> **Cognitive Level**—*Applying*
> **Client Needs Category**—*Physiological integrity*
> **Client Needs Subcategory**—*Reduction of risk potential*

67. 1, 3, 4, 5, 6. Assessment of a client's fall risk is a National Patient Safety Goal set by The Joint Commission and should be completed on admission, periodically during the hospitalization according to hospital policy, and when the client's status changes. Men are more likely to take risks or not ask for help, which makes them more at risk for falls. Clients who are confused become disorganized, are less likely to follow or remember instructions, have poor judgment, and are more likely to forget their limitations. Vertigo or dizziness makes clients unsteady on their feet, which also poses a risk for falls. Clients with sensory deficits such as hearing loss or visual impairment are more at risk for falls related to environmental hazards. Altered elimination, such as incontinence, urinary or bowel frequency, nocturia, or needing assistance to go to the toilet, also are risk factors that frequently cause falls. Taking antibiotics is not considered a risk factor for falls.

> **Test Taking Strategy**—*Analyze to determine what information the question asks for, which is risk factors for falls. Alternative-format "select all that apply" questions require considering each option independently to decide its merit in answering the question. Most accredited agencies have developed a focus assessment form listing various risk factors for falls with a numerical score. Familiarity with a focus assessment for falls enhances the selection of risk factors. Review techniques for fall risk assessment if you had difficulty with this question.*
> **Cognitive Level**—*Analyzing*
> **Client Needs Category**—*Physiological integrity*
> **Client Needs Subcategory**—*Reduction of risk potential*

68. 2, 3, 4, 5, 6. Medications that cause drowsiness or sleep or lower blood pressure place the client at higher risk for falls. Benzodiazepines are antianxiety drugs, such as alprazolam (Xanax), chlordiazepoxide (Librium), diazepam (Valium), and lorazepam (Ativan), which cause a tranquilizing effect. Sedatives and hypnotics also produce drowsiness and sleep. Some common examples of sedatives and hypnotics include flurazepam (Dalmane), triazolam (Halcion), zolpidem tartrate (Ambien), and secobarbital sodium (Seconal). Opiate narcotics such as morphine, fentanyl, codeine, and meperidine (Demerol) also cause drowsiness and sleep and affect judgment. Anticonvulsants containing barbiturates such as phenobarbital cause central nervous system (CNS) depression, resulting in sedation and dizziness. Antihypertensives, on the other hand, can cause orthostatic hypotension on rising, resulting in dizziness, vertigo, and unsteady gait. These drugs also put the client at risk for falls. Use of antihyperlipidemics does not pose a fall risk for the client.

> **Test Taking Strategy**—*Analyze to determine what information the question asks for, which is medications that increase risk for falls. Alternative-format "select all that apply" questions require considering each option independently to decide its merit in answering the question. Look at each classification*

and evaluate the drug's impact on a client who is at risk for falls. Consider any classification that affects balance, judgment, orientation, or blood pressure status. Review the categories of medications in the options to determine those that pose a risk for falls if you had difficulty answering this question.
Cognitive Level—*Analyzing*
Client Needs Category—*Physiological integrity*
Client Needs Subcategory—*Pharmacological therapies*

69. **1, 2, 4, 5.** Preventing a client from falling is of utmost importance. Instructing the client to ask for help before getting up, turning on the bed alarm, advising the client's family to inform staff when they are leaving the room, and placing the bed in its lowest position are all appropriate nursing activities to prevent falls. Applying restraints to prevent a client from falling should be used as a last resort when all other alternative interventions have been attempted. Obtaining an order for a physical therapy consult may help with strengthening the lower extremities and providing stamina, but this would be a long-term goal and not one that would prevent falls initially.
Test Taking Strategy—*Analyze to determine what information the question asks for, which is preventing a fall assessment. Alternative-format "select all that apply" questions require considering each option independently to decide its merit in answering the question. When considering a risk for falls, think safety. Associate all of the information about the client with each option and determine if this option would help maintain client safety. Applying restraints (option 3) is not appropriate in this situation because it violates the Omnibus Reconciliation Act (OBRA). Review fall precautions if you had difficulty answering this question.*
Cognitive Level—*Applying*
Client Needs Category—*Physiological integrity*
Client Needs Subcategory—*Reduction of risk potential*

70. **4.** A client with hemiplegia is best assisted from bed to a wheelchair by bracing the disabled foot and knee. The client with hemiplegia is unable to use a walker unless there is some residual strength in the paralyzed arm. The wheelchair is placed parallel to the bed. The nurse stands in front of the client to facilitate bracing and balancing.
Test Taking Strategy—*Use the process of elimination to identify the option that describes a principle that applies to proper transfer skills for a hemiplegic client. Begin by thinking of the physical weakness and how that impacts the client's ability to transfer. Eliminate any option in which use of the affected side would be required or the client's safety would be jeopardized. Considering the weakened side and the additional support needed to transfer leads to selecting option 4 as the correct answer. Review*

positioning and transfer skills if you had difficulty with this question.
Cognitive Level—*Applying*
Client Needs Category—*Physiological integrity*
Client Needs Subcategory—*Basic care and comfort*

71. **1, 3, 5.** Passive range-of-motion (ROM) exercises are performed on a routine basis (usually three times per day) to prevent paralyzed extremities from forming contractures. Passive ROM exercises should be performed on all of the joints that the client does not move actively; each joint exercise should be performed three times each. It is not necessary for the client's spouse to take the pulse, but the spouse should be instructed to watch for signs of pain, color changes, and respiratory distress. The client's spouse should also be instructed to watch for signs of fatigue and to allow rest periods between exercises to promote optimal joint functioning. Passive ROM exercises should be conducted slowly in a systematic sequence, starting at the head and working downward toward the lower extremities.
Test Taking Strategy—*Analyze to determine what information the question asks for, which is accurate performance of ROM exercises. Alternative-format "select all that apply" questions require considering each option independently to decide its merit in answering the question. Select all the options that are accurate statements regarding ROM exercises. Eliminate any choices that are inaccurate or of no importance, such as options 2, 4, and 6. Review how to perform ROM exercises if you had difficulty answering this question.*
Cognitive Level—*Applying*
Client Needs Category—*Physiological integrity*
Client Needs Subcategory—*Basic care and comfort*

72. **2.** To ensure the maximum potential use of the feet, they are maintained in a functional position, which correlates with a person's position when standing. When standing, the soles of the feet are flat against the supporting surface. Therefore, the soles of the client's feet should be parallel to the footboard when in bed. The legs should be straight (knees not bent) and the ankles not extended more than 90 degrees.
Test Taking Strategy—*Use the process of elimination to select the option that accurately describes use of the footboard. Because the footboard is used to maintain dorsiflexion of the foot, the best option for accomplishing that goal is option 2. Eliminate options 3 and 4 because they do not apply to positioning of the feet. Option 1 is not an achievable anatomic position. Review the purpose and method for using a footboard if you had difficulty answering this question.*
Cognitive Level—*Applying*
Client Needs Category—*Physiological integrity*
Client Needs Subcategory—*Reduction of risk potential*

73. 2. Expressive aphasia means that the client can understand what is said but cannot respond using spoken language. An appropriate alternative is to use some nonverbal method by which the client can communicate, such as pointing to a written or printed list of key words. Encouraging the client to practice key words is likely to cause frustration because the loss of language is not from a lack of effort or practice. Despite the client's inability to respond verbally, it is still appropriate for the nurse to speak to the client, but it should be done in a normal tone of voice, allowing the client ample time to complete thoughts. Completing the client's sentences serves no therapeutic benefit.

> *Test Taking Strategy—Use the process of elimination to identify the option that is "best for communicating" with the client's type of aphasia. The key concept is that the client can understand but cannot verbally respond. Option 2 is the only option that allows the client to communicate his or her thoughts by means of printed words. Review the difference between expressive and receptive aphasia if you had difficulty answering this question.*
> **Cognitive Level**—*Applying*
> **Client Needs Category**—*Psychosocial integrity*
> **Client Needs Subcategory**—*None*

74. 2. The long-term outcomes after a stroke are often determined by aggressive nursing efforts to maintain musculoskeletal function. Rehabilitation begins on admission with functional positioning, active and passive exercises, and early physical and occupational therapies. Managing bowel and bladder elimination does not have the same impact as preventing the development of musculoskeletal deformities. Helping the client cope with altered body image, depression, and grieving from loss of health and independence are appropriate nursing responsibilities; however, even if those concerns are positively resolved, the client's rehabilitation would be delayed if contractures and joint immobility develop.

> *Test Taking Strategy—Use the process of elimination to choose the option that relates to the "most important" goal for rehabilitation after a stroke. Although more than one option may be a component of rehabilitation, use Maslow's hierarchy of needs to select the single most important measure from among the options. Dealing with an altered body image and relieving depression relate to needs for self-esteem and self-actualization. Regulating bowel and bladder elimination relates to a physiologic need, but it is not as likely to affect rehabilitation as much as the development of contractures and joint deformities. Option 2 emerges as the most important goal of rehabilitation. Review the care of a client experiencing a stroke and Maslow's hierarchy of needs if you had difficulty answering this question.*

Cognitive Level—*Analyzing*
Client Needs Category—*Physiological integrity*
Client Needs Subcategory—*Reduction of risk potential*

75. 2. After a stroke, emotional fluctuations, also called lability, which can consist of inappropriate laughing or crying, are a common manifestation. Crying is the most common symptom. Family members need to be advised that this frequently occurs from the effects of the stroke. This manifestation is not a ploy to regain control of the client's life nor does it occur from the destructive effects in the brain. Emotional fluctuations do not occur in all stroke clients and do not always relate to having a major event in one's life.

> *Test Taking Strategies—Use the process of elimination to identify the best nursing response. The best response is to accurately answer the question when possible. Options 1 and 4 offer vague and unfounded answers. Option 3 can be eliminated as inaccurate because the emotional center of the brain may be damaged but not destroyed. Review therapeutic and nontherapeutic communication techniques if you had difficulty answering this question.*
> **Cognitive Level**—*Applying*
> **Client Needs Category**—*Psychosocial integrity*
> **Client Needs Subcategory**—*None*

76. 1, 4, 5, 6. One of the National Patient Safety Goals set by the Joint Commission states that clients who are being discharged on anticoagulants must have discharge teaching. Warfarin (Coumadin) is an orally administered anticoagulant that reduces the clotting time by causing a deficiency of prothrombin. It is used in stroke clients to reduce the risk of clot formation that could lead to further strokes. Discharge instructions should cover the following: dietary restrictions (foods high in vitamin K, including avocado, green leafy vegetables, and broccoli, can reverse or reduce drug effects); missed doses (the client should not double the dose if missed, but should call the physician); and bruising or blood in the urine (if the client experiences signs of bleeding, the physician should be notified immediately). In addition, the client and spouse should be aware of the need to follow physician orders to have frequent International Normalized Ratio (INR) levels determined until therapeutic levels can be obtained and periodically thereafter. There are no restrictions associated with warfarin use regarding the avoidance of heavy lifting or staying out of the sun.

> *Test Taking Strategy—Analyze to determine what information the question asks for, which is correct client teaching topics for a client receiving warfarin (Coumadin). Alternative-format "select all that apply" questions require considering each option independently to decide its merit in answering the question. Recall the information that clients taking warfarin (Coumadin), an anticoagulant, should be taught. Topics include evidence of unusual bleeding, food and drug interactions, the need for laboratory tests*

on a regular basis, and actions to take if one or more doses are missed. Review anticoagulant therapy with warfarin (Coumadin) if you had difficulty with this question.
Cognitive Level—*Applying*
Client Needs Category—*Physiological integrity*
Client Needs Subcategory—*Pharmacological therapies*

77. 3. Hemianopia is a visual field defect in which the client is unable to see the left or right half of an image. It is the result of the stroke affecting the client's visual pathway. In short, it is blindness in one-half of the visual field and may be temporary or permanent. To accommodate the client's residual peripheral vision, it is best to approach the client from the unaffected side. Placing food in a pattern resembling a clock will serve no therapeutic benefit, because the client will not be able to see half of the plate. The interventions listed in the other options have no therapeutic value when caring for a client with hemianopia.
Test Taking Strategy—*Analyze to determine what information the question asks for, which involves knowledge of hemianopia. Breaking down the word hemi- (related to half) and -opia (related to the eye) can be helpful in determining the definition. Options 1 and 2 may be eliminated as not helpful interventions for assisting with visual field deficits. Option 4 does not assist in minimizing the visual field deficit. Review the condition known as hemianopia and its implications for nursing care if you had difficulty answering this question.*
Cognitive Level—*Applying*
Client Needs Category—*Safe and effective care environment*
Client Needs Subcategory—*Safety and infection control*

78. 1. Coughing increases intracranial pressure and thereby increases the potential for cerebral bleeding. The other identified problems require the nurse's attention, but reducing or eliminating coughing should be the highest priority.
Test Taking Strategy—*Use the process of elimination to select the option that is "most important to address" when assessing the disease process. Consider the consequences that may occur in relation to a leaking aneurysm to select the best answer. Options 2, 3, and 4 can be readily eliminated because they are not likely to affect a leaking aneurysm. Option 1 emerges as the symptom of highest priority. Review the nursing care of a leaking aneurysm if you had difficulty with this question.*
Cognitive Level—*Analyzing*
Client Needs Category—*Physiological integrity*
Client Needs Subcategory—*Reduction of risk potential*

79.

| 6. Level of consciousness (LOC) |
| 2. Motor strength |
| 3. Vital signs |
| 5. Urine output |
| 1. Bowel elimination |
| 4. Skin integrity |

The first assessment that the nurse should make is to evaluate the client's LOC. This is the best indicator of brain function; any deterioration in the client's condition would alter LOC. Motor strength, the second assessment performed, is an indication of the brain's ability to control voluntary actions. Any changes in the ability to follow commands might signify deterioration. Vital signs are measured next (they should be measured frequently in a client with a cerebral aneurysm). Signs of a leaking aneurysm include increased pulse rate, respiratory changes, and elevated blood pressure. Urine output, bowel elimination, and skin integrity are assessed last. Decreased urine output may signal decreased kidney perfusion. Bowel movements are assessed regularly to ensure that the client is not straining to defecate. Skin integrity must be assessed for evidence of breakdown caused by the client's limited activity.
Test Taking Strategy—*Analyze to determine what information the question asks for, which involves sequencing assessments from most important to those of less importance for a client with a cerebral aneurysm. Begin with the assessments that will indicate a change of neurologic status or bleeding from the cerebral aneurysm. This ensures the safety of the client. Once you have identified neurologic assessments, consider what other general physical assessments are important to the client's status. Review assessments that are pertinent to a client with a cerebral aneurysm if you had difficulty answering this question.*
Cognitive Level—*Analyzing*
Client Needs Category—*Physiological integrity*
Client Needs Subcategory—*Physiological adaptation*

80. 4. Using nondrug interventions such as guided imagery in combination with an analgesic increases the drug's therapeutic effect. Most oral analgesics are administered at 3- or 4-hour intervals; giving another dose sooner or rearranging the medication times would be contraindicated. The goal of pain management is to relieve the symptoms of pain, thereby making the client more comfortable. Opioid analgesics are generally avoided in most neurologic conditions because they can alter the client's pupillary response, level of consciousness, bowel elimination pattern, and breathing. Mild nonopioid analgesics can be safely used to treat pain experienced by neurologic clients.

Test Taking Strategy—Use the process of elimination to identify the option describing the "most appropriate" nursing action that addresses the client's statement of unrelieved pain. Eliminate options 1 and 2 as not being in the nurse's scope of practice (administering medications earlier than prescribed and rearranging medication times) and in need of a physician's order. Before consulting the physician (option 3), the most appropriate action is to use a nondrug intervention. Review pain management techniques if you had difficulty answering this question.
Cognitive Level—Applying
Client Needs Category—Physiological integrity
Client Needs Subcategory—Basic care and comfort

Nursing Care of Clients with Tumors of the Neurologic System

81. 1, 5, 6. A positron emission tomography (PET) scan uses computed cross-sectional images of an organ to provide facts about benign and malignant cell activity. It is used primarily for lung, colon, liver, pancreatic, and brain tumors. The client should be instructed to eliminate caffeine, alcohol, tobacco, tranquilizers, and sedatives for 24 hours before a PET scan. Diuretics, shellfish, and shampoos do not affect PET results.

Test Taking Strategy—Analyze to determine what information the question asks for, which is substances that can interfere with a PET scan. Alternative-format "select all that apply" questions require considering each option independently to decide its merit in answering the question. An understanding of the protocol before a PET scan is important to successfully answering the question. Review substances such as central nervous system stimulants or depressants that should be avoided because they may affect the results of the test if you had difficulty answering this question.
Cognitive Level—Understanding
Client Needs Category—Physiological integrity
Client Needs Subcategory—Reduction of risk potential

82. 2. Consuming extra fluids helps excrete the radioisotope used during the examination. There is no specific reason to recommend taking a sedative, avoiding excessive sitting, or reporting signs of a fever.

Test Taking Strategy—Use the process of elimination to select the discharge instruction that is most appropriate in relation to the positron emission tomography (PET) scan procedure. A PET scan produces few adverse effects unless the radioisotope is not fully excreted. Eliminate option 1, which suggests that the client may have postprocedure restlessness or pain; option 3, which suggests that the client may have musculoskeletal or spinal effects; and option 4, which suggests that the client may have a break in skin or an infection. Review appropriate instructions to give after a PET scan if you had difficulty answering this question.
Cognitive Level—Applying
Client Needs Category—Physiological integrity
Client Needs Subcategory—Physiological adaptation

83. 1. The nurse must frequently monitor the neurologic status of a client who has had a craniotomy. One of the most important assessments involves checking the client's extremities for movement and motor strength (not for pulses). Any decrease in strength or ability to move usually indicates that the intracranial pressure is increasing. Although the other assessments are appropriate to note, they are not as significant to the client's critical condition.

Test Taking Strategy—Use the process of elimination to identify the option that describes a "preoperative assessment" and "postoperative comparison" indicating neurologic deficits after a craniotomy. Neurologic checks, including tests for motor strength (option 1), are always vital to assess the postoperative status. Review neurologic assessments performed postsurgically if you had difficulty answering this question.
Cognitive Level—Applying
Client Needs Category—Physiological integrity
Client Needs Subcategory—Physiological adaptation

84. 3. When catheterizing an adult male, the catheter is usually inserted at a distance of 6″ to 8″ (15 to 20 cm) or until urine begins to flow. A catheter that is inserted less than 6″ or inflated before urine flows might not be properly located in the bladder. Urethral damage may occur if the tip of the catheter and the bulb are not fully within the bladder.

Test Taking Strategy—Analyze to determine what information the question asks for, which is a principle that relates to catheterization of a male or a standard of care. Knowledge of male urologic anatomy is essential to successfully answering the question. Refer to the procedure for inserting a urinary catheter in a male client if you had difficulty with this question.
Cognitive Level—Understanding
Client Needs Category—Physiological integrity
Client Needs Subcategory—Physiological adaptation

85. 4. To preserve the client's dignity and to reduce the potential for infection, the hair of someone undergoing a craniotomy is usually clipped after the client has been transferred from the nursing unit to the surgical department. Clipping hair the night before facilitates colonization of microorganisms within the skin abrasions. If skin preparation is done on the nursing unit, it is best done before administering sedation. The hair is clipped before a shower so loose hair can be rinsed away.

> *Test Taking Strategy—Use the process of elimination to identify the best time for removing a client's hair before cranial surgery. Recall that the current practice is to remove hair just before beginning any surgical procedure. Consider all of the physical and psychological implications that contradict shaving hair from the scalp, which leaves option 4 as the best answer. Review preoperative care, especially as it relates to cranial surgery, if you had difficulty answering this question.*
> *Cognitive Level—Applying*
> *Client Needs Category—Physiological integrity*
> *Client Needs Subcategory—Reduction of risk potential*

86. 3. Clipping the hair as a routine skin preparation rather than shaving an area is performed primarily because of the risk of microscopic cuts and abrasions that can occur with shaving. These microscopic cuts and abrasions may pose a risk for infection if bacteria were to colonize them.

> *Test Taking Strategy—Use the process of elimination to identify the option that describes the best rationale for clipping scalp hair versus shaving the head. Option 1 can be eliminated because it does not offer a response that reflects evidence-based practice. Option 4 can be eliminated because superficial bleeding would not justify the cancellation of surgery. Option 2 is somewhat accurate, but it is vague and not likely to have as much merit as option 3. Review the standards of practice for preoperative skin preparation if you had difficulty answering this question.*
> *Cognitive Level—Applying*
> *Client Needs Subcategory—Safe and effective care environment*
> *Client Needs Subcategory—Safety and infection control*

87. 2. To reduce the potential for a wound infection, it is best to reinforce a moist dressing. Usually, the surgeon performs the first dressing change unless otherwise specified in the medical orders. The condition of the dressing and the action taken are important information to document. Removing or changing the dressing would be inappropriate.

> *Test Taking Strategy—Use the process of elimination to select an option that is most appropriate for the nurse to perform "first" after an "immediate postoperative assessment" finding of a moist dressing. The question asks for a priority action. At this time, options 1 and 3 can be eliminated because generally the surgeon initially changes the dressing. If the nurse assesses a moist dressing, the dressing must*

> *be reinforced to prevent wicking pathogens in the direction of the incision. Reinforcing the dressing is a greater priority than documenting the findings at this time. Review the principles that apply to the management of a dressing covering an open wound if you had difficulty answering this question.*
> *Cognitive Level—Applying*
> *Client Needs Category—Physiological integrity*
> *Client Needs Subcategory—Reduction of risk potential*

88. 4. Reorientation is appropriate during periods of confusion. It may be necessary to repeat information several times. Explaining the nature of the confusion to the client or withholding communication would be inappropriate. Reading to the client may help to raise the level of consciousness, but would not necessarily correct confusion.

> *Test Taking Strategy—Use the process of elimination to help in selecting the "best" intervention when interacting with a confused client. Considering that the goal of the intervention is reorientation, select the option that would be most effective for accomplishing that goal. Eliminate options 1, 2, and 3 because they do not promote achieving the goal. Option 4 "best" accomplishes the goal. Review techniques for reorientation if you had difficulty answering this question.*
> *Cognitive Level—Applying*
> *Client Needs Category—Psychosocial integrity*
> *Client Needs Subcategory—None*

89. 4. Clear liquids are given postoperatively to keep the mouth moist and to stimulate peristalsis of the GI system. However, before the client receives any oral fluids, it is essential that the nurse assess the client's ability to swallow. Clients undergoing neurologic surgery may have residual muscular weakness, which creates the potential for aspiration. It is an expectation that bowel sounds will return to all four quadrants postoperatively, but may not be totally functional by the time clear liquids are started. Ice chips are usually given before other types of clear liquids; the nurse should assess whether the client has any nausea or vomiting before starting broth, juice, or gelatin rather than obtaining information about food preferences. The ability to raise the head to drink is not as important to assess as the ability to swallow.

> *Test Taking Strategy—Use the process of elimination to select an option that ensures safety for the client. Preventing aspiration is a life-threatening consequence of providing oral fluids before a client can protect his or her own airway when swallowing. Therefore, assessing the client's ability to swallow is a priority. Eliminate options 1 and 2 as lower priorities. Both options 3 and 4 are important; however, the client must be able to swallow or risk aspiration. Review techniques for preventing aspiration in a client with dysphagia if you had difficulty answering this question.*
> *Cognitive Level—Applying*
> *Client Needs Category—Physiological integrity*
> *Client Needs Subcategory—Reduction of risk potential*

90. 4. Beneficence expresses acts of mercy, kindness, and charity. Although all of the options provide aspects of good nursing care. The best representation of beneficence is advocating for the wishes of the client.

Test Taking Strategy—Use the process of elimination to identify the best answer comparing nursing actions to the definition of beneficence. Recall that beneficence is the moral principle and ethical standard of the act of kindness. Select the best nursing action demonstrating those actions, which, most often, are actions between a nurse and client. Review the ethical principle of beneficence and actions related if you had difficulty answering this question.
Cognitive Level—*Analyzing*
Client Needs Category—*Safe and effective care environment*
Client Needs Subcategory—*Coordinated care*

Nursing Care of Clients with Nerve Disorders

91. 4. Cranial nerve XI is the spinal accessory nerve, which innervates the sternocleidomastoid and trapezius muscles. If the client can shrug his or her shoulders, the nurse understands that the client has an intact spinal accessory nerve. Wrinkling of the forehead and puffing out the cheeks tests cranial nerve VII function. Sticking out the tongue tests cranial nerve XII function.

Test Taking Strategy—Analyze to determine what information the question asks for, which is the cranial nerve XI assessment technique that best represents normal function. Knowledge of the cranial nerves and their functions is essential in answering the question. Cranial nerves come directly from the brain. Recall that there are 12 pairs of cranial nerves that begin with cranial nerve I (olfactory) innervating the nose (sense of smell) and cranial nerve II (optic) innervating the eyes (vision), and so on. Shrugging the shoulders is a function controlled by cranial nerve XI, the spinal accessory nerve. Review the functions of the cranial nerves, especially cranial nerve XI, if you had difficulty with this question.
Cognitive Level—*Applying*
Client Needs Category—*Physiological integrity*
Client Needs Subcategory—*Physiological adaptation*

92. 2. Trigeminal neuralgia is a painful condition involving cranial nerve V, the trigeminal nerve. The cause of this condition is unknown, but it produces problems with chewing, facial movement, and sensation. The client may describe the pain as sudden, severe, and burning. The pain, which comes and goes quickly, may occur several times per day. The client's care plan, therefore, must include measures to prevent any stimulation to trigger points that could provoke pain along the ophthalmic, mandibular, and maxillary branches of

the trigeminal nerve. Therefore, all contact with the face—including heat, cold, and drafts—should be avoided.

Test Taking Strategy—Use the process of elimination to identify the best intervention for preventing paroxysmal pain secondary to trigeminal neuralgia. The trigeminal nerve affects muscular and sensory activities involving the jaw, cheeks, and corneas. The term neuralgia describes pain that travels along the course of a nerve. Directing a fan toward the face or applying facial compresses, as identified in options 1 and 4, would produce pain in this client. Providing ice chips (option 3) may or may not affect the client's sensation of pain. Avoiding physical stimulation of the nerve (option 2) emerges as the most appropriate intervention for preventing pain when planning this client's care. Review trigeminal neuralgia and methods for preventing pain if you had difficulty answering this question.
Cognitive Level—*Applying*
Client Needs Category—*Physiological integrity*
Client Needs Subcategory—*Physiological adaptation*

93. 1. Because the liver produces prothrombin, a substance important to clot formation, signs of unusual bleeding in a client taking carbamazepine (Tegretol) indicate adverse effects to the liver. This drug also causes hematologic changes that may be evidenced as abnormal bleeding. Clay-colored stools and dark brown urine, not black stools or cloudy urine, are associated with liver disturbances. Mottled skin is not a sign of liver impairment.

Test Taking Strategy—Analyze to determine what information the question asks for, which is important information to provide a client who will be taking a drug that affects liver function. Recall that the physiologic functions of the liver include the production of prothrombin, a substance that promotes clotting. Liver dysfunction can contribute to bleeding, as identified in option 1, the only option that relates to the function of the liver. Review the functions of the liver and methods for detecting its dysfunction if you had difficulty answering this question.
Cognitive Level—*Applying*
Client Needs Category—*Health promotion and maintenance*
Client Needs Subcategory—*None*

94. 3. Directing the flow of the eye irrigant across the conjunctiva from the nasal to the temporal corners of the eye helps keep the solution from dripping down the client's nose. It also keeps debris from entering the nasolacrimal duct.

Test Taking Strategy—Use the process of elimination to select the option that best describes the technique for performing an eye irrigation. Recall that the correct procedure for eye irrigation avoids instilling fluid into the nasolacrimal ducts that originate in the lacrimal punta (opening) in the inner canthus of each eye. Therefore, option 3 describes the correct

procedure. Review eye irrigation technique if you had problems with this question.
Cognitive Level—*Understanding*
Client Needs Category—*Physiological integrity*
Client Needs Subcategory—*Pharmacological therapies*

95. 4. There are 12 cranial nerves, the seventh of which is the facial nerve. The cause of Bell's palsy is unknown, but inflammation occurs around the facial nerve, resulting in sudden paralysis of the skeletal muscles about the face. The paralysis is usually unilateral and affects the muscles of the eyelids and face, making speaking, chewing, and blinking difficult.

> **Test Taking Strategy**—*Use the process of elimination to identify the assessment finding most indicative of Bell's palsy. Recall the function of cranial nerve VII to determine the "most indicative" finding. Consider that the seventh of the 12 cranial nerves has motor and sensory functions in the facial area. With that knowledge, eliminate options 2 and 3. Because there is paralysis in the disease process, the most appropriate option is 4. Review the function of the cranial nerves and assessment findings associated with their dysfunction, focusing in particular on cranial nerve VII, if you had difficulty answering this question.*

Cognitive Level—*Applying*
Client Needs Category—*Physiological integrity*
Client Needs Subcategory—*Physiological adaptation*

96. 3. Bell's palsy involves impairment of cranial nerve VII, which affects the face, speaking, and chewing. Food may become trapped in the buccal pouch of a client with Bell's palsy. Therefore, the nurse should inspect this area after each meal, assess for mechanical trauma, and remove any oral debris. Controlling light has no therapeutic value. Bell's palsy affects the nerves of the face and does not affect motor involvement of the lower extremities. Therefore, instructing the client how to walk with a cane is unwarranted.

> **Test Taking Strategy**—*Use the process of elimination to select the option that identifies the most appropriate intervention for a client with a disorder involving cranial nerve VII. Focus on the consequences of facial motor dysfunction. Because this is the facial nerve, eliminate option 4. Eliminate option 1 because there is no structural visual impairment. Drinking from a straw is not indicated for a client with Bell's palsy. Option 3 is best because it directly relates to impairment of the nerve. Review the function of cranial nerve VII and managing the effects of its dysfunction if you had difficulty answering this question.*

Cognitive Level—*Applying*
Client Needs Category—*Physiological integrity*
Client Needs Subcategory—*Physiological adaptation*

97.

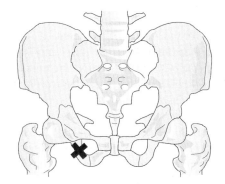

The correct placement of the X is the right ischium or near the right hipbone. Starting at lumbar segment 3 in the lower back, the sciatic nerve is the largest in the body. Pressure on the sciatic nerve from a herniated disk is typically the cause of sciatica. The client may experience pain, burning, tingling, or numbness in the leg or buttocks, often accompanied by a shooting pain that makes it hard for the client to stand up.

> **Test Taking Strategy**—*Analyze to determine what information the question asks for, which is the location of the sciatic nerve. Knowledge of the distribution of the sciatic nerve is essential to answering this question. Use knowledge of anatomy and physiology to determine the placement of the sciatic nerve. Use the symptoms of discomfort to suggest placement of the X.*

Cognitive Level—*Understanding*
Client Needs Category—*Physiological integrity*
Client Needs Subcategory—*Physiological adaptation*

98. 1. To allow room for instilling dye or air within the vertebral column, approximately 15 mL of spinal fluid is withdrawn via a lumbar puncture. The client is instructed to lie prone on the examination table. The table, however, is tilted to promote movement of the dye. Local anesthesia is used at the site of the lumbar puncture, but no other forms of anesthesia are commonly given.

> **Test Taking Strategy**—*Use the process of elimination to identify the statement that describes the "most accurate" information about a myelogram, a diagnostic test used to determine pathology within the spinal canal. Options 2, 3, and 4 are incorrect. The most accurate statement is option 1, which indicates that a myelogram involves injecting dye into the spinal column. Review the manner in which a myelogram is performed if you had difficulty answering this question.*

Cognitive Level—*Understanding*
Client Needs Category—*Physiological integrity*
Client Needs Subcategory—*Reduction of risk potential*

99. **2.** Bending the knees while keeping the back straight is an excellent technique for good body mechanics. The back is often strained by lifting objects with the waist bent. Heavy objects are carried close to the center of gravity. Clients should be placed on a firm mattress rather than a soft one.

> *Test Taking Strategy—Use the process of elimination to identify the option that best describes teaching that is appropriate for a client with low back pain. Recall that a herniated intervertebral disk is commonly caused by poor body mechanics. Apply knowledge of proper body mechanics—bending from the knees to lift, carrying heavy objects close to the center of gravity, and spreading the feet to distribute weight being borne by the spine—which will lead to selecting option 2. Review the principles of good body mechanics if you had difficulty answering this question.*

> **Cognitive Level**—*Applying*
> **Client Needs Category**—*Health promotion and maintenance*
> **Client Needs Subcategory**—*None*

100. **2.** Until healing takes place, logrolling is used to turn clients after spinal surgery. Logrolling involves moving the client's shoulders and hips as a unit to avoid twisting the spine.

> *Test Taking Strategy—Use the process of elimination to select the best technique for changing the position of a client who has undergone a spinal fusion. Recall that after a client has spinal surgery, there is an area of temporary weakness. Select the option that is most likely to stabilize the surgical area. Because the surgical area is the spine, logrolling (option 2) is the best choice. Review logrolling and its purpose if you had difficulty answering this question.*

> **Cognitive Level**—*Applying*
> **Client Needs Category**—*Physiological integrity*
> **Client Needs Subcategory**—*Reduction of risk potential*

101. **1, 3, 5, 6.** A diskectomy with spinal fusion involves the removal of the herniated disk followed by grafting a piece of bone onto the vertebrae. Clients should be instructed to avoid twisting or jerking the back, sit in a chair with a straight back, avoid sitting for prolonged periods, and avoid picking items up from the floor. If bending is necessary, the client should bend from the knees and hips, not the waist. Furthermore, clients should be instructed to monitor urine output for the first week and report color, temperature, and mobility changes of the lower extremities to the physician because surgery may have resulted in edema or hemorrhage at the operative site.

> *Test Taking Strategy—Analyze to determine what information the question asks for, which is discharge instructions for the client after diskectomy. Alternative-format "select all that apply" questions require considering each option independently to decide its merit in answering the question. Focus on the nature and placement of the surgery to independently select each option that would be included in the instructions. Determine if the instruction would have a direct correlation to the surgery. Review discharge instructions for a client who has undergone a diskectomy and spinal fusion if you had difficulty answering this question.*

> **Cognitive Level**—*Applying*
> **Client Needs Category**—*Physiological integrity*
> **Client Needs Subcategory**—*Reduction of risk potential*

102. **3, 4, 5.** The nurse would note the following findings in a client who is brain dead: nonreactive dilated pupils and nonreactive or absent corneal and gag reflexes. The client may still have spinal reflexes, such as deep tendon and Babinski reflexes, in brain death. Decerebrate or decorticate posturing would not be seen. Signs of dehydration, such as poor skin turgor and dry mucous membranes, would not be present unless the client was dehydrated from a previous disease process.

> *Test Taking Strategy—Analyze to determine what information the question asks for, which is assessment findings in brain death. Alternative-format "select all that apply" questions require considering each option independently to decide its merit in answering the question. Analyze the options, looking for assessment findings that are consistent with a client who has been pronounced brain dead. Focus on the neurologic status as the signs that would be present. Eliminate options 1 and 6 as not associated with the neurologic status. Eliminate option 2 because decerebrate posturing is associated with signs of brain injury. Review assessment findings in brain death if you had difficulty answering this question.*

> **Cognitive Level**—*Analyzing*
> **Client Needs Category**—*Physiological integrity*
> **Client Needs Subcategory**—*Physiological adaptation*

103. **2.** Placing a rolled towel under the client's chin allows the mouth to form a more natural appearance. This look is more aesthetically pleasing for family viewing the face of the deceased. Placing the arms at the side is a natural position. Bathing the client diminishes odors. While tubes are removed from the body, dressing may remain intact to absorb drainage from wound sites.

> *Test Taking Strategy—Analyze to determine what the question asks for, which is action by the nurse that makes the client more aesthetically pleasing for the family. Consider each option as promoting the most peaceful appearance. Review postmortem care if you had difficulty answering this question.*

> **Cognitive Level**—*Applying*
> **Client Needs Category**—*Physiological integrity*
> **Client Needs Subcategory**—*Basic care and comfort*

TEST

3

The Nursing Care of Clients with Disorders of Sensory Organs and the Integument

- Nursing Care of Clients with Eye Disorders
- Nursing Care of Clients with Disorders of Accessory Eye Structures
- Nursing Care of Clients with Ear Disorders
- Nursing Care of Clients with Nasal Disorders
- Nursing Care of Clients with Disorders of the Skin and Related Structures
- Correct Answers, Rationales, and Test Taking Strategies

Directions: With a pencil, blacken the space in front of the option you have chosen for your correct answer.

Nursing Care of Clients with Eye Disorders

A high-school chemistry student is sent to the school nurse after being splashed in the eyes with a chemical.

1. Which information is most important for the school nurse to obtain from the client initially?
[ ] **1.** Whether safety glasses were worn
[ ] **2.** The name of the splashed chemical
[ ] **3.** The treatment already provided
[ ] **4.** Whether the client's vision is impaired

The school nurse prepares to irrigate the student's irritated eye.

2. Assuming the following solutions are available, which one is best for the school nurse to use at this time?
[ ] **1.** Tap water
[ ] **2.** Sodium bicarbonate
[ ] **3.** Normal saline
[ ] **4.** Magnesium sulfate

3. The nurse is preparing to irrigate the student's eye. What steps are appropriate in completing the irrigation? Select all that apply.
[ ] **1.** Place the solution directly into the center of the eye.
[ ] **2.** Tilt the head toward the opposite eye.
[ ] **3.** Perform hand hygiene and put on gloves.
[ ] **4.** Offer the client a paper tissue.
[ ] **5.** Place the solution into the conjunctival sac.
[ ] **6.** Continue eye irrigations until all redness is resolved.

4. When irrigating the client's eyes, which technique describes the best way to direct the flow of irrigating solution?
[ ] **1.** Directly onto the corneal surface
[ ] **2.** Away from the inner canthus
[ ] **3.** Within the anterior chamber
[ ] **4.** Toward the nasolacrimal duct

5. After the student has been treated, which one of the following professionals is best for providing follow-up care?
[ ] **1.** An optician
[ ] **2.** An ophthalmologist
[ ] **3.** An optometrist
[ ] **4.** An orthoptist

6. When a foreign body becomes embedded in a client's eye, which nursing action should be taken first before referring the client for emergency treatment?
[ ] **1.** Remove the object with forceps.
[ ] **2.** Ask the person to blink rapidly.
[ ] **3.** Instill antibiotic ointment.
[ ] **4.** Loosely patch both eyes.

Before the physician performs an examination on the client, the nurse uses a Snellen chart to assess the client's visual acuity.

7. When describing the examination procedure to the client, which statement by the nurse is most accurate?
[ ] **1.** "You'll read words that are the size of newsprint."
[ ] **2.** "You'll read letters from a distance of 20 feet (6 meters)."
[ ] **3.** "You'll look at a color picture and identify an image."
[ ] **4.** "You'll look at a screen and tell me when an object appears."

To obtain a more definite refractive error measurement, a retinoscopic examination is ordered.

8. Before the examination can be completed, which type of eye medication would the nurse instill in the client's eye to dilate the pupil and temporarily paralyze the ciliary muscle?
[ ] **1.** Pilocarpine (Pilocar)
[ ] **2.** Dipivefrin (Propine)
[ ] **3.** Gentamicin (Genoptic)
[ ] **4.** Cyclopentolate solution (Cyclogyl)

9. A client comes to the eye clinic and tells the nurse that glasses have been ordered to correct nearsightedness. Which of the following terms would the eye clinic nurse use to document that a client has nearsightedness?
[ ] **1.** Presbyopia
[ ] **2.** Amblyopia
[ ] **3.** Hyperopia
[ ] **4.** Myopia

A nursing assistant confides to the nurse that a family member needs eyeglasses but cannot afford them.

10. Which organization can the nurse suggest as a community resource to the nursing assistant?
[ ] **1.** The Loyal Order of Moose
[ ] **2.** The American Legion
[ ] **3.** Lions Clubs International
[ ] **4.** The Knights of Columbus

The nurse reads in the medical record that a client has astigmatism.

11. Which statement would the nurse expect the client to report when looking at an object without wearing corrective glasses or contact lenses?
[ ] **1.** "I see near objects more clearly."
[ ] **2.** "I see a blurry area in front of me."
[ ] **3.** "I see far objects more clearly."
[ ] **4.** "I see two of the same object."

12. After cleaning a client's prescription eyeglasses with soap and warm water or a commercial glass cleaner, which nursing action is best for drying the moist lenses?
[ ] **1.** Rub the lenses with a paper tissue.
[ ] **2.** Wipe the lenses with a soft cloth.
[ ] **3.** Blot the lenses with a paper towel.
[ ] **4.** Blow on the lenses to promote air drying.

13. Which nursing intervention is most appropriate to include in the care plan of an anxious client who is blind or has both eyes patched?
[ ] **1.** Touch the client before speaking.
[ ] **2.** Explain what you plan to do beforehand.
[ ] **3.** Stand in front of the client when speaking.
[ ] **4.** Leave the room lights on at all times.

The nurse observes a nursing assistant ambulating a blind client.

14. Which instruction to the nursing assistant is best for maintaining the client's safety and security?
[ ] **1.** Let the client take your arm while walking.
[ ] **2.** Take the client's arm while walking.
[ ] **3.** Position the client in front of you and to your side.
[ ] **4.** Have the client walk independently by your side.

15. Which plan best promotes a blind client's feeling of self-reliance when eating?
[ ] **1.** Help the client locate food by comparing its placement to clock positions.
[ ] **2.** Ask a hospital volunteer to feed the client so the client does not have to ask for help.
[ ] **3.** Order foods that can be sipped from containers rather than eaten with utensils.
[ ] **4.** Ask the dietary department to serve the client's food on paper plates and in cups.

The nurse is assigned to care for an older client who has bilateral cataracts.

16. When the nurse reviews the client's health history, which symptom is directly related to the development of cataracts?
[ ] **1.** Gradual loss of vision
[ ] **2.** Feeling of fullness within the eye
[ ] **3.** Ocular pain or discomfort
[ ] **4.** Flashes of light

17. When the nurse inspects the client's eyes, which clinical finding is most indicative of cataracts?
[ ] **1.** Ruptured blood vessels in the eye
[ ] **2.** An irregularly shaped iris
[ ] **3.** A white spot behind the pupil
[ ] **4.** A painless corneal lesion

18. Which statement made by the client to the nurse best indicates an understanding of when cataract surgery is needed?
[ ] **1.** "I'll need surgery when my loss of vision really interferes with my activities."
[ ] **2.** "I'll need surgery when I can't control the pain anymore with eyedrops."
[ ] **3.** "I'll need surgery when I start to feel self-conscious about my appearance."
[ ] **4.** "I'll need surgery when my cataracts are at their maximum density."

The client with bilateral cataracts is scheduled to have a cataract removed from the right eye. Preoperative orders include the following: wash the face for 10 minutes on the morning of surgery, withhold anticoagulant therapy, and instill dilating drops every 15 minutes for 1 hour before surgery.

19. After reviewing the medical orders, which of the following is essential for the nurse to assess preoperatively?
[ ] **1.** The client's face for skin lesions
[ ] **2.** The time of the last dose of anticoagulant
[ ] **3.** The client's right eye for drainage
[ ] **4.** The client's left eye for signs of strain

One hour before surgery, the nurse instills eyedrops as per the physician's orders.

20. The nurse should instill the eyedrops into which part of the client's eye?
[ ] **1.** Onto the cornea
[ ] **2.** At the inner canthus
[ ] **3.** At the outer canthus
[ ] **4.** In the lower conjunctival sac

The nursing team meets to individualize a standardized postoperative nursing care plan for a client who is scheduled for a cataract extraction.

21. Which standing nursing order should be eliminated from this client's care plan?
[ ] **1.** Keep the client's bed in a low position at all times.
[ ] **2.** Reapply antiembolism stockings twice daily.
[ ] **3.** Urge the client to cough every 2 hours while awake.
[ ] **4.** Assist the client when ambulating in the hall or room.

22. After cataract surgery, the client tells the nurse of severe pain in the operative eye. Which nursing action is most appropriate?
[ ] **1.** Report the finding to the charge nurse.
[ ] **2.** Give the client a prescribed analgesic.
[ ] **3.** Assess the client's pupil response with a penlight.
[ ] **4.** Reposition the client on the operative side.

Before the client is discharged from the hospital, the physician instructs the client to wear a metal shield over the operative eye while sleeping.

23. When the client asks the nurse about the purpose of the eye shield, which explanation is best?
[ ] **1.** "The shield keeps foreign substances out of the eye."
[ ] **2.** "The shield protects the eye from accidental trauma."
[ ] **3.** "The shield reduces rapid eye movement when dreaming."
[ ] **4.** "The shield promotes dilation of the pupil at night."

24. Which information is most appropriate to include in the discharge instructions for the client who has undergone a cataract extraction?
[ ] **1.** Avoid bending over from the waist.
[ ] **2.** Keep both eyes patched at all times.
[ ] **3.** Sleep with the head slightly elevated.
[ ] **4.** Expect bleeding to decrease in 1 week.

A nurse is assigned to care for an older client with chronic open-angle glaucoma.

25. Priority nursing instruction should be focused on the development of which visual symptom?
[ ] **1.** Itching and burning eyes
[ ] **2.** Headaches while reading
[ ] **3.** Seeing halos around lights
[ ] **4.** Loss of peripheral vision

The nurse prepares to assist the physician during the client's examination.

26. When preparing the examination room, which instrument is placed within physician's reach to assess the client's intraocular pressure (IOP)?
[ ] **1.** Ophthalmoscope
[ ] **2.** Tonometer
[ ] **3.** Retinoscope
[ ] **4.** Speculum

27. Which symptom related to the chronic progression of untreated glaucoma will a client most likely report to the nurse?
[ ] **1.** Tunnel vision
[ ] **2.** Double vision
[ ] **3.** Bulging eyes
[ ] **4.** Bloodshot eyes

28. The nurse has been instructed to administer eye ointment to the client with glaucoma. On the drawing below, identify with an *X* the correct area to begin applying the ointment.

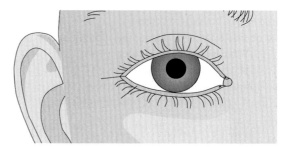

The client with chronic open-angle glaucoma is to administer timolol maleate (Timoptic) 1 gtt in each eye daily.

29. Which comment made to the nurse strongly suggests that the client with glaucoma needs more teaching?
[ ] **1.** "I must wash my hands before instilling the drops."
[ ] **2.** "This drug decreases the formation of fluid in my eye."
[ ] **3.** "I'll need to take this until my eye pressure is normal."
[ ] **4.** "The cap on the container should be replaced after use."

30. The nurse is reviewing current medications prescribed in addition to the Timoptic eye drops. Which medication is most important for the nurse to call to the physician's attention?
[ ] **1.** Atropine sulfate (Sal-Tropine)
[ ] **2.** Morphine sulfate (Roxanol)
[ ] **3.** Magnesium sulfate (Epsom salts)
[ ] **4.** Ferrous sulfate (Feosol)

31. Which assessment finding is commonly noted when the intraocular pressure (IOP) of a client with angle-closure glaucoma becomes dangerously high?
[ ] **1.** Spots in the visual field
[ ] **2.** Severe eye pain
[ ] **3.** Pinpoint pupils
[ ] **4.** Bulging eyes

32. The nurse compares the characteristics of open-angle glaucoma with those of angle-closure glaucoma. Which of the following statements describe ways they are similar? Select all that apply.
[ ] **1.** "The symptoms appear suddenly."
[ ] **2.** "The visual field examination demonstrates a loss of vision."
[ ] **3.** "Clients are initially treated with medications."
[ ] **4.** "Blurred vision is a common manifestation."
[ ] **5.** "Attacks are self-limited but are more harmful with each episode."
[ ] **6.** "Surgery is often required."

Once the intraocular pressure has been temporarily reduced, the physician performs an iridectomy on a client with angle-closure glaucoma.

33. When the nurse assesses the client's operative eye after surgery, which finding is most expected?
[ ] **1.** The pupil appears cloudy and gray.
[ ] **2.** The pupil is a fixed size and shape.
[ ] **3.** The entire iris lacks color.
[ ] **4.** A section of the iris appears black.

The nurse documents the health history of a client with a retinal detachment.

34. Of the following information provided by the client to the nurse, which factor is most likely to cause a retinal detachment?
[ ] **1.** The client is younger than age 40.
[ ] **2.** The client fell and struck the head.
[ ] **3.** The client has multiple allergies.
[ ] **4.** The client is being treated for glaucoma.

The nurse applies patches to both of the client's eyes, as instructed by the physician.

35. Which of the following would be the most appropriate action for the nurse to take when applying eye patches to the client?
[ ] **1.** Occluding all sources of room light
[ ] **2.** Ensuring that both patches exert tight pressure on the eyes
[ ] **3.** Maintaining the client's eyelids in a closed position
[ ] **4.** Making sure the client can see while the patches are in place

The nurse delivers a phone message to the client with a retinal detachment whose eyes are now patched. The client is on strict bed rest with the head of the bed slightly elevated.

36. Before leaving the room, which of the following nursing actions best preserves the client's dignity?
[ ] **1.** The nurse straightens the client's linens.
[ ] **2.** The nurse informs the client when leaving the room.
[ ] **3.** The nurse offers to give the client a back rub.
[ ] **4.** The nurse shares some current events with the client.

After a few days of continual bed rest, the client tells the nurse, "I'm not having any pain, and I'm not dying. Why can't I just get up once to go to the bathroom?"

37. Which response by the nurse is best in this situation?
[ ] **1.** "Gravity helps to reattach the separated retina."
[ ] **2.** "You don't want to be permanently blind, do you?"
[ ] **3.** "I can get you a sedative if it's hard to lie still."
[ ] **4.** "I am closely following your doctor's orders."

The client with a detached retina undergoes a scleral buckling procedure.

38. Postoperatively, which of the following client concerns should be the nurse's highest priority?
[ ] **1.** Pain
[ ] **2.** Vomiting
[ ] **3.** Anxiety
[ ] **4.** Fatigue

A client with myopia undergoes a laser keratotomy (LASIK) procedure.

39. Which statement made to the nurse is the best evidence that the client understands the anticipated outcome of this procedure?
[ ] **1.** "I'll have better night vision."
[ ] **2.** "I'll correctly identify colors."
[ ] **3.** "I'll see well without glasses."
[ ] **4.** "I'll use both eyes when reading."

A nurse is asked to assess a person who potentially has "pinkeye."

40. On inspecting the client's eye, the nurse will note which symptom of conjunctivitis in addition to erythema?
[ ] **1.** Dried drainage along the eyelid
[ ] **2.** Lack of pupil response to light
[ ] **3.** Bulging of the eye from the orbit
[ ] **4.** Loss of moisture on the cornea

41. Which health teaching instruction given by the nurse is most important for a client with conjunctivitis?
[ ] **1.** "Eat a well-balanced, nutritious diet with plenty of fluids."
[ ] **2.** "Always wear dark sunglasses when in bright light."
[ ] **3.** "Do not share towels or washcloths with family members."
[ ] **4.** "Avoid all aspirin-containing products."

The physician asks the nurse to assist with applying a stain to the eye of a client to determine if a foreign body is embedded in the cornea or if the cornea is injured.

42. During the examination, the nurse correctly hands the physician which solution?
[ ] **1.** Povidone-iodine (Betadine)
[ ] **2.** Gentian violet
[ ] **3.** Methylene blue
[ ] **4.** Fluorescein

43. What images will a client with macular degeneration most likely describe seeing?

[ ] **1.**
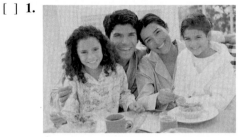
A

[ ] **2.**
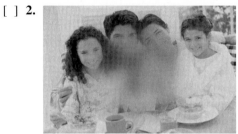
B

[ ] **3.**
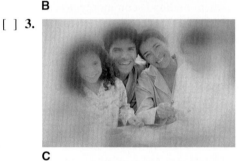
C

[ ] **4.**
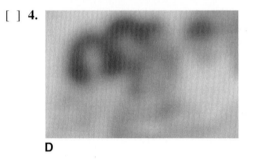
D

A nurse makes home visits to several older adult clients with chronic health problems.

44. To identify problems that may compromise the client's vision, the nurse recommends regular eye examinations by an ophthalmologist to which client?
[ ] **1.** A client who takes aspirin daily
[ ] **2.** A client who has diabetes mellitus
[ ] **3.** A client who is lactose intolerant
[ ] **4.** A client who has a pacemaker

A client with a malignant eye tumor has consented to undergo enucleation of the eye.

45. Which statement provides the best evidence that the client understands the postoperative outcome of this surgery?
[ ] **1.** "My vision will be restored with a plastic prosthesis."
[ ] **2.** "The prosthetic eye will be inserted during surgery."
[ ] **3.** "I will have to remove my prosthesis for cleaning."
[ ] **4.** "I will have a permanently empty eye socket."

46. Which symptom, expressed to the nurse, most suggests that a client who had a corneal transplant is experiencing rejection of the donor tissue?
[ ] **1.** Excessive tearing
[ ] **2.** Change in vision
[ ] **3.** Itching of the eye
[ ] **4.** Frequent blinking

Nursing Care of Clients with Disorders of Accessory Eye Structures

An older client's lower eyelid margins droop outward, exposing the conjunctival membrane and the lower portion of the eye.

47. On the basis of the anatomic changes in the tone of the eyelid, the nurse would expect the client to experience which problem?
[ ] **1.** Double vision
[ ] **2.** Photophobia
[ ] **3.** Lid spasms
[ ] **4.** Dry eyes

The nurse observes that a client has inflamed eyelid margins and patchy dandruff-like flakes that cling to the eyelids and eyelashes.

48. Which recommendation by the nurse is most appropriate if the client's condition is caused by hypersecretion of the sebaceous glands?
[ ] **1.** Increasing attention to hygiene
[ ] **2.** Limiting consumption of dietary fat
[ ] **3.** Switching to fluorescent lighting
[ ] **4.** Eating more deep yellow vegetables

49. When a client with a stye (hordeolum) asks a nurse to suggest measures to relieve the discomfort, what is the best advice the nurse can offer?
[ ] **1.** Squeeze the lesion to express the exudate.
[ ] **2.** Apply warm, moist compresses to the area.
[ ] **3.** Pierce the lesion with the tip of a pin.
[ ] **4.** Cover the lesion with a dry gauze dressing.

The physician diagnoses swelling within the inner surface of a client's eyelid as a chalazion, a gland obstructed with sebum.

50. Which of the following is correct information for the nurse to provide the client about the consequences if the tissue continues to proliferate?
[ ] **1.** Blindness may occur.
[ ] **2.** Lashes may fall out.
[ ] **3.** Surgery may be necessary.
[ ] **4.** Pain may be severe.

Nursing Care of Clients with Ear Disorders

While performing a nursing admission interview, the nurse notes that a client continues to ask that questions be repeated.

51. If the client worked at the following occupations, which one is most likely to have contributed to the hearing loss?
[ ] **1.** Telephone operator
[ ] **2.** Computer programmer
[ ] **3.** Musician
[ ] **4.** Teacher

After inspecting a client's ears, the nurse notes a large amount of cerumen.

52. What information is best for the nurse to tell the client about cleaning ears?
[ ] **1.** "It's best to use the corner of a soapy washcloth."
[ ] **2.** "Do you prefer a short or long cotton-tipped applicator?"
[ ] **3.** "Have you ever tried removing earwax with a hairpin?"
[ ] **4.** "I can refer you to a physician who will clean them."

53. Which instrument is most appropriate for the nurse to use to test a client's hearing acuity?
[ ] **1.** Otoscope
[ ] **2.** Tuning fork
[ ] **3.** Reflex hammer
[ ] **4.** Stethoscope

A client tells the nurse about experiencing continuous ringing in the ears.

54. Which question is most appropriate for the nurse to ask at this time?
[ ] **1.** "What childhood diseases have you had?"
[ ] **2.** "What's your present occupation?"
[ ] **3.** "Do you eat a well-balanced diet?"
[ ] **4.** "How much aspirin do you take?"

A client who wears a hearing aid is frustrated by the loud and shrill noise (feedback) that is heard occasionally.

55. Which nursing action is most helpful for reducing or eliminating feedback from the client's hearing aid?
[ ] **1.** Repositioning the hearing aid within the ear
[ ] **2.** Cleaning the hearing aid with a soft cloth
[ ] **3.** Replacing the battery in the hearing aid
[ ] **4.** Turning down the volume in the hearing aid

56. If a client who has recently experienced diminished hearing takes medications from each of the following drug categories, which one is most likely to have affected the client's hearing?
[ ] **1.** Nonsteroidal anti-inflammatory drug
[ ] **2.** Beta-adrenergic blocker
[ ] **3.** Aminoglycoside antibiotic
[ ] **4.** Histamine-2 (H$_2$) antagonist

57. When instilling prescribed medication into the ear of an adult, which is the correct technique for the nurse to use to straighten the ear canal?
[ ] **1.** Pull the ear upward and backward.
[ ] **2.** Pull the ear downward and forward.
[ ] **3.** Pull the ear upward and forward.
[ ] **4.** Pull the ear downward and backward.

58. After instilling medication into the client's ear, which nursing instruction is most appropriate?
[ ] **1.** Keep your head tilted for 5 minutes.
[ ] **2.** Pack a cotton ball tightly in your ear.
[ ] **3.** Do not blow your nose for at least 1 hour.
[ ] **4.** Wipe the excess medication from the ear.

When inspecting a client's ear, the nurse finds that the ear canal is red, swollen, and tender. The tympanic membrane is intact.

59. Which additional assessment finding provides evidence of an infection in the external ear?
[ ] **1.** Foul-smelling drainage
[ ] **2.** Scarred tympanic membrane
[ ] **3.** Diminished hearing
[ ] **4.** Enlarged lymph nodes

Parents bring their 3-year-old child to the pediatrician for a possible ear infection. They ask the nurse why their 18-year-old teenager does not seem to get ear infections.

60. Which response demonstrates that the parents understand the nurse's explanation of why organisms travel more easily from the nasopharynx to the middle ear in a child?
[ ] **1.** A child's eustachian tube is shorter and straighter.
[ ] **2.** A child's eustachian tube is longer and straighter.
[ ] **3.** A child's eustachian tube is shorter and more curved.
[ ] **4.** A child's eustachian tube is longer and more curved.

A middle ear infection is diagnosed in the 3-year-old child.

61. The nurse uses an illustration to explain to the child's parents the structure of the ear and the area of infection. Place an *X* to identify the location of the middle ear.

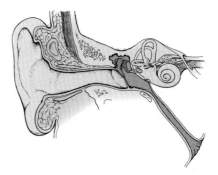

62. What is the best evidence that the antibiotic the nurse is administering for the treatment of acute otitis media is having a therapeutic effect?
[ ] **1.** The ear feels less warm to the touch.
[ ] **2.** Ringing sounds within the ear stop.
[ ] **3.** Ear drainage is thin and watery.
[ ] **4.** Ear discomfort is relieved.

63. If a client with a middle ear infection reports the following symptoms, which one is most indicative that the infection has spread to the inner ear?
[ ] **1.** Temporal headaches
[ ] **2.** A sore throat
[ ] **3.** Nasal congestion
[ ] **4.** Postural dizziness

Because of repeated episodes of otitis media despite antibiotic therapy, the physician intends to perform a myringotomy on the child with a middle ear infection.

64. When the nurse prepares the client for the myringotomy, which statement best explains the purpose of the procedure?
[ ] **1.** A myringotomy prevents permanent hearing loss.
[ ] **2.** A myringotomy provides a pathway for drainage.
[ ] **3.** A myringotomy aids in administering medications.
[ ] **4.** A myringotomy maintains motion of the ear bones.

65. When planning the child's discharge, what nursing instruction is most appropriate for the nurse to provide the parent concerning the cotton ball in the client's ear canal?
[ ] **1.** "Leave the cotton ball in place until it is saturated."
[ ] **2.** "Keep the cotton ball placed loosely within the ear canal."
[ ] **3.** "Soak the cotton ball in peroxide before insertion."
[ ] **4.** "Remove the cotton ball when the cotton becomes dry."

A middle-aged client is seen in the physician's office for diminished hearing caused by otosclerosis.

66. Which finding in the health history would the nurse expect of a client with otosclerosis?
[ ] **1.** Hearing loss beginning in childhood
[ ] **2.** Upper respiratory infections with high fevers
[ ] **3.** History of tonsils and adenoid removal
[ ] **4.** One or more relatives similarly diagnosed

The client asks the nurse to explain what the physician meant by noting a conductive hearing loss.

67. Which statement by the nurse most accurately explains the location of impairment?
[ ] **1.** "Sound waves do not travel to the inner ear."
[ ] **2.** "There is a malfunction of inner ear structures."
[ ] **3.** "The eighth cranial nerve is permanently damaged."
[ ] **4.** "Electric conversion of sound is not produced."

The team leader responsible for the client's initial care plan makes a nursing diagnosis of Risk for impaired verbal communication related to hearing loss.

68. When the team leader asks the admitting nurse to assist with developing a goal for the identified diagnosis, which goal correlates best with the diagnosis?
[ ] **1.** The client will respond appropriately to communication by staff.
[ ] **2.** The staff will improve verbal communication techniques.
[ ] **3.** The client will demonstrate the ability to express emotions.
[ ] **4.** The client will be able to communicate basic needs.

The nurse helps the team leader plan appropriate interventions to ensure effective communication with the client.

69. Which intervention is most appropriate to include in the care plan?
[ ] **1.** Speak directly into the client's ear.
[ ] **2.** Face the client directly when speaking.
[ ] **3.** Drop your voice at the end of each sentence.
[ ] **4.** Raise the pitch of your voice an octave higher.

The client is scheduled for a stapedectomy but does not seem to understand the verbal information the physician provided about the surgery.

70. Which nursing intervention is the best alternative for helping the client to comprehend the details of the procedure at this time?
[ ] **1.** Providing the client with a printed pamphlet on the topic
[ ] **2.** Asking another stapedectomy client to talk with the client
[ ] **3.** Providing someone proficient in sign language
[ ] **4.** Writing all the information in longhand

The client expresses concerns about the impending stapedectomy and says to the nurse, "There are so many awful complications that can happen with this surgery."

71. Which response by the nurse is most therapeutic to the client in this situation?
[ ] **1.** "You've got the best surgeon on the staff."
[ ] **2.** "Tell me more about how you're feeling."
[ ] **3.** "Don't worry. Those things hardly ever happen."
[ ] **4.** "Let's think positively about the outcome."

72. After the stapedectomy, which is the most appropriate technique for assessing whether the client's facial nerve function is intact?
[ ] **1.** Ask the client to identify familiar odors.
[ ] **2.** Ask the client to smile or raise the eyebrows.
[ ] **3.** Ask the client to stick out the tongue.
[ ] **4.** Ask the client to read printed information.

73. How should the nurse position the client for the first 24 hours after a stapedectomy?
[ ] **1.** Flat with the head elevated and tilted toward the nonoperative ear.
[ ] **2.** Facing forward with the head raised and the knees in a flexed position.
[ ] **3.** Supine with the head of the bed elevated and the head resting on the occiput.
[ ] **4.** Prone with the head positioned toward the operated side.

The day after the stapedectomy, the client is discouraged because hearing is more impaired than it was preoperatively.

74. Which is the most accurate rationale by the nurse that explains the client's current hearing deficit?
[ ] **1.** The client will have a temporary hearing loss until edema in the operative ear is relieved.
[ ] **2.** The client will have a temporary hearing loss until the nerve regenerates.
[ ] **3.** The client will have a temporary hearing loss until fitted with a molded plastic hearing aid.
[ ] **4.** The client will have a temporary hearing loss until the prosthesis becomes stabilized with new bone.

75. Which instruction by the nurse is best for preventing the dislodgement of the client's internal prosthesis after a stapedectomy?
[ ] **1.** "When chewing food, keep your mouth closed."
[ ] **2.** "When blowing your nose, use a paper tissue."
[ ] **3.** "When sneezing, keep your mouth wide open."
[ ] **4.** "When coughing, turn your head to the side."

76. The licensed practical nurse is coordinating client care with a nursing assistant. When reviewing the postoperative plan of care, which potential symptom places the client at a risk for injury?
[ ] **1.** Fatigue
[ ] **2.** Diplopia
[ ] **3.** Vertigo
[ ] **4.** Pain

77. The nurse knows that the client who underwent a stapedectomy understands the discharge instructions when the client identifies which activity to avoid for the next 6 months?

[ ] **1.** Listening to music
[ ] **2.** Flying in an airplane
[ ] **3.** Driving an automobile
[ ] **4.** Singing in the choir

78. Which common ailment should the nurse instruct the client who underwent a stapedectomy to immediately report to the physician?

[ ] **1.** The common cold
[ ] **2.** A sore throat
[ ] **3.** Productive cough
[ ] **4.** Conjunctivitis

The nurse is assessing a client who was admitted to the hospital for possible Ménière's disease.

79. Which subjective symptom is the client most likely to report to the nurse?

[ ] **1.** Burning
[ ] **2.** Pressure
[ ] **3.** Vertigo
[ ] **4.** Pain

The physician orders a caloric test for the client.

80. Which information provided by the nurse will best prepare the client for what to expect with caloric testing?

[ ] **1.** Cold water and warm water will be instilled into each of the ears.
[ ] **2.** You will wear earphones through which sounds are transmitted.
[ ] **3.** The room will be darkened, and scalp electrodes will be attached to the head.
[ ] **4.** Your blood will be drawn from a vein and examined microscopically.

81. Which response will the nurse most likely observe during the caloric test if the client has Ménière's disease?

[ ] **1.** Onset of severe symptoms
[ ] **2.** No response or change in symptoms
[ ] **3.** Nystagmus and slight dizziness
[ ] **4.** Aphasia and loss of consciousness

The client is positively diagnosed with Ménière's disease. During rounds, the nurse observes that the client seems anxious whenever a member of the nursing staff enters the room.

82. The nurse suspects that the client's anxiety is due to fear that nursing care will intensify symptoms. Which nursing intervention is most appropriate to add to the care plan at this time?

[ ] **1.** Let the client suggest ways to carry out care.
[ ] **2.** Discontinue nursing care measures at this time.
[ ] **3.** Restrict care to nutrition and elimination only.
[ ] **4.** Carry out nursing activities quickly and efficiently.

The client asks the nurse to clarify the physician's explanation about the cause of Ménière's disease.

83. The nurse is most accurate in stating that the cause of Ménière's disease is unknown but that the symptoms are related to which disorder?

[ ] **1.** An electrolyte deficit
[ ] **2.** An excess of fluid
[ ] **3.** A vitamin deficiency
[ ] **4.** An anatomic defect

84. When caring for a client with Ménière's disease, which nursing action is most helpful in preventing nausea and vomiting?

[ ] **1.** Increasing the client's intake of oral fluids
[ ] **2.** Changing the client's position frequently
[ ] **3.** Keeping the room lights dim
[ ] **4.** Avoiding jarring the bed

The client with Ménière's disease responds to conservative treatment and will be discharged.

85. The nurse should stress to the client the importance of adhering to which dietary restriction?

[ ] **1.** Fats
[ ] **2.** Sodium
[ ] **3.** Potassium
[ ] **4.** Cholesterol

86. Which statement by the client to the nurse indicates a need for additional teaching about Ménière's disease?

[ ] **1.** "I'll feel well between attacks."
[ ] **2.** "Future attacks may last minutes or days."
[ ] **3.** "My hearing will gradually improve."
[ ] **4.** "Ménière's disease is incurable."

Nursing Care of Clients with Nasal Disorders

87. When the nurse assesses a newly admitted client, which finding is most suggestive that the client may have had a fractured nose in the past?

[ ] **1.** Polyps are noted on nasal mucous membranes.
[ ] **2.** The nose is red, unusually large, and bulbous.
[ ] **3.** The septum deviates to the side, narrowing one naris.
[ ] **4.** There is serous drainage within the nares and pharynx.

An older client arrives at the emergency department with a severe nosebleed.

88. On the basis of the following data, which assessment finding most likely caused or contributed to the client's nosebleed?

[ ] **1.** Pulse rate of 110 beats/minute
[ ] **2.** Blood pressure of 200/104 mm Hg
[ ] **3.** Temperature of 97.6°F (36.4°C) orally
[ ] **4.** Respirations of 24 breaths/minute

89. Which nursing action is best for controlling the client's nosebleed?
[ ] **1.** Have the client lie down slowly and swallow frequently.
[ ] **2.** Have the client lie down and breathe through the mouth.
[ ] **3.** Have the client lean forward and apply direct pressure to the nose.
[ ] **4.** Have the client lean forward and clench the teeth.

The client's fear is heightened by observing the shirt that is extensively stained with blood from the nosebleed.

90. How can the nurse best relieve the client's fear and anxiety?
[ ] **1.** Recline the client so as to avoid seeing the blood.
[ ] **2.** Give the client a popular magazine to read.
[ ] **3.** Replace the client's clothing with a hospital gown.
[ ] **4.** Cover the client's eyes with a bath towel.

The physician uses silver nitrate to chemically cauterize the client's nasal area to stop the nosebleed.

91. Before the client leaves the emergency department, which nursing instruction is essential for preventing another nosebleed?
[ ] **1.** Advise the client to limit dietary intake of fluids.
[ ] **2.** Tell the client to sleep in a recliner or with the head up.
[ ] **3.** Show the client how to take the carotid pulse at hourly intervals.
[ ] **4.** Warn the client to avoid blowing the nose for several hours.

A client consults the physician concerning nasal polyps.

92. During the initial assessment, the nurse can assist the physician in determining the etiology of the client's problem by assessing if there is a history of which condition?
[ ] **1.** Recent nasal injury
[ ] **2.** Respiratory allergies
[ ] **3.** Previous nasal surgery
[ ] **4.** A past tonsillectomy

The client undergoes a nasal polypectomy and has nasal packing in place when returning from surgery.

93. Aside from blood on the anterior end of the packing, what other sign or symptom would suggest that the client is bleeding from the operative area?
[ ] **1.** Frequent swallowing
[ ] **2.** Impaired appetite
[ ] **3.** Slight hoarseness
[ ] **4.** Diminished hearing

A middle-aged client is having a rhinoplasty procedure to improve the appearance of the nose. After the rhinoplasty, the client asks the nurse how the repaired nose looks.

94. Which response by the nurse is best at this time?
[ ] **1.** "I'm sure you will look absolutely gorgeous."
[ ] **2.** "I didn't think you were unattractive before."
[ ] **3.** "Your face is swollen with bruises around the eyes."
[ ] **4.** "Your personality is more important than your looks."

Nursing Care of Clients with Disorders of the Skin and Related Structures

A nurse stops to give first-aid to a burn victim who is seen running from a home. The victim's clothing is on fire.

95. Which action is the nurse's immediate priority?
[ ] **1.** Rub petroleum jelly into the burned areas.
[ ] **2.** Wrap the affected areas with a clean cloth.
[ ] **3.** Apply ice to the affected burned areas.
[ ] **4.** Roll the victim to smother the flames.

The nurse notes that the victim's chest and neck are burned.

96. Which nursing action is most appropriate at this time?
[ ] **1.** Obtaining the client's pulse and blood pressure
[ ] **2.** Monitoring the client for respiratory distress
[ ] **3.** Identifying the client's next of kin
[ ] **4.** Determining the extent of the burn

The client is brought to the emergency department with partial-thickness and full-thickness burns.

97. Which immediate nursing interventions are appropriate for this client? Select all that apply.
[ ] **1.** Place ice packs on the burned areas.
[ ] **2.** Pour normal saline over the burned areas before dressing care.
[ ] **3.** Begin an I.V. infusion of lactated Ringer's solution.
[ ] **4.** Administer a tetanus injection.
[ ] **5.** Administer pain medication.
[ ] **6.** Administer oxygen therapy.

In the emergency department, it is determined that the burn victim has deep partial-thickness and full-thickness burns over 35% of the upper body.

98. The nurse who documents the burn injury is accurate in identifying the full-thickness burns as having what appearance?
[ ] **1.** White and leathery
[ ] **2.** Pink and blistered
[ ] **3.** Red and painful
[ ] **4.** Mottled and wet

99. Once the victim's blood pressure is stabilized, the best indication of successful response to the initial burn treatment is which assessment finding?
[ ] **1.** Normal body temperature
[ ] **2.** Minimal level of pain
[ ] **3.** Adequate urine output
[ ] **4.** Ability to perform exercises

Once the burn area is cleansed, the burn regimen is prescribed. The client's treatment plan includes using the open exposure method and using a topical agent without a dressing.

100. It is most appropriate for the nurse to monitor a client being treated by the open exposure method for which potential problem?
[ ] **1.** Infection
[ ] **2.** Hyperthermia
[ ] **3.** Depression
[ ] **4.** Malnutrition

The physician orders the application of mafenide acetate (Sulfamylon) to the burn wound.

101. When the nurse applies mafenide acetate cream to the burn wound, the nurse should recognize which of the following as its chief disadvantage?
[ ] **1.** Skin discoloration
[ ] **2.** Pain on application
[ ] **3.** Unpleasant odor
[ ] **4.** Contact dermatitis

The burn wound is periodically debrided using hydrotherapy.

102. Shortly before each debridement, which nursing intervention is essential?
[ ] **1.** Keeping the client in a fasting state
[ ] **2.** Witnessing a signed consent form
[ ] **3.** Administering a prescribed analgesic
[ ] **4.** Weighing the client on a bed scale

The health care team is informed that skin autografting is planned for the burn client.

103. Which action is most appropriate to include in the postoperative care plan when a client has skin grafts?
[ ] **1.** Minimize movement to prevent graft disruption.
[ ] **2.** Change the dressing over the graft every 8 hours.
[ ] **3.** Reinforce the graft dressing if drainage occurs.
[ ] **4.** Apply wet soaks to the graft every 4 hours.

Before discharge, the client is fitted for an elasticized pressure garment that covers the burned areas of skin.

104. Which statement is the best indication that the client understands the purpose of wearing the pressure garment?
[ ] **1.** It prevents subsequent wound infection.
[ ] **2.** It prevents exposure to the sun.
[ ] **3.** It reduces the severity of scar formation.
[ ] **4.** It reduces the potential for social rejection.

Another burn victim is brought to the emergency department with an electrical burn.

105. When examining the electrical burn on the victim, which assessment is most important for the nurse to determine?
[ ] **1.** The entry and exit wound sites
[ ] **2.** Degree of skin discoloration
[ ] **3.** Amount of eschar on the wound bed
[ ] **4.** Characteristics of wound drainage

During the nurse's initial physical assessment of an older client who was just transferred from a nursing home, the nurse notes that the client has a pressure ulcer on the left hip and sacrum.

106. On assessing the client's pressure ulcer (see photo), the nurse would document this as which stage?

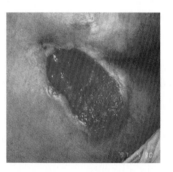

107. On the basis of the nurse's understanding of the etiology of pressure ulcers, the nurse should plan for which intervention to promote the client's skin integrity?
[ ] **1.** Apply a skin-toughening agent to susceptible areas.
[ ] **2.** Massage skin areas that remain persistently red.
[ ] **3.** Keep the head of the bed elevated 30 degrees.
[ ] **4.** Reposition the client every 2 hours.

The elderly bedridden client is frequently found at the bottom of the bed with the feet hanging over the end of the bed.

108. Because the immobile client slides down in bed, the nurse is correct to assess for which type of skin injury?
[ ] **1.** One that results from continuous pressure
[ ] **2.** One that results from a shearing force
[ ] **3.** One that results from friction
[ ] **4.** One that results from agitation in bed

An elderly client has been approved for admission to a long-term care facility for recuperation after open-heart surgery. The charge nurse receives the client's health history, which includes cardiovascular disease, recent coronary artery bypass graft surgery, arthritis, and a sacral pressure ulcer.

109. Before the client's arrival, which services should the nurse anticipate will facilitate this client's recovery? Select all that apply.
[ ] **1.** Nutritional consult
[ ] **2.** Physical therapy
[ ] **3.** Enterostomal therapy
[ ] **4.** Psychiatric therapy
[ ] **5.** Physician consult
[ ] **6.** Occupational therapy

A home health nurse visits the home of a family being treated for pediculosis (head lice).

110. Which of the parent's statements indicates a need for more teaching?
[ ] **1.** "Lice are gone if I don't see any one day after treatment."
[ ] **2.** "I've washed all the bed linens in soap, hot water, and bleach."
[ ] **3.** "None of my children shares each other's combs or brushes."
[ ] **4.** "Once there is an outbreak, all students should be inspected."

A biopsy reveals that a scalp lesion on a Caucasian male client is a basal cell carcinoma.

111. Which finding of the client's biographical data most likely contributed to developing skin cancer?
[ ] **1.** The client is a chronic cigarette smoker.
[ ] **2.** The client has male pattern baldness.
[ ] **3.** The client works for a drug manufacturer.
[ ] **4.** The client bathes with a deodorant soap.

The nurse is instructing a client about potential skin disorders and is discussing malignant melanomas.

112. What is the most common profile of a client with malignant melanoma?
[ ] **1.** An African American client with dark skin and dark hair
[ ] **2.** A Scandinavian client with freckles and blue eyes
[ ] **3.** A Mexican client with tan skin and dark brown hair
[ ] **4.** A Caucasian client with brown hair and brown eyes

113. Which area of health teaching is essential when a female client is prescribed isotretinoin (Accutane) for treating acne vulgaris?
[ ] **1.** Breast self-examination techniques
[ ] **2.** Techniques for avoiding pregnancy
[ ] **3.** Methods for predicting ovulation
[ ] **4.** Information on preventing sexual transmission

114. What is the best nursing advice for individuals who have frequent outbreaks of tinea pedis (athlete's foot)?
[ ] **1.** Never go barefoot when outdoors.
[ ] **2.** Cut toenails straight across.
[ ] **3.** Wear different shoes each day.
[ ] **4.** Avoid wearing white cotton socks.

A client with shingles (herpes zoster) is admitted to the hospital and is given acyclovir (Zovirax).

115. When the client asks about the cause of shingles, what is an accurate nursing response?
[ ] **1.** The reactivation of a dormant virus
[ ] **2.** A vector insect such as a tick
[ ] **3.** A toxin from a bacterial infection
[ ] **4.** An antibody response to a drug allergen

116. The nurse is outlining the typical progression of the clinical manifestation of shingles to the family. Arrange the clinical manifestations from earliest symptoms to late as the disease progresses. Use all the options.

1. Pain develops and severe itching follows.	
2. Low-grade fever and malaise.	
3. Dermatome area develops a red, blotchy appearance.	
4. Unilateral vesicles appear.	
5. Scarring or permanent skin discoloration is noted.	

117. Which health teaching information is most appropriate for a client with a herpes simplex virus type 1 infection?
[ ] **1.** Apply petroleum jelly to the lesions to prevent spreading the virus to adjacent areas.
[ ] **2.** Use good personal hygiene to prevent spreading the virus to other body parts.
[ ] **3.** Avoid using soap and water on open lesions.
[ ] **4.** Remove the scabs daily by soaking with hot compresses.

A nurse assesses a client with psoriasis at a dermatology clinic.

118. When examining the client's skin, which finding would the nurse expect to observe?
[ ] **1.** Weeping skin lesions on the trunk of the body.
[ ] **2.** Red skin patches covered with silvery scales.
[ ] **3.** Fluid-filled blisters surrounded by crusts.
[ ] **4.** A red rash containing raised pustules.

The client expresses self-consciousness about the patches of psoriasis on the lower arms and asks, "What's causing this condition?"

119. The nurse correctly teaches the client that psoriasis is an inflammatory dermatosis that results from which skin condition?
[ ] 1. A superficial skin infection
[ ] 2. The effects of dermal abrasion
[ ] 3. A proliferation of epidermal cells
[ ] 4. An infection of the hair follicles

A nursing assistant with an allergy to latex asks the nurse for advice on carrying out standard precautions for preventing the transmission of blood-borne viruses.

120. What is the best advice the nurse can offer the nursing assistant?
[ ] 1. "Rinse your latex gloves with running tap water before putting them on."
[ ] 2. "Apply a petroleum ointment to both hands before putting on latex gloves."
[ ] 3. "Don't wear gloves, but wash your hands vigorously with alcohol after client contact."
[ ] 4. "Wear two pairs of vinyl gloves when there's a potential for contact with body fluids."

By mistake, the nursing assistant donned a pair of latex gloves.

121. Which signs and symptoms indicate that the nursing assistant has had an allergic reaction to the latex gloves? Select all that apply.
[ ] 1. Raised areas and blisters on the hands
[ ] 2. Itchy, red, watery eyes
[ ] 3. Runny nose
[ ] 4. Nausea and vomiting
[ ] 5. Hives
[ ] 6. Chest tightness

A client who had prolonged exposure to cold weather consults a nurse about first-aid measures for treating frostbite.

122. Which measure is best for the nurse to recommend?
[ ] 1. Soak affected body parts in a warm solution that is approximately 100°F (37.8°C).
[ ] 2. Begin the rewarming process by first applying cold skin compresses.
[ ] 3. Apply a heating pad on the highest setting to the affected body parts.
[ ] 4. Flood the affected skin surface with hot water at a temperature of approximately 140°F (60°C).

123. A client comes to the clinic and complains of pruritus from dry skin. Which nursing instruction is most appropriate to convey to the client?
[ ] 1. Use hypoallergenic or glycerin soap for bathing.
[ ] 2. Apply lotion to the affected skin every other day.
[ ] 3. Take showers rather than tub baths.
[ ] 4. Rub the skin dry after bathing.

A nurse is working in a wound clinic and treats different types of wounds daily.

124. When developing nursing care plans, the nurse is careful to classify which type of wound as a chronic wound?
[ ] 1. A gunshot wound with tissue damage
[ ] 2. A slow-healing diabetic foot ulcer
[ ] 3. A stage I pressure ulcer on the coccyx
[ ] 4. A 7-day-old infected surgical wound

A client presents to the clinic with a rash. The nurse collects information related to the cause of the rash.

125. Which questions should the nurse ask to investigate the cause of the client's rash? Select all that apply.
[ ] 1. "Have you eaten foods that are different from your normal diet?"
[ ] 2. "Have you taken any new medications?"
[ ] 3. "Have you changed your laundry detergent?"
[ ] 4. "Have you been exposed to excessive sunlight?"
[ ] 5. "Have you been exercising in a gym?"
[ ] 6. "Have you gotten any new pets?"

Correct Answers, Rationales, and Test Taking Strategies

Nursing Care of Clients with Eye Disorders

1. 3. Immediate action is important when treating chemical injuries to the eyes. Therefore, it is important for the school nurse to determine what treatment was given at the time of injury. This information provides a baseline for further treatment. Diluting and removing the chemical reduces the potential for corneal damage. Identifying the chemical is important; however, taking time to determine what, if anything, will neutralize the chemical does not supersede immediate treatment. Liability is affected if safety glasses are not worn, but the priority is treating the chemical splash if that has not already been done. It is too soon to evaluate the extent of sensory damage.

Test Taking Strategy—Look for the key words "most important," which indicates a priority. Recall that diluting and removing the chemical by flushing the eyes with plain water should be done as soon as possible after the chemical injury (option 3). Review first-aid measures for managing a caustic chemical splash if you had difficulty answering this question.
Cognitive Level—*Applying*
Client Needs Category—*Physiological integrity*
Client Needs Subcategory—*Physiological adaptation*

2. 1. Water is typically used in an emergency to flush the eyes and dilute the chemical. Tap water from a faucet or shower is generally available. The other chemical solutions may be appropriate depending on the specific chemical that caused the trauma, but they may need to be diluted to a specific strength to prevent additional damage to the eye. Delaying first-aid measures wastes valuable time. Ideally, the student's eyes should have been flushed in the classroom at an appropriate eye wash station before seeing the nurse.

Test Taking Strategy—Use the process of elimination to help select the option that describes the best solution to irrigate the student's eyes. Although solutions that neutralize a chemical are preferred, options 2 and 4 can be eliminated because at this time the substance that splashed in the student's eyes is unknown. Option 3 can be eliminated because plain tap water (option 1) is readily available, most likely in sufficient quantity to provide a flush lasting at least 15 minutes. Review the management of a chemical burn to the eyes if you had difficulty answering this question.
Cognitive Level—*Applying*
Client Needs Category—*Physiological integrity*
Client Needs Subcategory—*Physiological adaptation*

3. 3, 4, 5. When irrigating the eyes, the nurse should perform hand hygiene and wear gloves to prevent the transmission of microorganisms. The nurse should offer the client a tissue or pad the shoulder area to absorb solution as it drains from the eye. The solution should not be directed into the center of the eye because this can harm the cornea. Instead, the irrigating solution should be instilled in the conjunctival sac, which is located by pulling the lower lid down. The client's head should be tilted toward the affected eye to facilitate drainage and prevent contamination of the unaffected eye. The eye will remain reddened after irrigation due to the irritant nature of the chemical. In a chemical exposure, the eye should be irrigated for at least 15 minutes.

Test Taking Strategy—Analyze to determine what information the question asks for, which is steps to take when irrigating an eye. Alternative-format "select all that apply" questions require considering each option independently to decide its merit in answering the question. Choose the options that correlate with the steps used when irrigating the eye. Review the procedure for performing an eye irrigation if you had difficulty answering this question.
Cognitive Level—*Applying*
Client Needs Category—*Physiological integrity*
Client Needs Subcategory—*Basic care and comfort*

4. 2. The irrigating solution is directed so that it flows from the inner canthus toward the outer canthus. This is an especially important principle to follow so that substances in one eye do not come in contact with the tissue of the other eye. It is best to instill the force of the water on the conjunctiva rather than onto the sensitive cornea, which may cause discomfort or reflex blinking. The anterior chamber is not an external eye structure. The nasolacrimal duct lies in the area of the inner canthus.

Test Taking Strategy—Use the process of elimination to select the best location for directing the irrigating solution when flushing the eye. Recall that the canthi (plural for canthus) are the angles where the upper and lower eyelids meet. Option 2 is the correct answer because instilling fluid away from the inner canthus avoids introducing the chemical into the unaffected eye through gravity flow. Review the recommended anatomic location when irrigating an eye if you had difficulty answering this question.
Cognitive Level—*Applying*
Client Needs Category—*Physiological integrity*
Client Needs Subcategory—*Basic care and comfort*

5. 2. An ophthalmologist is a physician who is licensed to diagnose and treat eye diseases and traumatic injuries. An optician fills prescriptions for corrective lenses. An optometrist tests vision and prescribes glasses or contact lenses to correct visual acuity. An orthoptist is a person who helps strengthen the extraocular muscles of the eye.

Test Taking Strategy—Use the process of elimination to select the best professional for providing follow-up care of a client who has incurred a chemical burn to an eye. Knowledge of the scope of practice for the professionals in options 1, 3, and 4 leads to their elimination as an answer. Option 2 remains as the correct answer because an ophthalmologist has a broader scope of medical practice than the others. Consult references that describe the practice areas provided by the professionals listed if you had difficulty answering this question.
Cognitive Level—Remembering
Client Needs Category—Health promotion and maintenance
Client Needs Subcategory—None

6. 4. The eyes are patched loosely with the lids closed to reduce further injury by blinking and eye movement. Instilling antibiotic ointment interferes with the medical examination, although antibiotic ointment may be prescribed after the object is removed. Attempts to remove an embedded object are left to those with specialized medical training.
Test Taking Strategy—Analyze to determine what information the question asks for, which is the initial action that should be taken when a client has a foreign body embedded in the eye. Recall that blinking the eyes is a reflex used to maintain moisture and clear debris from the cornea and conjunctiva. However, the muscular action involved in blinking may drive a foreign body even further within the eye or injure the posterior surface of the eyelid. Therefore, patching the eyes reduces the potential for more serious or secondary injuries to the eye and accessory structures until emergency medical care is provided. Review first-aid measures when a foreign body is within an eye if you had difficulty answering this question.
Cognitive Level—Applying
Client Needs Category—Physiological integrity
Client Needs Subcategory—Physiological adaptation

7. 2. A Snellen chart is used to test far vision and visual acuity by having the client read a series of block letters from a chart. Visual acuity is the ability to see detail in focus at a certain distance. Typically, clients stand 20 feet (6 m) from the chart and are asked to read letters that progressively become smaller. Normal visual acuity is 20/20. This means that a client can see an object at a distance of 20 feet that normally can be seen at 20 feet. Jaeger's chart is used to test near vision. Ishihara's plates are used to test color vision. A tangent screen, which is used to assess the peripheral visual field, requires the client to indicate when a stimulus is seen in the peripheral field of vision.
Test Taking Strategy—Note the key words "most accurate," and use them when looking for an option that provides the best description of a test involving a Snellen chart. Recall that a Snellen chart displays letters of the alphabet, or other symbols for young children or those who are illiterate, in sequential lines that become progressively smaller (option 2). Review the manner in which far vision and visual acuity are assessed using a Snellen chart if you had difficulty answering this question.
Cognitive Level—Applying
Client Needs Category—Health promotion and maintenance
Client Needs Subcategory—None

8. 4. Cyclopentolate solution (Cyclogyl) is used as a mydriatic (pupil-dilating) and cycloplegic (paralysis of ciliary muscle) drug, which prevents accommodation. Accommodation is the contraction or relaxation of the ciliary muscle to change the shape of the lens to focus on near or far objects. This drug is used for eye examinations or to treat uveal tract inflammatory conditions that benefit from pupillary dilation. Pilocarpine (Pilocar) is a direct-acting parasympathomimetic used to produce miosis (constriction of the pupil). Dipivefrin (Propine) is a sympathomimetic prodrug that is biotransformed into epinephrine within the eye. It is used to decrease intraocular pressure by enhancing aqueous outflow. Gentamicin (Genoptic) is an ophthalmic antibacterial drug used to treat various infections.
Test Taking Strategy—Analyze to determine what information the question asks for, which is a drug that dilates the pupil and temporarily paralyzes the ciliary muscle. Doing so interferes with accommodation and temporarily allows the physician to examine the interior of the eye. Consult a drug reference for the action of each drug listed in the options if you had difficulty answering this question.
Cognitive Level—Applying
Client Needs Category—Physiological integrity
Client Needs Subcategory—Pharmacological therapies

9. 4. The term for nearsightedness is *myopia*. Clients with myopia hold objects closer to their eyes to see them well. *Presbyopia* is a type of farsightedness associated with aging. It is caused by loss of elasticity in the lenses. Amblyopia is commonly referred to as *lazy eye*. Untreated, amblyopia results in the loss of vision in one eye from lack of use. *Hyperopia* is farsightedness.
Test Taking Strategy—Analyze to determine what information the question asks for, which is the medical term for nearsightedness. If you know the derivation of prefixes and suffixes of words, you may understand that the term myopia (option 4) stems from the Greek word my+ops (myops), meaning "near-sighted eye." Review definitions of these terms if you had difficulty answering this question.
Cognitive Level—Understanding
Client Needs Category—Health promotion and maintenance
Client Needs Subcategory—None

10. 3. The Lions Clubs International organization has vision and hearing improvements as its major goal. Local or state chapters can provide information and assistance to those who need but cannot afford glasses, a guide dog, hearing aid, or surgery. The other organizations are both fraternal and philanthropic, but they have not named vision or hearing assistance as their projects.

> *Test Taking Strategy—Analyze to determine what information the question asks for, which is a service organization that provides glasses to underserved clients. Recall that the International Lions Clubs (option 3) collects donated eyeglasses, which are then matched with recipients who lack the ability to obtain corrective lenses. Review the mission and service projects of the organizations listed if you had difficulty answering this question.*
> *Cognitive Level—Applying*
> *Client Needs Category—Health promotion and maintenance*
> *Client Needs Subcategory—None*

11. 2. Owing to an irregularly shaped cornea or lens, a person with astigmatism has unequal refraction of images on the retina. Therefore, there will be an area where objects appear more blurred or distorted (wider or taller) than they actually are. People with hyperopia see far objects more clearly. People with myopia can see near objects more clearly. No visual acuity disorder causes objects to appear unusually small.

> *Test Taking Strategy—Analyze to determine what information the question asks for, which is a statement describing the visual image caused by uncorrected astigmatism. Clients with astigmatism often describe seeing a blurred image that is distorted, similar to looking in a carnival mirror (option 2). Review the visual defect caused by astigmatism if you had difficulty answering this question.*
> *Cognitive Level—Applying*
> *Client Needs Category—Physiological integrity*
> *Client Needs Subcategory—Physiological adaptation*

12. 2. Glasses are washed first and wiped with a soft cloth to avoid scratching the surface with dirt and dust. Paper products such as paper tissues or towels should not be used for drying corrective lenses because they are made from wood pulp that can scratch the lens material. Plastic lenses scratch easily. Blowing to promote air drying is tedious and likely to leave streaks on the lenses.

> *Test Taking Strategy—Use the process of elimination to select the option that describes the best method for drying the lenses of eyeglasses after they have been washed. Options 1, 3, and 4 can be eliminated because they may scratch the lenses or would take too much time. Using a soft cloth (option 2) is the option that remains as the correct answer. A soft cloth contains fibers that are not abrasive. Review*

recommendations for cleaning and drying eyeglasses if you had difficulty answering this question.
> *Cognitive Level—Remembering*
> *Client Needs Category—Safe and effective care environment*
> *Client Needs Subcategory—Coordinated care*

13. 2. Anxiety occurs because a person feels threatened by an unexpected or unfamiliar situation. Hearing an explanation of care beforehand prepares a person for what is about to take place. The nurse should always speak before touching a blind client or one whose vision is obstructed by eye patches. Standing in front of a person when speaking may help a client who has a hearing disorder but not one who is blind. Having adequate light helps partially sighted clients, not those who cannot see.

> *Test Taking Strategy—Use the key words "most appropriate" to select the best option when communicating with a sightless client. Recall that telling a client what to expect (option 2), regardless of whether the anxious client is sighted or not, helps to decrease a stress response. Review communication techniques that reduce anxiety if you had difficulty answering this question.*
> *Cognitive Level—Applying*
> *Client Needs Category—Psychosocial integrity*
> *Client Needs Subcategory—None*

14. 1. A blind person feels safer and more secure by following the lead of someone who is sighted. This is best accomplished by having the blind person stand slightly behind and to the side while taking the sighted person's arm just above the elbow. Safety is a higher priority than total independence in an unfamiliar environment.

> *Test Taking Strategy—Use the process of elimination to help select the option that describes the best method for accompanying a blind client when ambulating. Options 2 and 3 can be eliminated immediately because they cause the client to feel pulled or pushed, a hazard to the client's safety. Option 4 can be eliminated because the client who walks independently is at risk for injury. Option 1 is the correct answer because letting the blind client take the sighted person's arm allows the client to remain about a half-step behind, which is a safer position. Recall that the optimum position is having the client walk slightly behind and to the side of the nurse if you had difficulty answering this question.*
> *Cognitive Level—Applying*
> *Client Needs Category—Safe and effective care environment*
> *Client Needs Subcategory—Safety and infection control*

15. 1. Using the imagery of a clock helps a blind client to locate food and self-feed. Feeding a client who has the ability to self-feed does not promote self-reliance.

Ordering liquid forms of nourishment without prior collaboration implies that the client is not capable of eating like an adult and may lower the client's self-esteem. Beverages in paper cups are more likely to spill during the client's attempts to eat independently and may reinforce a feeling of inadequacy.

Test Taking Strategy—Use the process of elimination to select the option that identifies the best way to preserve a blind client's self-reliance when eating. Recall that a blind client may continue to eat independently if the location of food is described by using clock imagery (option 1). Review techniques for preserving a blind client's independent self-care when performing activities of daily living if you had difficulty answering this question.
Cognitive Level—Applying
Client Needs Category—Psychosocial integrity
Client Needs Subcategory—None

16. **1.** A cataract is a clouding of the lens inside the eye which, to the client, is like looking through a frosty or fogged-up window. The visual change is due to degeneration of the eye lenses as a result of aging. A feeling of fullness and ocular pain or discomfort are more likely due to trauma or an inflammatory process. Seeing flashes of light is a symptom described by someone with a detached retina.

Test Taking Strategy—Analyze to determine what information the question asks for, which is a symptom in the client's health history that correlates with the development of cataracts. Recall that the function of the lens is to focus light on the retina. As cataracts, an opacity of the lens, become progressively worse, the client experiences diminished vision (option 1), which some describe as looking through a dirty window. Review the signs and symptoms associated with cataracts if you had difficulty answering this question.
Cognitive Level—Applying
Client Needs Category—Physiological integrity
Client Needs Subcategory—Physiological adaptation

17. **3.** When the eyes of someone with cataracts are examined, the usually black pupil appears white, gray, or yellow. This is due to an opacity of the lens, which lies behind the pupil, the opening in the center of the iris. Ruptured blood vessels on the eye are associated with conditions in which the blood pressure has been suddenly elevated, such as when performing Valsalva's maneuver while vomiting or defecating. An irregularly shaped iris can be the result of surgery performed for the treatment of glaucoma. Abnormal tissue may appear as a growth on the cornea.

Test Taking Strategy—Use the key words "most indicative" when selecting an option that describes an assessment finding that more closely relates to the appearance of a cataract than the other options. Recall that the lens, which is located behind the pupil, will change from transparent to cloudy (option 3) as the protein in its structure becomes

altered due to age-related changes. Review the clinical manifestations of cataract formation if you had difficulty answering this question.
Cognitive Level—Applying
Client Needs Category—Physiological integrity
Client Needs Subcategory—Physiological adaptation

18. **1.** The time for cataract removal is left to the client. It largely depends on the person's tolerance of the condition and the degree to which vision impairment interferes with the quality of life. Cataracts are painless. Feeling self-conscious about one's appearance is not necessarily a medically justifiable reason for pursuing surgery. Postponing surgery until a cataract reaches maximum density or "ripens" is no longer considered a standard of care.

Test Taking Strategy—Use the process of elimination to select the option that identifies a client's accurate understanding about when cataract surgery is indicated. Recall that the time to consider cataract surgery is relative to when it affects the client's quality of life (option 1). Review the conditions that indicate surgical removal of cataracts is appropriate if you had difficulty answering this question.
Cognitive Level—Analyzing
Client Needs Category—Health promotion and maintenance
Client Needs Subcategory—None

19. **2.** On reviewing the preoperative orders, it is especially important to note the time when anticoagulant medication was stopped. This is essential to reduce the risk of retrobulbar hemorrhage. Reviewing the last dose and time of medication allows the nurse to assess if the client has withheld the medication for the appropriate amount of time. Assessing for facial lesions and right eye drainage is appropriate to document preoperatively, but they are not as critical as documenting the last dose of anticoagulant medication. Eyestrain is a subjective finding that may also be documented preoperatively.

Test Taking Strategy—Analyze to determine what information the question asks for, which is the preoperative information that is more essential than any others. Recall that ensuring that the anticoagulant was stopped (option 2) is essential to the client's safety. Review the consequences that anticoagulant therapy can have on the outcome of surgery if you had difficulty answering this question.
Cognitive Level—Applying
Client Needs Category—Physiological Integrity
Client Needs Subcategory—Reduction of risk potential

20. **4.** Eyedrops and ointments are placed in the exposed lower conjunctival sac. The nurse should pull downward below the eye on the lower eyelid to form the conjunctival sac. If the eyedrops are placed on the cornea, they may cause discomfort and reflex blinking. Medication is systemically absorbed when instilled at the inner canthus. Placing eyedrops and ointments at the outer canthus makes it difficult to distribute them in the eye.

> *Test Taking Strategy*—*Analyze to determine what information the question asks for, which is the proper technique for instilling eyedrops. Recall that eyedrops are administered by pulling the lower eyelid down and instilling the medication in the conjunctival sac (being careful not to touch the dropper to the eye). Review the procedure for instilling medication in the eye if you had difficulty answering this question.*
> *Cognitive Level*—*Applying*
> *Client Needs Category*—*Physiological integrity*
> *Client Needs Subcategory*—*Pharmacological therapies*

21. 3. Coughing, vomiting, and other activities, such as straining or squeezing the eyelids together, are avoided to prevent an increase in intraocular pressure. Raising intraocular pressure strains the delicate sutures and may dislodge an implanted intraocular lens. All other interventions are appropriate for this client.

> *Test Taking Strategy*—*Analyze to determine what information the question asks for, which is an item in a standardized care plan that is inappropriate after a cataract extraction. Read the choices carefully because you are selecting the option that is contraindicated in this scenario. Recall that any activity, such as coughing, that increases intraocular pressure (option 3) may cause postoperative complications after cataract surgery. Review precautions that should be taken after a cataract extraction if you had difficulty answering this question.*
> *Cognitive Level*—*Applying*
> *Client Needs Category*—*Physiological integrity*
> *Client Needs Subcategory*—*Physiological adaptation*

22. 1. Severe pain is an indication that intraocular hemorrhage is occurring. It is essential to report this finding to the charge nurse or surgeon immediately. Giving an analgesic will mask the symptom, thereby diminishing its significance as a serious complication. Assessing the pupils will not reveal the cause of the symptom. The pupils will most likely be dilated and not respond to light. Postoperatively, cataract clients are not positioned on their operative side.

> *Test Taking Strategy*—*Look at the key words "most appropriate," indicating a priority. Recall that severe ocular postoperative pain is not normal and should be reported immediately. Review signs and symptoms of complications after cataract surgery if you had difficulty answering this question.*
> *Cognitive Level*—*Applying*
> *Client Needs Category*—*Physiological integrity*
> *Client Needs Subcategory*—*Physiological adaptation*

23. 2. A metal eye shield called a *Fox shield* is applied at night or before naps to prevent accidental injury to the operative eye. Although the shield is a mechanical barrier between the environment and the eye, its primary purpose is to prevent traumatic injury. Patching the eyes will not prevent the rapid eye movements that occur during sleep. If pupil dilation is necessary, drugs will be used to paralyze the ciliary muscle.

> *Test Taking Strategy*—*Analyze to determine what information the question asks for, which is the purpose for applying an eye shield postoperatively. Recall that an eye shield does what the name implies; it shields the eye from objects or movements that may injure the eye (option 2). Review methods for protecting the eye from injury after cataract surgery if you had difficulty answering this question.*
> *Cognitive Level*—*Applying*
> *Client Needs Category*—*Safe and effective care environment*
> *Client Needs Subcategory*—*Safety and infection control*

24. 1. Bending over is contraindicated for approximately 2 weeks after eye surgery because it puts strain on the operative sutures. It is unnecessary to keep both eyes patched at all times. The client may sleep with or without a pillow, but should be instructed to sleep only on the unaffected side for approximately 1 week to prevent pressure on the operative eye and reduce tissue edema. External bleeding is not expected at any time postoperatively. Intraocular bleeding, indicated by sudden eye pain, is considered a complication that necessitates immediate examination.

> *Test Taking Strategy*—*Note the key words "most appropriate," and apply them to select the option that identifies a discharge instruction that is more pertinent to a client having had cataract surgery than any of the others. Recall that any activity that increases intraocular pressure should be avoided. This includes straining at stool, coughing, sneezing, or bending from the waist (option 1). Review teaching that is appropriate before discharging a client who has had a cataract extracted if you had difficulty answering this question.*
> *Cognitive Level*—*Applying*
> *Client Needs Category*—*Safe and effective care environment*
> *Client Needs Subcategory*—*Coordinated care*

25. 4. Glaucoma is a progressive eye disease characterized by increased intraocular pressure resulting in atrophy of the optic nerve and possibly leading to blindness. The increased pressure is due to excessive fluid accumulation inside the eye. There are two types of glaucoma: angle-closure and open angle. Angle-closure glaucoma usually presents suddenly and is painful; open-angle glaucoma has a slower onset and few or no symptoms, until a gradual loss of the visual field occurs. Priority instruction includes information on the decreased visual field. Although open-angle glaucoma is not likely to cause significant symptoms, those who are affected generally describe a decrease in their peripheral vision. Itching and burning are most likely allergic responses. Headaches may occur when a client in need of corrective lenses strains to read. Clients with angle-closure glaucoma report seeing halos around lights.

Test Taking Strategy—Analyze to determine what information the question asks for, which is a symptom experienced by those with open-angle glaucoma. Recall that open-angle glaucoma causes a slow, progressive loss of peripheral vision (option 4) due to irreversible damage to the optic nerve. Review the signs and symptoms of both types of glaucoma if you had difficulty answering this question.
Cognitive Level—Analyzing
Client Needs Category—Physiological integrity
Client Needs Subcategory—Physiological adaptation

26. 2. The symptoms of glaucoma occur as a result of increased intraocular pressure. This condition is diagnosed using an instrument called a *tonometer*. There are many types of tonometers; one of the more common types is a Schiotz tonometer, which measures the depth of the impression made when a plunger is placed on the surface of the cornea. An ophthalmoscope is used for viewing the fundus or back portion of the eye. A retinoscope is used to measure visual acuity and determine refractory errors. A speculum is an instrument that widens a cavity.

Test Taking Strategy—Analyze to determine what information the question asks for, which is the instrument the nurse should have available when the physician wants to measure a client's intraocular pressure. Recall that a tonometer (option 2) measures tension or pressure, which in this case is the pressure resulting from excess fluid within the eye. Review the purpose for the instruments listed in the options if you had difficulty answering this question.
Cognitive Level—Remembering
Client Needs Category—Safe and effective care environment
Client Needs Subcategory—Coordinated care

27. 1. Chronic glaucoma causes a gradual loss of peripheral vision. If untreated, the visual field is reduced to only the image that is focused directly on the macula. Clients typically describe this as looking through a tube or tunnel. Double vision is due to neurologic diseases or a weakness in eye muscles. Bulging eyes, also called *exophthalmos*, accompanies hyperthyroidism. Inflamed eyes can be attributed to various irritating substances.

Test Taking Strategy—Look for the key words "most likely," which indicate the need to select an option that exclusively applies to the topic of the question. In this case, the answer is option 1 because as peripheral vision continues to be lost, the client will see only a narrow portion of the visual field. Remember that untreated glaucoma can cause a loss of peripheral vision that leads to tunnel vision if you had difficulty answering this question.

Cognitive Level—Applying
Client Needs Category—Physiological integrity
Client Needs Subcategory—Physiological adaptation

28.

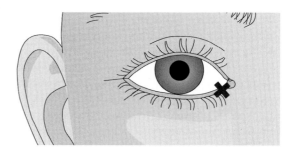

The correct technique is to apply a thin ribbon of ointment into the conjunctival pocket beginning at the inner canthus and moving to the outer canthus.

Test Taking Strategy—Analyze to determine what information the question asks for, which is the area where the application of eye ointment should begin. Recall that the medication is applied along the inner aspect of the lower eyelid medially to the nose and follows the length of the lid laterally. Review the procedure for applying eye ointment if you had difficulty answering this question.
Cognitive Level—Understanding
Client Needs Category—Health promotion and maintenance
Client Needs Subcategory—None

29. 3. Glaucoma can potentially lead to blindness and requires lifelong treatment with medication unless the condition is treated surgically. Hand washing and replacing the cap of the prescription container are aseptic measures that prevent the transmission of organisms within the eye. Timolol maleate (Timoptic) is a beta-adrenergic blocker that decreases aqueous humor formation without constricting the pupil.

Test Taking Strategy—Analyze to determine what information the question asks for, which is a statement by the client that demonstrates a need for additional teaching. Recall that increased intraocular pressure (IOP) can be managed with medications so that further damage to the optic nerve and loss of vision do not progress, but those medications must be self-administered throughout the client's lifetime (option 3). Even after IOP has been returned to a normal range, it will gradually increase if the client stops taking the prescribed medication. Review the prognosis for clients with glaucoma if you had difficulty answering this question.
Cognitive Level—Applying
Client Needs Category—Health promotion and maintenance
Client Needs Subcategory—None

30. 1. Atropine sulfate (Sal-Tropine) and other anticholinergic drugs dilate the pupil. This blocks the drainage of aqueous fluid. If administered, it may cause an acute attack by precipitating high intraocular pressure (IOP), which if left untreated can cause permanent blindness. Morphine sulfate (Roxanol) is an opioid analgesic. Magnesium sulfate is known as *Epsom salts* and is used for several purposes, especially to soothe musculoskeletal ailments and for relaxation. Ferrous sulfate (Feosol) is an iron preparation. None of these last three medications is contraindicated for clients with glaucoma.

> *Test Taking Strategy—Analyze to determine what information the question asks for, which is the drug that should be withheld if ordered for a client with glaucoma. Recall that any drug that dilates the pupil, such as atropine sulfate (option 1) or other anticholinergic or sympathomimetic drugs, will cause the lens to obstruct the flow of intraocular fluid moving through the canal of Schlemm, a circular drainage channel for aqueous fluid that leads to the venous circulation. Obstruction of fluid drainage raises IOP, which is already increased above normal range. Review the actions of each medication listed, looking for a reason one should be withheld if prescribed for a client with glaucoma if you had difficulty answering this question.*
> *Cognitive Level—Applying*
> *Client Needs Category—Physiological integrity*
> *Client Needs Subcategory—Pharmacological therapies*

31. 2. A client who experiences an acute increase in intraocular pressure (IOP) will have severe eye pain, nausea, vomiting, and loss of vision. Dangerously high ocular pressure is an emergency. A client with retinal detachment or hypertension typically describes seeing spots in the visual field. During an acute attack of angle-closure glaucoma, the pupils are widely dilated; treatment involves administering drugs that both constrict the pupils and eliminate intraocular fluid. The eyes appear normal in size even during an acute attack of angle-closure glaucoma, but the cornea and conjunctive become red and steamy in appearance.

> *Test Taking Strategy—Analyze to determine what information the question asks for, which is an assessment finding associated with increased IOP. Recall that the sudden obstruction of fluid drainage sends the pressure skyrocketing, causing severe eye pain (option 2). Review the signs and symptoms that develop in acute angle-closure glaucoma if you had difficulty answering this question.*
> *Cognitive Level—Applying*
> *Client Needs Category—Physiological integrity*
> *Client Needs Subcategory—Physiological adaptation*

32. 2, 3, 6. In both open-angle glaucoma and angle-closure glaucoma, the visual field examination indicates a loss of vision. Also, clients with either type of glaucoma are initially treated with medication. Surgical

management is required if medication therapy is unsuccessful.

In some cases, clients with open-angle glaucoma (a chronic form of the disease) are asymptomatic and may not realize that they have glaucoma until undergoing a routine eye examination. However, many clients experience eye discomfort, temporary blurred vision, and reduced peripheral vision. Clients with angle-closure glaucoma (an acute condition also known as narrow-angle glaucoma) experience sudden onset of symptoms. The eyes become rock hard and painful, and nausea and vomiting may occur. Each subsequent attack harms the eye.

> *Test Taking Strategy—Analyze to determine what information the question asks for, which are characteristics common to both types of glaucoma. Alternative-format "select all that apply" questions require considering each option independently to decide its merit in answering the question. Choose the options that identify symptoms shared by those who have either type of glaucoma. Compare the signs and symptoms of glaucoma in a reference, looking for similarities among the two types, if you had difficulty answering this question.*
> *Cognitive Level—Analyzing*
> *Client Needs Category—Physiological integrity*
> *Client Needs Subcategory—Physiological adaptation*

33. 4. An iridectomy involves removing a piece of the iris to allow aqueous fluid to flow from the posterior chamber into the anterior chamber through the trabecular meshwork and out the canal of Schlemm. Intense heat is used to create this opening for drainage. The iris no longer appears perfectly round postoperatively; the missing section appears black.

> *Test Taking Strategy—Analyze to determine what information the question asks for, which is the appearance of the eye after an iridectomy. Recall that the lens lies behind the iris, the center of which is the dark pupil. When a portion of the iris is removed, it changes the round appearance of the pupil; a section of the iris also appears black (option 4). Review the anatomic change in structure and appearance after a portion of the iris is removed if you had difficulty answering this question.*
> *Cognitive Level—Applying*
> *Client Needs Category—Physiological integrity*
> *Client Needs Subcategory—Physiological adaptation*

34. 2. The retina is the neurosensory layer of tissue on the innermost posterior surface of the eye. The retina contains rods and cones, which are necessary for color and black and white vision. Light that comes into the eye via the lens is focused onto the retina. The retina's photoreceptors convert the light into electrical impulses that are relayed to the optic nerve and ultimately to the brain for interpretation. Retinal detachment, the separation of retinal pigment epithelium from the sensory layer, has multiple etiologies. Common causes include trauma (such as occurs with a fall or a blow to the head), myopia, and degenerative changes. Aging is a factor, but the most common period for retinal detachment is between ages 50 and 60. Glaucoma may result in retinal detachment, but the opposite is not generally true. There is no causal relationship between retinal detachment and glaucoma

> *Test Taking Strategy—Look for the key words "most likely," indicating that one answer is better than the others. Recall that trauma to the head (option 2) may create sufficient force at the moment of impact to cause compression followed by decompression within the orbit of the eye, resulting in a retinal tear. Review etiologies of retinal detachment if you had difficulty answering this question.*
> **Cognitive Level**—*Applying*
> **Client Needs Category**—*Physiological integrity*
> **Client Needs Subcategory**—*Reduction of risk potential*

35. 3. The purpose for patching the eyes of a client with a detached retina is to keep the eyes at rest; therefore, patches are applied to both eyes with the eyelids closed. Keeping the eyelids closed also protects the eyes from contact with dust or fibers and prevents the eyes from becoming dry because blinking is difficult once the eyes are patched. Light is not necessarily harmful, but it may cause the client to look about rather than resting the eyes. Gravity rather than pressure has some therapeutic value when treating a detached retina. Patching the eyes but facilitating vision is a contradiction in therapeutic principles.

> *Test Taking Strategy—Look for the key words "most appropriate," indicating that one answer is better than the others. Until surgical treatment is performed, contact between the retina and choroid is promoted preoperatively through bed rest and patching both eyes. This prevents unnecessary head movement (option 3) and worsening of the detachment. Review the preoperative management of a client with a retinal detachment if you had difficulty answering this question.*
> **Cognitive Level**—*Applying*
> **Client Needs Category**—*Physiological integrity*
> **Client Needs Subcategory**—*Reduction of risk potential*

36. 2. It is important for the nurse to indicate when leaving because the client whose eyes are patched has no visual cue as to whether the nurse is still in the room. The client would find it frustrating and embarrassing to carry on a conversation if no one is there to respond. Straightening the client's linens, offering a back rub, and sharing current events are acts of kindness and good nursing care but do not specifically help to maintain the client's dignity.

> *Test Taking Strategy—Use the process of elimination to select the option that identifies the best nursing action for preserving the client's dignity before leaving the room. Options 1, 3, and 4 are good nursing care but do not specifically address the emotional needs of this*

client. *Review appropriate communication techniques when caring for a client whose vision is impaired if you had difficulty answering this question.*
> **Cognitive Level**—*Applying*
> **Client Needs Category**—*Psychosocial integrity*
> **Client Needs Subcategory**—*None*

37. 1. Bed rest and bilateral patching is a conservative treatment that relies on the principle of gravity to help reattach the separated retina. This approach is common before surgical alternatives are considered. Explaining the purpose of bed rest may help the client to comply with the prescribed therapy. Asking whether the client wants to be permanently blind may heighten anxiety. Although sedatives are sometimes prescribed, this situation does not warrant the added risks caused by sedation. Responding in a superficial, belittling manner, as in the last option, implies that the client's question is frivolous.

> *Test Taking Strategy—Use the process of elimination to select the option that provides the best response to the client's question. Options 2 and 4 can be eliminated because they are examples of nontherapeutic communication techniques. Option 3 can be eliminated because it describes an unnecessary and inappropriate nursing action. Recall that providing information that is accurate and honest helps facilitate a client's understanding and ultimately his or her cooperation. Review therapeutic and nontherapeutic communication techniques if you had difficulty answering this question and does not answer the question that the client asked.*
> **Cognitive Level**—*Applying*
> **Client Needs Category**—*Psychosocial integrity*
> **Client Needs Subcategory**—*None*

38. 2. Scleral buckling is a surgical procedure that takes a tuck in the sclera, thereby ultimately decreasing the size of the eyeball. This facilitates contact between the choroid and the retina, repairing a detachment. An increase in intraocular pressure, which occurs with vomiting, could damage the surgical repair; therefore, vomiting requires prompt treatment. The client requires an antiemetic; if one was not ordered, the nurse must notify the charge nurse or physician immediately. Pain is expected after surgery for a detached retina. Although pain causes discomfort, its treatment should not affect the outcome of the surgical procedure. Anxiety and fatigue are not physiologic problems and therefore do not rank as high on the list of priorities.

> *Test Taking Strategy—Use the process of elimination to select the postoperative problem that represents the highest priority for nursing action. Recall that vomiting (option 2) is a nursing priority because if not controlled, it can raise intraocular pressure and the risk for postoperative complications. Review the postoperative risks caused by vomiting, hiccupping, heavy lifting, or strenuous exercise after retinal surgery if you had difficulty answering this question.*

Cognitive Level—Applying
Client Needs Category—Physiological integrity
Client Needs Subcategory—Reduction of risk potential

39. 3. Radial keratotomy is performed to reshape the cornea so visual images converge directly on the retina. If the procedure is successful, the client should no longer require corrective lenses. Radial keratotomy does not improve night vision, correct color blindness, or facilitate binocular vision.

Test Taking Strategy—Use the process of elimination to select the option that provides the best evidence that the client understands the outcome of a LASIK procedure. Option 1 can be eliminated because night vision is facilitated by rhodopsin, a protein that requires an adequate intake of food containing vitamin A. Option 2 can be eliminated because color blindness is primarily a genetically inherited defect. Option 4 can be eliminated because the lack of binocular vision may be due to amblyopia (lazy eye) or strabismus (crossed eyes), which is corrected with eye exercises or surgery. Option 3 remains as the correct answer because radial keratotomy changes the shape of the cornea and corrects refractive errors. Review the purpose for performing laser keratotomy (LASIK) if you had difficulty answering this question.
Cognitive Level—Applying
Client Needs Category—Physiological integrity
Client Needs Subcategory—Physiological adaptation

40. 1. A client with pinkeye, a common name for viral or bacterial conjunctivitis, will have an obviously inflamed conjunctiva, sticky or crusty drainage that collects on the lid, itching or burning of the eyes, and possible edema of the eyelid. The disorder does not affect pupil response. The eyelid may be swollen, but the eye itself should not protrude. Tearing may be excessive.

Test Taking Strategy—Analyze to determine what information the question asks for, which is a sign of conjunctivitis (pinkeye) besides an inflamed appearance. If bacteria cause conjunctivitis, yellow or green drainage that tends to crust overnight (option 1) will be present. Viral conjunctivitis is more likely to be accompanied by a watery discharge that adheres to the lids as it dries. Allergies and exposure to irritating substances may also cause conjunctivitis. Review the signs and symptoms associated with conjunctivitis if you had difficulty answering this question.
Cognitive Level—Applying
Client Needs Category—Physiological integrity
Client Needs Subcategory—Physiological adaptation

41. 3. Using individual bath linens and performing frequent hand washing are techniques for preventing the transmission of infectious microorganisms present in the inflammatory secretions of a client with conjunctivitis.

Eating a nutritious diet and wearing sunglasses to filter ultraviolet light are healthful behaviors, but they are unrelated to the client's disorder. The use of aspirin is not contraindicated; in fact, a mild analgesic may relieve some of the client's discomfort.

Test Taking Strategy—Look for the key words "most important," indicating a priority. Recall that viral or bacterial conjunctivitis is quite contagious, especially among young children, who are not conscientious about hand hygiene. To prevent transmission of the infectious agent, anything that has been handled or used to clean the eyes such as wash cloths or towels (option 3) should be dedicated for use by the infected individual and not used in common with others. Review the etiologies of infectious conjunctivitis and methods for controlling the transmission of the causative organisms if you had difficulty answering this question.
Cognitive Level—Applying
Client Needs Category—Health promotion and maintenance
Client Needs Subcategory—None

42. 4. Fluorescein is a tissue-staining substance that is applied topically to assess the condition of the cornea, including the presence of foreign bodies or lesions. Povidone-iodine (Betadine) and gentian violet are used for their antimicrobial properties rather than for diagnostic purposes. Methylene blue is used to stain pathology slides.

Test Taking Strategy—Analyze to determine what information the question asks for, which is the substance that is used to examine the cornea to locate a foreign body. Recall that fluorescein (option 4) is an orange dye that will cause a foreign body or superficial scratches on the surface of the cornea to appear green when a blue light is directed at the eye. Review how a foreign body within the eye is detected if you had difficulty answering this question.
Cognitive Level—Understanding
Client Needs Category—Physiological integrity
Client Needs Subcategory—Pharmacological therapies

43. 2. The macula is a part of the retina that helps people see images in fine detail. Macular degeneration is an eye disorder that results in a change in blood supply to the macula, the point where light rays converge to provide the clearest and most distinct visual image. Having lost macular function, the client is left with what appears to the client as a bull's eye visual defect. Peripheral vision remains, but it is insufficient to read or perform other activities that require acute vision.

Test Taking Strategy—Note the key words "most likely," and use them to select an option that best describes the type of vision a person with macular degeneration develops. Recall that when the macula degenerates, only images in the peripheral field of vision (option 2) can be seen. Review the function

of the macula, focusing on the outcome of macular degeneration, if you had difficulty answering this question.
Cognitive Level—*Applying*
Client Needs Category—*Physiological integrity*
Client Needs Subcategory—*Physiological adaptation*

44. 2. Clients with diabetes mellitus are at risk for developing vascular pathology in the retina. Their retinal blood vessels tend to weaken and bleed. Loss of vision is delayed or prevented when weakened and bleeding retinal blood vessels are treated early with photocoagulation using a laser or by having a vitrectomy performed. Clients who take aspirin, are lactose intolerant, or have an artificial pacemaker are not at any higher risk for ophthalmologic complications than the general population.

> **Test Taking Strategy**—*Analyze to determine what information the question asks for, which is the condition that puts a client at risk for developing pathology involving the eye. Recall that one of the complications of diabetes mellitus is diabetic retinopathy, which may lead to blindness. Review the complications of diabetes mellitus, especially retinopathy, if you had difficulty answering this question.*
> **Cognitive Level**—*Applying*
> **Client Needs Category**—*Health promotion and maintenance*
> **Client Needs Subcategory**—*None*

45. 3. Enucleation is the removal of the eyeball from the eye socket, but the muscles surrounding the eyeball are usually left intact. After an enucleation, clients are taught how to remove, clean, and replace the shell-shaped prosthetic eye. The prosthetic eye is only cosmetic, not functional. A conformer, which is a round implant, is inserted during surgery to maintain the shape of the eye and prevent shrinkage of the surrounding tissue. The conformer remains permanently in place; the prosthesis is not inserted until healing takes place, which typically is approximately 4 to 6 weeks postoperatively.

> **Test Taking Strategy**—*Look for the key words "best evidence," indicating that one answer is better than the others. Recall that even though the contents of the eye socket are removed, a permanent conformer is implanted to maintain the shape and contour of the eye socket. A prosthesis that occupies the space between the eyelids lies on the surface of the conformer; it is removed for cleaning (option 3) on a weekly, monthly, or bi-monthly schedule. Review the care of an ocular prosthesis if you had difficulty answering this question.*
> **Cognitive Level**—*Applying*
> **Client Needs Category**—*Health promotion and maintenance*
> **Client Needs Subcategory**—*None*

46. 2. The cornea serves the eye in two ways. First, it protects the eye from dust, debris, and pathogens. Second, it controls and focuses the light that enters the eye. Corneal transplants are performed when the cornea is thinning, scarring because of infection or injury is present, or the cornea is cloudy. Signs of corneal transplant rejection include redness, loss of vision, and sensitivity to light. Tearing, blinking, and itching would require medical assessment; however, they are not the most significant symptoms that indicate corneal tissue rejection.

> **Test Taking Strategy**—*Use the process of elimination to select the option that is most suggestive of corneal transplant rejection. Option 3 can be immediately eliminated because itching correlates more with a minor allergic response to an airborne antigen. Although a corneal rejection may be accompanied by eye irritation such as tearing and frequent blinking (options 1 and 4), they are not as ominous as diminished vision (option 2). Review the symptoms that accompany rejection of a corneal transplant if you had difficulty answering this question.*
> **Cognitive Level**—*Applying*
> **Client Needs Category**—*Physiological integrity*
> **Client Needs Subcategory**—*Reduction of risk potential*

Nursing Care of Clients with Disorders of Accessory Eye Structures

47. 4. Incomplete closure of the eyelids leads to dry eyes. The tarsal muscles within the lids are generally atonic due to age and loss of superficial fat in the face; consequently, lid spasms are unlikely. Topical medications are used to treat the symptoms, but surgery or injections of botulinum toxin may provide a more permanent cosmetic and functional solution. Neither double vision nor light sensitivity is a common manifestation of structural disorders of the lids.

> **Test Taking Strategy**—*Analyze to determine what information the question asks for, which is a problem that results from an eyelid that droops. Recall that the eyelids protect the eye from external debris and keep the eye moist; the cornea and conjunctiva become dry (option 4) and the client may object to the change in appearance. Review the effect of incomplete eyelid closure on external structures of the eye if you had difficulty answering this question.*
> **Cognitive Level**—*Applying*
> **Client Needs Category**—*Physiological integrity*
> **Client Needs Subcategory**—*Physiological adaptation*

48. **1.** Blepharitis, an inflammation of the eyelid margin, is commonly associated with excessive oiliness of the skin, face, and scalp. In most cases, more frequent washing of the face and hair relieves the symptoms. In chronic or severe conditions, clients improve with the additional use of a topical antibiotic ointment. Limiting dietary fat, using fluorescent lighting, and eating more deep yellow vegetables are good lifestyle choices, but they will not decrease or remove secretions from the sebaceous glands in the eyelids.

> *Test Taking Strategy—Look at the key words "most appropriate," indicating that one option is better than the others. Option 1 is the best choice because keeping the face and hair clean will reduce and remove excessive oil. Review methods for managing blepharitis if you had difficulty answering this question.*
> *Cognitive Level—Applying*
> *Client Needs Category—Physiological integrity*
> *Client Needs Subcategory—Basic care and comfort*

49. **2.** A stye (hordeolum) is a bacterial infection within a meibomian gland, a special type of sebaceous gland at the rim of the eyelids. Warm, moist heat improves circulation to the area that is inflamed and swollen. Vasodilation relieves the edema and promotes a reduction in exudate via absorption or phagocytosis. Incision and drainage may become necessary, but a physician should do this, not the client. Covering the lesion disguises the appearance of the stye, but it does not provide any therapeutic benefit.

> *Test Taking Strategy—Use the process of elimination to select the option that provides the best nursing advice for relieving the discomfort caused by a stye. Options 2 and 3 can be eliminated immediately because squeezing or piercing the stye may introduce additional pathogens into the impaired skin. Option 4 can be eliminated because it conceals the stye but will not reduce its discomfort. Option 2 remains as the correct answer because warm, moist applications will relieve the symptoms and facilitate healing. Review the manner in which a stye is treated, focusing on measures for relieving discomfort, if you had difficulty answering this question.*
> *Cognitive Level—Applying*
> *Client Needs Category—Physiological integrity*
> *Client Needs Subcategory—Physiological adaptation*

50. **3.** A chalazion, a cyst that forms in an obstructed meibomian gland within the eyelid, tends to be minor. If gentle massage fails to relieve the obstruction, office surgery is performed to excise the cystlike growth of tissue. A chalazion is more likely to produce a sensation of pressure than of pain. The eyelashes are lost from seborrheic blepharitis, not a chalazion. Blindness is not commonly associated with a chalazion.

> *Test Taking Strategy—Analyze to determine what information the question asks for, which is correct information about a persistent chalazion. Recall that*

as a chalazion continues to increase in size, it may eventually impair the client's vision, necessitating surgical removal (option 3). Review how a chalazion is managed if you had difficulty answering this question.
> *Cognitive Level—Applying*
> *Client Needs Category—Physiological integrity*
> *Client Needs Subcategory—Reduction of risk potential*

Nursing Care of Clients with Ear Disorders

51. **3.** Musicians and others who are exposed to excessively loud sounds without ear protection can acquire sensorineural hearing loss. There is no significant evidence that occupations involving computer programming, using the telephone, or teaching in a classroom are associated with impaired hearing.

> *Test Taking Strategy—Note the key words "most likely," indicating that one answer is better than the others. Recall that the hair cells of the organ of Corti in the inner ear are sensitive to loud sounds. Sound is measured in decibels (dB). Ear protection should be worn if exposed to sounds that exceed 85 dB. The sound at a rock concert is generally between 120 dB and 150 dB, which can cause permanent hearing loss to musicians (option 3). Compare the sound levels to which persons in each of the occupations listed are exposed if you had difficulty answering this question.*
> *Cognitive Level—Applying*
> *Client Needs Category—Physiological integrity*
> *Client Needs Subcategory—Basic care and comfort*

52. **1.** The accumulation of normal cerumen is best removed by washing the ears with soapy water and a soft cloth. Hard and sharp objects can injure the ear canal or tympanic membrane. A medical referral is appropriate only if the cerumen is excessively hard or impacted.

> *Test Taking Strategy—Use the process of elimination to select the option that identifies the best method for cleaning the ears. Cleaning the ears with a soapy washcloth (option 1) is the best method because it is preferable hygienically and will not cause ear trauma. Review recommendations for removing accumulated cerumen if you had difficulty answering this question.*
> *Cognitive Level—Applying*
> *Client Needs Category—Health promotion and maintenance*
> *Client Needs Subcategory—None*

53. **2.** A tuning fork is used to test for conductive and sensorineural hearing loss. Weber's test is performed by striking the tuning fork and placing it centrally on the forehead. The Rinne test is performed by striking the tuning fork and placing it on the mastoid bone and beside the ear. An otoscope is used to inspect the physical structures in the external ear. A reflex hammer is used to test deep tendon responses. A stethoscope is used to auscultate body sounds.

> *Test Taking Strategy—Note the key words "most appropriate," which indicate that one option is better than the others. Select the option that identifies the instrument a nurse uses to test a client's ability to hear sound. Recall that a tuning fork (option 2) is used to determine how well or poorly a client hears sound, whether sound is perceived equally in both ears or is heard better in one ear than the other. Review the purpose for using the instruments listed, focusing on the one that is best for testing a client's ability to hear, if you had difficulty answering this question.*
> **Cognitive Level**—*Applying*
> **Client Needs Category**—*Health promotion and maintenance*
> **Client Needs Subcategory**—*None*

54. 4. Tinnitus, ringing or buzzing in the ears, is a common symptom experienced by people who take repeated, high dosages of aspirin. Although tinnitus is associated with many ear disorders and a few occupations, the other questions posed by the nurse do not necessarily help to establish a cause-and-effect relationship with the client's symptom.

> *Test Taking Strategy—Note the key words "most appropriate," and select the option that identifies a question that correlates with determining an etiology for the client's symptom better than the others. Recall that tinnitus may develop in clients from prolonged self-administration of high doses of aspirin (option 4), but the condition can be relieved once aspirin is discontinued. Review the side effects associated with aspirin therapy if you had difficulty answering this question.*
> **Cognitive Level**—*Applying*
> **Client Needs Category**—*Physiological integrity*
> **Client Needs Subcategory**—*Reduction of risk potential*

55. 1. Feedback, a loud shrill noise, occurs when a hearing aid is positioned incorrectly within the ear. Cleaning, replacing the battery, and regulating the volume are important considerations for the client with a hearing aid, but they do not affect feedback.

> *Test Taking Strategy—Look at the key words "most helpful," indicating that one answer is better than the others. Recall that feedback is generally due to a malposition of the hearing aid within the ear. Removing and replacing the hearing aid so it is more compatible with the ear anatomy tends to eliminate the problem. Review the causes of hearing aid feedback and how it can be managed if you had difficulty answering this question.*
> **Cognitive Level**—*Understanding*
> **Client Needs Category**—*Health promotion and maintenance*
> **Client Needs Subcategory**—*None*

56. 3. The aminoglycoside family of antibiotics, of which gentamicin sulfate (Garamycin) is one example, is ototoxic and nephrotoxic. Beta-adrenergic blockers cause vertigo but do not affect hearing acuity. Neither nonsteroidal anti-inflammatory drugs nor H_2 antagonists are known to be ototoxic.

> *Test Taking Strategy—Analyze to determine what information the question asks for, which is a category of drugs that is known to cause hearing loss. Recall that ototoxicity is among the side effects caused by aminoglycoside antibiotics (option 3). Review the side effects of the drug categories listed, focusing on their potential for ototoxicity, if you had difficulty answering this question.*
> **Cognitive Level**—*Analyzing*
> **Client Needs Category**—*Physiological integrity*
> **Client Needs Subcategory**—*Pharmacological therapies*

57. 1. The external ear canal is a curved tube that is about 1" (2.5 cm) long and extends from the auricle, the flared end of the ear, to the tympanic membrane. The ear canal lies within the temporal bone, the growth of which is not complete in an infant and child; thus, the angle for straightening the canal differs depending on the client's age. The correct technique for straightening the ear canal of an adult is to pull the ear upward and backward. For a child, the ear is pulled downward and backward.

> *Test Taking Strategy—Analyze to determine what information the question asks for, which is an accurate description of the method for straightening the ear canal of an adult. Recall that pulling the auricle up and back (option 1) straightens the ear canal of an adult. Review the anatomic differences between the ears of an adult versus those of a child and the manner in which each is manipulated to straighten the ear canal if you had difficulty answering this question.*
> **Cognitive Level**—*Understanding*
> **Client Needs Category**—*Physiological integrity*
> **Client Needs Subcategory**—*Pharmacological therapies*

58. 1. Keeping the head tilted to the side for at least 5 minutes or maintaining a side-lying position facilitates the movement of the medication to the lowest area of the ear canal. Cotton is loosely inserted within the ear to collect drainage and any excess volume of medication; therefore, wiping away remnants of the drug is unnecessary. The eustachian tube does connect the middle ear with the pharynx. However, if the tympanic membrane is intact, blowing the nose will not displace the medication.

> *Test Taking Strategy—Note the key words "most appropriate," which should alert you to the fact that one option is preferable to the others. Select the option that identifies the best instruction after instilling medication within the ear. Recall that before administering the medication, the client tilts his or her head away from the affected ear. Keeping the head tilted tempo-*

rarily (option 1) facilitates gravity flow of the medication to the end of the ear canal. Review the procedure for administering medication within the external ear if you had difficulty answering this question.
***Cognitive Level**—Applying*
***Client Needs Category**—Physiological integrity*
***Client Needs Subcategory**—Reduction of risk potential*

59. 1. *Otitis externa* is the medical term for an inflammatory process that involves the external ear. The presence of drainage, called *otorrhea*, is most suggestive that an inflammation is the underlying problem. Because the drainage is foul-smelling, the inflammation is most likely due to a pathogen. Hearing is diminished from swelling and drainage that block the transmission of sound on air currents, but other preinfectious factors can also cause a loss of hearing. Scarring of the tympanic membrane is not an indication that there is a current infection. It may, however, indicate that the tympanic membrane ruptured during a prior middle ear infection and is now healed. Enlarged lymph nodes are indicative of a systemic inner ear infection.

> *Test Taking Strategy—Use the process of elimination to select the option that identifies the assessment finding that is most indicative of an infection in the external ear. Recall that redness, swelling, and tenderness are classic signs of an inflammation. Drainage that is present in or from the external ear (option 1) suggests that the exudate contains white blood cells that are localizing the source of the infection and removing debris. Review the significance of foul-smelling drainage from the ear if you had difficulty answering this question.*
> ***Cognitive Level**—Applying*
> ***Client Needs Category**—Physiological integrity*
> ***Client Needs Subcategory**—Physiological adaptation*

60. 1. Microorganisms travel more easily through a pathway between the nose and eustachian tube that is short and straight, which is the case in infants and young children. With growth, the ear canal changes to a 45-degree angle. This natural curved angle provides a barrier against ascending pathogens.

> *Test Taking Strategy—Analyze to determine what information the question asks for, which is the reason young children have more ear infections than older persons. Recall that the anatomic difference between the ear canals of young children and adults explains why pathogens migrate more easily to the middle ear in young children. The ear canals of young children are shorter and straighter than those of adults (option 1). Review the anatomy of the eustachian tube and middle ear, comparing a young child's with that of an adult, if you had difficulty answering this question.*
> ***Cognitive Level**—Applying*
> ***Client Needs Category**—Health promotion and maintenance*
> ***Client Needs Subcategory**—None*

61.

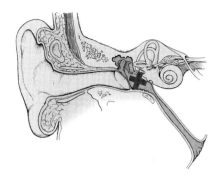

The middle ear, which is the site of the client's infection, is a small, air-filled cavity in the temporal bone. The eustachian tube extends from the floor of the middle ear to the pharynx and is lined with mucous membrane. A chain of three small bones—the malleus, the incus, and the stapes—stretches across the middle ear cavity from the tympanic membrane to the oval window.

> *Test Taking Strategy—Analyze to determine what information the question asks for, which is the location of the middle ear. Review the structures of the middle ear and their locations in relation to the external and inner ear if you had difficulty answering this question.*
> ***Cognitive Level**—Applying*
> ***Client Needs Category**—Physiological integrity*
> ***Client Needs Subcategory**—Physiological adaptation*

62. 4. Antibiotic efficacy is most evident when the client's ear discomfort is relieved. The inflamed area in the middle ear is beyond the reach of the fingers; therefore, assessing the temperature of the tissue by touch is impossible. Tinnitus, or disturbing sounds, is not generally a problem for a person during the acute phase of a middle ear infection. Watery or purulent drainage is an indication that the eardrum is perforated.

> *Test Taking Strategy—Use the process of elimination to select the option that identifies the best evidence that antibiotic therapy is having a therapeutic effect. The best evidence of effectiveness from among the four options is when the pain due to pressure from an accumulation of inflammatory exudates has been relieved (option 4). Review the desired outcome when antibiotics are used to treat an infection in the middle ear if you had difficulty answering this question.*
> ***Cognitive Level**—Applying*
> ***Client Needs Category**—Physiological integrity*
> ***Client Needs Subcategory**—Pharmacological therapies*

63. 4. The labyrinth, which is another name for the inner ear, contains structures that are responsible for both hearing and balance. Balance and equilibrium are maintained by receptors that sense rotation, acceleration, and deceleration of the body as it responds to gravitational changes. Structures in the vestibular pathway of the inner ear carry impulses via the eighth cranial nerve to the cerebellum in the brain. The cerebellum restores balance and postural stability by facilitating a correction from the motor cortex to skeletal muscles. When the labyrinth becomes infected, its functions are disrupted. Signs of labyrinthitis (inflammation of the labyrinth of the inner ear) include dizziness, nausea, vomiting, and nystagmus. Headaches indicate that the infection has extended to the meningeal area of the brain. Sore throat and nasal congestion are more likely caused by the primary upper respiratory infection, which commonly precedes a middle ear infection.

> *Test Taking Strategy*—Look at the key words "most indicative," indicating that one answer is better than any of the others. Recall that a disturbance in vestibular function interferes with balance, which some describe as a spinning sensation (option 4). Review the structures and function of the inner ear, especially those that promote balance, if you had difficulty answering this question.
> *Cognitive Level*—Understanding
> *Client Needs Category*—Physiological integrity
> *Client Needs Subcategory*—Physiological adaptation

64. 2. A *myringotomy*, which is the term for incising the tympanic membrane or eardrum, provides a pathway for drainage from the middle ear. As the exudate drains, the client's discomfort is reduced. A surgical incision is preferable to spontaneous rupture of the eardrum because a surgical incision heals better. In most situations, a *tympanoplasty*, the insertion of plastic tubes within the incised eardrum, is performed at the same time. The plastic tubes, which may remain in the ear for several months, equalize the air pressure within the middle ear when the natural pathway between the eustachian tube and middle ear is impaired. Although hearing may be permanently diminished by repeated middle ear infections, the potential for infection and the severity of future infections is reduced after the tympanic membrane is incised. Systemic antibiotics rather than topical drugs are more effective in treating a middle ear infection. Incising the eardrum is not done to preserve the motion of the ossicles in the middle ear.

> *Test Taking Strategy*—Use the process of elimination to select the option that identifies the best explanation for a myringotomy procedure. Recall that a myringotomy reduces excessive fluid pressure and discomfort by providing a pathway for drainage from the middle ear (option 2). Review the purpose for performing a myringotomy if you had difficulty answering this question.
> *Cognitive Level*—Applying
> *Client Needs Category*—Physiological integrity
> *Client Needs Subcategory*—Physiological adaptation

65. 2. Loosely packed cotton is more likely to absorb drainage than tightly packed cotton. The cotton ball should be replaced when it is moist, not totally saturated. The ear canal is generally cleaned using soap and water before inserting another dry cotton ball.

> *Test Taking Strategy*—Look at the key words "most important," indicating one answer is significantly better than the others. Recall that a compacted cotton ball will reduce the capacity of the fibers to absorb drainage, so positioning it loosely within the ear (option 2) is more effective. Review the procedure for replacing a cotton ball after a myringotomy if you had difficulty answering this question.
> *Cognitive Level*—Applying
> *Client Needs Category*—Physiological integrity
> *Client Needs Subcategory*—Reduction of risk potential

66. 4. Otosclerosis is the result of bony overgrowth of the stapes, a bone of the middle ear, and is a common cause of hearing impairments in adults. Although the cause of otosclerosis is unknown, most of those affected have a family history of this condition. The onset of this disorder usually becomes apparent when clients are in their 20s or 30s. High fever and removal of the tonsils or adenoids have no relationship to the development of otosclerosis.

> *Test Taking Strategy*—Analyze to determine what information the question asks for, which is an etiology that relates to otosclerosis. Recall that there is a familial predisposition for developing otosclerosis (option 4). Review the etiology and pathophysiology of otosclerosis if you had difficulty answering this question.
> *Cognitive Level*—Applying
> *Client Needs Category*—Physiological integrity
> *Client Needs Subcategory*—Physiological adaptation

67. 1. A conductive hearing loss occurs when there is a barrier in the transmission of vibrating sound waves from the external and middle ear to the inner ear. Common causes of conductive hearing loss include otosclerosis, otitis media, and a ruptured tympanic membrane. In otosclerosis, if the ossicles (the bones in the middle ear) are fused by a bony overgrowth, they no longer vibrate freely against the oval window (the membrane between the middle and inner ear) to transmit sound. The other options all describe the causes of sensorineural hearing loss.

> *Test Taking Strategy*—Note the key words "most accurately," which indicate that one option provides a better explanation than the others. Recall that a conductive hearing loss means that there is a disturbance in the transmission of sound waves entering the outer ear and moving through the middle and inner ear (option 1). Review the differences between conductive hearing loss and sensorineural hearing loss if you had difficulty answering this question.
> *Cognitive Level*—Applying
> *Client Needs Category*—Physiological integrity
> *Client Needs Subcategory*—Physiological adaptation

68. 1. Responding appropriately to communication with staff indicates an ability to understand the information that is being discussed despite impaired hearing. Accomplishing this goal indicates that the approaches used by the staff to communicate with the hearing-impaired client are effective. The goal should not indicate what the nursing team hopes to accomplish. The client with normal speech but decreased hearing does not have difficulty verbally communicating to staff or expressing emotions.

> *Test Taking Strategy—Use the process of elimination to select the option that identifies the best goal for the nursing diagnosis that has been identified. Option 2 can be eliminated because this does not describe a client-centered goal. Options 3 and 4 can be eliminated because these are not difficulties of the hearing-impaired client. Recall that the goal must show how the problem is ultimately reduced or eliminated. Review the principles for establishing goals for nursing diagnoses if you had difficulty answering this question.*
>
> **Cognitive Level**—*Analyzing*
> **Client Needs Category**—*Safe and effective care environment*
> **Client Needs Subcategory**—*Coordinated care*

69. 2. It is best to face a hearing-impaired client so that lip movements and facial expressions are seen because most hearing-impaired persons learn to adapt by lip reading or speech reading. Speaking into the client's ear distorts the words and masks visual cues. Dropping the voice causes some of the words to be missed. Raising or lowering the voice pitch helps persons with hearing loss in one or the other vocal registers. High tones are generally more difficult to hear.

> *Test Taking Strategy—Look at the key words "most appropriate," indicating one option has precedence over the others. Recall that facing a person (option 2) helps to project the sound toward the listener, allows for reading lips, and facilitates the listener's ability to observe nonverbal communication, which improves understanding. Review techniques for communicating with a client who has a hearing deficit if you had difficulty answering this question.*
>
> **Cognitive Level**—*Applying*
> **Client Needs Category**—*Physiological integrity*
> **Client Needs Subcategory**—*Basic care and comfort*

70. 1. As long as the client is literate and not visually impaired, reading a descriptive pamphlet is an appropriate alternative. Another stapedectomy client should not be the primary resource for explaining technical information. The client with otosclerosis probably is not so profoundly deaf that sign language is necessary. Writing short sentences or words is appropriate, but writing lengthy technical information is too tedious and time-consuming.

> *Test Taking Strategy—Use the process of elimination to select the option that identifies the best alternative from among those listed for providing the client with an explanation of the proposed surgical procedure. Option 1 remains as the best answer because it provides written rather than verbal information. Documenting the method used to help the client understand is also important. Review methods other than spoken information for providing health teaching for hearing-impaired clients if you had difficulty answering this question.*
>
> **Cognitive Level**—*Applying*
> **Client Needs Category**—*Safe and effective care environment*
> **Client Needs Subcategory**—*Coordinated care*

71. 2. Encouraging a discussion of feelings is therapeutic. Endorsing or defending the surgeon's expertise will not relieve the client's fears about the risks. Giving advice, offering a reassuring cliché, and changing the subject even to positive thoughts are nontherapeutic.

> *Test Taking Strategy—Look at the key words "most therapeutic," indicating one answer is better than the others. Recall that giving a client the opportunity to talk about his or her fears and feelings (option 2) and being an active listener are extremely therapeutic for relieving anxiety and clarifying the significance of a pending procedure. Review communication techniques that are therapeutic when a client indicates a concern about the method for treating a disorder if you had difficulty answering this question.*
>
> **Cognitive Level**—*Applying*
> **Client Needs Category**—*Psychosocial integrity*
> **Client Needs Subcategory**—*None*

72. 2. The facial nerve, which is cranial nerve VII, is assessed by having the client smile or raise the eyebrows. Facial asymmetry suggests damage to this nerve. The olfactory nerve is assessed by asking the client to identify familiar odors. The hypoglossal nerve is tested by having the client stick out the tongue. The optic nerve is tested by determining if the client can see.

> *Test Taking Strategy—Look at the key words "most appropriate," which indicate the necessity to select the best option for assessing the function of the facial nerve, which may have been damaged during the stapedectomy. Recall that the facial nerve facilitates contracting muscles in the face, promoting such actions as the ability to smile and raise the eyebrows (option 2). Review the function of cranial nerve VII and how its function is assessed if you had difficulty answering this question.*
>
> **Cognitive Level**—*Applying*
> **Client Needs Category**—*Physiological integrity*
> **Client Needs Subcategory**—*Physiological adaptation*

73. 1. Keeping the client flat with the head of the bed elevated and the operative ear up helps to maintain the placement of the prosthetic stapes and reduce the occurrence of vertigo. The client should not lie on the operative ear but should be positioned with the head toward the nonoperative ear. None of the other positional choices accomplishes this goal.

> *Test Taking Strategy—Analyze to determine what information the question asks for, which is a postoperative position indicated for a client after a stapedectomy. Recall that using gravity by keeping the operative ear up (option 1) helps maintain the prosthetic stapes in place until tissue healing affixes it to the incus. Review the nursing care of a client who has had a stapedectomy if you had difficulty answering this question.*
> *Cognitive Level—Applying*
> *Client Needs Category—Physiological integrity*
> *Client Needs Subcategory—Reduction of risk potential*

74. 1. Both rebound swelling and packing within the ear contribute to diminished hearing acuity after a stapedectomy. This setback is only temporary and eventually subsides in the absence of any complications. The success of the surgery is evident in a matter of weeks. If the surgery is successful, the client will not need a hearing aid. The prosthetic stapes is secured to the incus by a fine wire loop or hook; it moves without any bone formation around it.

> *Test Taking Strategy—Note the key words "most accurately," indicating one answer is more correct than the others for explaining the diminished hearing experienced by the client postoperatively. Recall that anything that acts as a barrier to sound conduction, such as edematous tissue, operative drainage, and dressing materials (option 1), will temporarily reduce the perception of sound. The expected hearing deficit should have been addressed with the client during preoperative teaching. Review the expectations for hearing in the immediate postoperative period after a stapedectomy if you had difficulty answering this question.*
> *Cognitive Level—Applying*
> *Client Needs Category—Physiological integrity*
> *Client Needs Subcategory—Physiological adaptation*

75. 3. To avoid displacing the device that replaces the stapes, the client should keep the mouth widely open when a sneeze is unavoidable. Aesthetically, chewing food with a closed mouth shows good etiquette. To prevent transmitting infectious organisms, it is best to enclose the exudate from the nose in a paper tissue and dispose of it in a lined refuse container. Turning the head also reduces the potential for droplet transmission of pathogens.

> *Test Taking Strategy—Use the process of elimination to help select the option that describes the nursing instruction that is best for preventing dislodgement*

of the prosthetic stapes. Resisting the desire to stifle a sneeze (option 3) or to avoid blowing the nose helps prevent pressure within the middle ear, which could dislodge the tenuous position of the prosthesis. Review precautions the client must take to avoid increasing pressure within the middle ear after a stapedectomy if you had difficulty answering this question.*
> *Cognitive Level—Applying*
> *Client Needs Category—Health promotion and maintenance*
> *Client Needs Subcategory—None*

76. 3. Stapedectomy clients commonly experience vertigo due to labyrinthitis or a loss of perilymph. To prevent injury, the nurse should ensure that the client's bedside rails are kept raised and that the client is assisted with ambulation. The client undergoing stapedectomy is generally young or middle-aged and is unlikely to feel exceptionally tired. Diplopia is not associated with the effects of this surgery. Although some discomfort is anticipated after surgery, this is not generally considered a major postoperative problem that predisposes the client to injury.

> *Test Taking Strategy—Analyze to determine what information the question asks for, which is a symptom that creates a risk for injury after a stapedectomy. Recall that clients often experience dizziness (option 3) temporarily after undergoing a stapedectomy. Review nursing care of clients who have undergone a stapedectomy if you had difficulty answering this question.*
> *Cognitive Level—Applying*
> *Client Needs Category—Safe and effective care environment*
> *Client Needs Subcategory—Coordinated care*

77. 2. Flying in an airplane is temporarily contraindicated after a stapedectomy because of the potential damaging effects that may occur with changes in air pressure. For the same reason, scuba diving is also avoided. None of the other activities is specifically contraindicated for a client who has had a stapedectomy.

> *Test Taking Strategy—Analyze the information about which the question asks, which in this case deals with an activity that the client should avoid temporarily. Recall that even though airplane cabins are pressurized to compensate for the low atmospheric pressure outside, passengers may experience barotrauma (option 2) when gases trapped within the middle ear or paranasal sinuses expand or contract when the plane climbs to a higher altitude or descends before landing. Review activities that the post-stapedectomy client must temporarily avoid if you had difficulty answering this question.*
> *Cognitive Level—Applying*
> *Client Needs Category—Physiological integrity*
> *Client Needs Subcategory—Reduction of risk potential*

78. 1. The client should be instructed by the nurse to report any signs of a common cold or condition that would contribute to congestion in the ears. A throat infection or productive cough is less likely than a common cold to involve the ears. Conjunctivitis is an infection of the conjunctiva of the eye, which does not include congestion of the ears as a symptom.

Test Taking Strategy—*Analyze to determine what information the question asks for, which is a condition that requires immediate reporting to the physician by the post-stapedectomy client. Recall that symptoms of the common cold (option 1) caused by rhinoviruses tend to be localized in the nose, sinuses, and nasopharynx, which could affect the pressure within the middle ear. Review the structures affected by the common cold, focusing on the ears, if you had difficulty answering this question.*

Cognitive Level—*Applying*
Client Needs Category—*Health promotion and maintenance*
Client Needs Subcategory—*None*

79. 3. Ménière's disease involves the inner ear, affecting balance and hearing, and is believed to be caused by excessive fluid in the inner ear but can be caused by a variety of conditions. The pressure from the fluid increases and causes the major symptom of Ménière's disease, which is severe vertigo. Typically, the client will describe this as a sensation of seeing and feeling motion or rotation, not just a case of dizziness. Ménière's disease encompasses a group of symptoms that includes progressive deafness, ringing in the ears, dizziness, and a feeling of pressure or fullness in the ears. The other symptoms are unrelated to Ménière's disease.

Test Taking Strategy—*Note the key words "most likely," and select the option that identifies a symptom that a client with Ménière's disease experiences more so than the others listed. Recall that the cause of Ménière's disease is unknown, but the symptoms include vertigo (option 3), hearing loss, and tinnitus. Review the pathophysiology of Ménière's disease if you had difficulty answering this question.*

Cognitive Level—*Applying*
Client Needs Category—*Physiological integrity*
Client Needs Subcategory—*Physiological adaptation*

80. 1. A caloric test, used to assess vestibular function, involves instilling cold and warm solutions separately into each ear. An audiometric test requires headphones. Electrodes are used for electroencephalography and electronystagmography. A specimen of blood is not used in a caloric test.

Test Taking Strategy—*Use the process of elimination to select the option that identifies the best explanation for how a caloric test will be performed. Recall that the term caloric implies temperature, which should provide a clue that option 1 is the correct answer. Review the purpose of a caloric test and how it is conducted if you had difficulty answering this question.*

Cognitive Level—*Applying*
Client Needs Category—*Physiological integrity*
Client Needs Subcategory—*Reduction of risk potential*

81. 1. A client with Ménière's disease will develop a sudden onset of severe symptoms, such as vertigo, nausea, vomiting, and tinnitus, during a caloric test. No response to the instillation of warm or cold solution within the ear indicates an auditory nerve tumor. People without Ménière's disease experience slight dizziness and nystagmus during a caloric test. Aphasia and loss of consciousness are unrelated to the mechanics or physiology of a caloric test.

Test Taking Strategy—*Look at the key words "most likely," and select the option that identifies the response to a caloric test that is more characteristic of a client with Ménière's disease than the others. Review diagnostic findings when a client has Ménière's disease if you had difficulty answering this question.*

Cognitive Level—*Applying*
Client Needs Category—*Physiological integrity*
Client Needs Subcategory—*Reduction of risk potential*

82. 1. Allowing the client to participate in the planning and implementation of nursing activities maintains an independent locus of control. The client, more than anyone, knows what movement will cause the least discomfort. Discontinuing or restricting nursing activities does not reflect a high standard of care. Performing nursing activities quickly heightens the client's anxiety because unexpected movements can induce or aggravate symptoms.

Test Taking Strategy—*Look for the key words "most appropriate," indicating that one answer is better than the others. Recall that the client should be a partner in planning nursing care. Therefore, allowing the client to suggest interventions (option 1), provided they are safe and appropriate, and implementing them ought to reduce the client's anxiety. Review the value of including the client in planning his or her own care if you had difficulty answering this question.*

Cognitive Level—*Applying*
Client Needs Category—*Psychosocial integrity*
Client Needs Subcategory—*None*

83. 2. Ménière's disease seems to be related to an increase in endolymphatic fluid within the spaces of the labyrinth in the inner ear. This may be from a hypersecretion, hypoabsorption, deficient membrane permeability, allergy, viral infection, hormonal imbalance, inherited abnormality, or mental stress. Electrolyte deficits and vitamin deficiencies do not play a role in the development of Ménière's disease. There are no anatomic differences between clients with Ménière's disease and those who do not have the disease. The pathology lies in the increased accumulation of fluid in the labyrinth, which interferes with neural impulses that regulate balance and hearing sent from the inner ear to the brain.

Test Taking Strategy—*Analyze to determine what information the question asks for, which is the possible etiology of the symptoms associated with Ménière's disease. Based on the hypothesis that excess fluid (option 2) is an underlying problem, treatment may include salt restriction and diuretic drug therapy. Review the pathophysiology of Ménière's disease if you had difficulty answering this question.*
Cognitive Level—*Applying*
Client Needs Category—*Physiological integrity*
Client Needs Subcategory—*Physiological adaptation*

84. 4. Sudden movement of the client's head or sudden body movements can precipitate an attack that includes nausea and vomiting. Decreasing the client's fluid intake is beneficial. Frequent changing of positions should be avoided. The intensity of room lights is not a factor in controlling the symptoms of Ménière's disease.

Test Taking Strategy—*Use the process of elimination to select the option that identifies the most helpful method for preventing nausea and vomiting when caring for a client with Ménière's disease. Recall that jarring the bed should be avoided (option 4) because it sets the endolymph in motion. The dizziness that occurs may be accompanied by nausea and vomiting. Review factors that can trigger symptoms experienced by the client with Ménière's disease if you had difficulty answering this question.*
Cognitive Level—*Applying*
Client Needs Category—*Physiological integrity*
Client Needs Subcategory—*Reduction of risk potential*

85. 2. Most clients with Ménière's disease can be successfully treated with diet and medication therapy. Many clients can control their symptoms by avoiding sodium and adhering to a low-sodium diet. The amount of sodium is one of the many factors that regulate the balance of fluid within the body. Sodium and fluid retention disrupts the delicate balance between endolymph and perilymph in the inner ear. Limiting the amount of fat intake and cholesterol in the diet is a good health practice but is not essential with Ménière's disease. Restriction of potassium is unnecessary.

Test Taking Strategy—*Analyze to determine what information the question asks for, which is a dietary restriction that should be followed by a client with Ménière's disease. Recall that sodium (option 2) and fluid volume are interrelated. Review measures that can reduce the occurrence of symptoms associated with Ménière's disease if you had difficulty answering this question.*
Cognitive Level—*Applying*
Client Needs Category—*Physiological integrity*
Client Needs Subcategory—*Reduction of risk potential*

86. 3. Hearing loss associated with Ménière's disease becomes progressively worse with each subsequent attack. The period of time that symptoms last is unpredictable. Between attacks, the client generally resumes normal activities and feels well. Surgery is performed in advanced cases to eliminate the vertigo, nausea, and vomiting. However, permanent deafness is a consequence of most surgical procedures.

Test Taking Strategy—*Analyze to determine what information the question asks for, which is evidence that the client requires additional teaching. Read the options carefully because an inaccurate statement must be selected. Recall that hearing loss increases with each attack, and the deficit is permanent (option 3). Review the manner in which hearing is affected for the client with Ménière's disease if you had difficulty answering this question.*
Cognitive Level—*Analyzing*
Client Needs Category—*Physiological integrity*
Client Needs Subcategory—*Physiological adaptation*

Nursing Care of Clients with Nasal Disorders

87. 3. Without proper medical attention, fractures and other nose injuries can displace the septum to one side or the other. Clients may or may not elect definitive treatment once localized swelling has subsided if satisfied with the atypical appearance and function of the nose. Nasal polyps are generally due to chronic inflammation. An enlarged, red, bulbous nose may be from a skin condition such as rosacea. Serous drainage indicates concurrent irritation from an allergen or pathogen.

Test Taking Strategy—*Note the key words "most suggestive," which indicate information that is more indicative of a previous nasal fracture than the information in the other options. Recall that a lateral force sufficient to cause a nasal fracture can twist and buckle the nose (option 3), resulting in cosmetic changes and impaired nasal breathing. Review the significance of finding a deviated septum during a client's assessment if you had difficulty answering this question.*
Cognitive Level—*Applying*
Client Needs Category—*Physiological integrity*
Client Needs Subcategory—*Physiological adaptation*

88. 2. Nosebleeds occur when the arterial blood pressure becomes high. The hypertension causes capillaries in the nasal membrane to rupture and bleed. Therefore, a pulse rate of 110 beats/minute is the result, not the cause, of blood loss. Anxiety causes a transient elevation in both the heart and respiratory rates. An oral temperature of 97.6°F (36.4°C) is slightly lower than normal. However, a low temperature is not likely to cause the nosebleed.

Test Taking Strategy—Look at the key words "most likely," indicating that one answer is better than the others. Select the option that identifies an assessment finding that correlates with the development of a nosebleed. Recall that when the pressure of blood within blood vessels becomes appreciably elevated (option 2), the vessel wall may rupture and cause observable bleeding. Review possible etiologies that are associated with nosebleeds if you had difficulty answering this question.
Cognitive Level—*Applying*
Client Needs Category—*Physiological integrity*
Client Needs Subcategory—*Physiological adaptation*

89. 3. The best first-aid measure for controlling a nosebleed is to apply direct pressure. Leaning forward allows blood to drain from the nose rather than down the nasopharynx into the throat. An upright position tends to lower the blood pressure. Swallowing, mouth breathing, and teeth clenching do not control bleeding.
Test Taking Strategy—Use the process of elimination to help select the option that describes the best nursing action for controlling a nosebleed. Options 1 and 2 can be eliminated because lying down can lead to aspiration, and swallowing blood can cause vomiting. Option 4 can be eliminated because clenching the teeth will not produce pressure on nasal blood vessels. Recall that any type of bleeding can be reduced or controlled by direct pressure (option 3). Review methods for controlling a nosebleed if you had difficulty answering this question.
Cognitive Level—*Applying*
Client Needs Category—*Physiological integrity*
Client Needs Subcategory—*Physiological adaptation*

90. 3. Fear is an emotional response to a real or imagined danger. It occurs when a person feels helpless or powerless to control the situation. Eliminating or reducing the fear-provoking stimulus—in this case the bloody clothing—will probably diminish fear. Having the client recline is inappropriate, because the first-aid treatment for a nosebleed involves having the client lean forward. A towel is unlikely to stay in place unless the client is reclining. An anxious or fearful person probably will not be able to concentrate on reading.
Test Taking Strategy—Use the process of elimination to select the option that identifies the best method for relieving the client's fear and anxiety. Recall that fear is the result of perceiving a threat to well-being, which in this case is represented by the blood on the client's shirt. Therefore, removing the bloody shirt from view (option 3) reduces the image that is triggering the client's fear. Review common responses that occur among individuals who see blood and how a fear response can be minimized if you had difficulty answering this question.
Cognitive Level—*Applying*
Client Needs Category—*Psychosocial integrity*
Client Needs Subcategory—*None*

91. 4. Blowing the nose retraumatizes the ruptured nasal capillaries, causing bleeding to recur. There is no need to restrict fluid intake. Taking the carotid pulse is unnecessary. Being told to keep the head up to help lower blood pressure is helpful, but it is not the most essential information the client requires in this situation.
Test Taking Strategy—Analyze to determine what information the question asks for, which is a nursing instruction that is essential for preventing a recurrence of nosebleed. Recall that vigorously blowing the nose (option 4) disrupts the tenuous clot that controls the bleeding and may lead to another bleeding episode. Review precautions that should be followed once a nosebleed (epistaxis) has been controlled if you had difficulty answering this question.
Cognitive Level—*Applying*
Client Needs Category—*Physiological integrity*
Client Needs Subcategory—*Physiological adaptation*

92. 2. Nasal polyps are benign growths found in the nasal passages. If large, they can affect breathing and the ability to smell, and can contribute to sinus infections. Nasal polyps are associated with chronic inflammation of the nasopharynx, which is caused by inhalant allergies or upper respiratory infections. Nasal injuries are more correlated with a deviated septum. A history of nasal surgery or tonsillectomy is incidental to the development of nasal polyps.
Test Taking Strategy—Analyze to determine what information the question asks for, which is data in a client's health history that relates to the development of nasal polyps. Recall that a chronic inflammatory response within the nose secondary to inhalant allergies (option 3) is believed to be a main cause of nasal polyps. Review the etiology associated with the formation of nasal polyps if you had difficulty answering this question.
Cognitive Level—*Applying*
Client Needs Category—*Physiological integrity*
Client Needs Subcategory—*Physiological adaptation*

93. 1. Swallowing at frequent intervals is common when blood accumulates posteriorly in the pharynx. The client feels the need to continue to swallow as the blood accumulates. Impaired appetite, hoarseness, and diminished hearing are abnormal assessment findings, but they are not directly related to nasal bleeding.
Test Taking Strategy—Analyze to determine what information the question asks for, which is an assessment finding that suggests the client is bleeding from the operative area after a nasal polypectomy. Because the nose is likely to have been packed to control bleeding, any blood loss will drain posteriorly down the throat. The client will swallow frequently (option 1) as blood accumulates in the oropharynx. Review the significance of frequent swallowing when a client has had nasal or pharyngeal surgery if you had difficulty answering this question.

Cognitive Level—*Applying*
Client Needs Category—*Physiological integrity*
Client Needs Subcategory—*Reduction of risk potential*

94. 3. Remaining objective and limiting the response to a description of the client's external appearance is the most appropriate approach. Predicting that the client will look gorgeous is considered false reassurance because body image is a personal concept. The client most likely felt unattractive before the surgery; contradicting an opinion might cause the client to mistrust the nurse. Telling the client that personality is more important also expresses the nurse's subjective opinion. It borders on giving advice, which is a nontherapeutic communication technique.

> *Test Taking Strategy*—*Use the process of elimination to select the option that identifies the best nursing response to the client's question concerning the appearance of the nose following a rhinoplasty. Options 1, 2, and 4 can be eliminated because they represent nontherapeutic responses. The client's face is likely to show evidence of swelling and blackened eyes. Therefore, option 3 is the best answer because it is an honest response without avoiding the question or providing comments that may or may not be accurate. Review principles of therapeutic communication if you had difficulty answering this question.*

Cognitive Level—*Applying*
Client Needs Category—*Psychosocial integrity*
Client Needs Subcategory—*None*

Nursing Care of Clients with Disorders of the Skin and Related Structures

95. 4. The first response in helping a victim who is in flames is to smother the fire either by rolling the victim on the ground or covering the flames with a blanket or some other dense material. Nothing but cool water is applied to the skin until the physician examines the victim. A clean cloth is used to cover the burn wound, but this would be done only after the flames are extinguished. The use of ice is contraindicated because it causes hypothermia or further thermal injury to the burned tissue.

> *Test Taking Strategy*—*Analyze to determine what information the question asks for, which is the nurse's immediate priority when helping a victim whose clothes are on fire. Recall that smothering the burning clothing (option 4) eliminates the oxygen that supports the combustion of flammable clothing and reduces the potential severity of a burn. Review methods for limiting the depth and extent of a burn if you had difficulty answering this question.*

Cognitive Level—*Analyzing*
Client Needs Category—*Physiological integrity*
Client Needs Subcategory—*Reduction of risk potential*

96. 2. Whenever a burn involves the head, neck, or chest, establishing and maintaining a patent airway is vitally important. Many burn victims, regardless of the area that is burned, inhale smoke, which irritates the air passages and results in increased respiratory secretions and edema of the air passages. Taking the pulse and blood pressure is important, but this assessment can be delayed until determining that the airway is patent. Identifying the next of kin and determining the extent of burns are less important than ensuring that the victim can breathe.

> *Test Taking Strategy*—*Look for the key words "most appropriate," indicating a priority. Because the client's neck and chest were burned, it is possible that breathing will become impaired. Monitoring breathing is a nursing action that is directed toward a physiologic need that is of greatest importance. Remember that the airway and breathing are factors that must be addressed whenever caring for a client, especially one predisposed to impaired ventilation.*

Cognitive Level—*Applying*
Client Needs Category—*Physiological integrity*
Client Needs Subcategory—*Physiological adaptation*

97. 3, 4, 5, 6. When a client with a burn arrives in the emergency department, the medical team works quickly to stabilize the body systems and assess the extent of the injury. Team members ensure adequate ventilation by administering oxygen or by inserting an endotracheal tube. Fluid resuscitation with lactated Ringer's solution and administration of pain medication are completed via an I.V. infusion. The client also receives a tetanus injection and antibiotics at this time. Ice and normal saline solution would not be placed on the wound because they may lead to hypothermia or further tissue damage.

> *Test Taking Strategy*—*Analyze to determine what information the question asks for, which is priority nursing interventions for a client with full-thickness and partial-thickness burns. Alternative-format "select all that apply" questions require considering each option independently to decide its merit in answering the question. Choose the options that correlate with components of nursing care of a client who is in the emergency department. Review nursing interventions that correlate with the early stage of burn care if you had difficulty answering this question.*

Cognitive Level—*Applying*
Client Needs Category—*Physiological integrity*
Client Needs Subcategory—*Physiological adaptation*

98. 1. Full-thickness burns include the epidermis, dermis, and subcutaneous layers of skin. Previously identified as third-degree or fourth-degree burns, these burns are generally white, cherry red, tan, dark brown, or black. The tissue is leathery and painless. Partial-thickness burns are pink to rosy red, dull white or tan, blistered, and painful.

> *Test Taking Strategy*—*Analyze to determine what information the question asks for, which is the appearance*

of a full-thickness burn. Recall that a full-thickness burn results in the greatest depth of a burn injury. The tissue is literally dead (white) or completely charred black and leathery (option 1). Review the characteristics of partial- and full-thickness burns if you had difficulty answering this question.
Cognitive Level—*Understanding*
Client Needs Category—*Physiological integrity*
Client Needs Subcategory—*Physiological adaptation*

99. 3. The first major complication of a burn is hypovolemic shock. Therefore, urine output is monitored hourly to evaluate the effectiveness of fluid replacement therapy. Burn clients initially receive massive volumes of fluid to replace what is lost from the intracellular space and what is transferred from the intravascular space to the interstitial space. Although body temperature is difficult to regulate during the initial stages after a burn injury, the client's temperature must be monitored to track the course of infection that typically occurs in later phases of burn management. Clients with full-thickness burns do not experience as much pain as those with partial-thickness burns over a similar percentage of body-surface area. Exercising is not an initial concern but becomes a priority when contractures develop during the healing phases of burn care.
Test Taking Strategy—*Use the process of elimination to select the option that identifies the assessment finding that provides the best evidence of the client's response to initial burn treatment. Recall that an adequate urine output (option 3) is evidence that the client's fluid replacement efforts are satisfactory. Review assessments that reflect adequate kidney perfusion if you had difficulty answering this question.*
Cognitive Level—*Analyzing*
Client Needs Category—*Physiological integrity*
Client Needs Subcategory—*Physiological adaptation*

100. 1. Infection is a common complication when the burn wound is exposed to microorganisms in the environment as well as those present and residing in the client's own tissues, secretions, and excretions. Hypothermia, rather than hyperthermia, occurs due to leaving the burn wound undressed. Depression about the potential change in body image and malnutrition occur regardless of the method used to manage the burn wound.
Test Taking Strategy—*Note the key words "most appropriate" used to ask about the problem that a nurse should monitor when caring for a burn client treated with the open method. Recall that impaired skin that is exposed to environmental pathogens is highly susceptible to infection (option 1). Review the disadvantages in using the open method of burn wound care if you had difficulty answering this question.*
Cognitive Level—*Applying*
Client Needs Category—*Physiological integrity*
Client Needs Subcategory—*Reduction of risk potential*

101. 2. Mafenide acetate (Sulfamylon) is an excellent antimicrobial for preventing and treating postburn wound infections. However, the pain it causes on application is an obvious disadvantage. It does not have an unpleasant odor. Another topical antimicrobial, silver sulfadiazine (Silvadene), does not cause pain but can cause a rash. Silver nitrate, which is used for burn wound management, stains tissue and everything else it contacts. It also causes stinging on application and increases the potential for electrolyte imbalance.
Test Taking Strategy—*Analyze to determine what information the question asks for, which is the chief disadvantage to applying mafenide acetate cream to the burn wound. Recall that mafenide acetate cream causes a transient burning sensation (option 2) when it is applied. Review the advantages and disadvantages of mafenide acetate cream as a topical antimicrobial medication if you had difficulty answering this question.*
Cognitive Level—*Applying*
Client Needs Category—*Physiological integrity*
Client Needs Subcategory—*Pharmacological therapies*

102. 3. Because debridement causes pain, it is essential to administer an analgesic no sooner than 30 minutes before the procedure. In the case of hydrotherapy when a whirlpool is used, the client does not need to refrain from ingesting food or fluids. If the client requires surgical debridement under anesthesia, a consent form must be obtained and the client needs to fast.
Test Taking Strategy—*Note the use of the key word "essential," which indicates a priority action. Recall that to reduce the pain that results from debridement, the nurse must administer an analgesic (option 3) before the procedure. Review the nursing care of a burned client who is undergoing wound debridement if you had difficulty answering this question.*
Cognitive Level—*Applying*
Client Needs Category—*Physiological integrity*
Client Needs Subcategory—*Physiological adaptation*

103. 1. Minimal movement of the grafted area is best for approximately 48 hours to ensure that the graft is not displaced. Disturbance of the graft may result in such problems as failure of the graft to adhere to underlying tissues, infection, and tissue necrosis. The graft dressing is only changed or reinforced by the physician. Wet soaks are not applied to the graft because this disturbs the contact between the graft and underlying tissues.
Test Taking Strategy—*Look at the key words "most appropriate," indicating that one answer is better than the others. Recall that the donor skin used for the graft is very thin and easily dislodged. Movement of the graft or shearing forces may lead to graft failure by disrupting the attachment of the graft*

to the wound bed. Reducing movement (option 1) helps avoid displacing the skin graft until it becomes established. Review the nursing care of a burn client after a skin graft if you had difficulty answering this question.
Cognitive Level—*Applying*
Client Needs Category—*Physiological integrity*
Client Needs Subcategory—*Physiological adaptation*

104. 3. Pressure garments are worn for as long as 2 years to promote a smooth appearance to the burn scar and help prevent or reduce wound contractures. An elastic garment reduces scarring by using pressure to align the skin's surface in a parallel plane, avoiding hypertrophic scarring and deformities. Pressure garments are not used to prevent wound infection, avoid exposure to sunlight, or prevent social rejection, although the latter two are considered secondary benefits.

> *Test Taking Strategy—Use the process of elimination to select the option that identifies the best indication that the client understands the purpose for wearing a pressure garment. Recall that to avoid a thickened, nodular, or buckling appearance to the skin (option 3), a pressure garment must be worn continuously for an extensive period of time. Review the purpose and regimen for the use of a pressure garment by a client who has been burned if you had difficulty answering this question.*
> **Cognitive Level**—*Applying*
> **Client Needs Category**—*Health promotion and maintenance*
> **Client Needs Subcategory**—*None*

105. 1. One of the most serious types of burns is an electrical burn. An electrical burn has an entry and exit wound site; it is essential to determine their locations. Typically, the entry wound is ischemic, charred, and depressed. Exit wounds may have an explosive appearance. The plan of care depends on the wound assessment. The degree of discoloration; amount of eschar, if any; and character of drainage, if any, are also noted but are not as important as assessing the primary wounds.

> *Test Taking Strategy—Note the key words "most important," indicating that one answer is better than the others. Select the assessment that takes precedence over the others when examining an electrical burn. Recall that determining the pathway the electrical current took through the body by looking for the entry and exit site (option 1) is a priority for identifying the extent of tissue and organ injury. Review assessment data that are unique to electrical burns if you had difficulty answering this question.*
> **Cognitive Level**—*Applying*
> **Client Needs Category**—*Physiological integrity*
> **Client Needs Subcategory**—*Physiological adaptation*

106. Stage III pressure ulcer.
Pressure ulcers are categorized in four stages by severity, with stage I being the least severe and the easiest to treat. Stage I is categorized by a nonblanchable reddened area on the skin but no skin breakdown. A stage II pressure ulcer involves a blistering effect and the skin becomes open. Stage II pressure ulcers are painful, and the edges of the skin may appear red and irritated. In a stage III ulcer (like the one illustrated), the underlying tissue is affected (usually down to the subcutaneous tissue) and the wound looks like a crater. Stage III pressure ulcers are very painful and can quickly deteriorate to stage IV pressure ulcers. Stage IV pressure ulcers are the most severe; typically bone, tendons, and ligaments are exposed. There is high risk for infections in stages III and IV pressure ulcers.

> *Test Taking Strategy—Analyze to determine what information the question asks for, which requires identifying the stage of the client's pressure ulcer based on the provided image. Note the shallow crater that extends to the subcutaneous tissue and may be accompanied by serous drainage, which is characteristic of a stage III pressure ulcer. Review the characteristics of the four stages of pressure ulcers if you had difficulty answering this question.*
> **Cognitive Level**—*Applying*
> **Client Needs Category**—*Physiological integrity*
> **Client Needs Subcategory**—*Physiological adaptation*

107. 4. Repositioning the client every 2 hours is the best method of restoring or maintaining skin integrity. Application of a skin-toughening agent would be ineffective if the client's position is not changed at frequent intervals. Keeping the head of the bed elevated is of no value in preventing skin breakdown; a sitting position creates a shearing force that contributes to skin impairment. Massaging skin that does not blanch when pressure is relieved is contraindicated because it causes further skin disruption and damage.

> *Test Taking Strategy—Analyze to determine what information the question asks for, which is a nursing intervention for restoring skin integrity when caring for a client who has a pressure ulcer. Recall that relieving pressure on the skin, especially over bony prominences, by frequently changing the client's position (option 4) increases capillary blood flow that will revitalize impaired tissue. Review nursing measures for managing the care of a client with a pressure ulcer if you had difficulty answering this question.*
> **Cognitive Level**—*Applying*
> **Client Needs Category**—*Physiological integrity*
> **Client Needs Subcategory**—*Reduction of risk potential*

108. **2.** Although all of the options could be a factor in causing injury to the client's skin, sliding down in bed most commonly results in a shearing force, thereby disrupting the integrity of the skin. The skin is separated from the underlying tissue; small blood vessels are stretched and torn in deeper areas under the skin. Friction occurs when two surfaces move across one another. Friction is usually, but not always, accompanied by shear. Friction causes surface abrasion, resulting in shallow injury to the epidermal layer of the skin. Pressure, friction, and shear all contribute to skin impairment.

Test Taking Strategy—Analyze to determine what information the question asks for, which is the type of skin injury caused by sliding down in bed. Recall that an injury caused by friction can be seen on the surface of the skin, whereas tissue injury from shearing forces (option 2) occurs more deeply beneath the skin and can result in tissue necrosis. Review the difference between shear and friction if you had difficulty answering this question.
Cognitive Level—Applying
Client Needs Category—Physiological integrity
Client Needs Subcategory—Reduction of risk potential

109. **1, 2, 3, 5, 6.** A dietary consult would be helpful to increase protein in the diet for wound healing for both the sacral pressure ulcer and the coronary artery bypass graft incision. Physical therapy and occupational therapy promote movement and activity, thereby eliminating continuous pressure on the sacral area and helping the client to return to a presurgical status more quickly. An enterostomal therapist, a specialist in skin and wound care, can be helpful in planning treatment for the pressure ulcer. Physician consultations are necessary as a follow-up to surgery and to monitor the client's general health and recovery. Nothing in the scenario provided indicates that the client requires psychiatric services.

Test Taking Strategy—Analyze to determine what information the question asks for, which is the services needed to facilitate recovery after cardiac surgery. Alternative-format "select all that apply" questions require considering each option independently to decide its merit in answering the question. To answer this question correctly, choose the options that correlate with the services needed to facilitate the client's recovery and preserve health. Review the functions of each of the services listed if you had difficulty answering this question.
Cognitive Level—Applying
Client Needs Category—Safe and effective care environment
Client Needs Subcategory—Coordinated care

110. **1.** Lice have a life span of approximately 30 days. Nits, eggs laid by adult females, hatch in 7 to 10 days and may not be affected by the first application of a pediculi-cide because they are attached tightly to the sides of hair shafts. The National Pediculosis Association opposes the use of strong chemicals such as lindane (Kwell) and benzene because they are neurotoxic. Other nonprescription pediculicides that contain pyrethrin, such as Nix, are effective. Although one use usually kills the initial infestation of lice, some adults and nits, small white lice eggs, may survive and be evident within 7 to 14 days of the initial treatment. If evidence of lice persists, a second application is necessary. As long as lice and nits are seen, shampooing must be repeated. The client's statements in the remaining options are essentially correct.

Test Taking Strategy—Analyze to determine what information the question asks for, which is a client's statement that requires clarification. Read the options carefully, looking for the statement that indicates a need for additional teaching. Recall that one application of a pediculicide may not eliminate all the head lice (option 1). Review the life span of lice, the instructions for using a pediculicide, and how nits can be removed mechanically if you had difficulty answering this question.
Cognitive Level—Applying
Client Needs Category—Health promotion and maintenance
Client Needs Subcategory—None

111. **2.** Basal and squamous cell carcinomas commonly occur in sun-exposed areas of the body, such as the scalp, ears, nose, and hands. Male-pattern baldness places fair-skinned individuals at risk for chronic exposure to ultraviolet radiation (sun exposure), which is a predisposing factor for developing malignant skin changes. Smoking cigarettes is a risk factor for other types of cancer. Working for a drug manufacturer does not provide sufficient information to determine if the client is exposed to ultraviolet radiation. Although exposure to chemicals is a factor in causing cancer, deodorant soap is considered a safe product.

Test Taking Strategy—Note the use of the key words "most likely," which indicates one answer is better than the others. Select the option that identifies a risk factor for developing skin cancer. Because the client is bald (option 2), skin cancer may develop on the exposed scalp after chronic exposure to sunlight. Review the etiology of the various types of skin cancer if you had difficulty answering this question.
Cognitive Level—Applying
Client Needs Category—Physiological integrity
Client Needs Subcategory—Physiological adaptation

112. **2.** Malignant melanoma, the least common form of skin cancer, but the one that causes the majority of deaths from skin cancer, is a malignancy involving darkly pigmented melanocytes. The common risk factors for malignant melanoma include fair-skinned or freckled, blue-eyed, light-haired clients of Celtic or Scandinavian origin, especially those who live in sunny climates and high altitudes. Such clients usually burn easily and do not tan; they may even have a significant history of severe sunburn.

> *Test Taking Strategy—Use the process of elimination to select the option that identifies the most common profile of persons who develop malignant melanoma. Options 1, 3, and 4 can be eliminated because darkly pigmented individuals are at lower risk for skin cancer. Recall that malignant melanomas arise from a pre-existing mole that undergoes changes when lightly pigmented skin (option 2) is exposed to ultraviolet radiation. Review the risk factors for developing malignant melanoma if you had difficulty answering this question.*

Cognitive Level—*Applying*
Client Needs Category—*Physiological integrity*
Client Needs Subcategory—*Physiological adaptation*

113. 2. Because birth defects are associated with isotretinoin (Accutane), a derivative of vitamin A, its use is contraindicated during pregnancy. It is classified in pregnancy risk category X, the most dangerous category, by the Food and Drug Administration because there are risks of miscarriage and congenital malformations, including nervous system defects, facial defects, and cleft palate. There is no known relationship between breast cancer or ovulation and increased vulnerability to the drug's adverse effects. Acne vulgaris, one condition for which this drug is prescribed, is not a sexually transmitted disease.

> *Test Taking Strategy—Note the key word "essential," which indicates a priority. Recall that isotretinoin is a teratogen, a substance that interferes with normal embryonic development. Therefore, women who are or may become pregnant (option 2) should not take this drug. Review precautions and side effects associated with isotretinoin if you had difficulty answering this question.*

Cognitive Level—*Applying*
Client Needs Category—*Physiological integrity*
Client Needs Subcategory—*Pharmacological therapies*

114. 3. Wearing a different pair of shoes each day provides time for shoe moisture to evaporate. The fungus growth that causes tinea pedis is supported in a dark, moist, and warm environment. Eliminating one or more of these factors may reduce the frequency of tinea pedis. Avoiding bare feet, cutting the nails straight across, and wearing colored socks will not promote or eliminate tinea pedis.

> *Test Taking Strategy—Use the process of elimination to select the option that identifies the best nursing advice for a client who has frequent outbreaks of tinea pedis. Option 1 can be eliminated, because instructing a client to never go barefoot is good advice for preventing foot trauma. Option 2 can be eliminated because cutting the nails straight across may help to prevent*

ingrown toenails. Option 4 can be eliminated because there is no health-related advantage to wearing colored socks. Option 3 is the correct answer because fungi will thrive and infect the feet of individuals who wear shoes that are damp from perspiration or inclement weather and do not dry sufficiently from day to day. Review methods for preventing tinea pedis if you had difficulty answering this question.

Cognitive Level—*Applying*
Client Needs Category—*Health promotion and maintenance*
Client Needs Subcategory—*None*

115. 1. Shingles results from a reactivation of the varicella-zoster virus, which lies dormant in the sensory ganglia after a previous infection with chickenpox. The individual with shingles usually reports a history of chicken pox in childhood. Shingles also occurs in those who have not had chicken pox but who come in contact with someone who has chicken pox or is immunocompromised. A one-time vaccine for shingles (Zostavax) is available for people age 60 years and older whether they have had chicken pox or not. Shingles is not caused by the bite of an insect, a bacterial toxin, or an antibody response.

> *Test Taking Strategy—Analyze to determine what information the question asks for, which is the etiology of shingles. Because shingles is a sequela, a condition that results from a disease, which is viral in this case, option 1 is the correct answer. Review the etiology of shingles if you had difficulty answering this question.*

Cognitive Level—*Applying*
Client Needs Category—*Physiological integrity*
Client Needs Subcategory—*Physiological adaptation*

116.

2. Low-grade fever, malaise develop.

3. Dermatome area develops a red, blotchy appearance.

4. Unilateral vesicles appear.

1. Pain develops and severe itching follows.

5. Scarring or permanent skin discoloration is noted.

Initial symptoms of shingles include a low-grade fever, headache, and malaise. The area of the skin along the nerve pathway or dermatome develops a red blotchy appearance. In 24 to 48 hours, vesicles appear on the skin along the nerve's pathway. The eruptions are typically unilateral and may include areas on the trunk, neck, and head. The eruptions become painful with intense itching. Scarring or permanent skin discoloration is possible.

Test Taking Strategy—Analyze to determine what information the question asks for, which requires sequencing the signs and symptoms as they develop when a client acquires shingles, using all the options. Review the initial symptoms of shingles and its progression if you had difficulty answering this question.
Cognitive Level—*Applying*
Client Needs Category—*Physiological integrity*
Client Needs Subcategory—*Physiological adaptation*

117. 2. Clients with herpes simplex virus type 1 lesions, also known as *cold sores* or *fever blisters*, are cautioned to use good personal hygiene to prevent the spread of the infection to other areas, such as the eyes and genitals. The application of petroleum jelly delays healing but does not prevent the spread of the infection. Any scabs that form should be allowed to dry and fall off. When cleaning the affected areas, clients should take care to use tissues or gauze to gently clean and remove any fluid that has formed on the lesions. The tissues or gauze should be used only once and then discarded.

Test Taking Strategy—Note the key words "most appropriate," which indicate that one option is better than the others. Recall that herpes simplex virus type 1 can be transferred to other body parts lined with mucous membranes. The most common method of transfer involves the hands. Therefore, hand hygiene (option 2) is particularly important. Review how the herpes simplex virus is transmitted if you had difficulty answering this question.
Cognitive Level—*Applying*
Client Needs Category—*Health promotion and maintenance*
Client Needs Subcategory—*None*

118. 2. Characterized by areas of redness covered with silvery scales, psoriasis is a common chronic disease of the skin in which erythematous papules form plaques with distinct borders. Areas affected usually include the elbows, knees, and scalp, although other areas may also be affected.

Test Taking Strategy—Analyze to determine what information the question asks for, which is the appearance of psoriatic lesions. Recall that the lesions associated with psoriasis appear as thick raised areas with well-defined borders. The raised areas are covered by white scales that easily flake off, revealing shiny red skin underneath (option 2). Review the development and appearance of psoriatic lesions if you had difficulty answering this question.
Cognitive Level—*Applying*
Client Needs Category—*Physiological integrity*
Client Needs Subcategory—*Physiological adaptation*

119. 3. Psoriasis is a chronic, noninfectious, inflammatory skin disease in which epidermal cells are produced at a rate about six to nine times faster than normal. The cells in the basal layer divide too quickly, and the newer formed cells move so rapidly to the skin surface that they become evident as profuse scales or plaques of epidermal tissue. Infections of the skin and hair follicles as well as dermal abrasion are not contributing factors to psoriasis.

Test Taking Strategy—Analyze to determine what information the question asks for, which is the underlying nature of psoriasis. Recall that the cause of psoriasis is essentially unknown, but the trigger for the disorder causes an aberrant, dysfunctional up-regulation of patchy skin cell regeneration (option 3). Review how epidermal cell proliferation contributes to the formation of lesions that are characteristic of psoriasis if you had difficulty answering this question.
Cognitive Level—*Applying*
Client Needs Category—*Physiological integrity*
Client Needs Subcategory—*Physiological adaptation*

120. 4. Vinyl gloves may be substituted for latex gloves; however, because vinyl is more permeable, two pairs should be worn. Most facilities now are providing latex-free gloves and equipment. Neither rinsing the gloves with tap water nor applying petroleum-based ointment eliminates an allergic reaction to latex. It is unsafe for nurses and other health care workers to care for clients without proper protection when there is a potential for contact with body fluids, especially those that contain blood.

Test Taking Strategy—Use the process of elimination to select the option that identifies the best advice for nursing personnel who have an allergy to latex, a substance that is common in examination gloves and other medical equipment. Recall that vinyl gloves (option 4) are a safe substitute for gloves that are made of latex. Review methods for avoiding an allergic reaction from latex when carrying out nursing care if you had difficulty answering this question.
Cognitive Level—*Applying*
Client Needs Category—*Safe and effective care environment*
Client Needs Subcategory—*Coordinated care*

121. 1, 2, 3, 5, 6. The protein in latex can cause some clients to experience an allergic response. Common signs and symptoms of a latex allergy include raised areas and blisters on the hands; itchy, red, watery eyes; runny nose; hives; and in extreme cases, chest tightness and anaphylactic shock. Nausea and vomiting are not usually associated with latex allergies.

Test Taking Strategy—Analyze to determine what information the question asks for, which is signs and symptoms of an allergic reaction to latex. Alternative-

format "select all that apply" questions require considering each option independently to decide its merit in answering the question. To answer this question correctly, choose the options that correlate with manifestations of an allergic reaction when a hypersensitive person dons gloves that contain latex. Review the signs and symptoms caused by contact with an allergen if you had difficulty answering this question.
Cognitive Level—*Applying*
Client Needs Category—*Physiological integrity*
Client Needs Subcategory—*Physiological adaptation*

122. 1. Frostbite is a condition in which there is damage and injury to parts of the body exposed to extreme cold. Frostbite usually occurs on fingers, toes, and body parts that are left uncovered. Soaking with a warm solution between 100°F and 106°F (37.7°C and 41.1°C) is recommended for the treatment of frostbite. Cold applications are contraindicated because this delays effective treatment. A heating pad or hot water is not used because either can cause further tissue damage.

> **Test Taking Strategy**—*Use the process of elimination to select the option that identifies the best measure the nurse can recommend to the client who has experienced frostbite. Recall that gradual warming (option 1) is the key to treating frostbite. Review first-aid measures for managing frostbite if you had difficulty answering this question.*
> **Cognitive Level**—*Applying*
> **Client Needs Category**—*Physiological integrity*
> **Client Needs Subcategory**—*Reduction of risk potential*

123. 1. Hypoallergenic or glycerin soap decreases skin irritation and therefore lessens itching (pruritus). Regular soap removes skin oils, which can contribute to or cause itching. Lotion should be applied more frequently than every other day. Tepid water, rather than hot or cold water, is recommended for bathing. Patting the skin dry, rather than rubbing, reduces skin irritation and itching.

> **Test Taking Strategy**—*Look at the key words "most appropriate," which indicates that one answer is better than the others. Select the option that identifies the best method for relieving itching associated with dry skin. Recall that bathing with commercial bar soap contributes to skin dryness, and an alternative that moisturizes the skin (option 1) should be substituted. Review methods for relieving dry skin*

and itching that may be associated with it if you had difficulty answering this question.
Cognitive Level—*Applying*
Client Needs Category—*Physiological integrity*
Client Needs Subcategory—*Physiological adaptation*

124. 2. Chronic wounds are long-standing wounds that are resistant to healing, such as a slow-healing diabetic foot ulcer. In many cases, such chronic wounds begin healing but characteristically fail to continue the healing process. Although the gunshot and surgical wounds mentioned may be slow to heal, the wounds are not necessarily considered chronic; their slow healing is secondary to infection or tissue damage. A stage I pressure ulcer involves only the first layer of skin and does not necessarily progress to a deeper wound.

> **Test Taking Strategy**—*Analyze to determine what information the question asks for, which is an example of a chronic wound. Recall that a chronic wound is one that is persistent and slow to heal (option 2). Review the definition of chronic and apply the term to the examples listed if you had difficulty answering this question.*
> **Cognitive Level**—*Applying*
> **Client Needs Category**—*Physiological integrity*
> **Client Needs Subcategory**—*Physiological adaptation*

125. 1, 2, 3, 6. When investigating the cause of a client's rash, it is important to ask about all aspects of the client's life. In this case, asking about food allergies; medication allergies; allergies related to soaps, detergents, or lotions; and allergies related to pets are important questions to include. Exposure to sunlight and exercising in a gym are not related to rashes.

> **Test Taking Strategy**—*Analyze to determine what information the question asks for, which is appropriate questions to determine the cause of a rash. Alternative-format "select all that apply" questions require considering each option independently to decide its merit in answering the question. Choose the options that correlate with questions that may identify the causes of the client's rash. Review substances that are considered common allergens if you had difficulty answering this question.*
> **Cognitive Level**—*Applying*
> **Client Needs Category**—*Physiological integrity*
> **Client Needs Subcategory**—*Physiological adaptation*

The Nursing Care of Clients with Endocrine Disorders

- Nursing Care of Clients with Disorders of the Pituitary Gland
- Nursing Care of Clients with Disorders of the Thyroid Gland
- Nursing Care of Clients with Disorders of the Parathyroid Glands
- Nursing Care of Clients with Disorders of the Adrenal Glands
- Nursing Care of Clients with Pancreatic Endocrine Disorders
- Correct Answers, Rationales, and Test Taking Strategies

Directions: *With a pencil, blacken the space in front of the option you have chosen for your correct answer.*

Nursing Care of Clients with Disorders of the Pituitary Gland

After suffering head trauma, a client develops signs and symptoms of diabetes insipidus.

1. Which characteristic symptom of the client's disorder would the nurse expect to find during an assessment?
[ ] **1.** Polyphagia
[ ] **2.** Polyuria
[ ] **3.** Glycosuria
[ ] **4.** Hyperglycemia

2. The physician orders a urinalysis. Which urine characteristic does the nurse anticipate?
[ ] **1.** Tea-colored
[ ] **2.** Pale yellow
[ ] **3.** Colorless
[ ] **4.** Light pink

3. Which nursing intervention is essential for monitoring the client's condition?
[ ] **1.** Measuring intake and output
[ ] **2.** Analyzing blood glucose levels
[ ] **3.** Inserting a Foley catheter
[ ] **4.** Sending urine samples to the laboratory

The nursing care plan indicates that the client must be weighed each day.

4. When directing the nursing assistant to weigh the client, which instruction is most important for obtaining accurate data?
[ ] **1.** Have the client stand on a bedside scale.
[ ] **2.** Weigh the client at the same time each day.
[ ] **3.** Ask that slippers be removed when being weighed.
[ ] **4.** Ask about the client's pre-disease weight.

The client is treated with intranasal lypressin (Diapid), 2 sprays q.i.d. and as needed.

5. The nurse observes the client self-administering the medication. Which action indicates that the client is using the medication correctly?
[ ] **1.** The client shakes the medication vigorously.
[ ] **2.** The client's head is tilted to the side.
[ ] **3.** The client inverts the drug container.
[ ] **4.** The client inhales with each spray.

6. Before the client is discharged, the physician orders lypressin (Diapid) to be administered p.r.n. When instructing the client about how to take this drug at home, the nurse tells the client to administer the drug when experiencing which sign or symptom?
[ ] **1.** Increased thirst
[ ] **2.** Onset of a headache
[ ] **3.** Dark yellow urine
[ ] **4.** A runny nose

The nurse is assessing a client who is experiencing signs and symptoms of acromegaly.

7. During physical assessment, which documented finding does the nurse identify as a clinical manifestation of acromegaly?
[ ] **1.** Shortened height
[ ] **2.** Enlarged hands
[ ] **3.** Gonadal atrophy
[ ] **4.** Loss of teeth

8. Which nursing diagnosis should the nursing team consider when developing this client's care plan?
[ ] **1.** Activity intolerance
[ ] **2.** Self-care deficit
[ ] **3.** Ineffective breathing
[ ] **4.** Impaired swallowing

Because medical treatment was unsuccessful, the client with acromegaly is scheduled for a trans-sphenoidal hypophysectomy. The night before surgery, the nurse provides the client with information about what to expect during the postoperative period.

9. Which statement by the client indicates a misunderstanding of the expected surgical outcome?

[ ] **1.** "My appearance will gradually become normal."
[ ] **2.** "I'll need to take replacement hormones."
[ ] **3.** "I'll need to see my physician regularly."
[ ] **4.** "The surgical incision will be inconspicuous."

10. When completing a postoperative assessment, which location is essential to ensure an absence of bleeding?

[ ] **1.** The skull
[ ] **2.** The nose
[ ] **3.** The ear canal
[ ] **4.** The tongue

Nursing Care of Clients with Disorders of the Thyroid Gland

A 35-year-old seeks medical attention to determine the reason menstruation has ceased. The physician orders a radioactive iodine uptake test.

11. After the test, the nurse provides the client with instructions. Which statement of the nurse is most accurate?

[ ] **1.** "You must remain isolated until the radiation level decreases sufficiently."
[ ] **2.** "You're free to go without further precautionary instructions."
[ ] **3.** "You must follow special precautions for a short period of time."
[ ] **4.** "You'll be given an antidote to reduce the radioactivity level."

The results of the diagnostic tests confirm that the client has myxedema.

12. In addition to amenorrhea, which other signs of myxedema is the nurse likely to observe in this client? Select all that apply.

[ ] **1.** Hoarse, raspy voice
[ ] **2.** Oily skin with large pores
[ ] **3.** Thin trunk and extremities
[ ] **4.** Extreme restlessness
[ ] **5.** Low body temperature
[ ] **6.** Decreased blood pressure

13. When the nurse conducts an admission history, which subjective symptom is the client likely to describe?

[ ] **1.** Difficulty urinating
[ ] **2.** Intolerance to cold
[ ] **3.** Profuse perspiration
[ ] **4.** Excessive appetite

The client with myxedema is treated with levothyroxine (Synthroid), one tablet P.O. every day.

14. Which statement provides the best evidence that the client understands the prescribed drug therapy?

[ ] **1.** "I must take this drug after meals."
[ ] **2.** "I should avoid driving when sleepy."
[ ] **3.** "I'll need to take this drug life-long."
[ ] **4.** "I can skip a dose if I'm nauseated."

15. Because the client is receiving levothyroxine (Synthroid) for the first time, the nurse recognizes the need to observe the client for adverse effects related to thyroid replacement therapy. For which signs and symptoms should the nurse assess? Select all that apply.

[ ] **1.** Dyspnea
[ ] **2.** Palpitations
[ ] **3.** Excessive bruising
[ ] **4.** Raised, red rash
[ ] **5.** Hyperactivity
[ ] **6.** Insomnia

A client seeks medical attention after noticing fullness in the neck. After several diagnostic tests, a large endemic goiter is diagnosed.

16. As the nurse provides care for the client newly diagnosed with a large goiter, which interventions should be implemented? Select all that apply.

[ ] **1.** Observe the client's respiratory status
[ ] **2.** Elevate the head of the client's bed
[ ] **3.** Provide a diet high in iodized salt
[ ] **4.** Obtain an order for a soft diet
[ ] **5.** Assess for high fever
[ ] **6.** Administer prescribed antibiotics

A client is undergoing treatment for Graves' disease.

17. Which characteristic facial feature would the nurse expect to note during a physical examination of this client?

[ ] **1.** Bulging eyes
[ ] **2.** Bulbous nose
[ ] **3.** Thick lips
[ ] **4.** Large tongue

The physician prescribes propylthiouracil (Propyl-Thyracil) to treat the client's condition.

18. Before administering this medication, what is essential for the nurse to ask the client?

[ ] **1.** "Do you have trouble swallowing?"
[ ] **2.** "Do you prefer a liquid form of medication?"
[ ] **3.** "Have you had digestive disorders in the past?"
[ ] **4.** "Is there a possibility you could be pregnant?"

19. Because propylthiouracil (Propyl-Thyracil) can cause agranulocytosis, the nurse advises the client to notify the physician if which problem occurs?
[ ] **1.** Persistent sore throat
[ ] **2.** Occasional heart palpitations
[ ] **3.** Fatigue on exertion
[ ] **4.** Prolonged bleeding with trauma

After diagnostic testing, a client with Graves' disease is informed that it is necessary to undergo a subtotal thyroidectomy. The physician prescribes potassium iodide (Lugol's solution) 4 gtt P.O. to be taken for 10 days before the scheduled surgery.

20. When the nurse teaches the client how to self-administer potassium iodide (Lugol's solution), which instruction is most appropriate?
[ ] **1.** Swallow the drug quickly.
[ ] **2.** Take the drug before meals.
[ ] **3.** Dilute the drug in fruit juice.
[ ] **4.** Chill the drug before taking it.

The client asks the nurse to explain the purpose of the preoperative drug therapy.

21. Which response by the nurse about potassium iodide (Lugol's solution) is correct?
[ ] **1.** It firms the gland so it is easily removed.
[ ] **2.** It decreases the postoperative recovery time.
[ ] **3.** It decreases the risk of postoperative bleeding.
[ ] **4.** It eliminates the need for hormone replacement.

22. Preoperatively, which information is most important to teach the client before the subtotal thyroidectomy?
[ ] **1.** Techniques for changing positions
[ ] **2.** Reasons for performing leg exercises
[ ] **3.** The necessity for daily dressing changes
[ ] **4.** Postoperative use of the incentive spirometer

23. To prepare for potential postoperative complications related to the thyroidectomy, which item is necessary to keep at the client's bedside?
[ ] **1.** Dressing change kit
[ ] **2.** Tracheostomy tray
[ ] **3.** Ampule of epinephrine
[ ] **4.** Mechanical ventilator

After surgery, the client is returned to the nursing unit in stable condition.

24. In which position should the client be maintained after the subtotal thyroidectomy?
[ ] **1.** Supine
[ ] **2.** Sims'
[ ] **3.** Semi-Fowler's
[ ] **4.** Recumbent

25. Postoperatively, the nurse should consult the physician before encouraging the client who has undergone a subtotal thyroidectomy to perform which activity?
[ ] **1.** Forced coughing
[ ] **2.** Deep breathing
[ ] **3.** Ambulating
[ ] **4.** Dangling legs

26. Which intervention is most appropriate to add to the client's care plan when monitoring for incisional bleeding after a subtotal thyroidectomy?
[ ] **1.** Observe for signs of hypovolemic shock.
[ ] **2.** Assess for dampness at the back of the client's neck.
[ ] **3.** Remove the dressing to directly inspect the wound.
[ ] **4.** Weigh all gauze dressings before and after changing.

27. Which assessment technique is most appropriate when checking for laryngeal nerve damage in a client who has had a thyroidectomy?
[ ] **1.** Turning the client's head from side to side
[ ] **2.** Observing the client swallowing
[ ] **3.** Looking for tracheal deviation
[ ] **4.** Asking the client to say "Ah"

28. The nurse should assess for hypocalcemia based on which client statements after a subtotal thyroidectomy? Select all that apply.
[ ] **1.** "I feel like I could vomit."
[ ] **2.** "My lips feel numb and tingly."
[ ] **3.** "Light seems to bother my eyes."
[ ] **4.** "I feel weak when I walk."
[ ] **5.** "I have cramps in my legs."
[ ] **6.** "I feel like my throat is constricting."

Because the client is exhibiting signs and symptoms of hypocalcemia after surgery, the nurse assesses for Chvostek's sign.

29. Place an *X* in the area of the head that the nurse should assess to determine a positive or negative Chvostek's sign.

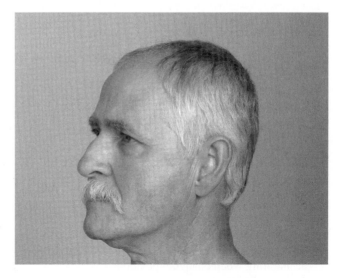

A day after a client undergoes subtotal thyroidectomy, the nurse suspects that the client is developing clinical manifestations related to thyroid crisis.

30. Which signs and symptoms related to thyroid crisis require immediate notification of the physician? Select all that apply.
[ ] **1.** High fever
[ ] **2.** Falling blood pressure
[ ] **3.** Regular noisy respirations
[ ] **4.** Hand spasms
[ ] **5.** Heart palpitations
[ ] **6.** Decreased urine output

Based on the client's clinical presentation, a diagnosis of thyroid crisis is made.

31. Which nursing interventions are most appropriate at this time? Select all that apply.
[ ] **1.** Take the client's vital signs at least every hour.
[ ] **2.** Assess Trousseau's sign every shift.
[ ] **3.** Limit the client's activity.
[ ] **4.** Administer antipyretics per order.
[ ] **5.** Encourage a diet high in iodized salt.
[ ] **6.** Make sure I.V. calcium gluconate is available.

32. At the beginning of thyroid replacement therapy after a thyroidectomy, the nurse must monitor the client closely for side effects. Which findings would the nurse expect to detect if the client is receiving more thyroid hormone replacement than required? Select all that apply.
[ ] **1.** Hyperglycemia
[ ] **2.** Tachycardia
[ ] **3.** Insomnia
[ ] **4.** Hirsutism
[ ] **5.** Tremors
[ ] **6.** Hypertension

Nursing Care of Clients with Disorders of the Parathyroid Glands

A client who develops a benign parathyroid tumor manifests signs of hyperparathyroidism.

33. When the nurse reviews the client's history, which assessment finding is closely associated with the client's diagnosis?
[ ] **1.** Nightly leg cramps
[ ] **2.** Recurrent kidney stones
[ ] **3.** Loose bowel movements
[ ] **4.** Excessive energy level

The nursing assistant assigned to this client asks why the care plan indicates that the client is at risk for falls and injury.

34. Which is the best explanation by the nurse concerning an effect of hyperparathyroidism?
[ ] **1.** The inability to maintain balance
[ ] **2.** The risk of developing seizures
[ ] **3.** Fainting when changing positions
[ ] **4.** Pathologic bone fractures

The client has three of the four lobes of the parathyroid gland surgically removed.

35. After the client returns from surgery and resumes eating, the nurse should encourage the client to eat foods from which food group?
[ ] **1.** Bread and cereals
[ ] **2.** Milk and cheese
[ ] **3.** Meat and seafood
[ ] **4.** Fruit and vegetables

A client diagnosed with hypoparathyroidism develops tetany and comes to the emergency department for treatment.

36. Which I.V. medication can the nurse expect the physician to order to treat the client's condition?
[ ] **1.** Calcium gluconate
[ ] **2.** Ferrous sulfate
[ ] **3.** Potassium chloride
[ ] **4.** Sodium bicarbonate

Nursing Care of Clients with Disorders of the Adrenal Glands

The nurse is caring for a client with a disorder of the adrenal glands.

37. The client and family speak very little English. To explain the location of the adrenal glands, the nurse uses a diagram. Place an X where the adrenal glands are located.

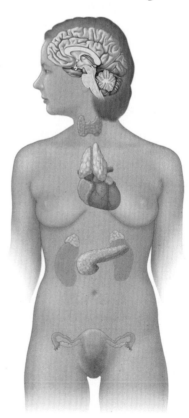

The nurse cares for a client with Addison's disease.

38. Which characteristic findings would the nurse expect to assess in a client with Addison's disease? Select all that apply.
[ ] **1.** Salt craving
[ ] **2.** Skin blemishes
[ ] **3.** Moon-shaped face
[ ] **4.** Bronzed skin
[ ] **5.** Hypoglycemia
[ ] **6.** Weight loss

39. Which nursing assessment is most helpful in evaluating the status of a client with Addison's disease?
[ ] **1.** Blood pressure
[ ] **2.** Bowel sounds
[ ] **3.** Breath sounds
[ ] **4.** Heart sounds

The client's care plan indicates that the nurse should assist the client in selecting foods that are good sources of sodium as part of the treatment for Addison's disease.

40. If the following foods are available, which one should the nurse recommend?
[ ] **1.** Graham crackers
[ ] **2.** Cheddar cheese
[ ] **3.** Raw carrots
[ ] **4.** Canned fruit

The nurse documents that the client has recurrent episodes of hypoglycemia.

41. If a regular diet is ordered, which between-meal snack should the nurse offer to help regulate the client's blood glucose level?
[ ] **1.** Lemonade and peanuts
[ ] **2.** Cola and potato chips
[ ] **3.** Coffee and a muffin
[ ] **4.** Milk and crackers

42. Because this client is at risk for developing addisonian crisis, which is also known as *acute adrenal insufficiency* and *adrenal crisis*, a life-threatening condition, what should the nurse instruct the client to avoid?
[ ] **1.** Stress-producing situations
[ ] **2.** Consuming alcoholic beverages
[ ] **3.** Eating complex carbohydrates
[ ] **4.** Getting too little sleep

43. A client with Addison's disease is admitted to the hospital with a history of nausea and vomiting for the past 3 days. The registered nurse (RN) administers methylprednisolone (Solu-Medrol), a glucocorticoid, intravenously. Which nursing action is most important for the licensed practical nurse (LPN) to implement in the client's plan of care?
[ ] **1.** Glucometer measurements
[ ] **2.** Intake and output volumes
[ ] **3.** Daily weights
[ ] **4.** Frequent oral care

A 38-year-old client is hospitalized after developing symptoms that resemble those of Cushing's syndrome. The nurse completes admission documentation.

44. Based on the client's condition, which findings will the nurse most likely document after completing the initial physical assessment? Select all that apply.
[ ] **1.** The client has very thin legs.
[ ] **2.** The client looks emaciated.
[ ] **3.** The client has bulging eyes.
[ ] **4.** The client's skin is pale.
[ ] **5.** The client has bruising.
[ ] **6.** The client's scalp hair is thin.

The nurse develops the care plan and documents an expected outcome that states, "The client will be free of infection during the hospital stay."

45. Based on the nurse's understanding of this disease process, for what reasons is the expected outcome justified? Select all that apply.
[ ] **1.** The client is at risk for skin breakdown related to thinning of the skin and edema.
[ ] **2.** Wound healing is prolonged in clients with this disorder.
[ ] **3.** The immunosuppressive effects of the disorder mask symptoms of infection.
[ ] **4.** The client is at risk for aspiration pneumonia related to laryngeal nerve damage.
[ ] **5.** The client's admission white blood cell count is elevated.
[ ] **6.** The client's admission temperature is within normal limits.

The physician orders a 24-hour urine collection to aid in the diagnosis of Cushing's syndrome.

46. The nurse is most accurate in telling the client that the urine collection will begin when?
[ ] **1.** With the client's next voiding
[ ] **2.** After the client's next voiding
[ ] **3.** After drinking a pitcher of water
[ ] **4.** With the first voiding in the morning

47. Which statement is correct concerning the collection of urine for a 24-hour specimen?
[ ] **1.** The volume of each voiding is measured and recorded.
[ ] **2.** The urine is placed in a container of preservative.
[ ] **3.** Each voiding is taken immediately to the laboratory.
[ ] **4.** The client voids directly into the specimen container.

After the health care team meets to discuss the client's nursing needs, the nursing diagnosis "Disturbed body image" is added to the care plan.

48. The best rationale for adding this nursing diagnosis to the care plan in the case of a female is that females with Cushing's syndrome typically experience which physiologic effect?
[ ] **1.** Masculine characteristics
[ ] **2.** Heavy menstrual flow
[ ] **3.** Extreme weight loss
[ ] **4.** Large, pendulous breasts

Diagnostic tests confirm that the client's adrenal glands are producing excessive amounts of adrenocortical hormones.

49. When the nurse explains the disorder to the client's spouse, it is accurate to stress that the client is also likely to experience which effect?
[ ] **1.** Anxiety and occasional panic attacks
[ ] **2.** Depression and suicidal tendencies
[ ] **3.** Impulsiveness and poor self-control
[ ] **4.** Forgetfulness and memory changes

The physician orders a low-sodium diet to help treat the client's Cushing's syndrome.

50. Which action by the nurse provides the best data for monitoring the client's therapeutic response to sodium restriction?
[ ] **1.** Monitoring sodium intake
[ ] **2.** Measuring pedal edema
[ ] **3.** Assessing skin turgor
[ ] **4.** Weighing the client

51. Which nursing interventions are most appropriate for managing the basic needs of a client with Cushing's syndrome? Select all that apply.
[ ] **1.** Have the client sleep on a convoluted (egg-crate) foam mattress.
[ ] **2.** Ambulate the client at frequent intervals.
[ ] **3.** Advise the client to ask for assistance when getting up.
[ ] **4.** Offer high-carbohydrate nourishment.
[ ] **5.** Check the client frequently for suicidal ideation.
[ ] **6.** Instruct the client to wear loose-fitting clothing.

Eventually, the client undergoes a bilateral adrenalectomy to correct Cushing's syndrome.

52. To detect complications of surgery in the immediate postoperative period, which assessment component is most important for the nurse to monitor?
[ ] **1.** Blood pressure
[ ] **2.** Urine output
[ ] **3.** Temperature
[ ] **4.** Specific gravity

53. Which documentation finding provides the best indication that the client has successfully avoided an adrenal (addisonian) crisis after surgery?
[ ] **1.** Urine output is approximately 2,000 mL/day.
[ ] **2.** The client's pedal edema has lessened.
[ ] **3.** Capillary blood glucose level is within normal limits.
[ ] **4.** Vital signs are within preoperative ranges.

54. Based on the knowledge that clients with Cushing's syndrome heal slowly, which nursing measure is most appropriate during the client's postoperative period?
[ ] **1.** Monitoring infusion of I.V. antibiotics
[ ] **2.** Removing tape toward the incision site
[ ] **3.** Increasing the client's dietary protein intake
[ ] **4.** Covering the wound with gauze

55. Which statement provides the best evidence that the client who has undergone a bilateral adrenalectomy understands the postoperative course?
[ ] **1.** "I should avoid people with infectious diseases."
[ ] **2.** "I need to limit my fluid intake to 1 quart per day."
[ ] **3.** "My appearance will never be the same as it was before."
[ ] **4.** "No other treatment is necessary after I recover from surgery."

Nursing Care of Clients with Pancreatic Endocrine Disorders

A 23-year-old client manifests symptoms of hyperinsulinism.

56. In response to a question about timing of symptoms during the nursing history, when is the client most likely to describe that symptoms typically occur?
[ ] **1.** After fasting more than 6 hours
[ ] **2.** About 2 hours after eating a meal
[ ] **3.** Late in the evening, before bedtime
[ ] **4.** Early in the morning, before breakfast

A glucose tolerance test is ordered to determine if the client has functional hypoglycemia.

57. Which instruction by the nurse concerning the test procedure is most accurate?
[ ] **1.** "You need to eat a large meal just before the test."
[ ] **2.** "Bring a voided urine specimen to the laboratory."
[ ] **3.** "You can drink coffee or tea in the morning before the test."
[ ] **4.** "You will be given a sweetened drink before the test."

58. To reduce or eliminate the symptoms that a client with functional hypoglycemia experiences, it is best for the nurse to recommend eating five or six small meals containing which nutrient?
[ ] **1.** Simple sugars
[ ] **2.** Complete proteins
[ ] **3.** Complex carbohydrates
[ ] **4.** Unsaturated fats

59. Which of the following provides the best evidence that the dietary measures to control functional hypoglycemia are therapeutic?
[ ] 1. The client experiences fewer incidences of weakness and tremors.
[ ] 2. The client experiences fewer incidences of thirst and dry mouth.
[ ] 3. The client experiences fewer incidences of muscle spasms and fatigue.
[ ] 4. The client experiences fewer incidences of hunger and abdominal cramps.

A nurse participates in a community-wide screening to identify adults who may have undiagnosed diabetes mellitus.

60. If the screening includes a measurement of postprandial blood glucose, the nurse is correct in explaining that blood will be drawn at which time?
[ ] 1. Approximately 2 hours before breakfast
[ ] 2. Approximately 2 hours after a meal
[ ] 3. Approximately 2 hours before bedtime
[ ] 4. Approximately 2 hours after fasting

61. Which statement indicates that a client with an elevated 2-hour postprandial blood glucose level understands the significance of the screening test?
[ ] 1. "I need to eat less frequently."
[ ] 2. "I need to stop eating candy."
[ ] 3. "I need to consult my physician."
[ ] 4. "I need to begin taking insulin."

62. Which signs and symptoms are most appropriate for the nurse to investigate when screening adults who have come to have their blood glucose tested?
[ ] 1. Diarrhea, anorexia, and weight gain
[ ] 2. Constipation, weight loss, and thirst
[ ] 3. Polycholia, polyemia, and polyplegia
[ ] 4. Polyuria, polydipsia, and polyphagia

After the screening test, one client is referred to a physician for additional follow-up. Further diagnostic tests confirm that the client has type 2 diabetes mellitus.

63. When given the news, the client denies the diagnosis and becomes angry, stating there has been a mistake in the tests. Which nursing action is most appropriate at this time?
[ ] 1. Emphasizing the importance of treatment
[ ] 2. Reassuring the client that the disease is easily managed
[ ] 3. Explaining that many people live with diabetes
[ ] 4. Listening as the client expresses current feelings

The client with newly diagnosed type 2 diabetes mellitus is referred to the diabetes clinic for teaching.

64. When the client asks the nurse why regular exercise is recommended for diabetic clients, the best answer is that exercise tends to facilitate which positive outcome?
[ ] 1. Regular exercise helps to control weight.
[ ] 2. Regular exercise helps to decrease appetite.
[ ] 3. Regular exercise helps to reduce blood glucose levels.
[ ] 4. Regular exercise helps to improve circulation to the feet.

A dietitian explains how to use the American Diabetes Association exchange list.

65. Which statement by the client provides the best evidence that the client understands the principle of an exchange list for meal planning?
[ ] 1. "I can eat one serving from each category on the exchange list per day."
[ ] 2. "Measured amounts of food in each category are equal to one another."
[ ] 3. "The number of servings from the exchange list is unlimited."
[ ] 4. "I need to use the exchange list to determine the nutrition in food."

66. The nurse knows the diabetic client understands what "free" foods on the exchange list means if the client excludes which one of the following from a meal plan?
[ ] 1. Iced tea
[ ] 2. Flavored water
[ ] 3. Light beer
[ ] 4. Club soda

67. Using the Dietary Exchange Plan for a 1,500 calorie diet in the chart below, which item is appropriate for the diabetic client to have in the midafternoon?

	Starch/bread	Meat	Vegetable	Fruit	Milk	Fat
Breakfast	2			1	1	1
Lunch	2	1	1	1		1
Snack				1		
Dinner	2	2	1	1		2
Bedtime	1			1	1	

[ ] 1. An 8-oz carton of milk
[ ] 2. Two graham crackers
[ ] 3. A medium apple
[ ] 4. A 2-oz slice of turkey

The physician prescribes glyburide (DiaBeta) orally for the client to treat diabetes.

68. When the client asks why a diabetic relative cannot take insulin orally, what is the best answer?
[ ] **1.** Insulin is inactivated by digestive enzymes.
[ ] **2.** Insulin is absorbed too quickly in the stomach.
[ ] **3.** Insulin is irritating to the gastric mucosa.
[ ] **4.** Insulin is incompatible with many foods.

69. The diabetic client tells the nurse that breakfast is always skipped. Which response by the nurse is most appropriate?
[ ] **1.** "If you drink a glass of milk and eat a breakfast bar, that will be sufficient for breakfast."
[ ] **2.** "You should eat each meal and snack at the same time each day."
[ ] **3.** "If you skip breakfast, eat a high-calorie snack at midmorning."
[ ] **4.** "Wait to take your medication until you eat your first meal of the day."

After the client is discharged from the hospital, the physician wants the client to continue to self-monitor the response to the diet and medication management.

70. Which monitoring approach is best for the nurse to recommend?
[ ] **1.** Testing the urine with a chemical reagent strip
[ ] **2.** Using a glucometer to check capillary blood glucose levels
[ ] **3.** Having laboratory personnel draw venous blood samples
[ ] **4.** Arranging for testing by a home health agency nurse

Emergency medical personnel bring a client who is lethargic and confused to the emergency department (ED). A tentative diagnosis of type 1 diabetes mellitus and diabetic ketoacidosis (DKA) is made.

71. Which assessment findings would the nurse expect to document if the client has DKA? Select all that apply.
[ ] **1.** The client is hypertensive and tachycardic.
[ ] **2.** The client is dyspneic and hypotensive.
[ ] **3.** The client breathes noisily and smells of acetone.
[ ] **4.** The client stares blankly and smells of alcohol.
[ ] **5.** The client has warm, flushed skin and has vomited.
[ ] **6.** The client complains of abdominal pain and is thirsty.

The nurse documents that Kussmaul's respirations were detected during the initial assessment.

72. Which respiratory pattern is the best description of the client's breathing?
[ ] **1.** Fast, deep, labored respirations
[ ] **2.** Shallow respirations, alternating with apnea
[ ] **3.** Slow inhalation and exhalation through pursed lips
[ ] **4.** Shortness of breath with pauses

The nurse plans to monitor the client's response to insulin therapy closely with an electronic glucometer and instructs the emergency department technician to take periodic capillary blood glucose measurements.

73. Which techniques are correct when using an electronic glucometer to monitor the client's capillary blood glucose level? Select all that apply.
[ ] **1.** Clean the client's finger with povidone-iodine (Betadine).
[ ] **2.** Take a set of vital signs before the test.
[ ] **3.** Pierce the central pad of the client's finger.
[ ] **4.** Apply a large drop of blood to a test strip or area.
[ ] **5.** Don gloves before piercing the client's finger.
[ ] **6.** Perform a quality control before the test.

After using the glucometer, the emergency department technician reports to the nurse that the client's capillary blood glucose measures 498 mg/dL.

74. Based on the client's blood glucose measurement, the nurse immediately reevaluates the client. Which physician orders should the ED nurse anticipate? Select all that apply.
[ ] **1.** STAT serum blood glucose
[ ] **2.** Intravenous regular insulin
[ ] **3.** Vital signs every 2 hours
[ ] **4.** A diet of six small, frequent meals
[ ] **5.** Electronic glucometer measurements before meals and at bedtime
[ ] **6.** Continuous cardiac monitoring

After stabilization in the emergency department, the client with diabetic ketoacidosis (DKA) is admitted to a step-down unit for further observation and treatment. After several episodes of hyperglycemia, the physician orders sliding-scale regular insulin administered subcutaneously for the client.

75. How soon after administering the client's dose of regular insulin subcutaneously should the nurse assess for signs of hypoglycemia?
[ ] **1.** 5 minutes later
[ ] **2.** 30 minutes later
[ ] **3.** 6 hours later
[ ] **4.** 10 hours later

76. The nurse teaches the client with newly diagnosed diabetes mellitus about the signs and symptoms of hypoglycemia. Which of the following should the nurse stress in teaching? Select all that apply.
[ ] **1.** Sleepiness
[ ] **2.** Shakiness
[ ] **3.** Thirst
[ ] **4.** Hunger
[ ] **5.** Diaphoresis
[ ] **6.** Confusion

During the midmorning after receiving insulin, the client reports feeling weak, shaky, and dizzy. The nurse asks the nursing assistant to obtain a capillary blood glucose measurement with a glucometer.

77. The nursing assistant reports to the nurse that the client's blood glucose reading is 58 mg/dL. What is the most appropriate nursing action at this time?
[ ] **1.** Administer the next scheduled dose of insulin.
[ ] **2.** Give the client ½ cup of sweet fruit juice.
[ ] **3.** Report the client's symptoms to the physician.
[ ] **4.** Perform a complete head-to-toe assessment.

The client with type 1 diabetes mellitus must learn to combine two insulins—regular and intermediate-acting—and self-administer the injection before being discharged.

78. Which action is the best indication that the client needs more practice in combining two insulins in one syringe?
[ ] **1.** The client rolls the vial of intermediate-acting insulin to mix it with its additive.
[ ] **2.** The client instills air into both the fast-acting and intermediate-acting insulin vials.
[ ] **3.** The client instills the intermediate-acting insulin into the vial of rapid-acting insulin.
[ ] **4.** The client inverts each vial before withdrawing the specified amount of insulin.

79. When the client practices self-administration of the insulin, which action is correct?
[ ] **1.** Piercing the skin at a 30-degree angle
[ ] **2.** Using a syringe calibrated in minims
[ ] **3.** Using a 22-gauge needle on the syringe
[ ] **4.** Rotating abdominal sites for each injection

80. The nurse receives an order to administer Novolin R 10 units with Novolin N 20 units to be given subcutaneously at 0730 hours. Place the following actions in correct sequence to show how the nurse would mix the medications. Use all the options.

1. Instill 20 units of air in the vial of Novolin N.	
2. Instill 10 units of air in the vial of Novolin R.	
3. Withdraw 20 units of insulin from the vial of Novolin N.	
4. Withdraw 10 units of insulin from the vial of Novolin R.	

The nurse implements a diabetes teaching plan in anticipation of the client's discharge.

81. Which statement indicates that the client has misunderstood the nurse's teaching?
[ ] **1.** "I may need more insulin during times of stress."
[ ] **2.** "I may need more food when exercising strenuously."
[ ] **3.** "My insulin needs may change as I get older."
[ ] **4.** "My dependence on insulin may stop eventually."

82. The nurse discusses the long-term effects of diabetes mellitus with the client and realizes that the client needs further teaching when the client identifies which occurrence as a complication of this disease?
[ ] **1.** Blindness
[ ] **2.** Stroke
[ ] **3.** Renal failure
[ ] **4.** Liver failure

83. When the client asks how to store an opened vial of insulin, which answer by the nurse offers the most correct instruction?
[ ] **1.** The best place for storing insulin is in the bathroom, close to the shower.
[ ] **2.** The best place to store insulin is in the refrigerator.
[ ] **3.** The best way to store insulin is at room temperature.
[ ] **4.** The best place for storing insulin is in a warm location but out of sunlight.

The nurse includes foot care as a component of diabetes teaching.

84. Which statement by the client about foot care indicates a need for further teaching?
[ ] **1.** "I need to inspect my feet daily."
[ ] **2.** "I should soak my feet each day."
[ ] **3.** "I need to wear shoes whenever I'm not sleeping."
[ ] **4.** "I need to schedule regular appointments with the podiatrist."

After 3 months, the client returns for a follow-up appointment with the physician to evaluate the progress of self-care.

85. Which information is most important for the nurse to elicit from the client to effectively evaluate compliance with the prescribed therapy?
[ ] **1.** The dosage and frequency of insulin administration
[ ] **2.** The client's glucose monitoring records for the past week
[ ] **3.** The client's weight and vital signs before the office interview
[ ] **4.** The symptoms experienced in the past month

86. Which laboratory test is most important for the nurse to monitor to determine how effectively the client's diabetes is being managed?
[ ] **1.** Fasting blood glucose
[ ] **2.** Blood chemistry profile
[ ] **3.** Complete blood count
[ ] **4.** Glycosylated hemoglobin (HbA1c)

During the physician's visit, the client reports researching the use of insulin pumps on the Internet and wants to know the possibility of being a candidate. After evaluating the client and discussing the request, the physician asks the nurse to provide instructions about management of the client's diabetes using a continuous insulin infusion pump.

87. The nurse teaches the client how the infusion pump operates and correctly points out that the infusion is typically administered in which location?
[ ] **1.** In a vein within the nondominant hand
[ ] **2.** In the muscular tissue of the thigh
[ ] **3.** In the subcutaneous tissue of the abdomen below the belt line
[ ] **4.** In an implanted I.V. catheter threaded into the neck

The nurse cares for an older client who is insulin dependent and lives in a long-term care facility.

88. When developing the client's care plan, which intervention is most appropriate to add?
[ ] **1.** Encourage the client to use an electric razor.
[ ] **2.** Tell the client to file rather than cut toenails.
[ ] **3.** Make sure that the client receives mouth care twice per day.
[ ] **4.** Advise the client to use deodorant soap when bathing.

89. The nurse has prepared 24 units of Humulin N insulin for subcutaneous administration. Identify with an X the preferred location for insulin administration to facilitate rapid absorption.

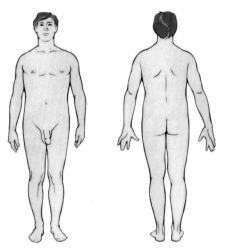

90. Which sign is most suggestive that a client with type 2 diabetes is developing hyperosmolar hyperglycemic nonketotic syndrome (HHNS)?
[ ] **1.** The client's serum glucose level is 650 mg/dL.
[ ] **2.** The client's urinary output is 3,000 mL/24 hours.
[ ] **3.** The client's skin is cool and moist.
[ ] **4.** The client's urine contains acetone.

A client with type 1 diabetes mellitus comes to the clinic complaining of persistent bouts of nausea, vomiting, and diarrhea for the past 4 days. The client has skipped insulin injections because of not being able to eat or keep anything down.

91. Which instruction should the nurse give the client about insulin administration during periods of illness?
[ ] **1.** Monitor blood glucose levels every 2 to 4 hours.
[ ] **2.** Eat candy or sugar frequently.
[ ] **3.** Attempt to drink a high-calorie beverage every hour.
[ ] **4.** Test urine daily for protein.

92. The nurse at the diabetic clinic is reviewing the electronic documentation of client lab work and physician notes. Which client does the nurse identify as needing extended assessment of diabetic management?
[ ] **1.** The client with a HbA1c of 12%
[ ] **2.** The client with fluctuating blood sugars of 97 to 165 mg/dL
[ ] **3.** The adolescent client who acquired type 1 diabetes as a child
[ ] **4.** The client who is moving from insulin via a vial to insulin from a prefilled pen

93. The nurse is instructing a client about using a prefilled insulin pen. Which statement, by the client, needs further clarification?
[ ] **1.** "I need to prime the pen before selecting the prescribed insulin dose."
[ ] **2.** "The insulin in the pen is the same as what I draw up in my vial."
[ ] **3.** "Since my spouse and I use the same type of insulin, we can share the insulin pen."
[ ] **4.** "Needle change is needed prior to administering the next insulin dosage."

94. During change of shifts, a nurse discovers that a hospitalized client with diabetes received two doses of insulin. After notifying the physician, which nursing action is most appropriate?
[ ] **1.** Completing an incident report
[ ] **2.** Calling the intensive care unit (ICU)
[ ] **3.** Performing frequent neurologic checks
[ ] **4.** Monitoring the client's blood glucose level

Correct Answers, Rationales, and Test Taking Strategies

Nursing Care of Clients with Disorders of the Pituitary Gland

1. 2. Diabetes insipidus is a disorder of the posterior lobe of the pituitary gland that results in excessive urination caused by inadequate amounts of antidiuretic hormone, or vasopressin. It can occur secondary to head trauma, brain tumors, or infections such as meningitis. Clients with diabetes insipidus may excrete as much as 20 L/day of very dilute urine; consequently, they need to compensate for fluid loss and may drink up to 20 to 40 L/day, resulting in frequent voiding that poses limits on activity. Weakness, dehydration, and weight loss will result. They also experience polydipsia (intense thirst) not polyphagia (excessive hunger) and hypernatremia. Hyponatremia, glycosuria, and hyperglycemia are not characteristic of this disorder.

> *Test Taking Strategy—Analyze to determine what information the question asks for, which is the most characteristic symptom of a client who has diabetes insipidus. Recall that the disease process is influenced by the pituitary gland's dysregulation of antidiuretic hormone (ADH), causing an excessive urine output (option 2). Review the functions of the posterior pituitary gland, focusing on the role of ADH if you had difficulty answering this question.*
> **Cognitive Level**—*Applying*
> **Client Needs Category**—*Physiological integrity*
> **Client Needs Subcategory**—*Physiological adaptation*

2. 3. The urine of someone with diabetes insipidus is so dilute that it appears colorless. The specific gravity may be 1.002 or less. The specific gravity measures the concentration of the urine; normal values of the urine are between 1.010 and 1.025. Dark tea- or cola-colored urine is commonly associated with glomerulonephritis (a renal disorder), not diabetes insipidus (an endocrine disorder). Normal urine appears pale yellow. Light pink urine indicates hematuria (blood in the urine), which can result from irritation, infection, or renal disorders.

> *Test Taking Strategy—Analyze to determine what information the question asks for, which is the appearance of urine excreted by a client with diabetes insipidus. Recall that the large volume of water that the kidney tubules are unable to reabsorb dilutes the urobilin, a yellow pigment excreted in urine. The urine becomes so diluted by the high volume of water that it appears colorless (option 3). Review the clinical manifestations of diabetes insipidus if you had difficulty answering this question.*
> **Cognitive Level**—*Applying*
> **Client Needs Category**—*Physiological integrity*
> **Client Needs Subcategory**—*Physiological adaptation*

3. 1. To prevent dehydration, it is essential to replace fluids based on the deficit between the client's intake and output. Glucose metabolism is unaffected in diabetes insipidus; therefore, monitoring blood glucose values is unnecessary. Although a client with diabetes insipidus might not eat well because of the constant drinking, maintaining an adequate fluid volume is the primary nursing concern; therefore, monitoring intake and output is critical in this situation. It is not necessary to insert an indwelling catheter to monitor urine output; however, urine does need to be measured. Sending urine to the laboratory is also unnecessary.

> *Test Taking Strategy—Analyze to determine what information the question asks for, which is the nursing intervention that is essential for monitoring the client with diabetes insipidus. Recall that the classic sign of the disorder is extreme polyuria, which leads to selecting option 1, measuring intake and output, as the correct answer. Review nursing assessment findings that are important to evaluate when caring for a client with diabetes insipidus if you had difficulty answering this question.*
> **Cognitive Level**—*Analyzing*
> **Client Needs Category**—*Physiological integrity*
> **Client Needs Subcategory**—*Reduction of risk potential*

4. 2. For the sake of comparison, clients are weighed at the same time each day, on the same scale, and wearing similar clothing each time. Nothing in the situation indicates whether a standing scale was used or whether the client wore slippers during previous weight assessments. The client's predisease weight has no bearing on the current condition except as a point of reference.

> *Test Taking Strategy—Note the key words "most important," indicating that more than one option may be correct, but one is essential for obtaining an accurate client weight. Recall that body weight fluctuates depending on a person's fluid intake and output. To accurately compare weight as an indicator of fluid gain or loss, it is most important to weigh a client at the same time each day (option 2), using the same scale, and with the client dressed similarly to other weight assessments. Review requirements for obtaining an accurate weight if you had difficulty answering this question.*
> **Cognitive Level**—*Applying*
> **Client Needs Category**—*Physiological integrity*
> **Client Needs Subcategory**—*Basic care and comfort*

5. 4. Lypressin (Diapid) is a synthetic hormone preparation of vasopressin and is prescribed because of its antidiuretic effects. It promotes reabsorption of water by acting on the collecting ducts in the kidneys, thereby decreasing urine excretion. The client's head should be maintained in an upright position when administering lypressin (Diapid) because the tip of the container is inserted upright into a nostril. The client then inhales while compressing the container and releasing the spray. Vigorous shaking does not improve the medication's effectiveness and, therefore, is unnecessary.

Test Taking Strategy—Analyze to determine what information the question asks for, which is evidence that a client who self-administers a nasal spray containing medication is doing so in a correct manner. Recall that to distribute the aerosolized spray to blood vessels within the nose where it will be absorbed, the client must inhale at the time the medication container is compressed (option 4). Review the procedure for administering medications in the form of a nasal spray if you had difficulty answering this question.
Cognitive Level—*Analyzing*
Client Needs Category—*Physiological integrity*
Client Needs Subcategory—*Pharmacological therapies*

6. 1. The need to administer additional doses of lypressin (Diapid) is based on increased thirst and frequency of urination. If more than the prescribed number of doses is required, the interval between routine administrations is generally decreased while the number of sprays at each dose remains the same. Someone with diabetes insipidus would have urine that is colorless, not dark yellow; a dark yellow color indicates that the urine is concentrated and has a high specific gravity. A runny nose is a side effect of excessive use of the nasal spray. Headaches are not typically associated with this disorder.

Test Taking Strategy—Analyze to determine what information the question asks for, which is the proper symptomatic use of lypressin. Recall that thirst (option 1) is a mechanism that triggers fluid consumption to compensate for a low circulating fluid volume. In the case of diabetes insipidus, thirst may be an early sign that excess fluid loss is occurring from copious urinary excretion. Consult a drug handbook for information on self-administering this drug on an as-needed basis if you had difficulty answering this question.
Cognitive Level—*Applying*
Client Needs Category—*Physiological integrity*
Client Needs Subcategory—*Pharmacological therapies*

7. 2. Acromegaly results from an overproduction of growth hormone. Growth hormone is secreted by the pituitary gland; if oversecreted, as in the case of a pituitary tumor, and left unchecked, it can lead to organ enlargement, increased blood glucose levels, hyperlipidemia, and lengthening and widening of the bones. When the disorder occurs in adulthood, the bones of the hands, jaw, feet, and forehead enlarge but do not lengthen. Acromegaly that develops at or before puberty generally results in gigantism. Undersecretion of growth hormone results in shortened height and dwarfism. Males with acromegaly are likely to experience impotence, but their testes are not unusually small. Although the disorder may cause wide gaps between the teeth due to jaw changes, acromegaly is not known to cause tooth loss.

Test Taking Strategy—Apply the key words "most likely" to each of the four options. Select the option

that correlates best with an assessment finding of a client with acromegaly. Recall that acromegaly is an endocrine disorder that occurs in adults after they have reached their full skeletal growth. Because the bones are no longer able to lengthen in response to excess growth hormone stimulation, they become enlarged (option 2). Review the clinical manifestations of persons who develop acromegaly if you had difficulty answering this question.*
Cognitive Level—*Applying*
Client Needs Category—*Physiological integrity*
Client Needs Subcategory—*Physiological adaptation*

8. 1. Despite the large size, a client with acromegaly is likely to suffer from *Activity intolerance* because of the client's size, muscle weakness, joint pain, and joint stiffness. There is no indication that the client with acromegaly will have difficulty providing self-care, although because of the large size, assistance may be needed. Pulmonary functions generally remain adequate. Clients with acromegaly have difficulty chewing because of the malformations in their jaw and teeth, but swallowing is unaffected.

Test Taking Strategy—Analyze to determine what information the question asks for, which is a nursing diagnosis that is appropriate when planning the care of a client with acromegaly. Because care plans represent high priority nursing problems, the nursing diagnosis should be one among those listed, that has the highest nursing concern. Recall that the client with acromegaly often lacks stamina and endurance despite having a large body size, making option 1 the best answer. Review the signs and symptoms associated with acromegaly, looking for defining characteristics that validate a nursing diagnosis of Activity intolerance, *if you had difficulty answering this question.*
Cognitive Level—*Applying*
Client Needs Category—*Safe and effective care environment*
Client Needs Subcategory—*Coordinated care*

9. 1. The treatment of choice for a pituitary tumor that is oversecreting growth hormone is a trans-sphenoidal hypophysectomy. This involves the surgical removal of the pituitary gland through the nasal passage through an incision under the upper lip. A belief that the client's appearance will return to normal reflects a misunderstanding of the outcome of surgery by the client. Unfortunately, a client with acromegaly will never regain a normal appearance despite successful treatment of the disease. Hormone replacement therapy is necessary after surgery or irradiation of the anterior pituitary gland. The client should wear a medical alert tag and see a physician regularly. The surgical incision is invisible.

Test Taking Strategy—Analyze to determine what information the question asks for, which is evidence of the client's lack of understanding of the surgical procedure. Read each of the options, looking for a statement

that reflects a misunderstanding—in other words, an inaccurate belief—regarding the outcome after a trans-sphenoidal hypophysectomy. After comparing all the options, select the one that is incorrect. Recall that removing the anterior lobe of the pituitary gland will not change the client's appearance, but it will elimi-nate further stimulation of the client's bone growth. Review the signs, symptoms, and treatment of pituitary tumors if you had difficulty answering the question.
Cognitive Level—*Analyzing*
Client Needs Category—*Physiological integrity*
Client Needs Subcategory—*Physiological adaptation*

10. 2. The surgical incision is made through the upper gingival mucosa in the mouth, along one side of the nasal septum and through the sphenoid sinus, or it is performed transnasally. Postoperatively, the nose is packed with gauze. In addition to checking the saturation and appear-ance of the gauze packing, the nurse inspects the pharynx, where blood or cerebrospinal fluid may drain posteriorly. Examining the client's skull, ear canal, or tongue will not help with the assessment.

Test Taking Strategy—Use the process of elimination to help select the option that identifies the best location for assessing the client for postoperative bleeding after a trans-sphenoidal hypophysectomy. If unsure, look at the word "trans-sphenoidal" and correlate the anatomic location of the sphenoid bone and its sinuses to the site of the surgical incision. Recall that the pituitary gland is located above the back of the nose, which leads to eliminating options 1, 3, and 4 and selecting option 2 as the best answer. Review a description of the surgical procedure and the anatomic landmarks that are involved if you had difficulty answering this question.
Cognitive Level—*Applying*
Client Needs Category—*Physiological integrity*
Client Needs Subcategory—*Reduction of risk potential*

Nursing Care of Clients with Disorders of the Thyroid Gland

11. 3. A radioactive iodine uptake test is used in diag-nostic scans and destroys thyroid tissue in disorders involving hyperthyroidism and thyroid malignancies. The amount of radiation used in a radioactive iodine uptake test is minute, but special precautions (such as flushing the toi-let twice after use, rinsing the bathroom sink and tub, and using separate bath linens) are generally suggested. These precautions are only needed for a few days. Although there is no antidote for radioactive iodine, there is no justifica-tion for isolating the client because of the minute exposure.

Test Taking Strategy—Apply the key terms "most accurate" to the instructions in each of the four options. Select the nursing statement that correctly identifies the client's care after a radioactive iodine

uptake test. *Recall that special precautions like those identified must be taken until the half-lives of the radioactive iodine are low enough to be considered safe. Review how the nursing care of a client under-going a radioactive iodine test is managed if you had difficulty answering this question.*
Cognitive Level—*Applying*
Client Needs Category—*Safe and effective care environment*
Client Needs Subcategory—*Safety and infection control*

12. 1, 5, 6. The severe form of hypothyroidism is called *myxedema*. Hypothyroidism is the result of insufficient production of thyroid-stimulating hormone that results in a slowing of metabolic processes. Myxedema is life-threaten-ing if left untreated. Common signs of myxedema include hypothermia, hypotension, a hoarse and raspy voice, slow speech, lethargy, expressionless face, protruding tongue, coarse and sparse hair, weight gain, and dry skin.

Test Taking Strategy—Analyze to determine what information the question asks for, which is signs of myxedema. Alternative-format "select all that apply" questions require considering each option independently to decide its merit in answering the question. Based on the location of the thyroid gland, which is anterior to the trachea, and the fact that thyroid hormones regulate metabolic processes, cor-rect signs include a change in a client's voice and altered vital signs. Review signs of myxedema if you had difficulty answering this question.
Cognitive Level—*Applying*
Client Needs Category—*Physiological integrity*
Client Needs Subcategory—*Physiological adaptation*

13. 2. Because of the lowered rate of metabolism, indi-viduals with myxedema do not generate the same amount of energy and body heat as those with a normal metabolism. Consequently, clients typically complain of being exces-sively cold. The disorder is not associated with difficulty in urination, profuse perspiration, or excessive appetite.

Test Taking Strategy—Analyze to determine what infor-mation the question asks for, which is a symptom that a client with myxedema is likely to report. Note the word "subjective," which indicates a manifestation that the client can identify, but one that is not obvi-ous during assessment by the nurse. Recall that this disorder results in slowed metabolism, which means that the client is not metabolizing nutrients to create calories at a normal rate. Calories are responsible for producing heat. Consequently, intolerance to cold (option 2) is the best answer. Review the symptoms of myxedema and the meaning of the term subjective symptoms if you had difficulty answering this ques-tion.
Cognitive Level—*Applying*
Client Needs Category—*Physiological integrity*
Client Needs Subcategory—*Physiological adaptation*

14. 3. Thyroid replacement therapy is maintained during the course of a client's lifetime. A low dose is given initially, then increased or decreased on the basis of the drug levels in the blood. Dosage adjustments are also made periodically during a client's lifetime based on the client's liver and kidney function, other medications that the client may be taking, and the client's clinical presentation of signs and symptoms. The physician prescribed the drug to be taken once per day, not after each meal. Levothyroxine (Synthroid) is more likely to cause insomnia than fatigue or sleepiness. The client should consult a physician before omitting or discontinuing the drug, regardless of the reason.

> *Test Taking Strategy—Use the process of elimination to help select the option that provides the best evidence that the client understands the drug therapy for managing myxedema. Options 1 and 4 can be eliminated because they do not reflect the dosage schedule for this medication. Option 2 can be eliminated because drowsiness is not a side effect of levothyroxine. Recall that thyroid replacement therapy is a lifelong component of treatment (option 3) when the thyroid gland no longer functions properly. Review the management of myxedema, focusing on the use of drug therapy, if you had difficulty answering this question.*
> *Cognitive Level—Applying*
> *Client Needs Category—Physiological integrity*
> *Client Needs Subcategory—Pharmacological therapies*

15. **1, 2, 5, 6.** Once the client is accurately diagnosed with hypothyroidism or myxedema, thyroid replacement therapy may be started. The nurse should watch for signs and symptoms related to *hyper*thyroidism, which could be an indication that the levothyroxine (Synthroid) dosage is too high. The adverse reactions include dyspnea, palpitations, hyperactivity, dizziness, insomnia, excessive hunger, rapid pulse, and GI complaints. Excessive bruising is not associated with thyroid replacement therapy; instead it is associated with anticoagulants. A rash is not associated with thyroid replacement therapy.

> *Test Taking Strategy—Analyze to determine what information the question asks for, which is assessments that are pertinent when a client begins thyroid replacement therapy. Alternative-format "select all that apply" questions require considering each option independently to decide its merit in answering the question. Recall that when thyroid hormones are replaced, the effects would be evidence of increased metabolic activity. Review the side effects associated with thyroid replacement therapy if you had difficulty answering this question.*
> *Cognitive Level—Applying*
> *Client Needs Category—Physiological integrity*
> *Client Needs Subcategory—Pharmacological therapies*

16. **1, 2, 3, 4.** An endemic goiter is caused by a deficiency of iodine in the diet resulting in an enlarged thyroid gland. As a consequence, the client feels a fullness in the neck. Appropriate nursing interventions include observing the client's respiratory status because the client may experience respiratory distress due to pressure on the trachea. Elevating the head of the bed can relieve respiratory symptoms. Because the endemic goiter is a result of iodine deficiency, providing a diet high in iodized salt is also appropriate. Obtaining an order for a soft diet is prudent because of the pressure of the enlarged thyroid on the esophagus, which makes swallowing difficult. There is no need to assess for fever or administer antibiotics because a goiter is not related to an infectious process.

> *Test Taking Strategy—Analyze the information the question asks, which is nursing interventions for a client with an endemic goiter. Alternative-format "select all that apply" questions require considering each option independently to decide its merit in answering the question. Select nursing interventions that reflect the etiology and physical consequences of an endemic goiter. Review the nursing care of a client with an endemic goiter if you had difficulty answering this question.*
> *Cognitive Level—Applying*
> *Client Needs Category—Physiological integrity*
> *Client Needs Subcategory—Physiological adaptation*

17. **1.** Graves' disease is due to hyperthyroidism. It is called by several names, including *toxic diffuse goiter, thyrotoxicosis, Basedow's disease,* and *exophthalmic goiter.* As the latter term indicates, exophthalmos (bulging or enlarged eyes) is a common characteristic. The other facial features described are not directly related to this thyroid disorder.

> *Test Taking Strategy—Analyze to determine what information the question asks for, which is a facial feature that is characteristic among persons who develop Graves' disease. Recall that exophthalmos, one of many clinical manifestations of hyperthyroidism, results from enlarged muscle and fatty tissue surrounding the rear and sides of the eyeball. Review the signs and symptoms of Graves' disease if you had difficulty answering this question.*
> *Cognitive Level—Understanding*
> *Client Needs Category—Physiological integrity*
> *Client Needs Subcategory—Physiological adaptation*

18. **4.** Propylthiouracil (Propyl-Thyracil), used in the medical treatment of hyperthyroidism, is given to block thyroid hormones preoperatively or for clients who are not candidates for surgery. It inhibits the manufacture of thyroid hormones but does not affect the hormones already circulating in the blood or those stored in the gland itself. Propylthiouracil can cause cretinism (hypothyroidism) in a developing fetus. Cretinism results in irreversible brain and skeletal abnormalities with mental retardation and dwarfism if thyroid replacement therapy is not initiated within the first 6 weeks after birth. Therefore, asking about the client's pregnancy status is essential. Although the client may have trouble swallowing and the drug may cause GI side effects, ensuring the safety of the client and a fetus is the nurse's priority. Propylthiouracil is not available in a liquid form, but the client may be instructed to crush the tablet and mix it with food.

Test Taking Strategy—*Analyze to determine what information the question asks for, which is an essential question the nurse should ask that affects the safe administration of propylthiouracil. Recall that this drug suppresses thyroid hormone production. However, if the client is pregnant, the drug can also suppress thyroid hormone production in a fetus, causing congenital hypothyroidism or cretinism. Review the action of propylthiouracil and its adverse effects on fetal development if you had difficulty answering this question.*
Cognitive Level—*Applying*
Client Needs Category—*Physiological integrity*
Client Needs Subcategory—*Pharmacological therapies*

19. 1. Agranulocytosis is a decrease in white blood cells (WBCs) produced to fight infections. A sore throat, fever, and malaise may indicate that the client has insufficient WBCs to prevent infection. Heart palpitations, a symptom of Graves' disease, become infrequent as treatment with propylthiouracil (Propyl-Thyracil) continues. Prolonged bleeding is evidence of thrombocytopenia (a decrease in platelets) and is not related to agranulocytosis. Fatigue can be caused by anemia related to a decreased number of circulating red blood cells.

Test Taking Strategy—*Analyze to determine what information the question asks for, which is an indication that agranulocytosis may be occurring in a client for whom propylthiouracil has been prescribed. Look for an option that relates to low numbers of WBCs. Because WBCs are necessary for fighting infections, having a sore throat (option 1) suggests a bacterial infection may be present. Review the definition of agranulocytosis and the health risks it creates if you had difficulty answering this question.*
Cognitive Level—*Applying*
Client Needs Category—*Physiological integrity*
Client Needs Subcategory—*Pharmacological therapies*

20. 3. Potassium iodide (Lugol's solution) is given in conjunction with an antithyroid drug such as propylthiouracil (Propyl-Thyracil) to curb thyroid activity before surgery and to decrease postoperative complications. Lugol's solution has a bitter, metallic taste and can cause burning in the mouth and sore teeth and gums. Diluting the strong solution in fruit juice or water tends to disguise its unpleasant taste. Although swallowing the drug quickly may ensure that all of the drug is taken, this is not the best advice. There is no real reason to recommend chilling the drug or taking it before meals.

Test Taking Strategy—*Apply the key words "most appropriate" to each of the four options to determine which nursing instruction is most applicable in regard to administering potassium iodide. Recall*

that diluting the drug in a substance like fruit juice (option 3) can mask its unpleasant taste. Review information on administering potassium iodide if you had difficulty answering this question.
Cognitive Level—*Applying*
Client Needs Category—*Physiological integrity*
Client Needs Subcategory—*Pharmacological therapies*

21. 3. Clients commonly receive antithyroid drugs several weeks before surgery to prevent excessive release of thyroid hormones during and after surgery. Preoperative therapy with antithyroid drugs reduces the potential for postoperative bleeding and the development of a thyroid crisis, or storm. Although the treatment reduces the size of the gland, this is not the underlying reason for the drug therapy. The postoperative recovery period is shortened if complications are prevented, but reducing the potential for bleeding is a more accurate answer. Thyroid replacement therapy may still be required after a subtotal thyroidectomy despite preoperative antithyroid drug therapy.

Test Taking Strategy—*Analyze to determine what information the question asks for, which is the purpose for administering Lugol's solution's preoperatively. Recall that handling the thyroid during its surgical removal can contribute to postoperative bleeding and excessive release of thyroid hormones. Administering potassium iodide in the form of Lugol's solution can reduce the risk for bleeding because it shrinks the thyroid gland. Review the action of potassium iodide, especially when given preoperatively to a client undergoing a thyroidectomy, if you had difficulty answering this question.*
Cognitive Level—*Applying*
Client Needs Category—*Physiological integrity*
Client Needs Subcategory—*Pharmacological therapies*

22. 1. Preoperative instructions must include how to support the head and neck when turning or rising to a sitting or standing position. This prevents tension on the sutures in the neck. The other information is important to include, but it is not as essential for the client to know.

Test Taking Strategy—*Apply the key words "most important" when evaluating the choices in the four options. Although there are similarities in all preoperative instructions, option 1 is most important for the particular type of surgery that this client will undergo. Review the preoperative teaching for a client who will have thyroid surgery if you had difficulty answering this question.*
Cognitive Level—*Applying*
Client Needs Category—*Physiological integrity*
Client Needs Subcategory—*Basic care and comfort*

23. 2. Airway obstruction is a potential postoperative complication for clients who undergo thyroidectomy. Therefore, a common standard of practice is to keep a tracheostomy tray in the client's room. A mechanical ventilator will probably be unnecessary once airway patency is reestablished. A dressing change kit can be easily obtained; it is not an emergency item. Epinephrine may be necessary if the client develops a life-threatening cardiac arrhythmia, but this drug is usually stocked in emergency crash carts.

Test Taking Strategy—Analyze to determine what information the question asks for, which is an item that should be kept at the bedside as preparation for a potential postoperative complication. Consider the nature and site of the surgery and that maintaining a patent airway is a priority for any client's care, but especially one in whom the surgical incision with the potential for swelling is adjacent to the trachea. Review the postoperative complications associated with thyroid surgery and nursing actions for managing their potential development if you had difficulty answering this question.
Cognitive Level—*Applying*
Client Needs Category—*Physiological integrity*
Client Needs Subcategory—*Reduction of risk potential*

24. 3. A subtotal thyroidectomy is the partial removal of the thyroid as treatment for an area that is overproducing thyroid hormones. Semi-Fowler's position, with the head elevated 30 to 45 degrees, is best for reducing postoperative incisional edema and facilitating ventilation. None of the other identified positions is therapeutic for accomplishing this goal.

Test Taking Strategy—Analyze to determine what information the question asks for, which is the body position that helps to prevent or reduce the potential for postoperative complications. Consider that the operative site is the neck, making breathing a nursing consideration. This leads to selecting option 3, a semi-Fowler's position with the head elevated, as the best choice for minimizing surgical complications. Review the postoperative nursing care of a client undergoing thyroid surgery if you had difficulty answering this question.
Cognitive Level—*Applying*
Client Needs Category—*Physiological integrity*
Client Needs Subcategory—*Reduction of risk potential*

25. 1. Coughing may precipitate bleeding in and around the surgical area and increase the risk of airway obstruction. Therefore, it is best to consult the physician before encouraging the client to cough postoperatively. The client is encouraged to take deep cleansing breaths, ambulate, and dangle the legs from the side of the bed, as tolerated. These activities will prevent pneumonia and postoperative thrombosis.

Test Taking Strategy—Analyze to determine what information the question asks for, which is an action that may potentially cause harm in this postoperative client. Although forced coughing helps to clear the airway postoperatively, it may contribute to bleeding in this particular client. Therefore, before encouraging
the client to cough, it is best to consult with the physician. Review factors that may contribute to bleeding in a postoperative client who has undergone thyroid surgery if you had difficulty answering this question.*
Cognitive Level—*Applying*
Client Needs Category—*Physiological integrity*
Client Needs Subcategory—*Reduction of risk potential*

26. 2. Gravity causes blood to pool in the back of the neck. This interferes with visual inspection of the neck dressing. Gently placing a gloved hand behind the client's neck and checking for dampness allows the nurse to determine if blood or drainage is oozing from the incisional wound. The pillow, bed linens, and dressing should also be inspected for fresh drainage each time the client is turned. Observing for hypovolemic shock is necessary; however, the nurse should be monitoring for blood loss long before hypovolemia becomes an issue. Initially, the physician removes the postoperative dressing to inspect the wound. Weighing the dressing is unnecessary because the physician asks for the number, not the weight, of soiled dressings.

Test Taking Strategy—Look at the key words "most appropriate" and apply them to select the best intervention among those listed for monitoring incisional bleeding after surgery on the thyroid gland. Although all of the options suggest methods for evaluating incisional bleeding, option 2 is the most appropriate technique because blood drains to the posterior of the neck under the influence of gravity. Review the nursing management of a client after having a thyroidectomy if you had difficulty answering this question.
Cognitive Level—*Analyzing*
Client Needs Category—*Physiological integrity*
Client Needs Subcategory—*Reduction of risk potential*

27. 4. Although hoarseness may be temporary after a subtotal thyroidectomy, laryngeal nerve damage is manifested by persistent voice changes or the inability to make vocal sounds. None of the other techniques is appropriate for assessing laryngeal nerve function.

Test Taking Strategy—Using the key words "most appropriate," look for an action that is best for detecting damage to the laryngeal nerve when assessing the client who has undergone thyroidectomy. Recall that the laryngeal nerve is a branch of the vagus nerve that provides motor and sensory functions to the larynx, the structure that facilitates making sounds and speaking. This leads to selecting option 4 as the correct answer because if the laryngeal nerve has been damaged, the client will not be able to say "Ah." Review the function of the laryngeal nerve and consequences if it becomes damaged if you had difficulty answering this question.
Cognitive Level—*Analyzing*
Client Needs Category—*Physiological integrity*
Client Needs Subcategory—*Reduction of risk potential*

28. 1, 2, 5, 6. Hypocalemia can occur after a subtotal thyroidectomy if the parathyroid glands, which regulate blood calcium levels, are accidentally removed. Signs and symptoms of hypocalcemia include nausea and vomiting, tingling and numbness around the mouth, muscle cramping in the lower extremities, and tightness of the throat (laryngeal spasms). These are commonly the first symptoms noted by a client after a subtotal thyroidectomy. The remaining complaints, weakness and sensitivity to light, are not usually associated with hypocalcemia.

Test Taking Strategy—Analyze to determine what information the question asks for, which is symptoms of hypocalcemia reported by the client. Alternative-format "select all that apply" questions require considering each option independently to decide its merit in answering the question. Consider the function of calcium and evidence of an insufficient level when choosing options. Review clinical manifestations of hypocalcemia if you had difficulty answering this question.
Cognitive Level—Analyzing
Client Needs Category—Physiological integrity
Client Needs Subcategory—Reduction of risk potential

29. Chvostek's sign is assessed by tapping the area over the facial nerve, which is about 1″ (2.5 cm) anterior to the earlobe, just below the zygomatic arch. A client with hypocalcemia will manifest Chvostek's sign, evidenced by facial muscle spasms such as twitching of the cheek, mouth, and nose.

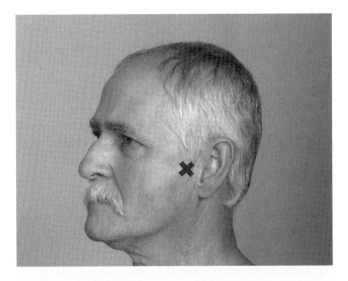

Test Taking Strategy—Analyze to determine what information the question asks for, which is the correct location to elicit Chvostek's sign. Recall that eliciting Chvostek's sign is a neurologic assessment that enables the examiner to determine if an insufficient blood calcium level is present. Review the purpose for assessing Chvostek's sign and the manner in which the assessment is performed if you had difficulty answering this question.

Cognitive Level—Applying
Client Needs Category—Physiological integrity
Client Needs Subcategory—Reduction of risk potential

30. 1, 5. Exaggerated signs of increased metabolism are a manifestation of thyroid crisis (also called *thyroid storm* or *thyrotoxicosis*). Some signs include hyperpyrexia (fever) as high as 41°C or 105.8°F, hypertension, severe tachycardia, chest pain, cardiac arrhythmias/palpitations, dyspnea, and an altered level of consciousness. Carpal spasms are a sign of hypocalcemia. Noisy respirations may indicate laryngospasm due to hypocalcemia or a partial airway obstruction. Hypotension is not a sign of thyroid crisis nor is decreased urine output.

Test Taking Strategy—Analyze to determine what information the question asks for, which is signs and symptoms of thyroid crisis. Alternative-format "select all that apply" questions require considering each option independently to decide its merit in answering the question. Recall that thyroid crisis is an emergency situation that results from an excessive level of thyroid hormone. Choose options that reflect increased metabolism. Review clinical manifestations of thyroid crisis if you had difficulty answering this question.
Cognitive Level—Analyzing
Client Needs Category—Physiological integrity
Client Needs Subcategory—Reduction of risk potential

31. 1, 3, 4. Thyroid crisis is a life-threatening situation and is triggered by manipulation during surgical removal of the thyroid gland, stress, infection, or physical examination of the thyroid gland. The nurse should monitor the client's vital signs at least hourly, paying close attention to the client's temperature (which is elevated), and heart rate and rhythm. Tachycardia and cardiac arrhythmias are common manifestations of this condition. Because of the increased metabolism, the heart has to work harder; unless managed, this could result in cardiac arrest. Therefore, limiting the client's activities decreases the workload on the heart and decreases the need for oxygen. Antipyretics decrease the client's temperature, so this is an important nursing activity. Eliciting Trousseau's sign is related to assessment for tetany, a consequence of hypocalcemia. Making sure I.V. calcium gluconate is available is related to treatment of hypocalcemia, not thyroid crisis. Encouraging a diet high in iodized salt is the treatment for goiter.

Test Taking Strategy—Analyze to determine what information the question asks for, which is nursing interventions for managing the consequences of thyroid storm. Alternative-format "select all that apply" questions require considering each option independently to decide its merit in answering the question. Choose nursing interventions that are appropriate when increased metabolism accelerates activities in all body systems. Review nursing measures used to

manage a client experiencing thyroid storm if you had difficulty answering this question.
Cognitive Level—Analyzing
Client Needs Category—Physiological integrity
Client Needs Subcategory—Physiological adaptation

32. **2, 3, 5, 6.** Thyroid replacement therapy can increase metabolism, causing symptoms similar to those of hyperthyroidism. Until the client adjusts to the replacement therapy or the optimum dosage is determined, the client may experience stimulation of the cardiovascular system, which is manifested by tachycardia and hypertension. Metabolic stimulation can also result in insomnia and tremors. Hyperglycemia and hirsutism are side effects of corticosteroid therapy.

Test Taking Strategy—Analyze to determine what information the question asks for, which is the assessment findings that correlate with a higher than necessary dose of thyroid replacement hormone. Alternative-format "select all that apply" questions require considering each option independently to decide its merit in answering the question. Select options that correlate with signs of hyperthyroidism, which is the consequence of administering thyroid hormone replacement in excess of what is appropriate for producing a euthyroid (normal thyroid) state. Review side effects of thyroid replacement therapy if you had difficulty answering this question.
Cognitive Level—Evaluating
Client Needs Category—Physiological integrity
Client Needs Subcategory—Pharmacological therapies

Nursing Care of Clients with Disorders of the Parathyroid Glands

33. **2.** When there is a disorder of the parathyroid gland, calcium and phosphorus levels are usually affected. In clients diagnosed with hyperparathyroidism, a parathyroid tumor usually causes hypercalcemia and a loss of calcium from the bones to the blood. This leads to the formation of kidney stones and other renal complications. Symptoms of hyperparathyroidism are described as "moans, groans, stones, and bones—with psychic overtones" because besides kidney stones, other signs and symptoms include loss of energy, skeletal tenderness, pain when bearing weight, brittle and fragile bones, emotional irritability, depression, and decreased memory. Cardiac arrhythmias are also common. Hypocalcemia or other etiologies cause leg cramps. Constipation, not loose stools, is more common among clients with hyperparathyroidism. Many clients experience chronic fatigue rather than having excessive energy.

Test Taking Strategy—Analyze to determine what information the question asks for, which is an assessment finding that correlates with hyperparathyroidism. Recall that parathormone increases blood calcium levels and that the excess calcium is excreted by the kidneys. Concentration of calcium in urine

contributes to the formation of renal calculi (option 2). *Review the consequences of hypercalcemia if you had difficulty answering this question.*
Cognitive Level—Applying
Client Needs Category—Physiological integrity
Client Needs Subcategory—Physiological adaptation

34. **4.** Loss of calcium from the bones weakens the skeletal system, which potentiates the risk of pathologic fractures. Impaired equilibrium, seizures, and syncope are not common among clients with hyperparathyroidism.

Test Taking Strategy—Analyze to determine what information the question asks for, which is an effect of hyperparathyroidism. Recall that to raise blood calcium levels, calcium is withdrawn from bones, making the client susceptible to osteopenia (low bone mass), osteoporosis (low bone density), and pathologic bone fractures (option 4). Review the consequences of hyperparathyroidism if you had difficulty answering this question.
Cognitive Level—Applying
Client Needs Category—Safe and effective care environment
Client Needs Subcategory—Safety and infection control

35. **2.** Postoperatively, it is therapeutic to include sources of calcium in the client's diet because the function of the parathyroid gland is suddenly and severely compromised. Foods that are good sources of calcium include milk and cheese. Calcium gluconate may be administered intravenously if the client experiences severe hypocalcemia.

Test Taking Strategy—Analyze to determine what information the question asks for, which is the food group a client who has had most of the parathyroid tissue removed should consume. Recall that the bones have been weakened by the hyperparathyroidism and a goal is to restore bone density. Consuming milk and cheese (option 2), which are excellent sources of calcium, supports the goal. Review the nutrients each of the four options provides, focusing on sources that increase calcium, if you had difficulty answering this question.
Cognitive Level—Applying
Client Needs Category—Physiological integrity
Client Needs Subcategory—Basic care and comfort

36. **1.** Hypoparathyroidism is caused by inadequate secretion of parathyroid hormone, which leads to increased phosphorus levels and a deficiency in blood calcium levels. This deficiency results in hypocalcemia and leads to tetany, the chief symptom of hypoparathyroidism. Tetany is a general muscular condition that results in tremors and spastic, uncoordinated movements. When tetany occurs, calcium gluconate or calcium chloride is the drug of choice for I.V. administration. Ferrous sulfate is a source of iron; it is administered orally to treat anemia. Potassium chloride is given to prevent or relieve hypokalemia. Sodium bicarbonate is administered to maintain normal acid-base balance.

Test Taking Strategy—Analyze to determine what information the question asks for, which is the medication used to treat the complication of tetany. Recall that tetany is a consequence of low levels of blood calcium. Consequently, calcium gluconate (option 1) is the best answer. Review how tetany is managed if you had difficulty answering this question.
Cognitive Level—*Applying*
Client Needs Category—*Physiological integrity*
Client Needs Subcategory—*Pharmacological therapies*

Nursing Care of Clients with Disorders of the Adrenal Glands

37.

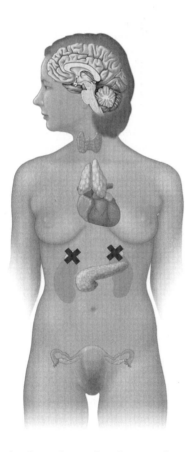

The adrenal glands are located at the top of each kidney, hence the name "ad- *renal*." The outer cortex and the inner medulla produce numerous hormones that affect the use of fats, proteins, and carbohydrates; suppress the inflammatory response; regulate the kidneys' excretion of sodium; supplement hormones that contribute to male secondary sexual characteristics; and promote physiologic activities that are helpful for responding to stressors.
Test Taking Strategy—Analyze to determine what information the question asks for, which is the location of the adrenal glands. Review the location of endocrine glands, with a focus on the adrenal glands, if you had difficulty answering this question.
Cognitive Level—*Remembering*

Client Needs Category—Physiological integrity
Client Needs Subcategory—Physiological adaptation

38. 1, 4, 5, 6. Addison's disease is caused by a deficiency of cortical hormones that develops from adrenal insufficiency. Clients appear unusually tan, bronze, or darkly pigmented. Other signs and symptoms include fatigue, weight loss/emaciation, hypotension, and decreased blood glucose. Decreased sodium levels result in a craving for salt. An increased potassium level is also a clinical manifestation of this disease. A moon-shaped face, skin blemishes, and obesity are more characteristic of a hyperfunctioning adrenal cortex or endogenous steroid therapy.
Test Taking Strategy—Analyze to determine what information the question asks for, which is signs and symptoms of Addison's disease. Alternative-format "select all that apply" questions require considering each option independently to decide its merit in answering the question. Review resources for the list of signs and symptoms associated with Addison's disease if you had difficulty answering this question.
Cognitive Level—*Applying*
Client Needs Category—*Physiological integrity*
Client Needs Subcategory—*Physiological adaptation*

39. 1. If inadequately treated, Addison's disease leads to dehydration and hypotension. If unresolved, it can lead to addisonian crisis, which is characterized by cyanosis, fever, and the classic signs of shock. Monitoring the blood pressure and its subsequent trends provides some of the best data for evaluating the client's health status. Bowel, breath, and heart sounds are not generally abnormal in Addison's disease.
Test Taking Strategy—Use the key words "most helpful" when analyzing which of the options is the best method for evaluating the status of a client with Addison's disease. Recall that this disease results in a decreased appetite, weight loss, and a low serum sodium level. These factors contribute to hypotension, which is assessed by monitoring the client's blood pressure. Review pertinent nursing assessments when caring for a client with Addison's disease if you had difficulty answering this question.
Cognitive Level—*Applying*
Client Needs Category—*Physiological integrity*
Client Needs Subcategory—*Reduction of risk potential*

40. 2. A client with Addison's disease has low sodium levels; therefore, replacing dietary sodium is important. Milk products, such as cheese, and other sources of animal protein are high in natural sodium content. Although baked goods also contain hidden sodium, two graham crackers have half the amount of sodium as 1 oz of cheddar cheese. Fruits and vegetables are considered low in sodium when compared with other food sources.
Test Taking Strategy—Analyze to determine what information the question asks for, which is the best choice

among the dietary items listed for raising the level of sodium in the blood. Recall that dairy products (option 2) are high in sodium as well as calcium. Consult references that identify the sodium content in the items listed if you had difficulty answering this question.
Cognitive Level—*Applying*
Client Needs Category—*Physiological integrity*
Client Needs Subcategory—*Basic care and comfort*

41. 4. Clients with Addison's disease are prone to developing low blood glucose levels (hypoglycemia). Snacks such as milk and crackers contain complex carbohydrates that take longer to metabolize than simple sugars. Therefore, they are more likely to help maintain a stable blood glucose level. To reduce episodes of hypoglycemia, it is appropriate to schedule at least six small meals per day or between-meal snacks. Although the other choices contain some complex carbohydrates, they also contain sources of quickly metabolized sugars.
Test Taking Strategy—Analyze to determine what information the question asks for, which is the best snack items among those listed for maintaining or raising the client's blood glucose level to normal or near-normal range. Recall the fundamental principle of raising and maintaining a consistent blood glucose level with complex carbohydrates (option 4) rather than producing spikes in blood glucose levels with simple sugars. Consult nutrition references for the amount of complex carbohydrate in each of the options if you had difficulty answering this question.
Cognitive Level—*Applying*
Client Needs Category—*Physiological integrity*
Client Needs Subcategory—*Basic care and comfort*

42. 1. Stress and any of the following factors—salt deprivation, infection, trauma, exposure to cold, or overexertion—can overwhelm the client's ability to maintain homeostasis. This imbalance can lead to the development of addisonian crisis, a life-threatening condition. Alcohol consumption, eating complex carbohydrates, and sleep deprivation are not relevant factors in Addison's disease.
Test Taking Strategy—Analyze to determine what information the question asks for, which is a method for avoiding the development of addisonian crisis. Recall that healthy adrenal glands secrete cortisol, a hormone that enables coping with stress, but cortisol is not sufficiently produced by clients who have Addison's disease. By avoiding stress-producing situations (option 1), which may overburden the status of a client with this disease, the client can prevent addisonian crisis. Review factors that contribute to addisonian crisis and methods for reducing the potential for its development if you had difficulty answering this question.
Cognitive Level—*Applying*
Client Needs Category—*Physiological integrity*
Client Needs Subcategory—*Reduction of risk potential*

43. 1. Administering a glucocorticoid raises blood glucose levels and often requires insulin coverage. It is important in clients receiving glucocorticoids to regularly monitor blood glucose levels using a glucometer. Intake and output and daily weights may be implemented, but these steps are not as important as monitoring blood glucose levels. There is no indication for frequent oral care.
Test Taking Strategy—Use the process of elimination to help select the option that identifies the most important nursing action to implement in relation to the administration of a glucocorticoid. Consider the effect of the medication and implications for monitoring for side effects. Option 4 can be immediately eliminated because there is no need for frequent mouth care in this client. Options 2 and 3 can be eliminated because they correlate more with administering parenteral fluid. Recall that glucocorticoids get their name from their effect on raising blood glucose levels. Thus, monitoring blood glucose via glucometer readings (option 1) is most important. Review nursing responsibilities when administering a glucocorticoid if you had difficulty answering this question.
Cognitive Level—*Analyzing*
Client Needs Category—*Physiological integrity*
Client Needs Subcategory—*Pharmacological therapies*

44. 1, 5, 6. Cushing's syndrome is the result of excessive corticosteroid production. When this occurs, the client develops several multisystem clinical manifestations, including thin extremities (from muscle wasting and weakness) and a heavy, obese trunk. Other common signs and symptoms include moon face, thinning scalp hair, buffalo hump, ruddy complexion, thin and fragile skin, bruising, striae, peripheral edema, hypertension, hirsutism (in women), mood changes, depression, and psychosis.
Test Taking Strategy—Analyze to determine what information the question asks for, which is typical assessment findings in a client with Cushing's syndrome. Alternative-format "select all that apply" questions require considering each option independently to decide its merit in answering the question. Choose options that correlate with signs that are common among persons with Cushing's syndrome. Review the clinical manifestations associated with Cushing's syndrome if you had difficulty answering this question.
Cognitive Level—*Applying*
Client Needs Category—*Physiological integrity*
Client Needs Subcategory—*Physiological adaptation*

45. 1, 2, 3. On admission to the hospital, the nurse should gather data from the physical assessment findings and from medical, drug, and allergy histories to develop a plan of care with expected outcomes based on the data collection. In this case, the nurse should observe for symptoms of an adrenal disorder. Because this disorder masks the signs of infection and there is a potential for prolonged wound healing and risk for skin breakdown, the expectation is that successful management will result in the client remaining infection-free during the hospitalization. Laryngeal nerve damage is not related to this disorder. An elevated white blood cell count is an indication that an infection already exists. A normal temperature on admission does not necessarily mean the client will remain afebrile during the hospitalization.

Test Taking Strategy—Analyze to determine what information the question asks for, which is the reasons that justify selecting an expected outcome of being infection free during hospitalization. Alternative-format "select all that apply" questions require considering each option independently to decide its merit in answering the question. Review factors that increase susceptibility to infection among persons with Cushing's syndrome if you had difficulty answering this question.
Cognitive Level—Analyzing
Client Needs Category—Physiological integrity
Client Needs Subcategory—Physiological adaptation

46. 2. To be precise, a 24-hour urine collection begins after a client empties the bladder and ends with a final voiding at the same time the following day.

Test Taking Strategy—Apply the key words "most accurate" to the choices listed. Choose the option that correctly describes when a 24-hour urine collection should begin. Recall that starting the collection immediately after a client voids (option 2) and discarding that voided urine ensures that the specimen does not contain urine that was formed prior to the start of testing. Review the procedure for collecting a 24-hour urine specimen if you had difficulty answering this question.
Cognitive Level—Applying
Client Needs Category—Physiological integrity
Client Needs Subcategory—Reduction of risk potential

47. 2. To avoid chemical changes in the contents of the urine, a 24-hour specimen is deposited in a container with preservative. Generally, the urine is refrigerated or placed on ice during the collection period. The collection container is usually kept in the client's room or bathroom. It is unnecessary to measure each voided volume; if this is done, it is for reasons other than specimen collection. Clients generally void into a urinal or container suspended in the toilet; the urine is then added to the collection container, but it is not taken to the laboratory until all the urine in 24 hours has been collected.

Test Taking Strategy—Use the process of elimination to help select the option that identifies a correct statement regarding the collection of a 24-hour urine specimen. Recall that chemical changes, such as becoming highly alkaline, may occur if urine is allowed to stand without being chemically preserved (option 2) or kept cool. Options 1, 3, and 4 can be eliminated because they do not meet the goals of

a 24-hour urine collection. Review the manner in which urine that is being collected for 24 hours is prevented from decomposing if you had difficulty answering this question.*
Cognitive Level—Applying
Client Needs Category—Physiological integrity
Client Needs Subcategory—Reduction of risk potential

48. 1. Female clients with Cushing's syndrome acquire masculine characteristics, such as a deep voice and excessive growth of body hair, including facial hair. If premenopausal, they may also develop amenorrhea. Large breasts, heavy menstruation, and severe weight loss are not characteristic of Cushing's syndrome.

Test Taking Strategy—Use the process of elimination to help select the option that identifies the best rationale for adding Disturbed body image to a female client's care plan. Option 3 can be eliminated immediately, because clients with Cushing's syndrome are likely to have fat distributed to various areas of the body, such as the upper back, abdomen, and face. Option 2 can be eliminated because irregular menstrual cycles are more common than heavy menses. Although striae may appear on the breasts, option 4 can be eliminated because breast size is more or less determined by a client's weight. Option 1 is the remaining and best answer, because female clients develop masculine characteristics such as facial hair from an excess of androgenic hormone production and a moon face. Review the changes in appearance that correlate with Cushing's syndrome, especially if the client is female, if you had difficulty answering this question.
Cognitive Level—Analyzing
Client Needs Category—Physiological integrity
Client Needs Subcategory—Physiological adaptation

49. 2. Depression is common among clients with Cushing's syndrome because of the severity of physical changes or excess cortisol from increased adrenal glucocorticoid production; this places clients at increased risk for suicide. The other emotional symptoms are not necessarily associated with Cushing's syndrome, although they may occur randomly in some clients for other psychophysiologic reasons.

Test Taking Strategy—Analyze to determine what information the question asks for, which is psychological or emotional changes that may be experienced by a person with Cushing's syndrome. Recall that there are many adverse mental effects, but depressive mood disorders (option 2) are a primary concern for individuals who have Cushing's syndrome as well as those who are prescribed endogenous corticosteroids. Review mental changes associated with excess adrenocortical hormones if you had difficulty answering this question.
Cognitive Level—Applying
Client Needs Category—Psychosocial integrity
Client Needs Subcategory—None

50. 4. A sodium-restricted diet is prescribed to reduce the potential for excess fluid volume and increased serum sodium levels. One of the best ways to monitor the effects of sodium restriction is by weighing the client daily. The client's skin turgor and pedal edema are unlikely to change as much as weight from one day to the next. Monitoring the amount of sodium that the client consumes from the dietary tray is appropriate to document, but it does not provide as objective an assessment as the daily weight.

Test Taking Strategy—Use the process of elimination to help select the option that identifies the best method for determining a therapeutic response to sodium restriction. Option 1 can be eliminated, because identifying sodium intake would be labor-intensive since it would require measuring the client's use of table salt as well as his or her consumption of dietary items that contain sodium. Options 2 and 3 have merit, but any changes in skin turgor or peripheral edema are likely to be subtle and trends difficult to identify. Weighing the client (option 4) is the best answer because it provides objective evidence of water loss that can be attributed to sodium restriction. Review physical assessments that are useful for monitoring a response to sodium restriction if you had difficulty answering this question.
Cognitive Level—*Analyzing*
Client Needs Category—*Physiological integrity*
Client Needs Subcategory—*Reduction of risk potential*

51. 1, 3, 5, 6. Clients with Cushing's syndrome have thin, fragile, easily traumatized skin that is susceptible to the effects of prolonged pressure. Therefore, it is appropriate to exercise gentleness when turning and repositioning the client and to use pressure-relieving devices such as a convoluted foam mattress. Loose-fitting clothing will also prevent skin breakdown and pressure. The client needs rest more than activity to accommodate for weakness and fatigue; because of the weakness, the client needs assistance when getting up from the chair or out of bed. Depression and suicidal tendencies are common in clients with Cushing's syndrome; therefore, it is prudent to keep close observation on the client. The client's carbohydrate intake should be limited because of the tendency for hyperglycemia.

Test Taking Strategy—Analyze to determine what information the question asks for, which is measures for managing the basic needs of a client with Cushing's syndrome. Alternative-format "select all that apply" questions require considering each option independently to decide its merit in answering the question. Select those nursing interventions that help manage the problematic symptoms a client with Cushing's syndrome is likely to have. Review nursing considerations when caring for a client with Cushing's syndrome if you had difficulty answering this question.
Cognitive Level—*Analyzing*
Client Needs Category—*Physiological integrity*
Client Needs Subcategory—*Basic care and comfort*

52. 1. Blood pressure is the best indicator of excessive blood loss or cardiovascular collapse, a sudden loss of effective blood flow, in the client who has an adrenalectomy. This manifestation would appear in the immediate postoperative period. Preoperative hypertension is likely to subside postoperatively, which would also be evidenced by lower blood pressure trends. Temperature would be an early indication of infection and would not present immediately in the postoperative period. Decreased urine output is a clinical manifestation; however, it would not occur in the immediate postoperative period. Specific gravity changes are indicative of other disorders.

Test Taking Strategy—Use the process of elimination to select the option that identifies the assessment component that is most important to monitor in the immediate postoperative period after a bilateral adrenalectomy. As with any type of surgery, assessing vital signs, including monitoring the blood pressure, is one of the standard methods for detecting postoperative complications. Because of this, vital signs are monitored every 15 minutes until they are somewhat stable. Review common complications that can potentially occur after bilateral adrenalectomy and the methods for detecting their development if you had difficulty answering this question.
Cognitive Level—*Analyzing*
Client Needs Category—*Physiological integrity*
Client Needs Subcategory—*Reduction of risk potential*

53. 4. Extreme hypotension, fever, vomiting, diarrhea, abdominal pain, profound weakness, headache, and restlessness are all signs of addisonian crisis, which occurs from a sudden drop in adrenocortical hormones. Therefore, the client's ability to maintain vital signs within preoperative ranges is the best indication that addisonian crisis has been avoided. An adequate urine output, normal blood glucose level, and lessening of pedal edema are all positive outcomes, but they are not the best evidence that addisonian crisis has been prevented.

Test Taking Strategy—Use the process of elimination to help select the option that identifies the best indication, from among other somewhat plausible options, that an addisonian crisis has been averted. Options 1, 2, and 3 have some merit because they are expected surgical outcomes. However, recall that severe hypotension is a life-threatening sign that an addisonian crisis is developing; maintaining stable vital signs that are within the preoperative range (option 4) is the best answer. Review the signs of addisonian crisis and methods for assessing client stabilization if you had difficulty answering this question.
Cognitive Level—*Evaluating*
Client Needs Category—*Physiological integrity*
Client Needs Subcategory—*Reduction of risk potential*

54. **2.** Because of the client's thin, fragile skin and tendency to heal slowly, it is best to pull tape toward the suture line rather than away from it when changing dressings. This will prevent the sutures from separating. Although it is true that protein promotes healing, and that the nurse needs to monitor I.V. antibiotics and cover the client's wound with gauze, these nursing measures are not as critical to the healing process as preserving an intact incisional site.

Test Taking Strategy—Apply the key words "most appropriate" when comparing the choices listed. Discriminate among the options to select an action that identifies a nursing measure that accommodates for the client's slow healing. Recall that pulling tape toward rather than away from the incision (option 2) keeps the wound edges approximated without interrupting the status of healing. This applies to removing a dressing on any client regardless of the type of surgery that was performed. Review the principles for changing a wound dressing that consists of gauze and adhesive tape if you had difficulty answering this question.

Cognitive Level—*Applying*
Client Needs Category—*Physiological integrity*
Client Needs Subcategory—*Basic care and comfort*

55. **1.** Postoperatively after a bilateral adrenalectomy, there is an increased risk for acquiring infections because of the anti-inflammatory effects of corticosteroid replacement hormones, which may mask the common signs of inflammation and infection. Therefore, avoiding people with infectious diseases is prudent for the client with Cushing's syndrome who has undergone a bilateral adrenalectomy. The client is also at risk for fluid volume deficits due to a deficit of aldosterone and should maintain an adequate fluid intake. The client's cushingoid appearance should slowly recede as hormone levels are reestablished at lower-than-preoperative levels. After a bilateral adrenalectomy, hormone replacement therapy is a lifelong necessity. In fact, a medical alert tag should be worn at all times.

Test Taking Strategy—Use the process of elimination to help select the option that identifies the best evidence that the client understands the postoperative course of his or her condition. Option 2 can be eliminated because a deficit of aldosterone impairs sodium reabsorption by the kidneys; without sodium, fluid volume is reduced. Option 3 can be eliminated because as the level of adrenocortical hormones is reduced, the client's appearance will become more normal. Option 4 can be eliminated because once the adrenal glands are removed, the client will require lifelong hormone replacement. Option 1 is the correct answer because the client will forever be susceptible to infections as a result of endogenous steroid replacement. Review the consequences faced by a client after bilateral adrenalectomy if you had difficulty answering this question.

Cognitive Level—*Analyzing*
Client Needs Category—*Health promotion and maintenance*
Client Needs Subcategory—*None*

Nursing Care of Clients with Pancreatic Endocrine Disorders

56. **2.** Hyperinsulinism, also known as *functional hypoglycemia*, is caused by an overproduction of insulin, which occurs about 2 hours after eating a meal, especially one containing refined sugar or simple carbohydrates. This results in a marked drop in blood glucose levels.

Test Taking Strategy—Apply the key words "most likely" when analyzing the choices listed. Identify the option that indicates the typical timing when symptoms of hyperinsulinism occur. Recall that symptoms associated with hyperinsulinism are triggered after consuming carbohydrates followed by a surge in insulin production. Pathologically, the amount of insulin is more than required to compensate for the level of ingested carbohydrates, causing the blood sugar to plummet about 2 hours after eating (option 2). Review the etiology of hyperinsulinism and the time when the client is most likely to experience symptoms if you had difficulty answering this question.

Cognitive Level—*Applying*
Client Needs Category—*Physiological integrity*
Client Needs Subcategory—*Physiological adaptation*

57. **4.** A container of 75 to 100 g of glucose is consumed orally or administered I.V. before the glucose tolerance test begins. Otherwise, the client fasts before and during the test and only water is allowed before the test. Urine specimens are collected before the glucose is administered and when subsequent blood samples are taken. The client is instructed to consume an adequate diet containing carbohydrates for at least 3 days before the diagnostic test, then fast for 12 hours before the test.

Test Taking Strategy—Using the key words "most accurate," select the option that provides correct information related to a glucose tolerance test. Recall that the test involves determining how well or poorly the pancreas is able to restore a normal blood sugar level after being challenged with a specific amount of oral glucose (option 4). Review how a glucose tolerance test is conducted if you had difficulty answering this question.

Cognitive Level—*Applying*
Client Needs Category—*Physiological integrity*
Client Needs Subcategory—*Reduction of risk potential*

58. **3.** To maintain stable blood glucose levels, it is best for clients with functional hypoglycemia to consume small, frequent meals that contain high-fiber complex carbohydrates. Some examples include fruits, vegetables, legumes, and whole grains. Simple sugars, such as glucose, fructose, and galactose, tend to stimulate the release of insulin and lower the blood glucose level drastically. Complete proteins and unsaturated fats in moderate amounts are components of a healthy diet, but they are not as therapeutic for stabilizing the blood glucose.

Test Taking Strategy—Use the process of elimination to help select the option that identifies the nutrient that aims to stabilize blood glucose levels. Consider that calorie-producing nutrients consist of carbohydrates, fats, and proteins. Eliminate option 1 because simple sugars are carbohydrates that are more likely to trigger symptoms in this client. Eliminate options 2 and 4 because they are not carbohydrates and do not trigger the release of insulin. Option 3 remains as the correct answer because complex carbohydrates take longer to digest and there is a slower release rather than a surge of insulin. Review the difference between the digestion and absorption of simple and complex carbohydrates if you had difficulty answering this question.
Cognitive Level—*Applying*
Client Needs Category—*Health promotion and maintenance*
Client Needs Subcategory—*None*

59. 1. If dietary measures are appropriate, clients experience fewer symptoms of hypoglycemia, such as weakness, tremors, headache, nausea, hunger, malaise, excess perspiration, confusion, and personality changes. The other choices do not relate to functional hypoglycemia.

Test Taking Strategy—Use the process of elimination to help select the option that provides the best evidence that dietary measures have achieved the goal of controlling functional hypoglycemia. After analyzing the options looking for signs or symptoms that are and are not associated with hypoglycemia, options 2, 3, and 4 can eliminated. Recall that among the symptoms of hypoglycemia, the client may experience weakness and tremors; thus, if there are fewer incidences of these (option 1), the client is experiencing a therapeutic dietary effect. Review the signs and symptoms of hypoglycemia and analyze the effect a client would experience if a therapeutic diet is followed if you had difficulty answering this question.
Cognitive Level—*Applying*
Client Needs Category—*Health promotion and maintenance*
Client Needs Subcategory—*None*

60. 2. The term *postprandial* means "after eating a meal." The meal acts as a glucose challenge. The blood glucose level normally increases in response to the intake of carbohydrates. Two hours later, the blood glucose level of nondiabetic patients should return to normal. If the blood glucose level remains elevated 2 hours after eating, it suggests a metabolic disorder such as diabetes mellitus.

Test Taking Strategy—Analyze to determine what information the question asks for, which is the timing of a blood specimen drawn to measure a client's postprandial blood sugar level. Recall that the term postprandial means "after eating," which leads to option 2 as the correct answer. Review the description of this test and the definition of postprandial if you had difficulty answering this question.
Cognitive Level—*Understanding*
Client Needs Category—*Health promotion and maintenance*
Client Needs Subcategory—*None*

61. 3. Positive screening test results are an indication that the client requires further evaluation by a physician. Because several factors and disease pathologies can cause hyperglycemia, it is always best to refer hyperglycemic individuals to a physician. Comments about taking insulin or avoiding candy should alert the nurse that the client requires further education about the condition.

Test Taking Strategy—Analyze to determine what information the question asks for, which is an accurate understanding about an abnormal postprandial blood sugar test. Recall that this is only a screening test and that further diagnostic testing may be required after the client consults his or her physician (option 3). Review the significance of an abnormal postprandial blood sugar test if you had difficulty answering this question.
Cognitive Level—*Analyzing*
Client Needs Category—*Health promotion and maintenance*
Client Needs Subcategory—*None*

62. 4. Polyuria (excessive secretion and voiding of urine), polydipsia (excessive thirst), and polyphagia (increased appetite) are the classic signs and symptoms of diabetes mellitus. Polycholia (increased secretion of bile), polyemia (increased amount of circulating blood), polyplegia (paralysis of several muscles), diarrhea, constipation, and anorexia are not considered signs and symptoms of this endocrine disorder. Weight gain or loss is seen in some people with diabetes.

Test Taking Strategy—Look at the key words "most appropriate" in reference to signs and symptoms that relate to testing blood glucose levels. Recall that an elevated blood glucose level is associated with diabetes mellitus. Of all the choices, option 4 identifies the most appropriate information to investigate because the signs and symptoms identified in that option are classic for diabetes mellitus. Review the signs and symptoms of diabetes mellitus if you had difficulty answering this question.
Cognitive Level—*Applying*
Client Needs Category—*Health promotion and maintenance*
Client Needs Subcategory—*None*

63. 4. The client needs time to accept the diagnosis, demonstrate anger, and talk about fears and concerns. Listening is the most therapeutic intervention at this point. Stressing the importance of treatment is likely to increase the client's fears. The client with type 2 diabetes may be required to take oral hypoglycemic agents, but telling the client that the disease is easily managed is false reassurance. Telling the client that others manage their diabetes ignores the fact that this disorder is unique to this client.

> *Test Taking Strategy—Apply the key words "most appropriate" to the choices in the four options. Recall that this diagnosis may create fear and anxiety. Denial and anger are methods used to cope when events threaten a person's well-being. Although all of the options describe plausible nursing actions, remember that it is always therapeutic and most appropriate for the nurse to listen as the client verbalizes his or her thoughts and feelings first (option 4) before proceeding further. Review nursing interventions that help clients cope with their fear if you had difficulty answering this question.*
> **Cognitive Level**—*Applying*
> **Client Needs Category**—*Psychosocial integrity*
> **Client Needs Subcategory**—*None*

64. 3. Exercise has many beneficial effects, such as controlling weight, reducing appetite, improving circulation, and lowering heart rate, regardless of a person's health status. For a client with diabetes, however, one of the primary benefits is a reduced blood glucose level. If the blood glucose level decreases with exercise, drug treatment with oral hypoglycemic agents or insulin may be delayed, reduced, or eliminated.

> *Test Taking Strategy—Use the process of elimination to help select the option that identifies the best outcome for including regular exercise in the diabetic treatment regimen. All of the options have merit. However, option 3 is the best answer because the primary reason a diabetic should exercise regularly is that it helps to reduce blood sugar levels. Review how diabetes mellitus is managed if you had difficulty answering this question.*
> **Cognitive Level**—*Analyzing*
> **Client Needs Category**—*Health promotion and maintenance*
> **Client Needs Subcategory**—*None*

65. 2. The main advantage of using an exchange list is that it eliminates the need to count calories. Instead, clients are prescribed the number of exchanges they may use in particular categories. They can choose among items of equal nutritional value, provided they consume the serving size the list specifies.

> *Test Taking Strategy—Use the process of elimination to select the option that identifies the best evidence that the client understands the principle for using a dietary exchange list. Option 1 can be eliminated because a healthy diet involves a variety of foods from among food groups. Option 3 can be eliminated because as in any diet, the number of servings is limited. Option 4 can be eliminated because the beauty of an exchange list is that the calories in the food choices have already been calculated for the client. Option 2 remains as the best answer because it reiterates that foods in each particular category can be "exchanged" for one another depending on what the client has available. Review information on using the American Diabetes Association exchange list if you had difficulty answering this question.*
> **Cognitive Level**—*Applying*
> **Client Needs Category**—*Health promotion and maintenance*
> **Client Needs Subcategory**—*None*

66. 3. "Lite" or "light" is a food-labeling term that means the product contains one-third fewer calories than a similar unaltered item. Thus, light beer contains calories or grams of nutrients that must be calculated in the diabetic client's diet and exchange list. The other selections are considered "free" and do not contain calories; therefore, these choices could be incorporated into the client's meal plan as "free."

> *Test Taking Strategy—Analyze to determine what information the question asks for, which is a food choice that is not considered a "free" food. "Free" foods include those in options 1, 2, and 4 because they do not contain calories nor have to be counted on the exchange. Because light beer (option 3) contains calories, excluding it shows evidence that the client understands the concept of "free" foods. Review the definition of "free" foods and examples on the American Diabetes Association's exchange list if you had difficulty answering this question.*
> **Cognitive Level**—*Analyzing*
> **Client Needs Category**—*Health promotion and maintenance*
> **Client Needs Subcategory**—*None*

67. 3. Given that the amounts in each option are correct, a medium apple is the most appropriate choice for this client. The 1,500-calorie Dietary Exchange Plan indicates that a client can have one fruit exchange as a midafternoon snack.

> *Test Taking Strategy—Analyze to determine what information the question asks for, which is the food that can be consumed as a midafternoon snack using the chart for a 1,500-calorie Dietary Exchange Plan. The chart identifies that the client can have one fruit exchange. Because option 3 is the only choice that lists fruit, it is the correct answer. Review the foods in various groups that are recommended to distribute the consumption of 1,500 calories over a full day if you had difficulty answering this question.*
> **Cognitive Level**—*Analyzing*
> **Client Needs Category**—*Physiological integrity*
> **Client Needs Subcategory**—*Basic care and comfort*

68. 1. Chemically, hormones generally belong to one of three groups: proteins and peptides, steroids (fat-soluble molecules), or those derived from tyrosine, an amino acid. Insulin belongs to the first group in the list. Insulin is administered parenterally because it is a protein substance that, if taken orally, would be altered by enzymes in the GI tract before it could be absorbed into the bloodstream. None of the other choices accurately describes the rationale for excluding insulin administration by the oral route.

> *Test Taking Strategy—Use the process of elimination to help select the option that identifies the best reason that insulin cannot be taken orally. Options 2, 3, and 4 can be eliminated because they are inaccurate statements. Option 1 is the correct answer because the protein structure of insulin can be destroyed by protease and peptidase enzymes like pepsin in the stomach. Review the rationale for administering insulin parenterally if you had difficulty answering this question.*

Cognitive Level—*Applying*
Client Needs Category—*Physiological integrity*
Client Needs Subcategory—*Pharmacological therapies*

69. 2. To maintain stable control of blood glucose levels, it is essential to take medication, eat, and exercise at regular, consistent times each day. Implying that the therapeutic regimen is flexible predisposes clients to develop unstable blood glucose levels and metabolic complications.

> *Test Taking Strategy—Apply the key words "most appropriate" when evaluating the choices in the four options. Remember that more than one option may seem reasonable, but only one is the best answer. Complying with the treatment regimen without deviating from the prescriber's recommendations for eating all meals regularly (option 2) helps to facilitate optimum control of blood sugar levels. Review factors that help to control blood sugar within consistent levels if you had difficulty answering this question.*

Cognitive Level—*Applying*
Client Needs Category—*Health promotion and maintenance*
Client Needs Subcategory—*None*

70. 2. Urine testing using reagent tablets or strips is the most economical of diabetic monitoring techniques and measures the amount of spilled glucose in the urine, but a home glucometer is more accurate and preferred for diabetic clients. Self-monitoring with a glucometer is costly but less expensive than the added charges for the services of laboratory personnel or a home health nurse.

> *Test Taking Strategy—Use the process of elimination to help select the option that identifies the best approach the client can use to monitor his or her efforts at controlling diabetes. Options 3 and 4 can be eliminated because these are not examples of self-monitoring. Although option 1 is inexpensive, it does not provide an "up to the minute" evaluation of symptom control;*

therefore, it can be eliminated. Option 2 remains as the correct answer because it provides very specific information at the time the capillary blood is tested. As a standard of care, diabetic clients are taught how to use a glucometer at home before being discharged. Review methods that diabetic clients use to self-monitor their progress in controlling blood sugar levels if you had difficulty answering this question.

Cognitive Level—*Applying*
Client Needs Category—*Safe and effective care environment*
Client Needs Subcategory—*Coordinated care*

71. 3, 5, 6. An acetone (sometimes described as sweet or fruity) breath odor, weakness, thirst, anorexia, vomiting, drowsiness, abdominal pain, rapid and weak pulse, hypotension, flushed skin, and Kussmaul's respirations (rapid, deep, and noisy) are manifested by persons with diabetic ketoacidosis (DKA). In severe cases, the client may be comatose or semi-comatose.

> *Test Taking Strategy—Analyze to determine what information the question asks for, which is assessment findings associated with DKA. Alternative-format "select all that apply" questions require considering each option independently to decide its merit in answering the question. Review the descriptions in each of the options, compiling a cluster that describes the clinical manifestations of DKA. Review the characteristics of DKA if you had difficulty answering this question.*

Cognitive Level—*Applying*
Client Needs Category—*Physiological integrity*
Client Needs Subcategory—*Physiological adaptation*

72. 1. Kussmaul's respirations, a common sign of diabetic ketoacidosis (DKA), are a compensatory mechanism to eliminate carbon dioxide from the body and prevent a further drop in pH. Respirations are typically fast, rapid, deep, and labored with a longer expiration. The other options are not characteristic of Kussmaul's respirations.

> *Test Taking Strategy—Use the process of elimination to help select the option that identifies the best description of Kussmaul's respirations. Recall that this pattern of breathing is characterized by an increase in the rate and depth of ventilation (option 1). Options 2 and 3 can be eliminated because this type of breathing is neither shallow nor slow. Option 4 can be eliminated because the breathing rhythm does not include pauses. Review the definition of Kussmaul's respirations and its purpose for restoring acid-base balance if you had difficulty answering this question.*

Cognitive Level—*Applying*
Client Needs Category—*Physiological integrity*
Client Needs Subcategory—*Physiological adaptation*

73. 4, 5, 6. Before the test, it is important that a quality control check be done on the machine to ensure an accurate reading, especially when a client has diabetic ketoacidosis (DKA). It is also mandatory that the technician don gloves when coming in contact with blood. It is best to let the blood flow passively by gravity onto the test strip or reflecting area of the electronic glucometer. Usually one large drop is sufficient to obtain an accurate reading. The skin is usually cleaned with soap and water, not Betadine. Piercing the central pad of a finger is avoided; the margin around the digit produces less pain. Vital signs may be taken at the same time in an attempt to coordinate care and save time, but they are not necessary for this test.

> *Test Taking Strategy—Analyze to determine what information the question asks for, which is the technique for electronic blood glucose monitoring. Alternative-format "select all that apply" questions require considering each option independently to decide its merit in answering the question. Review the procedure for testing capillary blood glucose levels with a glucometer if you had difficulty answering this question.*
> *Cognitive Level—Applying*
> *Client Needs Category—Physiological integrity*
> *Client Needs Subcategory—Reduction of risk potential*

74. 1, 2, 3, 6. For clients who have an extremely elevated capillary blood sugar as well as signs and symptoms of diabetic ketoacidosis (DKA), the blood glucose measurement must be validated. To verify that the blood glucose measurement is accurate, a STAT serum glucose level must be obtained before beginning insulin treatment. The nurse should also anticipate that the client's serum blood glucose levels will be acquired periodically, but because the critically ill client will not be eating regular meals, glucometer measurements would not be performed before meals and at bedtime. The nurse should anticipate that the intravenous administration of regular insulin will be ordered because it is the drug of choice to lower critically high blood glucose levels. Correcting fluid and electrolyte imbalance is another goal. Potassium is given to help the glucose reenter the cell, thereby lowering glucose levels. The nurse should connect the client to a cardiac monitor to observe changes in cardiac rate and rhythm related to hyperkalemia and peaked T waves and because the client has respiratory changes related to Kussmaul's (rapid, deep, and noisy) respirations. Vital signs are taken at least every 2 hours or more often during this critical period. After the client is stabilized and admitted to the hospital, dietary orders and orders for glucometer measurements can be written at that time.

> *Test Taking Strategy—Analyze to determine what information the question asks for, which is physician's orders the nurse can anticipate for a client with a blood glucose level of 498 mg/dL. Alternative-format "select all that apply" questions require considering each option independently to decide its merit in answering the question. Choose the medical orders that provide critical data and methods for stabilizing the client's condition. Review the medical management of DKA if you had difficulty answering this question.*
> *Cognitive Level—Analyzing*
> *Client Needs Category—Physiological integrity*
> *Client Needs Subcategory—Physiological adaptation*

75. 2. The onset of action of most rapid-acting insulins (regular insulin in particular) is within 30 to 90 minutes after administration. Hypoglycemia is even more likely to occur when insulin reaches its peak effect. For regular insulin, this peak is approximately 2 to 5 hours later. The duration of regular insulin is approximately 8 hours.

> *Test Taking Strategy—Analyze to determine what information the question asks for, which is the time that hypoglycemia may occur after administering a subcutaneous injection of regular insulin. Recall that regular insulin is a rapid-acting insulin with a short onset time of approximately 30 minutes. Because of the short time of onset, a client should be served his or her meal within ½ hour or less of administering regular insulin. Review the onset, peak, and duration of action of various types of insulin, focusing on regular insulin, if you had difficulty answering this question.*
> *Cognitive Level—Applying*
> *Client Needs Category—Physiological integrity*
> *Client Needs Subcategory—Pharmacological therapies*

76. 2, 4, 5, 6. A client with diabetes must learn to recognize the signs of hypoglycemia. Shakiness and disturbed cognition/confusion—two classic signs—occur when the central nervous system, which relies entirely on glucose for energy, receives insufficient glucose from the blood. The body releases epinephrine in response to low blood glucose, causing such symptoms as palpitations and diaphoresis. Hunger, a homeostatic response, promotes the consumption of calories. Signs of hyperglycemia (not hypoglycemia) include thirst and sleepiness.

> *Test Taking Strategy—Analyze to determine what information the question asks for, which is signs and symptoms of hypoglycemia. Alternative-format "select all that apply" questions require considering each option independently to decide its merit in answering the question. Select options that are characteristic of hypoglycemia. Review the signs and symptoms that may occur when the blood sugar level falls below normal range if you had difficulty answering this question.*
> *Cognitive Level—Applying*
> *Client Needs Category—Physiological integrity*
> *Client Needs Subcategory—Physiological adaptation*

77. 2. A blood glucose reading below 70 mg/dL is a sign of hypoglycemia. Assuming the glucometer reading is accurate and the client is symptomatic, the best action is to implement some means of increasing the client's blood glucose level. If the client is able to swallow or there is access to the GI tract, the standard for initial treatment is to administer 15 to 20 g of simple carbohydrate. This may be done with a variety of substances, such as ½ cup (4 ounces) of fruit juice, glucose tablet(s) that contain 15 g, 1 tube of glucose gel, or ¾ cup (6 ounces) of nondiet soda. The client may be reassessed in 15 minutes. If the blood glucose level remains below 70 mg/dL, the protocol is repeated two more times. If the blood glucose continues to measure less than 70 mg/dL, the physician is contacted. Insulin will drop the blood glucose level further; therefore, administering additional insulin is inappropriate in this case. A complete head-to-toe assessment may be done but will prolong onset of treatment. The physician is usually notified, but only after the nurse implements some method to increase the blood glucose level. The physician may prescribe parenterally administered glucose or glucagon if the client is unresponsive.

> *Test Taking Strategy—Use the key words "most appropriate" when analyzing the choices in the four options. Remember that more than one option may seem reasonable, but only one is the best answer. Recall that the primary objective is to raise the client's blood glucose level above 70 mg/dL, making option 2 the correct choice. Research the definition of hypoglycemia by the American Diabetes Association and the current treatment protocol if you had difficulty answering this question.*
> **Cognitive Level**—*Analyzing*
> **Client Needs Category**—*Physiological integrity*
> **Client Needs Subcategory**—*Physiological adaptation*

78. 3. The client needs to take care to avoid mixing the intermediate-acting insulin, which contains an additive, with the additive-free insulin. The additive-free insulin is always withdrawn first. The actions described in the other options are safe and appropriate for mixing two different types of insulins.

> *Test Taking Strategy—Use the process of elimination to help select the option that indicates that the client needs more practice for combining two types of insulin in one syringe. Read the options carefully, looking for an incorrect technique. Options 1, 2, and 4 describe correct actions and can, therefore, be eliminated. Option 3 is the answer because it describes an incorrect technique. Review the procedure for combining two types of insulin in one syringe if you had difficulty answering this question.*
> **Cognitive Level**—*Applying*
> **Client Needs Category**—*Safe and effective care environment*
> **Client Needs Subcategory**—*Safety and infection control*

79. 4. To prevent lipodystrophy and lipoatrophy and promote appropriate absorption of insulin, it is correct to rotate insulin injection sites; insulin is preferably administered in the abdomen. Insulin is prepared in an insulin syringe calibrated in units. A 25 to 30 gauge needle may be used to inject insulin. Insulin is injected at a 45- or 90-degree angle, depending on the client's size.

> *Test Taking Strategy—Use the process of elimination to select the option that identifies correct information about the self-administration of insulin injections. Rotating injection sites (option 4) is the best answer. Options 1, 2, and 3 can be eliminated because they contain incorrect information. Review principles that apply to administering insulin injections if you had difficulty answering this question.*
> **Cognitive Level**—*Applying*
> **Client Needs Category**—*Physiological integrity*
> **Client Needs Subcategory**—*Pharmacological therapies*

80.

| 1. Instill 20 units of air in the vial of Novolin N. |
| 2. Instill 10 units of air in the vial of Novolin R. |
| 4. Withdraw 10 units of insulin from the vial of Novolin R. |
| 3. Withdraw 20 units of insulin from the vial of Novolin N. |

When insulins are mixed, air is instilled in the vial with the longer-acting insulin first. The syringe is removed, and then air is added to the short-acting insulin. The prescribed amount of the short-acting insulin is immediately withdrawn into the syringe after instilling the air. The syringe is then returned to the vial of longer-acting insulin, and the prescribed amount is withdrawn into the syringe. The principle is "clear to cloudy," which means the clear insulin (Novolin R, in this example) is placed in the syringe first before adding the cloudy insulin (Novolin N, in this example) to the syringe.

> *Test Taking Strategy—Analyze to determine what information the question asks for, which involves placing the actions required for mixing two types of insulin in one syringe in their correct sequence. Consult references that describe how different types of insulins are combined in one syringe if you had difficulty answering this question.*
> **Cognitive Level**—*Applying*
> **Client Needs Category**—*Physiological integrity*
> **Client Needs Subcategory**—*Pharmacological therapies*

81. 4. Insulin-dependent clients are likely to remain so for the rest of their lives. Therefore, further instruction is needed if the client believes that it may eventually be unnecessary to take the medication. Even some clients with type 2 diabetes eventually become insulin-dependent. The client is correct in understanding that insulin needs increase during times of stress, such as infections and emotional crises. Although exercise is beneficial, clients may need additional calories to prevent symptoms of hypoglycemia.

Test Taking Strategy—Analyze to determine what information the question asks for, which is an incorrect statement about insulin use in type 1 diabetes mellitus. Keep in mind that the answer requires selecting an option that contains incorrect information. Because options 1, 2, and 3 are accurate statements, option 4 remains as the answer. Review the management of diabetes mellitus if you had difficulty answering this question.
Cognitive Level—*Applying*
Client Needs Category—*Safe and effective care environment*
Client Needs Subcategory—*Coordinated care*

82. 4. Clients with diabetes are prone to many systemic vascular and neurologic complications. These include a higher incidence of premature cataract formation, retinal hemorrhage and blindness, stroke, myocardial infarction, renal failure, peripheral neurovascular disease and amputations, and sexual dysfunction. Liver disease is atypical among clients with diabetes mellitus.

Test Taking Strategy—Analyze to determine what information the question asks for, which is a complication that is unrelated to diabetes mellitus. Recall that common complications include retinopathy, nephropathy, and vascular pathology. Liver failure (option 4) does not generally occur among clients with diabetes mellitus. Review the pathophysiology of diabetes and complications that may occur if you had difficulty answering this question.
Cognitive Level—*Applying*
Client Needs Category—*Physiological integrity*
Client Needs Subcategory—*Physiological adaptation*

83. 3. Insulin deteriorates if exposed to excessive heat or light. An opened vial of insulin is best stored at room temperature or in a cool, unrefrigerated area. Injecting cold insulin may cause unnecessary pain. The bathroom is not the best location for storing insulin because the temperature in the area may become excessively warm when a client or family members shower or bathe. Unopened vials may be kept refrigerated.

Test Taking Strategy—Apply the key words "most correct" when analyzing the four options. Choose the option that identifies the best manner or location for storing an opened vial of insulin. Recall that after opening a vial of insulin, it may be kept at room temperature for up to a month. Consult references concerning the storage of opened vials of insulin if you had difficulty answering this question.
Cognitive Level—*Applying*
Client Needs Category—*Physiological integrity*
Client Needs Subcategory—*Pharmacological therapies*

84. 2. Soaking the feet tends to soften the skin subjecting them to potential trauma. The feet are washed daily with soap and water, and then dried thoroughly before the client dons clean socks and supportive shoes. Clients with diabetes should inspect their feet daily for signs of injury or poor circulation. Going barefoot is contraindicated because this predisposes the client to foot injuries. The client should see a podiatrist regularly to have toenails cut and filed.

Test Taking Strategy—Analyze to determine what information the question asks for, which is an incorrect statement indicating that the client needs further teaching. Look for an option that contains an inaccurate statement. Recall that diabetics are prone to vascular complications and are slow to heal. Consequently, softening the skin on the feet by soaking them daily creates a risk for complications, making option 2 the statement that requires clarification. Review complications of diabetes involving the feet and lower extremities, focusing on methods that reduce those risks, if you had difficulty answering this question.
Cognitive Level—*Applying*
Client Needs Category—*Health promotion and maintenance*
Client Needs Subcategory—*None*

85. 2. The most objective evidence for evaluating how well the client is managing therapy is a record of glucose monitoring values. Some glucometers store the data so that results can be retrieved and evaluated. Otherwise, clients are asked to keep a written record of their monitoring results. Identifying the dosage and frequency of insulin administration does not indicate that the client is actually self-administering the insulin. Maintaining or gradually losing weight is good evaluative information, but it is not as specific as glucose monitoring values. Some clients are not as self-aware of symptoms, and some have an exaggerated awareness of their body functions. Therefore, subjective symptoms are not as valuable as hard objective data.

Test Taking Strategy—Apply the key words "most important" when evaluating the choices in the four options. Look for information that is better than the other three for helping to objectively determine the quality of the client's compliance. Recall that the trend in glucometer measurements (option 2) helps to evaluate how well or poorly the client is carrying out the therapeutic regimen. Review methods for assessing a diabetic client's compliance with the prescribed diet, medication, and exercise if you had difficulty answering this question.
Cognitive Level—*Evaluating*
Client Needs Category—*Health promotion and maintenance*
Client Needs Subcategory—*None*

86. 4. A glycosylated hemoglobin (HbA1c) test reveals the effectiveness of diabetic therapy for the preceding 8 to 12 weeks. A fasting blood glucose provides information on the blood glucose status for the immediate period of time. Blood chemistry includes a blood glucose measurement as well as several other diagnostic test results. A complete blood count indicates the status of the client's hematopoietic functions.

> *Test Taking Strategy—Using the key words "most impor-tant," look for a laboratory test that is used to moni-tor the effectiveness of the client's diabetic regimen. Recall that an HbA1c (option 4) provides valuable information about the success or failure to control the blood glucose level over a significant amount of time. Based on this test result, the treatment plan may be modified or the client may be counseled to use more effort at remaining compliant. Review the purpose for each test listed, focusing on the value of HbA1c results, if you had difficulty answering this question.*

Cognitive Level—*Applying*
Client Needs Category—*Physiological integrity*
Client Needs Subcategory—*Reduction of risk potential*

87. 3. Continuous insulin infusions are administered by the subcutaneous route, usually in abdominal tissue. However, any common subcutaneous sites (such as the buttocks, thighs, arms, and sections of the back) may be used. An insulin infusion pump delivers regular insulin at a carefully regulated rate. Insulin is absorbed too quickly when instilled intravenously.

> *Test Taking Strategy—Analyze to determine what informa-tion the question asks for, which is the anatomic area in which an insulin pump is located. Recall that the abdomen (option 3) is the preferred, but not exclusive, site for locating the infusion needle that is attached to the tubing and pump mechanism. Review information about insulin pumps, focusing on a location that is con-venient as well as easy to conceal and manually care for, if you had difficulty answering this question.*

Cognitive Level—*Applying*
Client Needs Category—*Health promotion and maintenance*
Client Needs Subcategory—*None*

88. 2. Clients with diabetes should consult their physician about trimming or cutting the toenails. An abrasive file may be used to keep the nails short, but it is best to refer clients to a podiatrist for nail maintenance or other foot problems. The other hygiene measures are good to implement, but they are not as pertinent to the care of a client with diabetes.

> *Test Taking Strategy—Use the key words "most appropri-ate" when analyzing the choices in the four options. Remember that more than one option may seem reasonable, but only one is the best answer. Although all of the options have merit, option 2 is the best answer because filing toenails reduces the potential for foot and nail problems that could lead to impaired healing or gangrene. Review the importance of foot care and prophylactic measures to prevent vascular complica-tions that may affect the feet and lower extremities if you had difficulty answering this question.*

Cognitive Level—*Applying*
Client Needs Category—*Health promotion and maintenance*
Client Needs Subcategory—*None*

89.

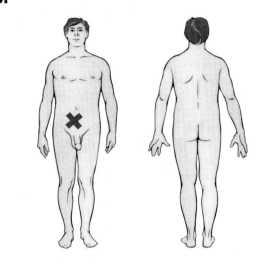

The abdomen is the preferred site for insulin administration to facilitate the most rapid rate of absorption. Absorption is somewhat slower in the arms, slower still in the legs, and slowest in the hip or buttocks area. The abdomen is also generally easier to access for self-administration, and the absorption rate is constant.

> *Test Taking Strategy—Analyze to determine what infor-mation the question asks for, which is the preferred location for injecting insulin subcutaneously. Review subcutaneous injection sites, focusing on the area of the fastest rate of insulin absorption, if you had dif-ficulty answering this question.*

Cognitive Level—*Applying*
Client Needs Category—*Physiological integrity*
Client Needs Subcategory—*Pharmacological therapy*

90. 1. Hyperosmolar hyperglycemic nonketotic syn-drome (HHNS) is an acute complication of diabetes characterized by extremely high blood glucose levels—between 600 and 1,000 mg/dL—without signs of ketoaci-dosis. The severe hyperglycemia causes fluid to shift from the intracellular space to the extracellular space, and urine elimination exceeds the upper limit of normal volumes. The skin would be warm and dry skin from dehydration, rather than cool and moist. Acetone is not present in the urine of clients experiencing HHNS; it is typically found in the urine of those with ketoacidosis.

> *Test Taking Strategy—Use the key words "most sugges-tive" when determining which option best correlates with HHNS. HHNS is characterized by a serum blood glucose level that measures an almost unbelievably high level, indicated in option 1. Review the cluster of signs and symptoms manifested by a client with HHNS if you had difficulty answering this question.*

Cognitive Level—Applying
Client Needs Category—Physiological integrity
Client Needs Subcategory—Physiological adaptation

91. 1. Insulin is a hormone that regulates glucose in the blood. During times of illness, dehydration (from persistent vomiting and diarrhea) and stress can cause the glucose level to increase significantly. This is especially critical for an insulin-dependent diabetic client who may have insufficient insulin to counteract the rising glucose level. Therefore, it is important for the nurse to teach the client about the effects of dehydration and the need for blood glucose monitoring when ill. Blood glucose levels should be monitored every 2 to 4 hours when factors interfere with eating and the usual schedule for administering insulin. Eating candy or drinking high-calorie beverages will cause the blood glucose level to rise, especially if there is insufficient insulin to counteract the glucose. Testing the urine daily for protein is not typically done during times of illness.

Test Taking Strategy—Analyze to determine what information the question asks for, which is how to control diabetic symptoms when unable to eat due to illness. Recall that many factors, including illness, cause fluctuations in blood glucose levels. Although the client in this scenario has withheld insulin administration to compensate for the fact that food is not being consumed, it is important to monitor blood glucose levels frequently (option 1) to ensure that neither dangerously high nor low blood glucose levels are developing and consult the physician if the nausea, vomiting, and diarrhea persist. Review strategies to identify and maintain blood glucose levels during illness if you had difficulty answering this question.
Cognitive Level—Applying
Client Needs Category—Health promotion and maintenance
Client Needs Subcategory—None

92. 1. The diabetic clinic nurse identifies the client with a HbA1c of 12% as a client in need of extended assessment and instruction in diabetic management. A HbA1c of 12% reflects a routine blood sugar of 300 mg/dL. The client with a blood sugar of 97 to 165 mg/dL is maintaining appropriate blood sugar levels. The adolescent type 1 diabetic has grown up with managing diabetes. The client switching to a new format of insulin administration will need instruction regarding technique only.

Test Taking Strategy—Analyze to determine what information the question asks for, which is the client who needs extended instruction on diabetic management, indicating a problem. Look at each client to identify the needed teaching on diabetic management. Note the abnormal lab value for a HbA1c leading to the correct answer. Review diagnostic testing for diabetic management if you had difficulty answering this question.

Cognitive Level—Analyzing
Client Needs Category—Physiological integrity
Client Needs Subcategory—Reduction of risk potential

93. 3. Prefilled insulin pens are a convenient way to administer insulin for individuals who travel, the visually impaired, or those who mix standard insulin types. Due to infection control concerns, each insulin pen is designed for only one person. It is correct that the insulin type is the same as the type in a vial, the needle is primed with insulin prior to use, and the needle is changed between injections.

Test Taking Strategy—Analyze to determine what information the question asks for, which is a client statement that needs further clarification. Look for the statement that is incorrect regarding the use of an insulin pen. If unsure, review directions for using an insulin pen and principles of infection control.
Cognitive Level—Analyzing
Client Needs Category—Physiological integrity
Client Needs Subcategory—Reduction of risk potential

94. 4. Insulin lowers blood glucose levels. The client who received two doses of insulin is at risk for developing hypoglycemia. Therefore, the nurse should monitor the client's blood glucose level immediately after the error is discovered and frequently thereafter. In addition, if the client is conscious, the nurse may offer fruit juice, a carbonated beverage, glucose tablets, or gel. If the client is unconscious, the nurse should prepare to start an I.V. dextrose infusion. Because a medication error was made, an incident report must be completed; however, this should not take priority over the client's well-being. Calling the intensive care unit (ICU) is unnecessary unless the client's glucose level drops dangerously low and treatment is ineffective. Performing neurologic checks and taking vital signs are prudent measures, but they are not as important as frequent blood glucose monitoring in this situation.

Test Taking Strategy—Analyze to determine what information the question asks for, which is the priority related to an overdose of insulin. Recall that this medication error will cause the blood sugar to fall well below normal levels. The client's blood sugar should be measured frequently (option 4); the physician should be kept informed; and treatment of hypoglycemia should proceed with oral glucose, an injection of 50% glucose, or an injection of glucagon. Review how to manage an overdose of insulin if you had difficulty answering this question.
Cognitive Level—Applying
Client Needs Category—Physiological integrity
Client Needs Subcategory—Pharmacological therapies

The Nursing Care of Clients with Cardiac Disorders

■ Nursing Care of Clients with Hypertensive Heart Disease
■ Nursing Care of Clients with Coronary Artery Disease
■ Nursing Care of Clients with Myocardial Infarction
■ Nursing Care of Clients with Congestive Heart Failure
■ Nursing Care of Clients with Conduction Disorders
■ Nursing Care of Clients with Valvular Disorders
■ Nursing Care of Clients with Infectious and Inflammatory Disorders of the Heart
■ Correct Answers, Rationales, and Test Taking Strategies

Directions: *With a pencil, blacken the space in front of the option you have chosen for your correct answer.*

Nursing Care of Clients with Hypertensive Heart Disease

A nurse volunteers to do blood pressure screenings at a local community hospital's annual health fair.

1. Which modification used by the nurse is most appropriate when taking the blood pressure of a client who weighs 250 pounds?
[ ] **1.** The nurse takes the blood pressure on the client's thigh.
[ ] **2.** The nurse has the client lie down during the assessment.
[ ] **3.** The nurse pumps the manometer up to 250 mm Hg.
[ ] **4.** The nurse uses an extra-large blood pressure cuff.

2. The nurse obtains adult blood pressure readings on four separate clients. Which client should have a follow-up blood pressure check within 2 months?
[ ] **1.** The client whose blood pressure is 138/88 mm Hg
[ ] **2.** The client whose blood pressure is 132/98 mm Hg
[ ] **3.** The client whose blood pressure is 120/80 mm Hg
[ ] **4.** The client whose blood pressure is 118/78 mm Hg

At the health fair, the nurse teaches the client's spouse how to take the blood pressure.

3. According to the nurse, when is the correct time to note the diastolic blood pressure reading?
[ ] **1.** When the loud knocking sounds become muffled
[ ] **2.** When the last loud knocking sound is heard
[ ] **3.** When the swishing sound becomes loud
[ ] **4.** When the swishing sound becomes faint

While getting the blood pressure checked, an African American client asks the nurse why it is important to control hypertension.

4. Which response by the nurse is most accurate?
[ ] **1.** Sustained hypertension decreases the life span of many blood cells.
[ ] **2.** Sustained hypertension leads to the formation of venous blood clots.
[ ] **3.** Sustained hypertension compromises blood flow to many vital organs.
[ ] **4.** Sustained hypertension predisposes to narrowing of the cardiac valves.

5. When obtaining a health history from this client, which finding strongly suggests that the client is hypertensive? Select all that apply.
[ ] **1.** Unexplained nosebleeds
[ ] **2.** Difficulty sleeping at night
[ ] **3.** Waking to urinate at night
[ ] **4.** Occasional heart palpitations
[ ] **5.** Dizziness
[ ] **6.** Pale skin color

The nurse advises the client to seek medical attention immediately following blood pressure readings of 206/110 mm Hg and 198/104 mm Hg.

6. Which finding is the best indication that the client's heart has been affected by sustained high blood pressure?
[ ] **1.** The client has a strong S_1 heart sound.
[ ] **2.** The client's heart rate is 100 beats/minute when active.
[ ] **3.** The client's heart is moderately enlarged.
[ ] **4.** The client has an irregular heart rhythm.

The physician of a client with hypertension recommends that the client follow a low-sodium diet.

7. The best evidence that the client understands the nurse's instructions regarding dietary restrictions is if the client states to avoid which item?
[ ] **1.** Soy sauce
[ ] **2.** Lemon juice
[ ] **3.** Maple syrup
[ ] **4.** Onion powder

8. If the client with hypertension is willing to implement lifestyle changes to reduce blood pressure, which changes, encouraged by the nurse, would be most beneficial? Select all that apply.
[ ] **1.** Eating a diet higher in fiber
[ ] **2.** Balancing rest with exercise
[ ] **3.** Taking time for more leisure activities
[ ] **4.** Giving up smoking cigarettes
[ ] **5.** Pursuing measures for losing weight
[ ] **6.** Assessing blood pressure in the morning and evening

The client with hypertension will begin taking furosemide (Lasix) 40 mg orally every day.

9. Which observation by the nurse is the best indication that the furosemide (Lasix) has had a desired effect?
[ ] **1.** The client's pulse becomes slower.
[ ] **2.** The client's blood pressure stabilizes.
[ ] **3.** The client's urine output increases.
[ ] **4.** The client's anxiety is diminished.

10. When preparing discharge instructions for this client, the nurse's instructions should include taking oral furosemide (Lasix) at what time of day?
[ ] **1.** Before bedtime
[ ] **2.** During the morning
[ ] **3.** With the main meal
[ ] **4.** In the late afternoon

11. When teaching the client about the side effects of furosemide (Lasix), the nurse's instructions should include the need to eat foods high in which mineral?
[ ] **1.** Potassium
[ ] **2.** Sodium
[ ] **3.** Calcium
[ ] **4.** Iron

12. The nurse instructs the client to monitor urine output while taking furosemide (Lasix) at home because use of the medication may lead to which condition?
[ ] **1.** Dehydration
[ ] **2.** Fluid overload
[ ] **3.** Hypernatremia
[ ] **4.** Hyperkalemia

Another client has an angiotension-converting enzyme (ACE) inhibitor, enalapril (Vasotec) 10 mg daily added to the medication regimen.

13. Which of the following client statements will the nurse recognize as a potential side effect of the medication?
[ ] **1.** "I have noticed that I am urinating more than normal."
[ ] **2.** "I have a dry, hacky cough throughout the day."
[ ] **3.** "I feel weak and lethargic in the afternoon."
[ ] **4.** "I feel that I am having heart palpitations."

14. When caring for the client who is prescribed the combination of a loop diuretic and beta blocker to control hypertension, which nursing considerations are essential? Select all that apply.
[ ] **1.** Assist the client to a standing position.
[ ] **2.** Maintain an intake and output record.
[ ] **3.** Maintain bed rest until blood pressure is normal.
[ ] **4.** Encourage keeping up with work as a diversional activity.
[ ] **5.** Monitor blood sugar readings.
[ ] **6.** Discuss sexual implications.

A 79-year-old client comes to the hospital for dizziness, light-headedness, fatigue, and dehydration. The client's blood pressure on admission is 92/48 mm Hg. As the nurse completes the admission assessment, a list of medications is obtained as part of the medication reconciliation process, a method of comparing the medications that the client has been taking with the current medication orders.

15. If the client reports taking the following medications, which are more than likely to have contributed to this client's signs and symptoms? Select all that apply.
[ ] **1.** Lisinopril (Zestril)
[ ] **2.** Valsartan (Diovan)
[ ] **3.** Metoprolol (Lopressor)
[ ] **4.** Warfarin (Coumadin)
[ ] **5.** Hydrochlorothiazide (HydroDIURIL)
[ ] **6.** Aspirin (Bufferin)

Nursing Care of Clients with Coronary Artery Disease

The nurse working on a medical-surgical unit identifies several clients who have been diagnosed with coronary artery disease (CAD).

16. Which of the following client risk factors is most significant for developing CAD?
[ ] **1.** Drinking a nightly cocktail
[ ] **2.** History of mitral valve repair
[ ] **3.** Rheumatic fever during childhood
[ ] **4.** Weighing 25 pounds (11.3 kg) above norm

The physician tells a client at risk for CAD that a high cholesterol level needs to be lowered and advises following a low-cholesterol diet.

17. When the client asks the nurse how cholesterol acts as a cardiac risk factor, what is the best explanation?
[ ] **1.** Excess fat in the blood expands the circulating blood volume.
[ ] **2.** Excess fat in the blood thickens the lining of the arteries.
[ ] **3.** Excess fat in the blood causes slower blood clotting.
[ ] **4.** Excess fat in the blood stimulates the heart to beat faster.

When the nurse makes inquiries about the client's diet, the client tells the nurse that breakfast usually includes sausage, eggs, hash browns, and white bread and butter.

18. When providing dietary instructions for this client, which healthful alternative should the nurse recommend?
[ ] **1.** Wheat toast for white bread
[ ] **2.** Margarine for butter
[ ] **3.** Cereal for eggs
[ ] **4.** Ham for sausage

Lifestyle changes prove insufficient for reducing the client's cholesterol level, and the physician prescribes the antihyperlipidemic drug atorvastatin calcium (Lipitor).

19. After providing medication instructions, the best evidence that the client knows this drug's potential side effects is when the client states it may cause which adverse effect?
[ ] **1.** Muscle pain
[ ] **2.** Palpitations
[ ] **3.** Visual changes
[ ] **4.** Weight loss

The client is scheduled for a stress electrocardiogram (ECG).

20. When the client asks why the physician ordered the ECG, how does the nurse correctly explain its purpose?
[ ] **1.** It will show how the heart performs during exercise.
[ ] **2.** It will determine the client's potential target heart rate.
[ ] **3.** It will verify how much the client needs to improve fitness.
[ ] **4.** It will help predict whether the client will have a heart attack soon.

A client with CAD experiences periodic chest pain and is diagnosed with angina pectoris.

21. If the client is typical of others who have angina pectoris, the nurse would expect the client to report that chest pain is best relieved by which nonpharmacological measure?
[ ] **1.** Taking a deep breath
[ ] **2.** Resting in a chair
[ ] **3.** Applying heat to the chest
[ ] **4.** Rubbing the chest

The client informs the nurse that the physician just prescribed sublingual nitroglycerin tablets to take whenever chest pain is experienced.

22. The nurse informs the client that the correct way to administer nitroglycerin is to place one tablet where?
[ ] **1.** Between the gum and cheek
[ ] **2.** At the back of the throat
[ ] **3.** Under the tongue
[ ] **4.** Between the teeth

23. Which side effects are most closely associated with the use of nitroglycerin tablets? Select all that apply.
[ ] **1.** Headache
[ ] **2.** Backache
[ ] **3.** Diarrhea
[ ] **4.** Jaundice
[ ] **5.** Dizziness
[ ] **6.** Pallor

The nurse explains to the client that nitroglycerin tablets lose their potency if exposed to light and air.

24. The nurse knows that the client understands how to determine when the nitroglycerin tablets need replacing when the client makes which statement?
[ ] **1.** "The tablets will smell like vinegar."
[ ] **2.** "The tablets will be discolored."
[ ] **3.** "They won't tingle in my mouth."
[ ] **4.** "They will disintegrate when I touch them."

25. If the chest pain is not relieved after taking one nitroglycerin tablet, the nurse should teach the client to take what action?
[ ] **1.** Take another tablet in 5 minutes.
[ ] **2.** Drive to the emergency department.
[ ] **3.** Call the physician immediately.
[ ] **4.** Swallow two additional tablets.

Because the client has repeated episodes of angina that have not been relieved with sublingual nitroglycerin, the physician prescribes a nitroglycerin transdermal patch (Nitrodisc).

26. Which nursing action is most appropriate when applying a new transdermal patch?
[ ] **1.** Rotate the application site.
[ ] **2.** Clean the skin with alcohol.
[ ] **3.** Tape the patch to the client's chest.
[ ] **4.** Take the blood pressure afterward.

27. Which assessment finding should signal the nurse to withhold applying the client's nitroglycerin patch and notify the physician?
[ ] **1.** Temperature of 99.8°F (37.6°C)
[ ] **2.** Respiratory rate of 24 breaths/minute at rest
[ ] **3.** Apical heart rate of 90 beats/minute
[ ] **4.** Blood pressure of 94/62 mm Hg

A client diagnosed with angina has been advised to reduce consumption of saturated fat and calories to control the progression of coronary artery disease (CAD).

28. The best evidence that the client is complying with the diet therapy is the report of using which type of fat for cooking?
[ ] **1.** Melted margarine
[ ] **2.** Clarified butter
[ ] **3.** Cooking spray
[ ] **4.** Liquid corn oil

When the client returns to the physician's office for a routine visit, the nurse reviews the client's weekly intake of food from the food diary. The client tells the nurse of being particularly fond of hot apple pies like those sold at a fast-food restaurant. The client reports eating several each week. The client asks the nurse how many calories are in one pie.

29. If the literature supplied by the fast-food chain indicates that one hot apple pie contains 2 g of protein, 14 g of fat, and 31 g of carbohydrates, how many calories are contained in one hot apple pie?

_____

Because this client has been experiencing an increased number of anginal episodes, the physician orders a cardiac catheterization and coronary arteriogram.

30. Which nursing action can best help reduce the client's anxiety in this situation?
[ ] **1.** Teach the client how coronary artery disease (CAD) is usually treated.
[ ] **2.** Listen to the client's feelings about this condition.
[ ] **3.** Explain that the procedure has been very helpful for other clients.
[ ] **4.** Avoid discussing the heart catheterization until the client has relaxed.

The nurse implements the teaching plan for cardiac catheterization and coronary arteriogram.

31. Which statement by the client indicates an understanding of what will happen during the testing procedure?
[ ] **1.** "I will be able to hear my heart beating in my chest."
[ ] **2.** "I will feel a heavy sensation all over my body."
[ ] **3.** "I will be anesthetized and will not feel any discomfort."
[ ] **4.** "I will feel a warm sensation as the dye is instilled."

32. Before the cardiac catheterization and coronary arteriogram, it is essential for the nurse to ask the client about any allergy to iodine or which other substance?
[ ] **1.** Penicillin
[ ] **2.** Morphine
[ ] **3.** Shellfish
[ ] **4.** Eggs

During the procedure, the physician threads the heart catheter through the femoral artery.

33. After the coronary arteriogram, the nurse must keep the client flat in bed with the affected leg in which position?
[ ] **1.** Extended
[ ] **2.** Flexed
[ ] **3.** Abducted
[ ] **4.** Adducted

34. After the femoral artery has been cannulated and the client is returned to the room, what should the nurse plan to do first?
[ ] **1.** Palpate the client's distal peripheral pulses.
[ ] **2.** Auscultate the client's heart and breath sounds.
[ ] **3.** Percuss all four quadrants of the client's abdomen.
[ ] **4.** Inspect the skin integrity in the client's groin.

35. The nurse provides discharge instructions for a client who has recovered after a cardiac catheterization. Which instructions should be included? Select all that apply.
[ ] **1.** Take a shower rather than a tub bath until the puncture site heals.
[ ] **2.** Perform leg exercises every 2 hours while awake.
[ ] **3.** Drink a generous amount of fluids for the next 24 hours.
[ ] **4.** Report worsening of pain in the leg that was catheterized.
[ ] **5.** Flush the toilet twice after eliminating urine and stool in the next 24 hours.
[ ] **6.** Change the dressing over the puncture site daily until it heals.

Based on the results of the coronary arteriogram, the physician recommends that the client undergo percutaneous transluminal coronary angioplasty (PTCA).

36. The nurse knows that the client understands the physician's explanation of the PTCA procedure when the client makes which statement?
[ ] **1.** "A balloon-tipped catheter will be inserted into my coronary artery."
[ ] **2.** "A Teflon graft will be used to replace an area of weakened heart muscle."
[ ] **3.** "A section of my leg vein will be grafted around a narrowed coronary artery."
[ ] **4.** "A battery-operated pacemaker will be implanted to maintain my heart rate."

While waiting to undergo percutaneous transluminal coronary angioplasty (PTCA), the client is given propranolol (Inderal).

37. When the client asks the nurse how propranolol helps to prevent angina, what is the best explanation?
[ ] **1.** Propranolol promotes excretion of body fluid.
[ ] **2.** Propranolol reduces the rate of heart contraction.
[ ] **3.** Propranolol alters pain receptors in the heart.
[ ] **4.** Propranolol dilates the major coronary arteries.

38. While the client takes propranolol (Inderal), what changes would the nurse expect to see in the client's pulse rate?
[ ] 1. Faster than usual
[ ] 2. Stronger than before
[ ] 3. Temporarily irregular
[ ] 4. Slower than in the past

The physician also advised the client to take 81 mg of aspirin daily while waiting for the scheduled percutaneous transluminal coronary angioplasty (PTCA).

39. What is the best explanation for the drug therapy in this situation?
[ ] 1. Aspirin tends to relieve chest pain.
[ ] 2. Aspirin tends to prevent blood clots.
[ ] 3. Aspirin tends to lower the blood pressure.
[ ] 4. Aspirin tends to dilate the coronary arteries.

40. When the client returns to the room after the percutaneous transluminal coronary angioplasty (PTCA) procedure, which assessment finding should be reported immediately to the physician?
[ ] 1. Urine output of 100 mL/hour
[ ] 2. Blood pressure of 108/68 mm Hg
[ ] 3. Dry mouth
[ ] 4. Chest pain

The client who previously had a percutaneous transluminal coronary angioplasty (PTCA) is now having coronary artery bypass graft (CABG) surgery. Shortly after the procedure, the client is returned to the room and assessed by the nurse.

41. The nurse checking the client's leg incision is aware that which is the most common blood vessel used in CABG surgery?
[ ] 1. The saphenous vein
[ ] 2. The femoral artery
[ ] 3. The popliteal vein
[ ] 4. The iliac artery

The nurse asks the nursing assistant to take the client's vital signs.

42. Which action by a newly hired nursing assistant indicates that the nurse needs to provide more instruction to the nursing assistant on how to accurately assess the client's pulse rate?
[ ] 1. The nursing assistant places a thumb over the radial artery.
[ ] 2. The nursing assistant counts the pulse rate for 1 full minute.
[ ] 3. The nursing assistant rests the client's arm on the abdomen.
[ ] 4. The nursing assistant presses the radial artery against the bone.

The client complains of having acute pain in the incisional area.

43. Based on the client's complaint, the nurse would expect the pain to have which possible effect on the vital signs?
[ ] 1. Temperature may be elevated.
[ ] 2. Pulse rate may become rapid.
[ ] 3. Respiratory rate may slow.
[ ] 4. Blood pressure may fall.

The physician orders a patient-controlled analgesia (PCA) infusion pump for the client after coronary artery bypass graft (CABG) surgery.

44. When the nurse informs the client about the use of the PCA pump, which instruction is most important to include?
[ ] 1. "Press the control button whenever you feel you need pain medication."
[ ] 2. "Call the nurse each time you need to use the PCA pump."
[ ] 3. "Use the PCA pump only when the pain is severe."
[ ] 4. "Do not use the PCA pump too frequently, because it can cause addiction."

45. What information about the client's use of a patient-controlled analgesia (PCA) pump is most important to communicate to the staff on the next shift?
[ ] 1. Name of the client's physician
[ ] 2. Purpose for using the pump
[ ] 3. Number of doses administered
[ ] 4. The client's need for further teaching

46. After the coronary artery bypass graft (CABG) surgery, which assessment finding provides the best evidence that collateral circulation at the donor graft site is adequate?
[ ] 1. The client is free from chest pain.
[ ] 2. The client's toes are warm and nonedematous.
[ ] 3. The client moves the operative leg easily.
[ ] 4. The client's heart rate remains regular.

Nursing Care of Clients with Myocardial Infarction

A 65-year-old client with severe chest pain is evaluated in the emergency department. A tentative diagnosis of myocardial infarction (MI) is made.

47. Which assessment finding is most closely correlated with an evolving MI?
[ ] 1. Profuse sweating
[ ] 2. Facial flushing
[ ] 3. Severe headache
[ ] 4. Productive cough

48. Which of the following electrocardiogram (ECG) changes supports the diagnosis that the client is experiencing a myocardial infarction (MI)?
[ ] **1.** Inverted P wave
[ ] **2.** Prolonged PR interval
[ ] **3.** Widened QRS complex
[ ] **4.** Elevated ST segment

49. When the nurse is obtaining this client's health history, which question about pain is least helpful?
[ ] **1.** "How long have you been in pain?"
[ ] **2.** "Where is your pain located?"
[ ] **3.** "What were you doing when your pain started?"
[ ] **4.** "What medications do you take for pain?"

50. If the client's severe chest pain is typical of other people who experience myocardial infarction (MI), the client is most likely to tell the nurse that the discomfort radiates to which area?
[ ] **1.** Flank
[ ] **2.** Groin
[ ] **3.** Abdomen
[ ] **4.** Shoulder

51. If the client makes the following statements regarding pain, which statement is most characteristic of a client experiencing a myocardial infarction (MI)?
[ ] **1.** "The pain comes and goes."
[ ] **2.** "The pain came on slowly."
[ ] **3.** "The pain is tingling in nature."
[ ] **4.** "The pain has remained continuous."

52. If the client's pain is due to a myocardial infarction (MI), which prescribed medication would be most helpful?
[ ] **1.** A nonsteroidal anti-inflammatory drug such as ibuprofen (Advil)
[ ] **2.** A nonsalicylate such as acetaminophen (Tylenol)
[ ] **3.** A salicylate such as aspirin
[ ] **4.** An opioid such as morphine sulfate

The client's spouse tells the nurse that medical attention for chest pain was delayed because the client thought the discomfort was due to strained muscles from doing yard work.

53. The nurse understands that the client's hesitation in going to the hospital is an example of which coping mechanism?
[ ] **1.** Regression
[ ] **2.** Projection
[ ] **3.** Denial
[ ] **4.** Undoing

54. Which risk factor is least likely to have predisposed the client to having a myocardial infarction (MI)?
[ ] **1.** Smoking cigarettes
[ ] **2.** Eating fatty foods
[ ] **3.** Working under emotional stress
[ ] **4.** Drinking an occasional cocktail

55. Which laboratory results would the nurse expect to be elevated if the client had a myocardial infarction (MI)?
[ ] **1.** Isoenzymes and troponin
[ ] **2.** Sodium and potassium
[ ] **3.** Red blood cells and platelets
[ ] **4.** Plasminogen and lactic acid

Based on the laboratory test results and the occurrence of symptoms for only a few hours, the physician instructs the nurse to admit the client to the intensive care unit (ICU) and administer streptokinase (Streptase). Once the client has been transferred and admitted to the ICU, the licensed practical nurse (LPN) attaches electrocardiogram (ECG) leads to the chest and connects the client to a cardiac monitor.

56. On the drawing below, place five leads (red, white, green, black, and brown) in the correct locations on the chest for monitoring the client in lead III.

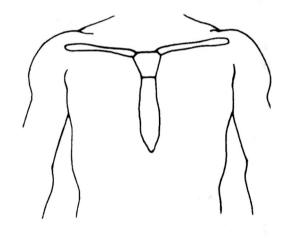

57. When the client is startled by an alarm caused by a loose lead, what is the best approach for the nurse to take to relieve the client's anxiety?
[ ] **1.** Describe the current heart rhythm.
[ ] **2.** Explain the reason why the alarm sounded.
[ ] **3.** Give the client a prescribed tranquilizer.
[ ] **4.** Allow the client to look at a rhythm tracing.

Shortly after the client arrives in the intensive care unit, the registered nurse (RN) prepares to administer streptokinase (Streptase). The licensed practical nurse (LPN) assists the RN in preparing the client for the treatment.

58. The LPN correctly explains to the client and the spouse that streptokinase (Streptase) is being given to achieve which effect?
[ ] **1.** To dissolve blood clots in a coronary artery
[ ] **2.** To slow the client's heart rate
[ ] **3.** To improve heart contraction
[ ] **4.** To lower the client's diastolic blood pressure

59. When a client receives streptokinase (Streptase), the nurse must monitor for which adverse effect?
[ ] **1.** Hypertension
[ ] **2.** Hyperthermia
[ ] **3.** Bleeding
[ ] **4.** Tachypnea

60. Which drug should the nurse have on hand in case the client develops an allergic reaction to streptokinase (Streptase)?
[ ] **1.** Vitamin K
[ ] **2.** Heparin
[ ] **3.** Diphenhydramine (Benadryl)
[ ] **4.** Warfarin (Coumadin)

61. Which symptom would the nurse expect to observe if the client is having an allergic reaction to streptokinase (Streptase)?
[ ] **1.** Urticaria
[ ] **2.** Dysuria
[ ] **3.** Hemoptysis
[ ] **4.** Dyspepsia

The client says to the intensive care unit (ICU) nurse, "Being here scares me. I almost died."

62. Which response by the nurse is most appropriate at this time?
[ ] **1.** "What are your concerns?"
[ ] **2.** "Why are you so scared?"
[ ] **3.** "Your doctor says you are doing just fine."
[ ] **4.** "You need to concentrate on getting well."

After recovering from a myocardial infarction (MI), the client is transferred to the medical-surgical unit for continued recovery and rehabilitation.

63. The nursing team develops a care plan and expected outcomes for the client's recovery. Which expected outcomes are most important? Select all that apply.
[ ] **1.** The client will not gain weight.
[ ] **2.** The client's activity tolerance will increase.
[ ] **3.** The client will comply with the dietary restrictions.
[ ] **4.** The client will avoid any alcoholic beverages.
[ ] **5.** The client will verbalize fears and anxieties freely.
[ ] **6.** The client will maintain pressure over the intravenous site.

Before discharge, the physician requests that the client receive dietary instructions about a calorie-restricted, low-fat, low-sodium diet as well as instructions about necessary activity restrictions.

64. Avoiding which of the following foods is the best evidence that the client understands the nurse's dietary instructions?
[ ] **1.** Pepperoni pizza
[ ] **2.** Vinegar and oil salad dressing
[ ] **3.** Liver and onions
[ ] **4.** Lemon-pepper chicken

65. After hearing the nurse's instructions about activity restrictions and the potentially dangerous consequences of certain activities, the client correctly states the importance for avoiding which of the following?
[ ] **1.** Carrying groceries from the car
[ ] **2.** Straining during a bowel movement
[ ] **3.** Bathing in warm water
[ ] **4.** Having sexual intercourse

At the client's follow-up clinic visit 1 week after discharge, the physician orders an echocardiogram to evaluate the damage done to the client's heart.

66. The nurse assumes that the client understands how an echocardiogram is performed when that client tells the nurse that this examination involves imaging the heart using which of one of the following?
[ ] **1.** Heat
[ ] **2.** Sound
[ ] **3.** Radiation
[ ] **4.** Electricity

A 65-year-old client collapses in the hospital elevator while coming to visit a family member. A nurse goes to the victim's aid.

67. Place the following list of resuscitation activities in the sequence in which they should be performed. Use all the options.

1. Open the victim's airway.	
2. Administer rescue breaths.	
3. Check responsiveness.	
4. Activate emergency assistance.	
5. Check for spontaneous breathing.	
6. Perform chest compressions.	

68. What is the most effective method for restoring circulation in a pulseless victim?
[ ] **1.** Performing chest compressions
[ ] **2.** Keeping the airway open
[ ] **3.** Using an automated external defibrillator (AED)
[ ] **4.** Positioning on a hard, flat surface

69. Which technique is most appropriate for the nurse to use to open the airway of a victim who is not breathing?
[ ] **1.** Elevate the neck.
[ ] **2.** Lift the chin.
[ ] **3.** Press on the jaw.
[ ] **4.** Clear the mouth.

70. Which is the best method for determining if the victim requires rescue breathing?
[ ] **1.** Observe the victim's skin color.
[ ] **2.** Feel for pulsations at the neck.
[ ] **3.** Check for absence of normal breathing.
[ ] **4.** Blow air into the victim's mouth.

71. How can the nurse deliver an effective volume of air into the lungs of a victim who is not breathing?
[ ] **1.** Press on the victim's trachea.
[ ] **2.** Remove the victim's dentures.
[ ] **3.** Pinch the victim's nose shut.
[ ] **4.** Squeeze the victim's cheeks.

The nurse further assesses the client, who is unresponsive and pulseless. The nurse begins chest compressions.

72. Where is the correct placement for the nurse's hands before administering cardiac compressions?
[ ] **1.** On the lower half of the sternum
[ ] **2.** Below the tip of the xiphoid process
[ ] **3.** Over the costal cartilage
[ ] **4.** Directly above the manubrium

73. During cardiopulmonary resuscitation (CPR), the nurse compresses the chest of an adult victim at which rate?
[ ] **1.** No less than 15 compressions per minute
[ ] **2.** No less than 40 compressions per minute
[ ] **3.** No less than 80 compressions per minute
[ ] **4.** No less than 100 compressions per minute

After the nurse calls for help, a second health care provider arrives to assist with cardiopulmonary resuscitation (CPR).

74. When two rescuers perform CPR on an adult, what is the ratio of compressions to ventilations?
[ ] **1.** 30 compressions to 2 breaths
[ ] **2.** 10 compressions to 1 breath
[ ] **3.** 1 compression for each breath
[ ] **4.** 1 compression to 5 breaths

75. Which finding best indicates that cardiac compressions can be discontinued?
[ ] **1.** The victim's color improves.
[ ] **2.** The pupils become dilated.
[ ] **3.** A pulse can be palpated.
[ ] **4.** The victim begins to vomit.

76. After the client has been successfully resuscitated by the nurse, which body position is most correct while awaiting transfer to the emergency department?
[ ] **1.** Supine with the head elevated
[ ] **2.** On the side upper knee flexed
[ ] **3.** Prone with the head lowered
[ ] **4.** Flat with the knees extended

As the client is being transported to the hospital, an observer comments, "I have had no training in CPR so I was not able to help."

77. Having heard the observer's comment, which statement by the nurse would be most helpful for an untrained individual to remember if a trained individual is not present?
[ ] **1.** An untrained person can always stay with the victim until help arrives.
[ ] **2.** Do not worry about compressions; just breathe regularly in the mouth.
[ ] **3.** Begin chest compressions in the center of the chest pressing down 2 inches (5 cm).
[ ] **4.** Place the client flat and elevate the feet to promote circulation.

Nursing Care of Clients with Congestive Heart Failure

78. Using the following cardiac structures, trace the normal pathway in which blood circulates on the left side of the heart. Use all the options.

1. Aorta	
2. Left ventricle	
3. Pulmonary veins	
4. Left atrium	
5. Mitral valve	

A 78-year-old client is admitted to the hospital with left-sided heart failure.

79. When obtaining a health history from the client, the nurse would expect to learn that which of the following was the client's earliest symptom?
[ ] **1.** Anorexia
[ ] **2.** Dyspnea
[ ] **3.** Nausea
[ ] **4.** Headaches

80. Because the client is exhibiting signs and symptoms of left-sided congestive heart failure (CHF), which position suggested by the nurse is most beneficial for the client at this time?
[ ] **1.** Supine with knees slightly bent
[ ] **2.** Side-lying on the right side
[ ] **3.** Side-lying on the left side
[ ] **4.** Semi-Fowler's position

81. The nurse anticipates that the client will most likely demonstrate which emotional response in relation to the development of heart failure?
[ ] **1.** Depression
[ ] **2.** Anxiety
[ ] **3.** Anger
[ ] **4.** Stoicism

After assessing the severity of the client's heart failure, the physician orders 2 l of oxygen per nasal cannula.

82. Which assessment finding is the best indication that oxygen therapy is effective?
[ ] **1.** The client's face is flushed.
[ ] **2.** Capillary refill is 6 seconds.
[ ] **3.** The client states, "I'm feeling better."
[ ] **4.** The apical pulse is less bounding.

The client's left-sided heart failure worsens with severe pulmonary edema. The nurse prepares to transfer the client to the intensive care unit (ICU).

83. The client tells the nurse of being extremely frightened. What is the most appropriate action for the nurse to take at this time?
[ ] **1.** Stay with the client.
[ ] **2.** Notify the physician.
[ ] **3.** Tell the client it will be fine.
[ ] **4.** Record the collected data.

84. To provide adequate care for the client with worsening left-sided heart failure, the intensive care unit (ICU) nurse should monitor which of the following on a daily basis?
[ ] **1.** Pupil response
[ ] **2.** Peripheral edema
[ ] **3.** Appetite
[ ] **4.** Weight

The nurse monitors the client's laboratory values because of the large doses of diuretics the client received to treat pulmonary edema.

85. Which value should the nurse report immediately to the physician?
[ ] **1.** Sodium: 137 mEq/L
[ ] **2.** Potassium: 2.5 mEq/L
[ ] **3.** Chloride: 97 mEq/L
[ ] **4.** Bicarbonate: 25 mEq/L

86. Which assessment finding would support the possibility of right-sided heart failure?
[ ] **1.** Jugular vein distention
[ ] **2.** Bradycardia
[ ] **3.** Dry, hacking cough
[ ] **4.** Flushed, red face

The physician orders digoxin (Lanoxin). After the digitalizing loading doses have achieved their therapeutic effect, the physician prescribes a daily maintenance dosage of 0.125 mg of digoxin P.O.

87. If each tablet of digoxin (Lanoxin) contains 0.25 mg, how much should the nurse administer to the client each day?

_____

88. Before administering the digoxin (Lanoxin) to the client, what nursing assessment is essential?
[ ] **1.** The client's heart rate
[ ] **2.** The client's blood pressure
[ ] **3.** The client's heart sounds
[ ] **4.** The client's breath sounds

89. If the client develops digoxin toxicity, what would the nurse expect the client to exhibit?
[ ] **1.** Anorexia and nausea
[ ] **2.** Dizziness and insomnia
[ ] **3.** Pinpoint pupils and double vision
[ ] **4.** Ringing in the ears and itchy skin

The nursing team establishes the nursing diagnosis Decreased cardiac output related to tachycardia, decreased stroke volume, and increased vascular volume, *and enters this into the client's care plan. The team also includes the following goal: The client will have an improvement in cardiac output by discharge.*

90. How can the nurse best measure whether the client has achieved the goal?
[ ] **1.** The client will have vital signs within normal parameters.
[ ] **2.** The client will lose no more than 5 lb/day.
[ ] **3.** The client will have decreased peripheral edema.
[ ] **4.** The client will have a 24-hour urine output of 1,000 mL.

Nursing Care of Clients with Conduction Disorders

The physician orders a 24-hour ambulatory electrocardiography using a Holter monitor for a client who has been experiencing brief fainting spells. The nurse provides instructions for the client regarding the purpose and use of the Holter monitor.

91. Which nursing instruction is most beneficial for helping the physician interpret the information collected by the Holter monitor?
[ ] **1.** "Record the times and types of physical activities you perform."
[ ] **2.** "Take your radial pulse rate every hour during the next day."
[ ] **3.** "Try to relax and limit your exercise as much as possible."
[ ] **4.** "Keep your lower extremities elevated while sitting."

92. To prevent electrical interference with the Holter monitor, it is most appropriate to recommend that the client avoid which action?
[ ] **1.** Standing close to a microwave oven
[ ] **2.** Driving under overhead power lines
[ ] **3.** Shaving with an electric razor
[ ] **4.** Using a cellular telephone

After evaluating the 24-hour Holter monitor tracings, the physician admits the client to the hospital for an abnormal heart rhythm. On admission, the nurse notes that the client has an irregularly fast heart rate and notifies the physician. The physician schedules the client for cardioversion.

93. The nurse knows that the client understands the cardioversion procedure when stating that it involves which action?
[ ] **1.** Administering an electrical current to the heart
[ ] **2.** Threading a thin, plastic catheter into the heart
[ ] **3.** Evaluating blood flow to areas of heart muscle
[ ] **4.** Scanning the heart after injecting a radioisotope

94. Before cardioversion is attempted, the nurse appropriately withholds which of the client's prescribed medication?
[ ] **1.** Diazepam (Valium)
[ ] **2.** Digoxin (Lanoxin)
[ ] **3.** Heparin
[ ] **4.** Warfarin (Coumadin)

95. Which finding would strongly indicate that the cardioversion procedure has been successful?
[ ] **1.** The client regains consciousness immediately.
[ ] **2.** Normal sinus cardiac rhythm is restored.
[ ] **3.** The apical heart rate equals the radial rate.
[ ] **4.** The pulse pressure is approximately 40 mm Hg.

Because the client continues to have an irregular heart rate, the physician schedules the insertion of an artificial pacemaker.

96. If the client understands the nurse's explanation of the heart's conduction system, which structure will the client identify as the site of the natural pacemaker? Place an X over the correct site.

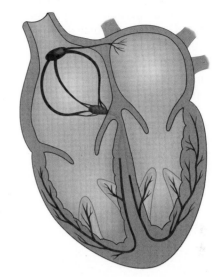

97. To assess the area where the permanent pacemaker battery has been implanted, the nurse knows to examine which area of the skin?
[ ] **1.** Beneath the left nipple
[ ] **2.** Near the brachial artery
[ ] **3.** In the midsternal area
[ ] **4.** Below the right clavicle

98. As part of the discharge instructions, the nurse correctly instructs the client that which symptom is a sign of artificial pacemaker malfunction?
[ ] **1.** Tingling in the chest area
[ ] **2.** Dizziness during activity
[ ] **3.** Pain radiating to the arm
[ ] **4.** Tenderness beneath the skin

A client is returning to the physician's office 2 days after having a cardiac ablation for an arrhythmia.

99. As the nurse updates the client's history, which client statement is most significant for the doctor to review?
[ ] **1.** "I have soreness at the incision site."
[ ] **2.** "I have had no cardiac palpitations."
[ ] **3.** "I have a bruise that extends down my leg."
[ ] **4.** "I have slight oozing at the insertion site."

Nursing Care of Clients with Valvular Disorders

During a routine preemployment physical examination, a physician discovers that a 28-year-old client has a heart murmur.

100. If the heart murmur is related to valve damage caused by a childhood infection, the nurse would expect the client to report having had which disease?
[ ] **1.** Varicella (chickenpox)
[ ] **2.** Rubella (German measles)
[ ] **3.** Rheumatic fever
[ ] **4.** Whooping cough

After a diagnostic workup, the physician informs the client that the client has mitral valve stenosis.

101. Indicate with an *X* the best anatomic area for the nurse to auscultate mitral valve sounds.

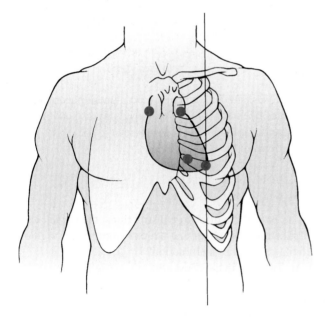

The physician prescribes 250 mg of nafcillin (Unipen) P.O. daily to treat the client's mitral valve stenosis.

102. Which statement by the nurse is the best explanation for why the client needs to take the prescribed medication?
[ ] **1.** "It may destroy the virus causing your disease."
[ ] **2.** "It may reduce the scar tissue on the valve."
[ ] **3.** "It may stop blood clots from forming."
[ ] **4.** "It may prevent future bacterial infections."

Over a period of 10 years, the client has been taking diuretics and digoxin for the long-term treatment of mitral valve stenosis. The client's condition has progressively worsened, and the client is now scheduled to have surgery for a mitral valve replacement.

103. Which statement is the best indication that the client understands the surgical procedure involving mitral valve replacement?
[ ] **1.** "My blood will be circulated through a heart-lung machine."
[ ] **2.** "The surgeon will enlarge my valve by inserting a stent."
[ ] **3.** "My chest will be opened during surgery, but my heart will not."
[ ] **4.** "A piece of my leg vein will be used to replace the diseased valve."

Postoperatively, the client experiences shortness of breath with moderate activity. The physician writes an order stating that the client may sit up in a chair if tolerating the increased activity.

104. Which nursing action would best reduce the client's energy expenditure?
[ ] **1.** Administering oxygen when the client is dyspneic
[ ] **2.** Staggering self-care activities over several hours
[ ] **3.** Providing analgesic medications when necessary
[ ] **4.** Restricting visitors to brief periods of time

105. Which assessment finding offers the best evidence that the client can tolerate the activity involved in getting out of bed?
[ ] **1.** The client's appetite has improved.
[ ] **2.** The client reports a more restful sleep.
[ ] **3.** The client's heart rate is stable.
[ ] **4.** The client can get out of bed without assistance.

The client is disappointed about not progressing quickly after the mitral valve replacement. One day, the frustrated client pushes away the lunch tray and it falls to the floor.

106. Which nursing response is most appropriate at this time?
[ ] **1.** Cleaning up the floor and saying nothing
[ ] **2.** Finding out what food would be preferred
[ ] **3.** Allowing the client to vent his or her feelings
[ ] **4.** Leaving the client alone until feeling better

107. When gathering nursing assessment data, which finding will adults with chronic cardiac diseases most frequently manifest?
[ ] **1.** Barrel-shaped chest
[ ] **2.** Flushed facial skin
[ ] **3.** Clubbed fingertips
[ ] **4.** Chest pain

Nursing Care of Clients with Infectious and Inflammatory Disorders of the Heart

A pulmonary artery catheter was used to monitor pressure within the heart of a client after cardiac surgery. The client is now suspected of having bacterial endocarditis.

108. Which assessment finding documented by the nurse provides the best evidence that the client has a bacterial infection?
[ ] **1.** Chest pain
[ ] **2.** Dry cough
[ ] **3.** Fever
[ ] **4.** Dyspnea

A 63-year-old client with liver cancer is admitted to the medical-surgical unit with a diagnosis of pericarditis.

109. When auscultating the client's heart and breath sounds during a routine shift assessment, which action by the nurse is most appropriate?
[ ] **1.** Asking the client to hold his or her breath
[ ] **2.** Turning off the television momentarily
[ ] **3.** Positioning the client flat in bed
[ ] **4.** Locating the xiphoid process

110. Which assessment finding best supports the assumption that the client's cardiac stroke volume is reduced?
[ ] **1.** The client faints with activity.
[ ] **2.** The client develops hypertension.
[ ] **3.** The client manifests bradycardia.
[ ] **4.** The client has a bounding pulse.

A 50-year-old client is scheduled for a heart transplant tomorrow. The night nurse is asked to review the surgical procedure with the client. Because of the client's anxiety, the client has difficulty comprehending the nurse's information.

111. Which nursing action is most appropriate to perform next?
[ ] **1.** The nurse notifies the physician, requesting a hypnotic or sedative.
[ ] **2.** The nurse provides a video of the surgery for the client to watch.
[ ] **3.** The nurse waits until the client's spouse is present to describe the surgery.
[ ] **4.** The nurse listens as the client talks about fears concerning surgery and rehabilitation.

112. During the postoperative period, what is the best rationale for the nurse frequently assessing the client's fluid status?
[ ] **1.** Urine retention is common after a heart transplant.
[ ] **2.** Urine output is an indication of perfusion to the kidneys.
[ ] **3.** Hydration determines when the client needs to be transfused.
[ ] **4.** Hydration indicates when fluids should be increased.

113. On the nursing unit, the nurse is a team member following a primary nursing care delivery model. Which activity is unique to this delivery system of nursing care?
[ ] **1.** The nurse shares the care of clients with assistive personnel.
[ ] **2.** The nurse oversees client care from admission to discharge.
[ ] **3.** The nurse is a liaison between the physician and client/family.
[ ] **4.** The nurse performs total care for a group of clients.

Correct Answers, Rationales, and Test Taking Strategies

Nursing Care of Clients with Hypertensive Heart Disease

1. 4. The nurse can assume that an obese client will need an extra-large adult cuff. A common guide is to select a cuff with a bladder that encircles at least two-thirds of the limb at its midpoint and is as wide as 40% of the midlimb circumference. If the cuff is too narrow, the blood pressure will be higher than its true measurement; if too wide, the measurement will be lower than the true pressure. A normal-sized cuff will not fit around the obese client's thigh. Having the client lie down would have no bearing on the cuff size, but it could affect a client's blood pressure measurement; in this case, the cuff is too small anyway. Pumping the manometer to 250 mm Hg is also incorrect. The blood pressure manometer should be pumped up to approximately 30 mm Hg above the baseline blood pressure. The American Heart Association recommends the following: Inflate the cuff while palpating the brachial artery, note when the pulse disappears, deflate the cuff, wait, and reinflate the cuff to 30 mm Hg above the point at which the pulse disappeared.

> *Test Taking Strategy—Look at the key words "most appropriate" in reference to a modification that is required when assessing the blood pressure of an obese client. Recall that the bladder within the blood pressure cuff must be larger than that within a normal adult-size cuff to avoid obtaining a falsely high measurement, which correlates with option 4. Review the equipment that is required when assessing a client's blood pressure if you had difficulty answering this question.*
> *Cognitive level—Applying*
> *Client Needs Category—Health promotion and maintenance*
> *Client Needs Subcategory—None*

2. 2. Blood pressure is determined by the cardiac output (amount of blood the heart pumps) and by the resistance of blood flow in the arteries. Normal blood pressure is less than 120/80 mm Hg. Prehypertension is a systolic measurement between 120 and 139 mm Hg or a diastolic measurement between 80 and 89 mm Hg. Stage 1 hypertension is a systolic measurement of 140 to 159 mm Hg or a diastolic measurement of 90 to 99 mm Hg. Stage 2 hypertension is a systolic measurement that exceeds 160 mm Hg or a diastolic measurement that exceeds 100 mm Hg. Of the four clients, The Joint National Committee on Prevention, Detection, Evaluation, and Treatment of High Blood Pressure (December 2003) recommends that an initial diastolic pressure

between 90 and 99 mm Hg be rechecked in 2 months even if the systolic pressure is less than 140 mm Hg; the higher the diastolic value, the greater the risk for complications due to hypertension. The blood pressure of the client in option 4 is considered normal.

> *Test Taking Strategy—Analyze to determine what information the question asks for, which is the client who needs a follow-up checkup in 2 months based on the assessed blood pressure measurement. The client in option 2 has Stage 1 hypertension, which requires reassessment within 2 months. Review recommendations for follow-up of blood pressure assessment established by the Joint National Committee for the Detection, Evaluation, and Treatment of High Blood Pressure if you had difficulty answering this question.*
> *Cognitive Level—Applying*
> *Client Needs Category—Health promotion and maintenance*
> *Client Needs Subcategory—None*

3. 2. The point at which the last sound is heard before a period of continuous silence (known as *Phase V of Korotkoff sounds*) is considered the best reflection of adult diastolic pressure. In some cases, two diastolic pressures are recorded: The pressure at which the loud knocking sound becomes muffled and the pressure when the last sound is heard.

> *Test Taking Strategy—Use the process of elimination to identify the option that best describes the sound at which the diastolic blood pressure measurement is identified. Option 1 can be eliminated because it describes the beginning of phase IV of Korotkoff sounds. Option 3 can be eliminated because it describes Phase II of Korotkoff sounds. Option 4 can be eliminated because it describes the beginning of Phase II Korotkoff sounds. Option 2 remains as the correct answer, because Phase V is identified as beginning when the last sound is heard. Review the phases of Korotkoff sounds, focusing on which sounds correspond to the systolic and diastolic blood pressure measurements, if you had difficulty answering this question.*
> *Cognitive Level—Applying*
> *Client Needs Category—Health promotion and maintenance*
> *Client Needs Subcategory—None*

4. 3. Sustained untreated hypertension tends to cause fibrous tissue formation in systemic arterioles. The fibrous tissue leads to decreased tissue perfusion, which is especially dangerous when it affects target organs, such as the heart, kidneys, and brain. Hypertension is not linked to a shortened life cycle of blood cells, venous clots, or stenosis of cardiac valves. The nurse should assess risk factors for hypertension at the time that the blood pressure is taken. Risk factors for hypertension include obesity, hypercholesterolemia, smoking, family predisposition, and ethnicity or race. In this case, African-American men are at greater risk for hypertension.

> *Test Taking Strategy—Apply the key words "most accurate" to the choices in the four options. Select the option that identifies the most correct reason for controlling hypertension. Recall that hypertension is the result of arterial constriction, which impairs blood flow to vital organs (option 3). Review the consequences of hypertension if you had difficulty answering this question.*
> *Cognitive Level—Applying*
> *Client Needs Category—Health promotion and maintenance*
> *Client Needs Subcategory—None*

5. **1, 5.** Hypertension is a serious disorder that is associated with stroke and heart disease. It may be classified as *primary* (without a known cause) or *secondary* (a known pathology). Some of the earliest signs and symptoms of hypertension include spontaneous nosebleeds, awakening with a headache, and blurred vision. Other symptoms include a persistent throbbing or pounding headache, dizziness, fatigue, and nervousness. Congestive heart failure, one of the complications of hypertension, can cause dyspnea when lying down, which may affect sleeping; insomnia, however, can have many causes. Nocturia and heart palpitations are not generally associated with hypertension. Usually clients with hypertension have flushed rather than pale skin.

> *Test Taking Strategy—Analyze to determine what information the question asks for, which is signs and symptoms of hypertension. Alternative-format "select all that apply" questions require considering each option independently to decide its merit in answering the question. Choose the options that best correlate to the signs and symptoms of hypertension. Review references that describe the clinical manifestations of hypertension if you had difficulty answering this question.*
> *Cognitive Level—Applying*
> *Client Needs Category—Physiological integrity*
> *Client Needs Subcategory—Physiological adaptation*

6. **3.** Myocardial hypertrophy (heart enlargement) is the direct consequence of the heart having to pump against increased peripheral vascular resistance due to hypertension. A strong S_1 heart sound is a healthy finding. A heart rate of 100 beats/minute is within normal limits, especially with activity. Hypertension is not usually associated with an irregular heart rhythm, which can have multiple causes.

> *Test Taking Strategy—Use the process of elimination to help select the option that describes a consequence of hypertension more accurately than other options. Recall that when the heart contracts against the resistance of narrowed arteries and arterioles, it requires more effort. Muscles increase in size when they are overworked. Consequently, option 3 is the*

best answer. Options 1 and 2 describe normal findings, and option 4 can have multiple causes. Review the consequences of hypertension, especially in relation to the heart, if you had difficulty answering this question.
> *Cognitive Level—Analyzing*
> *Client Needs Category—Physiological integrity*
> *Client Needs Subcategory—Physiological adaptation*

7. **1.** The Department of Health and Human Services recommends that adults should not consume more than 2,300 mg of sodium a day (1 tsp); the recommendations also say that African Americans, people with hypertension, and people who are middle-aged and older should not consume more than 1,500 mg of sodium a day, making their diets low in sodium. Limiting salt will also reduce fluid retention. Less circulating fluid in blood will decrease the volume the heart must pump and lower blood pressure. Soy sauce is high in sodium and, therefore, is restricted on a low-sodium diet. Lemon juice and onion powder (not onion salt) may be used liberally. Maple syrup is not restricted for its sodium content but may be limited if the client needs to monitor blood glucose levels or lose weight.

> *Test Taking Strategy—Use the process of elimination to identify the option that identifies the item that should be avoided by someone on a low-sodium diet. Options 2, 3, and 4 can be eliminated because they are not high in sodium. Recall that soy sauce is made from a salty broth of brewed or fermented grains of wheat and soy, which makes option 1 the correct answer. Review the sodium content of the items listed in the four options if you had difficulty answering this question.*
> *Cognitive level—Understanding*
> *Client Needs Category—Health promotion and maintenance*
> *Client Needs Subcategory—None*

8. **4, 5.** Smoking cessation is the single most therapeutic health change for anyone who has, or is at risk for, cardiopulmonary disease. Losing weight decreases the workload of the heart and therefore decreases blood pressure. Although increasing the intake of complex carbohydrates (such as fiber-containing oatmeal and other whole grains) has healthy benefits in lowering blood cholesterol, smoking cessation provides dramatic results in less time. Striking a healthy balance between rest and exercise and taking advantage of more leisure activities are beneficial, but any one of these cannot compare with the beneficial effects on arterioles achieved by smoking cessation and weight loss. Although it is important to document trends in blood pressure, taking the blood pressure more than once a day is excessive.

> *Test Taking Strategy—Analyze to determine what information the question asks for, which is lifestyle changes to reduce hypertension. Alternative-format "select all that apply" questions require considering each option independently to decide*

its merit in answering the question. Although some options may have merit, choices must be limited to the actions that are best for reducing blood pressure. Review techniques for lowering blood pressure if you had difficulty answering this question.
***Cognitive Level**—Applying*
***Client Needs Category**—Health promotion and maintenance*
***Client Needs Subcategory**—None*

9. 3. Furosemide (Lasix) is a loop diuretic often prescribed in conjunction with antihypertensives to lower blood pressure. It decreases excess fluid in the body. Therefore, an increase in urine output indicates that the drug is achieving its desired effect. Eliminating excessive water from the blood volume reduces the work of the heart. Furosemide (Lasix) may lower blood pressure due to the change in fluid volume, but stabilizing the blood pressure rather than lowering it does not offer the best evidence of the effectiveness of the medication. Pulse rate does not change appreciably when furosemide is given. Although decreasing anxiety can reduce vasoconstriction, it is not an effect that can be achieved with furosemide.

*   ***Test Taking Strategy**—Use the process of elimination to help select the option that identifies the best indication that furosemide is having a desired effect. Options 1 and 4 can be eliminated because these effects are not related to furosemide. Option 2 is not the primary purpose of furosemide therapy. Recall the relationship between excess circulating volume and increased blood pressure, which validates that increasing urine output (option 3) is the desired effect when administering furosemide. Review the evidence for evaluating how furosemide is producing a desired effect if you had difficulty answering this question.*
*   ***Cognitive Level**—Applying*
*   ***Client Needs Category**—Physiological integrity*
*   ***Client Needs Subcategory**—Pharmacological therapies*

10. 2. When given once daily, furosemide (Lasix) is generally administered in the early morning to avoid disturbing the client's sleep with the need to urinate. If the medication is ordered for twice a day, the first dose is usually given early in the morning at about 6 A.M., and the other dosage in the early afternoon at about 1 P.M.

*   ***Test Taking Strategy**—Analyze to determine what information the question asks for, which is a time of day to recommend for self-administering furosemide. Recall that the onset of diuresis occurs within 1 hour of taking the drug, with the peak effects occurring within 1 to 2 hours. Option 2 is the best answer because if the drug is taken on arising, urinary frequency would be more prevalent during the day and decrease over time as the drug is eliminated, resulting in a greater potential for uninterrupted sleep. Review recommended dosing schedules for clients who take diuretics if you had difficulty answering this question.*

***Cognitive Level**—Applying*
***Client Needs Category**—Physiological integrity*
***Client Needs Subcategory**—Pharmacological therapies*

11. 1. Furosemide (Lasix) typically depletes potassium levels; therefore, the client should eat foods that replace this electrolyte. One banana contains approximately 10 mEq of potassium. Other fruits that are rich sources of potassium include oranges and orange juice, cantaloupe, and nectarines. Although furosemide (Lasix) can also alter sodium levels, the unwanted effect causes potassium depletion. Unless dehydration occurs, the drug will not affect calcium and iron levels.

*   ***Test Taking Strategy**—Analyze to determine what information the question asks for, which is a mineral that the client should consume in relation to a side effect of furosemide. Recall that this drug inhibits the reabsorption of sodium in the loop of Henle. Chloride ions that usually pair with sodium ions combine with molecules of potassium that also pass into the urine, creating a potential for hypokalemia. Some physicians prescribe a potassium supplement to ensure that a deficit does not occur. Review potassium-depleting diuretics, focusing on the pharmacodynamics of furosemide, if you had difficulty answering this question.*
*   ***Cognitive Level**—Applying*
*   ***Client Needs Category**—Physiological integrity*
*   ***Client Needs Subcategory**—Pharmacological therapies*

12. 1. Diuretics are administered to prevent or treat fluid volume overload. They work by increasing the urine output; therefore, dehydration is a potential complication. The client should monitor urine output as a way of evaluating the effectiveness of the medication. A loop diuretic, such as furosemide (Lasix), increases sodium excretion, which can lead to hyponatremia, not hypernatremia. It is also a potassium-depleting drug, which can lead to low levels of potassium (hypokalemia). Many clients who take a loop diuretic replace the lost potassium by eating foods that contain appreciable amounts of this electrolyte or by taking potassium supplements.

*   ***Test Taking Strategy**—Analyze to determine what information the question asks for, which is a problem that can be identified by monitoring urine output. Note that the purpose of furosemide is to increase urination; if excessive, this could cause dehydration (option 1). Review the reasons dehydration can develop, focusing on untoward effects of diuretic drug therapy, if you had difficulty answering this question.*
*   ***Cognitive Level**—Applying*
*   ***Client Needs Category**—Physiological integrity*
*   ***Client Needs Subcategory**—Pharmacological therapies*

13. 2. A dry, hacky cough is a side effect of angiotensin-converting enzyme (ACE) inhibitors. The cough is attributed to the drug's increase in bradykinin, an inflammatory substance, which causes sensitization of sensory nerves in the airway and an enhancement of the cough reflex. If this occurs, the client should inform the health care provider because the medication may need to be changed. Switching to an angiotensin II receptor blocker (ARB) such as losartan (Cozaar) relieves the cough and lowers blood pressure. Angioedema (swelling of the face) also is a side effect of ACE inhibitors. Urinating more than normal is a therapeutic effect of a diuretic. Feeling weak and lethargic can be a symptom of many disease processes or anemia and is not characteristic of ACE inhibitors. Heart palpitations are not characteristic of potential side effects of ACE inhibitors.

Test Taking Strategy—Analyze to determine what information the question asks for, which is a side effect of ACE inhibitors. Although about 20% of individuals who take ACE inhibitors develop a dry hacky cough (option 2), it is considered more annoying than dangerous. Review the side effects of ACE inhibitors if you had difficulty answering this question.
Cognitive Level—Applying
Client Needs Category—Physiological integrity
Client Needs Subcategory—Pharmacological therapies

14. 1, 2, 5, 6. Caring for a client on multiple medications to treat hypertension requires that the nurse understand the side effects of antihypertensive medications. Because blood pressure is determined by cardiac output and peripheral vascular resistance, in general, first-line treatment of hypertension aims to eliminate fluid from the system, such as with a loop diuretic. Beta blockers are added as another treatment option. Nursing considerations include assisting the client to a standing position to prevent falls due to hypotension, assessing intake and output to document the therapeutic effect of fluid elimination, and monitoring blood glucose because hyperglycemia may be a side effect of diuretic therapy and beta blockers. Many antihypertensive medications such as beta blockers have the side effect of erectile dysfunction; therefore, sexual implications should be discussed. Maintaining the client on bed rest until the blood pressure stabilizes is inappropriate because this may take some time. Instruction on hypotension is important to maintain safety during early medication therapy. Working is typically not recommended as diversional therapy. Diversional therapy typically includes leisure activities such as reading a magazine, watching television, or exercising to relieve stress.

Test Taking Strategy—Analyze to determine what information the question asks for, which is nursing actions to take for a client receiving combination drug therapy for hypertension. Alternative-format "select all that apply" questions require considering each option independently to decide its merit in answering the question. Choose the options that best correlate with the nursing care of a client for whom a diuretic and a beta blocker have been prescribed to control hypertension. Review side effects of

antihypertensive drug therapy, focusing on the drug categories listed here, if you had difficulty answering this question.
Cognitive Level—Applying
Client Needs Category—Physiological integrity
Client Needs Subcategory—Pharmacological therapies

15. 1, 2, 3, 5. When a client has not reached a blood pressure goal, multiple drugs in various categories may be prescribed. In this case, the client is taking a multitude of medications to lower blood pressure. The combination of antihypertensive drugs has the potential for causing side effects such as dizziness, light-headedness, fatigue, hypotension, and dehydration. Lisinopril (Zestril), an angiotensin-converting enzyme (ACE) inhibitor, and valsartan (Diovan), an angiotensin II receptor blocker (ARB), promote vasodilation, which lowers blood pressure and could contribute to hypotension and dizziness. Metoprolol (Lopressor), a beta blocker, slows the heart rate, reducing cardiac output and circulating volume, which lowers blood pressure but may cause fatigue because it inhibits an increase in heart rate to compensate for activity. Hydrochlorothiazide (HydroDIURIL) is a loop diuretic that promotes the excretion of water by inhibiting the reabsorption of sodium in the nephrons, thus lowering blood pressure, but has the potential for causing dehydration. Neither warfarin (Coumadin), which is an anticoagulant, nor aspirin, an antiplatelet drug, is known to cause side effects like those described in the question.

Test Taking Strategy—Analyze to determine what information the question asks for, which is medications that could cause side effects of dizziness, light-headedness, low blood pressure, fatigue, and dehydration. Alternative-format "select all that apply" questions require considering each option independently to decide its merit in answering the question. Choose the options that correlate with drugs that cause the manifestations experienced by this client. Review the drugs listed, focusing on those whose effects could contribute to the client's presenting signs and symptoms, if you had difficulty answering this question.
Cognitive Level—Analyzing
Client Needs Category—Physiological integrity
Client Needs Subcategory—Pharmacological therapies

Nursing Care of Clients with Coronary Artery Disease

16. 4. Obesity, which is often linked with hyperlipidemia, is a risk factor for developing coronary artery disease (CAD). Drinking a nightly cocktail and undergoing surgery to repair the mitral valve are unrelated to development of CAD. Rheumatic fever is more likely to cause valvular disease than CAD.

Test Taking Strategy—Apply the key words "most signifi-cant" when evaluating the information in each of the options. Select the option that correlates most as a risk factor for developing CAD. Recall how obesity (option 4) is linked to atherosclerosis due to the accumulation of low-density lipoprotein (LDL) in the blood. Review various risk factors that predispose individuals to CAD if you had difficulty answering this question.
Cognitive Level—*Applying*
Client Needs Category—*Health promotion and maintenance*
Client Needs Subcategory—*None*

17. 2. A buildup of cholesterol in the blood vessels causes a condition known as *atherosclerosis*. As fat becomes deposited within the lining of arteries, the deposits enlarge to form plaque, which thickens the arterial walls and causes the blood vessels to narrow. Eventually the plaque is infiltrated with calcium, which causes the vessel to become hard and rigid. When a normal volume of blood is forced through these narrowed, inelastic vessels, the pressure within the vessels increases. The heart is prone to failure because it must work hard to pump against the vascular resistance. Cholesterol neither expands the circulating blood volume nor causes the heart to beat faster. Blood clots may form quicker due to the narrowing blood vessel. This narrowing can also cause stagnation of the blood.
Test Taking Strategy—Use the process of elimination to help select the option that identifies the best explanation for how cholesterol acts as a CAD risk factor. Recall that cholesterol is a saturated dietary animal fat that is transported in the blood by lipoproteins. Low-density lipoprotein (LDL) in particular enhances the deposition of cholesterol within the endothelium of arteries (option 2), causing atherosclerosis from an accumulation of fatty plaque. When the process involves the coronary arteries, it contributes to impaired circulation to heart muscle. Options 1, 3, and 4 can be eliminated because they provide incorrect explanations. Review the correlation of hypercholesterolemia and hyperlipidemia with CAD if you had difficulty answering this question.
Cognitive Level—*Applying*
Client Needs Category—*Physiological integrity*
Client Needs Subcategory—*Physiological adaptation*

18. 3. In keeping with a low-cholesterol diet, the healthiest change is to eat cereal rather than eggs for breakfast. Egg yolk is a rich source of cholesterol. There is not much, if any, appreciable change in cholesterol levels by substituting the foods listed in the other options. Whole-grain wheat toast, however, provides additional fiber, which is healthier than white bread.
Test Taking Strategy—Analyze to determine what information the question asks for, which is the healthiest substitution for a component that contains cholesterol in the client's diet. Recall that cereal (option 3),

preferably consumed with skim or reduced fat milk, would be better than consuming eggs. Review the sources of dietary cholesterol, focusing on those listed, if you had difficulty answering this question.
Cognitive Level—*Applying*
Client Needs Category—*Health promotion and maintenance*
Client Needs Subcategory—*None*

19. 1. Atorvastatin (Lipitor), one of many drugs that are referred to as *statins*, lowers low-density lipoprotein and total triglyceride levels and increases the amount of high-density lipoproteins. In doses large enough to lower blood fat components, this drug may cause back pain and muscle pain (myalgia). Although the link between statin drugs and myalgia as well as other muscle pathology continues to be speculative, some believe the side effect is due to a disruption in the lipid membrane layer of muscle cells caused by a depletion of cholesterol. The nurse must assess for muscle pain, tenderness, or weakness along with monitoring the client's cholesterol levels. Palpitations, visual changes, and weight loss are not known side effects of this drug.
Test Taking Strategy—Use the process of elimination to help select the option that identifies the best evidence that the client knows a potential adverse effect of atorvastatin. By identifying muscle pain (option 1), the client demonstrates knowledge of an adverse effect associated with statin therapy. Because the side effects identified in options 2, 3, and 4 are unrelated to statin drugs, these options can be eliminated. Review the side and adverse effects of statin medications, focusing on myopathy, myalgia, and rhabdomyolysis, if you had difficulty answering this question.
Cognitive Level—*Applying*
Client Needs Category—*Physiological integrity*
Client Needs Subcategory—*Pharmacological therapies*

20. 1. A stress electrocardiogram (ECG) demonstrates the extent to which the heart tolerates and responds to the additional demands placed on it during exercise. The ability of the heart to continue adapting is related to the adequacy of blood supplied to the myocardium through the coronary arteries. If the client develops chest pain, dangerous cardiac rhythm changes, or significantly elevated blood pressure, the diagnostic testing is stopped. Although the test may indicate that further exercise is needed, this is not the primary purpose of testing. An ECG does not predict the occurrence of a heart attack or determine the target heart rate.
Test Taking Strategy—Analyze to determine what information the question asks for, which is the purpose of a stress ECG. Recall that the difference between a resting ECG and a stress ECG is that the latter shows how exercise affects the heart's rate and rhythm (option 1). Review how a stress ECG is performed and its diagnostic advantages if you had difficulty answering this question.

Cognitive Level—*Applying*
Client Needs Category—*Physiological integrity*
Client Needs Subcategory—*Physiological adaptation*

21. 2. Angina, or chest pain, is caused by an inadequate supply of oxygenated blood to the myocardium due to narrowed coronary arteries. Rest generally relieves angina. Once the myocardium's demand for additional oxygen is reduced through inactivity or rest, the chest pain is relieved. Taking a deep breath and applying heat to the chest or rubbing the chest will not alleviate the pain of angina pectoris. One main difference between stable angina pectoris and a myocardial infarction is that rest relieves the chest pain associated with stable angina.

> *Test Taking Strategy*—*Use the process of elimination to help select the option that identifies the best nonpharmacological measure that typically relieves chest pain associated with angina pectoris. Options 1, 3, and 4 can be eliminated because they are not methods that will subsequently improve oxygenating cardiac muscle. Option 2 is the best answer because rest reduces the heart muscle's demand for oxygen. Once cardiac muscle has a sufficient amount of oxygen in relation to the work it must perform, chest pain is reduced or relieved. Review the pathophysiology of angina pectoris and methods used to manage its characteristic symptom if you had difficulty answering this question.*

Cognitive Level—*Applying*
Client Needs Category—*Physiological integrity*
Client Needs Subcategory—*Physiological adaptation*

22. 3. Nitroglycerin is a vasodilator. It dilates both veins and arteries. Some believe the best explanation for how nitroglycerin relieves chest pain is that peripheral vasodilation results in decreased venous return to the heart and vascular resistance to ventricular ejection, reducing the work of the heart and its need for oxygen. The sublingual form of nitroglycerin is one of the common routes for administering nitroglycerin on an as-needed basis. When administered, a tablet is placed under the tongue. The drug is then quickly absorbed through the rich supply of blood vessels beneath the tongue. Clients who take sublingual nitroglycerin for angina are instructed not to chew or swallow the tablets and not eat, drink, smoke, or chew tobacco until the tablet dissolves. Tablets for buccal administration are placed between the gum and cheek. A tablet intended for swallowing is placed on the tongue at the back of the throat. A chewable tablet is placed between the teeth.

> *Test Taking Strategy*—*Analyze to determine what information the question asks for, which is the location where nitroglycerin tablets should be placed when the client experiences chest pain. Recall that the tablet form of this drug is placed sublingually, meaning under the tongue (option 3). Review the various forms of nitroglycerin that are available and how they are administered, focusing on the sublingual route, if you had difficulty answering this question.*

Cognitive Level—*Applying*
Client Needs Category—*Physiological integrity*
Client Needs Subcategory—*Pharmacological therapies*

23. 1, 5. Side effects of nitroglycerin include headache, flushing, hypotension and dizziness. These effects are the direct result of vasodilation. The other choices are not associated with nitroglycerin.

> *Test Taking Strategy*—*Analyze to determine what information the question asks for, which is side effects of nitroglycerin. Alternative-format "select all that apply" questions require considering each option independently to decide its merit in answering the question. Choose the options that correlate with potential side effects of nitroglycerin. Review untoward responses to this drug if you had difficulty answering this question.*

Cognitive Level—*Applying*
Client Needs Category—*Physiological integrity*
Client Needs Subcategory—*Pharmacological therapies*

24. 3. The client should experience a fizzing or tingling in the mouth if nitroglycerin tablets are still fresh. Another possibility of lost tablet potency is a failure to experience relief of chest pain similar to that experienced when the prescription was originally filled. If potent, chest pain should be reduced or relieved in 1 to 5 minutes after administering a tablet. To ensure that tablets remain potent, they should be stored in a cool location, tightly capped to avoid moisture, and replaced every 3 months. They do not discolor or disintegrate when they have lost their potency. Old aspirin tablets, not nitroglycerin tablets, tend to smell like vinegar.

> *Test Taking Strategy*—*Analyze to determine what information the question asks for, which is the best evidence that the client understands that the supply of nitroglycerin tablets needs to be replaced. The ability to experience a burning or tingling sensation (option 3) is not a totally reliable method for assessing tablet potency, but it is the best choice from the list of options. Review the recommended frequency for replacing nitroglycerin tablets if you had difficulty answering this question.*

Cognitive Level—*Applying*
Client Needs Category—*Physiological integrity*
Client Needs Subcategory—*Pharmacological therapies*

25. 1. The dose of nitroglycerin may be repeated in 5 minutes, for a total of three doses. However, the client is told to call the physician if the pain is unrelieved after three successive doses because other treatment may be necessary. A client having chest pain should never drive to the hospital alone. Sublingual tablets are never swallowed.

> *Test Taking Strategy*—*Analyze to determine what information the question asks for, which is an action the client should take if chest pain is not relieved shortly after taking one nitroglycerin tablet. Recall that a sublingual tablet may be readministered at 5-minute*

intervals (option 1) after the first dose for a total of three tablets. If chest pain continues to be unresolved after three doses, the client or a support person should call 911 and request ambulance transport to an emergency department to rule out the possibility of a myocardial infarction. Review the dosing recommendations for sublingual nitroglycerin tablets if you had difficulty answering this question.
Cognitive Level—Applying
Client Needs Category—Physiological integrity
Client Needs Subcategory—Pharmacological therapies

26. 1. When topical nitroglycerin ointment or transdermal patches are used, application sites are rotated and the medication may be placed on the chest, back, upper abdomen, or arms. The drug reservoir should not be touched, squeezed, or manipulated in any way. The patch is self-adhering when the adhesive backing is removed. Ointment application papers are covered with plastic wrap and taped in place to prevent soiling and promote drug absorption. It is not necessary to clean the skin with alcohol before applying. Clipping the chest hair may be necessary, especially if the client is particularly hairy. After removing the old patch or paper, the old ointment should be removed with a dry cloth. It is not standard practice to take the client's blood pressure after application unless the client becomes symptomatic.
Test Taking Strategy—Apply the key words "most appropriate" to the four options. Look for the choice that is best at identifying a nursing action when applying a transdermal nitroglycerin patch. Remember that more than one option may have some merit, but the best answer must be selected. To avoid skin irritation, the standard of care is to rotate the application site (option 1) when applying a fresh patch. Review information on applying a transdermal nitroglycerin patch if you had difficulty answering this question.
Cognitive Level—Applying
Client Needs Category—Physiological integrity
Client Needs Subcategory—Pharmacological therapies

27. 4. Nitroglycerin dilates arterial vessels, especially the coronary vessels. This action lowers the blood pressure. Therefore, if the client's blood pressure is already low (as with a pressure of 94/62 mm Hg), the nurse should check with the physician before applying the patch. It is not unusual for a client with a myocardial infarction (MI) to have a slightly elevated temperature. This is probably due to the inflammatory response from the injury to the myocardium. A respiratory rate of 24 breaths/minute and an apical heart rate of 90 beats/minute are within normal limits.
Test Taking Strategy—Analyze to determine what information the question asks for, which is an assessment finding that could be potentiated by applying a nitroglycerin patch. Recall that a side effect of nitroglycerin is hypotension due to the dilation of blood vessels. If the client is currently hypotensive (option 4), the hypotension could be compounded

by applying a nitroglycerin patch. Review the effect nitroglycerin has on vital signs if you had difficulty answering this question.
Cognitive Level—Applying
Client Needs Category—Physiological integrity
Client Needs Subcategory—Pharmacological therapies

28. 3. Cooking spray adds no calories or fat to the food that is being cooked. Cutting calories will help weight loss and lessen the progression of coronary artery disease (CAD). Corn oil is an example of a polyunsaturated fat and is a good second choice. Using unsaturated fats helps lower blood cholesterol. In limited amounts, it is healthier to consume polyunsaturated fats made from vegetable products than saturated fats, such as butter, from animal sources, or hydrogenated fats, such as solid vegetable shortenings and hard margarines even in a melted form.
Test Taking Strategy—Use the process of elimination to help select the option that identifies the item that demonstrates the best evidence of client compliance with dietary measures for limiting the progression of CAD. Options 1 and 2 can be eliminated immediately because even in a liquid form, butter and margarine are examples of saturated fats that contribute to CAD. Option 4 has some merit because it is derived from a vegetable source and is classified as unsaturated fat when in a liquid form. However, option 3 is the best answer because there are zero grams of fat in a serving size, which is the equivalent of a ⅓ second spray. Review the differences between saturated and unsaturated fats and their relationship to CAD if you had difficulty answering this question.
Cognitive Level—Applying
Client Needs Category—Health promotion and maintenance
Client Needs Subcategory—None

29. 258 calories.
Protein and carbohydrates both have 4 cal/g; fat contains 9 cal/g. Thus, the total calorie count for a pie containing 2 g of protein, 14 g of fat, and 31 g of carbohydrate is 258 calories.
Test Taking Strategy—Analyze to determine what information the question asks for, which is a calculation of the total calories based on equivalents for protein, fat, and carbohydrate identified in the rationale. Check your mathematical calculation for errors if you had difficulty answering this question.
Cognitive Level—Applying
Client Needs Category—Health promotion and maintenance
Client Needs Subcategory—None

30. 2. A cardiac catheterization is a test in which a catheter is placed into the heart (usually through a vessel in the groin) to evaluate the anatomy and function of the heart and its blood vessels. Dye is injected through the catheter and images are taken as the dye fills the coronary arteries. Most clients are concerned about the test and more importantly, what the findings will be. When a client is worried and fearful, the nurse should encourage an expression of feelings and then listen attentively. Most clients feel alone, overwhelmed, and helpless during a crisis; being able to verbalize fears and concerns can help ease their emotional burden. Listening is an active process, even if the nurse does not make many verbal contributions. Teaching the client about the treatment of coronary artery disease (CAD) is inappropriate because learning is impaired during times of mild to severe anxiety. How others have responded to a diagnostic test or procedure disregards the uniqueness of the client's situation. Avoiding the subject communicates that the nurse does not care.

> *Test Taking Strategy—Use the process of elimination to help select the option that identifies the best method for reducing the client's anxiety. Options 1, 3, and 4 can be eliminated because they are examples of nontherapeutic communication as described in the rationale. Option 2 remains as the correct answer because providing an opportunity for an anxious client to verbalize feelings is always a therapeutic nursing action. Review communication techniques that help to relieve a client's fears and anxiety if you had difficulty answering this question.*
> **Cognitive Level**—*Applying*
> **Client Needs Category**—*Psychosocial integrity*
> **Client Needs Subcategory**—*None*

31. 4. The contrast dye used during the coronary arteriogram causes vasodilation and is experienced as a brief flush or warmth that spreads over the skin surface. Some clients feel fluttering or what is described as "butterflies" as the catheter is passed into the heart, disturbing its rhythm. Heaviness or chest pain, if experienced, is generally treated with nitroglycerin. The client receives sedation but is not anesthetized before the diagnostic testing.

> *Test Taking Strategy—Analyze to determine what information the question asks for, which is evidence that the client understands the nurse's teaching about what will happen during the cardiac catheterization. Recall that when the contrast dye is injected, it causes a warm sensation (option 4) throughout the body like a "hot flash" that lasts approximately 10 to 20 seconds. Review the method for performing a cardiac catheterization and preparation for a client who will undergo this test if you had difficulty answering this question.*
> **Cognitive Level**—*Applying*
> **Client Needs Category**—*Physiological integrity*
> **Client Needs Subcategory**—*Pharmacological therapies*

32. 3. People who are allergic to shellfish may also be sensitive to iodine. The radiopaque dye used during the arteriogram is iodine based. The physician must be notified if the client indicates a history of allergies to either substance. At this point, the physician will determine whether to cancel the procedure or prepare to administer an antihistamine or other emergency drugs. Morphine and penicillin are not associated with allergic reactions caused by the dye. Allergy to eggs is related to certain types of vaccines given as immunizations.

> *Test Taking Strategy—Use the process of elimination to identify the allergen that is most essential to determine before a cardiac catheterization. Options 1, 2, and 4 can be eliminated because these substances are not used during the procedure. Option 3 remains as the best answer because shellfish are a source of iodine. A client who is allergic to iodine or shellfish may also be hypersensitive to the iodine-based contrast medium. Review the correlation between shellfish, iodine, and contrast dye if you had difficulty answering this question.*
> **Cognitive Level**—*Applying*
> **Client Needs Category**—*Physiological integrity*
> **Client Needs Subcategory**—*Reduction of risk potential*

33. 1. If the femoral artery was the site used for inserting the heart catheter, the nurse must position the client so that the catheterized leg is extended (not bent) to prevent flexing the hip for 6 to 8 hours after the procedure. Flexing the hip may lead to bleeding and clot formation. Abduction and adduction have no bearing on the affected leg. Sandbags may be placed over the pressure dressing to decrease discomfort and control bleeding.

> *Test Taking Strategy—Analyze to determine what information the question asks for, which is the leg position required after a client undergoes a cardiac catheterization. Recall that circulating blood flow has been affected by placement of the catheter in the femoral artery, which is located in the groin. The leg must be placed in an extended position that facilitates blood flow (option 1) and does not contribute to clot formation. Review the potential complications that can occur at the site of cannulation and how the nurse can reduce or eliminate their development if you had difficulty answering this question.*
> **Cognitive Level**—*Applying*
> **Client Needs Category**—*Physiological integrity*
> **Client Needs Subcategory**—*Reduction of risk potential*

34. 1. Peripheral pulses distal to the catheter insertion site are assessed frequently after arteriography. This is performed because the injury to the artery and subsequent bleeding can lead to clot formation. A thrombus could totally occlude the flow of oxygenated blood through the vessel, resulting in the absence of a distal pulse—a medical emergency that must be reported immediately. After checking the client's pulses, the nurse inspects the skin integrity in the groin because bleeding, hemorrhage, or hematoma formation may occur. Assessing the heart, lungs, and abdomen should be done regardless of whether the arteriogram is performed.

Test Taking Strategy—Analyze to determine what information the question asks for, which is the nursing care of the client after cardiac catheterization. Recall that because the femoral artery in the groin was used as the site for inserting the catheter, assessing the distal pulses (option 1) provides the best indication that arterial circulation is being maintained or impaired. Review the nursing care of a client who has undergone a cardiac catheterization if you had difficulty answering this question.
Cognitive Level—*Applying*
Client Needs Category—*Physiological integrity*
Client Needs Subcategory—*Reduction of risk potential*

35. **1, 3, 4, 6.** After cardiac catheterization, a shower is preferred because it reduces the risk of infection at the puncture site. Consuming fluid promotes the excretion of dye that was instilled intravenously during the procedure. An increase in leg pain may indicate formation of an arterial thrombus and arterial occlusion, which requires immediate intervention. The puncture site should be covered with a dressing until it heals. The client should rest for 3 days and avoid strenuous activity; therefore, leg exercises are contraindicated. There is no need to flush urine or stool twice because excreted waste products contain no toxic or biological hazardous substances.

Test Taking Strategy—Analyze to determine what information the question asks for, which is discharge instructions after cardiac catheterization. Alternative-format "select all that apply" questions require considering each option independently to decide its merit in answering the question. Choose the options that correlate with discharge instructions that are pertinent to the client's self-care after cardiac catheterization. Review references that describe actions the client who has undergone a cardiac catheterization must perform after his or her discharge if you had difficulty answering this question.
Cognitive Level—*Applying*
Client Needs Category—*Physiological integrity*
Client Needs Subcategory—*Reduction of risk potential*

36. **1.** Percutaneous transluminal coronary angioplasty (PTCA) involves dilating narrowed or occluded coronary arteries with a double-lumen balloon catheter. The pressure from the inflated balloon compresses the fatty plaque that has narrowed the artery. Leg veins are used in coronary artery bypass grafting (CABG) surgery to bypass narrowed coronary arteries. A pacemaker is used when it is difficult to maintain a normal heart rate or rhythm with drug therapy. Grafting skeletal muscle, not Teflon, over scarred areas of the myocardium is now in experimental stages.

Test Taking Strategy—Analyze to determine what information the question asks for, which is a statement that provides evidence that the client understands

the PTCA procedure explained by the physician. Recall that a PTCA procedure involves the insertion of a balloon-tipped catheter into the coronary artery for the purpose of widening its lumen. Review the description of a PTCA and its purpose if you had difficulty answering this question.
Cognitive Level—*Applying*
Client Needs Category—*Physiological integrity*
Client Needs Subcategory—*Physiological adaptation*

37. **2.** Propranolol (Inderal) is a beta-adrenergic blocker (beta blocker). It blocks the sympathetic receptors for epinephrine. Epinephrine speeds the heart rate, which requires a great deal of oxygen. By blocking the effect of epinephrine, the heart rate is slowed and the myocardium does not need as much oxygen. In addition, at a slower rate, the heart fills with a greater volume of blood. Thus, each time the heart contracts, it delivers a substantial amount of blood to the coronary arteries. As long as the coronary arteries deliver an adequate amount of oxygenated blood to the myocardium, chest pain is prevented. Propranolol (Inderal) does not dilate major coronary arteries, nor does it help with the excretion of urine. Pain receptors are not altered by the use of this drug.

Test Taking Strategy—Use the process of elimination to help select the option that identifies the best explanation for the manner in which propranolol (Inderal) prevents angina. Recall that propranolol is a nonspecific beta-adrenergic antagonist that blocks beta receptors from responding to stimulation from the sympathetic nervous system. In doing so, propranolol reduces heart rate (option 2) and the force of heart muscle contraction, thereby reducing the heart's need for oxygen. Review propranolol's mechanism of action and the reasons for which it is prescribed if you had difficulty answering this question.
Cognitive Level—*Applying*
Client Needs Category—*Physiological integrity*
Client Needs Subcategory—*Pharmacological therapies*

38. **4.** Beta-adrenergic blockers such as propranolol (Inderal) interfere with the action of epinephrine. They reduce heart rate. Therefore, the pulse rate tends to be slower than in the nonmedicated period. Some clients develop bradycardia while taking the drug. Propranolol does not produce a stronger heartbeat or irregular heart rhythms.

Test Taking Strategy—Analyze to determine what information the question asks for, which is the effect of propranolol on the pulse. Recall that blocking beta$_1$ receptors in the heart slows the heart rate (option 4). Review how the sympathetic nervous system affects heart rate, and from that deduce the effect that would occur if the effect is blocked if you had difficulty answering this question.
Cognitive Level—*Applying*
Client Needs Category—*Physiological integrity*
Client Needs Subcategory—*Pharmacological therapies*

39. 2. Aspirin is recommended in low daily doses to reduce the potential for forming a blood clot, which could occlude the narrowed opening in a diseased coronary artery. It interferes with platelet aggregation or clumping and, therefore, acts as a prophylactic antithrombotic agent. Aspirin is more useful in relieving headaches and musculoskeletal pain than chest pain. Aspirin will not lower the blood pressure or cause vasodilation of the coronary arteries.

Test Taking Strategy—Use the process of elimination to help select the option that identifies the best explanation for taking low-dose aspirin before a percutaneous transluminal coronary angioplasty (PTCA) procedure. Options 1, 3, and 4 can be eliminated because aspirin does not relieve chest pain, lower blood pressure, or dilate coronary arteries. Option 2 remains as the best answer because aspirin has an antiplatelet action that reduces the potential for developing a thrombus in one or more coronary arteries. Review the actions for which aspirin may be prescribed, focusing on a reason that correlates with its use in a client with compromised coronary artery circulation, if you had difficulty answering this question.

Cognitive Level—Applying
Client Needs Category—Physiological integrity
Client Needs Subcategory—Pharmacological therapies

40. 4. Despite dilating one or more coronary arteries with a balloon-tipped catheter, it is possible for clients to experience chest pain after percutaneous transluminal coronary angioplasty (PTCA). Chest pain after PTCA should never be ignored or dismissed as being inconsequential. It can occur for a variety of reasons: sudden collapse of a previously dilated coronary artery, thrombus formation within a coronary artery, or a change in the diameter of an arterial lumen due to the presence of a stent, for example. Whatever the reason, chest pain should be reported immediately to the physician because it may indicate a life-threatening complication. If a thrombus in a coronary artery is untreated, a myocardial infarction (MI) could occur. An hourly urine output of 30 to 50 mL or more is considered adequate. A blood pressure of 108/68 mm Hg is within the low ranges of normal. A dry mouth is a consequence of fluid restriction and medication administered before the procedure. As long as the blood pressure continues to remain within normal ranges, the nurse relieves the discomfort of a dry mouth by giving oral care and administering oral fluids.

Test Taking Strategy—Analyze to determine what information the question asks for, which is an assessment finding after a PTCA procedure that should be reported immediately. Recall that chest pain (option 4) suggests myocardial ischemia; if unrelieved, it may result in damage to the heart muscle. Review potential complications after PTCA and indications of their development if you had difficulty answering this question.

Cognitive Level—Applying
Client Needs Category—Physiological integrity
Client Needs Subcategory—Reduction of risk potential

41. 1. Coronary artery bypass graft (CABG) surgery is performed when more than one blood vessel is partially or totally occluded. During CABG surgery, a healthy vein or artery is grafted to the diseased coronary artery to bypass the narrowed area, creating a new passageway for oxygen-rich blood to the heart muscle. The saphenous vein, which is located in the leg, is commonly harvested for grafting. The nurse should assess pulses and the incisional site in the affected leg immediately after surgery. The internal mammary artery, located in the chest, is another vessel sometimes used for CABG surgery. The other vessels mentioned are not typically used for this type of surgery.

Test Taking Strategy—Use the process of elimination to select the option that identifies the blood vessel most commonly used for a CABG. Option 4 can be eliminated immediately, because the iliac artery is a division of the abdominal aorta and is located in the pelvic area. Option 3 can be eliminated, because the popliteal vein is located in the posterior of the leg, making it difficult to surgically access during CABG surgery. Option 2 can be eliminated, because the femoral arteries are large blood vessels that are essential for delivering oxygenated blood to the lower extremities. Option 1 remains as the correct answer, because the saphenous vein is the longest human vein. It lies close to the surface within the lower extremity, making it more accessible for harvest. Review the blood vessels that are used when performing CABG surgery if you had difficulty answering this question.

Cognitive Level—Applying
Client Needs Category—Physiological integrity
Client Needs Subcategory—Physiological adaptation

42. 1. Using the thumb to obtain a pulse rate can yield inaccurate data because the health care worker's pulse may be felt rather than the client's. It is best to rest or support the client's arm and compress the artery against the bone using the fingertips. Counting the pulse for 1 full minute seems prudent immediately after major cardiovascular surgery.

Test Taking Strategy—Analyze to determine what information the question asks for, which is an incorrect technique that is being used by a nursing assistant when assessing a client's pulse. Recall that the radial pulse is assessed by lightly pressing the first and second fingertips against the radius. An inaccurate assessment may result if the thumb (option 1) is used because the nursing assistant may be confused by feeling her or his pulse. Review the correct technique for pulse assessment if you had difficulty answering this question.

Cognitive Level—Applying
Client Needs Category—Safe and effective care environment
Client Needs Subcategory—Coordinated care

43. 2. A client in acute pain is most likely to have a rapid pulse rate, rapid respiratory rate, and rising blood pressure. Pain is least likely to influence body temperature.

Test Taking Strategy—*Analyze to determine what information the question asks for, which is the effect pain has on vital signs. Recall that pain increases the heart rate (option 2), perhaps because it causes anxiety and sympathetic nervous system stimulation. Review factors that affect vital signs, focusing on the effect pain has on the pulse rate if you had difficulty answering this question.*
Cognitive Level—*Applying*
Client Needs Category—*Physiological integrity*
Client Needs Subcategory—*Physiological adaptation*

44. 1. With a patient-controlled analgesia (PCA) pump, the client presses a control button to release a very low dose of an opioid when feeling the need for medication. The dose is low enough to allow for frequent administration. Usually, this results in the client using less total medication because the discomfort rarely falls below a tolerable level. It is best to use the PCA pump before pain becomes severe. PCA pumps are used for only a few days postoperatively, making addiction unlikely. Because the client can use the machine independently, it frees the nurse to tend to other responsibilities.

Test Taking Strategy—*Use the process of elimination to help select the option that identifies the most important instruction for the client who will be using a PCA pump. Recall that one of the advantages of using a PCA pump is that the client can self-administer an analgesic medication intravenously when it is needed (option 1) without waiting for the nurse to respond. Review the purpose for providing a client with a PCA pump and nursing instructions that relate to its use if you had difficulty answering this question.*
Cognitive Level—*Applying*
Client Needs Category—*Physiological integrity*
Client Needs Subcategory—*Pharmacological therapies*

45. 3. The number of doses the client administered during the current shift is the most important information to communicate to the nurses on the next shift. This serves as a measure of how much pain the client is experiencing. The name of the client's physician is readily available on multiple records. The only reason to use a patient-controlled analgesia (PCA) pump is to relieve pain. The PCA pump allows the client to control the drug dosage, promoting a sense of independence and control over pain. If the client demonstrates a lack of understanding about the pump's function, this should be communicated to the next shift as well; however, it is not the most important information to convey.

Test Taking Strategy—*Apply the key words "most important" when evaluating which information is most significant to report. Recall that reporting the number of doses a client has self-administered*

(option 3) provides nurses on the next shift with data about the client's need for pain relief. Review information that is pertinent to a client's use of a PCA pump if you had difficulty answering this question.
Cognitive Level—*Applying*
Client Needs Category—*Safe and effective care environment*
Client Needs Subcategory—*Coordinated care*

46. 2. The saphenous vein is the most common blood vessel used for coronary artery bypass graft (CABG) surgery. Removing a portion of this leg vein can temporarily impair the return of venous blood to the heart. Impaired venous return is manifested by cool skin and edema in the toes, foot, or ankle of the operative leg. Therefore, the fact that the toes are warm and nonedematous is the best evidence that venous blood is adequately returning to the heart through other blood vessels in the leg. The ability to move the leg indicates that neurologic function is intact. A regular heart rate and absence of chest pain are evidence that the newly attached graft is supplying the heart muscle with adequate oxygenated blood.

Test Taking Strategy—*Use the process of elimination to help select the option that identifies the best evidence that circulation in the extremity from which the graft was taken is adequate. Recall that harvesting a section of the saphenous vein may temporarily impair venous circulation in the leg. Noting that the client's toes are warm and there is no evidence of edema (option 2) suggests that venous circulation is adequate. Review signs of adequate and disturbed venous circulation in a lower extremity if you had difficulty answering this question.*
Cognitive Level—*Evaluating*
Client Needs Category—*Physiological integrity*
Client Needs Subcategory—*Reduction of risk potential*

Nursing Care of Clients with Myocardial Infarction

47. 1. Another name for a heart attack is a *myocardial infarction* (MI) or *acute myocardial infarction* (AMI). An MI is the interruption of blood supply to the myocardium, causing heart cells to die. The cellular death is most commonly due to the occlusion of one or more of the coronary arteries. The chest pain accompanying an MI is usually so severe that the client becomes extremely diaphoretic. Hypotension is apt to make the client's skin appear pale or ashen, not flushed. Headache is more closely associated with stroke. Coughing is not characteristic.

Test Taking Strategy—*Analyze to determine what information the question asks for, which is assessment findings for a client suffering from an MI. Recall the signs and symptoms of an MI if you had difficulty answering this question.*

Cognitive Level—Applying
Client Needs Category—Physiological integrity
Client Needs Subcategory—Physiological adaptation

48. 4. When a client has a myocardial infarction (MI), the ST segment in the electrocardiogram (ECG) becomes elevated. This finding may be accompanied by T-wave inversion and occasionally a definite Q wave. Aside from these findings, other diagnostic findings include elevated levels of CK-MB, a cardiospecific enzyme, and elevated cardiac markers of myoglobin and troponin.

> *Test Taking Strategy—Analyze to determine what information the question asks for, which is ECG changes associated with an MI. Recall that the ST segment is normally isoelectric, but becomes elevated (option 4) when the myocardium is injured during an MI. Review normal ECG waveforms and changes that correlate with an MI if you had difficulty answering this question.*
> *Cognitive Level—Remembering*
> *Client Needs Category—Physiological integrity*
> *Client Needs Subcategory—Physiological adaptation*

49. 4. The most pertinent data to assess concerning a client's chest pain are its onset, quality, intensity, location, and duration and what makes the pain better or worse. In this case, chest pain is rarely relieved by medications used over the counter for other types of pain.

> *Test Taking Strategy—Look at the key words, "least helpful" and apply them to the statements in each of the four options. Select the option that requests health information that is irrelevant to the current situation. Consider that the questions in options 1, 2, and 3 are more important than asking the client to name pain medications (option 4) that are normally taken. Review assessment information that will be beneficial to the physician when diagnosing the problem if you had difficulty answering this question.*
> *Cognitive Level—Applying*
> *Client Needs Category—Health promotion and maintenance*
> *Client Needs Subcategory—None*

50. 4. A client experiencing a myocardial infarction (MI) is most likely to describe the pain as being substernal or radiating to the shoulder, arm, teeth, jaw, or throat. Other signs and symptoms of an MI include tachycardia, increased blood pressure, arrhythmias, cold and mottled skin, tachypnea, dyspnea, anxiety, elevated temperature, increased white blood cell count, and a rise in cardiac enzymes. Women may experience similar symptoms but may also have breast pain, pain in the upper back between the scapulae, and extreme fatigue. Older adults and diabetic clients may also present with atypical signs and symptoms.

> *Test Taking Strategy—Apply the key words "most likely" when considering the locations in the body where radiating pain associated with an MI may*

occur. Recall that only one answer is correct. The area of radiating pain that is commonly identified is the shoulder (option 4) and arm, although other locations are named in the rationale as well. Review the characteristics of pain experienced by clients having an MI if you had difficulty answering this question.
> *Cognitive Level—Applying*
> *Client Needs Category—Physiological integrity*
> *Client Needs Subcategory—Physiological adaptation*

51. 4. Unlike angina pectoris, in which the pain is relieved in a relatively short time, the pain caused by an acute myocardial infarction (MI) is continuous and is unrelieved by rest, sublingual nitroglycerin, or other oral nitrate drugs. Many clients describe the pain associated with an MI as "squeezing," "suffocating," or "crushing." The pain comes on suddenly and usually is not tingling in nature.

> *Test Taking Strategy—Apply the key words "most characteristic" when analyzing the four options. Select the option that typically applies to the pattern of pain experienced by a client having an MI. Recall that a distinguishing characteristic is that the discomfort tends to be continuous (option 4) and unrelieved. Review the pain manifestations associated with an MI if you had difficulty answering this question.*
> *Cognitive Level—Applying*
> *Client Needs Category—Physiological integrity*
> *Client Needs Subcategory—Physiological adaptation*

52. 4. An opioid analgesic, such as morphine sulfate, is usually required to relieve the severe pain associated with a myocardial infarction (MI). Because the pain is so severe and triggers fear of dying, the heart is tachycardic. Tachycardia increases the oxygen demands and places extra stress on dying tissue. Morphine sulfate decreases pain and relieves anxiety, thus slowing the heart rate. Nonsteroidal, nonsalicylate, and salicylate analgesics are generally prescribed for minor pain that is not cardiac in origin.

> *Test Taking Strategy—Apply the key words "most helpful" when looking for a pain medication in the four options that will relieve the pain experienced by a client having an MI. Recall that morphine sulfate is a drug that is used to relieve acute pain, whereas the drugs in the other options relieve pain of a lesser intensity. Review the type of pain for which morphine sulfate is prescribed if you had difficulty answering this question.*
> *Cognitive Level—Applying*
> *Client Needs Category—Physiological integrity*
> *Client Needs Subcategory—Pharmacological therapies*

53. 3. Denial is a coping mechanism used to control anxiety and fear. Denial diverts awareness of reality. The client refuses to believe that an event, such as a heart attack, is really happening. Regression occurs when a client resorts to a pattern of behavior characteristic of an earlier age. Projection involves blaming a negative situation on someone or something else. Undoing often takes on the form of offering a verbal apology or gift to make up for unacceptable behavior.

> *Test Taking Strategy—Analyze to determine what information the question asks for, which is a coping mechanism that is characterized by believing that the experienced symptoms are due to a condition that is less serious than a life-threatening myocardial infarction. Recall that denial (option 3) is a coping mechanism that protects the psyche by dismissing the potential reality that is occurring. Review common coping mechanisms, focusing on a description of denial, if you had difficulty answering this question.*
> **Cognitive Level**—*Applying*
> **Client Needs Category**—*Psychosocial integrity*
> **Client Needs Subcategory**—*None*

54. 4. Of the factors listed in this question, having an occasional alcoholic beverage is least likely to predispose a client to a myocardial infarction (MI). One drink of alcohol per day may increase the client's so-called good cholesterol (high-density lipoprotein) and will elevate triglyceride levels; however, the relationship of elevated triglyceride levels to heart disease has not been conclusively established. Smoking, working under stress, and eating a diet high in fat and "bad" cholesterol (low-density lipoprotein) are definite risk factors in developing an MI.

> *Test Taking Strategy—Apply the key words "least likely" when analyzing the choices in the four options. Note that when the phrase "least likely" is used, it means that three options are correct. Choose the option that presents the lowest risk for experiencing an MI. Recall that an occasional alcoholic cocktail (option 4) does not increase a person's risk for an MI, whereas the other three options represent high-risk factors. Review the risk factors that predispose to developing an MI if you had difficulty answering this question.*
> **Cognitive Level**—*Applying*
> **Client Needs Category**—*Health promotion and maintenance*
> **Client Needs Subcategory**—*None*

55. 1. Cardiac enzyme studies are the major tests used to diagnose myocardial infarction (MI). Cardiac enzymes and isoenzymes are released into the bloodstream when organs such as the heart are damaged. Isoenzymes include CK-MB, CK-BB, and CK-MM. CK-MB, the isoenzyme most commonly used to diagnose an MI, is found in high concentrations in the heart and skeletal muscles and in much smaller amounts in brain tissue. The creatine kinase (CK) blood level, especially its isoenzyme CK-MB, becomes elevated within 2 hours after an infarction. CK enzymes correlate to the size of the infarct—in other words, the higher the serum CK-MB, the greater the damage to the heart. If an MI is suspected, cardiac enzymes are drawn on admission and at periodic intervals (every

8 hours) for the next 2 days. Troponin, a protein necessary for heart conduction, is also quickly elevated during an MI. Therefore, it can be used to rule out or confirm an MI. Troponin levels are usually drawn in the emergency department or even in the ambulance on the way to the hospital. Sodium and potassium are electrolytes; they are not used to diagnose an MI. Red blood cell and platelet counts also are not considered diagnostic indicators of an MI. Plasminogen is a protein that, when activated, dissolves clots. Lactic acid is a waste product of cellular metabolism and causes sore skeletal muscles. Neither is used to diagnose an MI.

> *Test Taking Strategy—Analyze to determine what information the question asks for, which is the laboratory test results that are diagnostic for MI. Options 2, 3, and 4 can be eliminated because these tests are not used to diagnose an MI. Review diagnostic tests that correlate with confirming or ruling out a diagnosis of an MI, focusing on blood tests that measure isoenzymes and troponin levels, if you had difficulty answering this question.*
> **Cognitive Level**—*Analyzing*
> **Client Needs Category**—*Physiological integrity*
> **Client Needs Subcategory**—*Reduction of risk potential*

56.

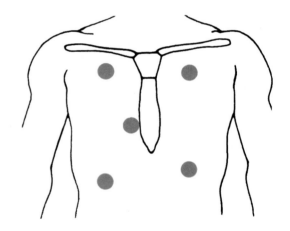

The correct locations for placement of leads in Lead III, the most common arrangement for monitoring clients who require cardiac care, are as follows:
WHITE (RA, right arm), 2nd intercostal space in the right midclavicular line
BLACK (LA, left arm), 2nd intercostal space in the left midclavicular line
RED (LL, left leg), on the lower rib cage at the 8th intercostal space chest, left midclavicular line
GREEN (RL, right leg), on the lower rib cage at the 8th intercostal space, right midclavicular line
BROWN (V1), at the fourth intercostal space, right sternal border.

> *Test Taking Strategy—Analyze to determine what information the question asks for, which is the correct locations for monitoring a client with a five lead wire system in Lead III. A method that helps to recall*

the correct placement is: White (sky) on the right; green (grass) under white on the lower right side, black (smoke) over red (fire) on the left side. Brown goes in the middle at the fourth intercostal space to the right of the sternal border. Review the colors and locations of each of the five leads for monitoring in Lead III if you had difficulty answering this question.
Cognitive Level—*Remembering*
Client Needs Category—*Physiological integrity*
Client Needs Subcategory—*Reduction of risk potential*

57. 2. Hospitalization, for most people, is a unique experience. Therefore, providing clients who are in an unfamiliar environment with information about hospital equipment, clinical procedures, and agency routines helps relieve anxiety. All explanations are given in simple, understandable terms. Once informed, clients have a basis for interpreting the reality of their experiences. A client is unlikely to understand a description of heart rhythm or interpret the pattern on a rhythm strip. Administering a tranquilizer at this time will not help prevent a similar reaction in the future.
Test Taking Strategy—*Use the process of elimination to identify the option that identifies the best nursing approach when a client becomes startled by a cardiac monitor alarm. Options 1 and 4 can be eliminated immediately because the information is most likely beyond the client's level of understanding and therefore may add to the client's anxiety. Option 3 can be eliminated because altering the client's sensorium with a tranquilizer interferes with the client's ability to deal with reality. Recall that knowledge is power. Option 2 remains as the best answer because a simple explanation that a loose lead can trigger an alarm can help relieve the client's emotional distress. Review techniques for relieving anxiety and fear if you had difficulty answering this question.*
Cognitive Level—*Applying*
Client Needs Category—*Psychosocial integrity*
Client Needs Subcategory—*None*

58. 1. In the case of a myocardial infarction (MI), a clot has occluded one of the coronary arteries, causing the heart muscle to be deprived of oxygen and permanently damaged. It is imperative to restore oxygenation to the myocardium by dissolving the clot. Streptokinase (Streptase), a thrombolytic enzyme, is most therapeutic if used within 6 hours after the onset of MI symptoms. It is used to dissolve deep vein and arterial thromboemboli. This and other thrombolytic agents, such as urokinase (Abbokinase), anistreplase (Eminase), alteplase (Activase), and tissue plasminogen activator (t-PA), activate plasminogen and convert it to plasmin. Plasmin breaks down the fibrin of a blood clot. Thrombolytic agents do not slow the heart rate, improve heart contraction, or lower blood pressure. Thrombolytics are contraindicated for clients who have bleeding disorders, a history of stroke, recent trauma, childbirth, or surgery.

Test Taking Strategy—*Analyze to determine what information the question asks for, which is the desired effect from administering streptokinase. Recall that the suffix -ase indicates this drug is an enzyme. Because it is a thrombolytic enzyme, its desired effect, as the name indicates, is to lyse (dissolve) a thrombus (blood clot). Review drug references that describe the mechanism of this drug's action and its uses if you had difficulty answering this question.*
Cognitive Level—*Applying*
Client Needs Category—*Physiological integrity*
Client Needs Subcategory—*Pharmacological therapies*

59. 3. Bleeding is the most common adverse reaction associated with thrombolytic drug therapy. Blood loss may be internal, involving the GI or genitourinary tract, or may result in bleeding within the brain. Most clients who receive streptokinase are placed in the intensive care unit for a period of very close observation. Bleeding may also be external or superficial, manifested as oozing from venipuncture or injection sites, nosebleeds, and skin bruising. Other side effects include hypotension, nausea and vomiting, and cardiac arrhythmias. Hypertension, hyperthermia, and tachypnea are not recognized side effects of this drug.
Test Taking Strategy—*Analyze to determine what information the question asks for, which is an adverse effect associated with administration of streptokinase. Recall that the function of thrombolytics is to dissolve existing clots; a major adverse effect, however, is bleeding or hemorrhage. Review the adverse effects of thrombolytic drugs like streptokinase if you had difficulty answering this question.*
Cognitive Level—*Applying*
Client Needs Category—*Physiological integrity*
Client Needs Subcategory—*Pharmacological therapies*

60. 3. The antihistamine drug diphenhydramine (Benadryl) is typically used when a client develops an allergic reaction to streptokinase (Streptase). Streptokinase is made from a nonhuman source and is antigenic; thus, it may provoke allergic reactions. Diphenhydramine inhibits most responses of smooth muscle to histamine, the chemical that is responsible for most allergic reactions. Vitamin K may be given as an antidote when prothrombin levels are beyond the therapeutic range, as in the case of oral anticoagulants such as warfarin (Coumadin). Both heparin and warfarin are administered to prevent future blood clots from developing.
Test Taking Strategy—*Analyze to determine what information the question asks for, which is a specific drug used to combat an allergic reaction to streptokinase. Recall that diphenhydramine (option 3) inhibits most responses of smooth muscle to histamine, the chemical that is responsible for allergic reactions. Refer to a drug reference for a description of the uses for the drugs listed if you had difficulty answering this question.*

Cognitive Level—*Applying*
Client Needs Category—*Physiological integrity*
Client Needs Subcategory—*Pharmacological therapies*

61. **1.** *Urticaria* is a term for hives. Hives, welts, and rashes are common manifestations of an allergic reaction to streptokinase (Streptase). In addition, the nurse may observe difficulty breathing, wheezing, and hypotension. *Dysuria* describes painful urination. Hemoptysis refers to coughing up bloody sputum. *Dyspepsia* is another word for indigestion. Dysuria, hemoptysis, and dyspepsia are not considered allergic reactions to streptokinase.

> *Test Taking Strategy*—*Analyze to determine what information the question asks for, which is a manifestation of an allergic reaction to streptokinase (Streptase). Urticaria, or hives (option 1), is a classic sign of an allergic reaction. Review the signs and symptoms of allergic reactions if you had difficulty answering this question.*

Cognitive Level—*Applying*
Client Needs Category—*Physiological integrity*
Client Needs Subcategory—*Pharmacological therapies*

62. **1.** Asking open-ended questions encourages the client to elaborate, which may eventually relieve emotional tension. The best approach is to listen actively, remain nonjudgmental, and avoid offering personal opinions. Asking a client a "why" question is usually nontherapeutic, because the client may not be consciously aware of what is motivating these feelings or behavior. Telling a client that the physician believes the client is doing fine implies that the client's fears are unfounded. A nonempathetic response may cause the client to terminate further discussion. Giving advice, as in "You need to concentrate on getting well," is also nontherapeutic because it blocks continued communication about the subject.

> *Test Taking Strategy*—*Apply the key words "most appropriate" when reviewing the options. Look for the option that identifies the response by the nurse that is more therapeutic than the other choices. Recall that asking open-ended questions (option 1) is a therapeutic communication technique that allows the client to reflect and answer honestly from his or her own perspective. Review examples of therapeutic communication techniques if you had difficulty answering this question.*

Cognitive Level—*Applying*
Client Needs Category—*Psychosocial integrity*
Client Needs Subcategory—*None*

63. **1, 2, 3, 5.** Heart failure is a common complication after myocardial infarction (MI). Gaining more than 2 lb/day is indicative of the heart's inability to pump fluids, which places additional work on the heart. Therefore, no additional weight gain is the goal. Throughout the recovery and rehabilitation phases, the goals of activity and exercise are accomplished by gradually increased conditioning;

therefore, increased tolerance to activity is an important outcome. A low-sodium diet decreases fluid volume, thereby reducing the workload of the heart, and a low-fat diet leads to weight reduction, which also decreases the heart's workload. Complying with such a diet is also an appropriate outcome.

A client with an MI is usually anxious for various reasons. During rehabilitation and just before discharge, the client may experience increased anxiety related to returning home, possible recurrence of an MI, and necessary health and lifestyle changes. Consequently, being able to verbalize fears and anxieties freely is an appropriate outcome.

Maintaining pressure over the intravenous site is indicated, but not during the recovery and rehabilitation phases. Other than a low-sodium, low-fat diet, there are usually no other dietary restrictions, and an occasional alcoholic beverage is allowed.

> *Test Taking Strategy*—*Analyze to determine what information the question asks for, which is appropriate goals for a client recovering from an MI. Alternative-format "select all that apply" questions require considering each option independently to decide its merit in answering the question. Choose the options that are the most important expected outcomes in this client's care to ensure a successful recovery. Review expected outcomes for recovery from MI if you had difficulty answering this question.*

Cognitive Level—*Analyzing*
Client Needs Category—*Physiological integrity*
Client Needs Subcategory—*Physiological adaptation*

64. **1.** Pepperoni pizza contains lots of calories, salt (processed meat), and fat (cheese). That makes this choice unsuitable for the client's low-calorie, low-fat, low-sodium diet. Vinegar and oil salad dressing is appropriate because it is low in sodium and calories. The oil, however, must be used sparingly. Liver and onions are acceptable for this client's dietary restrictions, and the liver may improve iron stores. However, liver contains some cholesterol and should be eaten sparingly. Lemon-pepper chicken is also acceptable on this client's diet because it is low in fat, and lemons and pepper are items that can be used freely with this type of diet.

> *Test Taking Strategy*—*Use the process of elimination to select the option that provides the best evidence that the client understands the diet teaching provided by the nurse. Options 2, 3, and 4 can be eliminated because they identify better food selections for the prescribed diet than option 1. Recall that the components included in a pepperoni pizza (option 1) are high in dietary substances the client should avoid. Consult nutritional tables that identify the amount of calories, fat, and sodium in the items listed if you had difficulty answering this question.*

Cognitive Level—*Applying*
Client Needs Category—*Health promotion and maintenance*
Client Needs Subcategory—*None*

65. 2. Straining during a bowel movement involves holding one's breath and bearing down against a closed glottis. This action, sometimes called *Valsalva's maneuver*, increases abdominal and arterial pressure. The increase in arterial pressure acts as resistance to the pumping action of the heart. The blood flow through the coronary arteries is temporarily reduced and can cause ischemia and chest pain. If the heart wall is necrotic, the pressure increase could cause the weakened muscle to rupture and the client to hemorrhage to death. Stool softeners are generally ordered prophylactically to eliminate straining when having a bowel movement. Clients who experience heart attacks can participate in their own self-care activities, such as bathing, provided they do not develop signs of activity intolerance. Signs that indicate the client should rest include becoming short of breath, developing a rapid or irregular heart rate, and experiencing increased blood pressure. Lifting heavy objects, such as groceries, and having sexual intercourse are permitted after discharge. However, clients must usually wait until they can climb two flights of stairs without chest pain before engaging in these activities. Some physicians recommend self-administering a nitroglycerin tablet prophylactically before intercourse.

> *Test Taking Strategy—Analyze to determine what information the question asks for, which is an activity that the client should avoid to reduce a potentially dangerous consequence. Recall that bearing down to eliminate stool (option 2) raises blood pressure and causes the heart to use greater force, and require more oxygen to the muscle, to eject blood. Review discharge instructions that aim to reduce complications after recovering from a myocardial infarction if you had difficulty answering this question.*
> *Cognitive Level—Applying*
> *Client Needs Category—Health promotion and maintenance*
> *Client Needs Subcategory—None*

66. 2. An echocardiogram uses ultrasonic (sound) waves to image the heart's structure. The sound waves are reflected back in various ways, depending on the density of the tissues, to produce a replication of the heart that is later evaluated. An X-ray uses radiation. An electrocardiogram (ECG) picks up electrical activity from the heart muscle. Thermography tests sense heat and variations in temperature to formulate images from body structures.

> *Test Taking Strategy—Analyze to determine what information the question asks for, which is an understanding of how the heart is imaged when an echocardiogram is performed. Consider the word "echo" to find a clue; an examination of the four options helps select option 2 as the correct answer. The echo from sound waves provides a structural image of the heart muscle and valves during cardiac cycles. Review the manner in which an echocardiogram is performed if you had difficulty answering this question.*

Cognitive Level—Applying
Client Needs Category—Physiological integrity
Client Needs Subcategory—Physiological adaptation

67.

3. Check responsiveness.
4. Activate emergency assistance.
6. Perform chest compressions.
1. Open the victim's airway.
5. Check for spontaneous breathing.
2. Administer rescue breaths.

The sequence of actions for resuscitation according to the American Heart Association's (AHA's) International Cardiopulmonary Resuscitation (CPR) and Emergency Cardiovascular Care (ECC) Guidelines of 2010 are as follows:

1. Check responsiveness.
2. Activate emergency assistance.
3. Perform chest compressions.
4. Open the victim's airway.
5. Check for spontaneous breathing.
6. Administer rescue breaths.

> *Test Taking Strategy—Analyze to determine what information the question asks for, which requires arranging the options in the order in which they should be performed when resuscitating a victim. To properly assess the need for resuscitation, the nurse's first action is to check for responsiveness by shaking the victim and shouting, "Are you OK?" If the victim remains unresponsive, the next step for the rescuer is to call loudly for additional help or activate emergency services personnel. If the victim cannot be aroused, the rescuer should begin compressions immediately. Current guidelines (2010) indicate that opening the airway, checking for breathing, and giving rescue breaths wastes valuable time and can be delayed until compressions are administered. Review the current guidelines for performing CPR if you had difficulty answering this question.*
> *Cognitive Level—Applying*
> *Client Needs Category—Physiological integrity*
> *Client Needs Subcategory—Physiological adaptation*

68. 3. An automated electronic defibrillator (AED) is a portable, battery-operated device that analyzes heart rhythms and delivers an electrical shock to restore a functional heartbeat. Early defibrillation within the first 3 to 5 minutes after a cardiac event, combined with early advanced care results in 50% or greater long-term survival rates. Successful resuscitation is reduced as the time to defibrillation is delayed.

Test Taking Strategy—*Use the process of elimination to help select the option that identifies the most effective method for restoring circulation in a pulseless victim. Option 2 can be immediately eliminated because a patent airway correlates more with providing effective rescue breathing. Although positioning a client on a hard, flat surface (option 4) is essential for effective chest compressions, positioning alone cannot restore circulation. Performing chest compressions (option 1) is vital, even before defibrillation is used, but recovery statistics are lower than when an AED (option 3) is used with measures identified in the other options. Review the algorithm for adult life support recommended by the American Heart Association's (AHA's) International Cardiopulmonary Resuscitation (CPR) and Emergency Cardiovascular Care (ECC) Guidelines of 2010 if you had difficulty answering this question.*
Cognitive Level—*Understanding*
Client Needs Category—*Physiological integrity*
Client Needs Subcategory—*Physiological adaptation*

69. 2. If the victim is not breathing and neck trauma is not suspected, the nurse would use the chin-lift/head-tilt method to open the airway. This is performed by using one hand to lift the chin upward to maintain position and placing the other hand across the victim's forehead. The jaw thrust method is used only if the chin-lift/head-tilt method does not open the airway adequately or if the victim might have a neck injury. Placing a hand under the neck is no longer recommended. After the airway is opened, the mouth is cleared with a finger sweep.

Test Taking Strategy—*Apply the key words "most appropriate" when considering each of the four options. Choose the option that describes the technique that is better than any of the others for opening a client's airway. Recall that the chin-lift technique (option 2) positions the tongue, which is the leading cause of an airway obstruction, away from the back of the throat. Review methods for opening the airway in preparation for checking for spontaneous breathing and administering rescue breaths if you had difficulty answering this question.*
Cognitive Level—*Applying*
Client Needs Category—*Physiological integrity*
Client Needs Subcategory—*Physiological adaptation*

70. 3. Once the airway is open, some victims begin breathing spontaneously. The nurse briefly assesses for spontaneous breathing, no breathing, or absence of normal breathing such as gasping for air. Leaning over the victim's head and listening or observing the chest rise and fall should be done as quickly as possible. Skin color is not a dependable indicator of breathing because hypotension is likely to cause the victim to appear pale or ashen. The nurse would check the carotid pulse to determine the need for

chest compressions, not rescue breathing. Administering rescue breathing is unnecessary if the victim is spontaneously breathing.

Test Taking Strategy—*Use the process of elimination to help select the option that identifies the best method for determining if a person requires rescue breathing. Option 3 is the correct answer because briefly assessing to determine the absence of breathing or an abnormal quality to breathing provides objective evidence that the client requires rescue breathing. The recommendation to look, listen, and feel for breathing is no longer followed because these steps require too much time. If normal breathing is absent, rescue breathing should begin after 30 compressions have been administered to the pulseless victim. Review criteria for determining if rescue breathing should be performed if you had difficulty answering this question.*
Cognitive Level—*Applying*
Client Needs Category—*Physiological integrity*
Client Needs Subcategory—*Physiological adaptation*

71. 3. Pinching the nose shut allows maximum ventilation with no loss of air through the nostrils. If the victim has a mouth injury or it is impossible to prevent air from leaking (in an adult victim), the rescuer may use the mouth-to-nose technique for giving ventilations. When resuscitating an infant or small child, the rescuer makes a seal by covering both the victim's nose and mouth with the rescuer's mouth. Once the breath is given, the rescuer allows the air to be exhaled passively. Pressing on the trachea may interfere with air passage. Removing dentures and squeezing the victim's cheeks may interfere with maintaining a tight seal during rescue breathing.

Test Taking Strategy—*Analyze to determine what information the question asks for, which is a description of how to deliver an effective volume of air into a victim who is not breathing. Recall that the principle is to seal any openings from which air could leak. Pinching the nose (option 3) and covering the adult victim's entire mouth when administering a rescue breath ensures that a full volume is delivered rather than only a partial amount. Review the technique for performing rescue breathing if you had difficulty answering this question.*
Cognitive Level—*Applying*
Client Needs Category—*Physiological integrity*
Client Needs Subcategory—*Physiological adaptation*

72. 1. The hands of the rescuer are on top of one another on the lower half of the sternum, two fingerbreadths above the xiphoid process. The costal cartilage connects the ribs to the sternum, so compressing over the costal cartilage could fracture the victim's ribs. The hands would be placed too high on the chest if positioned above the manubrium, which is the upper portion of the sternum. The hands would be too low if they are placed below the tip of the xiphoid process, a position that could damage the stomach, lacerate the liver, or cause vomiting.

Test Taking Strategy—*Analyze to determine what information the question asks for, which is the correct hand placement when performing chest compressions. Recall that placing the hands on the lower half of the sternum (option 1) is the correct location for hand placement because it allows safer compression of the heart against the vertebrae. Review the technique for performing chest compressions when resuscitating a victim if you had difficulty answering this question.*
Cognitive Level—*Applying*
Client Needs Category—*Physiological integrity*
Client Needs Subcategory—*Physiological adaptation*

73. 4. During cardiopulmonary resuscitation (CPR), the victim's chest is compressed at a rate of 100 times per minute. The American Heart Association's (AHA's) International CPR and Emergency Cardiovascular Care (ECC) Guidelines of 2010 indicate that an adult's sternum should be depressed approximately 2 inches (5 cm) or more with each compression. Rates below 100 per minute are unlikely to circulate blood adequately.

Test Taking Strategy—*Analyze to determine what information the question asks for, which is the rate of chest compressions for a pulseless victim. Recall that chest compressions should be performed at least 100 times per minute (option 4) regardless of the age of the victim. Review the rate and depth of chest compressions when performing CPR if you had difficulty answering this question.*
Cognitive Level—*Applying*
Client Needs Category—*Physiological integrity*
Client Needs Subcategory—*Physiological adaptation*

74. 1. The American Heart Association recommends that when two rescuers perform cardiopulmonary resuscitation (CPR), the ratio is 30 compressions to 2 breaths—the same as it is for one rescuer. CPR is never interrupted for longer than 7 seconds.

Test Taking Strategy—*Analyze to determine what information the question asks for, which is the ratio of chest compressions to breaths when two rescuers perform CPR on an adult. Recall that the ratio of 30 compressions to 2 breaths (option 1) for two-rescuer adult CPR is the same as it is for one-rescuer CPR. Review the guidelines for combining compressions and rescue breathing when performing CPR on an adult if you had difficulty answering this question.*
Cognitive Level—*Applying*
Client Needs Category—*Physiological integrity*
Client Needs Subcategory—*Physiological adaptation*

75. 3. If the pulse returns, cardiac compressions are stopped. The carotid pulse is assessed for a full 5 seconds after the first minute of resuscitation and every few minutes thereafter unless consciousness is restored. The victim's color may improve as a consequence of effective resuscitative efforts. Dilated and fixed pupils are an indica-

tion that the brain is inadequately oxygenated. Vomiting can occur in a nonbreathing and pulseless victim because of stomach distention with air.

Test Taking Strategy—*Use the process of elimination to help select the option that identifies the best evidence that chest compressions can be discontinued. Option 2 can be eliminated immediately because dilated pupils are an ominous sign suggesting brain death. Option 4 can be eliminated because vomiting indicates that rescue breaths are entering the stomach rather than the lungs or that the stomach is being compacted during chest compressions. Although option 2 has merit, it is not the best method for determining if chest compressions can be discontinued because the victim's color will improve as oxygenated blood is circulated. Option 3 remains as the correct answer because a palpable pulse is evidence that the heart is beating spontaneously. Review evidence that a victim is responding to resuscitation efforts if you had difficulty answering this question.*
Cognitive Level—*Applying*
Client Needs Category—*Physiological integrity*
Client Needs Subcategory—*Physiological adaptation*

76. 2. The recovery position after successful cardiopulmonary resuscitation (CPR) is a side-lying position with the upper leg flexed. This position helps protect and maintain the airway and prevents aspiration if the client should vomit. The other choices do not adequately maintain the airway.

Test Taking Strategy—*Use the process of elimination to help select the option that describes the best position for a victim after successful resuscitation. Option 1 can be eliminated because lying supine increases the potential for aspirating gastric fluids. Option 3 can be eliminated because lying prone does not facilitate breathing. Option 4 can be eliminated because the term "flat" is vague and could apply to either a supine or prone position. Option 2 remains as the correct answer because a lateral position facilitates keeping the airway free of vomitus. Flexion of the uppermost knee prevents the client from rolling onto his or her abdomen. Review a description or image of the recovery position if you had difficulty answering this question.*
Cognitive Level—*Applying*
Client Needs Category—*Physiological integrity*
Client Needs Subcategory—*Physiological adaptation*

77. 3. According to the American Heart Association's (AHA's) International Cardiopulmonary Resuscitation (CPR) and Emergency Cardiovascular Care (ECC) Guidelines of 2010, bystanders untrained in CPR may assist with CPR by calling 911 and performing chest compressions only in the center of the chest. The bystander is instructed to push down 2 inches (5 cm) at a rate of 100 beats/minute and continue until help arrives. Staying with the victim is helpful; however, circulating blood in the victim promotes oxygenation of the tissues. Promoting oxygenation of the tissues is the most important factor during this time to prevent tissue damage. Respirations are not as crucial as compressions, so rescue breathing is not required for the untrained bystander, who may be unwilling to provide rescue breathing. Placing the client flat and elevating the feet is important for a client in shock.

> *Test Taking Strategy—Apply the key words "most helpful" when considering the statements in each of the four options. Select the option that describes the role of an untrained person in resuscitation efforts. Recall that lay individuals may be hesitant to perform mouth-to-mouth resuscitation but can still perform chest compressions. Untrained laypersons also can receive instructions from emergency dispatch phone operators. Review the AHA's International CPR and ECC Guidelines of 2010 in reference to the emphasis on lay bystander chest compressions if you had difficulty answering this question.*
> **Cognitive Level—Applying**
> **Client Needs Category—Physiological integrity**
> **Client Needs Subcategory—Physiological adaptation**

Nursing Care of Clients with Congestive Heart Failure

78.

| 3. Pulmonary veins |
| 4. Left atrium |
| 5. Mitral valve |
| 2. Left ventricle |
| 1. Aorta |

Oxygenated blood enters the left side of the heart from the pulmonary veins. The oxygenated blood is then deposited into the left atrium. As the mitral valve opens, blood from the left atrium moves into the left ventricle. Then, blood is ejected through the aortic valve into the aorta when the left ventricle contracts.

> *Test Taking Strategies—Analyze to determine what information the question asks for, which is the sequence in which blood enters and leaves the left side of the heart. Recall that the pulmonary veins carry oxygen-rich blood to the heart itself, and that the aorta is the vessel that delivers oxygenated blood to systemic arteries and arterioles. Review the structures located on the left side of the heart if you had difficulty answering this question.*
> **Cognitive Level—Remembering**
> **Client Needs Category—Physiological integrity**
> **Client Needs Subcategory—Physiological adaptation**

79. 2. Heart failure refers to the heart's ineffective ability to pump blood to the tissues and organs to meet the body's metabolic needs. Congestive heart failure (CHF) is the accumulation of blood and fluids in the tissues and organs related to poor circulation. CHF is divided into two types: left-sided, which produces respiratory distress and pulmonary edema, and right-sided, which causes congestion of blood throughout the venous circulatory system. Left-sided heart failure often precedes right-sided heart failure. Early left-sided heart failure is manifested by dyspnea and fatigue. Other classic signs and symptoms include a moist cough, orthopnea, tachycardia, restlessness, and confusion. Signs and symptoms of right-sided heart failure include shortness of breath, edema of feet and ankles, pronounced neck veins, palpitations, tachycardia, weakness and fatigue, and fainting or light-headedness. Anorexia and nausea may have many causes and are not closely associated with CHF. Headaches are related to hypertension and not CHF.

> *Test Taking Strategy—Analyze to determine what information the question asks for, which is a symptom that is associated with left-sided heart failure. Recall that when the left side of the heart fails, the lungs become congested with blood, leading to dyspnea (option 2). Review the path of pulmonary circulation to the left side of the heart if you had difficulty answering this question.*
> **Cognitive Level—Remembering**
> **Client Needs Category—Physiological integrity**
> **Client Needs Subcategory—Physiological adaptation**

80. 4. A client with congestive heart failure (CHF) is usually most comfortable and has the least amount of difficulty with breathing when placed in either a semi-Fowler's, mid-Fowler's, high-Fowler's, or standing position. Sitting and standing positions cause organs to fall away from the diaphragm, giving more room for the lungs to expand. Right-side lying, left-side-lying, or back-lying positions, even with the knees bent, are inappropriate because they impede good lung expansion.

> *Test Taking Strategy—Use the process of elimination to help select the option that describes the most therapeutic position for a client with CHF who is having difficulty breathing. Options 1, 2, and 3 can be eliminated because none of these reduces the fluid that congests the lungs in left-sided heart failure, nor alleviates the pressure on the diaphragm from abdominal organs distended with fluid in right-sided heart failure. Recall that sitting (option 4) and standing relieve dyspnea because they reduce pulmonary hydrostatic pressure and congestion by pooling blood in lower anatomic levels and increase the potential for pulmonary expansion. Review the rationale for placing a client in semi-Fowler's or high Fowler's position if you had difficulty answering this question.*

Cognitive Level—*Remembering*
Client Needs Category—*Physiological integrity*
Client Needs Subcategory—*Physiological adaptation*

81. 2. Clients who are having difficulty breathing, a common symptom in left-sided heart failure, typically feel anxious, apprehensive, and fearful. Appropriate nursing interventions relate to decreasing the client's anxiety and promoting adequate oxygenation. Clients are much less likely to feel depressed, angry, or stoic during this time.

Test Taking Strategy—*Apply the key words "most likely" when analyzing the options, and select the option that identifies the emotional response experienced by a client with heart failure better than any of the others. Recall that anxiety (option 2) develops when a person senses a real or imagined threat to well-being. In the case of the client with congestive heart failure, struggling for air and feeling as though suffocating creates a sense of a life-threatening situation. Review the factors that contribute to anxiety if you had difficulty answering this question.*
Cognitive Level—*Applying*
Client Needs Category—*Psychosocial integrity*
Client Needs Subcategory—*None*

82. 4. Supplemental oxygen is commonly ordered to decrease the workload of the heart and increase the amount of oxygen in the blood. The cardiac workload is decreased when the apical pulse becomes less bounding and less rapid. Facial flushing can be a sign of fever or hypertension. Normal capillary refill is less than 3 seconds, so a 6-second capillary refill indicates that circulation is impaired. Subjective data related to the client's statement are important to collect, but objective data are more accurate indicators of the effectiveness of this treatment.

Test Taking Strategy—*Use the process of elimination to identify the option that is the best indication that oxygen therapy is effective. Option 1 can be eliminated because this is not a symptom of heart failure. Option 2 indicates that circulation is not improved. The subjective data indicated in option 3 are not as important as the objective data shown by option 4. Recall that the heart responds to hypoxemia by increasing the rate and force of heart contraction. Consequently, when the level of blood oxygenation improves as a result of supplemental oxygen, the apical pulse will be less forceful (option 4). Review the homeostatic mechanisms that result when the amount of blood oxygen is decreased, using deductive reasoning to determine the physiologic changes that occur when oxygenation improves, if you had difficulty answering this question.*
Cognitive Level—*Applying*
Client Needs Category—*Physiological integrity*
Client Needs Subcategory—*Physiological adaptation*

83. 1. The presence of another person, especially a health care provider, does much to relieve a client's anxiety. This is especially true when the client's perception is one of being helpless or powerless. It is essential for the nurse to make sure that the client is not left alone. Notifying the physician of the client's fear is inappropriate because the physician probably will not be able to do anything more in this situation. Telling the client that everything will be okay is meaningless reassurance and nontherapeutic. Recording of data can be temporarily postponed or verbally reported if needed.

Test Taking Strategy—*Apply the key words "most appropriate" when analyzing the actions in the four options, and select the option that is best for responding to a client who feels frightened. Recall that fear intensifies when it is experienced in isolation; fear is reduced when there is a supportive person available. Review techniques for minimizing fear and anxiety if you had difficulty answering this question.*
Cognitive Level—*Applying*
Client Needs Category—*Psychosocial integrity*
Client Needs Subcategory—*None*

84. 4. Significant weight gain or loss, such as a difference of 2 lb (0.9 kg) or more in 24 hours, indicates major changes in body fluid distribution. Weight gain indicates fluid retention and impaired renal excretion. Weight loss indicates a therapeutic response to medical and drug therapy. Pupil response and appetite are appropriate to monitor in the daily assessments, but heart failure is not likely to cause major changes in these findings. Edema of the lower extremities is a sign of right-sided heart failure; also, lower extremities should be monitored more often than once per day.

Test Taking Strategy—*Analyze to determine what information the question asks for, which is the nursing assessment that should be monitored daily when caring for a client with left-sided heart failure. Recall that diuretic therapy is used to reduce excess circulatory volume. Monitoring the client's weight (option 4) helps to assess a client's response to the therapeutic regimen. Review outcome assessments that correlate with the care of a client with congestive heart failure if you had difficulty answering this question.*
Cognitive Level—*Applying*
Client Needs Category—*Physiological integrity*
Client Needs Subcategory—*Basic care and comfort*

85. 2. Diuretics such as furosemide (Lasix) are potassium depleting. Therefore, it is important for the nurse to monitor for signs of hypokalemia. Normal serum potassium levels are between 3.5 and 5.0 mEq/L, so a potassium level of 2.5 mEq should signal the need for immediate attention. Normal serum sodium levels are between 135 and 145 mEq/L, making this choice within the normal range. Normal chloride levels are between 90 and 110 mEq/L, also making this value within normal limits. Bicarbonate is a blood gas value. Normal bicarbonate values are between 21 and 28 mEq/L; therefore, this value is also within the normal range.

Test Taking Strategy—*Analyze to determine what information the question asks for, which is an abnormal electrolyte level that could be life-threatening if left untreated. Recall that many diuretics are potassium-wasting; a serum potassium level of 2.5 mEq/dL could result in lethal cardiac arrhythmias. Review the listed laboratory values, comparing them with normal and abnormal levels, if you had difficulty answering this question.*

Cognitive Level—*Analyzing*
Client Needs Category—*Physiological integrity*
Client Needs Subcategory—*Reduction of risk potential*

86. 1. If jugular veins distend with the head elevated 45 degrees or more, this indicates that an increased volume of blood is not circulating well through the right side of the heart. Tachycardia—not bradycardia—is associated with heart failure. A dry, hacking cough is an indicator of left-sided heart failure and not right-sided heart failure. A flushed, red face is not commonly associated with heart failure; it is related to hypertension.

Test Taking Strategy—*Analyze to determine what information the question asks for, which is a sign or symptom of right-sided heart failure. Recall that if the right side of the heart fails to pump effectively, blood volume increases in the venous blood vessels delivering blood to the right atrium. Consequently, jugular vein distention (option 1) is an indication of right-sided heart failure. Review the signs and symptoms of right-sided heart failure if you had difficulty answering this question.*

Cognitive Level—*Remembering*
Client Needs Category—*Physiological integrity*
Client Needs Subcategory—*Physiological adaptation*

87. ½ tablet.
Half of a 0.25-mg tablet is the correct amount of drug to administer if the prescription is for 0.125 mg. The formula for determining the correct number of tablets is as follows:

$$\frac{\text{Dosage Desired}}{\text{Dosage on Hand}} \times \text{Quantity} = \text{Amount to Administer}$$

$$\frac{0.125}{0.25} \times 1 \text{ tablet} = 0.5 \text{ or } \frac{1}{2} \text{ tablet}$$

Test Taking Strategy—*Analyze to determine what information the question asks for, which involves calculating how many tablets are required to supply 0.125 mg when the supplied dose contains 0.25 mg*

per tablet. Review the calculation and consult references that explain how to calculate oral doses of medication if you had difficulty answering this question.

Cognitive Level—*Remembering*
Client Needs Category—*Physiological integrity*
Client Needs Subcategory—*Pharmacological therapies*

88. 1. Because digoxin (Lanoxin) affects cardiac automaticity and the conduction system, it is essential that the nurse monitor the client's apical or radial pulse for 1 full minute before administration of each dose of the drug. If the heart rate is below 60 beats/minute, the dose of digoxin is withheld. If the pulse rate is significantly decreased or if other arrhythmias develop secondary to the administration of this drug, digoxin immune Fab (Digibind) may be prescribed for its antidigoxin effect. Assessments of blood pressure, heart sounds, and breath sounds are part of a comprehensive cardiopulmonary assessment, but they are not directly affected by the administration of digoxin.

Test Taking Strategy—*Analyze to determine what information the question asks for, which is an essential assessment before administering a digoxin dose. Recall that digoxin slows the conduction of cardiac impulses through the atrioventricular (AV) node, slowing the heart rate (option 1). This action improves cardiac output by allowing a greater volume of blood to fill the heart before its contraction. A typical sign of toxicity to digitalis drugs is a pulse rate less than 60 beats/minute. Review the actions and side effects of digoxin if you had difficulty answering this question.*

Cognitive Level—*Remembering*
Client Needs Category—*Physiological adaptation*
Client Needs Subcategory—*Pharmacological therapies*

89. 1. GI symptoms associated with digoxin (Lanoxin) toxicity include anorexia, nausea, vomiting, and diarrhea. The client may also become drowsy and confused or have visual changes, such as blurred vision, disturbance in seeing yellow and green colors, and a halo effect around dark objects. Toxic doses of digoxin can also increase cardiac automaticity, causing a rapid heart rate, or depress the conduction of cardiac impulses, causing a slow heart rate. Serum drug levels are used to monitor the client's metabolism of digoxin. Pinpoint pupils are associated with opiate toxicity. Double vision is associated with myasthenia gravis. Ringing in the ears is a symptom of salicylate toxicity. Itching is a common side effect of many drugs, but it is not related to digoxin toxicity.

Test Taking Strategy—*Analyze to determine what information the question asks for, which is a clinical manifestation of digoxin toxicity. Although anorexia, nausea, vomiting, and diarrhea (option 1) are seemingly nonspecific, they may be caused by digoxin toxicity. A serum digoxin level that is greater than*

2 ng/mL (normal range, 0.5 to 2.0 ng/mL) would confirm that the manifestations are due to digoxin toxicity. Review the toxic effects of digoxin if you had difficulty answering this question.
Cognitive Level—*Remembering*
Client Needs Category—*Physiological integrity*
Client Needs Subcategory—*Pharmacological therapies*

90. 1. For the client who exhibits signs and symptoms of heart failure, the main goals include decreasing the heart's workload, improving circulation, and managing fluid retention. The identified goal of improved cardiac output can be measured by assessing the stability of vital signs. Rapid weight loss of 5 lb/day is too much and is inappropriate for this goal. Having a decrease in peripheral edema is too subjective and not easily measured. A 24-hour urine output of 1,000 mL is inadequate; an adequate urine output should be about 2,000 mL/day.

> **Test Taking Strategy**—*Use the process of elimination to help select the option that identifies the best measurement for evaluating whether the identified goal has been achieved. Options 2 and 4 can be eliminated because these findings are inappropriate for this goal. Option 3 can be eliminated because it is too subjective. Recall that normal vital signs, especially a normal heart rate, are indications that the cardiac output is improved. Review methods for evaluating effective cardiac output if you had difficulty answering this question.*
> **Cognitive Level**—*Applying*
> **Client Needs Category**—*Physiological integrity*
> **Client Needs Subcategory**—*Physiological adaptation*

Nursing Care of Clients with Conduction Disorders

91. 1. A Holter monitor is used for 24 hours or longer to gather data about a client's heart rhythm patterns during normal daily activity. For an accurate interpretation, it is important to correlate the recorded data with the performance of physical activity. Instructing the client to keep a log is a good way to do this. The client need not assess the radial pulse; the heart rate is determined from the rhythm strip. The client should not alter usual activities of daily living to obtain pertinent data. There is no reason that the client's lower extremities should be elevated while the Holter monitor is in place.

> **Test Taking Strategy**—*Apply the key words "most beneficial" to the choices in the four options. Select the option that is best for promoting the diagnostic value when a client wears a Holter monitor. Recall that keeping a log of physical activities (option 1) helps the physician correlate when and how the cardiac rhythm changes in relation to the client's activities of daily living. Review the purpose of a Holter monitor*

and the client's role during its use if you had difficulty answering this question.
Cognitive Level—*Applying*
Client Needs Category—*Physiological integrity*
Client Needs Subcategory—*Reduction of risk potential*

92. 3. Using electrical devices, such as electric razors and toothbrushes, may alter the data recorded with a Holter monitor. The other activities are not known to cause electrical interference with a Holter monitor.

> **Test Taking Strategy**—*Correlate the key words "most appropriate" with the items in the four options, looking for one that should be avoided to reduce electrical interference when a client wears a Holter monitor. Recall that electrical devices such as an electric razor (option 3) applied to or on the body interfere with the electrocardiogram signal that is being recorded on the monitor. Review client instructions that are pertinent to using a Holter monitor if you had difficulty answering this question.*
> **Cognitive Level**—*Applying*
> **Client Needs Category**—*Physiological integrity*
> **Client Needs Subcategory**—*Reduction of risk potential*

93. 1. Cardioversion is similar to defibrillation, except that cardioversion is a planned procedure, whereas defibrillation is used in emergency situations. Cardioversion involves administering a mild electric shock to the heart to correct rapid arrhythmias. Cardiac catheterization and angiography involve threading a catheter into the heart. Several types of cardiac imaging, such as multigated acquisition and thallium-201 scans, can be used to assess blood flow to the heart muscle.

> **Test Taking Strategy**—*Analyze to determine what information the question asks for, which is a statement that reflects an accurate understanding of cardioversion. Recall that when cardioversion is used, an electrical current is applied to the chest (option 1) to interrupt an arrhythmia and facilitate normal pacemaker initiation of cardiac conduction. Review how cardioversion is performed if you had difficulty answering this question.*
> **Cognitive Level**—*Applying*
> **Client Needs Category**—*Physiological integrity*
> **Client Needs Subcategory**—*Physiological adaptation*

94. 2. Digoxin (Lanoxin) and diuretics are withheld for 24 to 72 hours before elective cardioversion. Withholding these medications will ensure that the heart's normal conduction will not be affected during the procedure. Diazepam (Valium) is generally prescribed as a preprocedural sedative. There are no contraindications for withholding heparin or warfarin (Coumadin) and anticoagulants.

> **Test Taking Strategy**—*Analyze to determine what information the question asks for, which is a drug that should be withheld when a client will undergo*

cardioversion. Recall that digoxin (option 2) slows the conduction of cardiac impulses through the atrioventricular node, and therefore, there is a potential for asystole unless the drug is temporarily withheld. Review drugs that are administered and those that are withheld prior to performing electrocardioversion if you had difficulty answering this question.
Cognitive Level—*Applying*
Client Needs Category—*Physiological integrity*
Client Needs Subcategory—*Pharmacological therapies*

95. 2. The purpose of cardioversion is to stop the rapid ectopic cardiac rhythm and reestablish the sinoatrial (SA) node as the pacemaker. If this occurs, the heart beats regularly between 60 and 100 beats/minute. Such drugs as diazepam (Valium) and midazolam hydrochloride (Versed) are used to produce moderate sedation. The client remains awake, but usually has no memory of the experience. Equal apical and radial pulse rates are desirable, but this is not an indication of successful cardioversion. The normal difference between the systolic and diastolic blood pressures, also known as the *pulse pressure*, is approximately 40 mm Hg. Adequate cardiac output is generally reflected in a normal blood pressure measurement. However, the primary expected outcome of cardioversion is the restoration of normal cardiac rhythm.

> *Test Taking Strategy*—*Analyze to determine what information the question asks for, which is evidence of a successful outcome after cardioversion. Recall that the purpose of cardioversion is to restore a normal electrical rhythm to the heart, making option 2 the correct answer. Review the desired result when cardioversion is performed if you had difficulty answering this question.*
> **Cognitive Level**—*Applying*
> **Client Needs Category**—*Physiological integrity*
> **Client Needs Subcategory**—*Physiological adaptation*

96.

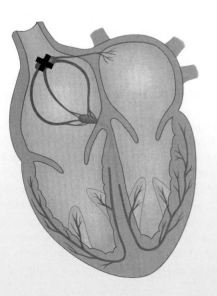

The sinoatrial (SA) node is the site of the heart's natural pacemaker. The SA node is called the pacemaker of the heart because it creates the electrical impulses that cause the heart to contract. This specialized tissue is located in the wall of the right atrium between the openings of the superior and inferior vena cavae. A properly functioning SA node initiates regular impulses at a rate of 60 to 100 beats/minute. Once an impulse is sent from the SA node, it then travels down several internodal pathways to the AV node, the bundle of His, the right and left bundle branches, and the Purkinje fibers.

> *Test Taking Strategy*—*Analyze to determine what information the question asks for, which is the location of the SA node. The SA node is located in the wall of the right atrium. Review the structures that make up the conduction system of the heart if you had difficulty answering this question.*
> **Cognitive Level**—*Remembering*
> **Client Needs Category**—*Physiological integrity*
> **Client Needs Subcategory**—*Physiological adaptation*

97. 4. A permanent pacemaker battery is usually implanted beneath the skin below the right clavicle. Sometimes the area below the left clavicle is used. The wire for a temporary pacemaker is inserted through a peripheral vein, not the brachial artery, and then threaded into the right atrium and the right ventricle. Pacemaker wires are placed during cardiac surgery in case a client needs pacing postoperatively. The wires are seen externally from the skin on the chest. The area beneath the nipple is too low for the pacemaker, and most pacemakers are not located in the sternal area.

> *Test Taking Strategy*—*Analyze to determine what information the question asks for, which is the location of an implanted pacemaker battery. Recall that the pacemaker is usually placed just under the right clavicle (option 4) and the electrical lead is either in the right atrium or right ventricle; dual leads are in both. Review where a permanent pacemaker is implanted if you had difficulty answering this question.*
> **Cognitive Level**—*Applying*
> **Client Needs Category**—*Physiological integrity*
> **Client Needs Subcategory**—*Physiological adaptation*

98. 2. If the artificial pacemaker does not support a heart rate high enough to maintain adequate cardiac output, the client feels dizzy and possibly faints. Tingling in the chest is unrelated to the artificial pacemaker. Pain that radiates to the arm is a symptom of angina pectoris or myocardial infarction. Tenderness may be caused by an infection.

> *Test Taking Strategy*—*Analyze to determine what information the question asks for, which is a symptom that suggests a pacemaker malfunction. Recall that an artificial pacemaker is designed to ensure*

cardiac conduction that facilitates an adequate cardiac output. If cardiac output is compromised, the client will experience symptoms of hypoperfusion. The brain is especially sensitive to an inadequate blood supply manifested by dizziness (option 2) and perhaps fainting. Review signs of decreased cardiac output secondary to pacemaker malfunction if you had difficulty answering this question.

Cognitive Level—*Applying*
Client Needs Category—*Safe and effective care environment*
Client Needs Subcategory—*Coordinated care*

99. 3. A cardiac ablation is an electrophysiological procedure used to destroy small aberrant areas of conductive tissue causing an arrhythmia. During the procedure, electrodes are threaded through a catheter inserted at the groin to within the heart. Once the electrodes identify the source of the arrhythmia, the tissue is destroyed. Localized soreness, some oozing of blood or serum, and bruising at the catheter insertion site are expected. Bruising that extends the length of the leg is unusual, and the nurse is correct to call the client's description of the bruising as needing further assessment by the physician.

> **Test Taking Strategy**—*Analyze to determine what information is atypical and requires a need for the physician's review. Bruising that travels down the leg potentially indicates continued venous bleeding. Review complications following a cardiac ablation if you had difficulty answering this question.*

Cognitive Level—*Analyzing*
Client Needs Category—*Physiological integrity*
Client Needs Subcategory—*Physiological adaptation*

Nursing Care of Clients with Valvular Disorders

100. 3. Rheumatic fever commonly causes permanent damage to the heart and valves and is often the result of a streptococcal infection (strep throat). About half of clients who had rheumatic fever have narrowed mitral valves. Varicella, rubella, and whooping cough (pertussis) are acute infections, but they are not known to cause damage to heart valves. Intrauterine rubella infection can cause congenital heart defects.

> **Test Taking Strategy**—*Analyze to determine what information the question asks for, which is a childhood disease that predisposes to valvular damage. Recall that streptococcal infections (option 3) cause rheumatic fever and rheumatic heart disease. Review the causes of rheumatic fever and its sequelae if you had difficulty answering this question.*

Cognitive Level—*Applying*
Client Needs Category—*Physiological integrity*
Client Needs Subcategory—*Physiological adaptation*

101.

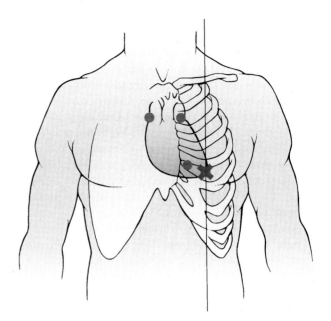

The sound from the mitral valve is best heard by auscultating the apical area, which is at the fifth intercostal space in the left midclavicular line. When assessing heart sounds, the auscultatory areas are not directly over the anatomic locations of the heart valves. The aortic valve is best heard at the second intercostal space to the right of the sternum. The pulmonic valve is best heard at the second intercostal space to the left of the sternum. The tricuspid valve is best heard at the fourth intercostal space to the left of the sternum.

> **Test Taking Strategy**—*Analyze to determine what information the question asks for, which is the location where sounds from the mitral valve can be heard best. Recall that the mitral valve is auscultated in the same location as the S_1 heart sound, which is at the fifth intercostal space in the left midclavicular line. Review the locations where heart sounds are auscultated if you had difficulty answering this question.*

Cognitive Level—*Understanding*
Client Needs Category—*Physiological integrity*
Client Needs Subcategory—*Physiological adaptation*

102. 4. A daily maintenance dose of penicillin, such as nafcillin sodium (Unipen), is prescribed to prevent future streptococcal infections for some people with a history of rheumatic heart disease. Subsequent streptococcal infections continue to damage the heart. If daily doses of antibiotic are not taken, they are generally prescribed before oral surgery, tooth extractions, or other invasive procedures are performed. Nafcillin will not destroy viruses, reduce scar tissue, or stop blood clots from forming.

> **Test Taking Strategy**—*Use the process of elimination to help select the option that identifies the best explanation for treating the client with nafcillin, an antibiotic*

in the penicillin family. Option 1 can be eliminated because antibiotics are not effective in treating viral infections. Although the mitral valve is damaged due to inflammation and scar tissue around its cusps, option 2 can be eliminated because antibiotic therapy will not reverse the damage that already exists. Option 3 can be eliminated because anticoagulants are used to prevent clots from forming. Option 4 remains as the correct answer because nafcillin is prescribed to reduce the potential for future infections caused by the streptococcal bacteria to which the client is susceptible. Review the cause of rheumatic fever and the reason for prophylactic antibiotic therapy if you had difficulty answering this question.
Cognitive Level—*Applying*
Client Needs Category—*Physiological integrity*
Client Needs Subcategory—*Pharmacological therapies*

103. 1. To maintain adequate perfusion of all the cells in the body during any open heart surgery, including mitral valve replacement, blood is oxygenated and circulated by cardiopulmonary bypass using a heart–lung machine. Porcine (pork) valves and mechanical valves, not harvested leg veins, are used for replacing diseased valvular tissue. Stents are not used to treat defective valves.
Test Taking Strategy—Use the process of elimination to help select the option that identifies the best evidence that the client understands how the surgical procedure to replace the mitral valve will be performed. Option 2 has some merit, because stenotic valves may be widened by performing a valvuloplasty using a balloon that is inflated within the narrowed valve; however, the natural valve is not replaced, which eliminates option 2. Although the mitral valve can be replaced endoscopically, the approach would not require opening the chest, thus eliminating option 3. Option 4 can be eliminated because it describes aspects of percutaneous transluminal coronary artery bypass. Option 1 remains as the correct answer, because the traditional method for replacing the mitral valve involves opening the heart while blood is circulated using a heart–lung machine. Review techniques for surgically replacing the mitral valve if you had difficulty answering this question.
Cognitive Level—*Applying*
Client Needs Category—*Physiological integrity*
Client Needs Subcategory—*Physiological adaptation*

104. 2. Ensuring adequate rest between routine self-care activities (such as bathing, oral hygiene, and ambulation) helps the client adapt to activity intolerance. Administering oxygen is appropriate to prevent hypoxemia, but it does not reduce energy expenditure. Analgesics help relieve pain, but they do not relieve shortness of breath. Visits from family and friends are likely to tire the client. However, because most clients benefit from the emotional support of signifi-

cant others, restricting the client's visitors would not be the first intervention implemented to reduce energy expenditure.
Test Taking Strategy—Use the process of elimination to help select the option that identifies the best method for reducing the client's energy expenditure postoperatively. Recall that staggering activities (option 2) will not tax the client's stamina and endurance as much as clustering the activities into a short amount of time. Review techniques for combating activity intolerance if you had difficulty answering this question.
Cognitive Level—*Applying*
Client Needs Category—*Physiological integrity*
Client Needs Subcategory—*Basic care and comfort*

105. 3. Evidence of activity intolerance includes rapid or irregular heart rate, hypotension, chest pain, dyspnea, and severe fatigue. If any of these are noted, the nurse is correct in limiting further activity. An improved appetite, restful sleep, and the ability to get out of bed without assistance are all positive signs, but they are not appropriate physiological criteria of a person's ability to tolerate activity.
Test Taking Strategy—Use the process of elimination to help select the option that provides the best evidence that the client is tolerating the activity involved in getting out of bed. Option 3 is the correct choice, because the heart rate generally increases to oxygenate tissues required for movement and exercise. A stable heart rate indicates that the energy is commensurate with the current level of oxygen supplied to tissues. Review homeostatic mechanisms that compensate for activities that exceed a client's tolerance if you had difficulty answering this question.
Cognitive Level—*Applying*
Client Needs Category—*Physiological integrity*
Client Needs Subcategory—*Reduction of risk potential*

106. 3. When a client is emotionally upset, it is most therapeutic to allow an opportunity to express feelings. Saying nothing or leaving the room is of little help because these actions are not supportive. In this case, the client is not unhappy with the food. Rather, the client is displacing anger and frustration onto an inanimate object. Finding out the food preferences avoids dealing with the emotional issues.
Test Taking Strategy—Apply the key words "most appropriate" when considering the actions described in the four options. Select the option that identifies the best nursing action for responding to the client's emotional outburst. Recall that listening (option 3) while the client verbalizes may help reduce the underlying cause of the client's distress. Review techniques for helping a client cope with disappointment and frustration if you had difficulty answering this question.
Cognitive Level—*Applying*
Client Needs Category—*Psychosocial integrity*
Client Needs Subcategory—*None*

107. 3. Clubbing of the fingertips is a physical change that occurs after years of poor oxygenation. It is found in people with long-term cardiopulmonary diseases. As the name suggests, the fingertips appear like clubs; they are wider than normal at the distal end. The angle at the base of the nail is greater than the normal 160 degrees. A barrel-shaped chest is most common in clients with chronic obstructive pulmonary disease. Flushed facial skin is seen in clients who are feverish or have hypertension or excess blood volume. Chest pain is a sign of impaired tissue oxygenation. It is not usually associated with chronic cardiac disease.

Test Taking Strategy—Apply the key words "most frequently" when looking for the option that identifies an assessment finding that occurs among clients with chronic cardiac disease. Recall that a chronic decrease in tissue oxygenation leads to an increased growth of fibrous tissue between the nail and distal portion of each digit, leading to a clubbed appearance (option 3) and subsequently alters the normal angle between the nail and the nail bed. Review the signs of chronic cardiac and pulmonary diseases if you had difficulty answering this question.
Cognitive Level—Applying
Client Needs Category—Physiological integrity
Client Needs Subcategory—Physiological adaptation

Nursing Care of Clients with Infectious and Inflammatory Disorders of the Heart

108. 3. A fever, one of the primary ways that the body fights an infection, tends to destroy or inhibit the growth and reproduction of microorganisms. Chemicals present in white blood cells, which fight infection, trigger a heat-producing response in the hypothalamus. Chest pain is usually caused by inadequate blood supply to the myocardium. Pneumonia is more likely to cause a moist cough. Dyspnea is a common finding in many cardiopulmonary diseases.

Test Taking Strategy—Use the process of elimination to help select the option that identifies the best evidence that a client has acquired a bacterial infection. Option 1 can be eliminated because chest pain is more likely due to myocardial ischemia. Options 2 and 4 can be eliminated because they could be due to a pulmonary infection rather than endocarditis. Option 3 remains as the correct answer because a fever is a common occurrence regardless of the location of an infection. Review clinical manifestations of an infectious process if you had difficulty answering this question.
Cognitive Level—Applying
Client Needs Category—Physiological integrity
Client Needs Subcategory—Physiological adaptation

109. 2. To enhance the ability to hear auscultated sounds, it is best to reduce or eliminate noise sources in the room, in this case the television. To auscultate the anterior, posterior, and lateral aspects of the chest, it is best for the client to be in a sitting position. Holding the breath may aggravate the client's already-compromised ventilation and would make assessment of lung sounds impossible. Locating the xiphoid process will not promote the auscultation of heart or breath sounds.

Test Taking Strategy—Apply the key words "most appropriate" when evaluating the choices in the four options. Select the option that enhances the assessment of heart and breath sounds better than any of the other choices. Recall that reducing noise within the environment (option 2) helps when attempting to identify and discriminate among heart and breath sounds. Review the technique for auscultating cardiac and breath sounds if you had difficulty answering this question.
Cognitive Level—Remembering
Client Needs Category—Physiological integrity
Client Needs Subcategory—Reduction of risk potential

110. 1. Fainting indicates that the volume of blood ejected from the left ventricle is inadequate to keep the brain oxygenated. Reduced stroke volume is also manifested by hypotension, tachycardia, and a weak pulse, which makes the other options inaccurate.

Test Taking Strategy—Use the process of elimination to help select the option that identifies the best evidence of reduced cardiac stroke volume. Option 2 can be eliminated because hypotension, not hypertension, is associated with reduced stroke volume. Option 3 can be eliminated because a slow heart rate allows greater cardiac filling, which promotes a normal or increased stroke volume. Option 4 can be eliminated because a bounding pulse, which is strong and forceful, is more likely detected when a client is anxious, has a fever, is exercising, or has excess circulating fluid. Option 1 remains as the correct answer because fainting indicates less than adequate blood flow to the brain. If you had difficulty answering the question, review the definition of cardiac stroke volume and the consequences if it is decreased.
Cognitive Level—Applying
Client Needs Category—Physiological integrity
Client Needs Subcategory—Physiological adaptation

111. 4. Fear of death is often a cause for increased anxiety in clients who undergo transplantation. Allowing the client to verbalize fears about death or concerns regarding personal finances, employment, length of rehabilitation, sexual performance, or immunosuppressive therapy helps decrease anxiety so that learning can take place. If the client's anxiety escalates to the point where the client is out of control, requesting an order for a sedative or hypnotic would be appropriate. Providing a video is inappropriate because there is no way to evaluate whether the client has learned anything. Also, the video may provide too much material to comprehend or be too graphic, causing further anxiety. Certainly the spouse should be included in the discussions about the procedure and length of rehabilitation. However, having the spouse at the bedside may not lessen the client's anxiety. Therefore, this choice is not the best option.

> ***Test Taking Strategy***—*Apply the key words "most appropriate" when discriminating among the four options. Select the option that describes the nursing action that is best for dealing with an anxious client preoperatively. Recall that providing an opportunity for the client to share fears (option 4) is a therapeutic measure for reducing anxiety. Review nursing techniques for relieving anxiety and fear if you had difficulty answering this question.*
> ***Cognitive Level***—*Applying*
> ***Client Needs Category***—*Psychosocial integrity*
> ***Client Needs Subcategory***—*None*

112. 2. Because the client has had a heart transplant, assessing urine output is a good indicator of the heart's ability to pump and perfuse the kidneys. Monitoring intake and output also helps the nurse determine whether the client has a fluid volume overload or deficit. Usually, recipients who undergo heart transplantation are fluid-restricted until their condition stabilizes; therefore, fluids are monitored. Hemoglobin values and hematocrit are used to help determine when the client needs transfusions. Urine retention is not common.

> ***Test Taking Strategy***—*Use the process of elimination to help select the option that identifies the best rationale for frequently assessing the client's fluid status postoperatively. Option 1 can be eliminated because clients are more likely to have a normal, but*

minimum, circulatory volume to reduce the workload on the new heart. Option 3 can be eliminated because the need for a transfusion is based on laboratory blood values. Option 4 has some merit, but option 2 is the best answer because an adequately pumping heart perfuses the kidneys, which in turn maintains fluid balance. Review the correlation between kidney function and heart function if you had difficulty answering this question.
> ***Cognitive Level***—*Applying*
> ***Client Needs Category***—*Physiological integrity*
> ***Client Needs Subcategory***—*Physiological adaptation*

113. 4. Primary nursing is a model for delivering nursing care in which one nurse individually manages assigned clients' care for the entire shift. Typically, the nurse is assigned a small group of clients, depending on the acuity and needs of the clients. All nursing care delivery models require the nurse to work as part of a multidisciplinary team and be a liaison for the family and physician. A group of nursing personnel that collectively care for a group of clients is a characteristic of a team nursing model. Case management is a delivery care model in which a nurse plans and coordinates the progress of clients through various phases of care to avoid delays, unnecessary testing, and overuse of expensive resources.

> ***Test Taking Strategy***—*Use the process of elimination to identify the key component of primary nursing. Note the word "primary" which indicates a responsibility of care by one nurse. Also, eliminate standards of care which all nursing delivery systems require. Review the components of primary care nursing if you had difficulty answering this question.*
> ***Cognitive Level***—*Applying*
> ***Client Needs Category***—*Safe and effective care environment*
> ***Client Needs Subcategory***—*Coordinated care*

The Nursing Care of Clients with Peripheral Vascular, Hematologic, and Lymphatic Disorders

■ Nursing Care of Clients with Venous Disorders
■ Nursing Care of Clients with Arterial Disorders
■ Nursing Care of Clients with Red Blood Cell Disorders
■ Nursing Care of Clients with White Blood Cell Disorders
■ Nursing Care of Clients with Bone Marrow Disorders
■ Nursing Care of Clients with Coagulation Disorders
■ Nursing Care of Clients with Inflammatory and Obstructive Lymphatic Disorders
■ Correct Answers, Rationales, and Test Taking Strategies

Directions: *With a pencil, blacken the space in front of the option you have chosen for your correct answer.*

Nursing Care of Clients with Venous Disorders

While helping a client onto the examination table, the nurse notes that the client has several large protruding leg veins.

1. Which risk factor revealed in the client's health history is most closely related to the development of varicose veins?
[ ] **1.** The client's mother also has varicose veins.
[ ] **2.** The client has smoked cigarettes for 20 years.
[ ] **3.** The client was a track athlete in high school.
[ ] **4.** The client is a 50-year-old corporate executive.

2. Which complaint made by the client to the nurse can best be attributed to varicose leg veins?
[ ] **1.** "My legs ache and feel tired after standing."
[ ] **2.** "My feet perspire heavily during the day."
[ ] **3.** "I wake up at night with a restless feeling in my legs."
[ ] **4.** "I have pain in my shins when I jog."

3. Which nursing instruction is most beneficial in helping relieve the client's symptoms caused by varicose veins?
[ ] **1.** Elevate your legs frequently during the day.
[ ] **2.** Keep the room temperature above 70°F (21°C).
[ ] **3.** Massage your calves when experiencing leg cramps.
[ ] **4.** Modify your lifestyle to include sedentary activities.

4. As the nurse provides discharge instructions to the client with varicose veins, which activity should the nurse suggest the client avoid?
[ ] **1.** Walking in athletic shoes.
[ ] **2.** Jogging a mile a day.
[ ] **3.** Sitting with crossed knees.
[ ] **4.** Wearing wool socks.

The client is scheduled for a ligation and vein-stripping procedure as treatment for varicose veins. After the surgeon explains the procedure, the client asks the nurse how the blood in the lower legs will circulate after surgery.

5. Which response by the nurse about blood circulation is most appropriate?
[ ] **1.** Some of the arteries begin to function as veins.
[ ] **2.** New veins grow to replace the ones that were removed.
[ ] **3.** Other veins take over the work of those removed.
[ ] **4.** The healthy vein ends are attached to other veins.

6. When the nurse is planning the client's postoperative care, which action is the highest priority?
[ ] **1.** Providing the client with protein-rich foods
[ ] **2.** Ambulating the client frequently
[ ] **3.** Monitoring for wound infection
[ ] **4.** Assessing for frequent leg cramping

Postoperatively, the client asks the nurse for pain medication. The physician orders ibuprofen (Motrin), 200 mg P.O. every 4 to 6 hours as needed for pain.

7. When offered the pain medication, the client says to the nurse, "If that's Motrin, I don't want it. It makes me sick to my stomach." What is the most appropriate nursing action at this time?

[ ] **1.** Tell the client that the drug is ibuprofen.
[ ] **2.** Explain that the prescribed medication must be taken.
[ ] **3.** Advise the client to take the drug with plenty of water.
[ ] **4.** Report the information to the charge nurse.

A 67-year-old client has developed venous stasis ulcers on the lower leg.

8. When assessing the client's lower leg, which findings characteristic of venous stasis ulcers is the nurse most likely to find? Select all that apply.

[ ] **1.** Purulent drainage from lesions
[ ] **2.** Blanched patches around open areas
[ ] **3.** Dark brown, dry, and crusty skin
[ ] **4.** Fluid-filled blisters
[ ] **5.** Edema in the lower legs
[ ] **6.** Fine red rash below the knee

The nurse caring for the client develops a nursing care plan.

9. When planning nursing care, which nursing intervention is most essential in promoting venous circulation?

[ ] **1.** Offer the client an analgesic for pain.
[ ] **2.** Apply elastic compression stockings.
[ ] **3.** Maintain a fluid intake of at least 2,500 mL.
[ ] **4.** Apply a heating pad to the lower extremity.

10. A client returns to the wound clinic for evaluation of a stasis ulcer. Which nursing observation confirms healing progress?

[ ] **1.** The wound is smaller, and more drainage is present.
[ ] **2.** The wound is smaller, and the client has less discomfort.
[ ] **3.** The wound is smaller, and the cavity appears pink.
[ ] **4.** The wound is smaller, and the margin is white.

The nurse covers the client's leg ulcer with a type of air-occlusive dressing.

11. The nurse informs the client that which of the following is the main advantage of this type of dressing?

[ ] **1.** It will reduce the formation of scar tissue.
[ ] **2.** It will relieve pain from skin irritation.
[ ] **3.** It will be less expensive than gauze dressings.
[ ] **4.** It will speed healing by keeping the wound moist.

12. Which of the following clients are at high risk for acquiring gangrene of the foot? Select all that apply.

[ ] **1.** An insulin-dependent diabetic client
[ ] **2.** An elderly man with impaired circulation
[ ] **3.** A woman who experiences trauma to the toes
[ ] **4.** A homeless person who has osteoarthritis
[ ] **5.** A client who is taking warfarin (Coumadin)
[ ] **6.** A client with a history of myocardial infarction

A nurse gathers admission history from a 57-year-old client who is scheduled to have abdominal surgery.

13. Which risk factors associated with thrombophlebitis should the nurse discuss with the physician? Select all that apply.

[ ] **1.** The client weighs 350 pounds (159 kg).
[ ] **2.** The client smokes two packs of cigarettes per day.
[ ] **3.** The client has been on bed rest due to heart failure.
[ ] **4.** The client complains of leg fatigue.
[ ] **5.** The client complains of cramping in the lower leg at night.
[ ] **6.** The client complains of pain in the joints.

The client is recovering from abdominal surgery that was performed 2 days earlier.

14. Upon nursing assessment, which finding is most likely to predispose this client to developing venous thrombosis in a lower extremity?

[ ] **1.** The client resists ambulation.
[ ] **2.** The client breathes shallowly.
[ ] **3.** The client requests analgesics frequently.
[ ] **4.** The client drinks coffee excessively.

The care plan indicates that the client should wear antiembolism stockings.

15. What is the best evidence that the prescribed antiembolism stockings are a correct size and fit for this client?

[ ] **1.** The stockings extend to midcalf.
[ ] **2.** The toes feel warm when touched.
[ ] **3.** The stockings are easily donned.
[ ] **4.** The heels are not reddened.

16. When the nurse assesses the client for Homans' sign, which technique is most accurate?

[ ] **1.** Have the client push each foot against the mattress.
[ ] **2.** Have the client extend the legs and flex each foot toward the head.
[ ] **3.** Ask the client to sit up in bed and point all the toes forward.
[ ] **4.** Ask the client to contract the thigh muscles.

17. If the client develops a thrombus in one of the leg veins, which client response would the nurse expect when eliciting Homans' sign?

[ ] **1.** Sharp, immediate calf pain
[ ] **2.** Sudden numbness in the foot
[ ] **3.** Inability to bend the knee when asked
[ ] **4.** Tingling throughout the affected leg

18. Aside from a positive Homans' sign, which additional assessment finding best supports the assumption that the client has a thrombus in a leg vein?
[ ] **1.** The foot on the affected leg is blue.
[ ] **2.** The affected leg is warmer than the other.
[ ] **3.** The capillary refill takes 2 seconds.
[ ] **4.** The lower affected leg is swollen.

On the basis of data collection, the client has been diagnosed with thrombophlebitis and is being treated with subcutaneous injections of heparin.

19. Which modification is most appropriate to add to the client's care plan at this time?
[ ] **1.** Ambulate twice each shift.
[ ] **2.** Massage the leg toward the heart.
[ ] **3.** Avoid elevating the client's legs.
[ ] **4.** Discourage active leg exercises.

The physician prescribes warm moist compresses to the affected leg.

20. Which nursing action is most appropriate when applying the warm moist compress?
[ ] **1.** Heating the water to 120°F (48.8°C)
[ ] **2.** Using sterile technique
[ ] **3.** Inspecting the skin every 4 hours
[ ] **4.** Covering the wet gauze with a towel

The physician orders heparin sodium 7,500 units subcutaneously.

21. Based on the physician's order, use the information on the drug label below to calculate the amount of heparin to administer to the client.

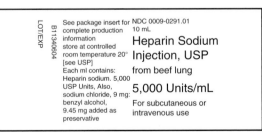

22. When the client wants to know why the physician prescribed this medication, which response by the nurse is correct?
[ ] **1.** "Heparin helps shrink blood clots."
[ ] **2.** "Heparin helps dissolve blood clots."
[ ] **3.** "Heparin prevents more clots from forming."
[ ] **4.** "Heparin prevents the clot from dislodging."

23. Which laboratory value should the nurse report to the physician before giving the heparin sodium injection?
[ ] **1.** Partial thromboplastin time (PTT)
[ ] **2.** Complete blood count (CBC)
[ ] **3.** Hemoglobin (Hb)
[ ] **4.** Prothrombin time (PT)

24. When the nurse withdraws the heparin sodium from the multidose vial, which technique is correct?
[ ] **1.** Remove the rubber stopper on the top of the vial.
[ ] **2.** Instill an equal volume of air as liquid to be withdrawn.
[ ] **3.** Mix the drug by rolling it between the palms.
[ ] **4.** Shake the drug vigorously to promote even distribution.

25. If the client is of average weight for the height, which action by the nurse is most appropriate when administering the heparin sodium subcutaneously?
[ ] **1.** Selecting the dorsogluteal site
[ ] **2.** Using a 22-gauge 1½" needle
[ ] **3.** Inserting the needle at a 45-degree angle
[ ] **4.** Massaging the site immediately afterward

26. Which assessment finding, noted several days after initiation of the client's daily heparin sodium injections, should be reported immediately to the physician?
[ ] **1.** The client develops abdominal tenderness.
[ ] **2.** The client notes tiny abdominal bruising from the needles.
[ ] **3.** The client's gums bleed after tooth brushing.
[ ] **4.** The client's stools are soft and light brown in color.

27. Which drug should the nurse plan to have available in case it becomes necessary to counteract the effects of heparin therapy?
[ ] **1.** Calcium lactate
[ ] **2.** Sodium benzoate
[ ] **3.** Protamine sulfate
[ ] **4.** Aluminum phosphate

A new graduate nurse applies prolonged pressure to the injection site of a client who is receiving anticoagulant therapy.

28. Which of the following is an accurate analysis of the nurse's action when performed after administering the injection to a client who is concurrently receiving heparin?
[ ] **1.** Prolonged pressure to the injection site is inappropriate as it promotes hematoma formation.
[ ] **2.** Prolonged pressure to the injection site is inappropriate because it delays drug absorption.
[ ] **3.** Prolonged pressure to the injection site is correct because it distributes the drug evenly.
[ ] **4.** Prolonged pressure to the injection site is correct because it diminishes blood loss.

The nurse prepares the client's discharge instructions. The client will continue to take warfarin (Coumadin) on a daily basis.

29. Which statement offers the best evidence that this client understands the risk for bleeding?

[ ] **1.** "I'll need to report having dark amber urine."
[ ] **2.** "I must report having tar-colored stools."
[ ] **3.** "I'll call the physician if I have green-tinged emesis."
[ ] **4.** "I'll call the physician if my skin looks yellow."

30. The nurse explains to the client that, because of taking warfarin (Coumadin), the client should avoid eating foods containing large amounts of vitamin K. Which foods should the client limit? Select all that apply.

[ ] **1.** Fresh spinach
[ ] **2.** Lettuce
[ ] **3.** Turnip greens
[ ] **4.** Brussels sprouts
[ ] **5.** Peas
[ ] **6.** Corn

31. The client asks the nurse if it is safe to resume taking dietary supplements and herbal medications after discharge. The nurse responds that much is unknown about dietary supplements and explores the types and dosages of these supplements. Considering the client's condition and medication regimen, which dietary supplements are likely to alter the client's International Normalized Ratio (INR) and prothrombin time (PT)? Select all that apply.

[ ] **1.** Gingko
[ ] **2.** St. John's wort
[ ] **3.** Willow bark
[ ] **4.** Ginger
[ ] **5.** Green tea
[ ] **6.** Creatine

A postoperative client has been receiving I.V. fluids through the same site for several days.

32. Which finding would the nurse expect to document if the client begins developing phlebitis at the I.V. site?

[ ] **1.** The vein is red and feels warm.
[ ] **2.** The vein looks dark and feels cool.
[ ] **3.** The vein is pale and feels hard.
[ ] **4.** The vein looks purplish and feels spongy.

33. What is the first nursing action to take when phlebitis at an I.V. site is suspected?

[ ] **1.** Elevate the affected extremity on pillows.
[ ] **2.** Apply pressure to the I.V. insertion site.
[ ] **3.** Administer the I.V. solution at a faster rate.
[ ] **4.** Remove the needle or catheter from the current site.

Nursing Care of Clients with Arterial Disorders

A 75-year-old client in a nursing home has arteriosclerosis.

34. Which assessment findings is the nurse most likely to observe when examining a client with arterial insufficiency secondary to peripheral arteriosclerosis? Select all that apply.

[ ] **1.** Thick, tough toenails
[ ] **2.** Flushed skin
[ ] **3.** Hyperactive knee jerk reflexes
[ ] **4.** Bounding peripheral pulses
[ ] **5.** Thin shiny skin
[ ] **6.** Decreased leg hair

35. Which sign or symptom would the nurse document when the client with arteriosclerosis actively exercises?

[ ] **1.** Cyanosis of the feet
[ ] **2.** Burning of the toes
[ ] **3.** Pain in both legs
[ ] **4.** Edema formation in the ankles

36. Which nursing intervention would be most appropriate if the client experiences cold feet as a result of impaired circulation?

[ ] **1.** Applying a commercial heat packet
[ ] **2.** Using an electric heating pad
[ ] **3.** Wrapping the feet in a warm blanket
[ ] **4.** Elevating the feet on a stool

The nurse prepares to use a Doppler ultrasound device to assess blood flow through the client's dorsalis pedis artery.

37. Place an *X* over the location where the nurse should place the Doppler ultrasound device.

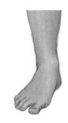

38. Which nursing technique is correct when using the Doppler device to assess the client's blood flow?

[ ] **1.** The nurse places the probe beside the ankle.
[ ] **2.** The nurse applies acoustic gel to the skin.
[ ] **3.** The nurse records the time of capillary refill.
[ ] **4.** The nurse measures the temperature of the skin.

A 36-year-old client with a 7-year history of Raynaud's disease comes to donate blood during a community blood drive.

39. Considering the client's diagnosis, in which part of the body would the nurse expect the client's symptoms to be chiefly located?
[ ] **1.** Legs
[ ] **2.** Hands
[ ] **3.** Chest
[ ] **4.** Neck

40. Which factor is the client with Raynaud's disease most likely to correlate with the onset of the discomfort?
[ ] **1.** Exposure to heat
[ ] **2.** Exposure to cold
[ ] **3.** Exposure to sun
[ ] **4.** Exposure to wind

41. When preparing this client's teaching plan, the nurse should include information on the importance of avoiding which one of the following?
[ ] **1.** Wearing gloves
[ ] **2.** Emotional stress
[ ] **3.** Drinking alcoholic beverages
[ ] **4.** Bathing with perfumed soap

A 32-year-old client has been diagnosed with thromboangiitis obliterans, also known as Buerger's disease.

42. When reviewing the health history, which early symptom of thromboangiitis obliterans would be identified in the record?
[ ] **1.** A heavy feeling in the lower extremities
[ ] **2.** Frequent problems with ingrown toenails
[ ] **3.** Leg pain accompanying walking or exercise
[ ] **4.** Swollen feet at the end of the day

43. While palpating the peripheral pulses in the lower extremities, the nurse would anticipate documenting which pulse characteristic?
[ ] **1.** Strong
[ ] **2.** Normal
[ ] **3.** Full
[ ] **4.** Weak

The nurse teaches the client how to perform Buerger-Allen exercises.

44. The nurse observes that the client performs the exercises correctly when the client lies flat with the legs elevated for several minutes and then performs which action?
[ ] **1.** Sits on the edge of the bed
[ ] **2.** Stands and touches the toes
[ ] **3.** Jogs in place at the bedside
[ ] **4.** Pretends to climb stairs

45. When preparing discharge instructions, what activity should the nurse warn the client with Buerger's disease to avoid?
[ ] **1.** Heavy lifting
[ ] **2.** Tobacco use
[ ] **3.** Airplane travel
[ ] **4.** Sexual activity

Abdominal X-rays reveal that a resident of a long-term care facility has an abdominal aortic aneurysm.

46. Which assessment findings, documented by the nurse in the client's history, are significant factors placing the client at risk for an abdominal aortic aneurysm? Select all that apply.
[ ] **1.** The client has type 1 diabetes mellitus.
[ ] **2.** The client has chronic hypertension.
[ ] **3.** The client has a sedentary lifestyle.
[ ] **4.** The client takes digoxin (Lanoxin).
[ ] **5.** The client is 80 years old.
[ ] **6.** The client smokes 2 packs of cigarettes per day.

47. During the client's physical examination, which assessment finding would the nurse expect to be most evident of the abdominal aortic aneurysm?
[ ] **1.** Edema of the feet
[ ] **2.** Hypoactive bowel sounds
[ ] **3.** Multiple abdominal petechiae
[ ] **4.** Pulsating abdominal mass

48. Which statement, made by the client to the nurse, shows an accurate understanding of the client's condition?
[ ] **1.** "An aneurysm is a weakened valve in the abdominal aorta."
[ ] **2.** "An aneurysm is a stationary blood clot in the abdominal vein."
[ ] **3.** "An aneurysm is a fatty deposit in the aorta wall."
[ ] **4.** "An aneurysm is an outpouching in the wall of the abdominal aorta."

The client refuses surgical treatment and wishes to stay in the long-term care facility.

49. Which symptom is the client most likely to exhibit if the aneurysm becomes larger or begins to dissect?
[ ] **1.** Hematuria
[ ] **2.** Indigestion
[ ] **3.** Rectal bleeding
[ ] **4.** Lower back pain

Several years ago, the client prepared an advance directive indicating that no heroic measures were to be performed to sustain life. At that time, the physician wrote a "do not resuscitate" (allow natural death) order.

50. If the client loses consciousness and remains unresponsive when the abdominal aortic aneurysm ruptures, which nursing action is most appropriate?
[ ] **1.** Have the client transferred to the hospital.
[ ] **2.** Call the local ambulance service.
[ ] **3.** Notify the attending physician.
[ ] **4.** Call the client's next of kin.

Nursing Care of Clients with Red Blood Cell Disorders

The complete blood count (CBC) of a 71-year-old client indicates that the erythrocytes are below normal.

51. Which of the following conditions most likely explains the client's reduced red blood cell count?
[ ] **1.** Mitral valve insufficiency
[ ] **2.** Arteriosclerotic heart disease
[ ] **3.** Peptic ulcer disease
[ ] **4.** Prostatic hypertrophy

52. Once the underlying cause of the client's low red blood cell count is treated, which nursing intervention is most appropriate for reducing the fatigue?
[ ] **1.** Advising the client to get at least 8 hours of sleep
[ ] **2.** Having the client exercise twice a day
[ ] **3.** Instructing the client to eat more simple carbohydrates
[ ] **4.** Encouraging periods of rest between activity

An 18-year-old college student has been feeling extremely tired and makes an appointment at the university's health office.

53. Which laboratory test would the nurse expect to have a lower than normal result if the cause of the client's fatigue is related to iron deficiency anemia?
[ ] **1.** Epstein-Barr virus (EBV) titer
[ ] **2.** Thyroid-stimulating hormone (TSH)
[ ] **3.** Fibrinogen level
[ ] **4.** Hemoglobin (Hb) level

54. Which information provided by the client is most relevant to the diagnosis of anemia?
[ ] **1.** The client has chronic back pain.
[ ] **2.** The client experiences frequent headaches.
[ ] **3.** The client feels cold most of the time.
[ ] **4.** The client had rheumatic fever as a child.

When taking the client's dietary history, the nurse learns that the client has been skipping meals.

55. The elimination of which food group has most likely contributed to the client's iron deficiency anemia?
[ ] **1.** Milk
[ ] **2.** Meat
[ ] **3.** Fruit
[ ] **4.** Vegetables

The physician orders ferrous sulfate (Feosol) 10 mg/day orally for the client.

56. When the nurse teaches the client regarding this medication, what time is best to take the medication?
[ ] **1.** 2 hours after a meal
[ ] **2.** With any meal of choice
[ ] **3.** Just before eating a meal
[ ] **4.** At bedtime with a snack

57. To maximize the absorption of the iron supplement, the nurse correctly advises the client to take the tablet with which beverage?
[ ] **1.** Milk
[ ] **2.** Tea
[ ] **3.** Soft drink
[ ] **4.** Orange juice

58. If the client understands the nurse's explanation about the side effects of iron, the client will indicate that this drug causes stools to turn which color?
[ ] **1.** Medium brown
[ ] **2.** Dark black
[ ] **3.** Clay-colored
[ ] **4.** Light green

Three days after going to the clinic, the client phones the health office and explains that it is difficult to swallow the large iron capsule. The physician orders a liquid iron preparation.

59. When instructing the client about the administration of the liquid iron preparation, what information should the nurse provide?
[ ] **1.** Use a straw when taking liquid iron.
[ ] **2.** Drink the liquid iron from a paper cup.
[ ] **3.** Pour the liquid iron over crushed ice.
[ ] **4.** Mix the liquid iron with whole milk.

A 42-year-old client develops anemia, but the etiology is unknown at this time.

60. During the initial interview, what information provided by the client is most likely related to the client's anemia?
[ ] **1.** The client fainted last week at work.
[ ] **2.** The client has occasional headaches.
[ ] **3.** The client's gall bladder has been removed.
[ ] **4.** The client's abdomen is somewhat tender.

61. During the client's physical assessment, which skin assessment finding would the nurse expect to document?
[ ] **1.** The skin appears mottled.
[ ] **2.** The skin is flushed.
[ ] **3.** The skin is pale.
[ ] **4.** The skin has a blue tinge.

A 50-year-old client is suspected of having pernicious anemia. The client is hospitalized for symptom management and diagnostic purposes.

62. Which is the most appropriate question to ask this client while collecting the admission history?
[ ] **1.** "Was all or a portion of your stomach removed?"
[ ] **2.** "Have you ever had any type of hepatitis?"
[ ] **3.** "Were you ever informed of other anemias?"
[ ] **4.** "Do you have severe allergic reactions?"

63. Which of the following nursing entries is least pertinent to include in the documentation after the nurse's initial interview of the client?
[ ] **1.** Client states, "I get nauseated when I eat."
[ ] **2.** The client is currently uninsured.
[ ] **3.** The skin over the back and buttocks is flushed.
[ ] **4.** The client has asked to see a minister.

64. If the client develops neurologic symptoms related to pernicious anemia, the nurse would expect the client to report having which symptom?
[ ] **1.** Numbness and tingling in the extremities
[ ] **2.** Morning headaches and sudden dizziness
[ ] **3.** Restlessness and sleep pattern disturbances
[ ] **4.** Periods of temporary amnesia and fainting

The physician orders a Schilling test for the client.

65. When instructing the client on the proper procedure to obtain the necessary specimen, which specimen container is provided?
[ ] **1.** A large urine container
[ ] **2.** A sterile cup for sputum
[ ] **3.** A fecal collection device for the toilet
[ ] **4.** A vial to obtain a venous blood sample

The Schilling test confirms that the client has pernicious anemia.

66. When the client asks the nurse how the disorder will be treated, which response by the nurse is most appropriate?
[ ] **1.** "The physician will probably prescribe blood transfusions."
[ ] **2.** "The physician will most likely prescribe iron medication."
[ ] **3.** "The physician will probably prescribe vitamin B$_{12}$ injections."
[ ] **4.** "The physician will probably prescribe vitamin K injections."

A 30-year-old client who is experiencing a sickle cell crisis is admitted to the hospital.

67. If this newly admitted client fits the profile of people in the United States with sickle cell anemia, the nurse would expect the client to be of which ethnic background?
[ ] **1.** Mexican American
[ ] **2.** Asian American
[ ] **3.** Native American
[ ] **4.** African American

68. During the admission assessment, which findings can the nurse attribute to the client's blood disease? Select all that apply.
[ ] **1.** The client's tongue is white.
[ ] **2.** The client's urine is cloudy.
[ ] **3.** The client is jaundiced.
[ ] **4.** The client is nauseated.
[ ] **5.** The client has pain.
[ ] **6.** The client is short of breath.

69. Which nursing intervention is the nurse's priority during the client's sickle cell crisis?
[ ] **1.** Improving nutrition
[ ] **2.** Controlling pain
[ ] **3.** Assisting ventilation
[ ] **4.** Relieving anxiety

70. If the nurse observes that the client's knee is edematous, which nursing measure is most appropriate to add to the care plan at this time?
[ ] **1.** Help the client to perform passive range-of-motion exercises.
[ ] **2.** Assist the client in changing positions to achieve comfort.
[ ] **3.** Ambulate the client at frequent intervals during the day.
[ ] **4.** Encourage the client to perform quadriceps-setting exercises.

The nurse is identifying nursing interventions for the nursing diagnosis, altered tissue perfusion.

71. Which nursing intervention is best for maintaining tissue perfusion during a sickle cell crisis?
[ ] **1.** Providing the client with a large quantity of fluids
[ ] **2.** Assisting the client with applying thigh-high elastic stockings
[ ] **3.** Elevating the client's lower extremities
[ ] **4.** Having the client dangle the legs over the side of the bed

The nurse reviews the hereditary implications and precipitating factors of sickle cell anemia with the client.

72. The nurse teaches the client that the sickle cell crisis was most likely triggered by which precipitating factors? Select all that apply.
[ ] **1.** Low blood glucose level
[ ] **2.** Fatigue
[ ] **3.** Overexertion
[ ] **4.** Overhydration
[ ] **5.** Fever
[ ] **6.** Smoking

73. When the client asks the nurse to elaborate on the significance of having the sickle cell trait, which response is best?
[ ] **1.** "People with sickle cell trait manifest the disease later in life."
[ ] **2.** "People with sickle cell trait have a milder form of disease symptoms."
[ ] **3.** "People with sickle cell trait do not develop symptoms of the disease."
[ ] **4.** "People with sickle cell trait have a much shorter life expectancy."

Nursing Care of Clients with White Blood Cell Disorders

A nurse caring for a 70-year-old client with chronic leukemia suspects that the client has an infection.

74. Which assessment finding by the nurse supports the possibility that the client has an infection?
[ ] 1. Blood in the stool
[ ] 2. Prolonged vomiting
[ ] 3. Cloudy urine
[ ] 4. Extreme fatigue

The nurse notes that the client's mouth bleeds after brushing the teeth.

75. Which alternative form of oral care is most appropriate at this time?
[ ] 1. Use foam mouth swabs.
[ ] 2. Use only dental floss.
[ ] 3. Use an antiseptic mouthwash.
[ ] 4. Eliminate the use of toothpaste.

76. When assisting the client with selecting foods from the menu, which food choice should the nurse suggest?
[ ] 1. Spaghetti with meatballs
[ ] 2. Grilled cheese sandwich
[ ] 3. Salad with French dressing
[ ] 4. Creamed potato soup

The client receives antineoplastic drugs to treat the leukemia.

77. The nurse provides client instruction on which common side effect of the medication therapy?
[ ] 1. Hair loss
[ ] 2. Rash
[ ] 3. Constipation
[ ] 4. Headaches

In addition to an abnormally low white blood cell count, laboratory test results indicate that the client has a platelet count of 75,000/mm³.

78. On the basis of the client's laboratory results, which nursing intervention is most appropriate at this time?
[ ] 1. Limiting the client's visitors to family
[ ] 2. Instituting neutropenic precautions
[ ] 3. Using small-gauge needles for injections
[ ] 4. Providing rest periods between activities

Several weeks later, the physician informs the client that the leukemia is in remission.

79. Which client statement indicates an understanding of the term *remission*?
[ ] 1. "I will never need cancer treatment again."
[ ] 2. "I will need medications again in a few months."
[ ] 3. "My disease has responded to treatment."
[ ] 4. "My disease is cured at the present time."

Two years after the client's initial treatment, the client is hospitalized again. Although the client's condition is stable, the physician has informed the client and the family that the client will probably not survive for more than 6 months.

80. Which of the following is the best example of the nurse in the role of client advocate?
[ ] 1. The nurse allows the client to direct wishes for personal care.
[ ] 2. The nurse discusses hospice care with the client's family.
[ ] 3. The nurse supports the client's wishes to have no further invasive procedures.
[ ] 4. The nurse decorates the client's room with cards from friends and family.

A high school student contracts infectious mononucleosis.

81. When the student asks the school nurse to explain how the disease was acquired, the nurse correctly responds that the virus causing this disease is transmitted by which route?
[ ] 1. Contact with microorganisms in blood
[ ] 2. Direct contact with an infected person
[ ] 3. Consuming contaminated food or water
[ ] 4. Being bitten by a mosquito

82. When reviewing the student's recent health, which symptom does the client state as experiencing first?
[ ] 1. Abdominal discomfort
[ ] 2. Aching joints
[ ] 3. Sore throat
[ ] 4. Intestinal upset

83. Which information is essential for the nurse to address when discussing self-care with this client?
[ ] 1. Compliance with antibiotic therapy
[ ] 2. The need to restrict physical activity
[ ] 3. The importance of taking supplemental vitamins
[ ] 4. Follow-up blood transfusions

A 32-year-old client with a diagnosis of Hodgkin's disease is admitted to the hospital.

84. If this client is typical of most clients who develop Hodgkin's disease, the nurse would expect to note which characteristic findings during the initial client assessment? Select all that apply.
[ ] 1. Weight gain, especially around the midsection
[ ] 2. A large lymph node in the client's neck
[ ] 3. Frequent headaches
[ ] 4. Chronic diarrhea
[ ] 5. Fine red, raised rash
[ ] 6. Night sweats

85. If the physical assessment is performed during the early stages of this client's disease, how will the nurse document the appearance of lymph nodes?
[ ] 1. Enlarged and painless
[ ] 2. Small and firm
[ ] 3. Enlarged and painful
[ ] 4. Fixed and hard

The client is scheduled to undergo external radiation of the cervical and axillary lymph nodes.

86. On admission, the client informs the nurse about using daily herbal therapy as a routine health practice. Which one of the following nursing actions is most appropriate?
[ ] **1.** Determine if herbal therapy is part of a naturalistic therapy regimen.
[ ] **2.** Recommend that the client suspend herbal use until after radiation therapy.
[ ] **3.** Assess what substances are being used and notify the physician.
[ ] **4.** Disregard the information as herbs do not interfere with radiotherapy.

87. Which nursing instruction should be included in the teaching plan when preparing the client for radiation therapy?
[ ] **1.** "Avoid getting the skin wet around your neck and under your arms."
[ ] **2.** "Avoid using any deodorants containing aluminum hydroxide."
[ ] **3.** "Shave the hair from your neck and underarms daily."
[ ] **4.** "Apply zinc oxide ointment to the radiated area after each treatment."

88. Which response by the nurse is most appropriate when the client becomes concerned that the skin is reddened?
[ ] **1.** Explain to the client that this is an expected outcome with radiation.
[ ] **2.** Instruct the client that the heat from radiation causes vasodilation.
[ ] **3.** Inform the client that the redness indicates superficial bleeding.
[ ] **4.** Reassure the client that the redness is hardly noticeable.

The client will continue radiation treatment as an outpatient after discharge from the hospital.

89. Which nursing instruction about being in the outdoor environment is most important to include in the client's discharge plan?
[ ] **1.** Be sure to wear several layers of warm clothing when outside.
[ ] **2.** Avoid becoming chilled or too warm.
[ ] **3.** Wear a mask when outdoors to filter dust and pollen.
[ ] **4.** Protect your irradiated skin from sunlight.

A client with advanced non–Hodgkin's lymphoma is being treated with antineoplastic drugs to control the disease.

90. Which finding should the nurse report immediately because it indicates that the client requires neutropenic precautions?
[ ] **1.** Anorexia and weight loss
[ ] **2.** Frequent diarrhea
[ ] **3.** Low white blood cell count
[ ] **4.** Disorientation and confusion

The client's disease fails to respond to medical treatment. The nurse is present in the room when the physician tells the client that the condition is terminal.

91. Which nursing action is most helpful in assisting the client to deal with impending death?
[ ] **1.** Providing literature on death and dying
[ ] **2.** Allowing privacy to reflect on the news
[ ] **3.** Encouraging communication regarding feelings
[ ] **4.** Suggesting a second opinion by another physician

A 24-year-old client makes an appointment with a clinic physician because of unexplained weight loss. When obtaining the client's history, the nurse suspects that the client's signs and symptoms are suggestive of human immunodeficiency virus (HIV) infection.

92. Which of the following signs and symptoms would lead the nurse to suspect HIV infection? Select all that apply.
[ ] **1.** Cough
[ ] **2.** Fever
[ ] **3.** Diarrhea
[ ] **4.** Fatigue
[ ] **5.** A blemish on the face
[ ] **6.** Swollen lymph nodes in the axillae and groin

93. Which of the following instructions about safer sex practices are appropriate for the nurse to discuss with the client? Select all that apply.
[ ] **1.** Brush teeth after oral intercourse.
[ ] **2.** Reduce the number of sexual partners to one.
[ ] **3.** Do not reuse condoms.
[ ] **4.** Avoid anal intercourse.
[ ] **5.** Engage in nonpenetrating sexual activities.

94. Which situation would place this client at highest risk for acquired immunodeficiency syndrome (AIDS)?
[ ] **1.** Recent cardiovascular surgery (6 months ago)
[ ] **2.** Recent vacation in Africa
[ ] **3.** Excessive alcohol consumption
[ ] **4.** Intravenous drug use

The physician orders several laboratory tests because of suspected acquired immunodeficiency syndrome (AIDS).

95. The physician asks to be notified when confirmation of antibodies to the human immunodeficiency virus (HIV) status is detected. Which diagnostic test will the nurse cite when notifying the physician?
[ ] **1.** Schick test
[ ] **2.** Dick test
[ ] **3.** Enzyme-linked immunosorbent assay (ELISA)
[ ] **4.** Venereal Disease Research Laboratory (VDRL) test

96. How can the nurse be best protected from acquired immunodeficiency syndrome (AIDS) when caring for a client with an unknown infectious status?
[ ] **1.** Wear a face mask when changing dressings.
[ ] **2.** Refrain from capping needles after injections.
[ ] **3.** Wear a cover-gown when giving a bed bath.
[ ] **4.** Put on gloves before taking the client's vital signs.

A client with acquired immunodeficiency syndrome (AIDS) is admitted to the hospital with an opportunistic respiratory infection. The client's statements to the nurse imply a sense of hopelessness.

97. When planning care for this client, which approach is most therapeutic?
[ ] **1.** Encourage the client to set small, daily goals.
[ ] **2.** Refer the client to the hospital chaplain.
[ ] **3.** Provide distractions such as watching television.
[ ] **4.** Recommend that the next of kin be contacted.

Nursing Care of Clients with Bone Marrow Disorders

A client with polycythemia vera has an enlarged spleen.

98. Which position suggested by the nurse would promote the most comfort for this client?
[ ] **1.** Sitting upright
[ ] **2.** Supine
[ ] **3.** Lateral
[ ] **4.** Legs elevated

99. Which nursing action is most appropriate to prevent the formation of blood clots in the client?
[ ] **1.** Administering diuretics as ordered
[ ] **2.** Increasing the client's fluid intake
[ ] **3.** Restricting dietary sodium
[ ] **4.** Encouraging the client to lose weight

The physician informs the client that phlebotomy is required and explains the procedure.

100. When speaking with the nurse later that day, which statement by the client provides the best evidence that the client understood the physician's explanation about the upcoming procedure?
[ ] **1.** "Blood will be removed from my vein."
[ ] **2.** "I'll have tourniquets applied to my arms."
[ ] **3.** "Some veins will be surgically occluded."
[ ] **4.** "I'll receive a blood transfusion."

101. Which symptom should the nurse recognize as a consequence of the client's polycythemia vera?
[ ] **1.** Angina
[ ] **2.** Dyspepsia
[ ] **3.** Dysuria
[ ] **4.** Anorexia

The physician plans to perform a bone marrow aspiration on a 67-year-old client who has had unexplained low counts of all blood cell components. The physician suspects aplastic anemia.

102. After the nurse explains the anatomic location for bone marrow aspiration to the client, the client correctly identifies the site where the specimen will be taken by pointing to which part of the body?
[ ] **1.** The posterior hip
[ ] **2.** The lower spine
[ ] **3.** The upper arm
[ ] **4.** The groin area

103. The nurse is assisting the physician during the client's bone marrow aspiration. Which nursing responsibility, during the procedure, is a priority?
[ ] **1.** Minimizing discomfort
[ ] **2.** Holding instruments
[ ] **3.** Regulating suction
[ ] **4.** Administering oxygen

104. Following the bone marrow aspiration procedure, which nursing assessment is a priority?
[ ] **1.** Assess fluctuations in blood pressure readings
[ ] **2.** Assess pressure dressing for bleeding at puncture site
[ ] **3.** Assess changes in cardiac rate and rhythm
[ ] **4.** Assess for any change in level of consciousness

The results of the bone marrow aspiration confirm that the client has aplastic anemia.

105. When the client is bathing, which nursing observation provides the best indication that the client is having difficulty tolerating the current level of activity?
[ ] **1.** Shortness of breath
[ ] **2.** Extreme nausea
[ ] **3.** Pulse of 60 beats/minute
[ ] **4.** Moist and cool skin

The physician and nurse are reviewing the client's complete blood count. The physician highlights a significantly low red blood cell count, low white blood cell count, and low platelet count.

106. When the nurse is assessing and providing personal care to the client, which assessment finding is most related to the client's low platelet count?
[ ] **1.** Multiple bruises
[ ] **2.** Pale skin color
[ ] **3.** Elevated body temperature
[ ] **4.** Cool extremities

107. The nurse is instructing the nursing assistant of precautions needed when a client has a white blood count of 2.4 cells/cmm (cubic millimeter). Which nursing measure is most important?
[ ] **1.** Performing conscientious hand hygiene
[ ] **2.** Wearing a gown when providing care
[ ] **3.** Applying direct pressure on all puncture wounds
[ ] **4.** Obtaining vital signs every 4 hours

The physician tells the client that 2 units of packed blood cells will be administered. The client verbalizes concern about becoming human immunodeficiency syndrome (HIV) positive from receiving transfusions of publicly donated blood.

108. Which response by the nurse is the most appropriate response to the client's comment?
[ ] **1.** "Blood donors are tested for HIV before their blood is accepted."
[ ] **2.** "Donated blood no longer contains the HIV virus."
[ ] **3.** "Donated blood is tested for HIV antibodies after collection."
[ ] **4.** "There's no way to identify the AIDS virus in blood yet."

109. When the client asks how packed cells are different from the usual blood transfusion, which response by the nurse is most accurate?
[ ] **1.** Packed cells contain the same blood cells in less fluid volume.
[ ] **2.** Packed cells contain more blood cells in the same fluid volume.
[ ] **3.** Packed cells are less likely to cause an allergic reaction.
[ ] **4.** Packed cells will stimulate the client's bone marrow to function.

The client has type A, Rh-positive blood. The licensed practical nurse is delegated by the registered nurse to obtain the blood from the facility laboratory.

110. When checking the label on the blood, which blood type would the nurses identify as being incompatible?
[ ] **1.** Type A, Rh-negative
[ ] **2.** Type O, Rh-positive
[ ] **3.** Type O, Rh-negative
[ ] **4.** Type AB, Rh-positive

111. During the first 15 minutes of the infusion, which assessment finding strongly suggests that the client is experiencing a transfusion reaction?
[ ] **1.** The client feels an urgent need to urinate.
[ ] **2.** The client's blood pressure becomes low.
[ ] **3.** The client has localized swelling at the infusion site.
[ ] **4.** The client's skin is pale at the site of the infusion.

The client reports having received corticosteroid treatment for more than 1 year in an effort to treat the disease.

112. While the nurse examines the client, which assessment finding is most likely related to the administration of corticosteroids?
[ ] **1.** The client's voice is quite husky.
[ ] **2.** The client's face is moon shaped.
[ ] **3.** The client's muscles are large.
[ ] **4.** The client's skin looks tanned.

113. Which statement made by the client best supports the nurse's suspicion of a complication resulting from the use of corticosteroids?
[ ] **1.** "I've experienced heartburn lately."
[ ] **2.** "I've been taking long naps daily."
[ ] **3.** "I've lost my appetite for food."
[ ] **4.** "I've noticed my urine is light yellow."

Because corticosteroid therapy has not effectively treated the aplastic anemia, the client has consented to have a bone marrow transplant. The client undergoes total body irradiation.

114. What is the highest nursing priority for this client immediately before, and for several weeks after, the bone marrow transplantation?
[ ] **1.** Relieving depression
[ ] **2.** Promoting nutrition
[ ] **3.** Preventing infection
[ ] **4.** Monitoring hydration

Nursing Care of Clients with Coagulation Disorders

A physician examines a client with purpura and makes a tentative diagnosis of idiopathic thrombocytopenia.

115. On the basis of the diagnosis, which finding would the nurse expect to note during a physical assessment of this client?
[ ] **1.** Small skin hemorrhages
[ ] **2.** Dark areas of cyanosis
[ ] **3.** Flushed red skin
[ ] **4.** Protruding veins

116. When the nursing team meets to develop a care plan for the client, which of the following would be considered a nursing priority?
[ ] **1.** Encouraging fluids
[ ] **2.** Promoting activity
[ ] **3.** Restricting visitors
[ ] **4.** Preventing injury

A client with hemophilia experienced a minor closed-head injury. Before discharge, the nurse reviews the signs and symptoms that indicate bleeding.

117. The nurse assumes that the client understands the discharge instructions based on an ability to name which symptom as an early indicator of intracranial bleeding?
[ ] **1.** Seizures
[ ] **2.** Drowsiness
[ ] **3.** Ringing in the ears
[ ] **4.** Diminished appetite

Nursing Care of Clients with Inflammatory and Obstructive Lymphatic Disorders

A 78-year-old client has just been admitted to a long-term care facility with lymphedema of the right arm.

118. Which finding in the client's medical history most likely contributed to the development of the client's lymphedema?
[ ] **1.** The client has a healed fracture of the humerus.
[ ] **2.** The client had a radical mastectomy years ago.
[ ] **3.** The client is being treated for pernicious anemia.
[ ] **4.** The client was immunized for smallpox as a child.

119. Which intervention is essential to include in the client's care plan?
[ ] **1.** Avoid giving injections in the right arm.
[ ] **2.** Avoid turning the client on the right side.
[ ] **3.** Avoid active exercise of the right arm.
[ ] **4.** Avoid trimming the fingernails on the right hand.

Correct Answers, Rationales, and Test Taking Strategies

Nursing Care of Clients with Venous Disorders

1. 1. Varicose veins are swollen, twisted, purple or blue, bulging veins that are most commonly found in the legs or ankles. Heredity is a predisposing factor in the development of varicose veins. Other contributing factors include occupations that require prolonged standing or sitting such as cashiers, clerks, or beauticians; congenital weakness of the vein structure; obesity; female gender; use of hormones (oral contraceptives or hormone replacement therapy [HRT]); increasing age; and pressure on veins from an enlarging uterus during the later months of pregnancy. Although smoking is definitely unhealthy, nicotine has a major vasoconstricting effect on arterioles, not veins. An active lifestyle or athletic exercise is beneficial for the cardiovascular system and probably had little to do with the client developing varicose veins.

> *Test Taking Strategy—Use the process of elimination to help select the option that identifies the risk factor that is more closely associated with the development of varicose veins than the others. Recall that having a blood relative (option 1) with varicose veins is a predisposing factor for this disorder. Review the risk factors for varicose veins if you had difficulty answering this question.*
> *Cognitive Level—Analyzing*
> *Client Needs Category—Health promotion and maintenance*
> *Client Needs Subcategory—None*

2. 1. Most clients with varicose veins state that their legs ache and feel heavy and tired, especially after prolonged standing. Because the impaired circulation is most prominent when the client sits or stands for long periods of time, symptoms are usually relieved during the night, especially when elevating the feet, or by walking. Restless legs are not a common manifestation of varicose veins. Perspiration is not associated with varicose veins. Leg pain during activity is more likely to be caused by inadequate arterial blood flow or a sports-related injury.

> *Test Taking Strategy—Use the process of elimination to select the option that identifies the sign or symptom that can be attributed to having varicose veins. Recall that stasis of venous blood results in engorgement of blood vessels in the lower extremities, causing discomfort (option 1) that becomes more noticeable at the end of the day. Review the signs and symptoms associated with varicose veins if you had difficulty answering this question.*
> *Cognitive Level—Applying*
> *Client Needs Category—Physiological integrity*
> *Client Needs Subcategory—Physiological adaptation*

3. 1. Elevating the legs periodically during the day relieves symptoms associated with varicose veins. Other techniques that improve venous circulation, such as isometric or isotonic exercise, are also helpful. Keeping the room temperature above 70°F (21°C) does provide comfort, but it will not appreciably affect venous circulation. Because circulation is already impaired, massaging the legs is not recommended because of the possibility of dislodging a clot. Sitting for long periods of time, as in a sedentary lifestyle, does not promote venous circulation.

Test Taking Strategy—Apply the key words "most beneficial" when considering the choices in the four options. Select the option that identifies the best method for relieving the symptoms caused by varicose veins. Recall that elevating the legs (option 1) uses gravity to promote the flow of venous blood back to the heart. Review interventions that provide symptomatic relief for clients with varicose veins if you had difficulty answering this question.
Cognitive Level—Applying
Client Needs Category—Physiological integrity
Client Needs Subcategory—Physiological adaptation

4. 3. Clients with varicose veins must avoid anything that promotes venous stasis, such as sitting with crossed knees, standing for long periods of time, and wearing tight undergarments or knee-high stockings. Walking and jogging, which are best performed while wearing athletic shoes, promote circulation. Wool socks absorb foot perspiration and provide warmth, but they are not any more effective for improving venous circulation than socks made of other fibers. Wearing elastic support hose is beneficial.

Test Taking Strategy—Analyze to determine what information the question asks for, which is an action that should be avoided by a person who has varicose veins. Recall that crossing the legs at the knees (option 3) interferes with venous circulation. Review interventions that promote the transport of venous blood to the right side of the heart if you had difficulty answering this question.
Cognitive Level—Applying
Client Needs Category—Safe and effective care environment
Client Needs Subcategory—Coordinated care

5. 3. After a vein-stripping procedure, blood returns to the right side of the heart through other veins deeper in the leg. Arteries cannot transport both oxygenated and unoxygenated blood. New veins do not form as replacements. The ends of the removed veins are sutured closed; they are not reconnected to other blood vessels.

Test Taking Strategy—Look at the key words "most appropriate" when considering the explanations described in the four options. Select the option that provides an accurate response to the client's question. Recall that venous blood will return to the right side of the heart via smaller collateral veins in the legs (option 3). Review the outcomes of surgical interventions used to treat varicose veins if you had difficulty answering this question.
Cognitive Level—Applying
Client Needs Category—Physiological integrity
Client Needs Subcategory—Physiological adaptation

6. 2. Early and frequent ambulation is essential after vein stripping and vein ligation surgery because it helps promote venous circulation, which is temporarily compromised by the removal of some leg veins. During the immediate postoperative period, walking is ordered hourly while the client is awake. Even during the night, the client is aroused and assisted to walk several times. Although adding protein to the client's diet will help with building and repairing tissue after surgery, this is not the priority intervention at this time. The nurse should always monitor for signs of infection, but this is not the priority after this type of surgery. Leg cramping is not usually associated with vein stripping.

Test Taking Strategy—Analyze to determine what information the question asks for, which is the nursing activity that has the highest priority during the postoperative care of a client who has had a vein ligation and stripping procedure. Unlike arterial blood, which is circulated by the contraction of the left ventricle, venous blood requires muscle contraction, which occurs during ambulation (option 2), to move blood toward the heart. Inactivity contributes to the formation of thrombi. Review the rationale for ambulating a client after vascular surgery involving veins if you had difficulty answering this question.
Cognitive Level—Analyzing
Client Needs Category—Safe and effective care environment
Client Needs Subcategory—Coordinated care

7. 4. If the client states that an unfavorable reaction occurred when taking a particular medication in the past, the nurse should withhold the medication and report the information to the charge nurse or the physician. It would be unethical to try to deceive a client by giving the generic name for a drug the client knows by the trade name. Telling the client that a medication must be taken is inappropriate; the physician will likely substitute another drug. Taking the drug with plenty of water is unlikely to reduce or prevent GI upset.

Test Taking Strategy—Look at the key words "most appropriate," which indicates that one nursing action listed is better than the others. Based on the Patient's Bill of Rights (1992), clients have the "right to make decisions … and refuse a recommended treatment." Reporting the client's previous unfavorable reaction to the medication to the charge nurse is a nursing responsibility. Review the client's legal rights if you had difficulty answering this question.
Cognitive Level—Applying
Client Needs Category—Physiological integrity
Client Needs Subcategory—Pharmacological therapies

8. 3, 5. Stasis ulcers appear darkly pigmented, dry, and scaly. Venous congestion causes edema, and this localized swelling interferes with adequate arterial blood flow, causing poor oxygenation and poor nourishment of skin tissue, usually below the knee. This, combined with the retention of metabolic wastes, leads to inflammation of the skin, sometimes referred to as *cellulitis*. The inflamed tissue chronically breaks open, forming craters that are difficult to heal. The remaining descriptions are not characteristic of such ulcers.

> *Test Taking Strategy—Analyze to determine what information the question asks for, which is the characteristics of a venous stasis ulcer. Alternative-format "select all that apply" questions require considering each option independently to decide its merit in answering the question. Choose the options that best characterize the appearance of stasis ulcers, recalling that their cause is impaired venous circulation. Review the causes and locations of venous stasis ulcers if you had difficulty answering this question.*
> *Cognitive Level—Applying*
> *Client Needs Category—Physiological integrity*
> *Client Needs Subcategory—Physiological adaptation*

9. 2. A major goal of therapy is to promote venous circulation. This is accomplished by applying elastic compression stockings, such as Jobst stockings, that maintain venous pressure at 40 mm Hg. These stockings are worn at all times except when lying down. Offering the client an analgesic for pain promotes the goal of pain control. Typically the client uses a mild analgesic for pain. Maintaining a fluid intake of at least 2,500 mL is important in wound healing and is a priority in accomplishing fluid maintenance. The nurse would not apply a heating pad to the lower extremity because heat dilates blood vessels, contributing to venous congestion.

> *Test Taking Strategy—Apply the key words "most helpful" when determining which nursing intervention is better than the others for promoting venous circulation. Recall that valves within the veins prevent pooling of blood in the veins. Supporting the valves using elastic compression stockings reduces the potential for venous stasis. Review interventions that promote venous circulation if you had difficulty answering this question.*
> *Cognitive Level—Applying*
> *Client Needs Category—Physiological integrity*
> *Client Needs Subcategory—Physiological adaptation*

10. 3. The appearance of pink tissue indicates that granulation tissue is forming. Granulation tissue consists of capillaries and fibrous collagen that seal and nourish the tissue. An increase in drainage suggests that cellular death is continuing or the wound is infected. Relief of discomfort is a positive sign; however, venous ulcers are not severely painful even in the acute stage. White or black wound margins suggest an extension of cell death.

> *Test Taking Strategy—Use the process of elimination to help select the option that identifies the best evidence that a stasis ulcer is healing. Recall that pink tissue (option 3) reflects adequate circulation and oxygenation to the tissue. Review how wound healing occurs and how the appearance of a wound changes as it heals if you had difficulty answering this question.*
> *Cognitive Level—Evaluating*
> *Client Needs Category—Physiological integrity*
> *Client Needs Subcategory—Physiological adaptation*

11. 4. A moist wound undergoes accelerated healing. An air-occlusive dressing prevents evaporation of wound moisture, thereby allowing the wound to heal by second intention at a more rapid rate. This may then decrease the amount of scar tissue, but this is a secondary benefit of using an air-occlusive dressing. Some also feel that healing is faster using an air-occlusive dressing because preventing oxygen from reaching the wound externally stimulates capillary growth to the wound. This type of dressing can remain in place for up to 7 days unless it loosens or the client develops signs of an infection. Air-occlusive dressings are initially more expensive than traditional gauze dressings; however, the need for less frequent changing tends to reduce the initial cost for some individuals. There is no evidence that this type of dressing will decrease pain related to skin irritation.

> *Test Taking Strategy—Analyze to determine what information the question asks for, which is the main advantage for using an air-occlusive dressing. Recall that a moist wound heals more rapidly and efficiently (option 4) than one that is exposed to conditions that dry the wound. Review the purposes of an air-occlusive dressing and its related benefits if you had difficulty answering this question.*
> *Cognitive Level—Applying*
> *Client Needs Category—Physiological integrity*
> *Client Needs Subcategory—Basic care and comfort*

12. 1, 2, 3. Gangrene (necrosis) of the toes and foot is a result of arterial insufficiency. Gangrene is preceded by arterial ulcers—small, circular, deep ulcerations on the tips of the toes or between the toes—that develop from a combination of ischemia and pressure and lead to tissue necrosis. Clients who have problems with circulation are at highest risk. These include clients with diabetes, clients with inadequate circulation, and those who have experienced trauma to the toes. Although homeless clients may have other risk factors, such as poor nutrition and hygiene issues, they are not at highest risk for acquiring gangrene. Taking warfarin (Coumadin) and having a history of myocardial infarction are not risk factors associated with arterial insufficiency and gangrene.

> *Test Taking Strategy—Analyze to determine what information the question asks for, which is clients at highest risk of developing gangrene. Alternative-format "select all that apply" questions require considering each option independently to decide its merit*

in answering the question. Choose the options that correlate with clients who are at risk for developing gangrene of the foot. Recall that there are several precipitating factors related to gangrene, but the underlying reason is arterial insufficiency. Review the causes of gangrene if you had difficulty answering this question.
Cognitive Level—*Analyzing*
Client Needs Category—*Physiological integrity*
Client Needs Subcategory—*Reduction of risk potential*

13. **1, 2, 3.** Thrombophlebitis is a condition in which a blood clot totally or partially occludes the venous blood flow. Several risk factors are associated with blood clot formation. They include obesity; smoking; immobilization and bed rest; history of myocardial infarction and congestive heart failure; multiple sclerosis; oral contraceptive use; and cancer of the breast, pancreas, prostate, or ovary. Leg fatigue is associated with varicose veins. Cramping in the lower leg is associated with a vitamin B deficiency. Pain in the joints is associated with sickle cell anemia.

Test Taking Strategy—*Analyze to determine what information the question asks for, which is risk factors for thrombophlebitis. Alternative-format "select all that apply" questions require considering each option independently to decide its merit in answering the question. For a correct answer to this question, choose the options that identify clients who are at risk for the development of thrombophlebitis. Review factors that predispose to forming blood clots if you had difficulty answering this question.*
Cognitive Level—*Applying*
Client Needs Category—*Physiological integrity*
Client Needs Subcategory—*Reduction of risk potential*

14. **1.** Thrombi typically form as a result of venous stasis. A common cause of venous stasis is inactivity. Postoperative clients are encouraged to perform active leg exercises and to ambulate frequently to promote venous circulation. Shallow breathing predisposes a client to pneumonia. Analgesics may make clients lethargic and less willing to ambulate, but pain is not a direct cause of thrombus formation. Caffeine constricts arteries and arterioles, which can impair oxygenated blood flow. Thrombi generally form in veins.

Test Taking Strategy—*Apply the key words "most likely" to the options when analyzing which client behavior predisposes to the formation of a thrombus. Recall that muscle contraction propels venous blood through valves in the path toward the right side of the heart. Resisting ambulation (option 1) allows venous blood to stagnate and clot. Review the roles that active leg exercises and ambulation play in preventing venous thrombi if you had difficulty answering this question.*
Cognitive Level—*Applying*
Client Needs Category—*Physiological integrity*
Client Needs Subcategory—*Physiological adaptation*

15. **2.** Aside from premeasuring the circumference of the calf from the heel to the popliteal space, the best evidence that antiembolism stockings fit correctly and provide adequate circulation is that the toes feel warm when touched and the capillary refill occurs in less than 3 seconds. Antiembolism stockings should cover the entire calf. Stockings that are easily donned indicate that they are too large for the client. Antiembolism stockings are not intended to prevent redness of the heels.

Test Taking Strategy—*Use the process of elimination to identify the option that identifies the best evidence that antiembolism stockings fit properly. Recall that warm toes (option 2) indicates that the constricting action of the stockings is not interfering with arterial circulation. Review the purpose of antiembolism stockings and how to measure and apply them if you had difficulty answering this question.*
Cognitive Level—*Applying*
Client Needs Category—*Physiological integrity*
Client Needs Subcategory—*Reduction of risk potential*

16. **2.** Although Homans' sign is used less today than in the past to assess thrombophlebitis, it is still used in some practices. To check for Homans' sign, an assessment used to detect venous thrombosis, the nurse would have the client extend each leg separately and dorsiflex the foot (pointing the toes toward the head). A positive Homans' sign is indicated by pain in the calf when the foot is dorsiflexed. None of the actions or positions described in the remaining options is correct.

Test Taking Strategy—*Use the process of elimination to help select the option that provides the most accurate description of the technique for assessing Homans' sign. Option 4 can be eliminated because it describes how a client would perform quadriceps setting exercises. Options 1 and 3 can be eliminated because they describe isotonic exercises. Option 2 remains as the correct answer because dorsiflexing the foot produces pain in the calf if a possible thrombus has developed. Review the purpose for assessing Homans' sign and how to perform it if you had difficulty answering this question.*
Cognitive Level—*Applying*
Client Needs Category—*Physiological integrity*
Client Needs Subcategory—*Reduction of risk potential*

17. **1.** If the client experiences pain in the calf immediately after dorsiflexing the foot (a positive Homans' sign), the discomfort may be due to a thrombus. Numbness, tingling, and impaired function are not classic signs of thrombophlebitis.

Test Taking Strategy—*Analyze to determine what information the question asks for, which is the client's response when assessing Homans' sign if a thrombus is present in a leg vein. Recall that a positive Homans' sign occurs when the client experiences immediate sharp calf pain (option 1). Review the*

cluster of signs and symptoms of thrombophle-bitis that may supplement the finding that results from assessing Homans' sign if you had difficulty answering this question.
***Cognitive Level**—Applying*
***Client Needs Category**—Physiological integrity*
***Client Needs Subcategory**—Physiological adaptation*

18. 4. If the client has a thrombus, the area distal to the thrombus would tend to swell due to the stasis of venous blood and the redistribution of plasma to the interstitial space from increased hydrostatic pressure in the capillaries. Below the thrombus, the leg would feel cool and appear pale. Capillary refilling time is normally less than 3 seconds.

> *Test Taking Strategy—Use the process of elimination to help select the option that identifies the best sign that correlates with a thrombus. Recall that the obstructed flow of blood through the vein with the thrombus will cause localized swelling (option 4). Review the signs and symptoms of a thrombus, particularly if it is located in the lower leg, if you had difficulty answering this question.*
> ***Cognitive Level**—Applying*
> ***Client Needs Category**—Physiological integrity*
> ***Client Needs Subcategory**—Physiological adaptation*

19. 1. Although ambulation was once contraindicated, current evidence-based practice now reports that early ambulation does not increase the risk for a pulmonary embolus in an anticoagulated client. In fact, it is beneficial for reducing swelling and pain. Active exercises can substitute for ambulation. When a thrombus is suspected, the legs must not be massaged. Massage can cause the blood clot to break away from the vessel wall and circulate, possibly to the lung. Although there is some controversy about elevating the legs, raising the legs 20 degrees or more may relieve local swelling; however, pillows should never be placed under the knees and the bed should not be gatched at the knees.

> *Test Taking Strategy—Recognize the key words "most appropriate," and look for an option that is better than the others in relation to the care of a client who has thrombophlebitis. Recall that bed rest is no longer required and has been found to be less beneficial than activity. Review complications of thrombophlebitis and nursing interventions that may prevent them if you had difficulty answering this question.*
> ***Cognitive Level**—Applying*
> ***Client Needs Category**—Safe and effective care environment*
> ***Client Needs Subcategory**—Coordinated care*

20. 4. A dry towel and a waterproof cover act as insulators, preventing rapid heat and moisture loss from the compress. To avoid burning the skin, the temperature of the compress solution is between 98°F and 105°F (36.6°C and 40.5°C). The skin is inspected at least every 30 minutes to monitor for thermal injury. Sterile technique is not necessary as long as the skin is intact.

> *Test Taking Strategy—Note the key words "most appropriate." Look for the option that identifies a standard of practice that applies to the therapeutic use of heat. Recall that covering the moist compress (option 4) helps to retain warmth and reduce evaporation of the moisture. Review how to apply warm moist compresses if you had difficulty answering this question.*
> ***Cognitive Level**—Understanding*
> ***Client Needs Category**—Physiological integrity*
> ***Client Needs Subcategory**—Basic care and comfort*

21. 1.5 mL. The drug label indicates that there are 5,000 units of heparin sodium per milliliter. Use the formula:

$$\frac{D\,(\text{Desired dose})}{H\,(\text{Dose on hand})} \times Q\,(\text{Quantity}) = X\,(\text{Amount to administer})$$

$$\frac{7{,}500\ \text{units}}{5{,}000\ \text{units}} \times 1\,\text{mL} = 1.5\,\text{mL}$$

> *Test Taking Strategy—Analyze to determine what information the question asks for, which requires calculating one dose of heparin sodium from a multidose vial that contains 5,000 units/mL. review how to calculate parenteral dosages if you had difficulty answering this question.*
> ***Cognitive Level**—Applying*
> ***Client Needs Category**—Physiological integrity*
> ***Client Needs Subcategory**—Pharmacological therapies*

22. 3. Heparin sodium prevents future clots from forming and prevents those that have formed from becoming larger. Heparin is an anticoagulant that inhibits the conversion of fibrinogen to fibrin. Only thrombolytic agents, such as streptokinase (Streptase), will shrink and dissolve clots already formed. The use of thrombolytic agents is extremely hazardous. The risks usually outweigh the benefits in the case of thrombophlebitis. Drug therapy will not prevent a thrombus from becoming dislodged.

> *Test Taking Strategy—Analyze to determine what information the question asks for, which is the reason heparin is prescribed for a client who has developed thrombophlebitis. Recall that heparin will not affect the clot that has already formed; the body's production of endogenous plasmin will eventually liquefy it. However, heparin will reduce the risk of forming additional clots. Review the action and purpose for administering heparin if you had difficulty answering this question.*
> ***Cognitive Level**—Understanding*
> ***Client Needs Category**—Physiological integrity*
> ***Client Needs Subcategory**—Pharmacological therapies*

23. 1. Partial thromboplastin time (PTT) is used to monitor the client's response to heparin therapy. The therapeutic range is 1.5 to 2.5 times the control time. A complete blood count (CBC) reports the number of blood cells, not blood clotting factors. Hemoglobin (Hb) relates to the blood's oxygen-carrying capacity and is unaffected by heparin sodium (Hepalean). Prothrombin time (PT) is a test used to monitor the response of a client who is receiving an oral anticoagulant such as warfarin (Coumadin). Another test used when clients are on warfarin therapy is the International Normalized Ratio (INR).

Test Taking Strategy—Analyze to determine what information the question asks for, which is the laboratory test result that is key to maintaining the safety of a client receiving heparin therapy. Recall that a PTT is used to monitor and prescribe the changing doses of heparin (option 1). One method for remembering the difference between a PT and PTT is that the two Ts in PTT resemble an H. H stands for heparin. Review the purpose of heparin administration and the laboratory value closely associated with heparin use if you had difficulty answering this question.
Cognitive Level—Understanding
Client Needs Category—Physiological integrity
Client Needs Subcategory—Pharmacological therapies

24. 2. When a drug is withdrawn from a vial, the nurse instills a volume of air equal to the amount of fluid that will be withdrawn. Adding air to the contents of a vial facilitates withdrawing the drug. If air is not instilled, the partial vacuum makes it difficult to remove solution. If too much air is instilled, solution will surge into the syringe and, in some cases, force the plunger from the syringe barrel. If the rubber stopper is removed, the drug will not remain sterile. Modified insulins, not heparin, are rotated gently before withdrawal to mix the additive and insulin. Heparin sodium (Hepalean) is not shaken before withdrawing it from the vial.

Test Taking Strategy—Analyze to determine what information the question asks for, which is the manner in which heparin is withdrawn from a multidose vial. Recall that adding air to the vial (option 2) increases the pressure within the container making it easier to fill the syringe with the parenteral medication. Review the procedure for withdrawing medication from a vial if you had difficulty answering this question.
Cognitive Level—Remembering
Client Needs Category—Physiological integrity
Client Needs Subcategory—Pharmacological therapies

25. 3. When the adult client is of average or thin size, it is acceptable practice to insert a needle intended for subcutaneous administration at a 45-degree angle to the skin. For obese adults, it is recommended that the nurse use a 90-degree angle to insert the needle. The dorsogluteal site is used for I.M. injections. The needle size for a subcutaneous injection is between ½″ and ⅚″ and 23- to 26-gauge. The injection site should not be massaged after heparin sodium (Hepalean) administration because this increases the tendency for localized bleeding.

Test Taking Strategy—Recognize the key words "most appropriate" and apply them to the four options. Select the option that accurately identifies the technique for administering a subcutaneous injection when the client is normal weight for height. Recall that the proper location of heparin administration is in the abdomen with the needle at a 45-degree angle (option 3). Review the technique for administering subcutaneous injections if you had difficulty answering this question.
Cognitive Level—Applying
Client Needs Category—Physiological integrity
Client Needs Subcategory—Pharmacological therapies

26. 3. Any sign of bleeding in a client receiving anticoagulant therapy must be reported. In this case, bleeding gums should be reported. Clients commonly complain about abdominal tenderness and tiny petechiae on the abdomen because of repeated subcutaneous needlesticks to the area. When this happens, the nurse should assess the abdomen for signs of a hematoma; however, abdominal tenderness and tiny points of intradermal bleeding secondary to needlesticks do not usually require immediate attention. Likewise, clients often complain about the number of times per day they are injected. Having stools that are light brown and soft is normal. Black, tarry stools would require immediate intervention because they could indicate bleeding.

Test Taking Strategy—Analyze to determine what information the question asks for, which is a symptom that represents a potential threat to the client's safety as a result of heparin therapy. Recall that significant bleeding, such as that which may occur during oral hygiene (option 3), should be reported. Review the side effects associated with the administration of heparin if you had difficulty answering this question.
Cognitive Level—Applying
Client Needs Category—Physiological integrity
Client Needs Subcategory—Pharmacological therapies

27. 3. Protamine sulfate, a heparin antagonist, is given to counteract the anticoagulant effects of heparin therapy and restore more normal clotting mechanisms. Calcium lactate is a mineral supplement. Sodium benzoate is used as a preservative. Aluminum phosphate is an ingredient in some antacid products.

Test Taking Strategy—Analyze to determine what information the question asks for, which is the drug that is used as an antidote for the anticoagulating effect of heparin. Although the exact mechanism is unknown, it is believed that protamine sulfate (option 3), which is a basic substance, combines with heparin,

which is strongly acidic, to form a stable complex that interferes with heparin's anticoagulant effect. Review how excessive anticoagulation secondary to heparin administration is managed if you had difficulty answering this question.
Cognitive Level—*Understanding*
Client Needs Category—*Physiological integrity*
Client Needs Subcategory—*Pharmacological therapies*

28. 4. When injections of anticoagulant medication cannot be avoided, it is appropriate for the nurse to apply pressure to the injection site for several minutes to prevent oozing of blood or localized bruising. Pressure is not applied to distribute the drug. Hematomas do not form as a result of applying pressure but can form if pressure is *not* applied. Drug absorption is not significantly affected by several minutes of local pressure.
Test Taking Strategy—*Analyze to determine what information the question asks for, which is whether the nurse's action of applying prolonged pressure after giving an injection to a client receiving anticoagulant therapy is appropriate or inappropriate and the basis for the analysis. Recall that applying pressure controls the potential for bleeding in and around an injection site (option 4). Review the potential for bleeding secondary to anticoagulant therapy and nursing measures that are appropriate when injections must be co-administered if you had difficulty answering this question.*
Cognitive Level—*Applying*
Client Needs Category—*Physiological integrity*
Client Needs Subcategory—*Pharmacological therapies*

29. 2. Black, sticky, tar-colored stools are a sign of bleeding from the upper GI tract. Dark amber urine is more indicative of low fluid volume. Emesis is usually green-tinged or clear. A coffee-ground appearance to emesis is more suggestive of GI bleeding. Jaundiced skin indicates a liver or biliary disorder or rapid hemolysis of red blood cells.
Test Taking Strategy—*Use the process of elimination to select the option that identifies the best evidence that the client understands a serious sign that anticoagulant therapy is having an adverse effect. Recall that bleeding in the upper GI tract correlates with having black stools (option 2). Review signs of blood loss secondary to anticoagulant therapy if you had difficulty answering this question.*
Cognitive Level—*Applying*
Client Needs Category—*Physiological integrity*
Client Needs Subcategory—*Pharmacological therapies*

30. 1, 2, 3, 4. Green leafy vegetables, such as spinach, lettuce, turnip greens, and Brussels sprouts, are among the best food sources of vitamin K. Vitamin K is associated with clotting factors in the blood. Half of the daily requirement of vitamin K comes from the diet, and the bacteria

from the intestine manufacture the remaining amounts. Warfarin (Coumadin) is an anticoagulant that prevents clot formation. If foods high in vitamin K are eaten, this will interfere with the main purposes of the drug.
Test Taking Strategy—*Analyze to determine what information the question asks for, which is foods high in vitamin K. Alternative-format "select all that apply" questions require considering each option independently to decide its merit in answering the question. In this question, select options that correlate with foods that should be avoided when taking warfarin (Coumadin). Recall that eating foods high in vitamin K will alter the effectiveness of the drug. Review food–drug interactions as they relate to warfarin if you had difficulty answering this question.*
Cognitive Level—*Applying*
Client Needs Category—*Physiological integrity*
Client Needs Subcategory—*Reduction of risk potential*

31. 1, 2, 3, 4. Many dietary supplements (including gingko, St. John's wort, willow bark, and ginger) can alter the client's International Normalized Ratio (INR) and prothrombin time (PT). Green tea and creatine, a supplement that increases muscle mass, are not known to alter these levels. The best policy for clients who are taking warfarin (Coumadin) is to avoid all dietary and herbal supplements unless the physician approves. Clients should also avoid vitamin and mineral supplements that contain vitamin K.
Test Taking Strategy—*Analyze to determine what information the question asks for, which is dietary supplements that affect INR and PT. Alternative-format "select all that apply" questions require considering each option independently to decide its merit in answering the question. Choose the options that correlate with dietary supplements that should be avoided when taking warfarin (Coumadin). Review each dietary supplement to determine if it alters warfarin's anticoagulant affect if you had difficulty answering this question.*
Cognitive Level—*Applying*
Client Needs Category—*Health promotion and maintenance*
Client Needs Subcategory—*None*

32. 1. Signs of phlebitis include redness, tenderness, warmth, and swelling of the vein. An inflamed vein also feels indurated (hard, not soft and spongy) or cordlike, but it does not appear pale, purple, or dark.
Test Taking Strategy—*Analyze to determine what information the question asks for, which is the appearance of a phlebitis developing at the site of an I.V. line. Recall that the cardinal signs of an inflammation include redness and localized warmth (option 1). Review the signs and symptoms of phlebitis as it relates to the site of an I.V. infusion if you had difficulty answering this question.*

Cognitive Level—*Applying*
Client Needs Category—*Physiological integrity*
Client Needs Subcategory—*Pharmacological therapies*

33. 4. The cause of the inflamed vein may be the presence of the foreign infusion device, the irritating solution, or trauma to the vein wall. In any case, the infusion should be discontinued and restarted in another site to prevent further injury to the vein and to promote healing. The standard of practice is to change an I.V. site at least every 72 hours regardless of whether it is exhibiting signs of phlebitis. Elevating the extremity is appropriate to relieve swelling after the needle or catheter has been removed. Applying pressure would not diminish the current problem; rather, it would slow the rate of infusion. Increasing the infusion rate is contraindicated because it has not been medically approved and places the client at risk for fluid volume excess.

> *Test Taking Strategy*—*Use the process of elimination to select the option that identifies the first action the nurse should take when suspecting phlebitis has developed. Recall that the goal is to eliminate the causative factor contributing to the phlebitis (option 4). Review the nursing action that is appropriate if phlebitis is suspected in a vein used for administering I.V. fluid if you had difficulty answering this question.*
> *Cognitive Level*—*Analyzing*
> *Client Needs Category*—*Physiological integrity*
> *Client Needs Subcategory*—*Physiological adaptation*

Nursing Care of Clients with Arterial Disorders

34. 1, 5, 6. Individuals with peripheral vascular disease develop trophic changes, consequences of chronically impaired delivery of nutritive substances to peripheral cells and tissues. This includes thick, hard nails; thin, shiny skin; and little hair growth on the extremities. Flushed skin may be a sign of hypertension, not peripheral vascular disease. The peripheral pulses are often weak and difficult to detect in a client with peripheral vascular disease. Hyperactive knee jerk reflexes are not characteristic of peripheral vascular disease.

> *Test Taking Strategy*—*Analyze to determine what information the question asks for, which is signs and symptoms of peripheral vascular disease. Alternative-format "select all that apply" questions require considering each option independently to decide its merit in answering the question. Choose the options that correlate with arterial insufficiency secondary to peripheral arteriosclerosis. Review the clinical manifestations of arteriosclerosis, particularly those affecting the integument, if you had difficulty answering this question.*

Cognitive Level—*Remembering*
Client Needs Category—*Physiological integrity*
Client Needs Subcategory—*Physiological adaptation*

35. 3. When the leg muscles become ischemic, the client with peripheral arterial insufficiency is most likely to report having pain in both legs. The pain goes away with rest, which is the reason the symptom is referred to as *intermittent claudication*. Cyanosis is more closely associated with venous congestion. Poor distal arterial circulation tends to heighten a person's sensation of being cold. A feeling that the toes are burning is not a common symptom of peripheral arterial insufficiency. Ankle edema is more likely to result because of poor circulation, not active exercise.

> *Test Taking Strategy*—*Analyze to determine what information the question asks for, which is the outcome a client with arteriosclerosis is likely to experience when actively exercising. Recall that cells and tissue require increased oxygenation when activity escalates. Without adequate oxygenation, leg pain (option 3) is likely to occur. Review the signs and symptoms of musculoskeletal ischemia secondary to arteriosclerosis if you had difficulty answering this question.*
> *Cognitive Level*—*Understanding*
> *Client Needs Category*—*Physiological integrity*
> *Client Needs Subcategory*—*Physiological adaptation*

36. 3. Extra clothing or blankets, rather than direct heat applications, are used whenever possible for individuals with peripheral arterial insufficiency. Because of the disease, such clients are typically insensitive to warm temperatures and are at high risk for being burned. Therefore, commercially prepared heat packets or heating pads are contraindicated. Instead, layers of loosely woven fibers, especially of natural material like cotton or wool, help hold pockets of warm air close to the body surface. This promotes a feeling of warmth. Elevating the feet relieves edema but does not necessarily make the feet feel warmer.

> *Test Taking Strategy*—*Apply the key words "most appropriate" when reviewing the four options. Select the intervention for warming the feet of a client with arteriosclerosis that is better than any of the others. Recall that older adults are more prone to thermal injury, so applying a warm blanket (option 3) is safer than using methods such as heating pads or heat packets. Review options and precautions for applying heat to a client if you had difficulty answering this question.*
> *Cognitive Level*—*Applying*
> *Client Needs Category*—*Physiological integrity*
> *Client Needs Subcategory*—*Basic care and comfort*

37.

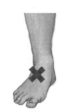

The dorsalis pedis artery is a blood vessel that supplies oxygenated blood and nutrients to the dorsum (top) of the foot. The pulse can be felt by palpating the skin surface halfway between the toes and the ankle. When a pulsation is difficult to feel, a Doppler ultrasound device can be positioned in the same location to transform arterial pulsation, if it is present, into an audible sound.

Test Taking Strategy—Analyze to determine what information the question asks for, which is the anatomic location for assessing the quality of blood flow through the dorsalis pedis artery. Review descriptions of the correct location of the dorsalis pedis artery if you had difficulty answering this question.
Cognitive Level—*Applying*
Client Needs Category—*Physiological integrity*
Client Needs Subcategory—*Reduction of risk potential*

38. 2. The nurse applies acoustic gel to the skin at the location of the dorsalis pedis artery when using a Doppler ultrasound device. Because air is a poor conductor of sound, the gel helps beam the ultrasound toward the blood vessel being assessed. Movement of red blood cells through an artery produces an intermittent, pulsating sound. Movement of blood through a vein makes a continuous sound, like whistling wind. The dorsalis pedis artery is on the top of the foot and is often used to assess the quality of blood flow to the foot. The posterior tibialis artery is beside the ankle and is used less frequently. When assessing capillary refill, the nurse releases a compressed nail bed and counts the number of seconds it takes for blood to return. A Doppler ultrasound device is not used to measure skin temperature.

Test Taking Strategy—Use the process of elimination to select the option that identifies the correct technique for assessing the dorsalis pedis artery with a Doppler ultrasound device. Recall that acoustic gel (option 2) helps reduce resistance to sound transmission so the nurse can better hear the pulsating sound made by the blood as it moves through the artery. Review the names and locations of peripheral pulses, especially what is called the pedal pulse, if you had difficulty answering this question.
Cognitive Level—*Applying*
Client Needs Category—*Physiological integrity*
Client Needs Subcategory—*Reduction of risk potential*

39. 2. Raynaud's disease is a condition that results in vasospasm of the small arteries and arterioles. Symptoms are generally confined to an individual's hands (most common) or feet and usually result when the client is exposed to cold or emotional upsets. The nose, ears, and chin are less commonly involved. The client experiences periodic episodes during which the affected areas feel cold, painful, numb, and prickly due to poor circulation. The hands usually turn white, then blue and, finally, red. As blood flow resumes, the deprived areas become flushed and warm. A throbbing sensation is then experienced.

Test Taking Strategy—Analyze to determine what information the question asks for, which is the location where a client with Raynaud's disease is likely to experience symptoms. Recall that the hands (option 2) are most commonly affected. Review the clinical manifestations associated with Raynaud's disease if you had difficulty answering this question.
Cognitive Level—*Applying*
Client Needs Category—*Physiological integrity*
Client Needs Subcategory—*Physiological adaptation*

40. 2. Conditions that lead to vasoconstriction, such as exposure to cold, emotional upsets, and use of tobacco, aggravate or exacerbate the symptoms experienced by individuals with Raynaud's disease. The effect of wind depends on the air temperature. Sun and heat are related to vasodilation and are not associated with this disease.

Test Taking Strategy—Apply the key words "most likely" to select the option that identifies the factor that correlates best with the onset of symptoms caused by Raynaud's disease. Recall that the symptoms of this disease are due to constriction of arteries and arterioles, which may be exacerbated by exposure to cold (option 2). Review factors that contribute to the signs and symptoms experienced by a person with Raynaud's disease if you had difficulty answering this question.
Cognitive Level—*Applying*
Client Needs Category—*Physiological integrity*
Client Needs Subcategory—*Physiological adaptation*

41. 2. Stress stimulates the sympathetic nervous system, causing vasoconstriction. When the arterioles narrow, blood flow is impaired, and the client experiences an episodic attack of pain, numbness, and pallor. Therefore, avoiding stressful situations is important in avoiding the onset of symptoms. Wearing warm gloves while outdoors in cold weather is beneficial and is recommended. Drinking alcoholic beverages and bathing with perfumed soap are not necessarily contraindicated for a person with Raynaud's disease.

Test Taking Strategy—Analyze to determine what information the question asks for, which is a behavior that a client with Raynaud's disease should be taught to avoid. Recall that the pathophysiology of this disorder involves vasoconstriction. Consequently,

avoiding stress (option 2), which is accompanied by the release of adrenaline, a vasoconstricting neurochemical, should be encouraged. Review interventions that reduce the occurrence of the signs and symptoms associated with Raynaud's disease if you had difficulty answering this question.
Cognitive Level—*Applying*
Client Needs Category—*Health promotion and maintenance*
Client Needs Subcategory—*None*

42. 3. Thromboangiitis obliterans (Buerger's disease) is an acute inflammation of the arteries and veins in the lower extremities. Consequently, a clot forms in the inflamed blood vessel. Smoking causes the disease to worsen. Individuals with the disease commonly report experiencing leg pain or muscle cramps (referred to as *intermittent claudication*) during periods of active movement. Rest can relieve this symptom; however, eventually the pain occurs even while the client is inactive. Clients with varicose veins, not Buerger's disease, report a feeling of heaviness in their legs. Ingrown toenails are not related to the disease. Although edema does occur among clients with Buerger's disease, it is more likely to occur when the disease is far advanced.
Test Taking Strategy—Analyze to determine what information the question asks for, which is an early symptom experienced by a person with thromboangiitis obliterans. Recall that pain is a cardinal symptom of inflammation. Because thromboangiitis obliterans involves inflammation of blood vessels in the lower legs, it is generally accompanied by pain (option 3), especially during active exercise. Review the signs and symptoms of thromboangiitis obliterans and factors that intensify discomfort if you had difficulty answering this question.
Cognitive Level—*Analyzing*
Client Needs Category—*Physiological integrity*
Client Needs Subcategory—*Physiological adaptation*

43. 4. Buerger's disease results in decreased blood flow to the legs and feet, although the hands are also sometimes affected. The distal peripheral pulses are frequently found to be weak, diminished, or absent because of impaired arterial circulation. A normal peripheral pulse feels strong or full and is easily felt with only moderate pressure.
Test Taking Strategy—Analyze to determine what information the question asks for, which is a characteristic of the pulse that is common in clients with Buerger's disease. Recall that the disease produces varying degrees of obstruction within the affected blood vessels, resulting in peripheral pulsations that are weak (option 4) or eventually absent as the disease progresses. Arterial obstruction may require amputation of the limb(s). Review assessment findings associated with Buerger's disease if you had difficulty answering this question.
Cognitive Level—*Understanding*
Client Needs Category—*Physiological integrity*
Client Needs Subcategory—*Physiological adaptation*

44. 1. Buerger-Allen exercises help improve and promote collateral circulation and should be done several times per day by the client with Buerger's disease. The client performs them by first lying down and elevating the legs above the heart for 2 to 3 minutes; then, sitting on the edge of the bed or couch, the client lowers the legs to a dependent position. When the legs flush, the client returns to lying flat in bed. After returning to bed, the client should move the feet and toes by dorsiflexion, plantar flexion, and internal and external rotation. Standing and touching the toes, jogging in place, and simulated stair climbing are not part of these exercises.
Test Taking Strategy—Analyze to determine what information the question asks for, which is the sequence involved in performing Buerger-Allen exercises. Recall that these exercises are meant to improve circulation by emptying vessels filled with stagnant blood that may form clots. Sitting (option 1) and lowering the legs helps reduce the potential for ischemia and pain. Review instructions on how Buerger-Allen exercises should be performed if you had difficulty answering this question.
Cognitive Level—*Remembering*
Client Needs Category—*Health promotion and maintenance*
Client Needs Subcategory—*None*

45. 2. A person with Buerger's disease should avoid tobacco because nicotine causes vasoconstriction. There are no contraindications for heavy lifting, traveling by air, or engaging in sexual activity based on the pathology involved in Buerger's disease.
Test Taking Strategy—Analyze to determine what information the question asks for, which is an activity that the client with Buerger's disease should avoid. Recall that smoking causes vasoconstriction. Smoking cessation (option 2) is the single most effective measure for preventing the progression of the disease and avoiding amputation. Review the disease process and interventions for treatment if you had difficulty answering this question.
Cognitive Level—*Applying*
Client Needs Category—*Safe and effective care environment*
Client Needs Subcategory—*Coordinated care*

46. 2, 5, 6. An aneurysm is an abnormal dilation (or bulging) of a blood vessel, usually an artery. The dilation typically results from weakness in a portion of the vessel and elevated blood pressure, which is higher in arteries. Several factors can predispose a client to develop an abdominal aortic aneurysm (AAA). These include hypertension (which may be secondary to arteriosclerosis), trauma, congenital weakness, smoking, and age. Although diabetes mellitus affects circulation, it is not considered a risk factor. A sedentary lifestyle predisposes clients to many cardiac risks, but it is not as highly correlated with aneurysm formation as hypertension or arteriosclerosis. Digoxin (Lanoxin) is a cardiac glycoside that increases the strength of myocardial contraction and lowers the heart rate. Its use, side effects, and indications have no bearing on aneurysm formation.

Test Taking Strategy—Analyze to determine what information the question asks for, which is risk factors for AAA. Alternative-format "select all that apply" questions require considering each option independently to decide its merit in answering the question. Choose the options that identify factors that place clients at risk for developing an AAA. Review predisposing factors associated with AAA if you had difficulty answering this question.
Cognitive Level—Applying
Client Needs Category—Physiological integrity
Client Needs Subcategory—Physiological adaptation

47. 4. When palpating the abdomen of a client with an abdominal aortic aneurysm (AAA), it may be possible to feel a pulsating mass. Edema of the feet is not commonly associated with AAAs. The extremities are more likely to exhibit signs of diminished circulation, such as paleness, feeling cool, and having faint peripheral pulses. Occasionally, thrombi may form and occlude blood flow to one or both legs, which then causes intense leg or foot pain. Bowel sounds are usually normal. Abdominal petechiae are usually associated with liver or blood disorders.

Test Taking Strategy—Note the key words "most evident" in relation to an assessment finding that is more prevalent than any identified in the other options. Recall that the abdominal aorta is a portion of the aorta, the largest artery in the body. It contains a massive volume of blood. Although an AAA may not cause symptoms before rupturing, it may be detected either at the time of an unrelated abdominal x-ray or by feeling a pulsating mass (option 4) near the center of the abdomen, just above the navel. Review clinical manifestations that relate to an AAA if you had difficulty answering this question.
Cognitive Level—Applying
Client Needs Category—Physiological integrity
Client Needs Subcategory—Physiological adaptation

48. 4. An aneurysm is a balloon-like outpouching in the wall of an artery, not a vein. Aneurysms commonly occur in the thoracic or abdominal aorta and in cerebral arteries because of the higher blood pressure in these vessels. Valves are usually seen in veins, and they keep the blood flowing in one direction, upward toward the heart. Weakened valves in veins cause blood vessels in the legs to appear distended and twisted. Weakened valves are not associated with abdominal aortic aneurysms (AAAs). A stationary blood clot (thrombus) may result from altered circulation, but it typically occurs in a vein, not an artery. A fatty deposit in the artery wall (plaque) may build up and lead to arteriosclerosis, which is a risk factor for AAAs.

Test Taking Strategy—Analyze to determine what information the question asks for, which is an accurate description of the pathology associated with an AAA. Recall that the portion of affected aorta, rather than remaining straight, bulges (option 4) due to a structural weakness caused by a reduction of elastin in the vessel wall. Review the changes in the aorta due to stretching and widening that increase over time if you had difficulty answering this question.
Cognitive Level—Applying
Client Needs Category—Physiological integrity
Client Needs Subcategory—Physiological adaptation

49. 4. Pressure from an enlarging or dissecting abdominal aortic aneurysm (AAA) is most likely to be manifested as lower back pain. The client will indicate that no position or nursing measure relieves the pain. The client will suffer internal hemorrhage, shock and, possibly, death if the aneurysm becomes so large that it ruptures. Rectal bleeding, hematuria, and indigestion are related to other conditions, not AAAs.

Test Taking Strategy—Use the key words "most likely" to narrow the selection among the options to one that identifies a symptom that is most characteristic of an aortic dissection. Recall that rupture may be the first indication that an AAA has formed. Clients generally report unrelenting pain that radiates through the abdomen to the back (option 4). Review clinical manifestations of a dissecting AAA if you had difficulty answering this question.
Cognitive Level—Applying
Client Needs Category—Physiological integrity
Client Needs Subcategory—Physiological adaptation

50. 3. If the client has an advance directive indicating a wish for no heroic efforts to sustain life, the nurse should notify the physician of the change in the client's condition. Pertinent assessments, such as vital signs and skin color, should also be reported at this time. If the client is not breathing and is pulseless, it would be unethical to violate the client's wishes (and the physician's written orders) by performing cardiopulmonary resuscitation (CPR). On the basis of the information the nurse communicates, the physician would decide if and when to transfer the client to the hospital. The physician generally notifies the client's next of kin, but this task may be delegated to the nurse.

Test Taking Strategy—Apply the key words "most appropriate" when reviewing the suggested actions in each of the four options. Select the option that identifies the nursing action that best complies with the client's instructions in the advance directive. Even though the nurse may feel hospitalization would extend the client's life, the nurse must defer any personal opinions and first contact the physician (option 3). Review the ethical obligations involved in following a client's advance directive if you had difficulty answering this question.

Cognitive Level—*Applying*
Client Needs Category—*Safe and effective care environment*
Client Needs Subcategory—*Coordinated care*

Nursing Care of Clients with Red Blood Cell Disorders

51. 3. Complications of peptic ulcer disease include chronic bleeding or hemorrhage. Blood loss occurs as the ulcer penetrates one or more blood vessels. If the bleeding is slight but continuous, it may go unnoticed until the client becomes weak and fatigued. Mitral valve insufficiency, arteriosclerosis, and an enlarged prostate are not usually associated with chronic or severe red blood cell (RBC) decreases.

Test Taking Strategy—*Note the key words "most likely" in relation to a condition that may be the etiology underlying a low number of RBCs. Recall that peptic ulcer disease (option 3), if untreated or ineffectively treated, may result in chronic blood loss that can eventually lead to anemia. Review the causes of a low RBC count and correlate them with peptic ulcer disease if you had difficulty answering this question.*
Cognitive Level—*Applying*
Client Needs Category—*Physiological integrity*
Client Needs Subcategory—*Physiological adaptation*

52. 4. Because the client is anemic, energy is compromised. Balancing rest with activity is one way of maintaining a consistent energy level and avoiding excessive energy expenditures. Adequate sleep, exercise, and eating foods that provide energy are all healthy behaviors, but they are not likely to make as significant an improvement as balancing energy use with rest.

Test Taking Strategy—*Look at the key words "most appropriate," and select the intervention that is best for reducing the client's fatigue. Recall that activity requires increased cellular demand for oxygen, which is delivered by hemoglobin on red blood cells; providing rest (option 4) limits the need for available oxygen and promotes endurance and stamina. Review interventions that relieve fatigue when a client is anemic if you had difficulty answering this question.*
Cognitive Level—*Applying*
Client Needs Category—*Physiological integrity*
Client Needs Subcategory—*Reduction of risk potential*

53. 4. Iron is necessary for the formation of hemoglobin (Hb). Therefore, a low Hb level reflects an iron deficiency. If the Hb level is below 12 g/dL in a woman or 14 g/dL in a man, the person is considered anemic. Because conditions other than iron deficiency can cause a low Hb level, additional diagnostic tests may be necessary. The Epstein-Barr virus (EBV) infects 80% of the U.S. population. Once the infection occurs, the virus becomes dormant but can reactivate later.

The EBV titer is used to make the determination of the presence of EBV. The thyroid-stimulating hormone (TSH) test is used to differentiate primary from secondary hypothyroidism. Fibrinogen levels are tests commonly performed when a client has a suspected clotting problem or is at high risk for bleeding. These tests are not typically performed on clients suspected of having nutritional anemia.

Test Taking Strategy—*Analyze to determine what information the question asks for, which is the laboratory test that correlates with detecting iron deficiency anemia. Recall that one of the components of heme in Hb is iron. Consequently, a blood test finding in which the Hb is low (option 4) supports a diagnosis of iron deficiency anemia. Review the composition of Hb and its function if you had difficulty answering this question.*
Cognitive Level—*Applying*
Client Needs Category—*Physiological integrity*
Client Needs Subcategory—*Physiological adaptation*

54. 3. An anemic person is likely to feel colder than usual most of the time. This symptom is most likely due to impaired cellular oxygenation from reduced hemoglobin levels. Without oxygen, the body's ability to produce calories during metabolism is affected. Frequent headaches, chronic back pain, and a history of rheumatic fever are unrelated to iron deficiency anemia.

Test Taking Strategy—*Look at the key words "most relevant" and apply them when selecting an option that correlates anemia with information the client provides. Recall that aerobic metabolism, which depends on oxygen, provides the highest yield of caloric energy via Kreb's cycle, also known as the citric acid cycle. The combustion of calories produces heat. If there is insufficient oxygen, as in anemia, there will be a reduced production of heat and energy. The client will feel cold (option 3) and tired. Review the signs and symptoms of anemia if you had difficulty answering this question.*
Cognitive Level—*Applying*
Client Needs Category—*Physiological integrity*
Client Needs Subcategory—*Physiological adaptation*

55. 2. Omitting meat from the diet can cause iron deficiency anemia. Good food sources of iron include meat, fish, certain beans, iron-enriched cereals, whole grain products, and green leafy vegetables such as spinach. However, iron is more poorly absorbed from vegetables. Milk does not contain iron but is a good source of calcium and protein. Likewise, most fruits do not contain large amounts of iron. Citrus fruits, however, aid in iron absorption and are good sources of potassium and vitamin C.

Test Taking Strategy—*Use the key words "most likely" to identify which food source, if omitted from the diet, correlates with developing iron deficiency anemia. Recall that omitting meat (option 2), which is a good food source of iron, predisposes to anemia if other sources of iron are not appreciably increased.*

Review foods that are high in iron if you had difficulty answering this question.
Cognitive Level—*Applying*
Client Needs Category—*Physiological integrity*
Client Needs Subcategory—*Basic care and comfort*

56. 1. Iron is absorbed poorly from the GI tract. Absorption occurs best when the drug is taken on an empty stomach with water. Taking the drug between meals or at least 1 hour before meals is the best routine for maximum benefit. Taking the drug just before eating or with the meal causes the drug to be present in the stomach with food. When food and other drugs such as antacids are taken simultaneously with iron, iron absorption is decreased. If a client experiences GI upset while taking iron, the discomfort may be reduced by taking the ferrous sulfate (Feosol) with food or milk rather than discontinuing the medication. If the client takes the ferrous sulfate (Feosol) only before bedtime, it would not be following the prescribed daily regimen, which is three times per day.

> *Test Taking Strategy*—*Analyze to determine what information the question asks for, which is the optimum time for the client to self-administer an iron supplement. Recall that iron is best taken when the stomach is empty because the undiluted hydrochloric acid in gastric secretions provides an optimum medium for iron absorption. Option 1 is the correct answer because food should no longer be in the stomach 2 hours after eating a meal. Unfortunately, some do not tolerate the GI side effects when taking the medication without food; enteric-coated forms also are available. Although taking iron with food is less desirable, it is better than totally omitting the iron supplement. Review the best time for administering ferrous sulfate if you had difficulty answering this question.*

Cognitive Level—*Applying*
Client Needs Category—*Physiological integrity*
Client Needs Subcategory—*Pharmacological therapies*

57. 4. The presence of vitamin C, found in orange or other citrus juices, improves the absorption of iron. For this reason, some pharmaceutical companies combine iron and vitamin C in the same capsule or tablet. Iron taken with milk interferes with its absorption. Taking iron with tea or a soft drink is not likely to be any more beneficial than taking it with water.

> *Test Taking Strategy*—*Analyze to determine what information the question asks for, which is the beverage that enhances the absorption of iron. Recall that increasing stomach acidity enhances absorption of many drugs, including an iron supplement. Because orange juice (option 4) contains ascorbic acid (vitamin C), it is the best answer from among the options for facilitating a greater absorption of iron. Review factors that support the absorption of ferrous sulfate if you had difficulty answering this question.*

Cognitive Level—*Applying*
Client Needs Category—*Physiological integrity*
Client Needs Subcategory—*Pharmacological therapies*

58. 2. Most individuals who take iron observe that their stools become black or dark green. Stool is normally a medium brown color. Clay-colored stools are associated with liver or biliary disease. The stool becomes light green with diarrhea, or it assumes this color from eating certain foods.

> *Test Taking Strategy*—*Analyze to determine what information the question asks for, which is the stool color that occurs when an iron supplement is consumed. Recall that at best only 10% to 30% of iron taken orally is absorbed. The residual remains in the lumen of the intestine, causing the feces to become a dark black color (option 2). Review the absorption and excretion of ferrous sulfate, particularly its effect on stool color, if you had difficulty answering this question.*

Cognitive Level—*Understanding*
Client Needs Category—*Physiological integrity*
Client Needs Subcategory—*Pharmacological therapies*

59. 1. Liquid iron preparations stain the teeth; therefore, drinking the medication through a straw minimizes drug contact with the teeth. Pouring the medication over ice or drinking it from a paper cup does not protect the teeth from unsightly staining. Mixing the medication with milk affects its absorption and does not protect the teeth. However, diluting the liquid iron with at least 2 to 4 ounces of water as well as using a straw reduces the potential for staining teeth.

> *Test Taking Strategy*—*Analyze to determine what information the question asks for, which is the manner in which a client should self-administer an iron supplement in liquid form. Recall that liquid iron temporarily stains the teeth. To avoid an unaesthetic appearance, liquid iron should be diluted and consumed through a straw (option 1). Brushing the teeth with baking soda once a week may also reduce the staining effect. Review health teaching for a client who has been prescribed liquid ferrous sulfate, focusing on interventions that prevent staining of the teeth, if you had difficulty answering this question.*

Cognitive Level—*Applying*
Client Needs Category—*Physiological integrity*
Client Needs Subcategory—*Pharmacological therapies*

60. 1. People who are anemic often experience dizziness and fainting. This is probably due to low blood volume or an inability to maintain adequate oxygenation to the brain. Anemia is also likely to cause an individual to feel tired and require more sleep. Headaches are not usually associated with anemia that is related to blood loss, but they may occur in a client with pernicious anemia. Having had the gallbladder removed does not relate to anemia because the function of the gallbladder is to aid fat digestion by releasing bile into the small intestine. Abdominal tenderness is unrelated to anemia but may occur with menstrual cramping.

> *Test Taking Strategy—Apply the key words "most likely" to each of the four options. Look for the option that identifies information in the client's health history that correlates more than the others with developing anemia. Recall that the brain is very sensitive to impaired oxygenation and low blood pressure, which may be manifested by light-headedness, dizziness, or fainting (option 1). Review the signs and symptoms of anemia if you had difficulty answering this question.*
> *Cognitive Level—Applying*
> *Client Needs Category—Physiological integrity*
> *Client Needs Subcategory—Physiological adaptation*

61. 3. The skin of an anemic client is typically pale. This is generally due to the fact that tissue oxygenation, which causes the skin and mucous membranes to appear pink, is impaired from reduced amounts of hemoglobin or red blood cells. Cyanosis, or a bluish color, is more likely caused by the buildup of carbon dioxide in the blood. A flushed appearance may be due to such factors as vasodilation, hypertension, increased blood volume, or thermal injury. Mottled skin is a condition characterized by generalized purplish, spotted areas. It is commonly seen in neonates who are chilled or inactive or in clients who are about to die.

> *Test Taking Strategy—Analyze to determine what information the question asks for, which is a skin color that correlates with anemia. Recall that anemic clients have a low red blood cell count or hemoglobin level. When the oxygen-carrying capacity is decreased, oxygenated blood is drawn away from the skin and directed to the brain and other vital organs, causing a pale appearance (option 3). Review the signs and symptoms of anemia if you had difficulty answering this question.*
> *Cognitive Level—Applying*
> *Client Needs Category—Physiological integrity*
> *Client Needs Subcategory—Physiological adaptation*

62. 1. Pernicious anemia, a condition in which the bone marrow produces larger than normal but fewer red blood cells, results from an inability to absorb vitamin B_{12}. This type of anemia is due to a lack of the intrinsic factor secreted by parietal cells in the stomach. The intrinsic factor normally binds with vitamin B_{12} in food allowing it to bypass stomach digestion. When vitamin B_{12} becomes absorbed from the ileum, it facilitates maturation of red blood cells. Therefore, clients who have had a total gastrectomy (removal of the stomach) eventually develop pernicious anemia unless prophylactically treated with injections of vitamin B_{12}. Intrinsic factor is not related to hepatitis, comorbidities of other anemias, or allergic reactions.

> *Test Taking Strategy—Based on the key words "most appropriate," look for an option that identifies*

a health-related question that is more pertinent than the others for establishing a relationship with pernicious anemia. Because of the stomach's role in providing the intrinsic factor, without which pernicious anemia develops, option 1 is the correct answer. Review the underlying cause of pernicious anemia if you had difficulty answering this question.

> *Cognitive Level—Applying*
> *Client Needs Category—Physiological integrity*
> *Client Needs Subcategory—Physiological adaptation*

63. 2. Personnel in the admissions or business office are responsible for obtaining information about the client's medical insurance or lack of health coverage. This information is not pertinent to nursing documentation. The nurse's narrative notes are used for documenting subjective and objective assessment data, nursing care, treatment interventions, and the client's responses. The remaining options are all appropriate to document.

> *Test Taking Strategy—Use the process of elimination to help select the option that identifies the least pertinent information in the nurse's documentation. Options 1 and 3 can be eliminated because subjective and objective assessment data are pertinent. Option 4 can be eliminated because nursing care involves accessing other disciplines to meet the client's needs. Option 2 remains as least pertinent to the scope of nursing documentation because the client will receive the same quality of care regardless of whether he or she is uninsured. Review the rationale for the information that is included in nursing documentation if you had difficulty answering this question.*
> *Cognitive Level—Applying*
> *Client Needs Category—Safe and effective care environment*
> *Client Needs Subcategory—Coordinated care*

64. 1. Pernicious anemia impairs peripheral and spinal cord nerve fibers, causing such symptoms as tingling and numbness in the extremities, loss of position sense, a staggering gait, and partial or total paralysis. Some speculate that these symptoms develop because vitamin B_{12} deficiency leads to a lack of methionine, an essential amino acid necessary for myelin, the insulation around nerves; contributes to an overabundance of fatty acids that are incorporated into nerves; or causes nerves to be more susceptible to damage by cytokines, tumor necrosis factor, and epidermal growth factor. Other symptoms include a smooth, sore, beefy red tongue and weakness. Headaches may occur, but they are not a classic complaint among those with pernicious anemia. Restlessness and sleep disturbances are not usually associated with this disorder. Some clients experience confusion, depression, personality changes, and memory loss, but not to the point of amnesia.

> *Test Taking Strategy—Analyze to determine what information the question asks for, which is neurologic symp-*

toms related to pernicious anemia. Recall that aside from anemia, vitamin B$_{12}$ deficiency can lead to nerve damage, resulting in tingling and numbness in the extremities (option 3). Review the signs and symptoms of pernicious anemia, focusing on neurologic manifestations, if you had difficulty answering this question.
Cognitive Level—*Applying*
Client Needs Category—*Physiological integrity*
Client Needs Subcategory—*Physiological adaptation*

65. 1. A Schilling test, which evaluates the absorption of radioactive vitamin B$_{12}$, is ordered for any client with suspected pernicious anemia. The test involves collecting all of the client's urine for 24 to 48 hours after oral and injected doses of vitamin B$_{12}$ are administered and measuring the radioactivity in the urine sample. To collect all of the urine throughout the 24 hour period, a large urine container is utilized. Blood, stool, and sputum specimens are not required for this test.
> *Test Taking Strategy—Use the process of elimination to help select the option that describes the specimen that is collected and examined to facilitate a diagnosis of pernicious anemia. Recall that one of the functions of the kidneys is to excrete water-soluble substances in urine (option 1). Review the Schilling test and how it is performed if you had difficulty answering this question.*
Cognitive Level—*Applying*
Client Needs Category—*Physiological integrity*
Client Needs Subcategory—*Reduction of risk potential*

66. 3. Pernicious anemia is incurable, but the manifestations of the disease can be treated by lifelong injections of vitamin B$_{12}$. Blood transfusions are administered to someone who has hemolytic anemia or severely low red blood cell counts and hemoglobin levels. Iron preparations are given when a client has nutritional anemia, or when blood cell counts or hemoglobin levels are low but the condition is not life-threatening. Vitamin K is administered for clotting disorders in which the client's prothrombin level is low.
> *Test Taking Strategy—Note the key words "most appropriate," and apply them when evaluating the nurse's response to the client's question. Select the option with the statement that identifies the usual treatment for pernicious anemia. Recall that if the intrinsic factor is not being produced, lifelong parenteral vitamin B$_{12}$ injections will be necessary. Review the treatment of pernicious anemia if you had difficulty answering this question.*
Cognitive Level—*Applying*
Client Needs Category—*Physiological integrity*
Client Needs Subcategory—*Physiological adaptation*

67. 4. Sickle cell anemia is a genetic condition that occurs when a person inherits two defective genes, one from each parent. If only one gene is inherited, the person carries the sickle cell trait. More people have sickle cell

trait than have sickle cell disease. The gene is found in 1 out of every 10 African Americans. Of those who inherit the disease, symptoms usually do not appear until after age 4 months. This disease is characterized by abnormal hemoglobin (HbS) found on the red blood cells (RBCs). HbS causes the RBCs to form a crescent (or sickle) shape within blood vessels and occlude blood flow. In Africa, the sickling effect developed as a genetic adaptation to protect against malaria; the genetic characteristic has continued from generation to generation. Because malaria in the United States is minimal, the genetic phenomenon is detrimental rather than protective. Sickle cell disease also occurs in smaller numbers among people of Mediterranean and Middle Eastern descent. It is not usually associated with Mexican Americans, Asian Americans, or Native Americans.
> *Test Taking Strategy—Analyze to determine what information the question asks for, which is the ethnic origin of persons who most often acquire sickle cell disease. Because African Americans are commonly affected, option 4 is the correct answer. Review characteristics of sickle cell disease, focusing on its inheritance, if you had difficulty answering this question.*
Cognitive Level—*Applying*
Client Needs Category—*Health promotion and maintenance*
Client Needs Subcategory—*None*

68. 3, 5, 6. Jaundice is commonly present in individuals with sickle cell anemia. It occurs because sickled red blood cells (RBCs) are destroyed more rapidly than normal RBCs. When RBCs are rapidly destroyed, bilirubin accumulates and causes the jaundiced skin color. Because of the abnormal shape of the RBC, the oxygen-carrying capacity is affected and clients are often short of breath. Pain is common when the crescent-shaped RBCs clump together, occluding the blood vessel. Pain can be acute or chronic, mild to severe. A white, coated tongue indicates a fungal infection or mouth breathing. Cloudy urine is a sign of a urinary tract infection. Nausea has multiple causes, but it is not usually a symptom of sickle cell anemia.
> *Test Taking Strategy—Analyze to determine what information the question asks for, which is signs and symptoms of sickle cell anemia. Alternative-format "select all that apply" questions require considering each option independently to decide its merit in answering the question. Choose the options that correlate with the signs and symptoms of sickle cell anemia. Review the pathophysiology and clinical manifestations associated with sickle cell anemia if you had difficulty answering this question.*
Cognitive Level—*Applying*
Client Needs Category—*Physiological integrity*
Client Needs Subcategory—*Physiological adaptation*

69. 2. Severe pain is the major problem for clients experiencing a sickle cell crisis. The pain is caused by tissue ischemia secondary to blockage of blood vessels by sickled red blood cells. Pain is most severe in the abdominal area; however, the chest, back, and joints may also be affected. Although the pain is likely to trigger anxiety, if the pain is controlled, anxiety is relieved as well. Adequate nutrition and ventilation are concerns for all clients. Usually, they are not a major concern in a sickle cell crisis unless complications, such as a cerebral or pulmonary infarction, develop.

Test Taking Strategy—Analyze to determine what information the question asks for, which is the nurse's priority focus when caring for a client experiencing a sickle cell crisis. Recall that vascular occlusion results in tissue ischemia and severe pain (option 2). Review the nursing care of the client in sickle cell crisis if you had difficulty answering this question.
Cognitive Level—Analyzing
Client Needs Category—Physiological integrity
Client Needs Subcategory—Physiological adaptation

70. 2. Because the client's activity is limited during a sickle cell crisis, it is important to change the client's position frequently to reduce discomfort and prevent complications of immobility. No specific position is ideal; the goal is to relieve pressure and promote comfort. Ambulation and any form of exercise are contraindicated because they increase the client's need for tissue oxygenation at a time when the oxygen-carrying capacity of red blood cells is limited.

Test Taking Strategy—Apply the key words "most appropriate" when selecting an answer among the four options. Choose the option that describes the best nursing measure when caring for a client with an edematous knee secondary to the effects caused by sickle cell crisis. Recall that during sickle cell crisis, the client has severe pain. Exercise and movement tend to contribute to discomfort, but helping the client change positions (option 2) may reduce pain. Review interventions that are appropriate for relieving joint pain in a lower limb if you had difficulty answering this question.
Cognitive Level—Analyzing
Client Needs Category—Physiological integrity
Client Needs Subcategory—Basic care and comfort

71. 1. Adequate hydration is a major goal for clients in sickle cell crisis. Increasing and maintaining high volumes of fluid by oral or I.V. routes promote the circulation and improve blood flow caused by sickled cells that have occluded the blood vessel. Although elastic stockings would also promote venous return of blood, the client's arterial blood contains the oxygen needed by cells and tissue. Elevating the legs relieves swelling associated with thrombus formation; however, in sickle cell crisis, the client is likely to have many microemboli. Neither elevating the legs nor dangling them helps move red blood cells that accumulate and form thrombi.

Test Taking Strategy—Use the process of elimination to help select the option that identifies the best intervention for maintaining tissue perfusion in the client experiencing a sickle cell crisis. Recall that a low volume of circulating fluid contributes to the clustering of sickled cells; therefore, increasing fluid intake (option 1) will help mobilize the bolus of cells and increase blood flow to the ischemic tissue. Review the need for adequate fluid intake and hydration in sickle cell anemia if you had difficulty answering this question.
Cognitive Level—Applying
Client Needs Category—Physiological integrity
Client Needs Subcategory—Physiological adaptation

72. 3, 5, 6. A sickle cell crisis occurs when the client has a high demand for oxygen. Factors that can trigger a crisis include overexertion, dehydration, fever, infection, alcohol ingestion, smoking, and exposure to cold weather or high altitudes. Although the client becomes fatigued during a crisis, this is not a precipitating cause. Low blood glucose levels are not known to trigger sickle cell crisis.

Test Taking Strategy—Analyze to determine what information the question asks for, which is precipitating factors in a sickle cell crisis. Alternative-format "select all that apply" questions require considering each option independently to decide its merit in answering the question. Select the options from among those provided that trigger sickling of the blood cells. Review resources that discuss factors contributing to an exacerbation of sickle cell anemia if you had difficulty answering this question.
Cognitive Level—Applying
Client Needs Category—Physiological integrity
Client Needs Subcategory—Physiological adaptation

73. 3. People with sickle cell trait inherit one defective gene and one normal gene for hemoglobin. Because the defective gene is a recessive trait, the disease (sickle cell anemia) is never manifested. Those who inherit a set of recessive genes (one defective gene from each parent) will have sickle cell anemia and manifest symptoms. A couple who both carry the recessive trait can produce a normal child (the child acquires a normal gene from both parents), a child who carries the trait (the child acquires one normal gene and one recessive gene), or a child with sickle cell anemia (the child acquires two recessive genes). Sickle cell anemia is usually diagnosed in childhood, not later in life. There is no evidence suggesting that clients who have sickle cell anemia have shorter life spans; however, some clients have died prematurely when they ignored the signs and symptoms of sickle cell crisis.

Test Taking Strategy—Use the process of elimination to help select the option that identifies the best response to the client's question about the significance of having sickle cell trait. Option 3 remains as the correct answer because a person with sickle cell trait does

not manifest symptoms but can pass on the defective gene to their children. Review the difference between sickle cell anemia and sickle cell trait and the genetics that relate to its inheritance if you had difficulty answering this question.
Cognitive Level—*Analyzing*
Client Needs Category—*Health promotion and maintenance*
Client Needs Subcategory—*None*

Nursing Care of Clients with White Blood Cell Disorders

74. 3. Cloudy urine is a common sign associated with a urinary tract infection. Other findings that suggest an infection include fever, cough, increased respirations and heart rate, and ulcerated oral mucous membranes. Blood in the stool is associated with GI bleeding or altered clotting mechanisms. Prolonged vomiting is a side effect of chemotherapy. Extreme fatigue accompanies reduced numbers of red blood cells, causing anemia.

> *Test Taking Strategy*—*Analyze to determine what information the question asks for, which is the assessment finding that supports the nurse's suspicion that the client has an infection. Recall that urine should be clear yellow and transparent. Cloudy urine (option 3) indicates the possibility that white blood cells, which increase during an infectious process, and debris are now present in the urine. Review the characteristics of urine when a urinary tract infection occurs if you had difficulty answering this question.*
> **Cognitive Level**—*Applying*
> **Client Needs Category**—*Physiological integrity*
> **Client Needs Subcategory**—*Physiological adaptation*

75. 1. Because the client's gums are bleeding, foam mouth swabs are less likely to traumatize the gums and oral mucous membranes. These swabs are substituted for the toothbrush temporarily. Because the mouth contains organisms that are a source of opportunistic infection, oral hygiene should not be discontinued. Antiseptic mouthwash may be used temporarily to eliminate bacteria, but this is not a permanent alternative to brushing. The risk for injury continues if the nurse eliminates toothpaste but continues to use the toothbrush. Using dental floss can cause further bleeding to the gums.

> *Test Taking Strategy*—*When analyzing the choices provided, use the key words "most appropriate" to determine the nursing approach for oral hygiene that is better than any of the others for a client with leukemia who develops bleeding gums. Recall that using a soft substance like foam swabs (option 1) will cause less trauma to gums that already bleed easily. Review alternatives to a toothbrush for providing oral hygiene and indications for their use if you had difficulty answering this question.*

Cognitive Level—*Applying*
Client Needs Category—*Physiological integrity*
Client Needs Subcategory—*Basic care and comfort*

76. 4. Soft, bland foods, such as creamed soups, cottage cheese, baked fish, macaroni and cheese, custard, and pudding, are recommended for clients with mouth ulcers. These types of foods help maintain nutrition and relieve oral discomfort. Spicy foods (such as spaghetti and French dressing) and coarse and irritating foods (grilled cheese sandwich) are avoided.

> *Test Taking Strategy*—*Analyze to determine what information the question asks for, which is a menu item that is best for a client who has bleeding gums. Recall that creamed potato soup (option 4) has minimum texture that would make it easier to chew compared to the other choices. Review dietary modifications that are appropriate to avoid causing further mouth trauma for a client with a disorder that affects chewing food if you had difficulty answering this question.*
> **Cognitive Level**—*Applying*
> **Client Needs Category**—*Physiological integrity*
> **Client Needs Subcategory**—*Basic care and comfort*

77. 1. Antineoplastic drugs are a classification of drugs used to kill cancer cells. The client who receives antineoplastic chemotherapy may experience hair loss. The hair loss is not permanent; hair growth returns when the drug therapy is discontinued. In the meantime, the nurse should allow the client to discuss feelings about the potential hair loss. If the client is troubled by the loss of hair, the nurse can offer suggestions for disguising the hair loss. Some possible alternatives include wearing a turban, baseball cap, scarf, or wig. Diarrhea, not constipation, is more closely associated with antineoplastic drugs. Other side effects of antineoplastic drugs include nausea, vomiting, and bone marrow suppression. Rashes and headaches are not related to this classification of drugs.

> *Test Taking Strategy*—*Analyze to determine what information the question asks for, which is a common side effect of antineoplastic drugs about which the client should be informed. Recall that antineoplastic drugs not only destroy cancer cells, but many also affect rapidly growing normal cells such as hair (option 1). Review the mechanism of action and common side effects of antineoplastic drugs if you had difficulty answering this question.*
> **Cognitive Level**—*Applying*
> **Client Needs Category**—*Physiological integrity*
> **Client Needs Subcategory**—*Pharmacological therapies*

78. 3. A low platelet count of less than 100,000/mm³ places the client at risk for bleeding. Using a small-gauge needle for injections reduces the amount of blood loss. Switching to oral medications when possible is even better. When the number of mature white blood cells (not platelets) is low, it is appropriate to place the client on neutropenic precautions and limit contact with visitors who may be infectious. Rest periods are appropriate to counteract the effects of a low red blood cell count.

> *Test Taking Strategy—Apply the key words "most appropriate" when reviewing the four options. Select the option that is better than any of the others for managing the care of a client with a low platelet count. Recall that an intervention that minimizes the potential for bleeding such as using small-gauge needles for injections (option 3) deals specifically with the client's potential risk. Review the function of platelets and nursing interventions that are necessary when a client has an impaired ability to control bleeding if you had difficulty answering this question.*
> *Cognitive Level—Analyzing*
> *Client Needs Category—Physiological integrity*
> *Client Needs Subcategory—Reduction of risk potential*

79. 3. The term *remission* means that the disease has responded to treatment and is not currently progressing; the original signs and symptoms of disease may even be absent. However, this does not mean the condition is cured. Although a remission is a good sign, the client's prognosis continues to be guarded because it is difficult to predict how long the remission will last. Treatment is reinstituted if the disease manifests again. For this reason, it is very important to stress that the client maintain regular checkups with the physician. In the meantime, the client should be encouraged to live as fully and normally as possible.

> *Test Taking Strategy—Analyze to determine what information the question asks for, which is a statement that correlates with an accurate interpretation of what the term remission implies. Recall that the term remission means that the disease process is under control (option 3) but is not necessarily cured. Review the definition of remission and how the term applies to a disease process if you had difficulty answering this question.*
> *Cognitive Level—Applying*
> *Client Needs Category—Health promotion and maintenance*
> *Client Needs Subcategory—None*

80. 3. An advocate performs duties on behalf of the client. To become a client advocate, the nurse must understand the client's rights. The nurse must uphold the client's right to be told the truth about his or her condition and the right to make an informed decision regarding his or her care. The best example of advocacy is upholding the client's decision to decline further invasive procedures. Allowing the client to refuse personal care promotes autonomy and client centered care. Discussing hospice without client input is not an example of client centered care. Decorating the room with cards is an act of kindness, especially with client input.

> *Test Taking Strategy—Analyze to determine what information the question asks for, which is a nursing action demonstrating the nurse as a client advocate.*

> *Consider the term advocate upholding the rights of others. Recall that as a client advocate, the nurse yields to the wishes of the client based on the nurse's understanding of client rights. An important component of client advocacy is demonstrated during end-of-life care decisions.*
> *Cognitive Level—Analyzing*
> *Client Needs Category—Safe and effective environment*
> *Client Needs Subcategory—Coordinated care*

81. 2. Mononucleosis, an acute viral disease caused by the Epstein-Barr virus, is transmitted by direct contact with the droplets or saliva of another infected person. Most common among 15- to 25-year-olds, this disease is referred to as *the kissing disease* because the virus passes from one individual to another orally. The incubation period is roughly 30 to 45 days. Sharing eating utensils, cups, and cigarettes are also ways of transmitting this disease. Disease transmission does not occur by eating contaminated food, being bitten by insects, or coming in contact with blood.

> *Test Taking Strategy—Analyze to determine what information the question asks for, which is the route by which mononucleosis is transmitted. Recall that the Epstein-Barr virus responsible for infectious mononucleosis is spread by any exchange of saliva (option 2) or using eating utensils on which saliva is still present. Although the virus remains in the body forever, its infectiousness diminishes over time. Review the etiology of mononucleosis and its mode of transmission if you had difficulty answering this question.*
> *Cognitive Level—Understanding*
> *Client Needs Category—Safe and effective care environment*
> *Client Needs Subcategory—Safety and infection control*

82. 3. One of the first signs of infectious mononucleosis is a severe sore throat. Onset of symptoms usually takes 1 to 2 weeks, and the client has flulike symptoms, such as fever, headache, anorexia, fatigue, and generalized aching. In severe cases, the lymph nodes—including the spleen—become enlarged. The symptoms last for 14 to 28 days. If complications develop, jaundice occurs. Abdominal discomfort, aching joints, and intestinal upset are not characteristic of the disorder.

> *Test Taking Strategy—Analyze to determine what information the question asks for, which is the initial symptom experienced by a person who acquires infectious mononucleosis. Infectious mononucleosis is also called glandular fever because its onset includes an elevated temperature accompanied by a sore throat (option 3). Review symptoms that accompany infectious mononucleosis if you had difficulty answering this question.*
> *Cognitive Level—Analyzing*
> *Client Needs Category—Physiological integrity*
> *Client Needs Subcategory—Physiological adaptation*

83. 2. Rest is essential for recovery from infectious mononucleosis. Therefore, activity should be restricted during the course of the illness. Physical activity is likely to intensify symptoms, prolong recovery, or contribute to complications involving the liver, spleen, heart, and nervous system. Nurses should instruct the client with an enlarged spleen or liver not to participate in contact sports, such as football or soccer, until the physician has released the client from treatment. Treatment is usually symptomatic, involving oral fluids, analgesics, and anti-pyretics. Because this is a viral infection, antibiotics are not warranted unless the client has a secondary bacterial infection. Taking vitamins may improve overall health if the client is anorexic, but this is generally unnecessary. Blood transfusions are not indicated for clients who have mononucleosis.

Test Taking Strategy—Use the process of elimination to help select the option that identifies essential information for the client's self-care. Recall that there is no specific treatment for infectious mononucleosis, but rest (option 2) will shorten the time for recovery. Review the symptomatic treatment for infectious mononucleosis if you had difficulty answering this question.
Cognitive Level—Applying
Client Needs Category—Phyciological integrity
Client Needs Subcategory—Reduction of risk potential

84. 2, 6. Hodgkin's disease is a malignant lymphatic condition chiefly characterized by one or more pain-lessly enlarged lymph nodes. Other signs and symptoms include pruritus (itching), anorexia, weight loss, fever, night sweats, fatigue, and enlargement of the lymphatic organs (such as the spleen). Bone pain may occur later as the disease progresses. Headaches, rashes, and diarrhea, if they occur, are not necessarily related to the primary disorder.

Test Taking Strategy—Analyze to determine what information the question asks for, which is signs and symptoms of Hodgkin's disease. Alternative-format "select all that apply" questions require considering each option independently to decide its merit in answering the question. Choose the options that correlate with the signs and symptoms of Hodgkin's disease. Review clinical manifestations of Hodgkin's disease in the rationale and similar information in other references if you had difficulty answering this question.
Cognitive Level—Analyzing
Client Needs Category—Physiological integrity
Client Needs Subcategory—Physiological adaptation

85. 1. During the early stages of Hodgkin's disease, the client's lymph nodes are typically enlarged and painless. Enlarged nodes are usually found first in the neck; if the client is untreated, the disease can spread throughout the lymphatic system. The physical change in cervical lymph nodes is generally one of the first abnormal signs of this disease. Later, the axillary and inguinal lymph nodes may also become involved. Regardless of the location in the body, cancerous growths are hardly ever painful in the early stages of the disease. This explains why early warning signs of cancer tend to be ignored. The other choices do not accurately describe the lymph nodes associated with Hodgkin's disease.

Test Taking Strategy—Analyze to determine what information the question asks for, which is a description of the findings of lymph node assessment that are characteristic of Hodgkin's disease. Recall that any type of cancer rarely causes pain in an early stage—including Hodgkin's disease. A person with Hodgkin's disease will most likely have painless lymph node enlargement (option 1). Review the initial signs and symptoms that accompany Hodgkin's disease if you had difficulty answering this question.
Cognitive Level—Applying
Client Needs Category—Physiological integrity
Client Needs Subcategory—Physiological adaptation

86. 3. On receiving the information that the client is using herbal therapy as a daily health practice, the nurse must assess the types of herbs being used and notify the physician. The physician will make the decision whether the client may obtain external radiation as scheduled or if the treatment will be delayed. Determining if the herbal therapy is part of a naturalist therapy regimen is good in order to understand the client's overall plan of care but is not a priority for the nurse at this time. Instructing the client to suspend or continue herbal therapy will be determined by the physician.

Test Taking Strategy—Apply the key words "most appropriate" when determining which nursing action in the list of options is better than the others. Even though herbs are plants, they contain active substances that can affect the medical treatment. The nurse's responsibility is to identity the herbal supplements the client uses and share that information with the physician. Review the definitions of alternative and complementary therapies and the precautions involved in their use if you had difficulty answering this question.
Cognitive Level—Analyzing
Client Needs Category—Physiological integrity
Client Needs Subcategory—Reduction of risk potential

87. 2. Deodorants or other skin preparations that contain metals are avoided because they absorb X-rays and increase skin irritation. The skin can be washed with tepid water, mild soap, and a soft washcloth. The hair in the area is not shaved. In fact, shaving may further impair the integrity of the skin, which is somewhat damaged temporarily by the radiation. Zinc oxide contains a metal; therefore, it should not be applied to the skin. If the skin does become dry, blistered, or begins to peel, the physician may prescribe a topical application of vitamin A and D ointment, lanolin, pure aloe vera gel, or cortisone ointment.

> *Test Taking Strategy—Analyze to determine what information the question asks for, which is information that should be included when preparing a client who will undergo radiation therapy. Recall that the client must be made aware of topical substances that may intensify the effect of radiation (option 2) as well as measures that will reduce damage to the skin. Review possible skin changes that may occur with external radiation and how they may be minimized if you had difficulty answering this question.*
> **Cognitive Level**—*Applying*
> **Client Needs Category**—*Physiological integrity*
> **Client Needs Subcategory**—*Reduction of risk potential*

88. 1. Skin reddening or bronzing is expected in the area that is irradiated. It is best to inform the client about anticipated skin changes before therapy begins and to stress that the red discoloration is only temporary. Although the ionizing radiation used in cancer therapy is a form of energy, it does not produce heat or cause bleeding under the skin. The client's concern is more likely related to a fear of adverse reactions to therapy than about the cosmetic change to the skin; therefore, reassuring the client that the redness is hardly noticeable is inappropriate.

> *Test Taking Strategy—Apply the key words "most appropriate" when discriminating among the statements in the options. Select the option that identifies an accurate nursing response to the client's concerns about reddened skin in the area targeted by external radiation. Recall that although the radiation is not felt, it has to go through the skin when it is beamed at its target. Varying degrees of redness and peeling skin are expected (option 1) but are not necessarily dangerous if measures are taken to ensure the integrity of the skin. Review the superficial effects of external radiation if you had difficulty answering this question.*
> **Cognitive Level**—*Applying*
> **Client Needs Category**—*Health promotion and maintenance*
> **Client Needs Subcategory**—*None*

89. 4. The most important information to give the client with irradiated skin is to protect it from direct sunlight. Advising the client to wear several layers of warm clothing is appropriate if the client has poor circulation. For comfort, any individual should avoid becoming chilled or too warm, so this choice is not as important as avoiding sunlight. Wearing a face mask is only warranted if the client has allergies to inhaled substances, has cardiovascular disease in which vasoconstriction causes ischemia, or needs a barrier to infectious microorganisms or environmental pollutants.

> *Test Taking Strategy—Use the process of elimination to select the option that identifies the most*

important information regarding exposure to the outdoor elements when receiving external radiation. Although all of the advice provided in the options has merit in various circumstances, preventing skin exposure to direct sunlight (option 4) is most critical and takes precedence over the other information. Review interventions that help prevent secondary skin damage when a client receives external radiation if you had difficulty answering this question.
> **Cognitive Level**—*Applying*
> **Client Needs Category**—*Physiological integrity*
> **Client Needs Subcategory**—*Reduction of risk potential*

90. 3. Non-Hodgkin's lymphoma is a malignant disease that primarily affects the lymphatic tissue of older adults. Like Hodgkin's disease, this condition begins with one lymph node and spreads to the rest of the body. Antineoplastic drugs (chemotherapy) can depress bone marrow function and decrease the body's ability to fight infection. If the white blood cell count drops to dangerously low levels, the client becomes susceptible to infection. Then neutropenic precautions (also known as *protective* or *reverse isolation*) are necessary to prevent exposure to microorganisms that can lead to infection. Periodic blood cell counts are monitored to assess for this potential complication. Anorexia, nausea, vomiting, weight loss, and diarrhea are also side effects of cancer treatment, but they are not indications that require the client to be placed on neutropenic precautions. Confusion and disorientation suggest that the client is experiencing neurologic problems and should be observed closely to protect the client's safety, but the symptoms do not justify implementing neutropenic precautions.

> *Test Taking Strategy—Analyze to determine what information the question asks for, which is information that should be reported immediately upon gathering data about a client with non-Hodgkin's lymphoma. Recall that the most abundant phagocytic white blood cells that attack microorganisms are neutrophils. If they are compromised (option 3), the client is susceptible to infection. As a safety precaution, health care workers follow neutropenic precautions. Review indications for neutropenic precautions if you had difficulty answering this question.*
> **Cognitive Level**—*Analyzing*
> **Client Needs Category**—*Safe and effective care environment*
> **Client Needs Subcategory**—*Safety and infection control*

91. 3. Discussing feelings with another person facilitates grieving. The client should not be left alone immediately after hearing this information. It is important to remain with the client until the information has been processed. The client would also benefit from talking with other supportive individuals, such as a spouse, family member, friend, or clergyman. Reading literature on the subject and thinking in private help some people, but most believe it is more effective to verbalize thoughts and feelings. If the client requests a second opinion, the request should not be denied; however, it would be inappropriate for the nurse to initiate the suggestion. Doing so is considered a form of false reassurance and could prolong the client's denial.

> *Test Taking Strategy—Use the key words "most help-ful" to identify the nursing response that is best for helping a client deal with his or her impending death. Recall that verbalizing one's feelings (option 3), especially with someone who is empathetic, is more therapeutic than internalizing them. Review therapeutic communication skills that help clients experiencing a crisis if you had difficulty answering this question.*
> *Cognitive Level—Applying*
> *Client Needs Category—Psychosocial integrity*
> *Client Needs Subcategory—None*

92. 1, 2, 3, 4, 6. Clients who exhibit the characteristic signs and symptoms of human immunodeficiency virus (HIV) infection will most likely exhibit coughing, fever, fatigue, diarrhea, and swollen lymph nodes. Other signs and symptoms include night sweats, unexplained weight loss, anorexia, and mouth lesions. Kaposi's sarcoma, which occurs in clients who are infected with HIV or are immunodeficient for other reasons, involves skin lesions of varying sizes and thicknesses that have a characteristic purple color. The lesions of Kaposi's sarcoma would not be characterized as a blemish.

> *Test Taking Strategy—Analyze to determine what information the question asks for, which is signs and symptoms of HIV infection. Alternative-format "select all that apply" questions require consider-ing each option independently to decide its merit in answering the question. Choose the options from the list provided that correlate with the signs and symptoms of HIV. Review the signs and symptoms manifested by a client infected with HIV if you had difficulty answering this question.*
> *Cognitive Level—Applying*
> *Client Needs Category—Physiological integrity*
> *Client Needs Subcategory—Physiological adaptation*

93. 2, 3, 4, 5. Practicing safer sex behaviors includes abstinence and reducing the number of sexual partners to one. The client should be encouraged to notify previous and present partners of the human immunodeficiency virus (HIV) status. Condoms should be used for each sexual encounter but should be discarded after one use. Anal intercourse should be avoided due to the risk of bleeding from injury to the rectum and anal tissues. Engaging in nonpenetrating sexual activities, such as mutual masturba-tion, demonstrates an understanding of safer sex behav-ior. Other safer behaviors include not sharing needles,

razors, toothbrushes, or objects used for sexual activities. Although the HIV has been identified in saliva, it has not been identified as a source of transmission. To be ulti-mately safe, oral intercourse should be avoided, and semen and urine should not be ingested.

> *Test Taking Strategy—Analyze to determine what infor-mation the question asks for, which is appropriate teaching about safer sex behaviors for the HIV-infected client. Alternative-format "select all that apply" ques-tions require considering each option independently to decide its merit in answering the question. For this item, select the options that correlate with safer sex practices. Review measures that promote safer sex if you had difficulty answering this question.*
> *Cognitive Level—Applying*
> *Client Needs Category—Health promotion and maintenance*
> *Client Needs Subcategory—None*

94. 4. I.V. drug users who share needles, male homo-sexuals, bisexuals, women who have intercourse with these males, and infants of infected mothers, including those who are breastfed, are at greatest risk for developing acquired immunodeficiency syndrome (AIDS). Haitians and Africans also have a high incidence of this disease among their native populations. Vacationing in Africa, drinking alcohol, or having had surgery does not place the client at any greater risk for AIDS than other individuals.

> *Test Taking Strategy—Use the process of elimination to select the option that correlates with the highest risk for acquiring human immunodeficiency virus (HIV) infection. Although alcohol abuse may interfere with good judgment and the potential for risky behaviors, I.V. drug use (option 4), especially when it involves circumstances in which needles are shared, has a high potential for transmitting HIV. Review the risk factors for AIDS and activities that may transmit HIV if you had difficulty answering this question.*
> *Cognitive Level—Analyzing*
> *Client Needs Category—Physiological integrity*
> *Client Needs Subcategory—Physiological adaptation*

95. 3. Enzyme-linked immunosorbent assay (ELISA) detects the presence of antibodies to viral antigens. A reactive ELISA is generally repeated. If it continues to be reactive, more specific tests for the human immunodefi-ciency virus (HIV) antibodies, such as the Western blot test or rapid enzyme immunoassay (Murex SUDS-HIV-1 anti-body test), are performed before making a definitive diag-nosis of acquired immunodeficiency syndrome (AIDS). The Venereal Disease Research Laboratory (VDRL) test is used as a screening test for syphilis. The Schick test is used to determine if a person has antibodies to the bacterial tox-ins of the organism that cause diphtheria. The Dick test is used to assess the immunologic status of a person who has been exposed to the toxins associated with scarlet fever.

Test Taking Strategy—Use the process of elimination to select the option that is most specific for diagnosing an HIV infection. Although the ELISA test (option 3) is used for screening and may be positive for reasons other than being infected with HIV, it is the most specific from among the options for detecting antibodies against HIV. Because there may be false positives, additional tests that can identify HIV infection more accurately may be performed subsequently. Review diagnostic tests currently available for identifying individuals who are infected with HIV if you had difficulty answering this question.
Cognitive Level—Applying
Client Needs Category—Safe and effective care environment
Client Needs Subcategory—Coordinated care

96. 2. Standard precautions are used when a person's infectious status is unknown. Standard precautions involve donning one or more protective garments—depending on the potential for coming into contact with blood or body fluids—and taking precautionary actions to avoid penetrating injuries with objects contaminated with blood or body fluid. In *all* situations, it is important to avoid recapping needles because this will prevent an accidental needle-stick injury. A face mask provides protection from being splashed with blood or body fluid; however, most dressings absorb liquid drainage, and wearing gloves is more appropriate. Wearing a cover gown is appropriate if blood and body fluid may potentially penetrate clothing; however, this measure is unnecessary when giving most clients a bed bath. Gloves are appropriate when touching areas of the body where there may be contact with blood or body fluids. Wearing gloves while taking vital signs is generally unnecessary.

Test Taking Strategy—Use the process of elimination to select the option that describes an action that provides the best protection from acquiring human immunodeficiency virus when caring for a client with an unknown infectious status. Options 1, 3, and 4 describe standard precautions, but the circumstances for their use are not valid. Because a client's blood may be in and on a used needle, needles should never be recapped (option 2). Review the rationale for leaving needles uncapped at the time of their disposal if you had difficulty answering this question.
Cognitive Level—Applying
Client Needs Category—Safe and effective care environment
Client Needs Subcategory—Safety and infection control

97. 1. Setting and reaching realistic daily goals is the most therapeutic approach and can help the client experience a sense of hope. Hope has a powerful influence on a dying person's will to live and can lift a depressed person's spirits. Referring the client to the chaplain is appropriate if the client requests contact with a clergyman. Distraction will not help a client deal with the feelings nor will it promote a sense of hope. Contacting the next of kin may be therapeutic, depending on the client's relationship with the family.

Test Taking Strategy—Use the key words "most therapeutic" when analyzing the choices in the four options. Select the option that is more beneficial than any of the others when caring for a client who has lost hope for improvement. Option 3 can be eliminated because it does not represent therapeutic communication. Options 2 and 4, although they may be therapeutic depending on the client, are not the best answers. Recall that setting and achieving a goal (option 1) provides evidence that progress is possible. Review nursing interventions that have the potential for fostering a sense of hope in persons who have become discouraged if you had difficulty answering this question.
Cognitive Level—Applying
Client Needs Category—Psychosocial integrity
Client Needs Subcategory—None

Nursing Care of Clients with Bone Marrow Disorders

98. 1. Polycythemia vera is a life-threatening disorder that results in the concentration of hemoglobin and an increase in the number of red blood cells. Symptoms include weakness, clotting, dizziness, painful extremities, and flushing of the face and extremities. If the client exhibits organ enlargement, sitting upright allows abdominal organs, such as the spleen, liver, and intestines, to fall away from the diaphragm. By reducing crowding of the diaphragm, dyspnea is reduced and the client feels more comfortable. Any other position will cause difficulty breathing.

Test Taking Strategy—Use the process of elimination to select the option that identifies a position that would provide the most comfort for a client with an enlarged spleen. Option 4 can be eliminated immediately because elevating the legs would increase pressure within the abdomen and contribute to the client's discomfort. Options 2 and 3 would not compress the abdominal organs, but neither of these choices is as beneficial as having the client sit upright (option 1). Review the rationale for placing clients with polycythemia vera in a Fowler's position if you had difficulty answering this question.
Cognitive Level—Applying
Client Needs Category—Physiological integrity
Client Needs Subcategory—Basic care and comfort

99. 2. Keeping a client with polycythemia vera well hydrated reduces the blood's viscosity, or thickness. Thrombi are less likely to form if the excessive numbers of blood cells are kept diluted within the plasma. In that way, they move more easily throughout the circulatory system, reducing the possibility of clumping together within a small blood vessel. Diuretics affect fluid balance and can cause dehydration, which may result in clot formation. Restricting dietary sodium and encouraging weight loss are healthful interventions, but they do not have a therapeutic effect on preventing the formation of blood clots.

> *Test Taking Strategy—Use the key words "most appropriate" to narrow the selection to an option that is better than the others for preventing blood clots in a client with polycythemia vera. Recall that blood cells aggregate (clump together) when there is a decrease in the fluid component of blood. Therefore, increasing fluid intake (option 2) prevents stagnation of blood cells. Review nursing interventions that prevent complications in a client with an excess of blood cells if you had difficulty answering this question.*
> *Cognitive Level—Applying*
> *Client Needs Category—Physiological integrity*
> *Client Needs Subcategory—Reduction of risk potential*

100. 1.   Treatment for polycythemia vera includes measures to remove blood. As much as 500 to 2,000 mL of blood is removed by performing a phlebotomy. This is similar to the technique for donating a unit of blood. Afterward, I.V. fluid is infused to dilute the remaining circulating cells. More aggressive therapy with radiophosphorus and radiation is used in an effort to decrease the bone marrow's cell production. A tourniquet may be used, but this choice does not provide the best evidence that the client understands the treatment. Receiving a blood transfusion will add more blood volume, which is already the cause of the problem. Surgically occluding blood vessels may result in further clot formation.

> *Test Taking Strategy—Use the process of elimination to select the option that provides the best evidence that the client understands the meaning of the term phlebotomy. Option 1 remains as the correct answer because the term phlebotomy means incising a vein, which is therapeutically necessary for removing blood when a client has polycythemia vera. Review the treatment for this disease process if you had difficulty answering this question.*
> *Cognitive Level—Analyzing*
> *Client Needs Category—Physiological integrity*
> *Client Needs Subcategory—Physiological adaptation*

101. 1.   Angina, pain or pressure in the chest, may occur as a result of inadequate blood flow and oxygenation to the heart caused by a thrombus in a coronary artery. Clots are more likely to form due to the thick nature of the circulating blood volume and the increased number of platelets as well as red and white blood cells. Indigestion, burning on urination, and loss of appetite should not be ignored by the nurse, but they are not commonly associated with polycythemia vera.

> *Test Taking Strategy—Analyze to determine what information the question asks for, which is a potential consequence for which the client with polycythemia vera is at risk. The increased volume of blood cells, which includes platelets, leads to greater viscosity of blood and thrombotic episodes such as myocardial infarction, which may be accompanied by angina (option 1); stroke; pulmonary embolism; and deep vein thrombo-*

sis. *Review complications associated with polycythemia vera if you had difficulty answering this question.*
> *Cognitive Level—Applying*
> *Client Needs Category—Physiological integrity*
> *Client Needs Subcategory—Physiological adaptation*

102. 1.   Bone marrow is aspirated from the iliac crest, the curved rim along the upper border of the ilium, felt in the hip area near the level of the waist. The sternum (breastbone), located in the center of the chest, is an alternate site for aspirating a sample of bone marrow. The iliac crest is generally the first choice because it contains more bone marrow than the sternum. The lower spine, upper arm, and groin area are not suitable sites for bone marrow aspiration.

> *Test Taking Strategy—Analyze to determine what information the question asks for, which is the anatomic location from which bone marrow will be aspirated. Recall that bone marrow is best removed from flat bones such as the iliac crest, which is in the posterior hip (option 1). Review the procedure for aspirating bone marrow if you had difficulty answering this question.*
> *Cognitive Level—Understanding*
> *Client Needs Category—Physiological integrity*
> *Client Needs Subcategory—Physiological adaptation*

103. 1.   The nurse's primary role in assisting with bone marrow aspiration is to help minimize the pain and discomfort the client is likely to experience. Despite the use of local anesthesia, the client typically feels pressure as the needle is driven into the bone, followed by brief but sharp pain as the needle finally enters the bone and marrow is withdrawn. Helpful measures include premedicating the client, providing distraction throughout the procedure, and offering encouragement and support. The physician generally needs no assistance with instruments during the procedure. A suction machine is not used, and oxygen is not usually needed under most conditions.

> *Test Taking Strategy—Analyze to determine what information the question asks for, which is a major nursing responsibility when assisting with a bone marrow aspiration. Recall that the client is likely anxious, which tends to intensify his or her actual or perceived discomfort. Using interventions that minimize the discomfort (option 1) is a major responsibility for the nurse. Review nursing responsibilities when a bone marrow aspiration is performed if you had difficulty answering this question.*
> *Cognitive Level—Analyzing*
> *Client Needs Category—Physiological integrity*
> *Client Needs Subcategory—Basic care and comfort*

104. 2.   Bleeding from the puncture site is one of the most common problems after bone marrow aspiration, especially if the platelet count is low. If bleeding is not controlled, a painful hematoma forms. Firm pressure or an ice pack is used to limit bleeding. Under usual circumstances, bone marrow aspiration does not cause shock. Though the blood pressure and pulse may fluctuate somewhat, any variation is usually due to pain, anxiety, and fear rather than loss of blood volume. Heart conduction can be expected to stay in normal sinus rhythm. The client remains awake and alert throughout and following the procedure.

Test Taking Strategy—*Use the process of elimination to select the nursing assessment that is essential to perform after bone marrow aspiration. Option 2 remains as the best answer because the physician uses a large-gauge needle to bore through the bone and withdraw marrow, which may result in bleeding from the site. Review the nursing care of a client after a bone marrow aspiration if you had difficulty answering this question.*
Cognitive Level—*Analyzing*
Client Needs Category—*Physiological integrity*
Client Needs Subcategory—*Reduction of risk potential*

105. 1. Aplastic anemia, commonly called *bone marrow depression anemia*, occurs when the bone marrow fails to produce red blood cells (RBCs). Platelets and white blood cells are also affected. The reduction in the number of circulating RBCs affects the blood's oxygen-carrying capacity. Consequently, clients with this problem have difficulty tolerating activities and may become short of breath with rapid or labored breathing. It is important for the nurse to provide the dyspneic client with frequent rest periods because rest decreases oxygen demands. Nausea is not generally associated with hypoxemia. The pulse rate typically increases with activity and poor oxygenation. Cool, moist skin accompanies a drop in blood pressure or other physical problems. It is not usually a classic sign of fatigue or activity intolerance.

Test Taking Strategy—*Use the process of elimination to select the option that identifies the best indication that the client is not tolerating activity well. Recall that tachypnea and labored breathing (option 1) are evidence of oxygen deprivation, which may be caused by a low RBC and hemoglobin count. Review the defining characteristics of the nursing diagnosis Activity intolerance if you had difficulty answering this question.*
Cognitive Level—*Applying*
Client Needs Category—*Physiological integrity*
Client Needs Subcategory—*Reduction of risk potential*

106. 1. A low number of platelets, also known as *thrombocytes*, increases the risk for bleeding. Bruises indicate bleeding into the skin. Pale skin color is associated with anemia, which is caused by a low red blood cell count. Elevated temperature may be a sign of infection or dehydration. Cool extremities are not associated with thrombocytopenia.

Test Taking Strategy—*Apply the key words "most likely" when analyzing the choices in the four options. Select the option that correlates more than any of the others with a low platelet count. Recall that when the ability to clot and control bleeding is compromised, bleeding into the skin and soft tissue will result in bruising (option 1). Review the function of platelets and a*

consequence of a reduced production of these cells if you had difficulty answering this question.
Cognitive Level—*Analyzing*
Client Needs Category—*Physiological integrity*
Client Needs Subcategory—*Physiological adaptation*

107. 1. A client with leukopenia, a low number of white blood cells (WBCs), is at high risk for infection. Hand hygiene is the best technique for reducing the spread of microorganisms and decreasing infection. Applying direct pressure to puncture wounds is necessary when the client has a low platelet count. Wearing a gown when providing care may help reduce the spread of infection, but it is not as effective as good hand washing. Monitoring baseline vitals signs is important because the red blood cells, WBCs, and platelets are all affected, but this choice does not address the client's risk for infection.

Test Taking Strategy—*Use the process of elimination to select the most important nursing measure when caring for a client with a reduced leukocyte count. Recall that leukocytes are WBCs, whose major function is to defend the body against infectious pathogens and remove cellular debris. When the WBC count is low, hand hygiene (option 1) reduces the potential for transferring disease and introducing microorganisms to the client. Review the nursing interventions that are appropriate when caring for a client with leukopenia if you had difficulty answering this question.*
Cognitive Level—*Analyzing*
Client Needs Category—*Safe and effective care environment*
Client Needs Subcategory—*Coordinated care*

108. 3. After it is collected, all donated blood is tested for human immunodeficiency virus (HIV) antibodies. Donated blood is the safest it has been since early 1985. However, it is still not 100% safe because some blood donors who have the virus in their blood have not produced sufficient antibodies to cause a positive reaction when the blood is tested. All potential blood donors are asked questions about lifestyle behaviors that indicate a risk for HIV infection, but some do not answer the questions honestly. Blood donors are encouraged to call the blood collection agency later and report an identifying number, not their name, if they feel someone is at risk by receiving a unit of their donated blood.

Test Taking Strategy—*Note the key words "most appropriate" when looking for an option that includes a response that is better than the others. Recall that all donated blood is tested for HIV (option 3) and discarded if the virus is present. Although this may not ensure total protection from HIV infection, the outcome has shown extremely positive results. Review procedures that are used to eliminate the potential for collecting and preserving donated blood that contains HIV if you had difficulty answering this question.*

Cognitive Level—*Applying*
Client Needs Category—*Health promotion and maintenance*
Client Needs Subcategory—*None*

109. 1. A unit of packed blood cells contains a similar number of blood cells found in a regular unit used in transfusions. However, when preparing the unit of packed blood cells, approximately two thirds of the plasma from a unit of whole blood is removed. The administration of packed cells is preferred for clients who need a blood transfusion but for whom additional fluid in the circulatory system is hazardous. Typically, the candidate for packed cells is someone who is prone to heart failure or who has poor kidney function and does not need the extra fluid. Packed cells pose the same risk for an allergic reaction as whole blood. They do not stimulate the bone marrow to produce blood cells.

Test Taking Strategy—*Use the process of elimination to select the option that identifies the most accurate explanation of how a transfusion of packed cells differs from one of whole blood. Option 2 can be eliminated because a main advantage of administering packed cells is that the total infused volume is reduced. Option 3 can be eliminated because a potential complication of administering both packed cells and whole blood is an allergic reaction. Option 4 can be eliminated because erythropoietin, a substance produced by the kidneys, stimulates the bone marrow to produce blood cells. Option 1 remains as the correct answer because after withdrawing some of the serum, what remains are packed cells. Review the differences between whole blood and packed cells if you had difficulty answering this question.*
Cognitive Level—*Understanding*
Client Needs Category—*Physiological integrity*
Client Needs Subcategory—*Reduction of risk potential*

110. 4. A person with type A, Rh-positive blood would have a reaction if transfused with type AB, Rh-positive blood. It is always best to administer the same blood type; however, a person with type O blood is referred to as the *universal donor*. In an emergency, anyone can receive type O, Rh-negative blood. People who are Rh-positive can receive compatible blood types that are either Rh-positive or Rh-negative. The reverse is *not* true; in other words, a person who is Rh-negative should never be given Rh-positive blood.

Test Taking Strategy—*Analyze to determine what information the question asks for, which is the blood type that is incompatible with that of the client if it is used in a blood transfusion. Recall that persons with type AB, Rh-positive are universal recipients, but their blood cannot be administered to those who have other blood types (option 4). Type A, Rh-positive blood is compatible with type A, Rh-negative; type O, Rh-positive; and type O, Rh-negative blood. Review blood types and their compatibilities if you had difficulty answering this question.*

Cognitive Level—*Applying*
Client Needs Category—*Safe and effective care environment*
Client Needs Subcategory—*Safety and infection control*

111. 2. Hypotension is one of the first signs of a serious blood transfusion reaction. In a serious transfusion reaction, urine formation is decreased. Swelling and pale skin at the infusion site are indications that there is a problem with the administration of the blood rather than a reaction to the blood product.

Test Taking Strategy—*Analyze to determine what information the question asks for, which is an assessment finding that correlates with a transfusion reaction. Recall that anaphylaxis, an allergic reaction to incompatible antigens in the donated blood, results in shock symptoms such as hypotension (option 2) almost immediately as the blood begins to infuse. Review signs and symptoms of an incompatibility reaction during a blood transfusion if you had difficulty answering this question.*
Cognitive Level—*Analyzing*
Client Needs Category—*Physiological integrity*
Client Needs Subcategory—*Reduction of risk potential*

112. 2. Long-term administration of corticosteroids causes body changes such as moon face and buffalo hump on the back of the neck. These resemble signs of Cushing's syndrome caused by a hyperfunctioning adrenal cortex. The voice is unaffected. Muscle wasting may occur with long-term corticosteroid use. Anabolic steroids cause muscle enlargement. Steroid administration causes the skin to appear thin and transparent, not tanned. Purple striae are found on the abdomen and hips. Owing to an inadequately functioning adrenal cortex, bronzed skin is found in individuals who have Addison's disease.

Test Taking Strategy—*Apply the key words "most likely" as a means of identifying the option that describes an effect of corticosteroid therapy. Recall that steroid therapy causes changes in appearance such as a moon face (option 2) when administered for an extended period of time. Review the side effects of corticosteroid therapy if you had difficulty answering this question.*
Cognitive Level—*Applying*
Client Needs Category—*Physiological integrity*
Client Needs Subcategory—*Pharmacological therapies*

113. 1. Steroids are known to cause peptic ulcers. For this reason, the physician may also prescribe drugs to protect the gastric mucosa from erosion. Clients who take corticosteroids usually do not experience drowsiness, anorexia, or light-colored urine.

Test Taking Strategy—*Use the process of elimination to select the option that provides the best evidence for the development of a complication from steroid therapy. The use of steroids is believed to erode the gastric mucosa (option 1) by inhibiting mucus-producing*

substances. Some believe that the development of an ulcer in someone for whom steroids have been prescribed results from high-dose therapy or co-administration of drugs that also irritate gastric mucosa such as nonsteroidal anti-inflammatory drugs. Review the side effects of oral corticosteroids if you had difficulty answering this question.
Cognitive Level—*Analyzing*
Client Needs Category—*Physiological integrity*
Client Needs Subcategory—*Pharmacological therapies*

114. 3. Total body irradiation destroys the client's bone marrow and places the individual at high risk for infection. Medical asepsis is scrupulously followed, prophylactic antibiotics and antifungal medications are administered, and visitors are restricted to prevent the client from acquiring an infection from which the client may not recover. The nurse never neglects to promote optimum nutrition and hydration and to help the client cope with fear and depression. However, if these problems occur, they are more easily treated than an infection.

> *Test Taking Strategy—Use the process of elimination to select the option that identifies the highest nursing priority when caring for a client who has recently received a bone marrow transplant. Recall that irradiating the bone marrow destroys the client's ability to manufacture blood cells, which makes the client susceptible to infection (option 3) that is potentially life threatening until the transplanted cells are reproduced in sufficient quantity. Review the risks associated with a bone marrow transplant and nursing measures when caring for the client who has undergone this procedure if you had difficulty answering this question.*

Cognitive Level—*Analyzing*
Client Needs Category—*Physiological integrity*
Client Needs Subcategory—*Physiological adaptation*

Nursing Care of Clients with Coagulation Disorders

115. 1. Idiopathic thrombocytopenia (ITP) is a bleeding disorder diagnosed by a low platelet count. This disorder has no known cause. ITP is characterized by small hemorrhages in the skin, mucous membranes, or subcutaneous tissues referred to as *purpura* or *petechiae*. Bleeding also occurs internally (from the nose, gums, in urine, and stools) when a person has thrombocytopenia, and women have unusually heavy menstrual flow. There is no other additional term for dark areas of cyanosis. The term for flushed, red skin is *erythema*. Protruding (distended) veins are referred to as *varicosities*.

> *Test Taking Strategy—Analyze to determine what information the question asks for, which is an assessment finding associated with ITP. Recall that one of the clinical manifestations of ITP is superficial bleeding into the skin (option 1) that appears like pinpoint-size spots resembling a reddish purple rash. Review the signs of idiopathic thrombocytopenia, recalling*

that ITP may not be accompanied by any symptoms, if you had difficulty answering this question.
Cognitive Level—*Applying*
Client Needs Category—*Physiological integrity*
Client Needs Subcategory—*Physiological adaptation*

116. 4. Preventing injury is a priority concern when caring for people with thrombocytopenia because they are prone to bleeding. The care plan specifies careful handling of the client, padding the side rails with soft material, using a soft toothbrush for mouth care, and using prolonged pressure when discontinuing I.V. infusions or injections. Activity is restricted to reduce the potential for injury. Generally, clients with thrombocytopenia are not at high risk for infection; therefore, visitors are not restricted. A normal intake of oral fluid is appropriate unless a client experiences a large loss of blood volume.

> *Test Taking Strategy—Analyze to determine what information the question asks for, which is the highest nursing priority when planning the care of a client with idiopathic thrombocytopenic purpura (ITP). Recall that a client with ITP has a potential for bleeding that may be difficult to control. Therefore, preventing injury (option 4) is the correct answer because it is more pertinent to safe care of the client than any of the others. Review the problems that a client with ITP is likely to develop and nursing measures for reducing their potential if you had difficulty answering this question.*

Cognitive Level—*Analyzing*
Client Needs Category—*Physiological integrity*
Client Needs Subcategory—*Reduction of risk potential*

117. 2. Hemophilia is a genetic disorder affecting clotting and is characterized by prolonged bleeding. Drowsiness, or a change in the level of consciousness, is one of the earliest signs of increased pressure from intracranial bleeding. Other signs of increased intracranial pressure include headache, visual problems, vomiting, motor weakness or paralysis, and personality changes. Seizures occur later as the bleeding progresses. Tinnitus, or ringing in the ears, is not commonly associated with active intracranial bleeding. The appetite should be unaffected, but the client may vomit with or without nausea.

> *Test Taking Strategy—Analyze to determine what information the question asks for, which is a manifestation of intracranial hemorrhage that a client with hemophilia should be able to name. Recall that when the contents of the cranium are increased by swelling, a mass, or fluid volume—bleeding in this case—one of the early signs is a decrease in the level of consciousness. A client with intracranial bleeding may appear to be sleepy (option 2) and difficult to arouse. Review the early signs of increased intracranial bleeding and pressure if you had difficulty answering this question.*

Cognitive Level—*Applying*
Client Needs Category—*Physiological integrity*
Client Needs Subcategory—*Physiological adaptation*

Nursing Care of Clients with Inflammatory and Obstructive Lymphatic Disorders

118. 2. When the axillary lymph nodes are removed during a radical mastectomy, lymph circulation is impaired. The lymph collects and pools within the arm on the side of the mastectomy. The condition is generally permanent once it develops. Elevating the affected arm and hand, applying an inflatable pressure sleeve or elasticized bandage, squeezing a rubber ball, and performing active range-of-motion exercises are immediate postoperative interventions designed to prevent, reduce, or eliminate the development of lymphedema. Fractures, pernicious anemia, and smallpox are not associated with lymphedema.

> *Test Taking Strategy—Note the key words "most likely" and apply them when searching the options to select a finding in the medical history that can be linked to lymphedema in the right arm. Recall that lymph circulates in a pathway of capillaries, lymph nodes, and lymphatic ducts before being returned to venous circulation. When axillary lymph nodes are removed during radical mastectomy (option 2), clients frequently develop lymphedema. Review the causes that can contribute to lymphedema if you had difficulty answering this question.*
> **Cognitive Level**—*Applying*
> **Client Needs Category**—*Physiological integrity*
> **Client Needs Subcategory**—*Physiological adaptation*

119. 1. Because circulation in the arm with lymphedema is impaired, certain nursing interventions (administering injections, taking a blood pressure, obtaining blood, or starting an I.V. infusion) are avoided. Prolonged pressure on the affected side during positioning is also avoided, but there is no contraindication to lying on the affected side for brief periods. Appropriate nursing interventions include performing active range-of-motion exercises and maintaining good nail hygiene such as trimming the nails.

> *Test Taking Strategy—Use the process of elimination to select the option that identifies a nursing action that is essential to avoid when providing care for a client with lymphedema. Recall that trauma from invasive procedures, such as an injection (option 1), may result in a wound that resists healing or is prone to infection due to compromised circulation. Review nursing precautions that are appropriate when caring for a client with lymphedema if you had difficulty answering this question.*
> **Cognitive Level**—*Applying*
> **Client Needs Category**—*Physiological integrity*
> **Client Needs Subcategory**—*Reduction of risk potential*

Directions: With a pencil, blacken the space in front of the option you have chosen for your correct answer.

Nursing Care of Clients with Upper Respiratory Tract Infections

During a visit to the physician's office, a client complains to the nurse that the physician would not prescribe an antibiotic for a head cold.

1. Which explanation to the client by the nurse regarding the use of antibiotics is best?
[ ] **1.** Antibiotics are ineffective in treating viral infections.
[ ] **2.** Antibiotics are ineffective after cold symptoms develop.
[ ] **3.** Antibiotics only prevent the spread of colds to others.
[ ] **4.** Antibiotics are used only for immunosuppressed individuals.

2. Which symptom reported by the client to the nurse is the best indicator that complications are developing from this cold?
[ ] **1.** Nasal stuffiness
[ ] **2.** Dry cough
[ ] **3.** High fever
[ ] **4.** Scratchy throat

3. Before recommending the use of a nonprescription decongestant to a client with a cold, which aspect of the medical history should be assessed? Select all that apply.
[ ] **1.** Arthritis
[ ] **2.** Asthma
[ ] **3.** Hypertension
[ ] **4.** Diabetes
[ ] **5.** Glaucoma
[ ] **6.** Arrhythmias

4. When teaching the client about topical nasal decongestant sprays, the nurse should warn that overuse of such medication is likely to result in which adverse effect?
[ ] **1.** Nasal irritation with rhinorrhea
[ ] **2.** Rebound congestion with nasal stuffiness
[ ] **3.** Ulceration of the nasal mucous membranes
[ ] **4.** Decreased ability to fight microorganisms

5. To prevent the client with a head cold from developing a secondary ear infection, which recommendation is most appropriate?
[ ] **1.** Sleeping with the head elevated
[ ] **2.** Blowing the nose very gently
[ ] **3.** Inserting cotton into the ears
[ ] **4.** Massaging the area behind the ears

A client with a prolonged upper respiratory infection seeks medical attention for symptoms of a low-grade fever, poor appetite, and malaise.

6. If the client has sinusitis in the maxillary sinuses, where will the client most likely report feeling pain?
[ ] **1.** Over the eyes
[ ] **2.** Near the eyebrows
[ ] **3.** In the cheeks
[ ] **4.** Above the ears

7. The nurse is teaching the client how to self-administer nose drops. When evaluating the client's technique, which method would the nurse identify as correct?
[ ] **1.** Bending the head forward, then instilling the drops
[ ] **2.** Pushing the nose laterally, then instilling the drops
[ ] **3.** Tilting the head backward, then instilling the drops
[ ] **4.** Turning the head to the side, then instilling the drops

An older client comes to the physician's office with a spouse who has symptoms of a respiratory tract infection. The spouse tells the nurse of having a cool-mist vaporizer at home and plans to use it to help relieve the nasal congestion.

8. The nurse instructs the client's spouse to empty and thoroughly clean the vaporizer after each use. Which rationale provides the basis for the nurse's instruction?
[ ] **1.** There is a potential for injury if the vaporizer is accidentally knocked off a nightstand.
[ ] **2.** Water left in the vaporizer can contribute to the growth of environmental pathogens.
[ ] **3.** The vaporizer can collect dust, which could affect the client's breathing.
[ ] **4.** Water evaporation causes calcium deposits that will obstruct the vaporizer.

Nursing Care of Clients with Inflammatory and Allergic Disorders of the Upper Airways

The physician orders a throat culture for a client with pharyngitis.

9. Which specimen collection technique should the nurse use to correctly obtain the throat culture from the client?
[ ] **1.** The nurse asks the client to expectorate sputum into a paper cup.
[ ] **2.** The nurse wipes the inner mouth and tongue with gauze.
[ ] **3.** The nurse swabs the throat with a sterile cotton applicator.
[ ] **4.** The nurse collects saliva in a sterile culture cup.

Laboratory results indicate that the client has an infection caused by group A streptococci. The physician prescribes oral potassium penicillin V (V-Cillin K).

10. The nurse advises the client to make sure to take the entire antibiotic prescription because an untreated or undertreated streptococcal infection may result in which of the following conditions?
[ ] **1.** Glomerulonephritis
[ ] **2.** Chickenpox
[ ] **3.** Shingles
[ ] **4.** Whooping cough

A nursing home resident is admitted to the hospital; in accordance with hospital protocol, a nasal swab is obtained to screen for methicillin-resistant Staphylococcus aureus *(MRSA).*

11. When the nurse obtains the nasal swab, which action is most accurate?
[ ] **1.** The nurse dons sterile gloves before obtaining the specimen.
[ ] **2.** The swab is placed in the anterior portion of the nare and swept superiorly.
[ ] **3.** The client is asked to blow the nose before the specimen is collected.
[ ] **4.** The nurse uses separate applicators for each nare.

A client calls the physician's office to schedule an appointment regarding laryngitis.

12. Until the client can be examined later that morning, which advice by the nurse would be most helpful?
[ ] **1.** "Sucking on ice chips should help."
[ ] **2.** "Rest your voice."
[ ] **3.** "Drink plenty of hot liquids."
[ ] **4.** "Massage your throat."

After 2 weeks of symptomatic treatment, the client still complains of hoarseness. The physician schedules a direct laryngoscopy.

13. Which statement by the client best indicates that the client understands the rationale for the direct laryngoscopy?
[ ] **1.** "The test will tell if my hoarseness is caused by tracheal polyps."
[ ] **2.** "The physician says that hoarseness can lead to bronchitis."
[ ] **3.** "I need to have the test because hoarseness is a symptom of laryngeal cancer."
[ ] **4.** "The physician wants to see if my hoarseness is because of enlarged tonsils."

A 23-year-old client experiences the following symptoms every fall: swollen nasal passages, endless sneezing, and red, watery, itchy eyes. The client makes an appointment with an allergist.

14. When the physician prescribes the first-generation antihistamine diphenhydramine (Benadryl) for the client's symptomatic relief, the nurse appropriately advises the client that first-generation antihistamines are associated with which side effect?
[ ] **1.** Weight loss
[ ] **2.** Constipation
[ ] **3.** Drowsiness
[ ] **4.** Depression

The physician recommends that the client undergo allergy skin testing.

15. When the client asks the nurse why skin testing is beneficial, which explanation is best?
[ ] **1.** The symptoms may be related to more than one substance.
[ ] **2.** Skin testing helps to build up blocking antibodies.
[ ] **3.** Allergic responses vary from person to person.
[ ] **4.** The allergy symptoms could become more serious.

16. The nurse is assessing and documenting the results of the skin testing. Which finding would the nurse document as a positive reaction?
[ ] **1.** The skin at the test site feels numb.
[ ] **2.** The skin at the test site feels painful.
[ ] **3.** The skin at the test site looks pale.
[ ] **4.** The skin at the test site looks red.

Based on the outcome of the skin tests, the client begins desensitization treatment. The client returns for weekly injections of diluted antigens of the allergic substances.

17. After the client receives the weekly injection, which nursing instruction is essential?
[ ] **1.** Take a couple of aspirin before leaving.
[ ] **2.** Wait at least 20 minutes before going home.
[ ] **3.** Make sure someone else drives the car.
[ ] **4.** Avoid getting the injection site wet.

18. When caring for a client with allergies, which nursing assessment finding is an early indication that the client is developing anaphylaxis?
[ ] **1.** Pain at injection site
[ ] **2.** Falling blood pressure
[ ] **3.** Decreased respirations
[ ] **4.** Loss of consciousness

19. If the client develops a severe allergic reaction, which drug should the nurse have available?
[ ] **1.** Codeine sulfate
[ ] **2.** Morphine sulfate (Roxanol)
[ ] **3.** Dopamine (Intropin)
[ ] **4.** Epinephrine (Adrenalin)

20. The client experiencing a severe allergic reaction becomes pulseless. The nurse shakes the client, shouts the client's name but gets no response, and activates the emergency medical response system. Which nursing action becomes the next priority?
[ ] **1.** Administer a single blow to the sternum.
[ ] **2.** Give two quick breaths that make the chest visibly rise.
[ ] **3.** Begin chest compressions at a rate of 100 per minute.
[ ] **4.** Administer an epinephrine (Adrenalin) injection.

21. When the nurse continues to assess a client being treated for a severe allergic reaction, which finding indicates improvement?
[ ] **1.** Temperature returns to 98.6°F
[ ] **2.** Blood pressure rises to 124/84
[ ] **3.** The client verbalizes feeling better
[ ] **4.** Redness at the site has not increased

Nursing Care of Clients with Cancer of the Larynx

The nursing team develops a care plan for a client who has been diagnosed with cancer of the larynx. The client is scheduled for a total laryngectomy. After surgery, the client is taken to the recovery room until stabilized.

22. Which assessment finding noted by the nurse on the client's return to the room is an early indication that the client's oxygenation status is compromised?
[ ] **1.** The client's dressing is bloody.
[ ] **2.** The client becomes restless.
[ ] **3.** The client's heart rate is irregular.
[ ] **4.** The client indicates feeling cold.

23. Because of this client's impaired speech, which nursing action facilitates optimum communication?
[ ] **1.** Lip-read the client's attempts at communication.
[ ] **2.** Inform the client to speak slowly when talking.
[ ] **3.** Listen attentively to the client's vocalizations.
[ ] **4.** Provide the client with paper and pencil.

The nursing team discusses the client's anger and depression related to the cancer diagnosis, the change in body image, and the loss of speech following a laryngectomy.

24. Which of the following best indicates that the client's grief is beginning to resolve?
[ ] **1.** The client wants only the spouse to visit.
[ ] **2.** The client says the physician made an incorrect diagnosis.
[ ] **3.** The client looks at the tracheostomy tube in a mirror.
[ ] **4.** The client asks the nurse for help with bathing.

Nursing Care of Clients with Inflammatory and Infectious Disorders of the Lower Airways

A client with a persistent upper respiratory infection develops acute bronchitis and is given a prescription for guaifenesin (Robitussin AC), an antitussive that contains codeine.

25. Aside from the characteristics of the client's cough, which other pertinent assessment finding should the nurse document?
[ ] 1. Family history of respiratory disease
[ ] 2. Current vital signs
[ ] 3. Appearance of respiratory secretions
[ ] 4. Any self-treatment measures used by the client

26. When the client asks why the physician prescribed this particular cough medicine, the nurse correctly responds that the guaifenesin liquefies mucus while the codeine is responsible for which action?
[ ] 1. Relieving discomfort
[ ] 2. Dilating the bronchi
[ ] 3. Suppressing coughing
[ ] 4. Reducing inflammation

27. Which instruction regarding the prescribed medication is most appropriate to tell this client?
[ ] 1. "Do not take the drug more frequently than prescribed."
[ ] 2. "Avoid taking the medication before going to sleep."
[ ] 3. "Drink more fluid throughout the day."
[ ] 4. "Warm the cough syrup to make it more palatable."

The nurse is caring for a client who must take a liquid cough syrup and several other oral tablets at the same time.

28. What nursing action is most appropriate when administering both types of oral medication to this client?
[ ] 1. Administer the cough syrup first, then the tablets.
[ ] 2. Wait 15 minutes after giving the cough syrup before giving the tablets.
[ ] 3. Give the cough syrup between administering the tablets.
[ ] 4. Administer the tablets first, then the cough syrup.

The prescribed dose of the client's liquid cough syrup is 5 mL.

29. Which household measurement should the nurse use when teaching the client how to self-administer the prescribed amount of liquid cough syrup?
[ ] 1. One ounce
[ ] 2. One tablespoon
[ ] 3. One teaspoon
[ ] 4. One capful

The client also receives a prescription for aerosol therapy to treat bronchitis.

30. Which statement by the client indicates an accurate understanding of the purpose of aerosol therapy?
[ ] 1. "Aerosol therapy relieves tissue irritation."
[ ] 2. "This therapy kills infectious organisms."
[ ] 3. "Aerosolization dries respiratory passages."
[ ] 4. "Aerosol therapy helps to slow breathing."

The nurse is preparing to administer penicillin G to a client. The prescription reads: penicillin G potassium 300,000 units I.M. q.i.d. The directions on the label state, "This vial contains 1,000,000 units of penicillin G potassium. Add 9.6 mL sterile water for injection to reconstitute the powder for a concentration of 100,000 units/mL."

31. How many milliliters of the reconstituted medication should the nurse administer to the client?

_____

When an adult client with a diagnosis of pneumonia is admitted to the unit, the nurse observes symptoms of shaking chills and a fever of 104.2°F (40.1°C). A chest X-ray and sputum specimens for culture and sensitivity are ordered.

32. To determine whether the pneumonia is caused by a bacteria or virus, the nurse asks the client about the onset of the symptoms. What is the rationale for the nurse's questioning?
[ ] 1. The symptoms of bacterial pneumonia usually come on rapidly and tend to be more severe.
[ ] 2. The symptoms of viral pneumonia usually come on rapidly and tend to be more severe.
[ ] 3. The symptoms of viral pneumonia begin a couple of weeks after a person has developed upper respiratory symptoms, such as congestion or a sore throat.
[ ] 4. The symptoms of bacterial pneumonia begin a couple of weeks after a person has developed upper respiratory symptoms, such as congestion or a sore throat.

33. Which nursing action is essential before the chest X-ray is taken?
[ ] 1. Make sure the client does not eat any food.
[ ] 2. Remove the metal necklace the client is wearing.
[ ] 3. Have the client swallow a contrast dye.
[ ] 4. Administer a parenteral analgesic.

The client who has been diagnosed with pneumonia has difficulty expectorating respiratory secretions.

34. Which nursing action is most appropriate when planning to obtain the ordered sputum specimen?
[ ] 1. Provide the client with a generous fluid intake.
[ ] 2. Encourage the client to change positions regularly.
[ ] 3. Ask the dietitian to send the client a clear liquid diet.
[ ] 4. Administer an antitussive before collecting the specimen.

35. Which time of day is best for the nurse to obtain a sputum specimen from the client?
[ ] **1.** Before bedtime
[ ] **2.** After a meal
[ ] **3.** Between meals
[ ] **4.** On awakening

36. Which statement best suggests that the client understands the nurse's instruction on how to handle the sputum specimen container?
[ ] **1.** "I should put gloves on before opening the container."
[ ] **2.** "I should wipe the container with an alcohol swab."
[ ] **3.** "I cannot put the lid on the container until the container is fairly full."
[ ] **4.** "I must not touch the inside of the container."

37. After collecting the sputum specimen from the client, which nursing action is most appropriate?
[ ] **1.** Administer oxygen
[ ] **2.** Provide mouth care
[ ] **3.** Offer nourishment
[ ] **4.** Encourage ambulation

38. Which assessment finding indicates that the client has most likely developed pleurisy as a result of the pneumonia?
[ ] **1.** Productive cough
[ ] **2.** Pain when breathing
[ ] **3.** Cyanotic nail beds
[ ] **4.** Rapid heart rate

The client is diagnosed as having pneumococcal pneumonia, and the physician orders penicillin (Bicillin) by I.M. injection.

39. When the client asks why the physician chose this particular drug to treat the pneumonia, which response by the nurse is best?
[ ] **1.** "The sensitivity report showed the organism is often killed by penicillin."
[ ] **2.** "Most viral infections respond well when treated with penicillin drugs."
[ ] **3.** "Penicillin is one of the safest yet most effective antibiotics."
[ ] **4.** "All antibiotics are similar; the choice of drug is not that important."

The nurse chooses to inject the prescribed dose of penicillin (Bicillin) into the ventrogluteal injection site.

40. Place an *X* at the correct location for the ventrogluteal injection.

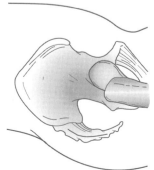

41. If a client is allergic to penicillin, the nurse should anticipate a hypersensitivity response to which other group of antibiotics?
[ ] **1.** Aminoglycosides such as kanamycin (Kantrex)
[ ] **2.** Tetracyclines such as doxycycline (Vibramycin)
[ ] **3.** Cephalosporins such as ceftriaxone (Rocephin)
[ ] **4.** Fluoroquinolones such as ciprofloxacin (Cipro)

A nurse volunteers to administer influenza vaccines to older adults during a community-wide immunization campaign.

42. Which question is essential for the nurse to ask before administering the influenza vaccine?
[ ] **1.** "Have you had influenza in the last year?"
[ ] **2.** "Did you receive pneumonia vaccine last year?"
[ ] **3.** "Are you allergic to eggs or egg products?"
[ ] **4.** "Do you have a history of respiratory disease?"

43. Other than obtaining a vaccination against influenza, which nursing advice is most helpful to high-risk clients who want to avoid getting influenza?
[ ] **1.** Consume adequate vitamin C.
[ ] **2.** Avoid crowded places.
[ ] **3.** Dress warmly in cold weather.
[ ] **4.** Reduce daily stress and anxiety.

A client is seen in the physician's office and is given oseltamivir (Tamiflu), an antiviral medication for the client's symptoms of fever, chills, muscle aches, rhinitis, and sore throat related to influenza.

44. When the nurse is instructing the client on the effectiveness of oseltamivir (Tamiflu), which of the following instruction points is essential?
[ ] **1.** Tamiflu must be started within 12 to 24 hours of the first symptoms.
[ ] **2.** Tamiflu must be taken on an empty stomach to aid in absorption.
[ ] **3.** Tamiflu affects the liver; liver enzymes are assessed before administration.
[ ] **4.** Tamiflu is most effective when administered intra-nasally.

45. When caring for a client with influenza, the nurse would expect to assess for which signs and symptoms of hypoxia? Select all that apply.
[ ] **1.** Cough
[ ] **2.** Restlessness
[ ] **3.** Fever
[ ] **4.** Tachypnea
[ ] **5.** Use of accessory muscles to breathe
[ ] **6.** Cyanosis

A nurse working in an assisted living facility notes that an elderly client with influenza has a fever of 104.6°F (40.3°C) and a dry cough. The client complains of sore muscles and a headache. The nurse instructs the nursing assistant to encourage the client to consume extra fluids.

46. If the client has normal cardiovascular and renal function, what is an appropriate goal for oral intake in the next 24-hour period?
[ ] **1.** 500 mL
[ ] **2.** 1,000 mL
[ ] **3.** 1,500 mL
[ ] **4.** 3,000 mL

The physician orders the nurse to give two acetaminophen (Tylenol) tablets orally every 4 hours, as needed, if the client has a temperature over 102°F (38.9°C) and to give a tepid sponge bath at the same time.

47. The nurse knows to discontinue the client's sponge bath if the client develops which symptom?
[ ] **1.** Nausea
[ ] **2.** Chills
[ ] **3.** Flushing
[ ] **4.** Confusion

48. Which finding best indicates that the sponge bath is having a therapeutic effect on the client?
[ ] **1.** The client feels more comfortable.
[ ] **2.** The client begins sweating profusely.
[ ] **3.** The client's temperature is 101°F (38.3°C).
[ ] **4.** The client's skin is flushed.

The nurse in a long-term care facility is required by the state's law to test all newly admitted clients for tuberculosis. The policy of the agency is to administer a Mantoux intradermal skin test.

49. The nurse's injection technique is correct if the needle is inserted into the client at a 10-degree angle in which location? Place an *X* over the appropriate location.

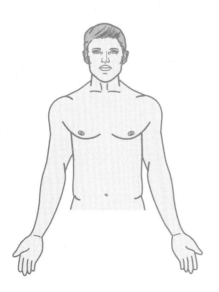

50. How long after administering a tuberculin skin test should the nurse inspect the client's injection site?
[ ] **1.** 1 week
[ ] **2.** 1 day
[ ] **3.** 48 hours
[ ] **4.** 5 days

51. The client asks the nurse, "What is the significance of a positive tuberculin skin test?" Which explanation is most accurate?
[ ] **1.** "You have an active tuberculosis infection."
[ ] **2.** "You have antibodies against tuberculosis."
[ ] **3.** "You are immune to tuberculosis."
[ ] **4.** "You require immediate isolation."

52. When a previously negative client has a positive reaction to a tuberculin skin test, which information about follow-up is most correct?
[ ] **1.** A skin test will be performed every 6 months.
[ ] **2.** A routine chest X-ray is required every year.
[ ] **3.** The client will need to live alone temporarily.
[ ] **4.** Antituberculosis drugs will be prescribed.

A client diagnosed with tuberculosis continues to have evidence of the tubercle bacilli in sputum after 6 weeks of drug therapy.

53. Which question is most important for the nurse to ask the client at this time?
[ ] **1.** "When did you last take your prescribed medications?"
[ ] **2.** "Have you taken all your medications as prescribed?"
[ ] **3.** "How many drug refills have you obtained?"
[ ] **4.** "Have you experienced any drug side effects?"

54. Which health measure is most important for the nurse to emphasize when instructing the client on how to prevent the transmission of tuberculosis while undergoing home drug therapy?
[ ] **1.** Wash plates and utensils in hot water.
[ ] **2.** Avoid sharing towels and wash cloths.
[ ] **3.** Cover your nose and mouth when coughing.
[ ] **4.** Wash your hands before and after meals.

Aware that the client must manage nutritional needs on a very low income, the nurse reinforces the dietitian's instructions.

55. If the client identifies that lunches often include the following foods, which meal is the most nutritious?
[ ] **1.** Tossed salad, rice, and iced tea
[ ] **2.** Jelly sandwich on whole wheat bread and coffee
[ ] **3.** Meatless chili with beans, corn bread, and milk
[ ] **4.** Chicken soup, gelatin, and sweetened lemonade

The physician prescribes a combination of rifampin (Rifadin) and isoniazid (INH) to treat this client's tuberculosis.

56. When the client asks the nurse about why the physician has prescribed two drugs, which response is most accurate?
[ ] **1.** One medication diminishes the side effects of the other.
[ ] **2.** One medication kills the live organism; the other, its spores.
[ ] **3.** Using combined medications can reduce the dosages of both drugs.
[ ] **4.** Using two or more drugs lowers the potential for bacterial resistance.

57. If the client complains of GI side effects associated with rifampin (Rifadin), which nursing action is best?
[ ] **1.** Administering the drug at night
[ ] **2.** Giving the drug with food or at mealtimes
[ ] **3.** Encouraging the client to drink plenty of water
[ ] **4.** Providing the client with an antacid

Nursing Care of Clients with Asthma

An adult client who has had asthma since early childhood comes to the emergency department in respiratory distress.

58. Which position is best for the client to be in while the nurse prepares to assess breath sounds?
[ ] **1.** Sitting
[ ] **2.** Standing
[ ] **3.** Lying on the back
[ ] **4.** Lying on the side

The nurse uses pulse oximetry to monitor the asthma client's oxygenation status.

59. Where on the client should the nurse position the sensor of the pulse oximeter to obtain an accurate measurement?
[ ] **1.** Apply it to the client's finger.
[ ] **2.** Apply it to the client's palm.
[ ] **3.** Clip it to the client's earlobe.
[ ] **4.** Wrap it around the client's leg.

60. Which pulse oximetry reading indicates to the nurse that the client has normal tissue oxygenation?
[ ] **1.** 80 to 90 mm Hg
[ ] **2.** 95 to 100 mm Hg
[ ] **3.** 80% to 85%
[ ] **4.** 95% to 100%

The client continues to have difficulty breathing with shortness of breath. The physician prescribes a levalbuterol hydrochloride (Xopenex) inhalation treatment.

61. After levalbuterol hydrochloride (Xopenex) administration, which client symptom does the nurse evaluate as a side effect of the medication?
[ ] **1.** Respiratory rate of 28 breaths/minute
[ ] **2.** Heart rate of 96 beats/minute
[ ] **3.** Blood pressure of 100/60 mm Hg
[ ] **4.** Drowsiness

A laboratory technician draws blood for an arterial blood gas (ABG) measurement from the client's radial artery before the physician's examination.

62. Immediately after the specimen is drawn, the registered nurse instructs the licensed practical nurse to perform which essential nursing action?
[ ] **1.** Apply direct pressure to the site for 5 minutes.
[ ] **2.** Warm the blood in the specimen tube for 5 minutes.
[ ] **3.** Assess the client's blood pressure in 5 minutes.
[ ] **4.** Elevate the client's arm for at least 5 minutes.

The physician orders administration of 60% oxygen with a partial rebreathing mask and reservoir bag to treat the client's asthma attack.

63. When administering oxygen to the client through a partial rebreathing mask, which observation is most important for the nurse to report to the respiratory therapy department?
[ ] **1.** Moisture is accumulating inside the mask.
[ ] **2.** The bag collapses during inspiration.
[ ] **3.** The mask covers the client's mouth and nose.
[ ] **4.** The strap around the client's head is snug.

The nurse is aware that oxygen toxicity occurs when oxygen concentrations of more than 50% are administered for longer than 48 hours.

64. Which of the following signs and symptoms would indicate that the client is experiencing oxygen toxicity? Select all that apply.
[ ] **1.** Nonproductive cough
[ ] **2.** Nausea
[ ] **3.** Hyperventilation
[ ] **4.** Headache
[ ] **5.** Substernal chest pain
[ ] **6.** Nasal stuffiness

The physician also orders 0.1 mg of epinephrine subcutaneously for the client. The label indicates that the epinephrine is a 1:1,000 dilution, which means that 1 g of epinephrine has been mixed with 1,000 mL of liquid.

65. Which is the correct volume needed for the nurse to administer the prescribed dose of 0.1 mg of epinephrine to the client?
[ ] **1.** 0.001 mL
[ ] **2.** 0.1 mL
[ ] **3.** 1.0 mL
[ ] **4.** 10 mL

66. Which nursing measure is most helpful in reducing the client's anxiety during an asthma attack?
[ ] **1.** Close the door to the examination room.
[ ] **2.** Remain within the client's view.
[ ] **3.** Pull the bedside privacy curtain.
[ ] **4.** Notify the client when the respiratory therapist arrives.

Upon discharge, the physician prescribes using a peak flow meter to judge asthma symptoms on a daily basis.

67. The nurse provides directions to the client on the proper use of a peak flow meter. Arrange the steps for the nurse's instruction to the client on the proper use of a peak flow meter in the correct sequence.

1. Record the highest rating after three attempts.	
2. Slide the marker or arrow to zero.	
3. Blow out as fast as you can.	
4. Take a deep breath.	
5. Put the mouthpiece of the flow meter into your mouth.	
6. Empty all of the air from your lungs.	

Nursing Care of Clients with Chronic Obstructive Pulmonary Disease

The physician orders pulmonary function tests (PFTs) for a client diagnosed with emphysema. The client has a history of smoking two packs of cigarettes per day for the past 40 years.

68. The best evidence that the client understands the procedure for a pulmonary function test is when stating that it involves which action?
[ ] **1.** Having an X-ray taken
[ ] **2.** Drawing a blood specimen
[ ] **3.** Breathing into a mouthpiece
[ ] **4.** Examining expectorated sputum

When the client develops a respiratory infection, the client's condition worsens, necessitating admission to the hospital. An arterial blood gas (ABG) analysis is ordered.

69. The ABG analysis results reveal that the client's partial pressure of arterial carbon dioxide ($PaCO_2$) is 65 mm Hg. The nurse recognizes that this is abnormal because normal $PaCO_2$ levels fall between which values?
[ ] **1.** 7.35 and 7.45
[ ] **2.** 80 and 100 mm Hg
[ ] **3.** 35 and 45 mm Hg
[ ] **4.** 22 and 26 mm Hg

Based on the arterial blood gas (ABG) results, the client is to receive supplemental oxygen. The nurse prepares to administer oxygen by nasal cannula.

70. When caring for a client with emphysema who is experiencing compromised breathing, which oxygen flow rate is most appropriate?
[ ] **1.** 2 L/minute
[ ] **2.** 5 L/minute
[ ] **3.** 8 L/minute
[ ] **4.** 10 L/minute

The client receives I.V. fluid containing aminophylline (Truphylline).

71. Which nursing explanation identifies the primary rationale for administering aminophylline?
[ ] **1.** Aminophylline relieves persistent coughing.
[ ] **2.** Aminophylline reduces sputum production.
[ ] **3.** Aminophylline dilates the bronchial airways.
[ ] **4.** Aminophylline thins respiratory secretions.

72. The nurse is planning care for the long-term management of a client with persistent asthma symptoms. Which type of medication would the nurse anticipate as a primary category of drug treatment?
[ ] **1.** Inhaled corticosteroid
[ ] **2.** Oral bronchodilator
[ ] **3.** I.V. sympathomimetic
[ ] **4.** Parenteral anti-inflammatory

73. The nurse performs postural drainage on the client. Which nursing intervention is most beneficial to loosen secretions?
[ ] **1.** Telling the client to take deep breaths
[ ] **2.** Striking the back with a cupped hand
[ ] **3.** Applying pressure below the diaphragm
[ ] **4.** Placing the client in a sitting position

74. Which nursing observation provides the best evidence that postural drainage is effective?
[ ] **1.** The client's respiratory rate is increased.
[ ] **2.** The client's heart rate is much improved.
[ ] **3.** The client's sputum culture is negative.
[ ] **4.** The client raises a large volume of sputum.

The physician orders two puffs of albuterol sulfate (Ventolin) twice a day as needed using a metered-dose inhaler.

75. After administering the first puff of medication, what client action demonstrates proper use of the inhaler?
[ ] **1.** The client depresses the canister a second time before exhaling.
[ ] **2.** The client holds his or her breath for up to 10 seconds before exhaling.
[ ] **3.** The client cleans the mouthpiece with a clean paper tissue or cloth.
[ ] **4.** The client bends from the waist to increase the exhaled volume.

Before discharge, the client with emphysema tells the nurse, "This disease makes me a prisoner in my own home."

76. Which is the best response from the nurse?
[ ] **1.** "Tell me more about how you are feeling."
[ ] **2.** "There are lots of things you can still do."
[ ] **3.** "You are just having a bad day today."
[ ] **4.** "What makes you say that?"

While preparing to return home, the client with emphysema verbalizes concern about continued fatigue and shortness of breath.

77. Which discharge instruction is most appropriate for reducing the client's fatigue and shortness of breath during mealtimes?
[ ] **1.** "Eat simple carbohydrates for quick energy."
[ ] **2.** "Eat fatty foods to get maximum caloric intake."
[ ] **3.** "Eat frequent, small meals to reduce energy use."
[ ] **4.** "Eat the largest meal late at night before sleep."

Nursing Care of Clients with Lung Cancer

The nurse is caring for an older client who is undergoing several diagnostic tests to determine a potential diagnosis of lung cancer.

78. If the client is typical of most others diagnosed with cancer of the lung, which early-warning sign was most likely ignored?
[ ] **1.** Difficulty swallowing
[ ] **2.** Gradual weight loss
[ ] **3.** Persistent cough
[ ] **4.** Coughing up blood

The client's preliminary diagnostic tests strongly suggest lung cancer. To make a definitive diagnosis, a bronchoscopy is scheduled.

79. Which action is most appropriate for the nurse to take before the bronchoscopy?
[ ] **1.** Keep the client from eating and drinking.
[ ] **2.** Have the client cough several times.
[ ] **3.** Ensure that the client gets adequate sleep.
[ ] **4.** Scrub the client's upper chest with an antiseptic.

80. After the bronchoscopy, what should the nurse closely monitor?
[ ] **1.** The client's level of consciousness
[ ] **2.** The client's oral status
[ ] **3.** The client's respiratory effort
[ ] **4.** The client's ability to speak

After the bronchoscopy, the nurse observes blood when suctioning secretions that have accumulated in the client's mouth.

81. To evaluate the significance of the client's bleeding, which additional assessment is most important for the nurse to make at this time?
[ ] **1.** Count the pulse rate.
[ ] **2.** Listen to heart sounds.
[ ] **3.** Check the pupillary response.
[ ] **4.** Measure the chest expansion.

82. Which assessment technique is essential before allowing a client food or fluids after a bronchoscopy?
[ ] **1.** Touch the arch of the palate with a tongue blade.
[ ] **2.** Listen to the abdomen for active bowel sounds.
[ ] **3.** Inspect the oral mucous membranes for integrity.
[ ] **4.** Palpate the throat while the client swallows.

After the bronchoscopy, the client is diagnosed with advanced lung cancer. Pleural effusion is also discovered. The nurse prepares the client for a thoracentesis.

83. When the nurse auscultates the client's lung sounds, which adventitious breath sounds are anticipated?
[ ] **1.** Wheezing in the upper lobes
[ ] **2.** A friction rub posterior to the affected area
[ ] **3.** Crackles over the affected area
[ ] **4.** Decreased sounds over the involved area

84. How should the nurse position the client while undergoing a thoracentesis?
[ ] **1.** Lithotomy position
[ ] **2.** Sitting
[ ] **3.** Prone
[ ] **4.** Supine

After the thoracentesis, the physician tells the client that a pneumonectomy is required. The physician explains the surgery and risk factors to the client.

85. Which statement by the client would indicate to the nurse that the client has an accurate understanding of the planned surgery?
[ ] **1.** "The surgeon is planning to remove one of my lungs."
[ ] **2.** "Only one lobe of my lung will be removed."
[ ] **3.** "The surgeon will take a sample of my lung tissue to be biopsied during the procedure."
[ ] **4.** "A lung will be opened and examined during surgery."

86. While developing the postoperative care plan for the client, it is essential to have the client lie in which position?
[ ] **1.** With the healthy lung uppermost
[ ] **2.** With the head lower than the heart
[ ] **3.** With the affected side upward
[ ] **4.** With the arms elevated on pillows

87. For the client who has just had a pneumonectomy, what is a temporary, expected outcome of thoracic surgery?
[ ] **1.** Persistent cough
[ ] **2.** Chest numbness
[ ] **3.** Impaired swallowing
[ ] **4.** Sore throat

The client requests pain medication after the pneumonectomy.

88. After administering morphine sulfate (Roxanol) to the client, which of the following is most important for the nurse to assess?
[ ] **1.** Rate and rhythm of the heart
[ ] **2.** Skin color and temperature
[ ] **3.** Presence of bowel sounds
[ ] **4.** Rate and depth of respirations

Nursing Care of Clients with Chest Injuries

A high school football player comes to the emergency department with signs and symptoms suggestive of two fractured ribs.

89. Before discharging a client with fractured ribs from the emergency department, which instruction is most important for the nurse to provide?
[ ] **1.** Breathe deeply several times every hour.
[ ] **2.** Breathe shallowly to avoid discomfort.
[ ] **3.** Breathe rapidly to promote ventilation.
[ ] **4.** Breathe into a paper bag every hour.

While on the way to work one morning, a nurse witnesses a motorcycle accident and stops to assist the victim.

90. When assessing the accident victim, which finding strongly suggests the presence of a flail chest?
[ ] **1.** Sucking air is heard near the chest.
[ ] **2.** The trachea deviates from midline.
[ ] **3.** A portion of the chest moves inward during inspiration.
[ ] **4.** The victim has severe chest pain during expiration.

On arrival at the emergency department, it is determined that the victim's lung collapsed during the accident. A hemothorax is diagnosed, and two chest tubes are inserted.

91. After chest tube insertion, where would the nurse expect to see bloody drainage?
[ ] **1.** From the victim's nose
[ ] **2.** From the victim's mouth
[ ] **3.** From the tube in the upper chest
[ ] **4.** From the tube in the lower chest

Both the victim's chest tubes are connected to a commercial water-seal drainage system.

92. When the nurse monitors the chamber with the water seal, which finding suggests that the system is functioning correctly?
[ ] **1.** The fluid rises and falls with respirations.
[ ] **2.** The fluid level is lower than when first filled.
[ ] **3.** The fluid bubbles continuously.
[ ] **4.** The fluid looks frothy white.

93. Which assessment finding indicates that air is leaking into the tissue around the victim's chest tube insertion site?
[ ] **1.** The tissue appears pale or almost colorless.
[ ] **2.** A hissing sound, like a leaking tire, can be heard.
[ ] **3.** The skin crackles when touched.
[ ] **4.** Air is felt as it escapes.

The victim is transported to another unit for a chest X-ray. The chest tubes and water-seal drainage system are still in place.

94. Which nursing action is most appropriate before transporting the client to have X-rays taken?
[ ] **1.** Clamp the chest tubes before leaving the room.
[ ] **2.** Keep the drainage system below the insertion sites.
[ ] **3.** Attach a portable suction machine to the chest tubes.
[ ] **4.** Provide mechanical ventilation during transport.

95. What is the best method for determining the amount of drainage from a chest tube when a closed water-seal system is used?
[ ] **1.** Empty the collection chamber, and measure the volume.
[ ] **2.** Subtract the client's fluid intake from drainage output.
[ ] **3.** Instill sterile irrigation solution, and measure the drainage.
[ ] **4.** Subtract the previously marked volume from the current amount.

The nurse is caring for a client who has a chest tube connected to a three-chamber water-seal drainage system.

96. Place an X on the chamber of the chest tube drainage system in which the nurse should observe continuous gentle bubbling when suction is used to facilitate drainage from the pleural space.

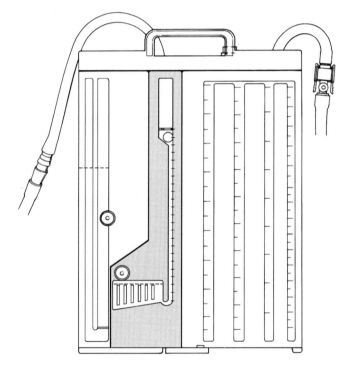

Nursing Care of Clients with Pulmonary Embolism

After abdominal surgery, a client suddenly experiences severe chest pain and dyspnea. A pulmonary embolism is suspected.

97. Where did the client's embolism most likely originate?
[ ] **1.** The deep veins of the legs
[ ] **2.** The pulmonary artery
[ ] **3.** The superior vena cava
[ ] **4.** The carotid artery

The client suddenly experiences chest pain and dyspnea and tells the nurse, "Nurse, I think I am dying."

98. Which response by the nurse is most appropriate at this time?
[ ] **1.** "The pain will lessen in a few minutes."
[ ] **2.** "I will stay with you until the physician comes."
[ ] **3.** "Why would you even think something like that?"
[ ] **4.** "Are your financial affairs in order?"

99. Which nursing intervention is most important in response to the client's physical symptoms at this time?
[ ] **1.** Administering oxygen by face mask
[ ] **2.** Assessing the client's capillary refill
[ ] **3.** Having the client rate the pain on a pain scale
[ ] **4.** Requesting a physician's order for cardiac enzymes

100. Based on the client's clinical presentation, which drug should the nurse anticipate will be administered intravenously?
[ ] **1.** Heparin
[ ] **2.** Aminophylline (Truphylline)
[ ] **3.** Nitroglycerin (Nitrodisc)
[ ] **4.** Aspirin

Nursing Care of Clients with Tracheostomies

101. Which assessment finding provides the best indication that the nurse needs to suction the client with a tracheostomy?
[ ] **1.** Respirations are low.
[ ] **2.** Pulse rate is slow.
[ ] **3.** Breath sounds are wet.
[ ] **4.** Blood pressure is elevated.

102. Which nursing action is essential before suctioning the client with a tracheostomy tube?
[ ] **1.** Preoxygenating the client
[ ] **2.** Moistening the catheter
[ ] **3.** Cleaning around the stoma
[ ] **4.** Removing the inner cannula

103. Before suctioning, the nurse attaches a pulse oximeter to the client's finger. Which nursing actions are appropriate at this time? Select all that apply.
[ ] **1.** Remove the client's fingernail polish.
[ ] **2.** Position the sensors so they are directly opposite to each other on the client's finger.
[ ] **3.** Connect the cable to the oximeter.
[ ] **4.** Set the SpO_2 alarms between 95% and 100%.
[ ] **5.** Notify the physician each time an alarm sounds.
[ ] **6.** Relocate the spring-loaded sensor periodically.

104. When suctioning a client with a tracheostomy, when is the best time to occlude the vent on the suction catheter?
[ ] **1.** Before inserting the catheter
[ ] **2.** When inside the inner cannula
[ ] **3.** While withdrawing the catheter
[ ] **4.** When the client begins coughing

105. When suctioning the airway of a client with a tracheostomy, the nurse applies suction for no longer than how many seconds?
[ ] **1.** 5 to 7
[ ] **2.** 10 to 12
[ ] **3.** 15 to 20
[ ] **4.** 25 to 30

106. While withdrawing the suction catheter from a client's tracheostomy tube, which nursing technique is correct?
[ ] **1.** Remove the catheter slowly.
[ ] **2.** Pinch and pull the catheter.
[ ] **3.** Plunge the catheter up and down.
[ ] **4.** Twist and rotate the catheter.

107. What is the best way to determine whether a client with a tracheostomy is becoming hypoxemic during suctioning?
[ ] **1.** Monitoring level of consciousness
[ ] **2.** Assessing skin color and temperature
[ ] **3.** Watching pulse oximetry levels
[ ] **4.** Counting the respiratory rate

108. When performing the client's tracheostomy care, which nursing action is correct?
[ ] **1.** Cut a gauze square to fit around the client's stoma.
[ ] **2.** Secure the ties at the back of the client's neck.
[ ] **3.** Attach new ties before removing old ones.
[ ] **4.** Replace the cannula after changing the ties.

109. Which nursing rationale best explains the reason for using a cuffed tracheostomy tube on the client?
[ ] **1.** The cuff prevents skin breakdown.
[ ] **2.** The cuff prevents aspiration.
[ ] **3.** The cuff is more comfortable.
[ ] **4.** The cuff reduces infection.

Nursing Care of Clients with Sudden Airway Occlusion

A nurse working in a physician's office receives a telephone call from a frantic person whose family member is choking on a piece of hard candy.

110. What information does the nurse need to know first before recommending further action?
[ ] **1.** Can the victim walk?
[ ] **2.** Can the victim cough?
[ ] **3.** How is the victim positioned?
[ ] **4.** Can the victim still swallow?

111. The nurse knows that the correct way to position the hands when performing the abdominal thrust maneuver is with the thumb side of the closed fist on which part of the victim's abdomen?
[ ] **1.** Directly on the manubrium
[ ] **2.** Above the xiphoid process
[ ] **3.** Below the navel
[ ] **4.** Below the sternum

Nursing Care of Clients Who Are Victims of Terrorist Agents

While attending an indoor event, several people become dyspneic and have burning, watery eyes. Terrorist activity is suspected. The victims are taken to the nearest emergency department for treatment.

112. Which agents should the nurse suspect as being the cause of the victims' symptoms? Select all that apply.
[ ] **1.** Anthrax
[ ] **2.** Sarin gas
[ ] **3.** Smallpox
[ ] **4.** Radiation
[ ] **5.** Cyanide
[ ] **6.** Ebola virus

113. As victims from the terrorist attack are arriving in the emergency department, a novice licensed practical nurse is caring for a client in cardiac arrest. Which type of leadership style is most beneficial to assist the novice nurse in caring for the client?
[ ] **1.** Lassez-faire
[ ] **2.** Autocratic
[ ] **3.** Democratic
[ ] **4.** Leader-follower

Correct Answers, Rationales, and Test Taking Strategies

Nursing Care of Clients with Upper Respiratory Tract Infections

1. 1. The common cold, called *rhinitis* or *coryza,* is a viral infection that affects the nasal passages and throat. A cold is spread by inhalation of droplets or through direct contact. Antibiotics are only useful in treating bacterial, not viral, infections. No drug cures the common cold. Antibiotics are started only when clients have a secondary bacterial infection; then, most individuals, regardless of their immune status, get a prescription for antibiotics.

> *Test Taking Strategy—Use the process of elimination to select the option that identifies the best explanation for excluding antibiotic therapy when treating a head cold. Options 2 and 3 can be eliminated immediately because they are not accurate statements. Option 4 may appear to have merit, but it is not the best answer because the common cold is caused by a virus and antibiotics are not effective when treating viral illnesses. Review drug therapy for viral infections if you had difficulty answering this question.*
> **Cognitive Level**—*Applying*
> **Client Needs Category**—*Health promotion and maintenance*
> **Client Needs Subcategory**—*None*

2. 3. A high fever suggests that the client with a common cold has acquired a secondary bacterial infection, such as bronchitis or pneumonia. Viral infections such as the common cold are associated with a low-grade fever. Symptoms of the common cold are generally confined to the head and throat. They include nasal congestion and discharge, nose and throat discomfort, sneezing, and watery eyes. The client may also have a headache, chills, fatigue, and loss of appetite. A dry cough is caused by irritation from nasal drainage passing into the pharynx. A productive cough indicates that the infection involves the lower respiratory tract.

> *Test Taking Strategy—Use the process of elimination to select the option that identifies the best indicator that a person with a cold is developing complications. Options 1, 2, and 4 can be eliminated because they are signs and symptoms that may accompany a cold. A high fever (option 3) suggests a more systemic rather than local problem is developing. Review the signs and symptoms of a cold and its secondary complications if you had difficulty answering this question.*
> **Cognitive Level**—*Applying*
> **Client Needs Category**—*Physiological integrity*
> **Client Needs Subcategory**—*Physiological adaptation*

3. 3, 5, 6. The common cold virus causes an inflammatory response within the nose and throat. Because one of the symptoms of a common cold is nasal stuffiness making it difficult to breathe, most clients can benefit from a decongestant. A decongestant decreases nasal edema by constricting blood vessels in the nose. Nonprescription decongestants that contain adrenergic drugs such as ephedrine sulfate or pseudoephedrine are contraindicated for clients with hypertension, heart disease, irregular heart rhythms, and narrow-angle glaucoma. Adrenergic drugs are not contraindicated for clients with arthritis, asthma, or diabetes unless they have cardiovascular disease.

> *Test Taking Strategy—Analyze to determine what information the question asks for, which is contraindications of decongestants. Alternative-format "select all that apply" questions require considering each option independently to decide its merit in answering the question. Recall that adrenergic drugs produce their effects by mimicking the sympathetic nervous system. Review the actions of decongestants and their side effects if you had difficulty answering this question.*
> **Cognitive Level**—*Applying*
> **Client Needs Category**—*Physiological integrity*
> **Client Needs Subcategory**—*Pharmacological therapies*

4. 2. Nasal decongestants have a vasoconstricting action. Using them more frequently than recommended tends to result in nasal stuffiness from rebound vasodilation. This means that the congestion worsens and recurs in less time after drug use. Decongestants do not cause microbial drug resistance. Ulceration of the nasal mucosa is more likely a consequence of irritation and trauma from blowing and wiping the nose. Most decongestants are adrenergic drugs, which cause vasoconstriction and an increase in heart rate and blood pressure. Decongestants, therefore, do not slow the heart rate. Decongestants do not cause mucosal ulceration; however, they can cause the mucous membranes to sting, burn, or feel dry. The immune system is unaffected by nasal decongestants.

> *Test Taking Strategy—Analyze to determine what information the question asks for, which involves health teaching regarding the use of topical nasal decongestant sprays. Recall that rebound phenomenon, also known as rhinitis medicamentosa, is an increase in localized edema and congestion when the ischemia and vasoconstrictive effects of the drug wear off. Review the consequences of using topical nasal sprays if you had difficulty answering this question.*
> **Cognitive Level**—*Applying*
> **Client Needs Category**—*Health promotion and maintenance*
> **Client Needs Subcategory**—*None*

5. **2.** The eustachian tube connects the nasopharynx with the middle ear. Excessive or forceful nose blowing can propel infectious secretions into the eustachian tube, causing a secondary ear infection. Keeping the head elevated when asleep, placing cotton in the ear canal, and massaging the area behind the ears will not reduce the risk of developing an ear infection.

> *Test Taking Strategy—Look for the key words "most appropriate" in reference to health teaching on how to avoid an ear infection during a cold. Recall the anatomy of the nasopharynx and ears, particularly the eustachian tubes, when considering the four options. Refer to references showing the anatomic relationships among these structures if you had difficulty answering this question.*
> *Cognitive Level—Applying*
> *Client Needs Category—Health promotion and maintenance*
> *Client Needs Subcategory—None*

6. **3.** Sinusitis, an inflammation of the sinuses (hollow cavities in the facial bones), usually follows an upper respiratory infection. The maxillary sinuses are located in the cheeks; therefore, pain from maxillary sinusitis would be felt in the cheek or upper teeth. If the frontal sinuses are infected, the pain would be felt near the eyes. Sinuses are not located above or behind the ears.

> *Test Taking Strategy—Use the process of elimination to select the option that correlates with the location of pain that is likely to occur when a client has maxillary sinusitis. Proper identification and location of each of the pairs of paranasal sinuses will help eliminate options 1, 2, and 4, leaving option 3 as the best answer because the maxillary sinuses are named for the maxilla, the cheek bone, where they interconnect. Review the anatomy of the paranasal sinuses if you had difficulty answering this question.*
> *Cognitive Level—Understanding*
> *Client Needs Category—Physiological integrity*
> *Client Needs Subcategory—Physiological adaptation*

7. **3.** Evidence that the client is self-administering nose drops correctly during a return demonstration to the nurse occurs when the client tilts his head backward enabling the liquid medication to settle within the nasopharynx by way of gravity. Bending forward would drain the medication from the nasal passages before it had a chance to provide a therapeutic effect. The other positions described would not help to distribute the nasal medication where it is intended for use.

> *Test Taking Strategy—Use the process of elimination to identify the option that best describes how to effectively instill nasal medications. Recall how gravity can help direct liquid medication toward the tissue on which it will act. This leads to eliminating options 1, 2, and 4, leaving option 3 as the best answer.*

> *Review the procedure for correctly instilling nasal medications if had difficulty answering this question.*
> *Cognitive Level—Evaluating*
> *Client Needs Category—Health promotion and maintenance*
> *Client Needs Subcategory—None*

8. **2.** Vaporizers disperse moistened air into the room and are used primarily by clients to help liquefy nasal secretions. Water sitting in a vaporizer for a prolonged time after use is likely to become stagnant, promoting the growth of microorganisms, especially *Pseudomonas* organisms. Vaporizers can disperse cool or warm mist. One that emits warm mist is more likely to cause scalding or injury if it is placed too close to the edge of a nightstand and is accidentally knocked over. Although dust can accumulate on the vaporizer if it is left sitting for a prolonged time, this is not as hazardous as the risk of the client developing an infection from pathogens. Calcium deposits may form because of the stagnant water, but they will not cause any ill effects.

> *Test Taking Strategy—Analyze to determine what information the question asks for, which is the rationale for emptying and cleaning a cool mist vaporizer after each use. Recall that vaporizers contain water, and standing water supports the growth of pathogens. Review the purpose of a cool mist vaporizer and the care that is required during and after its use if you had difficulty answering this question.*
> *Cognitive Level—Understanding*
> *Client Needs Category—Safe and effective care environment*
> *Client Needs Subcategory—Safety and infection control*

Nursing Care of Clients with Inflammatory and Allergic Disorders of the Upper Airways

9. **3.** Pharyngitis, also known as a *sore throat,* can be caused by bacteria (such as streptococci) or by viruses. When obtaining a culture, the nurse swabs the back of the client's throat with a sterile swab to obtain a sample of infectious organisms in the inflamed tissue of the pharynx. A throat culture is obtained from the posterior pharynx rather than the mouth and tongue. A sputum specimen is obtained by expectoration from the lower respiratory tract. Organisms in saliva would not necessarily indicate the pathogen causing pharyngitis.

> *Test Taking Strategy—Use the process of elimination to identify the option that best describes how to collect a specimen for a throat culture. Recall that the equipment for obtaining and storing the specimen must be sterile, and the specimen must contain secretions from the infected tissue, in this case the*

throat. These facts help to eliminate options 1, 2, and 4 because sputum, saliva, and pathogens inside the mouth or tongue are not the intended specimens. Having eliminated these options, option 3 emerges as the best answer. Review the procedure for obtaining a throat culture if you had difficulty answering this question correctly.
Cognitive Level—*Understanding*
Client Needs Category—*Physiological integrity*
Client Needs Subcategory—*Reduction of risk potential*

10. 1. Glomerulonephritis, rheumatic fever, and rheumatic heart disease are a few of the consequences of untreated or undertreated infections caused by beta-hemolytic streptococci. To ensure that the organism is destroyed, the American Heart Association recommends treating streptococcal infections with a 10-day course of penicillin V (V-Cillin K) or erythromycin (E-Mycin). Chickenpox and shingles are viruses, which are not treated with antibiotics. *Bordetella pertussis*, not streptococci, causes whooping cough.

> **Test Taking Strategy**—*Analyze to determine what information the question asks for, which is the consequences of untreated or undertreated streptococcal infections. Recall that streptococci can migrate and cause inflammation of other organs, in this case the glomeruli of the nephrons, if they are not completely eradicated. Review the etiology of the disorders listed if you had difficulty answering this question correctly.*

Cognitive Level—*Applying*
Client Needs Category—*Health promotion and maintenance*
Client Needs Subcategory—*None*

11. 2. MRSA stands for methicillin-resistant *Staphylococcus aureus*, and describes an *S. aureus* infection that is resistant to methicillin and a range of other antibiotics. To control the spread of MRSA in the community, those people at risk for being colonized with the pathogen, such as nursing home residents, are screened on admission. The most common site of colonization is the anterior nares. When a specimen is collected, a swab is placed in the anterior portion of a nostril and swept to the top. The nurse dons clean, rather than sterile gloves when collecting the specimen, which complies with standard precautions. Having the client blow the nose before collecting the specimen is not necessary because the bacteria will still be present on the surface of the nostril. The same swab is used for both nares. It would be rare that just one would be colonized.

> **Test Taking Strategy**—*Analyze to determine what information the question asks for, which is the correct technique for swabbing the nose to collect a screening specimen. Recall that when obtaining a screening specimen from the nose, the tip of the swab is placed within the anterior portion of the nostril, then*

angled superiorly, and rotated against the tissue as it is withdrawn. The action is repeated in the opposite nostril with the same swab. Review the procedure for obtaining a nasal specimen if you had difficulty answering this question correctly.
Cognitive Level—*Applying*
Client Needs Category—*Health promotion and maintenance*
Client Needs Subcategory—*None*

12. 2. Speaking in a normal voice or whispering prolongs laryngitis. Therefore, resting swollen vocal cords allows the local edema to subside and relieves hoarseness. Because the larynx is found between the throat and the trachea, sucking on ice chips will not be beneficial but may soothe the sore throat. Likewise, drinking hot liquids may help soothe the throat but will not help the larynx. Massaging the throat provides comfort for some people, but it does not relieve hoarseness.

> **Test Taking Strategy**—*Look at the key words "most helpful" in reference to advice for helping a client relieve symptoms associated with laryngitis. Recall that laryngitis, an inflammation of the voice box that results in hoarseness, can be relieved by totally resting the voice. Review health teaching for managing laryngitis if you had difficulty answering this question correctly.*

Cognitive Level—*Applying*
Client Needs Category—*Health promotion and maintenance*
Client Needs Subcategory—*None*

13. 3. Persistent hoarseness is the earliest symptom of cancer of the larynx. Nagging cough or hoarseness is one of the seven early warning signs of cancer identified by the American Cancer Society. Other symptoms of cancer of the larynx include a lump in the neck, difficulty swallowing, dyspnea, weight loss, and pain radiating to the ear. The other disorders mentioned cause respiratory symptoms but are not associated with hoarseness.

> **Test Taking Strategy**—*Use the process of elimination to select the option that identifies the rationale for performing a direct laryngoscopy on a client experiencing hoarseness. Recall that the vocal cords can be visualized with a laryngoscope, facilitating the detection of possible causes for the client's hoarseness, one of which may be cancer of the larynx (option 3). Options 1, 2, and 4 can be eliminated because they identify structures that are unrelated to causing hoarseness. Review the anatomy of the larynx and the purpose of a direct laryngoscopy if you had difficulty answering this question.*

Cognitive Level—*Applying*
Client Needs Category—*Physiological integrity*
Client Needs Subcategory—*Physiological adaptation*

14. 3. Histamine, a chemical released from mast cells at the time of an allergic response, causes symptoms such as watery eyes, sneezing, and coughing. Antihistamines are drugs that counteract these symptoms. Diphenhydramine (Benadryl), a first-generation antihistamine, commonly causes drowsiness and a tendency to fall asleep easily. Anyone taking a first-generation antihistamine is warned to use caution if driving or operating machinery. If there is any effect on weight, it is more likely to be weight gain as a result of reduction in activity. GI side effects include increased appetite, nausea, and diarrhea, but not constipation.

> *Test Taking Strategy*—*Analyze to determine what information the question asks for, which involves identifying a side effect of a first-generation antihistamine such as Benadryl. Recall that a major side effect of this class of drugs is decreased alertness, slowed reaction time, drowsiness, and sleepiness. Review the side effects of first-generation antihistamines if you had difficulty answering this question.*
> *Cognitive Level*—*Applying*
> *Client Needs Category*—*Physiological integrity*
> *Client Needs Subcategory*—*Pharmacological therapies*

15. 1. Many hypersensitive people are allergic to more than one substance. Testing does not promote the production of blocking antibodies. Skin testing is considered a standard practice among allergy specialists, and insurance companies partially or completely pay for this service. Allergy symptoms do vary from person to person, but this is not the main reason skin testing is done. Skin testing is not usually performed because of the threat of complications.

> *Test Taking Strategy*—*Use the process of elimination to select the option that identifies the best reason that skin testing is beneficial. Option 2 can be eliminated immediately because testing does not create blocking antibodies. Although options 3 and 4 are true, they are not reasons for undergoing skin testing. Option 1 remains the best answer because it supports the purpose of skin testing using the scratch test, intradermal test, or patch test to identify the allergen(s) to which the client is symptomatic. Once one or more allergens are identified, it may lead to more specific treatment to relieve or reduce allergic symptoms. Review the purpose for allergy skin testing if you had difficulty answering this question correctly.*
> *Cognitive Level*—*Applying*
> *Client Needs Category*—*Health promotion and maintenance*
> *Client Needs Subcategory*—*None*

16. 4. An area of local erythema (redness) indicates a positive reaction to the antigen applied to the scratched skin. Swelling, known as *induration*, may also accompany a reaction. A positive reaction does not appear pale or feel especially painful or numb.

> *Test Taking Strategy*—*Use the process of elimination to identify the option describing the best indication of a positive reaction to an allergen used during a scratch test. Recall that an allergic response is accompanied by redness (option 4) due to the vasodilating effect of histamine. Options 1 and 3 can be immediately eliminated because numbness and paleness are not characteristic of an allergic response. Option 2 may look appealing, but pain that may be experienced is more likely due to the scratch itself rather than a reaction to the allergen. If you had difficulty answering this question, review how a scratch test is performed and the manifestations that indicate sensitivity to a tested allergen.*
> *Cognitive Level*—*Applying*
> *Client Needs Category*—*Physiological integrity*
> *Client Needs Subcategory*—*Reduction of risk potential*

17. 2. The client undergoing desensitization stays in the physician's office for observation for at least 20 minutes after the injection. Occasionally, a person has a severe allergic reaction to even the small amount of antigen used in the desensitization injection. The client's safety is endangered if a severe reaction occurs and medical assistance is not immediately available. Antihistamines may reduce allergic symptoms, but aspirin has no direct effect. If a client waits 20 minutes, driving is not contraindicated. Clients may shower or bathe after such injections.

> *Test Taking Strategy*—*Look at the key word "essential," which implies a priority. Recall that the dangers of desensitization treatment can result in anaphylactic shock very shortly after being exposed to an allergen. Therefore, having the client wait for 20 minutes (option 2) is an essential nursing action because it ensures that staff will be available to respond if there is a potentially fatal allergic reaction. Review the causes and manifestations of anaphylactic shock if you had difficulty answering this question.*
> *Cognitive Level*—*Applying*
> *Client Needs Category*—*Physiological integrity*
> *Client Needs Subcategory*—*Reduction of risk potential*

18. 1. An anaphylactic reaction is a systemic hypersensitivity reaction that occurs within seconds to minutes after exposure to certain medications, foods, or insect stings. Vital signs provide significant data of impending anaphylaxis with decreasing blood pressure and an elevated heart rate. Later signs of anaphylaxis include labored breathing/chest tightness/coughing, hives/pruritus, loss of consciousness as blood pressure falls, and tachycardia. It is normal to experience some discomfort at the injection site.

> *Test Taking Strategy*—*Analyze to determine what information the question asks for, which is an early*

indication of anaphylaxis. Recall that anaphylactic shock occurs very quickly following contact with the allergen with early symptoms reflected in the vital signs. Anaphylactic shock includes severe hypotension, labored breathing (increased respiratory rate), gasping for air, skin color changes, anxiety (increase heart rate), and panic. Review the signs and symptoms of anaphylactic shock if you had difficulty answering this question. Review the signs and symptoms of anaphylactic shock if you had difficulty answering this question.
Cognitive Level—*Analyzing*
Client Needs Category—*Physiological integrity*
Client Needs Subcategory—*Physiological adaptation*

19. 4. Epinephrine (Adrenalin) is the drug of choice when a client experiences a severe allergic reaction. This drug helps raise the blood pressure by constricting blood vessels and dilating the bronchi, thereby facilitating breathing. Without emergency treatment, persons experiencing severe allergic reactions can die in 5 to 10 minutes. Key goals are to establish a patent airway and ventilate the client. Codeine and morphine sulfate (Roxanol) are central nervous system depressants, which potentiate hypotension. Dopamine (Intropin) is an adrenergic drug in the same family as epinephrine (Adrenalin), but it is not the drug of choice during anaphylaxis. It is commonly given later to maintain the blood pressure of individuals in shock.
Test Taking Strategy—*Analyze to determine what information the question asks for, which is the drug classically used to relieve symptoms of a severe allergic reaction. Recall that epinephrine is an adrenergic agent that raises blood pressure and dilates bronchi by mimicking the actions of the sympathetic nervous system. Review uses and actions of each of the drugs listed if you had difficulty answering this question.*
Cognitive Level—*Understanding*
Client Needs Category—*Physiological integrity*
Client Needs Subcategory—*Pharmacological therapies*

20. 3. After shaking the pulseless client, shouting the client's name, and calling for help, the next step in the Chain of Survival protocol is to begin administering chest compressions. After 30 chest compressions the nurse should open the airway and begin rescue breathing. A precordial thump is not administered in the case of a severe allergic reaction. Epinephrine (Adrenalin) is an emergency drug, but its administration would be at the direction of the physician or emergency services personnel.
Test Taking Strategy—*Analyze to determine what information the question asks for, which is the next nursing action after activating emergency services to facilitate survival of a pulseless client. Guidelines for resuscitation were recently revised. Airway, breathing, circulation, or the ABCs, have now been changed to circulation, airway, breathing (CAB).*

Review the steps in cardiopulmonary resuscitation if you had difficulty answering this question.
Cognitive Level—*Applying*
Client Needs Category—*Physiological integrity*
Client Needs Subcategory—*Physiological adaptation*

21. 3. Because shock is one of the major problems during a severe allergic reaction, monitoring blood pressure is the most important assessment for evaluating treatment effectiveness as blood flow returns to the periphery. A rising blood pressure indicates client improvement. A normal temperature, verbalization of feeling better (subjective data), and no further increasing redness at the site are suggestive that the client's condition is stable, but they are not as significant following treatment of an allergic reaction as the client's current blood pressure.
Test Taking Strategy—*Use the process of elimination to select the option that identifies the most important nursing action when caring for a client with a severe allergic reaction. Consider the development and symptoms related to shock (option 2). Eliminate option 1 as temperature is not usually affected by an allergic reaction. Eliminate options 3 and 4, though both reassuring, feeling better is subjective and levels of redness are difficult to confirm. Review the signs of a severe allergic reaction of you had difficulty answering this question.*
Cognitive Level—*Evaluating*
Client Needs Category—*Physiological integrity*
Client Needs Subcategory—*Physiological adaptation*

Nursing Care of Clients with Cancer of the Larynx

22. 2. Of the options provided, restlessness is most indicative of early hypoxia. Other signs of inadequate oxygenation include rapid, shallow breathing; nasal flaring; use of accessory muscles for breathing; hypertension; confusion; stupor; coma; and cyanosis of the skin, lips, and nail beds. Blood loss is expected after a laryngectomy; however, profuse or prolonged loss will eventually affect the red blood cells' oxygen-carrying capacity. Clients with compromised oxygenation are more likely to exhibit tachycardia than an irregular heart rhythm. Feelings of being cold are common after surgery and are generally related to the environmental temperature of the operating and recovery rooms.
Test Taking Strategy—*Analyze to determine what information the question asks for, which is an early indication of compromised oxygenation. Recall that restlessness (option 2) is an early sign of hypoxia that may be caused in this case from an impaired airway. Review the early and late signs of hypoxia if you had difficulty answering this question.*
Cognitive Level—*Applying*
Client Needs Category—*Physiological integrity*
Client Needs Subcategory—*Physiological adaptation*

23. 4. Until the laryngectomy client learns esophageal speech or the use of a mechanical vibrator, providing paper and pencil or a magic slate is the best alternative for communication. Lipreading is often frustrating for nursing personnel who are unaccustomed to this technique. The client has a permanent loss of natural voice as a result of a total laryngectomy. The client may be able to produce random sounds but will have difficulty verbalizing needs.

Test Taking Strategy—Analyze to determine what information the question asks for, which is a nursing action that promotes communication with a client whose larynx has been removed. Recall that a client who has had a total laryngectomy cannot ever speak normally, which eliminates options 2 and 3. Lipreading (option 1) can be tedious. Using paper and pencil (option 4) is the best alternative. Review nursing care of a client undergoing a total laryngectomy if you had difficulty answering this question.
Cognitive Level—*Applying*
Client Needs Category—*Physiological integrity*
Client Needs Subcategory—*Physiological adaptation*

24. 3. Looking at the tracheostomy tube is interpreted as dealing with the reality of the loss. This is a positive step toward acceptance and adaptation. Grieving follows a cycle of denial or disbelief, anger, depression, bargaining, and acceptance. Believing that the physician misdiagnosed the condition is an example of denial. Social isolation indicates a state of depression characterized by withdrawal from human interaction. Asking the nurse for help with bathing suggests that the client perceives himself or herself as helpless.

Test Taking Strategy—Use the process of elimination to select the option identifying the best indication that a client's postoperative depression and grief are becoming resolved. Looking at the tracheostomy tube (option 3) is a clue that the client is beginning to deal with the reality of the situation. Options 1, 2, and 4 describe actions that represent isolation, denial, and helplessness, all of which are examples of ineffective coping. Consult references that describe how acceptance may be manifested by a client with a change in body image if you had difficulty answering this question.
Cognitive Level—*Applying*
Client Needs Category—*Psychosocial integrity*
Client Needs Subcategory—*None*

Nursing Care of Clients with Inflammatory and Infectious Disorders of the Lower Airways

25. 3. When assessing a cough, the nurse first determines if the cough is productive or nonproductive. If the cough is productive, the nurse should document the color, odor, amount, and viscosity of sputum that is raised. Other

data that may aid the physician in making a diagnosis include the onset, duration, precipitating factors, and relief measures. Although family history is important, it does not relate to the cough itself. The client's vital signs may be affected by persistent coughing, but this does not address the characteristics of the cough. Self-treatment and medications used to control the cough are important to know, but they are not as pertinent as the presence and appearance of the sputum.

Test Taking Strategy—Analyze to determine what information the question asks for, which is additional information to document besides the characteristics of the client's cough. Recall that the appearance of expectorated secretions may help in the differential diagnosis of the respiratory condition. Review the physical findings used to describe sputum if you had difficulty answering this question correctly.
Cognitive Level—*Applying*
Client Needs Category—*Physiological integrity*
Client Needs Subcategory—*Physiological adaptation*

26. 3. Codeine depresses the cough center in the brain and is used to suppress coughing. Antitussives that contain codeine or a similar synthetic chemical, dextromethorphan, are called *sedative antitussives*. Antitussives are indicated for coughing when a person's lungs are clear or when persistent coughing adversely affects recovery from other conditions. Suppressing a cough is contraindicated if the client needs to expectorate sputum. Bronchodilators open respiratory passages. Salicylates are used to relieve discomfort, and steroids reduce inflammation.

Test Taking Strategy—Analyze to determine what information the question asks for, which is the reason the physician prescribed guaifenesin (Robitussin AC), an antitussive that contains codeine. Refer to pharmacology references for the reason sedative antitussives are prescribed if you had difficulty answering this question.
Cognitive Level—*Applying*
Client Needs Category—*Physiological integrity*
Client Needs Subcategory—*Pharmacological therapies*

27. 1. A client taking an opioid (codeine) is warned not to exceed the recommended dosage. Extra self-administration leads to sedation and habituation. Opioid antitussives can cause drowsiness but do not interfere with sleep patterns. Many clients take the medication before bed to suppress coughing so they can sleep. Expectorants, not opioid antitussives, are taken with extra fluids to thin mucoid secretions and facilitate their expectoration. Chilling medications, rather than warming them, would help to disguise an unpleasant taste.

Test Taking Strategy—Look at the key word "most appropriate" in reference to the health teaching that relates to the prescribed cough medication. Recall that self-administering more than the prescribed dosage of the cough medication containing codeine may decrease alertness. Review the side effects and precautions associated with codeine if you had difficulty answering this question.
Cognitive Level—*Applying*
Client Needs Category—*Physiological integrity*
Client Needs Subcategory—*Pharmacological therapies*

28. 4. Syrups are given after other oral medications and are not followed by water or other liquids for a period of time because they are intended to have a soothing effect on the mucosa of the pharynx. Waiting 15 minutes after giving the syrup shortens the time of local effectiveness. The remaining alternatives involve swallowing water immediately after administering the cough syrup and, therefore, are inappropriate.

> *Test Taking Strategy*—Analyze to determine what information the question asks for, which is the best nursing action to take when administering cough medication and oral tablets at the same time. Recall that medications that must be swallowed with water should be given before the cough syrup. Review the nursing implications when administering cough syrups if you had difficulty answering this question.
> **Cognitive Level**—*Applying*
> **Client Needs Category**—*Physiological integrity*
> **Client Needs Subcategory**—*Pharmacological therapies*

29. 3. The approximate equivalent of 5 mL in household measurements is 1 teaspoon. Some manufacturers of nonprescription cough medications include a dosing cup marked with various household equivalents. However, to ensure safety, the nurse should include an explanation of the equivalents during discharge instructions. One ounce equals 30 mL. One tablespoon equals about 15 mL. A capful is not an accurate measure because it can vary depending on the size of the bottle. Also, pouring medication into, then drinking from, the cap is unsanitary and can contaminate the remaining medication.

> *Test Taking Strategy*—Analyze to determine what information the question asks for, which is the household equivalent of 5 mL. Recall that 5 mL equals 1 teaspoon and eliminate all options but option 3. Review the household equivalents for metric measurements if you had difficulty answering this question.
> **Cognitive Level**—*Understanding*
> **Client Needs Category**—*Physiological integrity*
> **Client Needs Subcategory**—*Pharmacological therapies*

30. 1. Aerosol therapy involves depositing small droplets of moisture onto respiratory tissue. The warmed, moist air soothes the respiratory passages, relieves tissue irritation, and liquefies secretions produced as a result of the inflammation. Other benefits are obtained by adding medications to the vaporized water. Individuals with acute bronchitis are generally bothered initially by a nonproductive cough aggravated by dry air. Oral or parenteral antibiotic therapy, not aerosol therapy, is used to kill infectious organisms. Respiratory mucosa is moist. The respiratory rate is lowered as ventilation is improved. However, this is a secondary benefit of aerosol therapy and is not its primary purpose.

> *Test Taking Strategy*—Use the process of elimination to help select the option that correctly describes the purpose of aerosol therapy. Recall that an aerosol is a fine mist that is inhaled for localized relief of respiratory symptoms. Review information on the purposes of aerosol therapy and the manner in which it is provided if you had difficulty answering this question.
> **Cognitive Level**—*Analyzing*
> **Client Needs Category**—*Physiological integrity*
> **Client Needs Subcategory**—*Pharmacological therapies*

31. 3 mL.
To calculate the drug dosage, use the following formula:

$$\frac{\text{Desired dose}}{\text{Dose on hand}} \times \text{Quantity} = X \text{ (amount to administer)}$$

The desired dose is 300,000 units, and the dose on hand, once reconstituted, is 100,000 units/mL; therefore, the correct amount for administration is 3 mL.

> *Test Taking Strategy*—Analyze to determine what information the question asks for, which is the volume of medication to administer. Recall that medications are reconstituted by adding a specified amount of liquid to powdered medication to yield the indicated concentration. Review the process of reconstituting medications and calculation of parenteral dosages if you had difficulty answering this question.
> **Cognitive Level**—*Applying*
> **Client Needs Category**—*Physiological integrity*
> **Client Needs Subcategory**—*Pharmacological therapies*

32. 1. Pneumonia is a potentially fatal infection involving one or both lungs. A major difference between bacterial and viral pneumonia is the onset of symptoms. In bacterial pneumonia, the onset of symptoms is rapid and more severe. Bacterial pneumonia has an incubation period of hours to 1 to 2 days. The fever that accompanies bacterial pneumonia is quite high. The onset of symptoms for viral pneumonia occurs gradually, and they are less severe.

Laypeople call this type of pneumonia *walking pneumonia*. The incubation period for viral pneumonia is 2 to 5 days; it typically is preceded 2 to 3 days (not weeks) by an upper respiratory infection or sore throat.

> *Test Taking Strategy—Analyze to determine what information the question asks for, which is the basis for the nurse's query as to when the client's symptoms first appeared. Review the differences between bacterial and viral pneumonia if you had difficulty answering this question.*
> ***Cognitive Level***—*Analyzing*
> ***Client Needs Category***—*Physiological integrity*
> ***Client Needs Subcategory***—*Physiological adaptation*

33. **2.** Any article containing metal is removed before a chest X-ray is performed. The image of a metal object that remains in place during an X-ray may be misinterpreted as diseased tissue. Fasting is not required before a chest X-ray. No radiopaque dye is given for this test. Analgesia is unnecessary because the client will not have any accompanying discomfort.

> *Test Taking Strategy—Analyze to determine what information the question asks for, which is the nursing action that is essential before a chest X-ray is performed. Recall that an X-ray images dense structures, substances, and objects. A metal necklace worn by the client may be mistaken as a pathologic lesion or may obscure a pathologic lesion within the chest. Therefore, it is important to remove anything metallic from the client's chest before the X-ray. Review how X-ray images are produced and precautions about removing objects that may cause artifacts if you had difficulty answering this question.*
> ***Cognitive Level***—*Applying*
> ***Client Needs Category***—*Physiological integrity*
> ***Client Needs Subcategory***—*Reduction of risk potential*

34. **1.** Increasing the fluid intake can help thin respiratory secretions that are difficult to expectorate. Increasing moisture in inspired air through humidification also helps. Changing positions improves circulation and prevents pooling of respiratory secretions. Physicians must write an order for dietary changes. A clear liquid diet may thin secretions, but it is not usually ordered when a sputum specimen is needed. Antitussives are cough suppressants. Suppressing the cough will not allow sputum to be coughed up. An expectorant is the drug of choice if the client has a weak cough or a condition warrants its use.

> *Test Taking Strategy—Use the process of elimination to help select the option that describes the most appropriate action for obtaining a sputum specimen. Recall that for easier expectoration, the client should be well hydrated. Option 3 can be eliminated because this is not a nursing action. Option 4 is contraindicated in this client because an antitussive will suppress the cough. Changing positions (option*

2) can prevent pooling of respiratory secretions, but the most appropriate action to thin secretions is to provide adequate fluid (option 1). Review techniques for promoting the expectoration of sputum if you had difficulty answering this question.
> ***Cognitive Level***—*Applying*
> ***Client Needs Category***—*Physiological integrity*
> ***Client Needs Subcategory***—*Reduction of risk potential*

35. **4.** It is easiest to obtain a sputum specimen when the client first awakens in the morning, because secretions tend to accumulate in the respiratory tract during the night. Pooled secretions are more easily raised, especially if the individual is not fatigued from activity. Sputum collection may also be done after an aerosol treatment, which helps to loosen secretions. Forced coughing after a meal can lead to vomiting.

> *Test Taking Strategy—Use the process of elimination to help select the option that identifies the best time to obtain a sputum specimen. Recall that efforts to cough in the morning are likely to be more successful for collecting a sputum specimen because there is a greater volume of respiratory secretions accumulating during the night. Review methods for facilitating the collection of a sputum specimen if you had difficulty answering this question.*
> ***Cognitive Level***—*Applying*
> ***Client Needs Category***—*Physiological integrity*
> ***Client Needs Subcategory***—*Reduction of risk potential*

36. **4.** The client must avoid touching the inside of the sputum specimen container and the inside of its lid. The inside of the container must be kept sterile so that no sources of microorganisms (such as pathogens found on the hands), other than those present in the sputum, are collected. Wearing gloves and wiping the outside of the specimen container are unnecessary because the outside surface is considered unclean anyway. The lid should be placed on the container as soon as sputum is deposited to prevent contamination from outside sources.

> *Test Taking Strategy—Use the process of elimination to help select the option that identifies a client's accurate understanding about collecting a sputum specimen. Recall that contamination of the specimen or the container in which it is held may cause the results of the culture to be inaccurate. Eliminate options 1 and 2 because these steps are unnecessary because the outside surface is considered unclean. Option 3 is incorrect because the lid should be placed on the container as soon as sputum is deposited to prevent contamination from outside sources. Review the techniques that preserve the sterility of a sputum specimen if you had difficulty answering this question.*
> ***Cognitive Level***—*Analyzing*
> ***Client Needs Category***—*Physiological integrity*
> ***Client Needs Subcategory***—*Reduction of risk potential*

37. **2.** Mouth care is an appropriate hygiene measure after obtaining a sputum specimen. Expectorating sputum often causes a residual foul taste in the mouth or an unpleasant odor to the breath.

> *Test Taking Strategy—Use the process of elimination to help select the option that describes the most appropriate nursing action after obtaining a sputum specimen. Recall that because microorganisms in the sputum often make the breath and mouth foul-smelling and foul-tasting, good oral hygiene is an appropriate nursing intervention. Oxygen (option 1) is appropriate if the client is short of breath. Eating (option 3) is usually delayed until the client is rested and unlikely to become nauseous. Walking (option 4) may cause further fatigue after the effort of coughing. Option 2 remains as the most appropriate action to take. Review indications for providing oral care in other than routine circumstances if you had difficulty answering this question.*
> **Cognitive Level**—*Applying*
> **Client Needs Category**—*Physiological integrity*
> **Client Needs Subcategory**—*Basic care and comfort*

38. **2.** Pleurisy is an inflammation of the pleural membranes surrounding the lungs. The most classic symptom associated with pleurisy is feeling a sharp, stabbing pain when taking a deep breath.

> *Test Taking Strategy—Look at the key words "most likely" in reference to the assessment finding that correlates with pleurisy. Recall that there is an inflammatory process occurring between the layers of the pleura and that pain is a classic component of inflammation; the pain is aggravated during inspiration. The presence of a cough (option 1) would be because of some other pulmonary problem. Cyanotic nail beds (option 3) and tachycardia (option 4) are caused by any number of cardiopulmonary diseases that interfere with tissue oxygenation. But pain is a cardinal sign of pleurisy, making option 2 the most likely finding. Review the signs and symptoms of pleurisy if you had difficulty answering this question.*
> **Cognitive Level**—*Applying*
> **Client Needs Category**—*Physiological integrity*
> **Client Needs Subcategory**—*Physiological adaptation*

39. **1.** Pneumococcal pneumonia is a bacterial infection, and the antibiotics used to treat it are selected on the basis of their effect on the infectious organism, demonstrated by performing a culture and testing drug sensitivity. The organism is first encouraged to grow in the laboratory medium. Then small disks of various drugs are placed in the growing colonies. If growth is inhibited around a certain disk, this indicates that the drug is effective.

> *Test Taking Strategy—Use the process of elimination to help select the option that identifies the best reason for using penicillin to treat the client's pneumonia.*

Recall that in this client's case, a culture identified pneumococcus, also known as Streptococcus pneumoniae, as the causative organism. Penicillin is effective against gram-positive strains of streptococci, staphylococci, and some gram-negative bacteria such as meningococcus. Option 2 can be eliminated because this statement is incorrect; antibiotics are effective in treating bacterial infections but ineffective in treating viral infections. Option 3 is also an incorrect statement; although widely used, penicillin, like any drug, has dangerous side effects. Option 4 is an inaccurate statement because various factors (including drug effectiveness, cost, route of administration, and the client's history of drug allergy) affect the physician's choice of which drug to use. Review the uses for various classes of antibiotics, particularly the penicillins, if you had difficulty answering this question.
> **Cognitive Level**—*Applying*
> **Client Needs Category**—*Physiological integrity*
> **Client Needs Subcategory**—*Pharmacological therapies*

40.

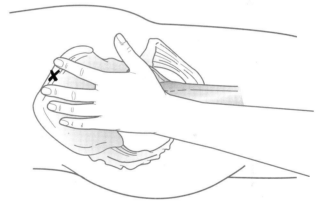

The ventrogluteal site, which is the most common site for adult intramuscular injections, lies in the area of the anterior and superior regions of the pelvic ilium. The site is identified by placing the palm of the hand on the greater trochanter and the index finger on the anterosuperior iliac spine. The middle finger is moved away from the index finger as far as possible. The injection is administered in the center of the space between the index and middle fingers.

> *Test Taking Strategy—Analyze to determine what information the question asks for, which is the correct location of the ventrogluteal injection site. Refer to sources that describe the technique for identifying the landmarks for this injection site if you had difficulty answering this question.*
> **Cognitive Level**—*Understanding*
> **Client Needs Category**—*Physiological integrity*
> **Client Needs Subcategory**—*Pharmacological therapies*

41. 3. Cephalosporins are chemically similar to the penicillins. Therefore, the nurse would expect that a client who is allergic to penicillin may also react adversely when given a cephalosporin-type of antibiotic. Before administering a cephalosporin to a client with a penicillin allergy, it is best to consult the physician and observe the client closely if the medical order is not changed. Although allergic reactions occur with the administration of any antibiotic, the other antibiotic groups do not demonstrate the same cross-sensitivity with penicillin.

Test Taking Strategy—Analyze to determine what information the question asks for, which is a category of antibiotic that can cause an allergic reaction in those hypersensitive to the penicillins. Recall that if a client has an allergic reaction to penicillin, he or she may also have one to the cephalosporins. Review the categories of antibiotics listed, looking particularly for a discussion of cross-sensitivities, if you had difficulty answering this question.
Cognitive Level—Applying
Client Needs Category—Physiological integrity
Client Needs Subcategory—Pharmacological therapies

42. 3. The influenza vaccine contains albumin from the eggs in which the virus is cultured. Some individuals who are allergic to eggs or egg products may react adversely and may require skin testing to determine how sensitive they are before receiving the flu vaccine. Influenza vaccinations, used to prevent flu symptoms caused by a virus, are repeated yearly to provide immunity against viral strains identified during the previous year. Pneumococcal pneumonia vaccine is given to prevent bacterial pneumonia; it is unrelated to the influenza vaccine. Influenza and pneumococcal vaccines are recommended for anyone older than age 65 years and those with chronic disease. Having a history of a respiratory disease is not an essential criterion for influenza vaccinations.

Test Taking Strategy—Analyze to determine what information the question asks for, which is the information that should be determined before administering the flu vaccine. Recall that administering flu vaccine to a person with a severe egg allergy may trigger symptoms that require emergency treatment. Review the flu vaccine protocol offered by the American College of Allergy, Asthma & Immunology if you had difficulty answering this question.
Cognitive Level—Applying
Client Needs Category—Physiological integrity
Client Needs Subcategory—Reduction of risk potential

43. 2. All of these options help reduce the potential for infection. However, because respiratory infections are spread primarily by direct contact with another sick individual, avoiding crowds is the best advice. The U.S. Public Health Service Advisory Committee on Immunization recommends annual vaccination against influenza for people older than age 65 years and those with chronic health problems.

Test Taking Strategy—Use the process of elimination to help select the option that identifies the intervention, other than receiving flu vaccine, that is most helpful for avoiding influenza. Recall that influenza is spread from infected people via respiratory droplets. Limiting exposure to infected individuals is superior to the interventions listed in the other options. Review techniques for limiting the transmission of infectious diseases transmitted by respiratory droplets if you had difficulty answering this question.
Cognitive Level—Applying
Client Needs Category—Health promotion and maintenance
Client Needs Subcategory—None

44. 1. Oseltamivir (Tamiflu) is typically ordered in 75-mg capsules or liquid suspension. Tamiflu is prescribed twice daily for 5 days and is most effective when administered within 12 to 24 hours of experiencing the first symptoms because the action of the medication is to prevent the spread of the virus. Tamiflu may be taken on an empty stomach or with food. No laboratory work is required before the initiation of the medication.

Test Taking Strategy—Analyze to determine what information the question asks for, which is a factor that affects the drug's effectiveness. Recall that Tamiflu is administered to reduce flu symptoms, making them less severe and shortening the course of the illness by several days. The longer the time between becoming infected and the initiation of drug treatment, the smaller the potential for modifying the symptoms and course of influenza. Review information on the use of Tamiflu and its mechanism of action if you had difficulty answering this question.
Cognitive Level—Applying
Client Needs Category—Physiological integrity
Client Needs Subcategory—Pharmacological therapies

45. 2, 4, 5, 6. Inadequate oxygenation causes the client to initially become restless and anxious. The respiratory rate accelerates in an effort to increase the diffusion of atmospheric oxygen from the lungs to the blood, causing tachypnea. When the increased respiratory rate is insufficient, accessory muscles compensate to increase the inspiratory volume. In the late stages of hypoxia, the client becomes confused as the brain suffers from oxygen deprivation. One of the last signs of hypoxia is cyanosis. Cough and fever may be signs of a respiratory infection that can lead to hypoxia, but they are not manifestations of a hypoxic state.

Test Taking Strategy—Analyze to determine what information the question asks for, which is the signs and symptoms of hypoxia. Alternative-format "select all that apply" questions require considering each

option independently to decide its merit in answering the question. Choose the options that relate best to the signs and symptoms of hypoxia. Review the signs and symptoms of hypoxia if you had difficulty answering this question.
Cognitive Level—*Applying*
Client Needs Category—*Physiological integrity*
Client Needs Subcategory—*Physiological adaptation*

46. 4. An intake of 3,000 mL per day is safe in the absence of any preexisting cardiovascular or renal problems. The additional fluid helps to keep the client hydrated and aids in temperature regulation. Less than 3,000 mL is insufficient because of the client's increased metabolic rate secondary to an extremely elevated body temperature.

Test Taking Strategy—Analyze to determine what information the question asks for, which is the appropriate fluid intake for a client with a high fever. Recall that evaporation of perspiration reduces fluid volume that should be replaced within a higher range of normal fluid intake. Review the safe range of daily fluid intake if you had difficulty answering this question.
Cognitive Level—*Applying*
Client Needs Category—*Physiological integrity*
Client Needs Subcategory—*Reduction of risk potential*

47. 2. Chilling is an indication that the body temperature is falling too rapidly. The muscle contraction that accompanies chilling produces heat and interferes with reducing body temperature. When chills occur, it is best to temporarily discontinue the sponge bath, dry the skin, and protect the client from any drafts. Nausea and confusion are not considered adverse effects associated with sponge bathing. A feverish individual is likely to have a flushed appearance that is unrelated to sponge bathing.

Test Taking Strategy—Analyze to determine what information the question asks for, which is the basis for discontinuing a sponge bath given for fever reduction. Recall that chilling increases body temperature, which is contrary to the purpose of the sponge bath. Review evidence of an adverse response when administering a sponge bath if you had difficulty answering this question.
Cognitive Level—*Applying*
Client Needs Category—*Physiological integrity*
Client Needs Subcategory—*Reduction of risk potential*

48. 3. A decrease in the client's temperature is the best evidence that the tepid sponge bath is having a therapeutic effect. Sweating may or may not be the result of sponge bathing; it may be an indication of another disease process. Although the client feels more comfortable, the statement reflects subjective information. Objective data, such as the client's temperature, are more reliable indicators. Flushed skin is a sign that accompanies an elevated temperature.

Test Taking Strategy—Use the process of elimination to select the option that identifies the best indication that a sponge bath is having a therapeutic effect. Recall that the primary goal for administering the sponge bath, in this case, is to reduce the client's fever, making option 3 the best answer. Options 1, 2, and 4 can be eliminated because they do not offer definitive evidence of a therapeutic effect of the sponge bath. Review the purpose for administering a sponge bath and criteria for evaluating its effectiveness if you had difficulty answering this question.
Cognitive Level—*Applying*
Client Needs Category—*Physiological integrity*
Client Needs Subcategory—*Physiological adaptation*

49.

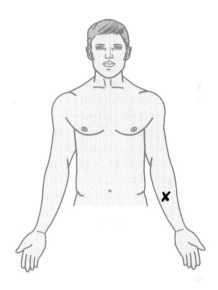

Typically when administering an intradermal injection, the needle is inserted between the layers of skin at approximately a 10- to 15-degree angle into the left forearm.
Test Taking Strategy—Analyze to determine what information the question asks for, which involves identifying the location for administering an intradermal injection. Recall that intradermal injections are used when administering tuberculin tests. Review the locations of injection sites, particularly the sites for intradermal injections, if you had difficulty answering this question correctly.
Cognitive Level—*Understanding*
Client Needs Category—*Physiological integrity*
Client Needs Subcategory—*Pharmacological therapies*

50. 3. The standard length of time for reading a tuberculin skin test is 48 to 72 hours after the test is administered. The nurse observes for redness and measures any evidence of an indurated (hard) area of tissue. Some individuals who are immunosuppressed do not always respond positively to the initial skin test, yet they are symptomatic. A second skin test that is more strongly concentrated is administered to immunosuppressed clients and additional diagnostic tests (such as a sputum examination and chest X-ray) are performed to definitively diagnose the disease.

> *Test Taking Strategy*—*Analyze to determine what information the question asks for, which is when a tuberculin test site should be assessed to determine if there was a reaction. The standard recommended time for assessment is 48 to 72 hours (option 3). Review the process for using a Mantoux test to screen for tuberculosis if you had difficulty answering this question correctly.*
> *Cognitive Level*—*Applying*
> *Client Needs Category*—*Health promotion and maintenance*
> *Client Needs Subcategory*—*None*

51. **2.** Tuberculosis is an infectious disease that is transmitted by inhaling moist droplets or dried spores containing the infectious organism. A positive tuberculin skin test indicates that, at some time, the person became infected with the microorganism that causes tuberculosis and developed antibodies. A positive skin test may or may not mean that an active infectious process is occurring. Isolation is not indicated on the basis of a positive skin test. Anyone with a positive tuberculin skin test without any known history of having had the disease must have a subsequent chest X-ray and sputum examinations. Drugs are administered prophylactically to individuals who suddenly test positive after having a history of being negative. A positive skin test does not indicate protective immunity.

> *Test Taking Strategy*—*Look at the key words "most accurate" in reference to the significance of a positive skin test. A positive skin test may indicate exposure or infection with the tuberculin bacillus, but does not suggest protective immunity (option 3), nor does it definitively indicate an active infection (option 1). Option 4 can also be eliminated because if an active infection is confirmed, clients can remain at home while taking medications. Clients who are hospitalized with confirmed or suspected tuberculosis are cared for using airborne precautions, isolation are recommended for clients with active infections. Review the interpretation and meaning of a positive tuberculin test if you had difficulty answering this question correctly.*
> *Cognitive Level*—*Applying*
> *Client Needs Category*—*Physiological integrity*
> *Client Needs Subcategory*—*Physiological adaptation*

52. **4.** Prophylactic drug therapy with isoniazid (INH) and rifampin (Rifadin) is initiated whenever a person with a previously negative tuberculin skin test demonstrates a positive reaction. INH is combined with other drugs if the disease is confirmed with additional diagnostic tests, such

as sputum examinations and chest X-rays. Chest X-rays are performed to diagnose tuberculosis and are repeated every 2 to 3 years thereafter. Once a skin test is positive, it remains positive lifelong. Therefore, skin tests every 6 months are not necessary. Most individuals with active tuberculosis become noninfectious within 2 weeks with appropriate drug therapy. Immediate family members and close contacts are also tested and treated prophylactically so that living separately is unnecessary.

> *Test Taking Strategy*—*Use the process of elimination to select the option that identifies the most correct information about actions that are taken when a person with a previously negative skin test has a positive reaction. Recall that tuberculosis is an infectious disease. Efforts are taken to eliminate the disease in the affected person and control its transmission among members of the community. Repeat skin tests (option 1) are not required, and X-rays are repeated every 2 to 3 years in clients with tuberculosis, not yearly (option 2). Option 3 can also be eliminated because close contacts should also be tested and treated if necessary. Review the regimen for drug therapy for tuberculosis and the time line for repeated chest X-ray if you had difficulty answering this question.*
> *Cognitive Level*—*Applying*
> *Client Needs Category*—*Physiological integrity*
> *Client Needs Subcategory*—*Reduction of risk potential*

53. **2.** Because noncompliance is one of the leading causes of treatment failures in tuberculosis, asking the client if all of the prescribed medication has been taken is appropriate. All clients who must take one or more drugs must be informed that their medications should be taken consistently throughout the treatment period. The remaining questions are appropriate but should not be asked until the nurse has determined that the client has been taking the medications appropriately.

> *Test Taking Strategy*—*Look at the key words "most important" in reference to information the nurse should ask when a client who has been on drug therapy for 6 weeks continues to have tuberculosis bacilli in a subsequent sputum specimen. Recall that most individuals with active tuberculosis become noninfectious within 2 weeks with appropriate drug therapy. Using a "cause and effect" rationale, the nurse needs to determine if the client has been compliant with drug therapy. Directly observed therapy (DOT), in which the nurse or public health employee delivers and watches the client swallow the drugs, may be necessary to ensure that the medications are being taken. If the client has been compliant, he or she may be infected with a drug-resistant strain. Review the factors that affect the course of treatment for clients with tuberculosis if you had difficulty answering this question.*

Cognitive Level—*Applying*
Client Needs Category—*Health promotion and maintenance*
Client Needs Subcategory—*None*

54. **3.** To prevent the transmission of infectious microorganisms that cause tuberculosis, it is most important to instruct the client to cover the nose and mouth when coughing or sneezing, dispose of paper tissues appropriately, and perform frequent hand washing. Although hand washing is important for everyone, there is no logical correlation between preventing tuberculosis, which is spread through airborne respiratory secretions, and washing hands before and after meals or avoiding sharing towels and wash cloths.

> *Test Taking Strategy*—*Use the process of elimination to select the option that correlates with the most important information for preventing the transmission of tuberculosis. Options 1, 2, and 4 are valid suggestions for hygiene. However, they are not as specific for preventing the spread of tuberculosis as option 3, covering the nose and mouth when coughing, which reduces the spread of airborne secretions containing the microorganism. Review the manner in which tuberculosis is transmitted and measures to control it if you had difficulty answering this question correctly.*
> *Cognitive Level*—*Applying*
> *Client Needs Category*—*Health promotion and maintenance*
> *Client Needs Subcategory*—*None*

55. **3.** Combining beans (chili) and a grain (corn bread) is an economical means of consuming all essential amino acids found in an animal source. Drinking milk also improves the nutrition of this meal choice. The alternative meals are economical. However, because they do not provide adequate sources of protein, they are not considered nutritious choices.

> *Test Taking Strategy*—*Use the process of elimination to help select the option that describes the food selections that provide the most nutrition for a client with a low income. Recall that there should be a variety of foods that contain protein, carbohydrates, and some fat. Review each of the foods individually and then in combination with others in the option to determine their nutritional composition as a whole if you had difficulty answering this question.*
> *Cognitive Level*—*Applying*
> *Client Needs Category*—*Health promotion and maintenance*
> *Client Needs Subcategory*—*None*

56. **4.** Rifampin (Rifadin) and isoniazid (INH) are commonly combined to treat tuberculosis (TB) because resistant strains of TB occur rapidly if either medication is used alone. Side effects are not reduced, they do not act at

different periods during the organism's life cycle, and their dosage is not altered when given in combination.

> *Test Taking Strategy*—*Analyze to determine what information the question asks for, which is the most accurate explanation for using a combination of drugs to treat tuberculosis. A drug regimen that uses only one drug results in the rapid development of resistance and treatment failure, making option 4 the best answer. Review the purpose for combination drug therapy when treating tuberculosis if you had difficulty answering this question.*
> *Cognitive Level*—*Applying*
> *Client Needs Category*—*Physiological integrity*
> *Client Needs Subcategory*—*Pharmacological therapies*

57. **2.** Giving medication with food protects the stomach from becoming upset. The potential for gastric upset is increased if irritating medications are administered on an empty stomach. Drinking water, providing an antacid, or giving the medication at night will not necessarily reduce GI side effects.

> *Test Taking Strategy*—*Use the process of elimination to select the option identifying the best action for preventing gastrointestinal side effects of rifampin drug therapy. Option 4 can be eliminated because lowering gastric pH may interfere with the drug's absorption. Option 1 has merit because sleep may interfere with the perception of nausea. Option 3, drinking plenty of water, would dilute the medication in the stomach, but the stomach distention may lead to vomiting. Option 2 remains as the best action because the presence of food in the stomach mixes with the medication and acts as a buffer, making the drug less irritating. Review techniques for relieving nausea, especially when it is a side effect of medications, if you had difficulty answering this question.*
> *Cognitive Level*—*Applying*
> *Client Needs Category*—*Physiological integrity*
> *Client Needs Subcategory*—*Pharmacological therapies*

Nursing Care of Clients with Asthma

58. **1.** A sitting position is preferred when auscultating the chest. This allows the nurse access to the anterior, lateral, and posterior chest areas. Changing positions during auscultation further taxes an already dyspneic client.

> *Test Taking Strategy*—*Use the process of elimination to help select the option that describes the best position for auscultating breath sounds. Options 2 and 3 can be eliminated because a client in respiratory distress generally cannot tolerate lying flat or on the side. Option 4 can be eliminated because standing is unsafe for a client who is having extreme difficulty breathing. Sitting (option 1) is preferred because it allows better access to the chest. Review*

the anatomy of the lungs and structures that may affect the transmission of sound to the ear pieces of a stethoscope if you had difficulty answering this question.

Cognitive Level—*Applying*
Client Needs Category—*Physiological integrity*
Client Needs Subcategory—*Physiological adaptation*

59. 1. Pulse oximetry is a noninvasive method for assessing oxygen saturation in the tissues. In most cases, the sensor of a pulse oximeter is applied to the finger, but it may also be applied to the earlobe, thumb, toe, or bridge of the nose. The leg is too dense to allow light to transilluminate from tissue to the sensor. Applying the sensor to the thickness of the palm of the hand is inappropriate.

Test Taking Strategy—*Analyze to determine what information the question asks for, which is the best location for the pulse oximeter sensor for collecting accurate data. Recall that the sensor uses light to detect blood flowing through the assessment site. The site must be thin enough to allow light to transilluminate from tissue to the sensor, which eliminates options 2 and 4. The sensor is generally applied to a finger (option 1). The earlobe (option 3), which is used less frequently, is a possible secondary location. Review the locations that are recommended when using a pulse oximeter if you had difficulty answering this question correctly.*

Cognitive Level—*Applying*
Client Needs Category—*Physiological integrity*
Client Needs Subcategory—*Reduction of risk potential*

60. 4. Normal oxygen saturation is 95% to 100%. Supplemental oxygen administration is appropriate if the oxygen saturation is sustained below 90%. The normal level of the partial pressure of oxygen (Pao_2), which is measured by arterial blood gas analysis, is 80 to 100 mm Hg.

Test Taking Strategy—*Analyze to determine what information the question asks for, which is the numerical value that corresponds to normal oxygen saturation. Recall that the amount of oxygen that is bound to hemoglobin is 95% or higher. Review the normal range for blood gas measurements, especially oxygen saturation, if you had difficulty answering this question correctly.*

Cognitive Level—*Applying*
Client Needs Category—*Physiological integrity*
Client Needs Subcategory—*Reduction of risk potential*

61. 2. Levalbuterol hydrochloride (Xopenex) is a bronchodilator used to treat narrowing of the airways by inhalation treatment in clients with asthma, especially those having difficulty breathing and shortness of breath. Side effects of the medication include several heart-related alterations, such as an elevated or irregular heart rate. Drowsiness is not a side effect of the medication.

A respiratory rate of 28 breaths per minute is not unusual for a client experiencing an asthma attack.

Test Taking Strategy—*Analyze to determine what information the question asks for, which involves identifying a side effect of levalbuterol (Xopenex). Recall that this drug is a beta-adrenergic agonist that stimulates bronchial receptors, resulting in the relaxation of smooth muscles in the bronchial tree. To a certain extent, receptors in the heart are also stimulated, mimicking responses like those produced by the sympathetic nervous system. Review the mechanism of action and side effects associated with beta-adrenergic agonists if you had difficulty answering this question.*

Cognitive Level—*Applying*
Client Needs Category—*Physiological integrity*
Client Needs Subcategory—*Pharmacological therapies*

62. 1. To avoid excessive blood loss and a painful hematoma from a punctured arterial site, it is essential to apply direct pressure for a minimum of 5 minutes. The specimen is cooled in ice after collection. The blood pressure is unlikely to be affected by the loss of a small amount of blood. Elevating the arm is one way to control bleeding from a vein, but it probably would be ineffective in the case of bleeding from an artery.

Test Taking Strategy—*Analyze to determine what information the question asks for, which is the nursing action that is essential to perform immediately after obtaining a sample of blood from an artery. Recall that arterial blood pressure is higher than that of venous blood, and arterial bleeding is less likely to stop on its own. Therefore, manual pressure must be applied by the nurse to prevent hematoma formation or blood loss. Review nursing responsibilities associated with obtaining an arterial blood specimen if you had difficulty answering this question.*

Cognitive Level—*Applying*
Client Needs Category—*Safe and effective care environment*
Client Needs Subcategory—*Safety and infection control*

63. 2. The reservoir bag of a partial rebreathing mask remains partially filled during inspiration. If the bag collapses completely, the equipment may be faulty. This information must be reported to the respiratory therapy department. A properly fitting mask should cover the mouth and nose, and the strap should fit the head snugly. Moisture is likely to accumulate because the oxygen is humidified; this information does not need to be reported. The nurse can wipe away the moisture and reapply the mask.

Test Taking Strategy—*Use the process of elimination to select the option identifying the most important information to report when using a partial*

rebreather mask. Recall that a partial rebreather mask conserves the first third of the client's exhaled air within the reservoir bag while the rest escapes through the side ports. The retained air keeps the bag inflated so as to facilitate rebreathing carbon dioxide, a respiratory stimulant. If the reservoir bag empties, it must be reported to the respiratory therapy department. Option 1 can be eliminated because moisture is a normal finding. Options 3 and 4 describe proper placement of the mask. Review the assessments that indicate correct functioning of this type of oxygen delivery system if you had difficulty answering this question.
Cognitive Level—*Applying*
Client Needs Category—*Safe and effective care environment*
Client Needs Subcategory—*Coordinated care*

64. **1, 2, 4, 5, 6.** Signs and symptoms of oxygen toxicity include a nonproductive cough, substernal chest pain, nasal stuffiness, nausea and vomiting, fatigue, headache, sore throat, and hypoventilation (not hyperventilation).
Test Taking Strategy—*Analyze to determine what information the question asks for, which is the signs and symptoms of oxygen toxicity. Alternative-format "select all that apply" questions require considering each option independently to decide its merit in answering the question. Choose the options that best demonstrate signs and symptoms of oxygen toxicity. Review the cause and effects of oxygen toxicity if you had difficulty answering this question.*
Cognitive Level—*Understanding*
Client Needs Category—*Physiological integrity*
Client Needs Subcategory—*Physiological adaptation*

65. **2.** The volume of epinephrine 1:1,000 needed to administer 0.1 mg is 0.1 mL. To solve the problem using a ratio-and-proportion method, use the following steps:

$$\frac{1{,}000 \text{ mg (1g)}}{1{,}000 \text{ mL}} = \frac{0.1 \text{ mg}}{X \text{ mg}}$$
$$1{,}000 \ X = 100 \text{ mL}$$
$$X = 0.1 \text{ mL}$$

Test Taking Strategy—*Analyze to determine what information the question asks for, which involves calculating a dosage. Refer to the ratio-and-proportion method and review the measurements to which the ratio 1:1,000 refers if you had difficulty with this question.*
Cognitive Level—*Remembering*
Client Needs Category—*Physiological integrity*
Client Needs Subcategory—*Pharmacological therapies*

66. **2.** Remaining with the client in respiratory distress provides support and reassurance that someone is available. This should help to ease the client's anxiety. Closing the door and pulling the privacy curtain are confining actions; they would most likely heighten the client's anxiety and feelings of suffocation.
Test Taking Strategy—*Use the process of elimination to help select the option that is most helpful in reducing the client's anxiety during an anxiety attack. Eliminate options 1 and 3 because these would most likely increase the client's anxiety. Notifying the client that the respiratory therapist has arrived (option 4) may decrease the anxiety somewhat but not as much as if the physician had arrived. Remaining with the client (option 2) is thus seen as the most helpful measure. Review methods for relieving anxiety if you had difficulty answering this question.*
Cognitive Level—*Understanding*
Client Needs Category—*Psychosocial integrity*
Client Needs Subcategory—*None*

67.

2. Slide the marker or arrow to zero.

5. Put the mouthpiece of the flow meter into your mouth

4. Take a deep breath.

3. Blow out as fast as you can.

6. Empty all of the air from your lungs.

1. Record the highest rating after three attempts.

Measurements from a peak flow meter can help the client and physician monitor the client's asthma symptoms. Instruction in the correct use of the peak flow meter include: Slide the marker or arrow to the zero in preparation of the breath measurement, put the mouthpiece of the meter in the mouth, take a deep breath, blow out (exhale) as fast as you can, empty all of the air from the lungs, and record the highest rating after three attempts.
Test Taking Strategy—*Analyze to determine what information the question asks for, which is the proper order of the steps to take when using a peak flow meter. Review the technique for using a peak flow meter if you had difficulty answering this question.*
Cognitive Level—*Understanding*
Client Needs Category—*Physiological integrity*
Client Needs Subcategory—*Reduction of risk potential*

Nursing Care of Clients with Chronic Obstructive Pulmonary Disease

68. 3. Pulmonary function tests (PFTs) assess the ventilation volume of the lungs by having the client breathe in and out through a mouthpiece. A tube connects the mouthpiece to an air-filled drum. The drum rises and falls with ventilation. A graphic recording of the air volume exchanged during breathing is obtained. X-rays, drawing blood, and analyzing sputum are not associated with PFTs.

> *Test Taking Strategy—Use the process of elimination to select the option that identifies the client's correct understanding of the manner in which a PFT is performed. Options 1, 2, and 4 can be eliminated because they do not describe the manner in which ventilation is assessed. Option 3 is correct because it describes breathing into a mouthpiece. Review how a pulmonary function test is performed if you had difficulty answering this question.*
> *Cognitive Level—Applying*
> *Client Needs Category—Physiological integrity*
> *Client Needs Subcategory—Physiological adaptation*

69. 3. Arterial blood gas (ABG) studies indicate the blood pH as well as the amounts of oxygen, carbon dioxide (CO_2), and bicarbonate (HCO_3^-) in the blood. The physician typically orders ABG studies when the client has an acute illness or a history of respiratory disease, or when the client's condition worsens. Normal $PaCO_2$ levels are 35 to 45 mm Hg. Clients who have emphysema usually have elevated CO_2 levels related to air trapping. A value of 7.35 to 7.45 is the normal pH of the blood. Normal partial pressure of arterial oxygen (PaO_2) is 80 to 100 mm Hg. Normal HCO_3^- is 22 to 26 mm Hg.

> *Test Taking Strategy—Analyze to determine what information the question asks for, which is the normal range of $PaCO_2$ in arterial blood. Refer to the rationale for normal values for blood gases and for $PaCO_2$ in particular. Review the data and values included in an ABG analysis if you had difficulty answering this question.*
> *Cognitive Level—Remembering*
> *Client Needs Category—Physiological integrity*
> *Client Needs Subcategory—Physiological adaptation*

70. 1. Giving oxygen at a rate greater than 2 L/minute to a client with chronic respiratory disease interferes with the brain's response to the hypoxic drive. In a client with chronic obstructive pulmonary disease (COPD), the stimulus to breathe comes from low levels of oxygen rather than high levels of carbon dioxide. Administering high concentrations of oxygen depresses the respiratory center.

> *Test Taking Strategy—Look at the key words "most appropriate" in reference to an oxygen flow rate that*

is safe to administer to a client with emphysema. Recall that the stimulus that causes clients with COPD to breathe is a low level of oxygen in their blood. Review the meaning of the "hypoxic drive to breathe" in reference to COPD if you had difficulty answering this question.
> *Cognitive Level—Applying*
> *Client Needs Category—Physiological integrity*
> *Client Needs Subcategory—Physiological adaptation*

71. 3. The therapeutic action of aminophylline (Truphylline) is the reduction of respiratory distress by dilating the airways. Aminophylline is classified as a bronchodilator. It does not relieve coughing, decrease sputum production, or thin secretions.

> *Test Taking Strategy—Use the process of elimination to help select the option that identifies the primary purpose for administering aminophylline. Option 1 can be eliminated because antitussives relieve coughing. Option 2 can be eliminated because anticholinergic medications reduce sputum production as well as other fluid secretions. Option 4 can be eliminated because mucolytics thin secretions. Option 3 remains as the best answer. Review the action and uses of aminophylline if you had difficulty answering this question correctly.*
> *Cognitive Level—Understanding*
> *Client Needs Category—Physiological integrity*
> *Client Needs Subcategory—Pharmacological therapies*

72. 1. When planning care for the long-term management of asthma symptoms, inhaled corticosteroids are the most common form of treatment. Inhaled corticosteroids such as fluticasone (Flonase), budesonide (Symbicort), and triamcinolone (Azmacort) are taken daily and enter the lungs directly. Oral bronchodilators such as montelukast (Singulair) and zileuton (Zyflo) are generally adjuvant medications to prevent asthma triggered by allergens. I.V. sympathomimetics such as methylxanthine (aminophyllin) are given when an acute asthmatic episode is in progress. Parenteral anti-inflammatory drugs such as ketorolac (Toradol) are administered cautiously to clients with asthma because they can contribute to an asthmatic attack in those who are sensitive to aspirin or nonsteroidal anti-inflammatory medications.

> *Test Taking Strategy—Analyze to determine what information the question asks for, which is the typical medication regimen for long-term management of asthma symptoms. The key words are "long term" indicating prevention of symptoms. Recall that clients with asthma self-administer inhaled corticosteroids on a daily basis. Review the prophylactic medications for management of asthma if you had difficulty answering this question.*
> *Cognitive Level—Analyzing*
> *Client Needs Category—Physiological integrity*
> *Client Needs Subcategory—Pharmacological therapies*

73. 2. Administering rhythmic gentle blows to the back with a cupped hand, known as *percussion*, causes thick secretions to break loose from within the airways. This technique is also combined with vibration. Vibration involves producing wavelike tremors to the chest by making firm, circular movements with open hands. For draining all but the upper lobes of the lung, the client is positioned so that the lower chest is elevated higher than the head.

> *Test Taking Strategy—Use the process of elimination to help select the option that is most beneficial for loosening respiratory secretions. Options 1, 3, and 4 are not as specific as percussing the chest (option 2) to loosen secretions. Deep breathing (option 1) improves ventilation, but it does not necessarily move secretions. Applying pressure below the diaphragm (option 3) is an emergency measure for relieving an obstructed airway. Sitting (option 4) does not mobilize the secretions. Review how percussion and vibration mobilize the secretions for easier expectoration if you had difficulty answering this question correctly.*
> *Cognitive Level—Applying*
> *Client Needs Category—Physiological integrity*
> *Client Needs Subcategory—Physiological adaptation*

74. 4. Expectorating a large volume of sputum is the best evidence that postural drainage is effective. The respiratory rate is lowered, not elevated, if hypoxia is relieved. An improved heart rate is not the best evidence that postural drainage is effective. A negative sputum culture only indicates that the client does not have an infection.

> *Test Taking Strategy—Use the process of elimination to help select the option that is most helpful in identifying the effectiveness of postural drainage for a client with chronic obstructive pulmonary disease (COPD). Recall that clients with COPD often have large amounts of thick drainage that is difficult to expectorate. Recall also that the purpose of postural drainage is to mobilize the secretions for easier removal. When that happens, the client has better oxygenation. Review the technique and indications for postural drainage if you had difficulty answering this question.*
> *Cognitive Level—Applying*
> *Client Needs Category—Physiological integrity*
> *Client Needs Subcategory—Physiological adaptation*

75. 2. To promote maximum distribution of inhaled medication, it is best to hold the breath for up to 10 seconds and then slowly exhale through pursed lips. If a second puff is ordered, the client should wait several minutes before self-administering another dose. The mouthpiece should be cleaned in warm water, rinsed, and allowed to air-dry at least once each day. Using pursed-lip breathing rather than bending from the waist is the preferred method for increasing exhaled volume.

> *Test Taking Strategy—Analyze to determine what information the question asks for, which is the action that should be taken after administering the first puff from a metered-dose inhaler. Recall that albuterol is considered a "rescue inhaler" because it is used when other prescribed medications fail to control asthma symptoms. To work effectively, albuterol must be distributed throughout the airways, which is accomplished by temporarily holding the breath. Review how to use a metered-dose inhaler if you had difficulty answering this question.*
> *Cognitive Level—Applying*
> *Client Needs Category—Physiological integrity*
> *Client Needs Subcategory—Pharmacological therapies*

76. 1. Encouraging the client to express his or her feelings is therapeutic. It shows that the nurse has empathy regarding the client's emotional condition and is willing to listen. Disagreeing with the client, belittling feelings, or using a reassuring cliché blocks the therapeutic effectiveness of communication.

> *Test Taking Strategy—Use the process of elimination to help select the option that represents the best response to the client's statement. Providing an opportunity for a client to express his or her thoughts and feelings (option 1) is always therapeutic. The other options illustrate nontherapeutic communication techniques. Review the principles of therapeutic communication and various techniques to use if you had difficulty answering this question.*
> *Cognitive Level—Applying*
> *Client Needs Category—Psychosocial integrity*
> *Client Needs Subcategory—None*

77. 3. Eating several small meals each day promotes adequate intake of calories without causing excess tiredness. Simple carbohydrates provide quick energy, but this recommendation is not better than eating various foods at frequent intervals. Dietary fats are higher in calories than carbohydrates and protein, but fat consumption contributes to hyperlipidemia and increases the risk of cardiovascular disease. Most people have more energy early in the day; consequently, eating the largest meal at night is counterproductive.

> *Test Taking Strategy—Look at the key words "most appropriate" in reference to a suggestion for combating fatigue and shortness of breath when eating. Recall that energy is needed for the process of consuming the food and its subsequent digestion. If the client does not overtax energy requirements by eating smaller, more frequent meals, he or she may*

experience less fatigue. Review mealtime techniques for reducing dyspnea if you had difficulty answering this question.
Cognitive Level—*Applying*
Client Needs Category—*Physiological integrity*
Client Needs Subcategory—*Basic care and comfort*

Nursing Care of Clients with Lung Cancer

78. 3. A cough and dyspnea are generally the earliest signs of lung cancer. Most people tend to ignore these signs, rationalizing that they are a consequence of chronic smoking. Therefore, early diagnosis and treatment of lung cancer are often delayed. Later signs of lung cancer include unexplained weight loss, blood-tinged sputum, fatigue, and respiratory distress.
> *Test Taking Strategy—Analyze to determine what information the question asks for, which is an early sign of lung cancer that is often ignored. Recall that a cough is an early-warning sign of cancer that also may be attributed to other causes, making it easy to ignore initially until other signs and symptoms become more evident. Review the clinical manifestations associated with lung cancer if you had difficulty answering this question.*
Cognitive Level—*Applying*
Client Needs Category—*Physiological integrity*
Client Needs Subcategory—*Physiological adaptation*

79. 1. A bronchoscopy is a diagnostic test that involves the direct visualization of the larynx, trachea, and bronchi. The physician passes a flexible tube through the client's nose or throat. Preparation for a bronchoscopy includes keeping the client from eating or drinking for at least 4 hours before the procedure. This reduces the risk of aspiration.
> *Test Taking Strategy—Look at the key words "most appropriate" used in reference to a nursing action to take before a client's bronchoscopy. Recall that the client's gag reflex will be impaired by the localized anesthetic, increasing the potential for aspiration if vomiting develops. Restricting food and fluids (option 1) reduces that risk. Coughing several times (option 2) has no effect on the bronchoscopy. Adequate rest (option 3) is desirable but not essential. The instrument used for bronchoscopy is introduced through the mouth; therefore, scrubbing the upper chest (option 4) is unnecessary. Review how a bronchoscopy is performed and the pretest and post-test nursing care if you had difficulty answering this question.*
Cognitive Level—*Applying*
Client Needs Category—*Physiological integrity*
Client Needs Subcategory—*Reduction of risk potential*

80. 3. Respiratory effort is the most critical assessment to make after a bronchoscopy because the bronchoscope is passed directly into the larynx, trachea, and bronchi. Respiratory effort is one of the first responses to change if the client experiences edema and trauma in the airway. All of the other assessment alternatives are appropriate but not as likely to indicate life-threatening consequences.
> *Test Taking Strategy—Analyze to determine what information the question asks for, which is a nursing assessment that is essential after a bronchoscopy. Recall that a compromised airway is life-threatening, making option 3 the best answer. Review the potential complications associated with a bronchoscopy if you had difficulty answering this question correctly.*
Cognitive Level—*Applying*
Client Needs Category—*Physiological integrity*
Client Needs Subcategory—*Reduction of risk potential*

81. 1. The pulse rate is the best indication of whether the nurse should be concerned about the presence of blood in the secretions at this time. Slight bleeding is expected following bronchoscopy as a result of trauma. If hemorrhage or impaired ventilation occurs, the pulse rate is rapid. Pupillary changes are an indication of brain function. Heart sounds indicate how effectively blood is circulating through the heart chambers. Chest expansion is more likely to change if one lung is not filling adequately with air.
> *Test Taking Strategy—Use the process of elimination to help select the option that is most important for determining the significance of blood that is present in suctioned oral secretions. Option 3 can be eliminated because the pupils will continue to react in spite of hemorrhage until the client expires. Option 4 can be eliminated because bleeding should not affect chest expansion. Option 2 has merit because if there is a large volume of bleeding, the nurse would find a rapid heart rate. However, option 1 is the best answer because the pulse rate is easily assessed, and it increases when there is an appreciable loss of blood such as during hemorrhage. Review the signs and symptoms that accompany hemorrhage if you had difficulty answering this question correctly.*
Cognitive Level—*Applying*
Client Needs Category—*Physiological integrity*
Client Needs Subcategory—*Reduction of risk potential*

82. 1. The nurse establishes that the gag reflex is present before the client is given food or oral fluids after a bronchoscopy. Stimulating the palatal arch causes the client to gag if the effects of the local anesthetic have worn off. The other choices are techniques of physical assessment but are unlikely to be affected by a bronchoscopy.
> *Test Taking Strategy—Use the process of elimination to help select the option that identifies an essential nursing action before allowing a client to take oral*

fluids and food after bronchoscopy. Recall that the client may not be able to protect his or her airway if it remains anesthetized. Therefore, the nurse must assess that the client's gag reflex is intact (option 1) to reduce the risk for aspiration. Review potential complications associated with undergoing a bronchoscopy if you had difficulty answering this question.

Cognitive Level*—Applying*
Client Needs Category*—Physiological integrity*
Client Needs Subcategory*—Reduction of risk potential*

83. 4. Pleural effusion is the accumulation of fluid between the pleural membranes. It is common in clients who have lung cancer, pneumonia, tuberculosis, pulmonary embolism, and heart failure. When auscultating the lungs, the nurse can expect to hear decreased breath sounds over the affected area and dullness when the area is percussed. The changes are related to the amount of fluid displacing the lung tissue. Wheezing is heard in clients with asthma. Crackles are sounds that result from the delayed openings of deflated airways; they sometimes clear when the client is coughing. Friction rubs may result from pleural effusion, but they are heard over the affected area, not posterior to it.

> ***Test Taking Strategy****—Analyze to determine what information the question asks for, which is the characteristic breath sounds associated with a pleural effusion. Recall that the density of fluid from the effusion will obscure the transmission of sound from the lung to the nurse's stethoscope, making them more difficult to hear, which correlates with option 4. Review the lung changes caused by a pleural effusion if you had difficulty answering this question.*

Cognitive Level*—Applying*
Client Needs Category*—Physiological integrity*
Client Needs Subcategory*—Physiological adaptation*

84. 2. Thoracentesis involves draining excess pleural fluid from the pleural space by inserting a needle into the chest wall. A client undergoing this procedure is best placed in a sitting position so that the physician has access to the eighth or ninth rib space. It is helpful for the seated client to rest the head and elevate the arms on the overbed table. If this position is impossible, the nurse may alternatively place the client on the unaffected side.

> ***Test Taking Strategy****—Analyze to determine what information the question asks for, which is the position in which the nurse should place a client before a thoracentesis. Recall that when a thoracentesis is performed, a needle will be placed within the pleural space. A sitting position (option 2) helps the physician gain access to the appropriate anatomic location. A lithotomy position (option 1) is used for procedures in which the clinician needs access to genitourinary structures, including the vagina,*

urinary meatus and, possibly, the rectum. A prone or supine position (options 3 and 4) is inappropriate for a thoracentesis. Review the manner in which a thoracentesis is performed if you had difficulty answering this question.

Cognitive Level*—Applying*
Client Needs Category*—Physiological integrity*
Client Needs Subcategory*—Reduction of risk potential*

85. 1. The prefix *pneumo-* refers to lung, and the suffix-*ectomy* means removal; therefore, the client would be correct in understanding that the procedure involves removal of the lung. A lobectomy involves the removal of only a lobe of the lung. Although a pneumonectomy may involve taking a lung sample or opening a lung for examination, these are not the primary reasons for performing the surgical procedure.

> ***Test Taking Strategy****—Analyze to determine what information the question asks for, which is the statement that reflects an accurate understanding of the surgical procedure. Although all the options have merit, option 1 is the best answer because it provides the explanation for the meaning of pneumonectomy. Review the definition of the word pneumonectomy and what the surgical procedure involves if you had difficulty answering this question.*

Cognitive Level*—Applying*
Client Needs Category*—Physiological integrity*
Client Needs Subcategory*—Physiological adaptation*

86. 1. The client with a pneumonectomy lies with the healthy, nonoperative lung uppermost. This position allows for better lung expansion and oxygenation. If the affected side were upward, ventilation would be compromised because of the compression of the remaining healthy lung between the mattress and body weight. Lying with the head lowered interferes with breathing because abdominal contents press against the diaphragm. Elevating the arms on pillows may be an optional position to use if the client's breathing becomes labored.

> ***Test Taking Strategy****—Analyze to determine what information the question asks for, which is the position in which it is essential to place a client after pneumonectomy. Recall that postoperatively the client will be ventilating with the lung that remains. To avoid further compromising the client's breathing, the nurse should position the client in a sitting position or on the operative side (option 1) when lying down. Review the effect positioning has on breathing with only one functioning lung if you had difficulty answering this question.*

Cognitive Level*—Applying*
Client Needs Category*—Physiological integrity*
Client Needs Subcategory*—Reduction of risk potential*

87. 2. Removal of the lung is often accompanied by interruption of the intercostal nerves. As a consequence, clients who undergo a pneumonectomy may experience temporary numbness in the operative area. Sore throat and impaired swallowing are related to endotracheal intubation and not the surgery itself. If the client has a persistent cough, it is more likely related to a preexisting disease rather than an expected outcome of the surgical procedure.

Test Taking Strategy—Analyze to determine what information the question asks for, which is a temporary consequence the client will experience after pneumonectomy. Recall that sensory nerves are involved in the perception of tactile stimuli. When the nerves in the chest are surgically disrupted, their function will be temporarily impaired. Review the outcomes associated with a pneumonectomy if you had difficulty answering this question.
Cognitive Level—Applying
Client Needs Category—Physiological integrity
Client Needs Subcategory—Physiological adaptation

88. 4. Morphine sulfate (Roxanol), an opioid analgesic, depresses respiratory rate and depth. If the respiratory rate is severely compromised, the client will have inadequate oxygenation. Morphine does slow peristalsis, and bowel sounds should be assessed frequently; however, this is not the most important assessment to make.

Test Taking Strategy—Use the process of elimination to help select the option that identifies the most important assessment to make when administering morphine sulfate. Recall that the side effects of morphine include respiratory depression and decreased peristalsis. Although option 3, presence of bowel sounds, seems to be a good choice, bowel sounds are likely to be present, but hypoactive. However, option 4 relates to breathing, which is a critical function that must be maintained, making it the best answer. Refer to the rationale for reasons. Option 1 is not the best answer because, although morphine indirectly affects heart rate by decreasing the pain that elevates it, heart rhythm is unaffected. Assessing the skin color and temperature (option 3) is not related to the use of morphine. Review nursing assessments that are pertinent when administering opioid analgesics if you had difficulty answering this question.
Cognitive Level—Applying
Client Needs Category—Physiological integrity
Client Needs Subcategory—Pharmacological therapies

Nursing Care of Clients with Chest Injuries

89. 1. To prevent the widespread collapse of alveoli known as *atelectasis,* clients with fractured ribs are instructed to breathe deeply several times every hour.

People with fractured ribs have a natural tendency to breathe shallowly to avoid discomfort; however, shallow breathing promotes atelectasis.

Test Taking Strategy—Use the process of elimination to select the option that identifies the most important instruction to provide a client with fractured ribs. Recall that breathing deeply (option 1) promotes effective lung expansion, thereby preventing atelectasis, which can impair oxygenation. Option 2 can be eliminated because it contradicts the correct answer. Breathing rapidly (option 3) leads to respiratory alkalosis. Breathing into a paper bag (option 4) promotes an increased level of carbon dioxide in the blood, which is appropriate for individuals who are hyperventilating and becoming light-headed. Review the physiology of external respiration, focusing on the role muscles play in filling the lungs and alveoli with air, if you had difficulty answering this question.
Cognitive Level—Applying
Client Needs Category—Safe and effective care environment
Client Needs Subcategory—Coordinated care

90. 3. Flail chest is a condition in which ribs are broken in two or more places, making the chest wall unstable. Paradoxical movement of the unstable section during inspiration and expiration characterizes this condition. In other words, when the client takes a breath, an area of the chest wall moves inward; when the client exhales, the area moves outward. A sucking chest wound and tracheal deviation are associated with a pneumothorax. Chest pain that is aggravated by breathing is not unusual when there is a traumatic injury, but it is more likely to increase during inspiration when the chest expands.

Test Taking Strategy—Analyze to determine what information the question asks for, which, in this case, is an assessment finding that suggests the client has a flail chest. Remember that when the ribs are intact or only fractured in one location, the chest wall moves out during inhalation and inward during exhalation. When a section of the ribs is broken free of any attachment, a portion of the chest moves opposite from what is expected. Review the signs and symptoms that accompany flail chest if you had difficulty answering this question.
Cognitive Level—Applying
Client Needs Category—Physiological integrity
Client Needs Subcategory—Physiological adaptation

91. 4. When a person experiences a hemothorax, blood collects and drains by gravity through the tube in the lower chest. Air in the chest rises and exits through the tube in the upper chest. It would be unusual to see blood coming from the victim's nose or mouth in this situation. If the client has a productive cough, the sputum may be blood tinged.

Test Taking Strategy—*Analyze to determine what information the question asks for, which is the location where the nurse would expect to observe bloody drainage. Refer to the scenario, which indicates that a chest tube was inserted. Remember that chest tubes are used to remove air and fluid (in this case, blood) from the pleural space. Blood accumulates low in the pleural space under the influence of gravity. Therefore, option 4 correlates with the best answer. Review the purpose of a drainage tube in the lower chest as well as one located in the upper chest if you had difficulty answering this question.*
Cognitive Level—*Applying*
Client Needs Category—*Physiological integrity*
Client Needs Subcategory—*Physiological adaptation*

92. **1.** The fluid in the water-seal chamber should rise and fall in synchrony with respirations or may bubble intermittently immediately after the tube has been inserted. If the lung has expanded, if the drainage system is connected to suction, or if the tubing is kinked or plugged, the rise and fall of fluid and intermittent bubbling would not be seen. If the fluid level falls below the filling line of 2 cm, more fluid should be added. Continuous bubbling indicates a leak in the system. The fluid in the water-seal chamber should be clear.

Test Taking Strategy—*Analyze to determine what information the question asks for, which is evidence a chest drainage system is functioning correctly. Recall that this type of drainage system has three chambers. A sign that correlates with correct functioning is the fluctuation of fluid up and down in the water seal chamber in synchrony with respirations until the lung re-expands. Continuous bubbling in this chamber (option 3) indicates a pleural leak or leak in the tubing system. Review nursing assessments that relate to a water-seal chest drainage system if you had difficulty answering this question.*
Cognitive Level—*Applying*
Client Needs Category—*Physiological integrity*
Client Needs Subcategory—*Physiological adaptation*

93. **3.** Air that is leaking and becoming trapped within the local tissue at the insertion site crackles when touched. The crackling sound, called *crepitus* or *subcutaneous emphysema*, resembles that of crisp rice cereal when mixed with milk. The nurse would not feel puffs of air or hear a hissing sound because the air does not escape into the atmosphere. The air tends to diffuse into the tissue and rise to the upper part of the body. Eventually, the client's face and neck may appear swollen and the tissue around the chest may appear pale; however, this is not a phenomenon directly linked to an air leak.

Test Taking Strategy—*Analyze to determine what information the question asks for, which is an assessment finding that indicates air accumulating in the tissue around the tube insertion site rather than escaping into the drainage system. The pockets of air in subcutaneous tissue have been compared to various familiar substances like crispy rice cereal or commercial bubble wrap in relation to how it feels and the crackling sound it makes when compressed (option 3). Review evidence of subcutaneous emphysema if you had difficulty answering this question.*
Cognitive Level—*Applying*
Client Needs Category—*Physiological integrity*
Client Needs Subcategory—*Physiological adaptation*

94. **2.** When transporting a client to another area of the hospital, the water-seal drainage collector is always kept below the tubes' insertion sites to facilitate drainage. As long as the water seal is maintained, the client's lung function should be unaffected. Suction may be added to the water-seal system, but the tube connecting to the suction source is disconnected when the client is ambulated or transported from the room. Mechanical ventilation is necessary only when a client cannot maintain adequate oxygenation even with supplemental oxygen. In that case, a portable X-ray may be ordered and taken to the client's room.

Test Taking Strategy—*Look at the key words "most appropriate" in reference to the nursing action to take before transporting a client with a drainage tube in place from his or her room to another area. Recall that if the drainage tube is connected to suction, it can be separated from the suction source and continue to function by gravity. Keeping the drainage system below the insertion sites (option 2) will facilitate that purpose. Options 1 and 3 are not only incorrect, but may be unsafe as well. Clamping the chest tubes (option 1) for an appreciable amount of time would lead to a tension pneumothorax. Option 3 can be eliminated because suction is not applied directly to the chest tubes. Mechanical ventilation (option 4) is not a usual step to take. Review the nursing care of a client with a water-seal chest drainage system if you had difficulty answering this question.*
Cognitive Level—*Applying*
Client Needs Category—*Physiological integrity*
Client Needs Subcategory—*Physiological adaptation*

95. **4.** At the beginning of each shift, the nurse should assess the color, consistency, and amount of drainage present in the water-seal system. The previous nurse marks the level of drainage on the calibrated collection chamber with the date and time. The drainage volume is calculated by subtracting the previously marked volume from the current total volume. The drainage compartment is never emptied while the chest tube is in place.

> *Test Taking Strategy—Use the process of elimination to help select the option that describes the best method for measuring drainage from a water-seal drainage system. Recall that the standard of practice is to mark the level in the drainage chamber at the end of each shift and add the date and time, but never empty it. Therefore, option 1 can be eliminated. The volume of drainage that occurred on each shift is calculated by subtracting the current from the former measured mark (option 4). Subtracting fluid intake from output (option 2) only helps in evaluating the status of the client's total fluid balance. Option 3 can be eliminated because chest tubes are not irrigated. Review the nursing management of a client with a chest tube drainage system if you had difficulty answering this question.*
> *Cognitive Level—Applying*
> *Client Needs Category—Physiological integrity*
> *Client Needs Subcategory—Physiological adaptation*

96.

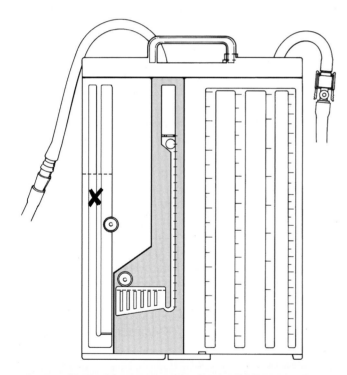

When suction is applied to a three-chambered chest drainage system, continuous gentle bubbling is observed in the column that is filled with water to the 20-cm mark. The level of water regulates the amount of suction applied to the system. The middle chamber contains the water seal, which fluctuates intermittently with the client's respirations until the lung reexpands. The remaining chamber, which is subdivided into three columns, collects air and

liquid drainage. The air exits from the chest tube, diffuses through the water in the middle compartment, and eventually escapes through a vent into the atmosphere; the liquid drainage remains in the collection chamber.

> *Test Taking Strategy—Analyze to determine what information the question asks for. Recall that when wall suction is applied to the system, it causes gentle bubbling in the chamber that has a greater amount of water than the water-seal chamber. Review the purposes of the various chambers that make up a chest tube drainage system if you had difficulty answering this question.*
> *Cognitive Level—Applying*
> *Client Needs Category—Physiological integrity*
> *Client Needs Subcategory—Physiological adaptation*

Nursing Care of Clients with Pulmonary Embolism

97. **1.** Pulmonary emboli are obstructions (clots) in one or more of the pulmonary vessels. The usual site for clot formation is in the deep veins of the legs or in the pelvis. Conditions that predispose a client to pulmonary emboli include recent surgery, bed rest, immobility, trauma, obesity, and postpartal status. Clots are more likely to form in the veins, where there is venous stasis, although they can form anywhere. They are less likely to form in the pulmonary artery or the carotid artery because the blood pressure is higher in those vessels.

> *Test Taking Strategy—Look at the key words "most likely" in reference to identifying the location where a pulmonary embolism commonly originates. Recall that the most common origin of a clot that travels to the lungs is a thrombus in the deep veins of the legs, where they develop from stasis of blood flow. Review the etiology of thrombus formation and pulmonary embolism if you had difficulty answering this question.*
> *Cognitive Level—Applying*
> *Client Needs Category—Physiological integrity*
> *Client Needs Subcategory—Physiological adaptation*

98. **2.** Staying with a frightened client is one of the best methods for relieving or reducing anxiety. Telling the client that symptoms will lessen in a few minutes is nontherapeutic because it offers false reassurance. Asking a "why" question is also nontherapeutic because this demands an explanation from the client rather than acceptance of his or her feelings. Asking if the client's finances are in order avoids the issue and, therefore, is nontherapeutic.

> *Test Taking Strategy—Look at the key words "most appropriate" as they refer to a nursing response that is supportive when a client senses a potential for dying. Leaving an anxious and fearful client alone escalates the panic being experienced. The nurse should remain with the client and commandeer*

additional assistance from other nurses or the emergency response team. Review anxiety-relieving principles, such as remaining calm, using a soft voice and confident attitude, using therapeutic touch, and staying with the client, if you had difficulty answering this question.
Cognitive Level—*Applying*
Client Needs Category—*Psychosocial integrity*
Client Needs Subcategory—*None*

99. 1. Administering oxygen is the most significant immediate action for reducing the client's dyspnea and chest pain. Maintaining the airway and breathing are priorities at this point. Assessing capillary refill is a good choice and can be a useful way to monitor tissue perfusion, but it is not the priority action when the client is experiencing chest pain and dyspnea. Having the client rate the pain on a pain scale is another good choice, but not the priority at this time. Cardiac enzymes are ordered for clients suspected of having a myocardial infarction, not a pulmonary embolism.

Test Taking Strategy—Use the process of elimination to select the option that describes the most important intervention to perform when caring for a client experiencing symptoms associated with a pulmonary embolism. Option 4 can be eliminated immediately because cardiac enzymes are not likely to be elevated unless there is a secondary injury to the heart. Options 2 and 3 have merit, but option 1 is the best answer because providing1 supplemental oxygen helps to reduce respiratory distress and chest pain. Review nursing care of a client at the time he or she experiences a pulmonary embolism if you had difficulty answering this question.
Cognitive Level—*Analyzing*
Client Needs Category—*Physiological integrity*
Client Needs Subcategory—*Physiological adaptation*

100. 1. Intravenous heparin is given to treat a pulmonary embolism. This drug prevents further clot development as well as the showering of mini emboli. Through the course of treatment, the client receives I.V. heparin followed by subcutaneous enoxaparin sodium (Lovenox) and heparin, and finally by warfarin (Coumadin), which is given orally. Clotting studies are drawn frequently during anticoagulant therapy.

Test Taking Strategy—Analyze to determine what information the question asks for, which is identifying the drug used to treat a pulmonary embolism. Recall that heparin is an anticoagulant that is given to prevent any further clots from forming. Aminophylline (Truphylline), a bronchodilator (option 2), is not used to treat pulmonary embolism. Nitroglycerin (Nitrodisc) is a vasodilator (option 3) commonly used to treat angina. Aspirin, while having anticoagulant properties (option 4), is not the drug of choice

for this disorder. Review the uses of these drugs if you had difficulty answering this question.
Cognitive Level—*Applying*
Client Needs Category—*Physiological integrity*
Client Needs Subcategory—*Pharmacological therapies*

Nursing Care of Clients with Tracheostomies

101. 3. Wet breath sounds indicate that secretions are accumulating within the airway. Because a client with a tracheostomy sometimes lacks the ability to cough effectively, the nurse protects and maintains an open airway.

Test Taking Strategy—Use the process of elimination to help select the option that identifies the best indication for suctioning a client's tracheostomy. Option 1 can be eliminated because a fast respiratory rate or labored respirations, rather than low respirations, indicate that oxygenation is impaired. A rapid pulse rate is more likely to indicate impaired ventilation, rather than a slow pulse rate (option 2). An elevated blood pressure (option 4) is unrelated to the need for oxygenation. Option 3, which remains, is the best answer because if the airway is patent, breathing should be noiseless and effortless. Wet breath sounds indicate secretions are occupying space within the airway and have the potential to impair oxygenation. Review the criteria for suctioning a natural or artificial airway if you had difficulty answering this question.
Cognitive Level—*Applying*
Client Needs Category—*Physiological integrity*
Client Needs Subcategory—*Physiological adaptation*

102. 1. Preoxygenating the client is a priority before suctioning the client. Many times the client feels that all of the oxygen is being "vacuumed" from the lungs. It is a safe practice to moisten the catheter by immersing it in sterile normal saline solution, then suctioning the solution through the lumen. This is completed in the preparation for suctioning. This tests the function of the suction machine and reduces the surface tension inside the plastic catheter. Although clients with artificial airways need frequent mouth care, this is not essential before performing tracheal suctioning. The stoma is cleaned from time to time, but this does not have to be done before suctioning the airway. The airway is suctioned before removing the inner cannula for cleaning.

Test Taking Strategy—Analyze to determine what information the question asks for, which is the essential action to perform before suctioning a client's tracheostomy. All of the actions listed in the options are components of tracheostomy care. However, preoxygenation (option 1) is essential, because providing supplemental oxygen reduces the risk of hypoxia as the suction catheter removes secretions and air from the airway.

Cognitive Level—Applying
Client Needs Category—Physiological integrity
Client Needs Subcategory—Physiological adaptation

103. **1, 2, 3, 6.** A client's fingernail polish or acrylic nails should be removed before monitoring with a pulse oximeter because they interfere with the transmission of light. The light emitting diode (LED) and photodetector must be aligned opposite each other on the monitoring site for an accurate reading. A pulse oximeter functions by delivering sensed data to the monitor via a cable. Some pulse oximeters are attached with an adhesive band. Others are spring-loaded; both types must be relocated periodically to avoid injuring the skin.

An arterial oxygen saturation (SpO_2) of at least 95% is clinically acceptable as normal; therefore, the SpO_2 alarm should be set to sound when it detects a level below 95%. (Many agencies suggest setting the alarm for a measurement below 85%.) An SpO_2 of 90% is equated with a partial pressure of oxygen of 60 mm Hg, an indication that the client could benefit from the supplemental administration of oxygen. When an alarm sounds, the nurse assesses the client to determine if the sensing device has become loose or has been removed, the client is restless and causing some artifacts that the machine is interpreting as significant changes, or the client is hypoxic. The nurse would notify the physician only if measures to improve the client's oxygenation status, such as administering supplemental oxygen, are ineffective.

Test Taking Strategy—Analyze to determine what information the question asks for. Alternative-format "select all that apply" questions require considering each option independently to decide its merit in answering the question. Choose the options that correlate with the use of a pulse oximeter. Consult references that discuss the use of a pulse oximeter if you had difficulty answering this question.
Cognitive Level—Applying
Client Needs Category—Physiological integrity
Client Needs Subcategory—Reduction of risk potential

104. **3.** The vent on a suction catheter is occluded after the catheter is fully inserted and is being withdrawn. This reduces the potential for hypoxemia. Closing the vent before insertion or when the catheter is just inside the inner cannula prolongs the time that oxygen is removed from the airway. Coughing may or may not coincide with the proper time to occlude the vent; therefore, it is not used as a criterion for this action.

Test Taking Strategy—Use the process of elimination to select the option that identifies the best time to occlude the vent when suctioning a client. Options 1 and 2 can be eliminated because occluding the vent at these times would remove an excessive amount of oxygen when combined with that removed as the catheter is

being withdrawn. Option 4 can be eliminated because coughing may occur with the vent open or occluded. Option 3 remains as the best answer because it creates the suction required to remove secretions while minimizing the amount of oxygen being removed. Review the procedure for suctioning a tracheostomy if you had difficulty answering this question.*
Cognitive Level—Applying
Client Needs Category—Physiological integrity
Client Needs Subcategory—Physiological adaptation

105. **2.** Suctioning should not extend beyond 10 to 12 seconds. Some suggest holding one's own breath during suctioning. This technique promotes awareness of the air hunger the client is experiencing. Suctioning for too little time will not effectively clear the airway. Suctioning for longer than 15 seconds causes hypoxemia.

Test Taking Strategy—Analyze to determine what information the question asks for, which is the maximum amount of time a suction catheter should be occluded while in the airway. Recall that the suctioning process removes oxygen as well as secretions. The potential for hypoxia increases the longer the vent is occluded. Standards of care indicate that the vent should be occluded no longer than 10 to 12 seconds (option 2). Reoxygenating the client is required if additional suctioning is required. Review the procedure for suctioning a tracheostomy if you had difficulty answering this question correctly.
Cognitive Level—Applying
Client Needs Category—Physiological integrity
Client Needs Subcategory—Physiological adaptation

106. **4.** Twisting and rotating the catheter during its withdrawal helps remove secretions located within the circumference of the airway. Withdrawing the catheter slowly causes the nurse to exceed the recommended time for suctioning. Neither pinching and pulling the catheter nor plunging it up and down is an acceptable technique during suctioning.

Test Taking Strategy—Analyze to determine what information the question asks for, which is the correct technique to use when withdrawing a suction catheter from the airway. Recall that the suction catheter has several ports. Twisting and rotating the catheter (option 4) enables greater contact between the ports and the retained secretions. Review the procedure for suctioning a tracheostomy, particularly the recommended action when withdrawing the catheter, if you had difficulty answering this question.
Cognitive Level—Applying
Client Needs Category—Physiological integrity
Client Needs Subcategory—Physiological adaptation

107. 3. Hypoxemia refers to a decreased amount of oxygen in the blood. Monitoring the pulse oximeter is useful for detecting the saturation of hemoglobin with oxygen. It takes a prolonged state of hypoxemia to alter a client's level of consciousness, skin color, and respiratory rate.

Test Taking Strategy—Use the process of elimination to help select the option that identifies the best method for determining that a client is becoming hypoxemic during suctioning. All of the options are appropriate assessment techniques for determining a client's oxygenation status. However, option 3, watching the oxygen saturation level displayed on the pulse oximeter, provides the most objective data concerning blood oxygenation. Review the purpose for pulse oximetry and the percent that reflects a compromise in oxygenation if you had difficulty answering this question.

Cognitive Level—*Analyzing*
Client Needs Category—*Physiological integrity*
Client Needs Subcategory—*Physiological adaptation*

108. 3. To prevent the possibility that the client may cough the tracheostomy tube out of the airway, the old ties are not removed until the replacement ties are secured. Special drain sponges or tracheostomy dressing materials are used, or gauze is folded rather than cut to fit around the stoma. The inner cannula is replaced as soon as it is cleaned, rinsed, and dried, or within at least 5 minutes.

Test Taking Strategy—Analyze to determine what information the question asks for, which is the correct nursing action when providing tracheostomy care. Recall that until new ties are secured, the soiled ties hold the tracheostomy tube in place preventing it from being accidentally displaced from the trachea. Eliminate options 1 and 2 because they are not correct. Gauze squares are not cut to fashion a stomal dressing because the cut threads may enter the airway and irritate the tissue. Eliminate option 4, because a delay in replacing the inner cannula may cause mucous secretions to accumulate and dry in the outer cannula. This alters the size of the opening and interferes with replacement. Review the procedure for tracheostomy care, particularly in relation to changing the dressing and ties, if you had difficulty answering this question.

Cognitive Level—*Applying*
Client Needs Category—*Physiological integrity*
Client Needs Subcategory—*Physiological adaptation*

109. 2. A cuff on a tracheostomy tube forms a tight seal, preventing liquid nasopharyngeal secretions, stomach contents, or tube-feeding formula from entering the lower respiratory passages. If the person is receiving mechanical ventilation, the cuff ensures that the oxygenated air does not escape before it is delivered to the lower areas of the lungs. An inflated cuff may lead to tissue breakdown if the pressure occludes capillary blood flow. Using a cuffed tracheostomy tube does not provide more comfort or reduce infection any better than an uncuffed tracheostomy tube.

Test Taking Strategy—Use the process of elimination to help select the option that identifies the best reason for using a cuffed tracheostomy tube. Option 1 can be eliminated because the cuff may actually contribute to tissue ischemia if it is overinflated. Option 3 can be eliminated because it neither contributes nor detracts from the client's comfort. Option 4 has some merit because if aspiration is prevented, it could also prevent a pulmonary infection. However, option 2 represents the best answer because sealing the two areas from each other prevents fluids from entering the lower airway. Consult references that identify the purpose for using a cuffed tracheostomy tube if you had difficulty answering this question.

Cognitive Level—*Applying*
Client Needs Category—*Physiological integrity*
Client Needs Subcategory—*Physiological adaptation*

Nursing Care of Clients with Sudden Airway Occlusion

110. 2. The ability to cough indicates that the foreign object in the airway is not totally obstructing the air passage. As long as the obstruction is only partial, the client is capable of coughing to clear his or her own airway. The victim's ability to walk is not important except to verify that the brain is still receiving oxygen and the client has not lost consciousness. The victim's position is not the most important data to obtain at this time. The ability to swallow will not dislodge an object that is in the victim's airway.

Test Taking Strategy—Analyze to determine what information the question asks for, which is information the nurse should determine before providing further instructions to a person assisting a client with an airway occlusion. Recall that if a client can cough (option 2), the airway is only partially occluded and continued efforts to cough may clear the obstruction. If the client cannot cough, the airway is totally occluded and further actions are required to prevent death from occurring. Review the actions that are necessary for relieving an obstruction from the airway if you had difficulty answering this question.

Cognitive Level—*Understanding*
Client Needs Category—*Physiological integrity*
Client Needs Subcategory—*Physiological adaptation*

111. 4. The thumb side of the fist is placed against the abdomen, below the sternum but above the navel. The xiphoid process is the tip of the sternum, and the manubrium is the upper portion of the sternum. Neither location is used when performing the abdominal thrust.

> *Test Taking Strategy—Analyze to determine what information the question asks for, which is the correct placement of the hands when attempting to relieve an airway occlusion. Recall that the process for relieving an airway obstruction is to move air that is trapped in the lungs with sufficient force to expel the foreign object. Option 4 is the best answer because it describes how the hand positions facilitate this objective. Review how to perform the abdominal thrust maneuver, particularly the correct hand placements, if you had difficulty answering this question.*

Cognitive Level—*Remembering*
Client Needs Category—*Physiological integrity*
Client Needs Subcategory—*Physiological adaptation*

Nursing Care of Clients Who Are Victims of Terrorist Agents

112. 1, 2, 5. Although the thought of terrorist activity is not pleasant, nurses should be aware of agents that may be used in a terrorist attack. Anthrax is a biological agent. With inhalation exposure to anthrax, the initial symptoms may resemble a common cold: sore throat, mild fever, muscle aches, and malaise. The symptoms can progress to severe breathing problems, respiratory arrest, and shock. Sarin gas is a chemical nerve agent that causes tachypnea, respiratory distress, chest tightness, and runny nose and eyes. Cyanide, a chemical agent, produces signs and symptoms such as tachypnea, dyspnea, restlessness, and redness on the palms of the hands and soles of the feet. Victims of biological agents such as smallpox and Ebola virus do not present with respiratory distress. They most generally develop GI symptoms and high fever. Victims of radiation poisoning also manifest GI symptoms, depending on the degree of exposure.

> *Test Taking Strategy—Analyze to determine what information the question asks for, which is the agents that may cause respiratory signs and symptoms. Alternative-format "select all that apply" questions require considering each option independently to decide its merit in answering the question. Choose the options that identify agents potentially used by terrorists that cause respiratory signs and symptoms. Consult references such as those provided by the Centers for Disease Control and Prevention's Web site that discuss these agents, focusing on the signs and symptoms experienced by victims of these agents, if you had difficulty answering this question.*

Cognitive Level—*Applying*
Client Needs Category—*Physiological integrity*
Client Needs Subcategory—*Physiological adaptation*

113. 2. During emergency situations, an autocratic leader provides clear expectations and directions on what needs to be done. These decisions are made independently with little input from the group/nurses. This type of leadership is most beneficial for a novice nurse as the nurse is directed to the priorities of care for the client in cardiac arrest. A laissez-fairre leader allows the group to make decisions with little input from the leader. A democratic leader allows the group to have input into the decision making process. Leader-follower is a theory that is based on how individuals interact.

> *Test Taking Strategy—Analyze to determine what information the question asks for, which is the leadership style that is best suited in an emergency situation. Consider the need for immediate direction, not discussion, which leads to the autocratic (self) option. Review the characteristics of various leadership styles and situations for which they are best suited if you had difficulty answering this question.*

Cognitive Level—*Applying*
Client Needs Category—*Safe and effective care environment*
Client Needs Subcategory—*Coordinated care*

The Nursing Care of Clients with Disorders of the Gastrointestinal System and Accessory Organs of Digestion

Directions: With a pencil, blacken the space in front of the option you have chosen for your correct answer.

Nursing Care of Clients with Disorders of the Mouth

A client develops mucositis of the oral cavity while receiving chemotherapy for cancer.

1. Which food items are best for the nurse to withhold from the client's dietary tray? Select all that apply.
[ ] **1.** Tomato soup
[ ] **2.** Lime gelatin
[ ] **3.** Canned peaches
[ ] **4.** Hot coffee
[ ] **5.** Toast
[ ] **6.** Vanilla ice cream

2. The nurse assesses the client's oral cavity and plans to assist with oral care. Which item should be obtained to accomplish the goal?
[ ] **1.** A pediatric toothbrush
[ ] **2.** A battery-operated toothbrush
[ ] **3.** Sponge-tipped swabs
[ ] **4.** Mint-flavored mouthwash

A nurse is assigned to care for several clients who require total care and is planning oral care for them.

3. The nurse should plan specialized oral care twice a day for which client?
[ ] **1.** The client who has full dentures
[ ] **2.** The client who is on fluid restrictions
[ ] **3.** The client who is on a low-residue diet
[ ] **4.** The client who sucks on ice chips

4. Which techniques are most appropriate when providing oral care for a client's dentures? Select all that apply.
[ ] **1.** Using hot water while brushing and rinsing the dentures
[ ] **2.** Holding the dentures over a basin of water or a soft towel
[ ] **3.** Applying solvent to remove oral adhesive from the dentures
[ ] **4.** Placing the dentures in a clean, dry container after brushing
[ ] **5.** Donning clean gloves before taking dentures from the client's mouth
[ ] **6.** Removing the lower plate from the mouth by turning it to a slight angle

5. When the nurse is brushing an unconscious client's teeth, how should the client be positioned?
[ ] **1.** Supine with the head elevated
[ ] **2.** Side-lying with the head lowered
[ ] **3.** In Trendelenburg's position with the head slightly raised
[ ] **4.** In a dorsal recumbent position with the head elevated

A client who has been taking an antibiotic for the past 2 weeks comes to the physician's office complaining of difficulty in eating and swallowing. A candidal infection is suspected.

6. If the client has candidiasis (thrush), which assessment finding is the nurse most likely to observe when inspecting the oral cavity?
[ ] **1.** Clear, shiny, domed vesicles on the tongue
[ ] **2.** Red, ulcerated patches at the gum margin
[ ] **3.** White, curdlike patches throughout the mouth
[ ] **4.** Dark brown, flat lesions in the oropharynx

The client asks the nurse about the source of the oral infection.

7. The nurse correctly explains that most individuals acquire candidiasis (thrush) by which means?
[ ] **1.** Transferring bacteria from unclean dental instruments
[ ] **2.** Having an overgrowth of normal mouth organisms
[ ] **3.** Inhaling moist droplets when someone sneezed
[ ] **4.** Using someone's unwashed eating utensils

The physician prescribes nystatin (Mycostatin) oral suspension to treat the client's candidiasis.

8. Which instruction should the nurse plan to give the client when administering the nystatin (Mycostatin) oral suspension?
[ ] **1.** Drink the medication through a straw.
[ ] **2.** Dilute the medication with cold water.
[ ] **3.** Swish the drug within the mouth, and then swallow it.
[ ] **4.** Brush the teeth after using the medication.

A 70-year-old client is referred for suspected cancer of the mouth after a routine dental examination.

9. If the client is typical of others with this diagnosis, which contributing factor is the nurse most likely to find when reading the medical history?
[ ] **1.** The client smoked marijuana occasionally as a teenager.
[ ] **2.** The client has used smokeless tobacco throughout adulthood.
[ ] **3.** The client has had exposure to asbestos as a construction worker.
[ ] **4.** The client has poor dental hygiene with several rotting teeth.

The client's oral cancerous lesion is surgically removed, and postsurgical radiation therapy is planned after discharge.

10. When the nurse plans postoperative nursing care, which nursing interventions should be implemented? Select all that apply.
[ ] **1.** Position the client with the head of the bed flat.
[ ] **2.** Assess the client's ability to speak clearly.
[ ] **3.** Irrigate the client's mouth when fully awake and alert.
[ ] **4.** Observe the client's ability to swallow.
[ ] **5.** Provide ice chips as tolerated.
[ ] **6.** Watch for signs of depression.

The client's discharge orders have been written and radiation therapy is scheduled the following week.

11. Before discharge, the nurse prepares the client about the expected side effects of radiation therapy. Which topics should the nurse include in the discharge plan? Select all that apply.
[ ] **1.** Alopecia
[ ] **2.** Pale skin at the site
[ ] **3.** Restlessness
[ ] **4.** Stomatitis
[ ] **5.** Xerostomia
[ ] **6.** Confusion

While being prepared for an annual gynecologic examination, a client discusses with the nurse a herpes simplex type 1 mouth lesion, which the client refers to as a "cold sore."

12. Which statement made by the client indicates that further instruction regarding herpes simplex is needed?
[ ] **1.** "My cold sore is caused by a virus."
[ ] **2.** "I got this by kissing someone who also has one."
[ ] **3.** "I have been under a lot of stress lately."
[ ] **4.** "The sores can only form on the lips."

The client is prescribed acyclovir (Zovirax) by the physician to treat the herpes lesions.

13. Which statement indicates that the client understands the purpose for the drug therapy?
[ ] **1.** "I know that this drug will kill all the virus causing the lesion."
[ ] **2.** "The drug shortens the duration of an outbreak."
[ ] **3.** "The drug prevents future outbreaks from occurring."
[ ] **4.** "I'll need to take the drug daily for the rest of my life."

Nursing Care of Clients with Disorders of the Esophagus

A 60-year-old client has been experiencing difficulty swallowing. The nurse in the ambulatory surgery department schedules the client for an esophagoscopy.

14. Which statement made by the client indicates an understanding of the preparations necessary for an esophagoscopy?
[ ] **1.** "I need to eat a light breakfast before the examination."
[ ] **2.** "I should consume a low-residue diet until the test has been completed."
[ ] **3.** "I need to avoid food and fluids after midnight before the test."
[ ] **4.** "I have to drink a quart of liquid before arriving for the test."

The esophagoscopy reveals that the client has a stricture near the end of the esophagus.

15. To help improve the client's ability to swallow, which recommendation made by the nurse is most appropriate?
[ ] **1.** Eat a variety of foods containing a thickener.
[ ] **2.** Thoroughly chew everything that is eaten.
[ ] **3.** Avoid drinking beverages while eating a meal.
[ ] **4.** Consume a full-liquid diet.

A 38-year-old client is admitted with bleeding esophageal varices and will require a blood transfusion.

16. As the nurse reviews the client's medical record, which factor is most likely related to the present condition?
[ ] **1.** There was a prior suicide attempt by ingesting lye.
[ ] **2.** The client has a history of oral cancer.
[ ] **3.** The client is a known hemophiliac.
[ ] **4.** There is a history of chronic alcohol consumption.

The registered nurse (RN) starts an infusion of whole blood and asks the licensed practical nurse (LPN) to continue monitoring the client during the blood transfusion.

17. According to the Joint Commission's National Patient Safety Goals, which nursing action regarding blood administration is most appropriate?
[ ] **1.** Two nurses must review the blood bag and client's arm bracelet before administration.
[ ] **2.** An indwelling (Foley) catheter must be placed during the transfusion.
[ ] **3.** An I.V. line using a 22-gauge needle should be started before administration.
[ ] **4.** Each unit of blood should be completed within 12 hours of starting it.

18. As the licensed practical nurse is monitoring the client receiving a blood transfusion, which assessment finding is the best indication of a transfusion reaction?
[ ] **1.** The client's urine is very dark yellow.
[ ] **2.** The client suddenly becomes dyspneic.
[ ] **3.** The client's skin is pale and cool.
[ ] **4.** The client experiences extreme thirst.

During a routine home visit, a client describes what the nurse believes may be symptoms related to gastroesophageal reflux disease (GERD).

19. The home care nurse updates the plan of care to include nursing interventions related to which chief complaint?
[ ] **1.** Vomiting
[ ] **2.** Nausea
[ ] **3.** Anorexia
[ ] **4.** Heartburn

20. While the client is awaiting an appointment with the physician, which nursing instruction is most helpful for providing some relief from the symptoms the client is experiencing?
[ ] **1.** "Eat three well-balanced meals a day."
[ ] **2.** "Eat foods that are easy to swallow."
[ ] **3.** "Avoid lying down after eating."
[ ] **4.** "Drink clear liquids at room temperature."

21. Which modification in the client's position is most appropriate to recommend at this time?
[ ] **1.** Have the client remain supine on a mattress that contains a bed board.
[ ] **2.** Advise the client to sleep on a water bed temporarily.
[ ] **3.** Tell the client to elevate the legs on pillows when retiring at night.
[ ] **4.** Have the client raise the head of the bed on 4-inch blocks.

A 75-year-old client with metastatic cancer of the esophagus is undergoing palliative treatment that includes total parenteral nutrition (TPN) administered through a central subclavian catheter.

22. Which nursing assessment is essential for evaluating the client's response to the TPN?
[ ] **1.** Test the urine specific gravity.
[ ] **2.** Monitor the capillary blood glucose level.
[ ] **3.** Measure the arterial pulse pressure.
[ ] **4.** Obtain an apical-radial pulse rate.

23. Which finding documented in the client's chart is the best evidence that the client is responding favorably to the administration of TPN?
[ ] **1.** The client's electrolytes are in balance.
[ ] **2.** The client is gaining weight.
[ ] **3.** The client's appetite is returning.
[ ] **4.** The client is voiding clear, yellow urine.

In anticipation of transferring the client to a nursing home, the physician inserts a gastrostomy tube for nourishment.

24. Immediately after the gastrostomy tube is inserted, which finding should the nurse consider normal when assessing the gastrostomy drainage?
[ ] **1.** Milky drainage
[ ] **2.** Serosanguineous drainage
[ ] **3.** Green-tinged drainage
[ ] **4.** Bright, bloody drainage

25. Which technique is the best way to determine if the gastrostomy tube has migrated after being inserted?
[ ] **1.** Testing the pH of aspirated secretions
[ ] **2.** Monitoring the results of stomach X-rays
[ ] **3.** Measuring the length of the external tube
[ ] **4.** Palpating the abdomen for distention

The nurse fills a tube-feeding bag with two 8-ounce cans of commercially prepared formula that will infuse continuously through the client's gastrostomy tube through a feeding pump.

26. If the client is to receive 120 mL of formula per hour, the nurse can expect that the entire bag of formula will be empty in how many hours?

_____

While the tube-feeding formula is infusing, the client tells the nurse about feeling full and nauseated.

27. Which nursing actions are most appropriate at this time? Select all that apply.
[ ] **1.** Measure the stomach residual.
[ ] **2.** Administer an antiemetic by gastrostomy tube.
[ ] **3.** Stop the infusion temporarily.
[ ] **4.** Add water to dilute the formula.
[ ] **5.** Turn the client onto the right side.
[ ] **6.** Request an order for a different type of formula.

28. After the tube-feeding formula has infused, which action should the nurse take next?
[ ] **1.** Place the client on the left side.
[ ] **2.** Lower the head of the client's bed.
[ ] **3.** Clamp the opening of the gastrostomy tube.
[ ] **4.** Instill several ounces of plain tap water down the tube.

The client with the gastrostomy is silent and withdrawn as the nurse cares for the insertion site.

29. Which statement made by the nurse is most appropriate for encouraging the expression of feelings?
[ ] **1.** "Are you depressed?"
[ ] **2.** "It must be tough for you."
[ ] **3.** "This may get better soon."
[ ] **4.** "Lots of people eat this way."

30. The client is being discharged. Which nursing instruction is best to provide the family if the gastrostomy tube becomes obstructed?
[ ] **1.** Irrigate the gastrostomy tube with cola.
[ ] **2.** Instill sterile water with a syringe.
[ ] **3.** Milk the gastrostomy tube.
[ ] **4.** Apply suction to the gastrostomy tube.

Nursing Care of Clients with Disorders of the Stomach

A 46-year-old client is hospitalized to determine the cause of intermittent gnawing epigastric pain. The admitting nurse obtains the client's health history and suspects a peptic ulcer.

31. On the basis of the suspected condition, the nurse would expect the client to report that the epigastric pain decreases with which activity?
[ ] **1.** When skipping meals
[ ] **2.** When going to bed
[ ] **3.** When eating food
[ ] **4.** When vomiting

32. In addition to the client's clinical presentation, which positive laboratory finding provides further evidence that the client's symptoms are related to a peptic ulcer?
[ ] **1.** Urine that is positive for albumin
[ ] **2.** Blood that is positive for glucose
[ ] **3.** Stool that is positive for blood
[ ] **4.** Emesis that is positive for pepsin

The client is scheduled for an X-ray of the upper GI tract.

33. After the nurse explains the procedure for performing an upper GI X-ray, which statement by the client best indicates an understanding of what this test involves?
[ ] **1.** "A flexible tube will be inserted into my stomach."
[ ] **2.** "Dye will be infused into my vein before the test."
[ ] **3.** "My body will be placed within an imaging chamber."
[ ] **4.** "I'll have to swallow a large amount of barium."

Diagnostic tests reveal that the client has a duodenal ulcer. The physician writes an order for clarithromycin (Biaxin) 500 mg t.i.d., metronidazole (Flagyl) 250 mg q.i.d., and omeprazole (Prilosec) 40 mg b.i.d.

34. Record the total number of milligrams for all three medications per day.

_____

The client asks the nurse why the physician has prescribed an antibiotic for the ulcer.

35. Which explanation by the nurse regarding the use of antibiotics for ulcer therapy is most accurate?
[ ] **1.** Antibiotics heal the irritated mucous membrane of the stomach.
[ ] **2.** Antibiotics eliminate a microorganism that depletes gastric mucus.
[ ] **3.** Antibiotics add a protective coating over the ulcerated mucosa.
[ ] **4.** Antibiotics prevent secondary GI infections.

The licensed practical nurse (LPN) assists the team leader in planning the client's discharge teaching. The goal is to provide the client with information that will help prevent further GI irritation.

36. The nurse instructs the client to follow the label directions when taking medications to relieve occasional pain and discomfort associated with the ulcer. Which medication is most appropriate for the client to take based on the medical history and current diagnosis?
[ ] **1.** Acetaminophen (Tylenol)
[ ] **2.** Aspirin (Anacin)
[ ] **3.** Ibuprofen (Advil)
[ ] **4.** Naproxen (Naprosyn)

The nurse prepares a client with a history of recurrent peptic ulcer disease for abdominal surgery.

37. As the nurse performs a head-to-toe physical assessment, which finding best indicates that the client's ulcer has perforated?
[ ] **1.** The client's skin is ecchymotic.
[ ] **2.** The client's abdomen feels boardlike.
[ ] **3.** The client's pupils are widely dilated.
[ ] **4.** The client's respirations are rapid.

The licensed practical nurse (LPN) assists the registered nurse (RN) in inserting a nasogastric (NG) tube in the client with a perforated ulcer.

38. To determine the length of tubing to insert, the nurse correctly places the tip of the tube at the client's nose and measures the distance from there to which area?
[ ] **1.** The jaw and then midway to the sternum
[ ] **2.** The mouth and then between the nipples
[ ] **3.** The midsternum and then to the umbilicus
[ ] **4.** The ear and then to the xiphoid process

39. Which instruction should the nurse give the client when the tube is in the oropharynx?
[ ] **1.** "Breathe deeply as the tube is advanced."
[ ] **2.** "Hold your head in a sniffing position."
[ ] **3.** "Press your chin to your upper chest."
[ ] **4.** "Avoid coughing until the tube is down."

40. Place the following nursing actions in order from first to last based on how the nurse would perform a nasogastric (NG) tube insertion. Use all the options.

1. Instruct the client to sip water as the tube is inserted.
2. Aspirate fluid from the stomach.
3. Have the client lower the chin.
4. Inspect the nares to determine which should be used.
5. Secure the NG tube to the nose.
6. Ask the client to tilt the neck to simulate a sniffing position.

41. Which setting is most appropriate to use when connecting the client's single-lumen nasogastric (NG) tube to suction preoperatively?
[ ] **1.** Low intermittent suction
[ ] **2.** Low continuous suction
[ ] **3.** High intermittent suction
[ ] **4.** High continuous suction

42. If the client turns blue and coughs as the nasogastric (NG) tube is inserted, which additional sign indicates that the tube has entered the respiratory tract?
[ ] **1.** Inability to speak
[ ] **2.** Inability to swallow
[ ] **3.** Sneezing
[ ] **4.** Vomiting

43. Which is the most appropriate technique for determining if the distal end of the nasogastric (NG) tube is in the stomach?
[ ] **1.** Requesting a portable X-ray of the stomach
[ ] **2.** Listening over the stomach as air is instilled
[ ] **3.** Adding 100 mL of tap water into the tube
[ ] **4.** Feeling for air at the proximal end of the tube

The client with the perforated ulcer senses the critical nature of the condition and asks the nurse, "Am I going to die?"

44. Which response by the nurse is most appropriate?
[ ] **1.** "We are doing everything we can right now to help you."
[ ] **2.** "That is something you'll have to ask your physician."
[ ] **3.** "Now what kind of a silly question is that?"
[ ] **4.** "I've seen patients with similar problems pull through."

A gastrojejunostomy, also called a Billroth II, is performed to treat the client's perforated ulcer. The client returns to the room after recovering from the anesthesia.

45. When the client does not adequately cough and deep-breathe postoperatively due to incisional pain, which nursing action is most appropriate at this time?
[ ] **1.** Explain about the high risk for developing pneumonia.
[ ] **2.** Have the client press a pillow against the incision when coughing.
[ ] **3.** Ask the physician to order some oxygen for the client.
[ ] **4.** Keep the head of the bed elevated at all times.

The nurse notes that the nasogastric (NG) tube placed during the client's gastrojejunostomy has stopped draining; the physician orders an irrigation.

46. Which technique is most appropriate when the nurse irrigates the NG tube?
[ ] **1.** Instilling 30 mL of sterile distilled water into the tube
[ ] **2.** Administering oxygen before the irrigation
[ ] **3.** Recording the volume instilled and removed
[ ] **4.** Asking the client to swallow frequently

The physician writes an order to discontinue the client's nasogastric (NG) tube and begin a full liquid diet. The nurse is recording the client's intake and output.

47. On the basis of the following list of food consumed within the past 8 hours, how many milliliters of intake should the nurse record? Use all in the list.
[ ] **1.** One cup of thin, cooked cereal
[ ] **2.** One 8-ounce carton of milk
[ ] **3.** ¼ cup of ice cream
[ ] **4.** 8 ounces of supplemental nutritional drink
[ ] **5.** 6 ounces of creamed soup
[ ] **6.** ½ cup of fruit-flavored gelatin

The nurse creates a teaching plan for a client who develops dumping syndrome after a gastrojejunostomy.

48. Which advice would the nurse offer to a client recovering from a gastrojejunostomy to prevent symptoms associated with dumping syndrome? Select all that apply.
[ ] **1.** Consume a generous amount of fluid during meals.
[ ] **2.** Avoid eating simple carbohydrates.
[ ] **3.** Restrict consumption of raw fruits and vegetables.
[ ] **4.** Eat several small meals throughout the day.
[ ] **5.** Lie down for 30 minutes after a meal.
[ ] **6.** Chew food thoroughly while eating.

A 74-year-old client experiences persistent indigestion, feeling of gastric fullness, and unexplained weight loss.

49. When reviewing the results of the client's diagnostic tests, which finding would strongly suggest to the nurse that the client's symptoms are related to stomach cancer?
[ ] **1.** Gastric analysis showing absence of hydrochloric acid
[ ] **2.** An elevated level of gastrin in the blood
[ ] **3.** Gastric irritation noted during a gastroscopy
[ ] **4.** A decrease in hemoglobin and hematocrit

The client is diagnosed with stomach cancer and scheduled for a total gastrectomy. After surgery, the client who has a single-lumen nasogastric (NG) tube informs the nurse about being very thirsty.

50. In response to the client's statement, which nursing intervention is most appropriate to add to the care plan?
[ ] **1.** Offer fluids at least every 2 hours.
[ ] **2.** Provide crushed ice in sparse amounts.
[ ] **3.** Increase oral liquids on the dietary tray.
[ ] **4.** Refill the water pitcher twice each shift.

One year after the gastrectomy, the client develops pernicious anemia. A home health nurse administers 1,000 mcg of vitamin B$_{12}$ intramuscularly every month.

51. If the label on the vial of vitamin B$_{12}$ indicates that there is 1 mg of drug per milliliter of solution, the nurse is accurate in withdrawing which amount?
[ ] **1.** 0.1 mL
[ ] **2.** 1 mL
[ ] **3.** 10 mL
[ ] **4.** 0.01 mL

The nurse chooses to use the vastus lateralis muscle as the site for the I.M. vitamin B$_{12}$ injection.

52. If the correct technique for administering the injection is followed, the nurse should give the injection in which location?
[ ] **1.** Upper arm at a 45-degree angle
[ ] **2.** Outer thigh at a 90-degree angle
[ ] **3.** Anterior thigh at a 90-degree angle
[ ] **4.** Outer buttock at a 45-degree angle

Nursing Care of Clients with Disorders of the Small Intestine

A 19-year-old client has been having up to five loose stools per day. The client is admitted to the hospital for diagnostic testing and symptomatic treatment.

53. When the nurse collects a stool specimen for ova and parasites, which action is correct?
[ ] **1.** The nurse holds a specimen container under the client's anus.
[ ] **2.** The nurse places the collected specimen in a sterile container.
[ ] **3.** The nurse refrigerates the covered specimen after collection.
[ ] **4.** The nurse immediately takes the specimen to the laboratory.

The physician has prescribed diphenoxylate hydrochloride (Lomotil) 5 mg orally q.i.d. for the client's diarrhea.

54. When the nurse checks the medication administration record, which military time schedule for administering this drug is most accurate?
[ ] **1.** 0730, 1130, 0430
[ ] **2.** 0600, 1200, 1800, 0000
[ ] **3.** 0900, 1300, 1700
[ ] **4.** 0400, 0800, 1200, 1600, 2000

The physician restricts the client's diet to include only clear liquids.

55. When the client asks for something to eat, which foods are most appropriate for the nurse to provide? Select all that apply.
[ ] **1.** Chicken broth
[ ] **2.** Ginger ale
[ ] **3.** Gelatin
[ ] **4.** Orange juice
[ ] **5.** Milkshake
[ ] **6.** Vanilla pudding

The nurse assesses the client for signs of fluid volume deficit related to the diarrhea.

56. Which assessment finding is most likely to indicate that the client is becoming dehydrated?
[ ] **1.** Elevated blood pressure
[ ] **2.** Irregular heart rate
[ ] **3.** Pink mucous membranes
[ ] **4.** Dark yellow urine

The physician orders a colonoscopy because of the client's persistent diarrhea. The nurse instructs the client to drink 250 mL of an electrolyte solution called GoLYTELY every 15 minutes over a 2-hour period.

57. Which observation by the nurse provides the best evidence that the solution has achieved its primary purpose?
[ ] **1.** The client's serum electrolyte levels are normal.
[ ] **2.** The client's intake approximates the output.
[ ] **3.** The client's stools become clear liquid.
[ ] **4.** The client's bladder fills with urine.

After drinking the prescribed dose of GoLYTELY and having numerous stools, the client reports feeling chest palpitations to the nurse. The nurse suspects an electrolyte imbalance and requests a physician order for laboratory work.

58. The client's laboratory report comes back. Which laboratory values would result in the nurse immediately recognizing that the client has an electrolyte imbalance? Select all that apply.
[ ] **1.** Sodium, 126 mEq/L
[ ] **2.** Potassium, 2.8 mEq/L
[ ] **3.** Chloride, 90 mEq/L
[ ] **4.** Calcium, 9.4 mEq/dL
[ ] **5.** Phosphorus, 3.5 mEq/dL
[ ] **6.** Blood urea nitrogen (BUN), 16 mg/dL

The client's electrolyte imbalance is corrected. Before the colonoscopy, the client is given moderate sedation using midazolam hydrochloride (Versed).

59. During the colonoscopy and in the immediate recovery period, for which potential adverse effect of midazolam hydrochloride (Versed) is it essential that the nurse assess the client closely?
[ ] **1.** Unstable blood pressure
[ ] **2.** Cardiac rhythm disturbance
[ ] **3.** Respiratory depression
[ ] **4.** Altered consciousness

The colonoscopy reveals that the client with diarrhea has Crohn's disease. The physician places the client on a fiber-controlled diet.

60. After talking with the dietitian, the client demonstrates an understanding of the therapeutic diet by indicating that fiber refers to which substance?
[ ] **1.** Foods that require chewing
[ ] **2.** The muscle found in red meat
[ ] **3.** The semisolid mass in the stomach
[ ] **4.** The indigestible parts of plants

The client eventually develops a draining fistula between a loop of the ileum and the skin. The nursing team meets to revise the client's care plan.

61. On the basis of this new complication, which problem should the nursing team consider the highest priority when planning the client's care?
[ ] **1.** Pain from complex dressing changes
[ ] **2.** Skin breakdown
[ ] **3.** Body image
[ ] **4.** Containment of the odor from the wound

Nursing Care of Clients with Disorders of the Large Intestine

A 52-year-old client is admitted to the ambulatory surgery department for repair of an inguinal hernia. The nurse takes the signed operative consent form to the client to confirm the procedure. The form states that the surgical procedure will be a right inguinal herniorrhaphy.

62. When the client states to the nurse, "I hope I can get along without that section of my bowel," which action should the nurse take next?
[ ] 1. Cancel the surgery.
[ ] 2. Notify the physician.
[ ] 3. Witness the client's signature.
[ ] 4. Clip the hair in the right groin.

63. According to the National Patient Safety Goals, surgical site verification and time-out processes must be performed. Place the statements in the order in which they should occur.

1. Time-out is done immediately before starting the procedure in the location where the procedure will be performed.

2. The surgeon verifies the surgical site with the client, initialing the correct site with an appropriate marking pen.

3. The nurse reviews the surgical consent, noting the correct procedure and site

4. The procedure begins after the time-out when staff is confident the correct procedure is being performed on the correct client.

5. Before positioning the client on the operating room table, the nurse identifies the client using the client's name and birth date on the identification band.

6. All staff stops what they are doing and participates in the final verification, answering verbally when verifying the surgical site.

The client returns from surgery, which was performed under spinal anesthesia.

64. When the nurse is reviewing postoperative orders, which order should the nurse question?
[ ] 1. Diet as tolerated
[ ] 2. Fluids as desired
[ ] 3. Vital signs until stable
[ ] 4. Fowler's position

65. Which postoperative assessment should the nurse consider a priority after the client's herniorrhaphy?
[ ] 1. Ability to urinate
[ ] 2. Coughing efforts
[ ] 3. Level of consciousness
[ ] 4. Pain tolerance

After surgery, the nurse brings a suspensory (slinglike support) for a male client to apply.

66. Which explanation regarding the use of the suspensory is most appropriate?
[ ] 1. It is used to prevent sexual impotence.
[ ] 2. It is used to prevent scrotal edema.
[ ] 3. It is used to prevent strain on the incision.
[ ] 4. It is used to prevent wound contamination.

The physician orders meperidine hydrochloride (Demerol) 50 mg I.M. every 4 hours as needed to help relieve the client's pain after surgery.

67. If the drug is supplied in ampules of 100 mg/mL, what amount should the nurse administer?
[ ] 1. 1.0 mL
[ ] 2. 0.5 mL
[ ] 3. 2.0 mL
[ ] 4. 0.2 mL

68. The nurse appropriately documents the administration of meperidine hydrochloride (Demerol) on the client's medical administration record and in which other area?
[ ] 1. Computer database
[ ] 2. Opioid control log
[ ] 3. Drug enforcement form
[ ] 4. Pharmacy access book

A 31-year-old client with a long history of ulcerative colitis is admitted to the hospital for a colectomy.

69. Aside from the client's report of severe diarrhea, which other characteristic signs or symptoms will most likely be identified when admitting this client? Select all that apply.
[ ] 1. Mucus and blood in the stool
[ ] 2. Hypoactive bowel sounds
[ ] 3. Striae on the abdomen
[ ] 4. Shallow ulcerations in the client's mouth
[ ] 5. Left lower abdominal pain
[ ] 6. Incontinence

The nurse assesses the client's abdomen for bowel sounds following the sequential anatomic areas of the bowel.

70.

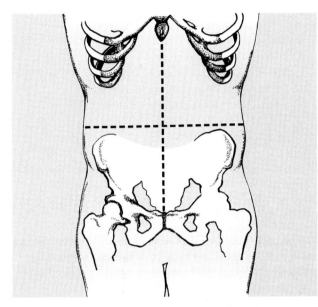

Place an X in the quadrant the nurse auscultates to assess the proximal portion of the ascending colon.

The nursing team includes the nursing diagnosis of "Bowel incontinence related to the loss of voluntary bowel control as evidenced by a sudden urgency for defecation" on the client's care plan.

71. Which intervention is most appropriate when managing this nursing diagnosis?
[ ] **1.** Keep the bedside commode nearby
[ ] **2.** Answer the client's signal for help promptly
[ ] **3.** Provide a disposable brief for the client
[ ] **4.** Assist the client to the bathroom frequently

The client tells the nurse about being hospitalized several times in the past few months without much improvement; this surgery is the last resort. The client is discouraged and states, "I'm sure this surgery will not help either."

72. Which response by the nurse is most therapeutic?
[ ] **1.** "You're saying that you doubt that you'll get better."
[ ] **2.** "Do you want to talk to your physician again before surgery?"
[ ] **3.** "I'd recommend a more positive attitude this time around."
[ ] **4.** "Of course surgery will work. Others wish they'd had it done sooner."

73. After giving the client preoperative medications, including meperidine hydrochloride (Demerol), hydroxyzine (Vistaril), and atropine sulfate, what is the most important action for the nurse to perform?

[ ] **1.** Raising the bed side rails
[ ] **2.** Helping the client to the toilet
[ ] **3.** Observing for a dry mouth
[ ] **4.** Placing an emesis basin by the bedside

After recovering from anesthesia after the colectomy, the client is transferred to the nursing unit.

74. When the nurse monitors the client postoperatively, which assessment finding is most indicative of shock?
[ ] **1.** Bounding pulse
[ ] **2.** Slow respirations
[ ] **3.** Low blood pressure
[ ] **4.** High body temperature

The client receives oxygen by nasal cannula at 2 L/minute (28%) postoperatively.

75. If the client is adequately oxygenated, the nurse knows that the pulse oximeter attached to the client's finger should measure oxygen saturation in which range?
[ ] **1.** 25% to 30%
[ ] **2.** 35% to 50%
[ ] **3.** 60% to 80%
[ ] **4.** 95% to 100%

The client's care plan includes providing measures for caring for the ileostomy created at the time of surgery.

76. Which of the following nursing interventions are appropriate for managing the care of a client with an ileostomy? Select all that apply.
[ ] **1.** Change the faceplate of the appliance and pouch daily.
[ ] **2.** Inspect the size, color, and condition of the stoma.
[ ] **3.** Clean the peristomal area with alcohol or acetone.
[ ] **4.** Attach the opening of the faceplate snugly around the stoma.
[ ] **5.** Empty the pouch of the appliance as soon as stool is expelled.
[ ] **6.** Apply a skin barrier substance to excoriated skin.

77. When implementing the client's care plan, when is the best time of day for the nurse to perform stomal care and to change the appliance?
[ ] **1.** After the client awakens in the morning
[ ] **2.** After the client has showered after breakfast
[ ] **3.** After the client has been ambulating in the hall
[ ] **4.** After the client finishes the evening meal

78. The oncoming nurse is receiving report which includes assessment findings of the client's ileostomy stoma. Which nursing description would the oncoming nurse interpret as a normal finding?
[ ] **1.** Pale pink with a red marginal border
[ ] **2.** Bright red with a shiny appearance
[ ] **3.** Dark tan with no drainage or bleeding
[ ] **4.** Dusky blue located slightly below the skin level

79. When the nurse cleans the skin around the client's stoma, which technique is most appropriate?
[ ] **1.** Cleaning the area with povidone-iodine (Betadine)
[ ] **2.** Swabbing the skin with 70% alcohol
[ ] **3.** Using water and mild soap
[ ] **4.** Scrubbing the skin with peroxide

80. Which technique is most accurate when changing the ileostomy appliance?
[ ] **1.** Placing the faceplate over the opening of the stoma so it occludes it
[ ] **2.** Cutting the appliance opening ⅛″ to ¼″ larger than the stoma
[ ] **3.** Adhering the appliance after the skin has air-dried for 30 minutes
[ ] **4.** Securing the appliance snugly at the waist or belt line

81. Which activity is unrealistic for a client with a conventional ileostomy?
[ ] **1.** Swimming
[ ] **2.** Jogging
[ ] **3.** Having sexual intercourse
[ ] **4.** Controlling defecation

A 20-year-old client comes to the emergency department with pain that is localized on the lower right side of the abdomen. The physician suspects appendicitis.

82. Which laboratory test ordered on admission is important for the nurse to monitor at this time?
[ ] **1.** Bilirubin level
[ ] **2.** Serum potassium level
[ ] **3.** Prothrombin time
[ ] **4.** Leukocyte count

83. If the client is typical of others with appendicitis, where can the nurse expect the client will experience tenderness when the abdomen is palpated? Indicate the site with an *X*.

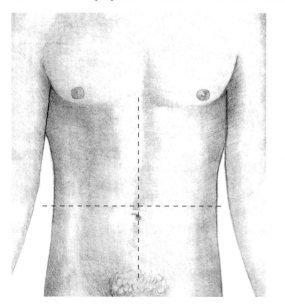

The physician considers removing the client's appendix with laparoscopic surgery.

84. When the client asks the nurse about the benefits of this type of procedure, which statements are accurate? Select all that apply.
[ ] **1.** The recovery period is shorter.
[ ] **2.** No anesthesia is necessary.
[ ] **3.** There will be a small surgical scar.
[ ] **4.** Exercise can be resumed immediately.
[ ] **5.** Sexual intercourse may be resumed quicker.
[ ] **6.** Soft, easy-to-digest foods are eaten immediately after surgery.

The client's condition worsens and the physician fears that the appendix has ruptured. The client is prepared for an emergency appendectomy. The laparoscopic approach for removing the appendix is no longer an option.

85. The nurse questions the client about activities just before coming to the hospital and suspects which of the following most likely contributed to rupturing the client's appendix?
[ ] **1.** The client ate tacos with spicy salsa.
[ ] **2.** The client continued usual activities.
[ ] **3.** The client applied a heating pad to the lower abdomen.
[ ] **4.** The client took acetaminophen (Tylenol) for discomfort.

The client returns from surgery with an open (Penrose) drain extending from the incision. A sterile dressing covers the drain.

86. In which position should the nurse place the client to promote drainage from the wound?
[ ] **1.** Lithotomy
[ ] **2.** Fowler's
[ ] **3.** Recumbent
[ ] **4.** Trendelenburg's

87. The physician orders the client's dressing to be changed daily. When changing the client's dressing, which nursing action is correct?
[ ] **1.** The nurse removes the soiled dressing with sterile gloves.
[ ] **2.** The nurse frees the tape by pulling it away from the incision.
[ ] **3.** The nurse encloses the soiled dressing within a latex glove.
[ ] **4.** The nurse cleans the wound in circles toward the incision.

The client requests medication to relieve pain from the appendectomy. The physician has ordered meperidine hydrochloride (Demerol) 60 mg I.M. q4h p.r.n.

88. If the label on the meperidine hydrochloride (Demerol) vial states 50 mg/mL, how much should the nurse administer to the client?

_____

A 68-year-old client has noted bloody stools for the past 6 months. One possible diagnosis is colorectal cancer.

89. Aside from rectal bleeding, which information in the client's medical history strongly suggests colorectal cancer? Select all that apply.
[ ] **1.** The client states that bowel habits have changed.
[ ] **2.** The client has insulin-dependent diabetes.
[ ] **3.** The client experiences chronic indigestion.
[ ] **4.** The client has had a history of hepatitis.
[ ] **5.** The client has dull abdominal pain.
[ ] **6.** The client has a history of drug abuse.

The nurse provides instructions about the client's scheduled outpatient sigmoidoscopy. The night before the procedure, the client will begin preparing for the test.

90. Which statement by the client indicates that additional teaching is needed before the sigmoidoscopy?
[ ] **1.** "I should plan to spend the night in the hospital."
[ ] **2.** "I should eat a light meal the evening before the examination."
[ ] **3.** "A flexible scope will be inserted into my rectum."
[ ] **4.** "I should take my prescribed medications in the morning."

91. The nurse assisting with the sigmoidoscopy places the client in which position?
[ ] **1.** Lithotomy
[ ] **2.** Sims'
[ ] **3.** Orthopneic
[ ] **4.** Fowler's

Based on the findings from the sigmoidoscopy, the client will need to undergo a bowel resection to remove the cancerous tumor.

92. If a low-residue diet is ordered for the client before surgery, which food would be contraindicated?
[ ] **1.** Ground meat
[ ] **2.** Bran cereal
[ ] **3.** Orange juice
[ ] **4.** Baked fish

Before colorectal surgery, the client will receive 1 g of neomycin sulfate (Mycifradin) orally every hour for four doses and then 1 g orally every 4 hours for the balance of the 24 hours.

93. If the neomycin sulfate (Mycifradin) tablets come in a dosage strength of 500 mg per tablet, how many tablets should the nurse administer each time?
[ ] **1.** ½ tablet
[ ] **2.** 1 tablet
[ ] **3.** 2 tablets
[ ] **4.** 4 tablets

94. When the client asks the nurse why neomycin sulfate (Mycifradin) was prescribed, the most accurate explanation in this case is that the drug is given for which reason?
[ ] **1.** To treat any current infection the client may have
[ ] **2.** To suppress the growth of intestinal bacteria
[ ] **3.** To prevent the onset of postoperative diarrhea
[ ] **4.** To reduce the number of bacteria near the incision

During the postoperative period, the client's abdominal incision separates and the bowel protrudes through the opening.

95. What is the first action that the nurse should take at this time?
[ ] **1.** Check the client's vital signs.
[ ] **2.** Call the client's physician.
[ ] **3.** Cover the bowel with moist gauze.
[ ] **4.** Push the bowel back through the opening.

A home health nurse visits a 71-year-old client and observes that the client's abdomen is quite distended. The client complains of nausea and reportedly has been vomiting for the past 48 hours.

96. Which question is important for the nurse to ask to determine if the client has a bowel obstruction?
[ ] **1.** "When did you last eat a full meal?"
[ ] **2.** "How much fluid are you vomiting?"
[ ] **3.** "Does the emesis appear to contain feces?"
[ ] **4.** "Has your appetite changed considerably?"

The client is hospitalized and a nasogastric tube is inserted. Unfortunately, the client's bowel obstruction is unrelieved by gastric decompression. The client is scheduled for a laparotomy, possible colon resection, and a temporary colostomy. The client's preoperative orders include meperidine hydrochloride (Demerol) and atropine sulfate I.M.

97. If the written order for the atropine sulfate says to administer 5 mg I.M. and the usual adult preoperative dose is 0.4 to 0.6 mg, which action is best for the nurse to take next?
[ ] **1.** Give the usual preoperative dose of atropine.
[ ] **2.** Administer just the meperidine hydrochloride (Demerol) at this time.
[ ] **3.** Withhold both the medications and notify the physician.
[ ] **4.** Consult the pharmacist on which action to take.

The surgeon creates a double-barrel colostomy in the transverse colon.

98. Place an *X* over the stoma from which the nurse can expect the elimination of stool.

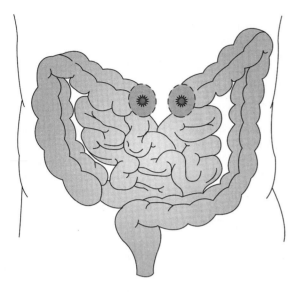

A few days after surgery, the physician orders daily colostomy irrigations.

99. Which position is best for the client when irrigating the colostomy?
[ ] **1.** Lying on the left side
[ ] **2.** Sitting on the toilet
[ ] **3.** Standing at the sink
[ ] **4.** Kneeling in the bathtub

During a conversation concerning the client's feelings about the colostomy, the client suddenly becomes silent and tearful.

100. Which nursing action is most appropriate at this time?
[ ] **1.** Change the subject to something more pleasant.
[ ] **2.** Refrain from interjecting comments or questions.
[ ] **3.** Provide information about colostomy care.
[ ] **4.** Offer a referral for psychological counseling.

The client says to the nurse, "I don't think I will ever learn to change this bag correctly."

101. Which nursing response is most appropriate at this time?
[ ] **1.** Encourage the client to express any concerns.
[ ] **2.** Reassure the client that adjustment will come with time.
[ ] **3.** Recommend that the client investigate care in a nursing home.
[ ] **4.** Say nothing, but quote the client's statement in the chart.

A nursing home resident is admitted to the hospital with diarrhea. A diagnosis of Clostridium difficile (C. difficile) *is made.*

102. To prevent C. difficile from being transmitted to other hospitalized clients, which nursing actions are most appropriate? Select all that apply.
[ ] **1.** Use alcohol foam to wash hands when providing client care.
[ ] **2.** Request an order to place the client in contact isolation.
[ ] **3.** Wash hands with soap and water on entering and exiting the client's room.
[ ] **4.** Apply a mask when coming in contact with the client's feces.
[ ] **5.** Place the client in a negative-pressure room.
[ ] **6.** Cohort clients with diarrhea to the same general location in the hospital.

Nursing Care of Clients with Disorders of the Rectum and Anus

A nurse assesses blood pressures at a senior citizens' community center during the lunch hour. An 80-year-old client discreetly asks the nurse for help with constipation.

103. Before recommending an over-the-counter laxative, the nurse asks which medications the client takes. If the medications include examples from each of the classifications listed here, which are known to cause constipation? Select all that apply.
[ ] **1.** Opiates
[ ] **2.** Iron preparations
[ ] **3.** Antacids containing calcium
[ ] **4.** Antibiotics
[ ] **5.** Antihypertensives
[ ] **6.** Nonsteroidal anti-inflammatory drugs (NSAIDs)

A nurse who works at a nursing home cares for several clients with bowel elimination problems.

104. When a nursing home resident informs the nurse about an inability to have a bowel movement without taking a daily laxative, which information is essential for the nurse to provide?
[ ] **1.** Long-term use of laxatives impairs natural bowel tone.
[ ] **2.** Stool softeners are likely to be less harsh.
[ ] **3.** Daily enemas are preferred to laxatives.
[ ] **4.** Dilating the anal sphincter may aid bowel elimination.

A nurse receives a report that one of the nursing home residents has not had a bowel movement for 3 days. On further investigation, the nurse suspects a fecal impaction.

105. Which of the following strongly indicates that a client has a fecal impaction?
[ ] 1. The client passes liquid stool frequently.
[ ] 2. The client has foul-smelling stools.
[ ] 3. The client requests medication for a stomach ache.
[ ] 4. The client hasn't been eating well lately.

Before removing the fecal impaction, the nurse reviews the client's medical history.

106. Which of the following conditions are contraindications for digitally removing a fecal impaction? Select all that apply.
[ ] 1. History of cardiac surgery
[ ] 2. History of reproductive surgery
[ ] 3. History of radiation to the abdomen
[ ] 4. Presence of hemorrhoids
[ ] 5. Dependence on laxatives
[ ] 6. Use of anticoagulants

107. Which technique is best for confirming that a client has a fecal impaction?
[ ] 1. Administering an oil-retention enema
[ ] 2. Inserting a gloved finger into the rectum
[ ] 3. Reviewing the results of the client's lower GI X-ray
[ ] 4. Listening to the client's bowel sounds every 4 hours

A nursing home resident who is receiving supplemental tube feedings is complaining of bloating and abdominal distention.

108. Before inserting a rectal tube, what nursing measure is most helpful for eliminating a client's intestinal gas?
[ ] 1. Ambulating the client in the hall
[ ] 2. Providing a carbonated beverage
[ ] 3. Restricting the intake of solid food
[ ] 4. Administering an opioid analgesic

109. If a rectal tube becomes necessary to relieve a client's abdominal distention and discomfort, what is the maximum length of time the nurse should plan to leave the tube in place each time it is used?
[ ] 1. 15 minutes
[ ] 2. 20 minutes
[ ] 3. 45 minutes
[ ] 4. 60 minutes

During the administration of a cleansing soapsuds enema, a client experiences cramping and has the urge to defecate.

110. Which nursing action is most appropriate at this time?
[ ] 1. Quickly finish instilling the remaining solution.
[ ] 2. Tell the client to stop breathing and bear down.
[ ] 3. Briefly stop the administration of the enema solution.
[ ] 4. Turn the client supine and elevate the feet.

111. When the nurse is inserting a rectal suppository to relieve constipation, which nursing action is most appropriate?
[ ] 1. The nurse dons a sterile glove on the dominant hand.
[ ] 2. The nurse positions the client on the right side.
[ ] 3. The nurse inserts the suppository approximately 2″ to 4″ (5 to 10 cm).
[ ] 4. The nurse instructs the client to retain the suppository for 5 minutes.

112. Which of the following should be planned first before beginning bowel retraining for a client experiencing bowel incontinence?
[ ] 1. Limit the client's daytime physical activity.
[ ] 2. Record the time of day when incontinence occurs.
[ ] 3. Decrease the amount of food eaten at each meal.
[ ] 4. Empty the client's bowel with a soapsuds enema.

A home health nurse reviews the health history of a client who has hemorrhoids.

113. Which factor most likely contributed to the development of the client's hemorrhoids?
[ ] 1. Taking a daily stool softener
[ ] 2. History of ulcerative colitis
[ ] 3. Frequent constipation
[ ] 4. Occupation of a computer programmer

114. Besides increasing the consumption of bulk-forming foods (such as whole grains, fresh fruits, and vegetables), what is the most appropriate instruction the nurse can give the client with hemorrhoids?
[ ] 1. Eat small meals frequently.
[ ] 2. Drink eight glasses of water per day.
[ ] 3. Take a daily laxative.
[ ] 4. Reduce the intake of refined sugar.

The client with hemorrhoids eventually has them surgically removed. The nurse assists with giving the client a sitz bath postoperatively.

115. What is the best way to evaluate the effectiveness of the sitz bath for this client?
[ ] 1. The client's rectum is less painful.
[ ] 2. The client's incision is clean and well approximated.
[ ] 3. The client feels refreshed.
[ ] 4. The client has no evidence of a hematoma.

The physician prescribes docusate sodium (Colace) for the client. The client asks the nurse to explain why the medication is needed.

116. Which explanation given by the nurse correctly states the purpose of the medication?
[ ] **1.** To ease bowel evacuation and its related discomfort
[ ] **2.** To irritate the bowel and promote stool elimination
[ ] **3.** To stimulate peristalsis to remove wastes after digestion
[ ] **4.** To reduce intestinal activity and decrease stool size

A client is admitted for surgical treatment of a pilonidal cyst.

117. When obtaining the client's health history, which characteristic findings would the admitting nurse expect the client to report? Select all that apply.
[ ] **1.** A history of intermittent rectal bleeding
[ ] **2.** An open area near the coccyx that is draining
[ ] **3.** Frequent episodes of diarrhea
[ ] **4.** Baby-fine anorectal hair
[ ] **5.** Pain and swelling at the base of the spine
[ ] **6.** Frothy, foul-smelling stool

Before discharging the client, the nurse explains how to apply a nonprescription anesthetic ointment.

118. Which instruction regarding medication administration is essential for promoting the drug's local effect?
[ ] **1.** Use gloves when applying the ointment.
[ ] **2.** Store the ointment in the refrigerator.
[ ] **3.** Apply the ointment just before defecating.
[ ] **4.** Clean the area before applying the drug.

Nursing Care of Clients with Disorders of the Gallbladder

A 45-year-old client is suspected of having cholecystitis.

119. When describing the discomfort to the nurse, the client is most likely to indicate that the pain worsens at which time?
[ ] **1.** Shortly after eating
[ ] **2.** When the stomach is empty
[ ] **3.** After periods of activity
[ ] **4.** Before rising in the morning

120. If this client is typical of others with cholecystitis, besides localized pain, the client may describe feeling pain that is referred to which area?
[ ] **1.** Right shoulder
[ ] **2.** Midepigastrium
[ ] **3.** Neck or jaw
[ ] **4.** Left upper arm

121. If the cause of the client's inflamed gallbladder is gallstones, the nurse would anticipate the laboratory data to indicate which finding?
[ ] **1.** Low red blood cell count
[ ] **2.** Low hemoglobin level
[ ] **3.** Elevated cholesterol level
[ ] **4.** Elevated serum albumin level

122. If gallstones obstruct the flow of bile, how would the nurse expect the client's stools to appear?
[ ] **1.** Black and tarry
[ ] **2.** Light clay-colored
[ ] **3.** Brown with bloody mucus
[ ] **4.** Greenish yellow

123. When the dietitian has finished instructing the client about a low-fat diet, the nurse knows that the client requires additional teaching based on which statement?
[ ] **1.** "I can eat chicken that has been broiled."
[ ] **2.** "Because fish is good for me, I'll still get to eat a lot of baked fish."
[ ] **3.** "I can have a hamburger and fries when I go out with friends."
[ ] **4.** "I guess I'll eat more roasted turkey for dinner."

Because the client's gallbladder was unable to concentrate and excrete bile, it could not be visualized by cholecystography. The physician orders an ultrasound of the gallbladder. The nurse explains the scheduled procedure to the client.

124. Which comment indicates that the client has an accurate understanding of the preparation necessary for the procedure?
[ ] **1.** "Preparation involves withholding food for approximately 8 to 12 hours."
[ ] **2.** "I'll need to drink a container of barium just before the X-ray."
[ ] **3.** "I'll be allowed to eat a large test meal the night before the X-ray."
[ ] **4.** "Just before the test, they'll insert a large needle into one of my arm veins."

Ultrasound of the client's gallbladder reveals several stones in the common bile duct. A laparoscopic cholecystectomy is scheduled.

125. Which statements made by the nurse provide the best explanations of this procedure? Select all that apply.
[ ] **1.** "The procedure will require moderate sedation."
[ ] **2.** "The surgery will require a long period of gastric decompression."
[ ] **3.** "The abdomen will be inflated with carbon dioxide to provide a maximum view."
[ ] **4.** "There will be four small puncture sites."
[ ] **5.** "Most clients return home the evening after the procedure."
[ ] **6.** "A T-tube is inserted to drain bile until the surgical wound heals."

Another client comes to the clinic with signs and symptoms related to gallbladder disease but is not a candidate for a laparoscopic cholecystectomy. The surgeon schedules an open cholecystectomy.

The client returns from surgery with a nasogastric tube, a T-tube for bile drainage, and a Jackson-Pratt tube for wound drainage in place.

126. Immediately after surgery, the nurse assesses the drainage from the T-tube. Which assessment finding best indicates that the drainage color is normal at this time?
[ ] **1.** The drainage is dark red or pale pink.
[ ] **2.** The drainage is clear or transparent.
[ ] **3.** The drainage is bright red or orange.
[ ] **4.** The drainage is greenish yellow or brown.

127. The nurse is required to take which actions when emptying the drainage receptacle of the client's Jackson-Pratt closed-wound drain? Select all that apply.
[ ] **1.** Empty the drainage into a measuring container.
[ ] **2.** Adjust the suction setting to low continuous suction.
[ ] **3.** Squeeze the receptacle to expel air.
[ ] **4.** Release the roller clamp.
[ ] **5.** Cover the vent.
[ ] **6.** Stabilize the drainage tube.

128. The nurse should anticipate implementing which interventions to manage this client's T-tube? Select all that apply.
[ ] **1.** Record the amount of drainage from the T-tube.
[ ] **2.** Unclamp the T-tube at hourly intervals.
[ ] **3.** Keep the T-tube drainage bag parallel with the incision.
[ ] **4.** Inspect the skin around the tube for irritation.
[ ] **5.** Maintain the client in Fowler's position.
[ ] **6.** Notify the physician if the drainage changes color.

129. When the nurse assesses the T-tube in the early postoperative period, which finding requires immediate action?
[ ] **1.** The drainage bag is hanging below the abdomen.
[ ] **2.** The drainage tubing is currently clamped.
[ ] **3.** The drainage tube is taped to the client's right side.
[ ] **4.** The drainage volume was 100 mL in the past 6 hours.

130. When the client begins to consume food again, which routine for clamping and unclamping the T-tube should the nurse plan to follow?
[ ] **1.** Unclamp the tube during the day.
[ ] **2.** Unclamp the tube during the night.
[ ] **3.** Unclamp the tube for 2 hours after eating.
[ ] **4.** Unclamp the tube for 2 hours before eating.

131. How would the nurse reestablish negative pressure within the Jackson-Pratt tube when emptying the drainage bulb reservoir?
[ ] **1.** By compressing the bulb reservoir and closing the drainage valve
[ ] **2.** By opening the drainage valve, allowing the bulb to fill with air
[ ] **3.** By filling the bulb reservoir with sterile normal saline solution
[ ] **4.** By securing the bulb reservoir to the skin near the wound

Nursing Care of Clients with Disorders of the Liver

A 20-year-old college student goes to the university health service after developing a sudden onset of flulike symptoms.

132. When the health nurse monitors the client's laboratory test results, which elevated level would strongly suggest a possible liver disorder?
[ ] **1.** Serum potassium
[ ] **2.** Serum creatinine
[ ] **3.** Blood urea nitrogen (BUN)
[ ] **4.** Alanine aminotransferase (ALT)

The physician determines that the college student has hepatitis A.

133. When the client asks the nurse how the hepatitis A was acquired, what is the best answer?
[ ] **1.** Fecal-oral route
[ ] **2.** Insect carriers
[ ] **3.** Infected blood
[ ] **4.** Wound drainage

An infection control nurse is consulted on measures for reducing the potential transmission of the hepatitis A virus to others.

134. On the basis of the routes of transmission for this disease, which infection control measure is essential to include in the client's care plan?
[ ] **1.** Wear gloves whenever entering the client's room.
[ ] **2.** Don a mask and gown when providing direct care.
[ ] **3.** Maintain the client in a private room at all times.
[ ] **4.** Perform vigorous hand washing after leaving the room.

Several of the college student's friends call the health service because they are concerned about their own risks for acquiring hepatitis A.

135. To prevent the spread of hepatitis A, the nurse correctly advises that close contacts receive which medication?
[ ] **1.** An antibiotic
[ ] **2.** Serum immunoglobulin
[ ] **3.** Hepatitis vaccine
[ ] **4.** An anti-inflammatory drug

A 23-year-old develops jaundice and goes to the public health department. Testing reveals that the cause of the client's jaundice is hepatitis B. The nurse gathers information regarding the client's social history.

136. What information from the client's history indicates a predisposition for acquiring hepatitis B? Select all that apply.
[ ] **1.** The client moved from Europe.
[ ] **2.** The client is a sexually active homosexual.
[ ] **3.** The client abuses alcohol.
[ ] **4.** The client works in a restaurant.
[ ] **5.** The client has had a blood transfusion.
[ ] **6.** The client was punctured with an unused needle.

137. Which measure is most appropriate if a nurse who has not received a series of vaccinations for hepatitis B experiences a needle-stick injury while caring for this client?
[ ] **1.** Obtain immediate immunization with hepatitis B vaccine.
[ ] **2.** Receive hepatitis B immunoglobulin within 1 week.
[ ] **3.** Take penicillin (Pentam) for a minimum of 10 days.
[ ] **4.** Scrub the puncture site with diluted household bleach.

138. The nurse informs the client that because of the disease, it is essential to avoid which activity for life?
[ ] **1.** Sexual activity
[ ] **2.** Donating blood
[ ] **3.** Drinking alcohol
[ ] **4.** Traveling to foreign countries

A 60-year-old client seeks medical attention with symptoms of vomiting blood and passing bloody stools. The tentative diagnosis is cirrhosis of the liver.

139. Which information in the client's health history most likely relates to the development of cirrhosis? Select all that apply.
[ ] **1.** The client drinks a fifth of whiskey daily.
[ ] **2.** The client smokes two packs of cigarettes per day.
[ ] **3.** The client has a history of pancreatitis.
[ ] **4.** The client has been taking antihypertensive medications for the past 15 years.
[ ] **5.** The client eats poorly as a consequence of being homeless for 5 years.
[ ] **6.** The client has been exposed to asbestos.

140. If the client's cirrhosis is advanced, what will the nurse expect to find during the initial health assessment? Select all that apply.
[ ] **1.** Laboratory results revealing an elevated serum cholesterol level
[ ] **2.** The presence of spiderlike blood vessels on the skin
[ ] **3.** An unusually large and edematous abdomen
[ ] **4.** An abnormally high blood glucose level
[ ] **5.** Skin that is jaundiced
[ ] **6.** Vein engorgement around the umbilicus

141. Which assessment finding indicates that the client is bleeding from somewhere in the upper GI tract?
[ ] **1.** The client has midepigastric pain.
[ ] **2.** The client states, "I feel nauseated."
[ ] **3.** The client's stools are black and sticky.
[ ] **4.** The client's abdomen is distended and boardlike.

The physician considers performing a liver biopsy to confirm a diagnosis of cirrhosis.

142. If the liver biopsy is performed, the nurse must monitor the client immediately after the procedure for which potential complication?
[ ] **1.** Hemorrhage
[ ] **2.** Infection
[ ] **3.** Blood clots
[ ] **4.** Collapsed lung

143. After a liver biopsy, which nursing order is most appropriate to add to the client's care plan?
[ ] **1.** Ambulate the client twice each shift.
[ ] **2.** Keep the client in high Fowler's position.
[ ] **3.** Position the client on the right side.
[ ] **4.** Elevate the client's legs on two pillows.

The physician orders magnetic resonance imaging (MRI) instead of the liver biopsy to confirm the diagnosis.

144. Before the magnetic resonance imaging (MRI) study is performed, which nursing action is essential?
[ ] **1.** Administering a pretest sedative
[ ] **2.** Removing the client's dental bridge
[ ] **3.** Asking if the client is allergic to opiates
[ ] **4.** Inserting a Foley retention catheter

The care plan indicates that the nurse should monitor the client with cirrhosis each day for signs and symptoms of ascites.

145. To implement this nursing order, which nursing action is most appropriate?
[ ] **1.** Reviewing the client's serum bilirubin levels
[ ] **2.** Monitoring the client for vomiting and diarrhea
[ ] **3.** Pressing on the client's abdomen testing for rebound tenderness
[ ] **4.** Measuring the client's abdominal circumference

Magnetic resonance imaging (MRI) confirms the diagnosis of hepatic cirrhosis and reveals a large amount of fluid in the peritoneal cavity. A paracentesis is planned.

146. Which nursing action is most appropriate before assisting with the paracentesis?
[ ] **1.** Asking the client to void
[ ] **2.** Withholding food and water
[ ] **3.** Clipping hair from the client's abdomen
[ ] **4.** Placing the crash cart outside the client's room

147. After the paracentesis has been performed, which nursing responsibility is essential?
[ ] **1.** Increasing the client's oral fluid intake
[ ] **2.** Recording the volume of withdrawn fluid
[ ] **3.** Administering a prescribed analgesic
[ ] **4.** Encouraging the client to deep-breathe

148. While the nurse is assisting with a bed bath, a large erythemic area that does not blanch with pressure relief is noted on the client's right buttock. Further nursing assessment reveals that the impaired skin is shallowly abraded with the appearance of a ruptured blister in the center. At which stage would the nurse document this wound?
[ ] **1.** Stage I
[ ] **2.** Stage II
[ ] **3.** Stage III
[ ] **4.** Stage IV

The client's I.V. line has infiltrated and has to be removed and restarted in a new site. The licensed practical nurse (LPN) collaborates with the registered nurse (RN) about assisting with these procedures.

149. Which nursing action is most appropriately delegated to the LPN?
[ ] **1.** Clean the new insertion site with an antiseptic.
[ ] **2.** Flush the I.V. line with no more than 1 mL at any given time.
[ ] **3.** Obtain a vial of vitamin K to keep at the bedside.
[ ] **4.** Apply pressure to the old insertion site after I.V. removal.

150. Which laboratory result, if elevated, is most indicative that the client may develop hepatic encephalopathy?
[ ] **1.** Serum creatinine
[ ] **2.** Serum bilirubin
[ ] **3.** Blood ammonia
[ ] **4.** Blood urea nitrogen

151. Which assessment finding best indicates that the cirrhotic client's condition is worsening?
[ ] **1.** The client is difficult to arouse.
[ ] **2.** The client's urine output is 100 mL/hour.
[ ] **3.** The client develops pancreatitis.
[ ] **4.** The client's breath smells fruity.

The seriousness of the client's condition is explained to the client's spouse. The spouse is prepared for the possibility of the client's death.

152. When the client's spouse begins crying while recalling various significant events they shared together, which nursing action is most therapeutic at this time?
[ ] **1.** Offer to call a close family member.
[ ] **2.** Listen to the spouse's expressions of thoughts.
[ ] **3.** Suggest calling a clergyman from their church.
[ ] **4.** Ask about the spouse's future plans.

Nursing Care of Clients with Disorders of the Pancreas

A 48-year-old client comes to the emergency department because of severe upper abdominal pain. The client reports that the pain came on suddenly a few hours ago and nothing so far has relieved it. The nurse observes that the client is curled in a fetal position and is rocking back and forth. A diagnosis of acute pancreatitis is made.

153. Which action would best assist the nurse in further assessing the client's pain?
[ ] **1.** Determining if the client can stop moving
[ ] **2.** Asking the client to rate the pain from 0 to 10
[ ] **3.** Observing whether the client is breathing heavily
[ ] **4.** Giving the client a prescribed pain-relieving drug

154. Which laboratory test result, if elevated, provides the best indication that the client's pain is caused by pancreatitis?
[ ] **1.** Serum bilirubin
[ ] **2.** Serum amylase
[ ] **3.** Lactose tolerance
[ ] **4.** Glucose tolerance

155. The nurse closely watches the client for complications related to acute pancreatitis. Which complications pose the greatest risk for the client? Select all that apply.
[ ] **1.** Hyperglycemia
[ ] **2.** Necrosis of the pancreas
[ ] **3.** Peritonitis
[ ] **4.** Development of jaundice
[ ] **5.** Portal hypertension
[ ] **6.** Thrombocytopenia

The physician orders the insertion of a nasogastric (NG) sump tube and the client's fluid and nutritional needs are temporarily met by I.V. fluid.

156. While assessing the I.V. infusion, the nurse should report which finding immediately to the charge nurse?
[ ] **1.** The tubing is coiled on the top of the mattress.
[ ] **2.** The container has approximately 100 mL of fluid left.
[ ] **3.** The fluid is infusing into a vein in the client's non-dominant hand.
[ ] **4.** Less fluid than ordered has infused at this time.

After the client has been maintained on NPO (nothing by mouth) status for several days, the nasogastric (NG) tube is removed and the client is placed on a bland, low-fat diet.

157. Which food should the nurse remove from the client's breakfast tray?
[ ] **1.** Stewed prunes
[ ] **2.** Skim milk
[ ] **3.** Scrambled eggs
[ ] **4.** Whole-wheat toast

158. Before the client with acute pancreatitis is discharged from the hospital, which information is essential for the client to receive?
[ ] **1.** The client must never donate blood again.
[ ] **2.** The client must avoid lifting heavy objects.
[ ] **3.** The client must not drink alcohol in any form.
[ ] **4.** The client must forego taking strong laxatives.

A 69-year-old client is admitted with a diagnosis of cancer of the pancreas.

159. If this client is typical of most others who develop pancreatic cancer, the nurse would expect which early problem to be the one the client sought treatment for?
[ ] **1.** Sharp pain
[ ] **2.** Weight loss
[ ] **3.** Bleeding
[ ] **4.** Fainting

The physician meets with the client to provide information that the pancreatic cancer has metastasized, making aggressive treatment unrealistic. The client's condition is terminal.

160. The client asks the nurse, "Am I dying?" What is the best response from the nurse?
[ ] **1.** "Yes, you have little time left."
[ ] **2.** "No, you're not going to die."
[ ] **3.** "Tell me about how you are feeling."
[ ] **4.** "Is there someone you would like me to call?"

The client has an advance directive that requests no aggressive treatment. The client is referred for hospice care.

161. If the client has pain medication ordered every 3 to 4 hours as necessary, which action by the hospice nurse is most appropriate to promote maximum comfort at this time?
[ ] **1.** Give the medication immediately on request.
[ ] **2.** Administer the medication every 3 hours.
[ ] **3.** Ask the physician to prescribe a high dose.
[ ] **4.** Give the medication when the pain is severe.

Nursing Care of Clients with Culturally Diverse Backgrounds

A Jewish client is admitted to the hospital for signs and symptoms related to diverticulitis. As the nurse takes the client's admission history, dietary preferences are discussed.

162. If the client is an Orthodox Jew, which foods would be prohibited on the dietary tray? Select all that apply.
[ ] **1.** Pork chops
[ ] **2.** Shrimp
[ ] **3.** Coffee
[ ] **4.** Iced tea
[ ] **5.** Ham and cheese pizza
[ ] **6.** Strawberries

A Hispanic American client comes to the clinic with complaints of intestinal cramping and constipation that alternates with diarrhea. The nurse performs a cultural assessment and learns that the client has a strong belief in the hot-cold theory of diseases.

163. If the nurse understands the client's beliefs regarding the hot-cold theory and its effect on health and illness, which statement describing those beliefs is most accurate?
[ ] **1.** When healthy, the human body displays a balanced blending of hot and cold characteristics. Sickness results if an excess of hot or cold foods are ingested.
[ ] **2.** The terms *hot* and *cold* refer to the temperature of foods or remedies used to treat illness.
[ ] **3.** The physician's orders should include treatments similar to the nature of a person's illness.
[ ] **4.** The concept of hot and cold as it relates to health and illness is practiced widely in France, Russia, Spain, and among Native Americans

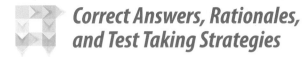

Correct Answers, Rationales, and Test Taking Strategies

Nursing Care of Clients with Disorders of the Mouth

1. 1, 4, 5. When the mucous membrane of the oral cavity is inflamed, it is best to eliminate foods that are acidic, salty, spicy, dry, or very hot. Cool, bland foods are more appropriate for clients with mucositis.

Test Taking Strategies—Analyze to determine what information the question asks for, which is foods that can irritate inflamed mucous membranes in the mouth. Alternative-format "select all that apply" questions require considering each option independently to decide its merit in answering the question. Choose options that identify food items that are likely to irritate or cause trauma to oral tissue that is already inflamed. Refer to a nutrition text and information about dietary recommendations for a client with mucositis if you had difficulty with this question.
Cognitive Level—Applying
Client Needs Category—Physiological integrity
Client Needs Subcategory—Basic care and comfort

2. 3. Oral swabs can clean plaque from the teeth, promote more comfort, and produce less irritation than a toothbrush—regardless of its size or type. Even a soft-bristled toothbrush may cause too much trauma. Normal saline mouth rinse is preferable to a flavored mouthwash. Flavoring may refresh the breath but irritate the mouth.

Test Taking Strategy—Use the process of elimination to choose the option that best identifies an item used to provide oral care that does not further injure the oral mucosa. Options 1 and 2 have bristles, which could lead to bleeding. Decide which is the better choice: option 3 or option 4. The sponge-tipped swab (option 3) would be gentle on the oral mucosa, making this choice the better option. Review oral care protocol if you had difficulty with this question.
Cognitive Level—Applying
Client Needs Category—Physiological integrity
Client Needs Subcategory—Basic care and comfort

3. 2. Clients who are limited in the amount of fluid they may consume need frequent mouth care. Limited hydration can reduce the volume of saliva, which helps keep the teeth clean and inhibits bacterial growth. A client with full dentures has the same oral hygiene needs as a person with natural teeth. A low-residue diet is one that reduces the volume of undigested substances in the bowel; the diet alone does not necessitate specialized oral hygiene. Sucking on ice chips is not an indication for modifying routine measures for oral hygiene.

Test Taking Strategy—Analyze to determine what information the question asks for, which is identifying the client who requires more frequent oral care from among the provided choices. A client whose fluid is restricted is likely to have dry mucous membranes, making frequent oral care a priority. Review indications for providing frequent oral care if you had difficulty answering this question.
Cognitive Level—Analyzing
Client Needs Category—Physiological integrity
Client Needs Subcategory—Basic care and comfort

4. 2, 5, 6. Gloves are always worn when coming in contact with a client's blood or body fluids (such as saliva). Holding dentures over a basin of water or a soft towel prevents them from breaking if they should slip from the nurse's hands. Turning the lower plate to a slight angle breaks the suction that holds the denture to the gum, making it easier to remove. Hot water may warp the plastic from which some dentures are made. Oral adhesives do not require a special solvent for removal. The adhesives usually rinse off easily with lukewarm water. When not being used, dentures are kept in water to retain their fit and color.

Test Taking Strategy—Analyze to determine what information the question asks for, which is appropriate steps to take when caring for dentures. Alternative-format "select all that apply" questions require considering each option independently to decide its merit in answering the question. Review oral and dental care procedures as they relate to dentures if you had difficulty with this question.
Cognitive Level—Applying
Client Needs Category—Physiological integrity
Client Needs Subcategory—Basic care and comfort

5. 2. When administering oral hygiene to an unconscious client, the nurse should place the client on the side with the head slightly lowered and tilted toward the mattress. This is the best position for preventing aspiration. Because the unconscious client cannot swallow, this position allows the fluid to run out of the mouth instead of pooling in the back of the throat. Trendelenburg's position, in which the client's legs and feet are higher than the head, is used for treating shock victims; it is inappropriate for oral hygiene. A client in the dorsal recumbent position is placed supine flat, with the knees bent and feet flat on the mattress. Because the client is flat, the risk for aspiration is greater in this position.

Test Taking Strategy—Analyze to determine what information the question asks for, which is the proper position for an unconscious client when providing oral care. When you think of the oral care of an unconscious client, think of the high risk for aspiration. Eliminate any option in which fluids could potentially enter the trachea and lungs (options 1, 3, and 4) due to safety concerns. Note that option 2,

a head-down position, makes use of gravity to keep liquids in the mouth. Review oral care for unconscious clients if you had difficulty answering this question.
Cognitive Level—*Applying*
Client Needs Category—*Safe and effective care environment*
Client Needs Subcategory—*Safety and infection control*

6. 3. Candidiasis (thrush) is a fungal infection that appears as small white patches resembling milk curds on the mucous membranes of the mouth and tongue. Candidiasis often occurs when antibiotic therapy destroys the normal flora of the body, which then allows yeast/fungi to grow. Immunosuppression, such as occurs in clients with acquired immunodeficiency syndrome (AIDS) or cancer, may also result in candidiasis. Red, ulcerated patches near the margin of the teeth and gums are characteristic of gingivitis. Herpes simplex lesions—clear, raised vesicles that transform into shallow ulcers—are not restricted to the tongue.
> **Test Taking Strategy**—*Analyze to determine what information the question asks for, which is the appearance of candidal lesions. Recall that the symptoms of candidiasis (thrush) are a result of a fungal infection caused by the organism Candida albicans. The word albicans is a derivative of the Latin word alba, which means "white." Fungal infections in both the oral cavity and vagina are characterized as having small white patches. Review the characteristics of mucosal infections involving Candida albicans if you had difficulty answering this question.*
Cognitive Level—*Applying*
Client Needs Category—*Physiological integrity*
Client Needs Subcategory—*Physiological adaptation*

7. 2. Antibiotic therapy can upset the balance of organisms in the body, allowing some natural microbes to grow unchecked. Candidiasis is considered an opportunistic infection because the source of the infection is usually the client. It is unlikely that the client would acquire candidiasis from soiled dental instruments because most dentists follow guidelines for sterilizing their equipment between uses. Candidiasis is usually not transmitted by eating or drinking from someone's unclean utensils, especially if the person has a normal immune system. Because the organisms are present in the mouth, it is possible, but highly improbable, that the infection could be acquired by inhaling respiratory droplets from another individual.
> **Test Taking Strategy**—*Analyze to determine what information the question asks for, which is the source of candidiasis. Knowledge of the subject and understanding of opportunistic infections are essential for answering the question correctly. Once that is understood, the basis for the candidiasis leads*

to selecting option 2 as the correct answer. Review common opportunistic infections if you had difficulty answering this question.
Cognitive Level—*Understanding*
Client Needs Category—*Physiological integrity*
Client Needs Subcategory—*Physiological adaptation*

8. 3. Because nystatin (Mycostatin) is poorly absorbed from the GI tract, holding the liquid suspension in the mouth as long as possible facilitates contact of the drug with the organism. The client is allowed to swallow the medication after swishing it around. There is no need to use a straw or to dilute the medication in this instance. Brushing the teeth will remove the medication from the mouth, causing the medication to be ineffective.
> **Test Taking Strategy**—*Analyze to determine what information the question asks for, which is the proper use of nystatin. Considering that the medication's intended action is within the oral cavity, options 1 and 4 can be eliminated because a straw would divert the medication away from the mucosa, as would brushing the teeth. Eliminate option 2 because diluting the medication would reduce its effectiveness. Option 3 keeps the medication in contact with the infection as long as possible and is the best choice. Review the recommendations for administering nystatin oral suspension if you had difficulty answering this question.*
Cognitive Level—*Applying*
Client Needs Category—*Physiological integrity*
Client Needs Subcategory—*Pharmacological therapies*

9. 2. Factors that predispose the client to cancer of the mouth include any source of chronic irritation, such as holding a pipe in the mouth, holding chewing or smokeless tobacco in the mouth, alcohol consumption, or prolonged contact with rough dental appliances. Lip cancer is related to prolonged sun or wind exposure. Smoking marijuana as a teenager is unlikely to be the cause of the client's mouth cancer at this time. Medical complications associated with marijuana use include an increased risk of chronic cough, bronchitis, and emphysema, as well as increased risk of cancer of the head, neck, and lungs. Likewise, exposure to asbestos is related to lung cancer rather than mouth cancer. Poor dental hygiene and decaying teeth are not usually risk factors predisposing the client to cancer of the mouth. However, poor oral and dental hygiene may worsen cancerous lesions.
> **Test Taking Strategy**—*Look at the key words "most likely" in reference to a contributing factor in the development of oral cancer. Recall that the chronic use of smokeless tobacco places carcinogens in direct contact with the oral mucosa. Over time, oral tissues can undergo neoplastic malignant changes. Of the four options, option 2 identifies a common risk factor for oral cancer. Review common etiolo-*

gies associated with oral cancer if you had difficulty answering this question.
Cognitive Level—*Analyzing*
Client Needs Category—*Physiological integrity*
Client Needs Subcategory—*Physiological adaptation*

10. **2, 3, 4, 6.** The three main objectives for clients who are recovering from oral cancer surgery include maintaining a patent airway, promoting nutrition, and supporting communication. The client should be positioned with the head of the bed elevated (not flat), making it easier to breathe and cough up secretions and reducing edema. Because the client's tongue may be affected or partially removed, assessing the client's ability to speak is important. The nurse may need to provide alternative forms of communication if the client's speech is unable to be understood. Irrigation of the oral cavity is essential to remove old blood and tissue debris and to keep the surgical site clean. Although providing ice chips is usually common after surgery, in the case of a client recovering from oral cancer surgery, hot and cold foods are to be avoided because of the sensitivity of the oral tissues and teeth. Before giving any fluids, the nurse must assess the client's ability to swallow because pooling of saliva in the mouth and drooling are common in the postoperative period. Clients recovering from oral cancer surgery should be observed for signs of depression related to disfigurement, loss of communication skills, inability to eat and drink normally, and loss of health related to the cancer itself and further cancer treatment.

> *Test Taking Strategy*—*Analyze to determine what information the question asks for, which is the priority nursing interventions after oral cancer surgery. Alternative-format "select all that apply" questions require considering each option independently to decide its merit in answering the question. Evaluate each option in relation to protecting the airway, incisional care, and the client's coping status. Review information about managing the care of a client undergoing oral surgery if you had difficulty with this question.*
> **Cognitive Level**—*Applying*
> **Client Needs Category**—*Physiological integrity*
> **Client Needs Subcategory**—*Reduction of risk potential*

11. **1, 4, 5.** Radiation therapy is used to destroy cancer cells. It can be external or internal. Common side effects related to radiation therapy include alopecia (hair loss), erythema/redness (not paleness) and inflammation at the site, fatigue rather than restlessness, and alterations of the oral mucosa, including stomatitis (inflammation of the mouth) and xerostomia (dry mouth). Confusion is not a side effect of radiation therapy. Other common side effects of radiation therapy include nausea, vomiting and diarrhea, loss of appetite, and bone marrow suppression.

> *Test Taking Strategy*—*Analyze to determine what information the question asks for, which are potential side effects of radiation therapy. Alternative-format "select all that apply" questions require considering each option independently to decide its merit in answering the question. Evaluate each option to determine if it is a potential side effect of radiation therapy. Select all options that are expected side effects; note those specific to the treatment area, in this case the mouth. Review the physiological effects of radiation therapy, especially that directed at the mouth, if you had difficulty answering this question.*
> **Cognitive Level**—*Applying*
> **Client Needs Category**—*Physiological integrity*
> **Client Needs Subcategory**—*Physiological adaptation*

12. **4.** The herpes simplex virus causes herpes simplex type 1 infection, and lesions can appear on the face, cheeks, nose, lips, or in the perioral (mouth) area. When erupting, these vesicles are painful, weep, and eventually crust over. Most nonclinicians refer to these lesions as *cold sores* or *fever blisters*. The herpes virus remains latent until activated or triggered by stress, sunlight, or fever. The incubation period is usually 2 to 12 days, and transmission is by direct contact. Therefore, hand washing and good personal hygiene are used during the time the virus is replicating and being shed. Usually, herpes simplex type 1 lesions heal in 10 to 14 days.

> *Test Taking Strategy*—*Analyze to determine what information the question asks for, which is characteristics of herpes simplex virus type 1 infection. This question indicates that the client made an incorrect statement regarding the herpes simplex virus infection that the nurse must correct; therefore, evaluate each option for misinformation. Option 4 incorrectly asserts that the lesions appear only on the lips. Review herpes simplex type 1 virus infections if you had difficulty answering this question.*
> **Cognitive Level**—*Analyzing*
> **Client Needs Category**—*Physiological integrity*
> **Client Needs Subcategory**—*Physiological adaptation*

13. **2.** Acyclovir (Zovirax) does not cure the herpes infection or prevent future outbreaks. It only shortens the time during which the virus is replicating and being shed. Some of the virus retreats within nerve fibers and escapes detection by the body's immune system, where it remains dormant until stimulated. The drug may be administered orally or topically. Oral acyclovir is taken when the client first becomes aware of symptoms, such as an area of itching, pain, or tingling on the mucous membrane. Oral doses are generally taken for 10 days.

> *Test Taking Strategy*—*Analyze to determine what information the question asks for, which is a correct statement regarding treatment with acyclovir. Recall that acyclovir inhibits DNA replication in the virus,*

thus shortening the duration of the outbreak. Review antiviral therapy, specifically therapy with acyclovir, if you had difficulty answering this question.
Cognitive Level—*Analyzing*
Client Needs Category—*Physiological integrity*
Client Needs Subcategory—*Pharmacological therapies*

Nursing Care of Clients with Disorders of the Esophagus

14. 3. An esophagoscopy is a diagnostic test that involves passing a flexible fiberoptic tube down the esophagus. Food and fluids are avoided to reduce the potential for aspiration. Therefore, the client should be NPO (nothing by mouth) after midnight. After the procedure, the nurse should wait for the gag reflex to return before giving the client any food or fluid.

Test Taking Strategy—Analyze to determine what information the question asks for, which is steps to take when preparing for an esophagoscopy. Identify the option that is a correct statement regarding test preparation. Recall that many diagnostic tests require that the client avoid food and fluids after midnight. Review preparation procedure for an esophagoscopy if you had difficulty with this question.
Cognitive Level—*Analyzing*
Client Needs Category—*Physiological integrity*
Client Needs Subcategory—*Reduction of risk potential*

15. 2. Taking smaller bites and chewing food thoroughly help the bolus slip through the narrowed stricture. Switching to thickened food or a full liquid diet is too drastic at this time. Drinking liquids throughout a meal is beneficial in thinning the bolus of food and should be encouraged.

Test Taking Strategy—Look at the key words "most appropriate" as they relate to promoting food consumption when there is a stricture in the esophagus. Eliminate option 1 because thickener is applied to fluids only, rather than a variety of foods. Options 3 and 4 are opposites and are both inappropriate because fluids help to thin foods to pass through the stricture, and the diagnosis does not require a fluid diet. Review nursing actions to improve client swallowing ability if you had difficulty with this question.
Cognitive Level—*Applying*
Client Needs Category—*Physiological integrity*
Client Needs Subcategory—*Basic care and comfort*

16. 4. Esophageal varices are dilated, twisted veins found in the lower esophagus. The condition is usually related to portal hypertension from cirrhosis of the liver. Chronic consumption of alcohol can damage the liver and interfere with blood flow from the esophagus and other abdominal organs. Esophageal veins distend and bleed because of the portal hypertension created by the stagnation of blood. Attempted suicide using lye will cause damage to the esophagus, but this damage is not called *esophageal varices*. Oral cancer has no correlation with esophageal varices. Hemophilia is a hereditary bleeding disorder; however, it is not the cause of the bleeding esophageal varices. Bleeding esophageal varices are life-threatening and can result in shock or death.

Test Taking Strategy—Look at the key words "most likely" in reference to a factor that relates to bleeding esophageal varices. Recall that esophageal varices, cirrhosis of the liver, and portal hypertension are commonly related to chronic alcohol consumption. Review the pathophysiology of esophageal varices if you had difficulty answering this question.
Cognitive Level—*Analyzing*
Client Needs Category—*Physiological integrity*
Client Needs Subcategory—*Physiological adaptation*

17. 1. The National Patient Safety Goals were developed by The Joint Commission as a way of ensuring safe client care in the clinical setting. One of the National Patient Safety Goals deals with client identification when administering blood. To be in compliance with the established goals, two licensed personnel must review the blood bag itself for the correct blood type, date, and time, as well as checking the client's individual blood tags and arm bracelet before any blood product can be administered. The process must take place at the client's bedside, not at the nurse's station. If there is a discrepancy, the blood cannot be given. In most circumstances, the registered nurse (RN) is responsible for starting the blood infusion while the licensed practical nurse (LPN) monitors the client during the procedure. None of the other options is related to the National Patient Safety Goals. An indwelling (Foley) catheter is not needed during a blood transfusion. Most blood should be infused with an 18- to 20-gauge needle so the blood cells will not be damaged during infusion. Blood transfusions should be completed within 4 hours of starting to prevent bacterial growth.

Test Taking Strategy—Look at the key words "most appropriate" in reference to patient safety goals and blood administration. Having two nurses identify the client and review the blood tag meets the safety goal. No other option meets a safety goal. Review the procedure for administering blood to a client if you had difficulty answering this question.
Cognitive Level—*Applying*
Client Needs Category—*Safe and effective care environment*
Client Needs Subcategory—*Safety and infection control*

18. 2. Dyspnea, hypotension, chest constriction, tachycardia, and back pain are some of the major symptoms associated with an incompatibility transfusion reaction—a life-threatening reaction. The other assessment findings are signs and symptoms associated with hypovolemia, most likely resulting from the client's blood loss.

> *Test Taking Strategy—Use the process of elimination and recall the signs of a transfusion reaction. If unsure, consider that blood incompatibilities are life-threatening, and critically think through potential systemic effects. Review the complications of blood administration and the signs of transfusion reactions, particularly an incompatibility reaction, if you had difficulty with this question.*
> **Cognitive Level**—*Analyzing*
> **Client Needs Category**—*Physiological integrity*
> **Client Needs Subcategory**—*Pharmacological therapies*

19. 4. Gastroesophageal reflux disease (GERD) results when a weakened area of the diaphragm enables a portion of the stomach to protrude into the esophagus. The acid contents of the stomach reflux into the esophagus, causing irritation and inflammation, which the client describes as heartburn. Other symptoms include belching, epigastric pressure, and pain after eating and when lying down.

> *Test Taking Strategy—Analyze to determine what information the question asks for, which is the most common complaint associated with GERD. Options 1 and 2 can be eliminated as being similar, and option 3 can be eliminated because it is not characteristic of GERD. Review the signs and symptoms of GERD if you had difficulty answering this question.*
> **Cognitive Level**—*Understanding*
> **Client Needs Category**—*Physiological integrity*
> **Client Needs Subcategory**—*Physiological adaptation*

20. 3. Sitting in an upright position for at least 2 hours after eating keeps swallowed food and gastric contents within the stomach by means of gravity. The client with a hiatal hernia should also be encouraged to sleep with the head of the bed elevated and to eat small, frequent meals to avoid overdistending the stomach. Drinking room-temperature liquids has no effect on relieving the discomfort associated with gastroesophageal reflux disease (GERD).

> *Test Taking Strategy—Analyze to determine what information the question asks for, which is the best instruction to relieve the chief symptom of heartburn. Eliminate options 1, 2, and 4 because they all suggest food or fluid interventions and are comparable. Review the pathophysiology of GERD if you had difficulty answering this question.*
> **Cognitive Level**—*Applying*
> **Client Needs Category**—*Health promotion and maintenance*
> **Client Needs Subcategory**—*None*

21. 4. Elevating the head of the bed helps to prevent gastric reflux. This is a therapeutic intervention in gastroesophageal reflux disease (GERD).

> *Test Taking Strategy—Look at the key words "most appropriate" in reference to a position that relieves symptoms of GERD. Because GERD is the backflow of gastric contents, option 4 is the only option that would accomplish the goal. Review the interventions that relieve GERD if you had difficulty answering this question.*
> **Cognitive Level**—*Applying*
> **Client Needs Category**—*Health promotion and maintenance*
> **Client Needs Subcategory**—*None*

22. 2. It is essential to monitor the blood glucose level frequently because total parenteral nutrition (TPN) solutions contain high concentrations of glucose. Insulin coverage may be needed to maintain the blood glucose level within an acceptable range. The specific gravity may become lower if the client begins to excrete large volumes of urine, but it is not generally monitored. Pulse pressure, the difference between the systolic and diastolic arterial pressure measurements, is usually unaffected by TPN. There is no need to monitor apical and radial pulses in relation to the TPN.

> *Test Taking Strategy—Analyze to determine what information the question asks for, which is the need to identify an essential assessment to evaluate the response of a client receiving TPN. Recall that blood glucose levels are directly affected by the components of TPN, making option 2 the best choice. Review the physiological effects of administering TPN if you had difficulty answering this question.*
> **Cognitive Level**—*Analyzing*
> **Client Needs Category**—*Physiological integrity*
> **Client Needs Subcategory**—*Reduction of risk potential*

23. 2. Gradual, steady weight gain is one of the best ways to tell that a client is responding favorably to total parenteral nutrition (TPN). If laboratory reports are monitored daily, the client's electrolytes should be adjusted based on the results; therefore, they should be in balance. However, a balance in electrolytes does not necessarily indicate that the client is responding favorably to TPN. Hunger is an emotional and physical phenomenon. Even well-nourished, satiated people can feel hungry when they see, smell, or even think about food. Therefore, return of the client's appetite does not indicate that TPN is successful. If the TPN is infusing according to the physician's orders, the client's fluids should be in balance with normal urine output. Voiding clear yellow urine, however, is not an indication of the TPN itself, but of the amount of fluids that is being infused.

> *Test Taking Strategy—Use the process of elimination to help select the option that provides the best outcome to TPN administration. Option 2, weight gain or at least preventing weight loss, reflects the goal of providing nutrition that meets the client's metabolic*

*needs. Review the purposes for administering TPN if
you had difficulty answering this question.*
Cognitive Level—*Evaluating*
Client Needs Category—*Physiological integrity*
Client Needs Subcategory—*Basic care and comfort*

24. **2.** Slight pinkish (serosanguineous) bleeding or clear
serous drainage at the gastrostomy site is a normal finding immediately after a gastrostomy has been performed.
Milky drainage suggests an infection; drainage occurring
after feedings have been initiated may indicate leakage of
formula. Intestinal secretions cause green-tinged drainage,
but the gastrostomy is located in the client's stomach, not
intestines. Bright, bloody drainage indicates arterial bleeding, which is not a normal finding.

> **Test Taking Strategy**—*Analyze to determine what
> information the question asks for, which is an
> expected characteristic of drainage immediately
> after insertion of a gastrostomy tube. Recall that a
> gastrostomy tube is inserted percutaneously and that
> there will likely be some temporary bleeding. Using
> this rationale, options 1, 3, and 4 can be eliminated;
> they are associated with either an infection or place-
> ment of the tube in an area other than the stomach.
> Review the procedure for gastrostomy tube insertion
> and care if you had difficulty with this question.*
> **Cognitive Level**—*Applying*
> **Client Needs Category**—*Physiological integrity*
> **Client Needs Subcategory**—*Reduction of risk potential*

25. **3.** Comparing the measured length of tubing extending from the gastrostomy site is an easy and appropriate
technique for determining tube migration. A change in
pH from acid to alkaline indicates intestinal migration,
but most gastrostomy tubes are too short to reach the
small intestine. X-rays are expensive and expose clients to
unnecessary radiation. A distended abdomen may indicate
many complications, but tube migration is not one of them.

> **Test Taking Strategy**—*Use the process of elimination to
> help select the option that identifies the best method
> for determining migration of a gastrostomy tube.
> The word migration indicates that the tube is either
> further inward or outward than when originally
> inserted. Option 3 is the best assessment finding
> because it determines the gastrostomy tube's length
> outside the abdomen. Review the nursing care of a
> client with a gastrostomy tube if you had difficulty
> answering this question.*
> **Cognitive Level**—*Applying*
> **Client Needs Category**—*Physiological integrity*
> **Client Needs Subcategory**—*Basic care and comfort*

26. **4 hours.**
Each ounce equals 30 mL. Therefore, 8 ounces equal
240 mL. It will take a total of 4 hours to instill 480 mL
(two 8-ounce cans) at a rate of 120 mL/hour.

> **Test Taking Strategy**—*Analyze to determine what
> information the question asks for; this is a dos-
> age calculation problem that requires converting
> equivalents of ounces to milliliters to determine the
> total time of the infusion. Refer to a pharmacology
> text for equivalent measurements if you had difficulty
> calculating the answer.*
> **Cognitive Level**—*Applying*
> **Client Needs Category**—*Physiological integrity*
> **Client Needs Subcategory**—*Basic care and comfort*

27. **3, 5.** It is important that the stomach not become
overdistended. Temporarily stopping the infusion will
allow the remaining formula in the stomach to be digested.
This will decrease the client's feeling of fullness. Repositioning the client onto the right side may also assist with
faster gastric emptying and decrease the client's feelings of
fullness. The stomach residual is checked before administering an intermittent feeding. As a general rule, the gastric
residual should be no more than 150 mL of the previous
intermittent feeding or, if continuous, no more than half
of the previous hour's infusion volume. Administering
an antiemetic will stop the nausea, but this is not the best
choice at this time. Adding water to formula adds more
volume and dilutes the nutrients. It is too early to request
a change in types of formula, but the nurse should closely
monitor the client's tolerance for the next day or so.

> **Test Taking Strategy**—*Analyze to determine what
> information the question asks for, which is nurs-
> ing actions to alleviate nausea in the client with a
> gastrostomy tube. Alternative-format "select all that
> apply" questions require considering each option
> independently to decide its merit in answering the
> question. Select options in which nursing actions
> diminish feelings of fullness and nausea. Review
> nursing actions related to the administration of for-
> mula through a gastrostomy tube if you had difficulty
> answering this question.*
> **Cognitive Level**—*Applying*
> **Client Needs Category**—*Physiological integrity*
> **Client Needs Subcategory**—*Basic care and comfort*

28. **4.** The nurse should rinse the feeding tube after each
use to maintain its patency and to meet the client's needs
for water. To prevent aspiration, the head of the bed should
always be elevated during and for at least a half hour after
a tube feeding. The client's head should also be turned to
the side to allow regurgitated formula and saliva to drain
from the mouth. Gastrostomy tubes may be clamped intermittently, but only after they have been rinsed with water.

> **Test Taking Strategy**—*Note the word "next" in the
> stem. Identify the correct action that should be
> completed first. Option 2 can be eliminated because
> it jeopardizes the client's safety. Options 1, 3, and
> 4 are appropriate actions, but option 4 represents
> the next action to perform in the sequence. Review*

nursing actions related to the care of a gastrostomy tube if you had difficulty with this question.
Cognitive Level—*Applying*
Client Needs Category—*Physiological integrity*
Client Needs Subcategory—*Basic care and comfort*

29. 2. In this case, sharing perceptions or validating the client's emotions is the best therapeutic communication technique for encouraging a discussion of feelings. Most clients tend to deny feeling angry or depressed if asked a direct question. Asking questions that have "yes-no" responses is not therapeutic because this does not encourage the client to elaborate on feelings. Telling the client that the situation may improve offers false reassurance and may cause the client to lose trust in the nurse's ability to be supportive. Knowing that many other clients are nourished by tube feedings will not necessarily make it easier for the client to cope with the situation.

> *Test Taking Strategy—Look at the key words "most appropriate" in relation to a communication technique that encourages the expression of feelings. Questions in which the nurse's goal is to promote a client's verbalization require therapeutic communication techniques such as sharing perceptions and open-ended questions. Review therapeutic and nontherapeutic communication techniques if you had difficulty with this question.*
Cognitive Level—*Applying*
Client Needs Category—*Psychosocial integrity*
Client Needs Subcategory—*None*

30. 1. Gastrostomy tubes may become obstructed with formula residue and remnants of medication, which is why the tube should be flushed with water after each use. Cola, a common household beverage, provides effervescence and acidity to break through the solidified substance interfering with the flow of fluid. Using sterile water is not necessary because the GI tract is not sterile, but instilling warm water is an alternative. Milking the tube may be attempted, but this is typically ineffective. Suction is never applied to a gastrostomy tube.

> *Test Taking Strategy—Use the process of elimination to help select the best instruction from among the options provided for eliminating an obstruction within a gastrostomy tube. Option 4 can be eliminated immediately because a gastrostomy tube is used to instill formula, water, and medications; it is not used to remove secretions. Option 2 can be eliminated because using sterile water is not appropriate. Discriminate between options 1 and 3. Option 1 is the best option because cola may disintegrate an obstructing substance. Review suggestions for eliminating an obstruction in a gastrostomy tube if you had difficulty answering this question.*
Cognitive Level—*Applying*
Client Needs Category—*Physiological integrity*
Client Needs Subcategory—*Physiological adaptation*

Nursing Care of Clients with Disorders of the Stomach

31. 3. Clients with peptic ulcers generally find that eating relieves their discomfort. The pain is caused by irritation of the eroded mucosa by hydrochloric acid and pepsin. Food tends to dilute the acid, thereby raising the pH of the secretions. This reduces irritation of the ulcerated tissue. Skipping a meal increases the pain because the acid secretions become concentrated. Many ulcer clients report awakening at night with pain. Vomiting does not cause or relieve the discomfort associated with an ulcer.

> *Test Taking Strategy—Analyze to determine what information the question asks for, which is an understanding of the source of the pain of a peptic ulcer. Recall that the gastric and duodenal mucosa is chemically eroded in a client with a peptic ulcer and that the presence of food provides something other than the mucosa for the hydrochloric acid and pepsin to act on. Review the pathophysiology of peptic ulcers if you had difficulty answering this question.*
Cognitive Level—*Applying*
Client Needs Category—*Physiological integrity*
Client Needs Subcategory—*Physiological adaptation*

32. 3. Blood in the stool is a significant finding of peptic ulcer disease. Its presence indicates that bleeding is occurring within the GI tract. If bleeding occurs in the upper GI tract, the stool appears thick, black, and tarry. This finding is called *melena*. However, blood may be present without an obvious change in the normal color of stool, a finding referred to as *occult blood*. Although identifying blood in the stool is not proof that the client has a peptic ulcer, it aids in the differential diagnosis. Albumin in the urine is associated with renal disease. An elevated blood glucose level may be due to diabetes mellitus. Emesis is not tested for the presence of pepsin.

> *Test Taking Strategy—Analyze to determine what information the question asks for, which is a laboratory finding that supports the hypothesis that the client's symptoms are ulcer related. Because a peptic ulcer is often associated with bleeding from the ulcer site, option 3 is the only option that indicates a relationship with the GI tract. Review tests used to diagnose peptic ulcers if you had difficulty answering this question.*
Cognitive Level—*Applying*
Client Needs Category—*Physiological integrity*
Client Needs Subcategory—*Physiological adaptation*

33. 4. An upper GI X-ray uses barium as a contrast medium. Once ingested by the client, this opaque substance fills the hollow structures of the esophagus and stomach, improving their imaging.

> *Test Taking Strategy—Use the process of elimination to help select the option that identifies correct*

information regarding an upper GI X-ray. Recall that contrast media, such as barium, are necessary to provide the best image of the hollow organs within the GI tract and that the medium can be delivered to the upper GI tract most easily by having the client swallow it. Option 1 can be eliminated because a flexible tube is used for a gastroscopy, not an upper GI procedure. Option 2 can be eliminated because the contrast is swallowed, not introduced through a vein, and option 3 describes a computed tomography scan, not an upper GI study. Review the upper GI X-ray procedure if you had difficulty answering this question.
Cognitive Level—*Analyzing*
Client Needs Category—*Physiological integrity*
Client Needs Subcategory—*Physiological adaptation*

34. **2,580 mg.**
The total number of milligrams per day for all three medications is 2,580. The calculation is as follows:

Biaxin 500 mg t.i.d.	=	$500 \times 3 = 1{,}500$ mg
Flagyl 250 mg q.i.d.	=	$250 \times 4 = 1{,}000$ mg
Prilosec 40 mg b.i.d.	=	$40 \times 2 = 80$ mg
Total	=	2,580 mg

Test Taking Strategy—*Analyze to determine what information the question asks for; this is a dosage calculation problem that first requires interpreting the abbreviations that indicate the frequency for administering the prescribed medications. Once the frequency is determined, the number of milligrams can be added together to find the total. Refer to a pharmacology text for the meaning of abbreviations denoting frequency if you had difficulty calculating the answer.*
Cognitive Level—*Understanding*
Client Needs Category—*Physiological integrity*
Client Needs Subcategory—*Pharmacological therapies*

35. **2.** Antibiotics such as clarithromycin (Biaxin) eliminate *Helicobacter pylori*, the bacterium that depletes gastric mucus and causes the majority of peptic ulcers. Although antibiotics may ultimately heal the irritated mucous membrane of the stomach, this is not the primary reason for giving such drugs. Antibiotics neither coat the stomach nor are prescribed to prevent secondary infections in the case of ulcers.
Test Taking Strategy—*Analyze to determine what information the question asks for, which is the relationship between antibiotics and the bacterium known to cause ulcers. Review the cluster of drugs used to eradicate peptic ulcers caused by a bacterial infection if you had difficulty answering this question.*

Cognitive Level—*Applying*
Client Needs Category—*Physiological integrity*
Client Needs Subcategory—*Pharmacological therapies*

36. **1.** Acetaminophen (Tylenol) is not associated with gastritis or ulcer formation; therefore, this drug would be safest to take. Salicylates such as aspirin (Anacin) and nonsteroidal anti-inflammatory drugs, such as ibuprofen (Advil) and naproxen (Naprosyn), are closely linked to gastric irritation and ulcer formation and should be avoided. This link is well documented.
Test Taking Strategy—*Look at the key words "most appropriate" in relation to an analgesic that has the least potential for harm when taken by a client who has an ulcer. Recall the side effects of the listed medications and their effects on the disease process. Because acetaminophen (option 1) is not associated with gastric irritation that could lead to bleeding, clients with ulcers can safely take it rather than the drugs listed in options 2, 3, and 4. Review the side effects of the medications listed if you had difficulty answering this question.*
Cognitive Level—*Analyzing*
Client Needs Category—*Physiological integrity*
Client Needs Subcategory—*Pharmacological therapies*

37. **2.** When the stomach or other GI structure perforates, the abdomen becomes very hard, rigid, and tender. The skin becomes pale, not ecchymotic, due to vasoconstriction associated with shock. Dilated pupils are due to a variety of causes and do not necessarily relate to perforation. Rapid respirations can be associated with pain but are not as significant as a tense abdomen.
Test Taking Strategy—*Use the process of elimination to help select the option that provides the best indication that an ulcer has perforated. Recall that a perforation releases GI contents into the abdomen, causing the abdomen to become hard, rigid, and tender, which corresponds to option 2. Option 1 can be eliminated because it is incorrect; the skin becomes pale rather than ecchymotic. Options 3 and 4 are not specifically related to perforation. Review the signs and symptoms of ulcer perforation if you had difficulty answering this question.*
Cognitive Level—*Applying*
Client Needs Category—*Physiological integrity*
Client Needs Subcategory—*Physiological adaptation*

38. **4.** The distance from the nose (N) to the earlobe (E) to the xiphoid (X) is called the *NEX measurement*. It is commonly used to determine the approximate distance to the stomach. None of the other landmarks is correct for approximating the length for nasogastric (NG) tube insertion.
Test Taking Strategy—*Analyze to determine what information the question asks for, which is the procedure for measuring the length to which an NG*

tube should be inserted. Recall the preliminary steps of measuring and marking the length of the tubing, beginning with the nose to the ear and ending at the xiphoid process; this will provide an estimate for the unique size of the client. Review the meaning of a NEX measurement if you had difficulty answering this question.
Cognitive Level—*Remembering*
Client Needs Category—*Physiological integrity*
Client Needs Subcategory—*Reduction of risk potential*

39. 3. Placing the chin to the chest helps to direct the tube into the esophagus rather than the lower airway. The client is given water to sip, which makes breathing deeply difficult. A sniffing position is appropriate when first inserting the tube into a client's nose. Coughing occurs as a reflex if the tube enters the airway; it is a helpful sign that the tube is in the wrong location.
Test Taking Strategy—*Analyze to determine what information the question asks for, which is the position that facilitates correct placement of an NG tube. Recall that flexing the chin (option 3) alters the passageway to the respiratory tract and avoids incorrectly placing the tube in that location. Review how to facilitate inserting an NG tube within the stomach rather than the airway if you had difficulty answering this question.*
Cognitive Level—*Applying*
Client Needs Category—*Physiological integrity*
Client Needs Subcategory—*Reduction of risk potential*

40.

4. Inspect the nares to determine which should be used.
6. Ask the client to tilt the neck to simulate a sniffing position.
3. Have the client lower the chin.
1. Instruct the client to sip water as the tube is inserted.
2. Aspirate fluid from the stomach.
5. Secure the NG tube to the nose.

The nares are inspected to determine which to use for tube insertion; in most cases, either may be suitable.
To minimize trauma to the nasal mucosa, the client's neck is then hyperextended to simulate a sniffing position. Once the tube is visualized in the oropharynx, the client is instructed to lower the chin to the chest to facilitate advancing the tube into the esophagus and stomach rather than into the airway. The client is instructed to sip water as the tube is advanced. To determine if the tube is within the stomach, fluid is aspirated. If the aspirated fluid is acidic

(indicating it has been obtained from the stomach), the tube is secured to the nose.
Test Taking Strategy—*Analyze to determine what information the question asks for, which is the correct sequence for NG tube insertion. Visualize the procedure and then place the steps in their sequential order. Review the procedure for inserting an NG tube if you had difficulty answering this question.*
Cognitive Level—*Applying*
Client Needs Category—*Physiological integrity*
Client Needs Subcategory—*Reduction of risk potential*

41. 1. Low intermittent suction is the best setting for a single-lumen nasogastric (NG) tube. This setting reduces trauma to the gastric mucosa and reduces the volume of electrolytes that are withdrawn from the client's gastric secretions. Low continuous suction is used for vented or double-lumen NG tubes.
Test Taking Strategy—*Look at the key words "most appropriate" in reference to the suction setting when using an NG tube. Low intermittent suction (option 1) is safer because it reduces the potential for pulling on the wall of the stomach and conserves some electrolytes that are present in gastric secretions. Review suction settings recommended for NG tubes if you had difficulty answering this question.*
Cognitive Level—*Applying*
Client Needs Category—*Physiological integrity*
Client Needs Subcategory—*Reduction of risk potential*

42. 1. One indication that the gastric tube has been incorrectly positioned in the respiratory tract is the client's inability to speak. This would occur if the tube was inadvertently located between the folds of the vocal cords, preventing the vibration necessary for speech. The tube would need to be withdrawn to the level of the oropharynx to reestablish the client's ability to breathe and speak. Swallowing would not be affected in this situation. Sneezing and vomiting are not appropriate signs to evaluate whether a gastric tube is in the wrong location.
Test Taking Strategy—*Analyze to determine what information the question asks for, which is an indication that a nasogastric (NG) tube has entered the respiratory tract. Recall that speech is the result of vibrations in the vocal cords. Therefore, a tube that lies within or beyond the vocal cords interferes with the ability to speak. Review clinical findings that suggest an NG tube has entered the respiratory tract if you had difficulty answering this question.*
Cognitive Level—*Applying*
Client Needs Category—*Physiological integrity*
Client Needs Subcategory—*Reduction of risk potential*

43. 2. Hearing a whooshing sound over the stomach as a bolus of air is instilled through the proximal end of the nasogastric (NG) tube is one method for determining placement. If the tube is in the esophagus, the client will belch. Another technique is to aspirate secretions from the tube and test the pH. If the secretions come from the stomach, the pH will be very acidic. A portable X-ray is an accurate method, but the cost and unnecessary radiation exposure make this method inappropriate. Liquids are never instilled through an NG tube until placement has been verified. In addition, instilling water before surgery places the client at risk for aspiration in the operation room. If the tip is not in the stomach, aspiration could occur. Feeling for air is an unacceptable technique for determining placement.

> *Test Taking Strategy—Look at the key words "most appropriate" in reference to the technique for determining that the distal end of an NG tube is within the stomach. Although option 1 is feasible and reliable, it is also costly. Auscultating over the stomach is safer and more time efficient. Review techniques for assessing distal location of an NG tube if you had difficulty answering this question.*
> **Cognitive Level**—*Applying*
> **Client Needs Category**—*Physiological integrity*
> **Client Needs Subcategory**—*Reduction of risk potential*

44. 1. The nurse offers the client some hope by validating the conscientious efforts being made. The response is objective without giving false reassurance. In the second option, the client may interpret the nurse's unwillingness to answer as an indication that the client's worst fear is confirmed. By implying that a serious question is silly or frivolous, as in the third option, the client may be discouraged from attempting further communication about any fears and feelings. The last option shows a disregard for the client's unique perception and fears.

> *Test Taking Strategy—Look at the key words "most appropriate" in relation to a response to the client's question about the possibility of dying shortly. Option 1 is most appropriate because it provides factual information specifically about the client's situation. It does not ignore or belittle the client's question, as in options 2 and 3, nor give false reassurance, as in option 4. Review therapeutic and nontherapeutic communication techniques if you had difficulty answering this question.*
> **Cognitive Level**—*Applying*
> **Client Needs Category**—*Psychosocial integrity*
> **Client Needs Subcategory**—*None*

45. 2. Splinting or supporting the incision promotes deeper inhalation and more forceful coughing. Explaining the risks for developing pneumonia is not likely to result in efforts to clear the airway. Oxygen would not be necessary unless ventilation is compromised. A high-Fowler's position facilitates the potential for a larger volume of air, but adequate lung expansion probably will not occur unless the client actively uses the respiratory muscles.

> *Test Taking Strategy—Look at the key words "most appropriate" in reference to a nursing action that is useful when a postoperative client fails to cough and deep-breathe. Recall that supporting the incision decreases pain transmission because it limits abdominal movement. If the potential for pain is reduced, the client may be more willing to cough and deep breathe. Review techniques for promoting coughing and deep breathing after abdominal surgery if you had difficulty answering this question.*
> **Cognitive Level**—*Applying*
> **Client Needs Category**—*Physiological integrity*
> **Client Needs Subcategory**—*Reduction of risk potential*

46. 3. Any fluid instilled or removed is recorded to maintain accurate intake and output. A nasogastric (NG) tube is usually irrigated with normal saline solution, not water, and the fluid does not have to be sterile. Oxygen is administered before tracheobronchial suctioning, not NG irrigation. Swallowing does not affect gastric tube irrigation.

> *Test Taking Strategy—Use the process of elimination to help select the option that is most appropriate when irrigating an NG tube. Options 2 and 4 do not apply to gastric tube irrigation so they may be eliminated immediately. Discriminate between options 1 and 3. Option 1 contains misinformation because the irrigation solution does not need to be sterile nor is plain water used. Option 3 provides a correct nursing action and a standard for NG tube irrigation, making it the correct choice. Review the procedure for irrigating an NG tube if you had difficulty answering this question.*
> **Cognitive Level**—*Applying*
> **Client Needs Category**—*Physiological integrity*
> **Client Needs Subcategory**—*Reduction of risk potential*

47. 1,080 mL. Fluid intake is the sum of all of the following: liquids the client drinks, the liquid equivalent of melted ice chips, foods that are liquid by the time they are swallowed (such as gelatin, ice cream, and thin, cooked cereal), I.V. infusions, and fluid instillations (such as the fluid used to flush a gastric feeding tube). The fluid volume for this client includes 1 cup (240 mL) of thin, cooked cereal; 1 carton (8 ounces, or 240 mL) of milk; ¼ cup (60 mL) of ice cream, 8 ounces (240 mL) of supplemental nutritional drink, 6 ounces (180 mL) of creamed soup, and ¼ cup (120 mL) of fruit-flavored gelatin.

> *Test Taking Strategy—Analyze to determine what information the question asks for, which requires converting liquid equivalents and math skills. Consult a pharmacology text if you had difficulty answering this question.*

Cognitive Level—Understanding
Client Needs Category—Physiological integrity
Client Needs Subcategory—Basic care and comfort

48. 2, 4, 5. Dumping syndrome is the rapid emptying of large amounts of concentrated dietary solids and liquids into the small intestine, resulting in a significant amount of glucose in intrajejunal contents and the consequential release of insulin that causes hypoglycemia. To prevent or manage the symptoms associated with this condition, the nurse teaches the client to limit the consumption of fluid and simple carbohydrates at mealtimes, eat at least six small meals a day, and lie down for 30 minutes after eating to slow gastric emptying.

Test Taking Strategy—Analyze to determine what information the question asks for, which is steps to take to prevent dumping syndrome. Alternative-format "select all that apply" questions require considering each option independently to decide its merit in answering the question. Choose options that identify techniques for preventing symptoms associated with the dumping syndrome and review similar information if you had difficulty answering this question.
Cognitive Level—Analyzing
Client Needs Category—Physiological integrity
Client Needs Subcategory—Reduction of risk potential

49. 1. Absence of free hydrochloric acid in the stomach is associated with stomach cancer. This finding distinguishes the etiology of the symptoms from other causes such as peptic ulcer. Gastrin is a hormone secreted by the mucosa of the pylorus and stomach that causes hypersecretion of gastric acid. Gastric irritation, or gastritis, and a decrease in hemoglobin and hematocrit are common findings with multiple etiologies; they are not usually related to stomach cancer.

Test Taking Strategy—Analyze to determine what information the question asks for, which is a diagnostic test result that correlates with gastric cancer. Recall that normal functioning of the stomach includes the secretion of hydrochloric acid. If cancer cells are present, an absence of hydrochloric acid occurs, making option 1 the correct answer. Review diagnostic testing and stomach cancer if you had difficulty answering this question.
Cognitive Level—Applying
Client Needs Category—Physiological integrity
Client Needs Subcategory—Reduction of risk potential

50. 2. Clients with nasogastric (NG) tubes that are connected to suction are generally placed on NPO (nothing by mouth) status. Providing a few ice chips helps moisten the mouth and quench the thirst. Giving larger amounts of water or other fluids would result in their removal from the stomach because of the suction. Removal of fluids also results in the removal of essential electrolytes.

Test Taking Strategy—Look at the key words "most appropriate" in reference to a nursing intervention for a client with an NG tube who is thirsty. Recall that an NG tube that, in this case, is connected to suction removes electrolytes along with gastric secretions. It is important to relieve the client's thirst without contributing to a deficit of electrolytes. Review the nursing management of a client with an NG tube connected to suction if you had difficulty answering this question.
Cognitive Level—Applying
Client Needs Category—Physiological integrity
Client Needs Subcategory—Basic care and comfort

51. 2. There are 1,000 mcg in 1 mg. The order is for the administration of 1,000 mcg, and there is 1 mg of drug per milliliter of solution. Therefore, the correct volume in this case is 1 mL.

Test Taking Strategy—Analyze to determine what information the question asks for, which involves dosage calculation. To compute the answer the supplied dose of 1 mg must be converted to micrograms. Review metric equivalents if you had difficulty answering this question.
Cognitive Level—Applying
Client Needs Category—Physiological integrity
Client Needs Subcategory—Pharmacological therapies

52. 2. I.M. injections are given at a 90-degree angle. The vastus lateralis muscle (the site for this injection) is located on the outer aspect of the thigh. The deltoid muscle is in the upper arm. The rectus femoris muscle is located on the anterior thigh, and the dorsogluteal muscle is in the upper outer quadrant of the buttock.

Test Taking Strategy—Analyze to determine what information the question asks for, which is the correct technique for an I.M. injection in the vastus lateralis muscle. Eliminate options 1 and 4, because I.M. injections require a 90-degree angle. Discriminate between whether the correct vastus lateralis site is the outer or anterior thigh. Review the administration of I.M. injections and the locations of appropriate sites if you had difficulty answering this question.
Cognitive Level—Applying
Client Needs Category—Physiological integrity
Client Needs Subcategory—Pharmacological therapies

Nursing Care of Clients with Disorders of the Small Intestine

53. 4. Stool specimens that may contain ova and parasites should be examined when the feces is fresh and warm. Ova and parasites will not survive for long if the feces is kept below body temperature. Drying and cooling destroy the organisms and result in invalid findings. The client can use a bedpan or toilet for bowel elimination and specimen collection. Holding the container under the client's anus would be inappropriate. Using a tongue blade, the nurse can transfer a portion of stool to a waxed, covered container. The specimen container need not be sterile.

Test Taking Strategy—Analyze to determine what information the question asks for, which is the correct action to take when the nurse collects a stool specimen for ova and parasites. Recall that keeping the stool at near body temperature will keep the parasite alive and facilitate its subsequent identification. Review the stool specimen collection procedure if you had difficulty with this question.
Cognitive Level—Applying
Client Needs Category—Physiological integrity
Client Needs Subcategory—Reduction of risk potential

54. 2. The abbreviation *q.i.d.* means that the drug is to be administered four times a day. Scheduled hours may differ depending on the predetermined timetable set by the health agency. However, in following the order as it is written, administration can be no less or no more than four times during a 24-hour period. The other choices contain too few or too many hours. Military time is based on a 24-hour clock. Each hour is numbered in continuous sequence.

Test Taking Strategy—Use the process of elimination to help select the option that accurately identifies a schedule for administering the medication as it was prescribed. Knowledge of the meaning of the abbreviation q.i.d. and military time is essential. Option 2 is the only option that identifies a medication administration schedule of four times a day. Refer to a pharmacology text if you had difficulty with this question.
Cognitive Level—Applying
Client Needs Category—Physiological integrity
Client Needs Subcategory—Pharmacological therapies

55. 1, 2, 3. A clear liquid diet includes bouillon, tea or coffee, flavored gelatin, fruit ices, clear carbonated beverages such as ginger ale, and some clear fruit juices such as apple or grape. Coffee and tea are clear liquids, but they are GI stimulants and therefore should be limited in clients who have diarrhea. Milk or milk products may cause further diarrhea and are not permitted on this type of diet.

Test Taking Strategy—Analyze to determine what information the question asks for, which is what foods constitute clear liquids. Alternative-format "select all that apply" questions require considering each option independently to decide its merit in answering the question. Recall that clear liquids are liquids or gelatins that are typically transparent. Review the components of a clear liquid diet if you had difficulty answering this question.

Cognitive Level—Applying
Client Needs Category—Physiological integrity
Client Needs Subcategory—Basic care and comfort

56. 4. A dark yellow color indicates that the client's urine is concentrated, a sign of dehydration. Pink mucous membranes are a normal finding. An elevated blood pressure and irregular heart rate are abnormal findings, but these signs are not associated with fluid volume deficit or dehydration.

Test Taking Strategy—Look at the key words "most likely" in reference to an assessment finding that relates to dehydration. Recall that dehydration results in a decrease of circulating blood volume from which the kidneys make urine. Consequently there is a concentration of urobilin, the yellow pigment in urine, making option 4 the best choice.
Cognitive Level—Applying
Client Needs Category—Physiological integrity
Client Needs Subcategory—Physiological adaptation

57. 3. GoLYTELY is given as a colonic lavage. Within 30 minutes of ingesting the first volume of the solution, the client should experience the first of many bowel movements. The bowel must be clear of feces for the colonoscopy to be effective. This solution is preferable to other forms of bowel cleansing because it is less likely to deplete electrolytes or cause water intoxication. The other choices are expected outcomes of administering an oral electrolyte solution, but they are not the main reason for administering a solution for the purpose of colonic lavage.

Test Taking Strategy—Use the process of elimination to help select the option that identifies the best evidence that GoLYTELY has achieved a therapeutic effect. Because this solution is a bowel cleansing agent used before a colonoscopy, option 3 emerges as the best answer. Review the purpose for administering GoLYTELY and the importance of emptying the large intestine before a colonoscopy if you had difficulty answering this question.
Cognitive Level—Applying
Client Needs Category—Physiological integrity
Client Needs Subcategory—Pharmacological therapies

58. 1, 2, 3. Sodium is the most abundant cation in the blood and functions in the body to maintain osmotic pressure and acid-base balance and to transmit nerve impulses. Very low values can result in seizures and neurologic symptoms. The normal adult range is between 135 and 146 mEq/L. Potassium is essential for maintaining proper fluid balance, nerve impulse function, muscle function, and cardiac (heart muscle) function. Very low values can cause cardiac arrhythmias. The normal range of potassium is between 3.5 and 5.5 mEq/L. Chloride is influenced by the extracellular fluid balance and acid-base balance. Chloride passively follows water and sodium. The normal adult range is 95 to 112 mEq/L. Calcium is involved in bone metabolism, protein absorption, fat transfer, muscular contraction, transmission of nerve impulses, blood clotting, and cardiac function. It is regulated by parathyroid hormone. The normal adult range is 8.5 to 10.3 mEq/dL. Phosphorus is generally inverse with calcium. The normal adult range is 2.5 to 4.5 mEq/dL. Blood urea nitrogen (BUN) increases can be caused by excessive protein intake, kidney damage, certain drugs, low fluid intake, intestinal bleeding, exercise, or heart failure. Decreased levels may be due to a poor diet, malabsorption, liver damage, or low nitrogen intake. The normal adult range is 7 to 25 mg/dL. BUN is not considered an electrolyte but an indicator of renal function.

Test Taking Strategy—Analyze to determine what information the question asks for, which is electrolyte levels that can be affected by illness. Alternative-format "select all that apply" questions require considering each option independently to decide its merit in answering the question. Choose options in which the serum electrolyte values are in an abnormal range; note that sodium, potassium, and chloride are electrolytes that are frequently imbalanced during illness. Review laboratory values for the listed substances if you have difficulty with this question.
Cognitive Level—Analyzing
Client Needs Category—Physiological integrity
Client Needs Subcategory—Reduction of risk potential

59. 3. Respiratory depression is a potential side effect when midazolam (Versed) is administered. This drug allows the client to communicate and cooperate during the procedure, but afterward the client will have no memory of doing so. The client does not lose consciousness. Although many drugs can cause unstable blood pressure and cardiac arrhythmias, these complications are not commonly associated with midazolam.

Test Taking Strategy—Analyze to determine what information the question asks for, which is an undesirable effect associated with midazolam. Recall that midazolam is a benzodiazepine used for conscious sedation during diagnostic tests. Its side effects include drowsiness, brief amnesia, and respiratory depression; thus, option 3 directly relates an undesirable side effect. Review the therapeutic use, side effects, and adverse effects of midazolam if you had difficulty answering this question.
Cognitive Level—Applying
Client Needs Category—Physiological integrity
Client Needs Subcategory—Pharmacological therapies

60. 4. Fiber is the undigested portion of fruits, vegetables, grains, and nuts that is not broken down and absorbed during the digestive process. Animal products are not a source of dietary fiber. Food that requires chewing is too limited a definition for fiber, and some foods do not contain fiber. The semisolid mass of food in the stomach is called chyme.

Test Taking Strategy—Analyze to determine what information the question asks for, which is evidence that the client understands the source of dietary fiber. Recall that raw fruits and vegetables, whole grains, nuts, and beans—all plant sources—are high in fiber, leading to the correct answer of option 4. Review sources of dietary fiber if you had difficulty answering this question.
Cognitive Level—Applying
Client Needs Category—Health promotion and maintenance
Client Needs Subcategory—None

61. 2. Ileal drainage contains enzymes and bile salts that are very damaging to the skin. Therefore, preserving skin integrity is most important at this time. Intact skin is the first line of defense against microorganisms. The nurse should monitor for fluid and electrolyte imbalances related to wound drainage. Pain management may need to be addressed, especially if dressings are necessary, but this is not as important as maintaining skin integrity. Clients with draining wounds sometimes experience foul-smelling odors, but odor containment also is not the priority at this time. Body image changes are also a complication, especially if the wound is foul-smelling and slow to heal; however, body image is a psychological issue and does not take priority over physiologic issues such as skin integrity.

Test Taking Strategy—Use the process of elimination to help select the option identifying the highest priority problem for a client with a draining intestinal fistula. Using Maslow's hierarchy, options 3 and 4 have a lower priority. Option 1 has merit, but it is a secondary problem and may resolve if skin breakdown (option 2) is aggressively managed. Review the nursing care of a client with a draining intestinal fistula if you had difficulty answering this question.
Cognitive Level—Evaluating
Client Needs Category—Safe and effective care environment
Client Needs Subcategory—Coordinated care

Nursing Care of Clients with Disorders of the Large Intestine

62. 2. The client's statement indicates a failure to understand the procedure; therefore, the consent to undergo the procedure is not valid. In this case, the nurse needs to inform the physician, who is responsible for providing an explanation of the surgery, its risks and complications, and then obtaining informed consent. The nurse should never allow a client to sign a consent form that is not fully understood. The nurse is responsible for witnessing the client's signature and ensuring that the legal aspects of the consent form are upheld. If the client's misinformation is clarified and corrected, the surgery need not be canceled. The nurse does not proceed with skin preparation until the discrepancy is settled.

Test Taking Strategy—Analyze to determine what information the question asks for, which is an action that should be taken in response to evidence of a client's misunderstanding of the scheduled surgical procedure. Legally, there must be informed consent, which is not evident based on the client's statement. The physician should be notified before the presurgical procedures proceed. Review the legal principle of informed consent and the nurse's responsibility when witnessing a client's consent for treatment if you had difficulty answering this question.
Cognitive Level—Applying
Client Needs Category—Safe and effective care environment
Client Needs Subcategory—Coordinated care

63.

3. The nurse reviews the surgical consent, noting the correct procedure and site.

2. The surgeon verifies the surgical site with the client, initialing the correct site with an appropriate marking pen.

5. Before positioning the client on the operating room table, the nurse identifies the client using the client's name and birth date on the identification band.

1. Time-out is done immediately before starting the procedure in the location where the procedure will be performed.

6. All staff stops what they are doing and participates in the final verification answering verbally when verifying the surgical site.

4. The procedure begins after the time-out when staff is confident the correct procedure is being performed on the correct client.

Before any surgery, a surgical consent must be obtained. It is the nurse's responsibility to review the surgical consent for completeness, noting the correct client, procedure, and site. The surgeon or person performing the procedure is responsible for marking the site; the site marking should occur with the client awake, aware, and free of any narcotics or anesthetics. When the client enters the surgical suite itself, before positioning on the surgery table, the circulating nurse identifies the client by name and date of birth (identifiers may vary from institution to institution) and compares the surgical consent form with the client's identification bracelet. Just before the surgery, time-out is called; all staff in the operating room should stop what they are doing and participate in the final verification of the correct client, site, and procedure. They must answer verbally. The procedure is then begun after the time-out process.

Test Taking Strategy—Analyze to determine what information the question asks for, which is the sequence in which National Patient Safety Standards mandate surgical site verification and time-out processes before surgery. Organize the options, beginning with reviewing the surgical consent and ending with the start of the surgical procedure. Refer to the Joint Commission's universal protocol for surgical site verification and time-out processes if you had difficulty with this question.
Cognitive Level—Applying
Client Needs Category—Safe and effective care environment
Client Needs Subcategory—Safety and infection control

64. 4. To help prevent headaches after spinal anesthesia, it is customary to keep the client's head flat for 6 to 12 hours postoperatively. Therefore, the nurse should question an order to place the client in Fowler's position. The remaining orders in this question are appropriate and should be implemented.

Test Taking Strategy—Analyze to determine what information the question asks for, which is the postoperative order that should be questioned. Option 4 indicates the client may be placed in Fowler's position, which is inappropriate after spinal anesthesia and would represent a questionable postoperative order. Review the postoperative nursing care of a client who has received spinal anesthesia if you had difficulty answering this question.
Cognitive Level—Analyzing
Client Needs Category—Safe and effective care environment
Client Needs Subcategory—Safety and infection control

65. 1. Although pain is important to assess, the client's safety and welfare are jeopardized if the client experiences undetected urine retention. Coughing is contraindicated after this type of surgery. When spinal anesthesia is administered, the client remains alert.

Test Taking Strategy—Analyze to determine what information the question asks for, which is a priority assessment on a client who has had a herniorrhaphy. Consider the nature of the surgery and possible complications. Option 2 is not a concern with spinal anesthesia. Option 3 is contraindicated, because there is a potential for developing an incisional hernia at the surgical site when the client coughs. Although relieving pain (option 4) is important, urine retention (option 1) represents a greater physiologic threat. Review the postoperative nursing care of a client undergoing a herniorrhaphy if you had difficulty answering this question.

Cognitive Level—Applying
Client Needs Category—Physiological integrity
Client Needs Subcategory—Reduction of risk potential

66. 2. A suspensory is used on a male client after a herniorrhaphy to help prevent scrotal swelling. This device will not prevent impotence, strain on the incision, or wound contamination.

Test Taking Strategy—Look at the key words "most appropriate" in reference to an explanation for the male client's use of a suspensory. Based on the name of the device, prevention of scrotal edema (option 2) is the only purpose for using this type of device. Review the male client's use of a suspensory if you had difficulty answering this question.
Cognitive Level—Applying
Client Needs Category—Physiological integrity
Client Needs Subcategory—Reduction of risk potential

67. 2. The order reads to give the client 50 mg of meperidine (Demerol). The ampule contains 100 mg/mL.

$$\frac{\text{Desired}}{\text{Have}} \times \text{quantity} = X$$

$$\frac{50 \text{ mg}}{100 \text{ mg}} \times 1 \text{ mL} = X \text{mL}$$

$$X = 0.5 \text{ mL}$$

Test Taking Strategy—Analyze to determine what information the question asks for, which involves dosage calculation. Refer to the mathematical formula and calculation in the rationale. Review the process for calculating a parenteral dosage if you had difficulty answering this question.
Cognitive Level—Applying
Client Needs Category—Physiological integrity
Client Needs Subcategory—Pharmacological therapies

68. 2. The federal government mandates that the manufacturing, distribution, and dispensing of addictive drugs such as meperidine hydrochloride (Demerol) be controlled. Therefore, an accurate accounting of its administration should be kept in an opioid control log, also known as a *narcotics record*. Some health care facilities may use computerized record keeping or other forms to internally track the use of opioids, but these types of medications still need to be recorded to ensure that the drugs have not been stolen or mishandled.

Test Taking Strategy—Analyze to determine what information the question asks for, which is documentation requirements when administering meperidine. Recall that meperidine is an opioid, a controlled substance, and that administration of this category of drugs must be accounted for in a narcotics record. Review the nursing responsibilities involved in administering a controlled substance if you had difficulty answering this question.

Cognitive Level—Applying
Client Needs Category—Physiological integrity
Client Needs Subcategory—Pharmacological therapies

69. 1, 5, 6. Ulcerative colitis is a chronic inflammation of the colon and rectum with an unknown cause and has exacerbations and remissions. It is seen most commonly in young adults. Clients with ulcerative colitis may have 12 to 20 diarrheal stools per day that contain blood and mucus along with fecal material. In addition, clients experience cramping and lower left abdominal pain, dehydration, fatigue, and weight loss; the urge to defecate is so urgent that the client is usually incontinent. Bowel sounds are most likely to be hyperactive related to the frequency of the stools. Striae are red or white streaks on the skin due to stretching. Because the client with ulcerative colitis suffers from weight loss and emaciation, striae do not typically occur. Ulcerated lesions in this disease are confined to the colon, not the mouth.

Test Taking Strategy—Analyze to determine what information the question asks for, which is the signs and symptoms of ulcerative colitis. Alternative-format "select all that apply" questions require considering each option independently to decide its merit in answering the question. Consider each option independently as a characteristic sign or symptom of ulcerative colitis. Review information about the manifestations of ulcerative colitis if you had difficulty answering this question.
Cognitive Level—Applying
Client Needs Category—Physiological integrity
Client Needs Subcategory—Physiological adaptation

70.

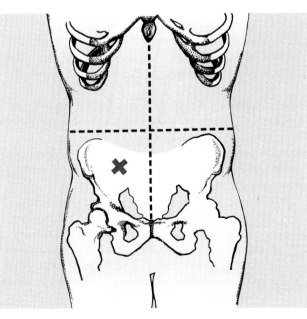

The nurse first assesses the right lower quadrant to listen to bowel sounds in the area of the ascending colon. The right and left upper quadrants of the abdomen are the locations of the transverse colon. The left lower quadrant is the area of the descending colon.

Test Taking Strategy—Analyze to determine what information the question asks for, which is the location of the proximal portion of the ascending colon. Knowing the anatomic location of the ascending colon and the meaning of proximal is essential for placing the X in the correct location. Consult an anatomy text if you had difficulty answering this question.
Cognitive Level—Understanding
Client Needs Category—Health promotion and maintenance
Client Needs Subcategory—None

71. 1. According to the scenario, the client is 31 years old. Keeping the commode next to the bedside is the most appropriate intervention because the client will probably be able to get in and out of bed with minimal assistance. This intervention would be less appropriate if the client was an older adult or too weak to get up. Answering the client's call light is always appropriate, but may be unnecessary if the client can get up alone. Providing a disposable brief for an able-bodied person with fecal incontinence is usually emotionally devastating. It is done only as a last resort, preferably with the client's permission. Assisting the client to the bathroom frequently may or may not be appropriate, depending on the client's last bowel movement.

Test Taking Strategy—Look at the key words "most appropriate" in relation to a nursing intervention for preventing or eliminating bowel incontinence. All of the options have merit, but because the client is a young adult, option 1 is the best answer. Review methods for managing the urge to defecate when a client has frequent stools if you had difficulty answering this question.
Cognitive Level—Applying
Client Needs Category—Physiological integrity
Client Needs Subcategory—Basic care and comfort

72. 1. Reflecting is a response that lets the client know that both the content and the feelings are understood. Offering to contact the physician avoids the chance to provide emotional support and, therefore, is inappropriate. Giving advice and disagreeing with a client are blocks to therapeutic communication.

Test Taking Strategy—Use the process of elimination to help select the option that provides a therapeutic response to the discouraged client's statement. Eliminate options 3 and 4 because they are examples of nontherapeutic communication techniques. Option 2 looks appealing as an answer, but referring the client to the physician is a poor substitute for personally interacting with the client. Review therapeutic and nontherapeutic communication techniques if you had difficulty with this question.

Cognitive Level—Applying
Client Needs Category—Psychosocial integrity
Client Needs Subcategory—None

73. 1. After giving the preoperative medication, the nurse should raise the bed side rails and instruct the client to remain in bed because meperidine (Demerol) and hydroxyzine (Vistaril) depress the central nervous system, making it difficult for the client to remain alert. Elimination is accomplished before giving the preanesthetic drugs. One of atropine sulfate's anticipated side effects is a dry mouth; however, this is not a priority nursing concern. Likewise, nausea is one of the side effects of meperidine, but placing an emesis basin at the bedside is not as important as ensuring the client's safety.

Test Taking Strategy—Use the process of elimination to help select the option that identifies the most important nursing action after administration of preoperative medications. When administrating preoperative medications that contribute to sedation, safety is always a concern. Option 1 is best for ensuring the client's safety. Review the nursing care of a client during the preoperative period if you had difficulty answering this question.
Cognitive Level—Applying
Client Needs Category—Safe and effective care environment
Client Needs Subcategory—Safety and infection control

74. 3. A dropping blood pressure is a common indicator that a client is going into shock. A systolic pressure of 90 to 100 mm Hg indicates impending shock; below 80 mm Hg, shock is present. Other signs of shock include a rapid, thready pulse; pale, cold, and clammy skin; rapid respirations; a falling body temperature; restlessness; and a decreased level of consciousness. None of the other choices is associated with the signs or symptoms of shock.

Test Taking Strategy—Use the process of elimination to select the option that represents the sign that is most indicative of shock. Knowledge of the pathophysiology underlying shock leads to the correct answer. Recall that hypovolemic shock is a loss of circulatory volume that is commonly caused by hemorrhage. Option 3 is the only option that correlates with the loss of circulatory volume, which in turn lowers the blood pressure. Options 1, 2, and 4 are not signs of shock. Review the signs and symptoms of shock if you had difficulty answering this question.
Cognitive Level—Applying
Client Needs Category—Physiological integrity
Client Needs Subcategory—Physiological adaptation

75. 4. Normal oxygen saturation is between 95% and 100%. The measurements in the other options indicate hypoxemia and should be reported immediately.

*Test Taking Strategy—Analyze to determine what infor-
mation the question asks for, which is the oxygen
value that represents adequate oxygenation. Pulse
oximetry reveals a client's arterial blood oxygen
saturation, or the percentage to which oxygen is
bound to hemoglobin. Recall that a range between
95% and 100% is optimal. Review oxygen saturation
levels and its assessment using a pulse oximeter if
you had difficulty answering this question.*
Cognitive Level—*Understanding*
Client Needs Category—*Physiological integrity*
Client Needs Subcategory—*Reduction of risk potential*

76. **2, 6.** When caring for an ileostomy, the nurse should
observe the characteristics of the stoma on a daily basis,
making sure to check its size, color, and general condition.
A skin protection barrier, such as karaya, should be applied
to any excoriated skin. The faceplate of the ileostomy is
generally left in place for 3 to 5 days, unless it becomes
loose or causes skin discomfort. The pouch is emptied,
rinsed, or detached and replaced on an as-needed basis.
It is unnecessary to empty the pouch as soon as stool is
expelled, but the pouch should be emptied when it is one
third to one half full to avoid pulling the faceplate from the
skin due to the excessive weight of semiliquid stool. The
stoma and peristomal area are cleaned with mild soap and
water, not alcohol or acetone, which can dry and irritate
the tissue. The faceplate should not fit snugly around the
stoma; it should be trimmed to allow room for the stoma
plus an extra ⅛″ to ¼″ to avoid compromising blood flow
to the stoma site.

*Test Taking Strategy—Analyze to determine what
information the question asks for, which is nursing
actions in the care of a client with an ileostomy.
Select or eliminate each option independently in
relation to a typical ostomy client's nursing care.
Review information about ostomy care if you had
difficulty answering this question.*
Cognitive Level—*Applying*
Client Needs Category—*Physiological integrity*
Client Needs Subcategory—*Physiological adaptation*

77. **1.** The best time for changing an appliance and providing stomal care is when the bowel is somewhat inactive.
This is usually in the morning before any food has been
eaten. Exercise and eating tend to increase bowel activity,
making it likely that intestinal contents will spill onto the
skin if the procedure is done afterward.

*Test Taking Strategy—Use the process of elimination
to help select the option that identifies the best time
of day to change the ileostomy appliance. Options
2, 3, and 4 can be eliminated because they represent
times during which the bowel is more active and
is likely to expel a higher volume of stool. Option
1 emerges as the best answer because the client's
dietary intake has been limited or absent during*

the night, reducing the rate of peristalsis and stool
elimination from the ileostomy. Review the gastrocolic reflex and its effect on bowel elimination if you
had difficulty answering this question.*
Cognitive Level—*Applying*
Client Needs Category—*Physiological integrity*
Client Needs Subcategory—*Physiological adaptation*

78. **2.** A normal healthy stoma is bright red or pink
because of its rich blood supply and has a shiny appearance. When cleaning, a healthy stoma may bleed slightly.
If the stoma is light pink or dusky blue, the blood supply
to the tissue is compromised. A tan stoma is atypical even
in those with a darker complexion; bleeding would be a
reassuring finding. If the stoma is pale pink or dusky blue,
the blood supply to the tissue is compromised. A normal
stoma is elevated above the surrounding tissue. A tan
stoma is atypical even in those with a darker complexion;
further assessments are necessary to determine the cause.

*Test Taking Strategy—Analyze to determine what infor-
mation the question asks for, which is the normal
color and characteristics of a stoma. Recall that the
stoma, which consists of a layer of mucous membrane, requires an adequate blood supply, giving it a
pink or red color. Review the physical characteristics
of a normal stoma if you had difficulty answering
this question.*
Cognitive Level—*Applying*
Client Needs Category—*Physiological integrity*
Client Needs Subcategory—*Physiological adaptation*

79. **3.** Mild soap and tepid water are most often recommended for cleaning the skin around the stoma. Povidone-
iodine (Betadine) is not recommended because it may
irritate the skin. Alcohol is also drying and irritating to
the skin. Scrubbing should be avoided because friction is
likely to interrupt the skin integrity.

*Test Taking Strategy—Look at the key words "most
appropriate" in reference to the technique for cleaning the peristomal skin. Eliminate the options that
would be irritating or harmful to a healing stoma.
Using mild soap and water (option 1) is the only
option that cleans the peristomal skin without traumatizing the tissue or causing discomfort. Review
recommended substances for cleaning peristomal
skin if you had difficulty answering this question.*
Cognitive Level—*Applying*
Client Needs Category—*Physiological integrity*
Client Needs Subcategory—*Physiological adaptation*

80. **2.** The appliance opening must be large enough to
avoid impairing circulation to the stoma but small enough
that ileal drainage will not damage the skin. There should
be only about a ⅛″ to ¼″ margin of skin exposed around
the stoma. This allows room to attach the faceplate to the
skin rather than to the stoma. The faceplate needs to cover

an adequate amount of skin to prevent excoriation due to contact with enzymes and bile salts in ileal drainage. The stomal opening must not be obstructed, or stool will not pass. Because defecation cannot be controlled and the feces are liquid, it is inappropriate to allow the skin to air-dry for 30 minutes. The appliance must cover the stoma; the bag may or may not be directly at the waist or belt line.

> *Test Taking Strategy—Note the key words "most accurate" when asked about the technique for changing an ileostomy appliance. Recall that the appliance must encircle the stoma without impairing its blood supply, which option 2 describes. Review how an ileostomy appliance is fitted over a client's stoma if you had difficulty answering this question.*

Cognitive Level—*Applying*
Client Needs Category—*Physiological integrity*
Client Needs Subcategory—*Physiological adaptation*

81. 4. Because there is no sphincter to control the watery discharge from a conventional ileostomy, it is difficult for most clients to gain control of bowel elimination. It is realistic for people with an ileostomy to jog, swim, have sexual relations, get pregnant, and generally pursue careers and enjoy all manner of social activities.

> *Test Taking Strategy—Analyze to determine what information the question asks for, which is an activity that is impossible for a client with a conventional ileostomy. Recall that the fecal effluent from the ileum is unformed and watery and there is no sphincter control, making control of defecation an unrealistic expectation. Review the activities that may or may not be compromised as a result of having an ileostomy if you had difficulty answering this question.*

Cognitive Level—*Applying*
Client Needs Category—*Physiological integrity*
Client Needs Subcategory—*Physiological adaptation*

82. 4. Appendicitis, inflammation of the appendix, is often accompanied by infection. The white blood cell (leukocyte) count increases when infection or inflammation is present; it is expected to rise in this case. These cells fight infection by walling off, destroying, or removing damaged tissues or pathogens. The bilirubin level is typically monitored closely in a client with liver or gallbladder disease. The serum potassium level would be important if the client has anorexia, vomiting, or diarrhea. The prothrombin time is generally monitored when a client is receiving the anticoagulant warfarin sodium (Coumadin).

> *Test Taking Strategy—Analyze to determine what information the question asks for, which is the laboratory test finding that supports a diagnosis of appendicitis. Recall that when the appendix becomes inflamed, there is a migration of leukocytes to the tissue and the bone marrow increases the number of white blood cells it produces. Consequently options 1, 2, and 3 can be eliminated because they are unrelated*

> *to the inflammatory process. Option 4 emerges as the best answer because it correlates with leukocytosis. Review the physiologic processes associated with the inflammatory response if you had difficulty answering this question.*

Cognitive Level—*Applying*
Client Needs Category—*Physiological integrity*
Client Needs Subcategory—*Reduction of risk potential*

83.

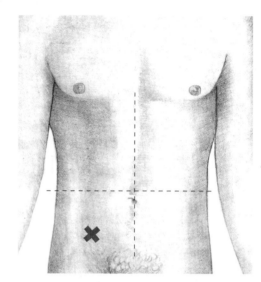

Appendicitis is characterized by pain and tenderness in the lower right quadrant, midway between the umbilicus and the crest of the ilium.

> *Test Taking Strategy—Analyze to determine what information the question asks for, which is the anatomic location of the tenderness experienced by a client with appendicitis. Recall that the classic sign of appendicitis is pain when pressure is applied and then released over what is known as McBurney's point, in the lower right quadrant. The phenomenon is known as rebound tenderness. Review the signs of appendicitis if you had difficulty answering this question.*

Cognitive Level—*Applying*
Client Needs Category—*Physiological integrity*
Client Needs Subcategory—*Physiological adaptation*

84. 1, 3. A shorter recovery period is only one of the many advantages of laparoscopic surgery. However, some form of anesthesia is used. There is a smaller than usual surgical scar but activity restrictions are still in place; these include no lifting, straining, or sexual intercourse for a minimum of 10 to 15 days postoperatively. After discharge from the hospital, the client may resume a diet as tolerated.

> *Test Taking Strategy—Analyze to determine what information the question asks for, which is the advantages of laparoscopic surgery. Alternative-format*

"select all that apply" questions require considering each option independently to decide its merit in answering the question. Choose any option that identifies a benefit of laparoscopic surgery. Review the advantages of laparoscopic surgery if you had difficulty answering this question.
Cognitive Level—Applying
Client Needs Category—Physiological integrity
Client Needs Subcategory—Reduction of risk potential

85. **3.** Heat applications should be avoided whenever there is a possibility that abdominal discomfort is due to appendicitis. Heat dilates blood vessels, increases swelling, and promotes rupture of the vermiform appendix. Withholding food and fluid is advantageous if the symptoms are due to gastroenteritis or if emergency surgery is necessary. Pain, nausea, and fever generally limit usual activity and dietary intake. Acetaminophen (Tylenol) is a nonsalicylate that lowers a fever and relieves discomfort but does not predispose to rupturing the appendix.
    Test Taking Strategy—Look at the key words "most likely" in reference to a factor that may have contributed to rupturing the appendix. Recall that local applications of heat (option 3) increase the blood supply to an area and that, in turn, contributes to edema of the tissue. As the tissue expands and swells, it is prone to rupturing. Review factors that increase the potential for rupturing an inflamed appendix if you had difficulty answering this question.
Cognitive Level—Analyzing
Client Needs Category—Physiological integrity
Client Needs Subcategory—Physiological adaptation

86. **2.** An open drain relies on gravity to remove secretions absorbed by the dressing. Therefore, Fowler's position is most appropriate for promoting wound drainage. None of the other positions promote the collection of wound drainage near the drain.
    Test Taking Strategy—Analyze to determine what information the question asks for, which is the best position for promoting drainage from an open drain. Understanding terminology relating to body positions is essential for answering the question; also recall that gravity is helpful in promoting drainage. Fowler's position, in which the torso is upright (option 2), is the best answer. Review the use of an open drain and respective nursing measures involved in client care if you had difficulty answering this question.
Cognitive Level—Applying
Client Needs Category—Physiological integrity
Client Needs Subcategory—Physiological adaptation

87. **3.** Soiled dressings are enclosed in a receptacle or container, such as the nurse's glove, to prevent the transmission of infectious microorganisms. A clean glove is

used to remove soiled dressings. Tape is pulled toward the wound to prevent separating the healing edges. Wound cleaning should always carry microorganisms and debris away from, not toward, the incision.
    Test Taking Strategy—Analyze to determine what information the question asks for, which is the correct nursing action when changing the client's abdominal dressing. Consider the aspects of wound/incisional care, including standards and infection control principles. Recall that a principle of medical asepsis is to enclose the soiled dressing in the glove and dispose of it properly. Review the procedure for changing a gauze dressing as well as principles of asepsis if you had difficulty answering this question.
Cognitive Level—Applying
Client Needs Category—Safe and effective care environment
Client Needs Subcategory—Safety and infection control

88. 1.2 mL.

Use the formula:

$$\frac{\text{Desired dose}}{\text{Dose on hand}} \times \text{Quantity} = X \text{(amount to administer)}$$

$$\text{Solve for } X\text{: } \frac{60\,\text{mg}}{50\,\text{mg}} \times 1\,\text{mL} = X\,\text{mL}$$

$$X = 1.2\,\text{mL}$$

    Test Taking Strategy—Analyze to determine what information the question asks for, which involves dosage calculation. Use a standard formula to determine the volume of medication to administer parenterally. Review the process for calculating parenteral doses if you had difficulty answering this question.
Cognitive Level—Applying
Client Needs Category—Physiological integrity
Client Needs Subcategory—Pharmacological therapies

89. **1, 5.** A change in bowel habits is one of the seven danger signals for cancer identified by the American Cancer Society. Bowel movements alternate between diarrhea and constipation. Other signs and symptoms of colorectal cancer include dull abdominal pain (pain is a late sign of cancer), melena (black, tarry stools), abdominal distention, rectal pain, and narrowing of the diameter of the feces. Jaundice related to hepatitis is not closely related to colorectal cancer but is related to diseases affecting the liver. Chronic indigestion is more closely related to stomach cancer than colorectal cancer. Being an insulin-dependent diabetic patient is not a risk factor related to cancer. However, diabetes can cause complications related to healing and recovery. There is no correlation between drug abuse and colorectal cancer, although lifestyle choices affect healing and recovery.

Test Taking Strategy—*Analyze to determine what information the question asks for, which is symptoms of colorectal cancer. Alternative-format "select all that apply" questions require considering each option independently to decide its merit in answering the question. Analyze each option one at a time and select any that applies to the disease process. Review factors in a client's health history that relate to colorectal cancer if you had difficulty answering this question.*
Cognitive Level—*Applying*
Client Needs Category—*Physiological integrity*
Client Needs Subcategory—*Physiological adaptation*

90. **1.** Unless there are complications, a client who has a sigmoidoscopy as an outpatient will be able to return home the same day. The client may eat lightly the evening before a sigmoidoscopy. A flexible scope is more commonly used than a rigid one. Medications are taken before the test and do not interfere with the test findings.

Test Taking Strategy—*Analyze to determine what information the question asks for, which is a statement indicating misinformation on the part of the client that the nurse should clarify. Recall that a sigmoidoscopy procedure can be performed in a physician's office or endoscopic outpatient unit. It does not require hospitalization. Review the procedure for performing a sigmoidoscopy if you had difficulty answering this question.*
Cognitive Level—*Applying*
Client Needs Category—*Physiological integrity*
Client Needs Subcategory—*Reduction of risk potential*

91. **2.** Sims' position, which is a left lateral side-lying position, is commonly preferred when a flexible sigmoidoscope is used. A knee-chest position is used with a rigid sigmoidoscope. A lithotomy position is used for cystoscopy and vaginal examinations. An orthopneic position is helpful for promoting rest in dyspneic individuals. Fowler's position is used for many reasons, including improving ventilation, but not for a sigmoidoscopy.

Test Taking Strategy—*Analyze to determine what information the question asks for, which is the client position that facilitates performing a sigmoidoscopy. This question requires an understanding of terms describing procedural positioning. Recall that the physician must have access to the anus to enter and advance the sigmoidoscope into the sigmoid area of the large intestine, making option 2 the best answer. Review the position used to perform a sigmoidoscopy if you had difficulty answering this question.*
Cognitive Level—*Applying*
Client Needs Category—*Physiological integrity*
Client Needs Subcategory—*Reduction of risk potential*

92. **2.** A low-residue diet is composed of foods that the body can absorb completely so that there is little residue to form feces. A low-residue diet contains no foods containing fiber (such as bran cereal), fruits, vegetables, or whole-grain breads. Fruit and vegetable juices, with the exception of prune juice, are allowed in minimal amounts. Tender or ground meat and refined carbohydrates such as pasta can be eaten.

Test Taking Strategy—*Analyze to determine what information the question asks for, which is a food that is not included on a low-residue diet. Bran cereal (option 2) contains fiber, which is avoided in a low-residue diet, and so is the best answer. Review the food items that are allowed and those that are excluded from a low-residue diet if you had difficulty answering this question.*
Cognitive Level—*Analyzing*
Client Needs Category—*Physiological integrity*
Client Needs Subcategory—*Basic care and comfort*

93. **3.** There are 1,000 mg in 1 g. The nurse gives the client two 500-mg tablets to administer 1 g of neomycin. Use the ratio and proportion method to solve for X.

$$\frac{500 \text{ mg}}{1{,}000 \text{ mg}} = \frac{1 \text{ tablet}}{X \text{ tablet}}$$
$$500\,X = 1{,}000$$
$$X = 2 \text{ tablets}$$

Test Taking Strategy—*Analyze to determine what information the question asks for, which involves calculating the number of tablets to administer based on the dose prescribed by the physician. Recall that the first step requires converting 1 g to its equivalent in milligrams. Once the measurements are the same, calculation can proceed using a standard formula, as shown in the example. Review the process for converting equivalents and calculating oral doses if you had difficulty answering this question.*
Cognitive Level—*Applying*
Client Needs Category—*Physiological integrity*
Client Needs Subcategory—*Pharmacological therapies*

94. **2.** During the operative procedure, the bowel is opened and some contents can leak within the peritoneum. Neomycin sulfate (Mycifradin) destroys intestinal bacteria and reduces the risk of a postoperative infection. Antibiotics commonly cause, rather than prevent, diarrhea. Surgery usually is not performed if the client has an ongoing infection.

Test Taking Strategy—*Look at the key words "most accurate" that are used in reference to the rationale for administering neomycin preoperatively. Recall that neomycin sulfate is an antibiotic and that the bowel contains many microorganisms. These organ-*

isms are nonpathogenic as long as they remain in the large intestine. However, they can cause an infection if they are transferred to peritoneal or abdominal tissue during the surgical procedure. Consequently, option 2 is the best answer. Review the use for neomycin, focusing on its administration before intestinal surgery, if you had difficulty answering this question.
Cognitive Level—*Applying*
Client Needs Category—*Physiological integrity*
Client Needs Subcategory—*Pharmacological therapies*

95. 3. Evisceration is the protrusion of the intestines through the abdominal wall. It usually occurs in a wound that is not healing because of an infection, excessive coughing or straining, abdominal distention, obesity, or poor wound healing due to malnutrition or corticosteroid therapy. The first action to take in the case of evisceration is to cover the bowel with sterile gauze moistened with sterile normal saline solution or povidone-iodine and a self-adhering plastic drape. This prevents the bowel from drying or becoming colonized with bacteria until it can be surgically repaired. The physician would be notified and vital signs taken only after taking emergency action. The bowel should not be manipulated, except by the physician. Evisceration is considered a medical emergency.

> *Test Taking Strategy*—*Analyze to determine what information the question asks for, which is the first nursing action to take when a wound eviscerates. Keeping the bowel moist and covered limits contamination of the tissues that will be returned to the abdominal cavity. Review the nursing actions that are necessary in the case of bowel evisceration if you had difficulty answering this question.*
Cognitive Level—*Analyzing*
Client Needs Category—*Physiological integrity*
Client Needs Subcategory—*Physiological adaptation*

96. 3. When an obstruction interferes with the movement of intestinal contents toward the rectum for elimination, the client begins to experience distention and vomiting. At first, the emesis contains gastric contents. As time passes, the vomitus may contain fecal matter and have a foul odor. The other questions are appropriate to ask, but they do not necessarily provide information associated with an intestinal obstruction.

> *Test Taking Strategy*—*Analyze to determine what information the question asks for, which is a sign or symptom of a bowel obstruction. Consider the consequence of an obstruction when choosing the answer. Recall that if the bowel becomes obstructed, fecal contents may be eliminated in a retrograde fashion in emesis. Review the signs and symptoms associated with a bowel obstruction if you had difficulty answering this question.*

Cognitive Level—*Applying*
Client Needs Category—*Physiological integrity*
Client Needs Subcategory—*Physiological adaptation*

97. 3. The nurse should always question any written order that is unclear or potentially unsafe. This includes a drug dosage that is higher or lower than the dosages given in approved references. The nurse should never administer a different dosage until consulting a physician about the discrepancy. Written orders for combined preoperative medications indicate that they are given together. Therefore, giving meperidine hydrochloride (Demerol) alone is inappropriate. The pharmacist is a reliable source for obtaining drug information; however, the only person who can revise the order is the physician.

> *Test Taking Strategy*—*Analyze to determine what information the question asks for, which is the nursing responsibility when a prescribed dosage of a medication is outside the usual range. According to the Code of Ethics for Nurses with Interpretive Statements, published by the American Nurses Association, the nurse must protect, advocate for, and protect the health, safety, and rights of the client. Therefore, option 3 is the best action because it protects the client from harm. Review the legal and ethical responsibilities of nurses if you had difficulty answering this question.*
Cognitive Level—*Analyzing*
Client Needs Category—*Safe and effective care environment*
Client Needs Subcategory—*Coordinated care*

98.

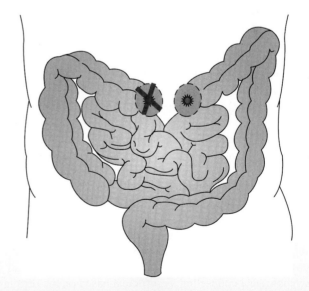

A double-barrel colostomy is created as a temporary measure; the two portions of the large intestine will be reconnected in the future. The proximal stoma eliminates fecal material; the distal stoma releases mucus. It is not necessary to put a drainage collection device over the stoma that releases mucus.

Test Taking Strategy—Analyze to determine what information the question asks for, which is the portion of the colostomy through which stool is eliminated. Recall that the proximal stoma remains connected to the small intestine and other structures in the upper GI tract. Consequently, it is the exit point for eliminating stool. Review information about various types of colostomies, focusing on the purpose and nursing management of a client with a double-barrel colostomy, if you had difficulty answering this question.
Cognitive Level—Applying
Client Needs Category—Physiological integrity
Client Needs Subcategory—Physiological adaptation

99. 2. The best position for performing colostomy irrigation is sitting on the toilet. This position and the environment simulate normal bowel elimination. The toilet is also convenient for hanging the distal end of the irrigating sleeve. The stool is easily flushed away along with the drained irrigating solution. Because it takes some time for the bowel evacuation to be complete, clients often appreciate the privacy of the bathroom. If sitting on the toilet is impossible or impractical for the client, ensure privacy by allowing the client to sit in bed with the end of the sleeve placed in a bedpan. Kneeling in the bathtub is not safe. Standing at the sink may be effective, but disposal of the feces and the irrigating solution in the sink would be a problem.

Test Taking Strategy—Use the process of elimination to help select the option that identifies the best client position when irrigating a colostomy. Recall that a sitting position provides the best position for the client to access the stoma, insert the irrigating tip, instill irrigating fluid, and expel the solution and stool. Review the procedure for irrigating a colostomy if you had difficulty answering this question.
Cognitive Level—Applying
Client Needs Category—Physiological integrity
Client Needs Subcategory—Reduction of risk potential

100. 2. Silence, when used appropriately, is a powerful means of communicating without verbalizing. Among other things, silence conveys acceptance, provides the client time to collect thoughts, allows relief from emotionally charged content, and gives the client the opportunity to proceed when ready. Changing the subject is nontherapeutic. It indicates that the nurse cannot handle the topic of conversation. Switching the discussion to physical care is a form of changing the subject. Active listening, rather than psychological counseling, is sufficient based on the data in the situation.

Test Taking Strategy—Look at the key words "most appropriate" in reference to a nursing action when a client stops talking and becomes tearful. Recall that silence on the part of the nurse is a therapeutic communication technique. Review therapeutic and

nontherapeutic communication techniques if you had difficulty answering this question.
Cognitive Level—Applying
Client Needs Category—Psychosocial integrity
Client Needs Subcategory—None

101. 1. Encouraging the expression of concerns provides the client with an opportunity to ventilate feelings without fear of retaliation. An open discussion can effectively lower the client's frustration level. Reassurance, in this case, is somewhat premature. The client needs to verbalize and clarify the specific perceived problems. With the assistance of the nurse and other health care professionals, the client ought to achieve the ability to accomplish self-care. Maintaining the client's independence is preferable to institutionalized care. Saying nothing indicates to the client that the nurse prefers to be uninvolved with emotional problems. Quoting a client, however, is always appropriate when documenting information.

Test Taking Strategy—Look at the key words "most appropriate" in reference to a client's statement describing doubt about becoming competent to manage the care of a colostomy. Recall that providing a client an opportunity to verbalize his or her feelings as well as being an active listener is always therapeutic. Review therapeutic and nontherapeutic communication techniques if you had difficulty answering this question.
Cognitive Level—Applying
Client Needs Category—Psychosocial integrity
Client Needs Subcategory—None

102. 2, 3. One of the most widespread and potentially serious of all health care–acquired illnesses is *Clostridium difficile* (*C. difficile*). *C. difficile* bacterial spores are located in soil, air, water, human and animal feces, and on most surfaces. The bacteria do not typically create problems until they grow in abnormally large numbers in the intestinal tract of people taking antibiotics or other antimicrobial drugs. Then, because the normal flora of the body is interrupted, *C. difficile* bacteria take over and can cause symptoms ranging from diarrhea to life-threatening inflammation of the colon. To prevent the spread of the bacteria, clients must be placed in contact isolation and meticulous hand hygiene performed by washing the hands with soap and water when entering and exiting the room. Gowns and gloves must be donned when coming in contact with feces. Generally, masks are not worn. Alcohol foam cleaner is not used because its use does not kill the spores of the *C. difficile* bacteria. Clients with tuberculosis (not *C. difficile*) require a negative-pressure room. Cohorting all clients with diarrhea to the same general location in the hospital is not appropriate because *C. difficile* may not be the cause of every client's diarrhea.

Test Taking Strategy—Analyze to determine what information the question asks for, which is steps to

prevent transmitting C. difficile. Alternative-format "select all that apply" questions require considering each option independently to decide its merit in answering the question. Read and consider each option independently; select one or more options that identify appropriate transmission precautions for C. difficile. Review transmission-based infection control practices if you had difficulty answering this question.
Cognitive Level—Applying
Client Needs Category—Safe and effective care environment
Client Needs Subcategory—Safety and infection control

Nursing Care of Clients with Disorders of the Rectum and Anus

103. 1, 2, 3. Drugs that commonly cause constipation include the opiates such as morphine, meperidine (Demerol), fentanyl, and codeine. These slow the peristalsis of the bowel. Iron preparations also cause constipation, causing the feces to become hard and dry. Antacids that contain calcium carbonate are known to cause constipation because of the calcium salts that are an active ingredient. Antibiotics can cause diarrhea. Antihypertensives and non-steroidal anti-inflammatory drugs (NSAIDs) are not known to cause constipation.

> *Test Taking Strategy*—Analyze to determine what information the question asks for, which involves identifying medication classifications that are prone to causing constipation. Alternative-format "select all that apply" questions require considering each option independently to decide its merit in answering the question. Review the potential side effects of the drug categories listed if you had difficulty answering this question.
> *Cognitive Level*—Analyzing
> *Client Needs Category*—Physiological integrity
> *Client Needs Subcategory*—Pharmacological therapies

104. 1. Long-term use of laxatives causes the bowel to become sluggish because it is repeatedly subjected to artificial stimulation. Stool softeners are less harsh than laxatives. However, it is best to determine the cause of the constipation and treat the etiology with lifestyle changes rather than continue to rely on pharmaceutical interventions. Daily enemas are just as habituating as laxative abuse. Dilating the anal sphincter is not usually an acceptable technique for promoting bowel elimination.

> *Test Taking Strategy*—Use the process of elimination to help select the option that identifies essential information to tell a client about taking a daily laxative. Option 3 can be immediately eliminated, because substituting a daily enema is no more therapeutic than the client's use of a daily laxative. Options 2 and 4 have merit because they can promote bowel

elimination, but the best approach would be to suggest lifestyle changes. Recall that daily use of a laxative contributes to laxative dependence, making option 1 the best answer. Review factors that contribute to chronic constipation and the adverse effects of self-administering a laxative on a daily basis if you had difficulty answering this question.
Cognitive Level—Applying
Client Needs Category—Physiological integrity
Client Needs Subcategory—Pharmacological therapies

105. 1. A fecal impaction is stool that is so hard and dry that it cannot be expelled. A client with a fecal impaction tends to expel liquid stool around the hardened mass that is located in the rectum. Common causes of a fecal impaction include immobility, paralysis, dehydration, and history of chronic bowel problems. Foul-smelling stools are not associated with fecal impactions. A stomach ache may be associated with constipation or other conditions, but this is not the main assessment finding associated with fecal impaction. Loss of appetite may be either the cause or the effect of impaired bowel elimination. Its presence is not necessarily an indication of a fecal impaction.

> *Test Taking Strategy*—Analyze to determine what information the question asks for, which is a sign of a fecal impaction. Options 3 and 4 may be inter-related; however, clients who experience a fecal impaction may pass liquid stool (option 1) despite having a large amount of dried stool within the rectum. Review the signs associated with a fecal impaction, particularly the passage of liquid stool, if you had difficulty answering this question.
> *Cognitive Level*—Applying
> *Client Needs Category*—Physiological integrity
> *Client Needs Subcategory*—Basic care and comfort

106. 1, 2, 3, 6. Clients who have had cardiac surgery should not have manual removal of the fecal impaction because digital manipulation can cause stimulation of the vagus nerve, causing bradycardia or arrhythmias. Furthermore, manual removal of fecal impactions is contraindicated in clients with a history of reproductive surgery or radiation to the abdomen because this method could further damage weakened tissue. Prolonged bleeding could occur in clients who routinely receive anticoagulants such as heparin, enoxaparin (Lovenox), or warfarin (Coumadin). The presence of hemorrhoids is not a contraindication when removing fecal impactions; however, caution should be used. If the client is dependent on laxatives, it is unlikely that the client will have a fecal impaction.

> *Test Taking Strategy*—Analyze to determine what information the question asks for, which is factors that contraindicate the digital removal of impacted stool. Alternative-format "select all that apply" questions require considering each option independently to decide its merit in answering the question. Review

factors that may be affected by manipulating rectal tissue if you had difficulty answering this question.
***Cognitive Level**—Analyzing*
***Client Needs Category**—Physiological integrity*
***Client Needs Subcategory**—Physiological adaptation*

107. 2. By inserting a lubricated, gloved finger within the rectum, it is possible to confirm the presence of a hard mass of stool. An X-ray may confirm the presence of a mass in the rectum but is expensive and relatively unnecessary. An oil-retention enema is a method for relieving the impaction after its presence is confirmed. Monitoring bowel sounds causes unnecessary delay in treating the problem.

* **Test Taking Strategy**—Use the process of elimination to help select the best technique for confirming the presence of a fecal impaction. Option 1 can be immediately eliminated because it is an intervention rather than an assessment. Option 4 can be eliminated because bowel sounds help identify normal, hypoactive, or hyperactive peristalsis, but if they are abnormal, it will not indicate the cause. Option 3 has merit, but physical assessment (option 2) is more time efficient and less expensive than radiographic assessment. Review the characteristics of a fecal impaction if you had difficulty answering this question.*
***Cognitive Level**—Applying*
***Client Needs Category**—Physiological integrity*
***Client Needs Subcategory**—Physiological adaptation*

108. 1. Activity promotes the movement of gas toward the anal sphincter, where it can be released. Restricting food may prevent additional gas from forming, but it will not help eliminate any gas that is already present. Opioid analgesics tend to slow peristalsis and contribute to constipation, stool retention, and intestinal gas.

* **Test Taking Strategy**—Look at the key words "most helpful" in reference to a nursing measure that promotes the expulsion of intestinal gas. Recall that ambulation (option 1) helps to direct gas toward the anus. Options 2 and 3 can be eliminated because carbonated beverages can increase gas accumulation and restricting food is inappropriate. Option 4 can be eliminated because opioid analgesics actually contribute to intestinal gas. Review methods for eliminating intestinal gas if you had difficulty answering this question.*
***Cognitive Level**—Applying*
***Client Needs Category**—Physiological integrity*
***Client Needs Subcategory**—Basic care and comfort*

109. 2. A rectal tube should remain in place only approximately 20 to 30 minutes at one time to help relieve distention from accumulating gas. Placement for only 5 minutes is unlikely to achieve an optimum effect, yet longer than 30 minutes is unnecessary. The tube is removed and replaced again in 1 to 2 hours if gas continues to accumulate.

* **Test Taking Strategy**—Analyze to determine what information the question asks for, which is the maximum time for keeping a rectal tube in place. Knowledge of nursing standards or nursing policy for rectal tube placement recommends a 20- to 30-minute period (option 2). Review the procedure for using a rectal tube or refer to the facility's policy if you had difficulty answering this question.*
***Cognitive Level**—Understanding*
***Client Needs Category**—Safe and effective care environment*
***Client Needs Subcategory**—Safety and infection control*

110. 3. Interrupting the instillation of enema solution allows time for the bowel to adjust to the distention. Rapidly instilling the remaining solution may cause the client to lose bowel control and fluid retention. Taking deep breaths or panting rather than holding the breath relieves some discomfort. Placing the client supine will not help the client's cramping or the sudden urge to defecate.

* **Test Taking Strategy**—Note the key words "most appropriate" and "at this time" in reference to an action that is indicated when a client experiences cramping and an urge to defecate while receiving an enema solution. Recall that ideally the nursing goal is to infuse an appreciable volume of the solution, have the client retain the solution within the bowel temporarily, and assist the client to a location where the solution and stool can be eliminated. Selecting the action described in option 3 helps reduce the client's discomfort before continuing to instill the remainder of the enema solution. Review the nursing procedure for administering a cleansing soap-suds enema, particularly how to manage untoward effects, if you had difficulty answering this question.*
***Cognitive Level**—Applying*
***Client Needs Category**—Physiological integrity*
***Client Needs Subcategory**—Basic care and comfort*

111. 3. A rectal suppository is inserted approximately 2″ to 4″ (5 to 10 cm). For the best effect, the suppository must be inserted beyond the internal sphincter. A clean glove, not a sterile one, is used to avoid contact with organisms in the rectum, stool, or blood. A right lateral position is not the correct anatomic position for suppository placement. Instead, the client should be positioned on the left side. Retaining the suppository until the client feels an urge to defecate ensures its effectiveness. Suppositories should be retained for at least 30 minutes.

* **Test Taking Strategy**—Look at the key words "most appropriate" in reference to a nursing action that relates to inserting a rectal suppository. Recall that to be effective, the suppository must be inserted beyond the internal anal sphincter (option 3). Options 2 and 4 can be eliminated because they*

offer incorrect actions; a clean glove, rather than a sterile one, is used; the client is positioned on the left side; and the suppository is left in place at least 30 minutes. Review the procedure for inserting a rectal suppository if you had difficulty answering this question.
Cognitive Level—*Understanding*
Client Needs Category—*Physiological integrity*
Client Needs Subcategory—*Pharmacological therapies*

112. 2. Bowel elimination tends to occur in a cyclic pattern. Assessing the bowel elimination pattern precedes other interventions. Limiting activity impairs rather than promotes bowel elimination. The diet should have adequate amounts of water and bulk-forming foods to help the client form soft, rather than dry, hard stool. The regular administration of enemas eventually may help to regulate bowel elimination, but it is not the first step in a bowel-retraining program.
> *Test Taking Strategy—Analyze to determine what information the question asks for, which is the first step in bowel retraining. Recall that assessing the client is the first step in planning any care. Options 1, 3, and 4 are interventions, some of which are inappropriate to include in any bowel-retraining regimen. Review recommended nursing actions for retraining a client to control bowel elimination if you had difficulty answering this question.*
Cognitive Level—*Analyzing*
Client Needs Category—*Physiological integrity*
Client Needs Subcategory—*Basic care and comfort*

113. 3. Chronic constipation, hereditary factors, and conditions that increase venous pressure in the abdomen and pelvic area, such as pregnancy, ascites, and liver disease, foster the development of hemorrhoids. Clients who take daily stool softeners are not usually prone to constipation. Clients diagnosed with ulcerative colitis have diarrhea, not constipation. Sedentary jobs, such as computer programming, may predispose the client to constipation but not necessarily hemorrhoids.
> *Test Taking Strategy—Look at the key words "most likely" as they relate to identifying a factor contributing to the development of hemorrhoids. Recall that chronically straining to expel hard stool (option 3) can distend veins in the rectal area, causing them to become dilated and filled with blood. Review factors that contribute to hemorrhoid formation if you had difficulty answering this question.*
Cognitive Level—*Applying*
Client Needs Category—*Physiological integrity*
Client Needs Subcategory—*Physiological adaptation*

114. 2. The cellulose that remains after eating high-fiber foods absorbs water in the bowel, increases bulk, and stimulates peristalsis. This prevents constipation, which

can lead to hemorrhoids. Lack of adequate fluid makes constipation more severe. Therefore, drinking eight glasses of fluid daily will keep the feces bulk moist and easier to expel. Although taking a daily laxative may help with constipation and the client's hemorrhoids, it can result in dependence on the drug, making it an inappropriate choice. Neither of the other recommendations aids in preventing or eliminating constipation.
> *Test Taking Strategy—Look at the key words "most appropriate" in reference to instructions that will be helpful to the client with hemorrhoids. Recall that preventing or relieving chronic constipation can greatly reduce the symptoms caused by hemorrhoids. Drinking sufficient fluids each day (option 2) helps to keep stool moist. Review methods for managing constipation if you had difficulty answering this question.*
Cognitive Level—*Applying*
Client Needs Category—*Health promotion and maintenance*
Client Needs Subcategory—*None*

115. 2. A sitz bath keeps the incisional area clean and promotes healing. This provides objective evidence that the incision is healing and the sitz bath is effective. Secondly, a sitz bath provides a comfort measure because the warm water soothes the discomfort and pain in the surgical area. Pain is subjective; therefore, a report of a less painful incision is less reliable than objective evidence. Because only the buttocks are submerged in water, evidence of personal hygiene is not an appropriate criterion for effectiveness. The presence or absence of a hematoma has no bearing on the effectiveness of the sitz bath.
> *Test Taking Strategy—Use the process of elimination to help select the option that describes the best method for evaluating the effectiveness of a sitz bath. Gathering objective assessment data, such as those identified in option 2, provides the best evidence that the purpose of the sitz bath is being accomplished. Review the purposes for administering a sitz bath if you had difficulty answering this question.*
Cognitive Level—*Analyzing*
Client Needs Category—*Physiological integrity*
Client Needs Subcategory—*Basic care and comfort*

116. 1. Docusate sodium (Colace) is a stool softener. Retaining water in the stool softens the mass and makes the stool easier and less painful to pass. Some categories of laxatives, including castor oil, stimulate bowel evacuation by irritating the intestinal mucosa. Bulk-forming laxatives such as psyllium (Metamucil) stimulate peristalsis by adding bulk and water to the stool. Drugs that reduce intestinal activity promote constipation rather than stool elimination.
> *Test Taking Strategy—Analyze to determine what information the question asks for, which is the purpose for administering docusate sodium. Recall that this*

medication is a stool softener, which correlates with the statement in option 1. Review the mechanism of action associated with docusate sodium if you had difficulty answering this question.
Cognitive Level—*Understanding*
Client Needs Category—*Physiological integrity*
Client Needs Subcategory—*Pharmacological therapies*

117. 2, 5. The word *pilonidal* means a nest of hair. The growth of stiff body hair in the anorectal area at puberty commonly precipitates irritation within the sinus tract. A pilonidal cyst is actually a sinus with one or more openings onto the skin. Once the integrity of the skin is impaired, microorganisms enter and cause subsequent infection near the coccyx, as evidenced by purulent drainage. Pain and swelling at the base of the spine are common findings. Pilonidal cysts are not related to rectal bleeding; frothy, foul-smelling stool; or diarrhea.

Test Taking Strategy—*Analyze to determine what information the question asks for, which is information in the client's health history that correlates with characteristic findings of a pilonidal cyst. Alternative-format "select all that apply" questions require considering each option independently to decide its merit in answering the question. Select one or more options that are associated with this condition. Review the signs and symptoms of a pilonidal cyst if you had difficulty answering this question.*
Cognitive Level—*Applying*
Client Needs Category—*Physiological integrity*
Client Needs Subcategory—*Physiological adaptation*

118. 4. Cleaning the area before applying a topical medication ensures that the drug is maximally absorbed. The client may wish to wear gloves for aesthetic and aseptic reasons, but their use will not affect the medication's action. For comfort, an ointment applied to a sensitive area is generally kept at room temperature unless otherwise directed by the manufacturer. It is more appropriate to apply this type of medication immediately after a bowel movement because pain is greater at that time. This drug can also be routinely applied in the morning and evening.

Test Taking Strategy—*Analyze to determine what information the question asks for, which is information that is essential to tell a client who will be self-administering anesthetic ointment to the rectal area. Recall that a topical drug's effectiveness is related to the cleanliness of the skin or mucous membrane to which it is applied, a fact that is verified by the statement in option 4. Review information on drug absorption in relation to topically applied medications if you had difficulty answering this question.*
Cognitive Level—*Applying*
Client Needs Category—*Physiological integrity*
Client Needs Subcategory—*Pharmacological therapies*

Nursing Care of Clients with Disorders of the Gallbladder

119. 1. The characteristic upper right quadrant pain of cholecystitis typically occurs after eating. Cholecystitis is especially aggravated when the meal has a high fat content, which impairs bile flow and causes nausea, vomiting, distention, and flatulence. Ulcers are more likely to cause pain when the stomach is empty. Activity is unlikely to influence the discomfort of cholecystitis. The volume and types of foods eaten, rather than the time of day they are consumed, are more significant in the development of gallbladder disease.

Test Taking Strategy—*Look at the key words "most likely" in reference to when the discomfort associated with cholecystitis generally occurs. Recall that the gallbladder contracts and releases bile into the small intestine in response to cholecystokinin, which is secreted when fatty substances are consumed. This correlates with option 1. Review the function of the gallbladder in the digestive process if you had difficulty answering this question.*
Cognitive Level—*Applying*
Client Needs Category—*Physiological integrity*
Client Needs Subcategory—*Physiological adaptation*

120. 1. The referred pain of cholecystitis is felt either in the right shoulder or in the back at the level of the shoulder blades. Ulcers and esophageal reflux cause pain in the midepigastric region. Angina pectoris may be experienced as pain in the neck or jaw or down the left arm.

Test Taking Strategy—*Analyze to determine what information the question asks for, which is the location of referred pain experienced by clients with cholecystitis. Recall that referred pain is felt in areas other than the affected organ or tissue. Refer to texts regarding the pain associated with cholecystitis if you had difficulty answering this question.*
Cognitive Level—*Applying*
Client Needs Category—*Physiological integrity*
Client Needs Subcategory—*Physiological adaptation*

121. 3. Evidence suggests that an elevated cholesterol level predisposes certain clients to gallstone formation. The majority of gallstones are thought to form when bile in the gallbladder is thick, high in cholesterol, and low in bile acids. A low red blood cell count or hemoglobin level is commonly found in people with bleeding disorders, nutritional deficiencies, and bone marrow disorders. An elevated serum albumin level is not generally associated with cholecystitis.

Test Taking Strategy—*Analyze to determine what information the question asks for, which is the laboratory test finding that correlates with cholecystitis. Recall that gallstones are composed of cholesterol, making option 3 the correct answer. Review the pathophysi-*

ology of gallstone formation or a laboratory test manual if you had difficulty with this question.
Cognitive Level—*Applying*
Client Needs Category—*Physiological integrity*
Client Needs Subcategory—*Reduction of risk potential*

122. **2.** Bile pigments cause the normal brown appearance of stool. If bile is prevented from entering the small intestine, the stool is likely to appear clay-colored. Black, tarry stools indicate bleeding high in the GI tract; such stools also result from the administration of oral iron therapy. Dark brown stool is normal; the shade may vary depending on the food eaten. Bloody mucus associated with brown stools may indicate hemorrhoids. Greenish yellow stool is more commonly associated with diarrhea.
Test Taking Strategy—*Analyze to determine what information the question asks for, which is the color of the stool when bile pigments are absent. Recall how bile pigments contribute to the color of stool or eliminate options that describe color characteristics caused by other disorders. Review information that discusses the physiology of stool characteristics if you had difficulty answering this question.*
Cognitive Level—*Applying*
Client Needs Category—*Physiological integrity*
Client Needs Subcategory—*Physiological adaptation*

123. **3.** Greasy fried foods and fatty meats are not allowed on a low-fat diet. Baked or broiled fish, poultry, and lean meat are permitted. Leaner cuts of beef, such as round steak, could be ground and used in recipes that call for hamburger. Hard cheese, cream, gravies, salad oil, rich desserts, and nuts are restricted. Whole milk, butter or margarine, and sometimes eggs can be used in limited amounts.
Test Taking Strategy—*Analyze to determine what information the question asks for, which is the statement indicating a client's misunderstanding about a low-fat diet that requires clarification. Recall that a hamburger and French fries (option 3) are high in fat and will contribute to symptoms for the client with cholecystitis. When analyzing the four options, note that options 1, 2, and 4 contain chicken, fish, and turkey, which are allowed on a low-fat diet, making option 3 more obviously a food to be avoided. Review information about a low-fat diet if you had difficulty answering this question.*
Cognitive Level—*Analyzing*
Client Needs Category—*Physiological integrity*
Client Needs Subcategory—*Basic care and comfort*

124. **1.** The person undergoing an ultrasound of the gallbladder must not eat food for approximately 8 to 12 hours before the test. Restricting food helps to eliminate the presence of gas. Intestinal gas interferes with the transmission of sound waves toward the gallbladder and the scan of the

structure's image. Water is permitted. Barium is used as a contrast medium for upper and lower GI X-rays, not a gallbladder ultrasound. Applying a water-soluble lubricant to a hand-held transducer and passing it across the abdomen during ultrasonography produces an image of the gallbladder. Insertion of needles is not part of the procedure.
Test Taking Strategy—*Analyze to determine what information the question asks for, which is a client's accurate understanding of the preparation for an ultrasound of the gallbladder. Recall that temporarily withholding food facilitates a better image during an ultrasound because the sound waves will not be distorted by gas and remnants of digested contents within the intestinal tract. Consequently, option 1 is the best answer. Review the preparation of a client for an ultrasound, particularly a cholecystography, if you had difficulty answering this question.*
Cognitive Level—*Applying*
Client Needs Category—*Physiological integrity*
Client Needs Subcategory—*Reduction of risk potential*

125. **3, 4, 5.** Laparoscopic cholecystectomy is the preferred surgical procedure for gallbladder removal in about 80% of cases. The procedure involves general (not moderate) sedation, and is performed using an endoscope inserted into one of four small sites in the abdomen. Carbon dioxide is used to inflate the abdomen to displace the abdominal structures and make visualization easier. Most clients return home the same evening after the procedure. Long periods of gastric decompression and the insertion of a T-tube are used when the client has an open cholecystectomy.
Test Taking Strategy—*Analyze to determine what information the question asks for, which involves identifying accurate statements about laparoscopic cholecystectomy. Alternative-format "select all that apply" questions require considering each option independently to decide its merit in answering the question. Recall the differences between a laparoscopic procedure and an open cholecystectomy as you analyze each option. Review both techniques for removing a gallbladder if you had difficulty answering this question.*
Cognitive Level—*Applying*
Client Needs Category—*Physiological integrity*
Client Needs Subcategory—*Reduction of risk potential*

126. **4.** The pigment found in bile is derived from hemoglobin. Depending on the concentration of pigment, the normal appearance of bile drainage is green-yellow to orange-brown. Bile is generally clear, but clear is not a color. Dark red drainage indicates that venous blood is mixed with the biliary drainage. Bright red drainage is a sign of fresh or arterial bleeding.
Test Taking Strategy—*Use the process of elimination to help select the option that provides the best*

description of normal drainage from a T-tube. The T-tube drains bile coming from the hepatic duct to the common bile duct, the cystic duct having been removed. Recall the color of normal bile or eliminate the options of those that are atypical. Review the characteristics of bile drainage if you had difficulty answering this question.
Cognitive Level—*Applying*
Client Needs Category—*Physiological integrity*
Client Needs Subcategory—*Physiological adaptation*

127. **1, 3, 5, 6.** A Jackson-Pratt closed-wound drain removes blood and exudates without using a suction machine. A vacuum or negative pressure is created by expelling air from the receptacle and replacing the cap that covers the vent while still compressing the receptacle. When emptying the receptacle, the cap that covers the vent is opened, the contents of the receptacle are emptied from the open vent and measured, air is expelled from the emptied receptacle, the vent is covered, and the tubing is stabilized to the client's gown or dressing to keep it from tugging at the insertion site. The tubing is kept unclamped at all times to allow fluid to enter the drainage receptacle. Jackson-Pratt drains do not have roller clamps.

> *Test Taking Strategy—Analyze to determine what information the question asks for, which involves selecting nursing actions when emptying a Jackson-Pratt closed-wound drainage system. Analyze each option individually and select one or more that apply. Recall that a Jackson-Pratt drain uses negative pressure, a vacuum, to pull fluid into the drainage receptacle. Review the differences between closed and open wound drains and how they are managed if you had difficulty answering this question.*
Cognitive Level—*Applying*
Client Needs Category—*Physiological integrity*
Client Needs Subcategory—*Reduction of risk potential*

128. **1, 4, 5, 6.** A T-tube is inserted to drain bile that is continuously formed by the liver and cannot be stored and concentrated in the gallbladder, which has been surgically removed. The tube is kept unclamped in the immediate postoperative period. The nurse connects the tube to a collection bag and facilitates drainage by keeping the client in Fowler's position with the drainage bag below the site of insertion. The nurse inspects the skin around the tube because bile may leak around the tube insertion site and irritate the skin. The nurse measures and records the volume of drainage from the T-tube. The color of the drainage may be blood-tinged initially, but it should eventually appear greenish brown.

> *Test Taking Strategy—Analyze to determine what information the question asks for, which is the correct management of a T-tube. Alternative-format "select all that apply" questions require considering each option independently to decide its merit in answer-*

ing the question. Visualize the nursing care that is involved, with consideration for pertinent assessments and the effect posture and gravity have on T-tube drainage. Read each option individually and select one or more that apply. Review information about managing the care of a client with a T-tube if you had difficulty answering this question.
Cognitive Level—*Applying*
Client Needs Category—*Physiological integrity*
Client Needs Subcategory—*Reduction of risk potential*

129. **2.** The client's T-tube should remain unclamped until beginning to resume oral feedings. Clamping the tube would cause reflux of bile toward the liver; immediate action is necessary if the nurse finds the tube clamped in the early postoperative period. It would be appropriate to support the tubing to prevent kinking or dislodgement. Placing the drainage bag in a dependent position facilitates drainage by gravity. A volume of up to 500 mL in 24 hours is not unusual.

> *Test Taking Strategy—Analyze to determine what information the question asks for, which is a T-tube assessment finding that requires immediate attention. Recall that if the T-tube is clamped, there will be a backflow of bile toward the hepatic duct and the liver that makes bile. Option 2 identifies this point of concern. Review the nursing care of a client with T-tube drainage if you had difficulty answering this question.*
Cognitive Level—*Applying*
Client Needs Category—*Physiological integrity*
Client Needs Subcategory—*Physiological adaptation*

130. **3.** Because bile is essential to digestion, the T-tube is generally unclamped for up to 2 hours after a meal is consumed. As healing takes place and edema is reduced, some bile begins draining into the small intestine even when the tubing is clamped.

> *Test Taking Strategy—Analyze to determine what information the question asks for, which is the schedule for clamping and unclamping a T-tube. Recall that bile facilitates the digestion of fat. Unclamping the T-tube after a meal (option 3) allows bile to enter the small intestine and mix with consumed fatty substances. Review the function of bile and the nursing care of a client with T-tube drainage if you had difficulty answering this question.*
Cognitive Level—*Applying*
Client Needs Category—*Physiological integrity*
Client Needs Subcategory—*Physiological adaptation*

131. **1.** To establish negative pressure, the vent is uncovered and the bulb is squeezed. Air and drainage are eliminated from the bulb reservoir. After the bulb is squeezed, the bulb is recapped. The Jackson-Pratt drain is an example of a closed drainage device. The device could drain by gravity, not negative pressure, if the drainage valve was left open. The bulb reservoir is never filled with normal saline solution. The reservoir is secured to the skin with tape. However, this is done to prevent tension on the tubing and possible dislodgement from the insertion site, not to reestablish negative pressure in the drainage system.

> *Test Taking Strategy—Analyze to determine what information the question asks for, which is the method for reestablishing negative pressure with a Jackson-Pratt wound drain. Review information about the use of a Jackson-Pratt wound drain if you had difficulty answering this question.*
> *Cognitive Level—Applying*
> *Client Needs Category—Physiological integrity*
> *Client Needs Subcategory—Physiological adaptation*

Nursing Care of Clients with Disorders of the Liver

132. 4. Alanine and aspartate aminotransferase, previously called *transaminase,* are blood tests performed to assess liver function. Liver and other organ diseases result in elevated levels of these particular enzymes. The tests are repeated periodically to evaluate the client's response to treatment. Serum potassium testing is performed to monitor electrolyte balance when a client's nutritional or fluid balance has been altered. Serum creatinine and blood urea nitrogen (BUN) tests are performed to monitor kidney, not liver, function.

> *Test Taking Strategy—Analyze to determine what information the question asks for, which is a laboratory test finding that indicates liver dysfunction. Recall that alanine aminotransferase (ALT) is an enzyme found in various organs, but especially the liver. Measuring ALT is helpful in diagnosing and monitoring liver diseases. Review the purposes for the laboratory tests listed if you had difficulty with this question.*
> *Cognitive Level—Applying*
> *Client Needs Category—Physiological integrity*
> *Client Needs Subcategory—Reduction of risk potential*

133. 1. Infectious hepatitis A is generally spread by the fecal-oral route. In other words, the stool contains the virus, and the pathogen is spread to the mouth of a susceptible individual. Transmission is direct after contact with the excrement of an infected person or indirect by ingesting fecally contaminated food or water or food handled by an individual with the virus. This virus is also present in the blood and saliva of infected individuals; however, transmission through these routes is rarer.

> *Test Taking Strategy—Use the process of elimination to help select the option that identifies the best answer for the manner in which hepatitis A is transmitted. Options 2 and 3 can be immediately eliminated*

because hepatitis A is not transmitted by an insect vector nor by the blood of an infected person. Option 4 has merit if the wound drainage contains fecal material, but it is not the best answer because this transmission method is less likely than option 1, especially when the nurse dons gloves. Review the modes of transmission of the various types of hepatitis if you had difficulty answering this question.
> *Cognitive Level—Understanding*
> *Client Needs Category—Safe and effective care environment*
> *Client Needs Subcategory—Safety and infection control*

134. 4. Conscientious hand washing is the best defense against disease transmission. Gloves are worn when nursing care involves direct contact with the client, any excrement, or other body fluids. Wearing gloves, though, does not eliminate the need for hand washing. A gown is used if soiling is possible, but a mask is not necessary. Only individuals who cannot be relied on to practice good hand washing are placed in a private room.

> *Test Taking Strategy—Analyze to determine what information the question asks for, which is an infection control measure to prevent the transmission of hepatitis A. Recall that hepatitis A is transmitted via the fecal-oral route, making handwashing an essential method of infection control even after removing gloves during the client's care. Review transmission-based precautions for managing clients with hepatitis A if you had difficulty answering this question.*
> *Cognitive Level—Applying*
> *Client Needs Category—Safe and effective care environment*
> *Client Needs Subcategory—Safety and infection control*

135. 2. Immunoglobulin, formerly known as *gamma globulin,* is made from pooled donor serum containing ready-made antibodies; it is recommended for postexposure to a person with hepatitis A. It is most effective if administered from 48 hours to 2 weeks of exposure. Antibiotic therapy is ineffective in preventing or eliminating hepatitis A, which is a viral infection. Hepatitis vaccinations are usually given to clients at risk for contracting hepatitis B. Anti-inflammatory drugs, such as salicylates, nonsalicylates, and steroids, are ineffective in preventing the spread of hepatitis A.

> *Test Taking Strategy—Use the process of elimination to help select the option identifying how an infection with hepatitis A may be prevented among exposed persons. Eliminate option 3 because vaccines are intended as a pre-exposure measure to actively develop antibodies to prevent infection. Options 1 and 4 can be eliminated because they do not have antiviral effects. Option 2 remains as the best answer*

because passive immunity with serum immunoglobulin is used when there is a high risk of infection and insufficient time for persons to develop their own immune response. Review the administration of serum immunoglobulin if you had difficulty answering this question.
***Cognitive Level**—Applying*
***Client Needs Category**—Safe and effective care environment*
***Client Needs Subcategory**—Safety and infection control*

136. 2, 5. Sexually active homosexual men are at particularly high risk for acquiring bloodborne infections. The source of the hepatitis B virus is the blood of infected people or carriers. The virus is present in semen, saliva, and blood. It is transmitted by sexual contact, contaminated blood products, or accidental or intentional puncture with objects or needles that contain traces of infected blood. The client living in Europe has no bearing on the disease. Alcohol abuse compounds, but does not cause, liver damage concurrent with hepatitis. Working in a fast food restaurant is more of a factor in acquiring hepatitis A than hepatitis B.

Test Taking Strategy—Analyze to determine what information the question asks for, which is risk factors for hepatitis B transmission. Alternative-format "select all that apply" questions require considering each option independently to decide its merit in answering the question. Consider each option individually as to its potential for causing a hepatitis B infection. Select one or more options that apply. Recall that hepatitis B is a bloodborne infection; focus on aspects of the client's history that elevate client risk. Review etiologies for hepatitis B infection if you had difficulty answering this question.
***Cognitive Level**—Applying*
***Client Needs Category**—Health promotion and maintenance*
***Client Needs Subcategory**—None*

137. 2. For anyone who has not been vaccinated for hepatitis B, the best action after exposure to the blood of someone with hepatitis B is to receive hepatitis B immunoglobulin within 24 hours but no later than 7 days. Vaccination immediately after exposure does not provide sufficient antibody protection. Viruses are unaffected by antibiotics such as penicillin (Pentam). Bleach is an effective antiseptic, but it is not the best prophylaxis to counter exposure to the hepatitis B virus.

Test Taking Strategy—Look at the key words "most appropriate" in reference to a postexposure intervention after a needle-stick injury. Focus on the action that best protects the nurse and the timeframe for effectiveness among the listed options. Immunoglobulin therapy (option 2) provides the best answer.

Review prophylaxis for hepatitis B if you had difficulty answering this question.
***Cognitive Level**—Applying*
***Client Needs Category**—Health promotion and maintenance*
***Client Needs Subcategory**—None*

138. 2. Donating blood is not recommended for people who have had hepatitis. The virus remains in the blood years after the person has had the acute illness and can be passed to others. Blood collection personnel are taught to screen and reject any potential donor who indicates having had jaundice. Safe sex may be practiced, which would include using a condom. Convalescence is prolonged after the acute phase of hepatitis, but eventually there are no permanent physical restrictions. Alcohol use has negative effects on the liver, but its use is not necessarily restricted. Individuals with hepatitis antibodies are not barred from foreign travel.

Test Taking Strategy—Analyze to determine what information the question asks for, which is an activity that must be avoided for the person's lifetime after acquiring hepatitis B. Recall that hepatitis B is a blood-borne viral infection, making blood donation (option 2) the best answer. Review the consequences of having been infected with the hepatitis B virus if you had difficulty answering this question.
***Cognitive Level**—Applying*
***Client Needs Category**—Health promotion and maintenance*
***Client Needs Subcategory**—None*

139. 1, 5. Cirrhosis is a degenerative liver disease characterized by damaged, nonfunctional liver cells. The etiology of Laënnec's portal cirrhosis, the most common form of cirrhosis in the United States, is chronic malnutrition and alcoholism. Chronic malnutrition is often a consequence of alcoholism and is evidenced by weight loss, muscle wasting, hair loss, and fatigue. Smoking is associated with lung cancer, not cirrhosis of the liver. Pancreatitis can cause jaundice as the gland autodigests itself and disrupts the flow of secretions through the adjacent ducts, but this is a complication of cirrhosis of the liver. The client's hypertension could be secondary to alcohol abuse. Asbestos exposure is associated with lung cancer.

Test Taking Strategy—Analyze to determine what information the question asks for, which is causative factors in the development of cirrhosis. Alternative-format "select all that apply" questions require considering each option independently to decide its merit in answering the question. Recall that a health history consists of biographical data, chief complaint, history of present illness, past history, family history, and social history Review risks that contribute to cirrhosis if you had difficulty answering this question.

Cognitive Level—*Applying*
Client Needs Category—*Physiological integrity*
Client Needs Subcategory—*Physiological adaptation*

140. **2, 3, 5, 6.** Clients who have cirrhosis typically experience chronic fatigue, nausea, vomiting, diarrhea, weight loss, jaundice, and a low-grade fever. The client also has an enlarged liver and spleen, edema of the legs, feet, and abdomen, bruising, and vein engorgement around the umbilicus. The skin of a person with cirrhosis usually manifests multiple vascular lesions with a central red body and radiating branches. These are known as *spider angiomas*. They are also referred to as *telangiectasia, spider nevi,* or *vascular spiders*. Clients with cirrhosis also usually have scant body hair. Elevated serum cholesterol levels and hyperglycemia are not usually associated with cirrhosis.

> *Test Taking Strategy*—*Analyze to determine what information the question asks for, which involves identifying assessment data that correlate with advanced cirrhosis. Alternative-format "select all that apply" questions require considering each option independently to decide its merit in answering the question. Consider the late signs of liver dysfunction and the manner in which they are physically manifested. Refer to common assessment findings in clients with cirrhosis if you had difficulty answering this question.*
>
> *Cognitive Level*—*Applying*
> *Client Needs Category*—*Physiological integrity*
> *Client Needs Subcategory*—*Physiological adaptation*

141. **3.** In the absence of the client taking an oral iron supplement, black or tarry stools indicate that a significant amount of blood is being lost from the stomach or somewhere in the proximal end of the intestine. If the bleeding were from the rectal or anal area, the blood would be bright red. Pain, nausea, and abdominal distention usually do not accompany gastric hemorrhage.

> *Test Taking Strategy*—*Analyze to determine what information the question asks for, which is an assessment that indicates upper GI bleeding. Recall that blood loss in the upper GI tract remains in the tract and travels through the small and large intestines. Review the causes of black tarry stools vs. stools that contain bright red blood if you had difficulty answering this question.*
>
> *Cognitive Level*—*Applying*
> *Client Needs Category*—*Physiological integrity*
> *Client Needs Subcategory*—*Physiological adaptation*

142. **1.** After a liver biopsy, the client is monitored closely for signs of hemorrhage. A person with cirrhosis is at especially high risk for bleeding or hemorrhage because liver disease results in diminished prothrombin. Prothrombinemia causes a prolonged delay in the time it takes for blood to clot; therefore, blood clots are not usually a prob-

lem. Although the client may acquire an infection from the biopsy, an invasive procedure, infection does not usually occur immediately after the procedure. A collapsed lung is not typically an issue unless extremely poor technique was used in the procedure.

> *Test Taking Strategy*—*Analyze to determine what information the question asks for, which is the complication that may occur immediately after a liver biopsy. Recall that a client with cirrhosis is prone to bleeding, especially from a percutaneous puncture, due to a decreased production of prothrombin. Review the nursing care of a client undergoing a liver biopsy if you had difficulty answering this question.*
>
> *Cognitive Level*—*Applying*
> *Client Needs Category*—*Physiological integrity*
> *Client Needs Subcategory*—*Reduction of risk potential*

143. **3.** By positioning the client on the right side, the weight of the body tends to put pressure on the puncture site. This compression helps to reduce or prevent bleeding. Ambulation is contraindicated because it promotes bleeding. Neither high Fowler's position nor elevating the legs is appropriate for controlling bleeding.

> *Test Taking Strategy*—*Look at the key words "most appropriate" in reference to a nursing order that is essential when planning the care of a client following a liver biopsy. Because bleeding is a significant potential problem, positioning the client so as to prevent or limit bleeding (option 3) should be added to the care plan. Review the nursing care of a client undergoing a liver biopsy if you had difficulty answering this question.*
>
> *Cognitive Level*—*Applying*
> *Client Needs Category*—*Physiological integrity*
> *Client Needs Subcategory*—*Reduction of risk potential*

144. **2.** Magnetic resonance imaging (MRI) produces detailed images, section by section, using magnetic fields to visualize soft-tissue structures such as tumors. Metallic objects present a safety hazard during an MRI. Consequently, internal metal objects such as a dental bridge should be removed. Jewelry, chains, and medallions are also removed. Sedation is not usually required except for clients who are severely claustrophobic. Asking if the client is allergic to opiates is inappropriate because clients are not given analgesics when undergoing an MRI. Giving the client an opportunity to void is a conscientious comfort measure.

> *Test Taking Strategy*—*Analyze to determine what information the question asks for, which is the preparation of a client before an MRI. Note the keyword "essential." Recall that an MRI uses magnets to obtain an image and that therefore metal in or on the body will distort the image. Whether the magnetic force is strong enough to pull metal in a dental bridge is debatable, but to reduce the potential, it*

should be removed. Review preparation and precautions associated with an MRI if you had difficulty answering this question.
Cognitive Level—*Applying*
Client Needs Category—*Physiological integrity*
Client Needs Subcategory—*Reduction of risk potential*

145. 4. Ascites is the collection of fluid within the peritoneal cavity and is a consequence of cirrhosis. It is caused by portal hypertension. Signs of ascites include visible and massive abdominal swelling. Dyspnea is secondary to the swelling. Vomiting and diarrhea are not associated with ascites but with cirrhosis. Serum bilirubin levels are assessed with jaundice related to cirrhosis, not ascites. Assessing for rebound tenderness is related to appendicitis, not ascites.

Test Taking Strategy—Look at the key words "most appropriate" in reference to a nursing assessment that relates to ascites. Recall that ascites is the result of fluid accumulation in the peritoneal cavity, which directly relates to option 4. Review assessment techniques for evaluating the progression or regression of ascites if you had difficulty answering this question.
Cognitive Level—*Applying*
Client Needs Category—*Physiological integrity*
Client Needs Subcategory—*Physiological adaptation*

146. 1. An abdominal paracentesis is performed to aspirate abdominal fluid caused by ascites. The bladder is emptied just before a paracentesis. A full bladder may be punctured as the needle is inserted through the abdominal wall. The client can eat and drink before the test. The physician usually prepares the skin with an antiseptic such as povidone-iodine (Betadine); therefore, hair removal is not indicated. There is no need for the crash cart to be outside the client's door because cardiac arrest is not a common occurrence related to this procedure.

Test Taking Strategy—Note the key words "most appropriate" in reference to preparing a client for a paracentesis. Consider the location and manner in which the procedure is performed. To ensure the safety of the client, having the client void (option 1) is the best answer because it reduces the risk of puncturing a bladder that is filled with urine. Review nursing care of a client undergoing a paracentesis if you had difficulty answering this question.
Cognitive Level—*Applying*
Client Needs Category—*Physiological integrity*
Client Needs Subcategory—*Reduction of risk potential*

147. 2. Documentation of the total volume of aspirated fluid is essential. Fluid replacement is determined more by the client's urine output and vital signs than by the volume of aspirated fluid. As a rule, clients do not require pain relief after a paracentesis. Ventilation is usually improved

after ascitic fluid has been removed; clients generally do not need additional encouragement to deep-breathe.

Test Taking Strategy—Analyze to determine what information the question asks for, which involves identifying an essential nursing action after a paracentesis is performed. Consider each option and decide which option is most important. Recall that it is the nurse's responsibility, rather than the physician's, to record the total volume of ascitic fluid that was removed. Eliminate options 1, 3, and 4 because these are unnecessary after paracentesis. Review the nursing responsibilities when caring for a client undergoing a paracentesis, especially in relation to the fluid that is removed, if you had difficulty answering this question.
Cognitive Level—*Applying*
Client Needs Category—*Physiological integrity*
Client Needs Subcategory—*Physiological adaptation*

148. 2. Stage II pressure sores are red similar to stage I, but also include broken or blistered skin that may have ruptured with evidence of serum. A stage III pressure sore involves a deeper crater extending into subcutaneous tissue. Stage IV pressure sores result in tissue necrosis that extends to muscle or bone.

Test Taking Strategy—Analyze to determine what information the question asks for, which is the stage of the described pressure sore. Recall pressure sores are staged from a reddened area through necrotic tissue extending to the bone. Based on the description of the pressure sore as a red superficially abraded area but no further impairment leads to the answer.
Cognitive Level—*Applying*
Client Needs Category—*Physiological integrity*
Client Need Subcategory—*Physiological adaptation*

149. 4. Because of the tendency for the client with cirrhosis to bleed, the licensed practical nurse (LPN) should apply sustained pressure for a longer period to prevent hematoma formation and bruising. Placing a vial of vitamin K at the bedside is unnecessary, even though vitamin K helps with clotting. Unless the LPN is credentialed to start I.V. lines in the state where he or she is practicing, starting an I.V. line is a function of the registered nurse (RN). This includes preparing the site with a bactericidal agent and flushing the I.V. line.

Test Taking Strategy—Look at the key words "most appropriate" in reference to an action that can be delegated to an LPN when discontinuing and restarting an I.V. line on a client with cirrhosis of the liver. After reviewing the listed options, option 1 could be performed by an LPN, but it is generally performed by the RN before inserting the venous access device. While the new infusion site is being accessed, the RN could delegate applying pressure to control bleeding from the site of the discontinued I.V. line to an LPN, which corresponds with option 4. Review responsibilities of an LPN, who has not been certified to perform a venipuncture, in relation to I.V. therapy if you had difficulty answering this question.

Cognitive Level—*Applying*
Client Needs Category—*Safe and effective care environment*
Client Needs Subcategory—*Coordinated care*

150. 3. Rising levels of ammonia in the blood are toxic to the central nervous system and can cause alterations in consciousness. Serum bilirubin is monitored to assess the liver's ability to form bile and transport it to the gallbladder for concentration. Bilirubin is not associated with hepatic encephalopathy but is seen in clients with cirrhosis. Serum creatinine and blood urea nitrogen levels are tests used to monitor renal function.

Test Taking Strategy—Analyze to determine what information the question asks for, which is a laboratory test that indicates a potential for encephalopathy when performed on a client with cirrhosis. Recall that ammonia levels increase in clients with hepatic encephalopathy, which leads to selecting option 3 as the correct answer. Research the indications for these laboratory tests and the abnormal results if you had difficulty answering this question.

Cognitive Level—*Applying*
Client Needs Category—*Physiological integrity*
Client Needs Subcategory—*Reduction of risk potential*

151. 1. Difficulty in arousing the cirrhotic client indicates a significant neurologic change. It is typically a sign that the client is progressing into hepatic coma. The client's physiologic and safety needs become even more important at this time. Jaundice is usually present in clients diagnosed with cirrhosis. Seizures may occur. The urine output is within normal limits. Pancreatitis is not associated with worsening cirrhosis. Fruity breath is related to diabetic ketoacidosis, not worsening cirrhosis.

Test Taking Strategy—Use the process of elimination to select the option that provides the best indication of worsening of the client's condition. Immediately eliminate option 2 because this finding is normal. Eliminate options 3 and 4 because they are indicative of other disease processes. Option 1 is a significant finding related to the development of hepatic coma. Review the signs of liver failure and hepatic coma if you had difficulty answering this question.

Cognitive Level—*Analyzing*
Client Needs Category—*Physiological integrity*
Client Needs Subcategory—*Physiological adaptation*

152. 2. Working through grief involves dealing with a loss. Reviewing one's life is often a task that takes place in anticipatory grieving. This is therapeutic and should

not be suppressed. Therefore, active listening is the most appropriate nursing measure. Suggesting that a close family member be called is a way of avoiding the situation. Calling the clergy at the church may or may not be appropriate, depending on the client's religious beliefs; however, the nurse can always take this step after listening to the client. It would be unrealistic to expect the client's spouse to think about future plans before dealing with the reality of the impending loss.

Test Taking Strategy—Use the process of elimination to select the option describing the most therapeutic nursing action in response to a crying spouse. Recall that listening (option 2) is therapeutic, especially in relation to the grieving process. Review nursing measures that support the grieving process if you had difficulty answering this question.

Cognitive Level—*Applying*
Client Needs Category—*Psychosocial integrity*
Client Needs Subcategory—*None*

Nursing Care of Clients with Disorders of the Pancreas

153. 2. Pain is a subjective experience. Asking the client to rate the pain helps to assess its intensity. A numeric rating scale can be used later to evaluate the effectiveness of the pain-relief techniques used. Noting whether the client is able to stop moving is an invalid assessment technique. A cooperative client may make an effort to stop moving despite the continuation of severe pain. Perspiration is a physiologic sign that may accompany pain; however, because many factors can cause perspiration, noting its presence or absence is not the best assessment technique. Administering an analgesic is a nursing intervention, not a form of assessment.

Test Taking Strategy—Use the process of elimination to select the option that is best for helping to assess the pain of a client with pancreatitis. Option 4 can be eliminated immediately because assessment should occur before implementing an intervention. Options 1 and 3 can be eliminated because they are not objectively related to assessing pain. Recall that a nursing standard is to assess pain intensity using a standard numeric 0 to 10 pain scale (option 2). Review pain assessment techniques if you had difficulty answering this question.

Cognitive Level—*Analyzing*
Client Needs Category—*Physiological integrity*
Client Needs Subcategory—*Basic care and comfort*

154. 2. An elevated serum amylase level is the most reliable evidence of pancreatitis. The bilirubin level becomes elevated if the pancreatitis is due to an obstruction of the common bile duct or pancreatic duct. Glucose tolerance test abnormalities indicate dysfunction of the endocrine functions of the pancreas, which is secondary to pancreatitis. Elevated bilirubin and abnormal glucose tolerance tests are not the best indicators of pancreatitis. Lactose tolerance test results have no relationship to pancreatitis.

> *Test Taking Strategy—Use the process of elimination to select the best option identifying a laboratory test that suggests pancreatitis. Recall that amylase, an enzyme that converts starches to sugars, is produced by the pancreas and salivary glands. An elevation of serum amylase (option 2) is a biochemical marker for pancreatitis. Refer to resources that discuss these laboratory tests if you had difficulty answering this question.*
>
> **Cognitive Level**—*Applying*
> **Client Needs Category**—*Physiological integrity*
> **Client Needs Subcategory**—*Reduction of risk potential*

155. **1, 2, 3.** Pancreatitis is the inflammation of the pancreas and can be acute or chronic. Causes of pancreatitis are structural abnormalities, abdominal trauma, metabolic disorders, infections, inflammatory bowel disease, alcoholism, and vascular disorders. One serious complication of acute pancreatitis includes hyperglycemia, in which there is an imbalance of glucagon, insulin, and somatostatin. This is why it is crucial for the nurse to get frequent blood sugar measurements. Another serious complication includes necrosis and hemorrhage of the pancreas. Peritonitis is another serious complication. Development of jaundice and portal hypertension are complications seen in clients with cirrhosis, not pancreatitis. Thrombocytopenia (low platelets) is a complication of many diseases, but is not typically associated with pancreatitis.

> *Test Taking Strategy—Analyze to determine what information the question asks for, which is identifying complications that a client with pancreatitis is at greatest risk for developing. Alternative-format "select all that apply" questions require considering each option independently to decide its merit in answering the question. Analyze each option individually and select one or more that represent complications of pancreatitis. Review the pathophysiology of pancreatitis if you had difficulty answering this question.*
>
> **Cognitive Level**—*Analyzing*
> **Client Needs Category**—*Physiological integrity*
> **Client Needs Subcategory**—*Physiological adaptation*

156. **4.** The nurse assigned to care for a client with an I.V. infusion has a responsibility to monitor the infusion to ensure that it is instilling the prescribed volume at the correct rate. Any volume more or less than prescribed must be reported to the nurse in charge. The infusion can flow by gravity with the tubing coiled on the bed. The nondominant hand is preferred for an I.V. infusion. There is ample time, with 100 mL left, to temporarily postpone reporting the information.

> *Test Taking Strategy—Analyze to determine what information the question asks for, which is the finding that must be reported immediately after inspecting the infusion of I.V. fluid. Recall that the nurse is responsible for ensuring that the infusion of I.V. fluids is at the prescribed rate. If there is a significant difference in infusion rates, as indicated by option 4, it is considered a medication error. Review nursing responsibilities that relate to the infusion of I.V. fluids if you had difficulty answering this question.*
>
> **Cognitive Level**—*Analyzing*
> **Client Needs Category**—*Physiological integrity*
> **Client Needs Subcategory**—*Physiological adaptation*

157. **3.** The nurse would be correct to remove scrambled eggs from the dietary tray of a client on a bland, low-fat diet. One scrambled egg made with milk and butter has approximately 8 g of fat. One cup of cooked, unsweetened prunes has only a trace of fat. One cup of nonfat skim milk has a trace of fat. One slice of unbuttered whole-wheat toast has only 1 g of fat.

> *Test Taking Strategy—Analyze to determine what information the question asks for, which is a food that is not included on a bland, low-fat diet. Consider both the spiciness and fat content of the items in the options. In this case the fat content of scrambled eggs makes option 3 the correct answer. Review the food items that are excluded on a bland, low-fat diet if you had difficulty answering this question.*
>
> **Cognitive Level**—*Applying*
> **Client Needs Category**—*Physiological integrity*
> **Client Needs Subcategory**—*Basic care and comfort*

158. **3.** There is an established relationship between the chronic consumption of alcohol and the incidence of pancreatitis. Once an acute attack of pancreatitis has occurred, the client is at risk for chronic pancreatitis. Use of alcohol leads to continued inflammation of the pancreas. It is essential to protect the pancreas from further irritation because serious complications (including destruction of the organ itself, peritonitis, shock, and even death) can occur. Having had pancreatitis does not disqualify a client from donating blood, doing heavy lifting, or taking laxatives.

> *Test Taking Strategy—Analyze to determine what information the question asks for, which is appropriate discharge instructions for a client with pancreatitis. Recall the relationship between exacerbations of pancreatitis when alcohol is consumed, which is identified in option 3. Review the long-term consequences of chronic pancreatitis if you had difficulty answering this question.*
>
> **Cognitive Level**—*Applying*
> **Client Needs Category**—*Physiological integrity*
> **Client Needs Subcategory**—*Physiological adaptation*

159. 2. Anorexia and weight loss appear early in the onset of cancer of the pancreas. Pancreatic cancer, like most other forms of cancer, does not usually cause acute pain in the early stages. If the client with pancreatic cancer experiences pain early on, it is usually dull and more apparent at night. In addition, bleeding is not typically a problem unless the cancer has also affected the liver. Fainting, unless from weight and fluid loss, is not a common sign of pancreatic cancer.

Test Taking Strategy—Analyze to determine what information the question asks for, which is the sign or symptom that commonly causes clients with undiagnosed pancreatic cancer to consult a physician. Recall that cancer of any kind generally begins with vague symptoms, such as unexplained weight loss (option 2). Review information on the early signs and symptoms of pancreatic cancer if you had difficulty answering this question.
Cognitive Level—Applying
Client Needs Category—Physiological integrity
Client Needs Subcategory—Physiological adaptation

160. 3. The most therapeutic response in this situation is to encourage the client to talk about thoughts and feelings. People who are dying often know without being told that they are terminal. It is more important to support a client's hope than to bluntly confirm suspicions. It would be unethical to say that the terminal client's condition will improve. The nurse would be appropriate in acting as a liaison in contacting someone who can help the client take care of unfinished business; however, this would not be the first or best nursing response in this case.

Test Taking Strategy—Analyze to determine what information the question asks for, which is the best nursing response to a client's question about his or her prognosis. Consider which option provides an opportunity for the client to express feelings, which is option 3. Although option 1 is an honest answer, it is brutally frank and thus nontherapeutic. Option 2 is a dishonest answer, and option 4, more or less, confirms the client's suspicion about being terminally ill without providing immediate support. Review therapeutic communication techniques if you had difficulty answering this question.
Cognitive Level—Applying
Client Needs Category—Psychosocial integrity
Client Needs Subcategory—None

161. 2. It is better to control pain before it escalates. When pain is intense, relief is more difficult to achieve. Peaks and valleys of pain are reduced by administering pain-relieving drugs on a routine schedule throughout the 24-hour period rather than just when it becomes absolutely necessary to do so. The goal is to keep the client free from pain yet not dull consciousness or the ability to communi-

cate. Asking the physician to order a high dose initially is premature. Tolerance is likely to develop later. It would be more appropriate to consult the physician about changing the medication order when the client's condition warrants it.

Test Taking Strategy—Look at the key words "most appropriate" in reference to a nursing action that will provide maximum comfort for a client receiving hospice care. Recall that giving narcotic analgesics on a scheduled basis, rather than prn, is most likely to provide sustained levels of comfort. Review the goals of hospice care, especially in relation to managing pain, if you had difficulty answering this question.
Cognitive Level—Applying
Client Needs Category—Physiological integrity
Client Needs Subcategory—Pharmacological therapies

Nursing Care of Clients with Culturally Diverse Backgrounds

162. 1, 2, 5. Orthodox Jewish clients have strict dietary laws called Kashrut, which include avoiding pork and pork products (ham), shellfish (shrimp, crab, lobster, escargot), and scavenger fish such as catfish. In addition, mixing dairy products and meat dishes (ham and cheese pizza) in the same meal is prohibited. Jewish law requires that foods must be properly supervised by a rabbi, making them "kosher," or "fitting," to eat. According to these dietary laws, Orthodox Jews must also avoid the flesh, organs, eggs, and milk of forbidden animals. All the birds and mammals Orthodox Jews are permitted to eat must be killed in accordance with Jewish law; that is, all blood must be drained from the meat or boiled out of it before it is eaten. In addition, fish, eggs, fruits, vegetables, and grains can be eaten with either meat or dairy; utensils that have come into contact with meat must be kept separate from those used with dairy food; and utensils that have come into contact with nonkosher food may not be used with kosher food. Grape products are prohibited if made by non-Jews. Coffee, tea, and strawberries are permitted in the kosher diet.

Test Taking Strategy—Analyze to determine what information the question asks for, which are dietary items that are contrary to the beliefs of Orthodox Judaism. Alternative-format "select all that apply" questions require considering each option independently to decide its merit in answering the question. Consider each option individually, comparing it with Jewish dietary practices. Review the cultural beliefs of Orthodox Jews if you had difficulty answering this question.
Cognitive Level—Applying
Client Needs Category—Psychosocial integrity
Client Needs Subcategory—None

163. 1. The concept of hot and cold as it relates to health and illness is also known as the humoral theory; it is based on the idea that four major fluids dominate the body: blood, phlegm, choler (yellow bile), and melancholy (black bile). An imbalance in the body's fluids (humors) is thought to lead to illness; likewise, when the body is in a state of health, the fluids are said to be balanced. Furthermore, it is believed that each food that is eaten has a dominant characteristic that promotes a particular fluid in the body. The classification of foods as hot or cold has nothing to do with the actual temperature of the food, nor to any other observable or taste-related factor. To achieve balance between health and illness, the physician should order treatments that are opposite to the nature of a person's illness (i.e., diseases caused by exertion should be treated by rest). The hot-cold concept of disease ranks among the most popular systems of contemporary folk medicine in the United States, especially in metropolitan areas with high populations of Asians. This concept is widely practiced in Chinese, Indian, Hong Kong, Filipino, and Latin American cultures by millions of people.

> ***Test Taking Strategy***—*Use the process of elimination to select the most accurate statement regarding the hot-cold theory from among the provided options. Recall that this theory applies to balancing hot and cold substances in the internal and external environment to preserve or restore health. Review cultural beliefs, especially as they relate to the hot-cold theory, if you had difficulty answering this question.*

Cognitive Level—*Applying*
Client Needs Category—*Psychosocial integrity*
Client Needs Subcategory—*None*

The Nursing Care of Clients with Urologic Disorders

Directions: *With a pencil, blacken the space in front of the option you have chosen for your correct answer.*

Nursing Care of Clients with Urinary Incontinence

A stroke victim is admitted to a long-term care facility for bladder retraining related to incontinence.

1. Which nursing assessment is most important before beginning bladder retraining for this client?
[ ] **1.** Recording the times at which the client is incontinent
[ ] **2.** Checking the specific gravity of the urine
[ ] **3.** Monitoring the extent of bladder distention
[ ] **4.** Weighing the client's incontinence pad

Several residents are sitting around the nurses' station when the nurse overhears a patient care technician (PCT) state in a loud, irritated voice, "He's wet again. Why can't he ever stay dry?"

2. On the basis of the nurse's knowledge of patient rights, which Federal law has the PCT violated?
[ ] **1.** Good Samaritan Act
[ ] **2.** Hippocratic Oath
[ ] **3.** Health Insurance Portability and Accountability Act (HIPAA)
[ ] **4.** Emergency Medical Treatment and Liability Act (EMTALA)

The client's niece comes to the long-term care facility for a visit and asks the nurse, "How is he doing? Is he making progress with his bladder retraining?"

3. Which response by the nurse is most appropriate?
[ ] **1.** "His bladder retraining is coming along, and before long he will be urinating like normal."
[ ] **2.** "He seems to have more incontinence in the afternoon and evening."
[ ] **3.** "In order to protect his privacy, I can't give you that information."
[ ] **4.** "Bladder retraining is slow work. We have to take him to the toilet every 2 hours."

During bladder retraining, the client tells the nurse that he intends to restrict his fluid intake to remain dry for longer periods of time.

4. Which response by the nurse is best?
[ ] **1.** Encourage the client to restrict fluid intake because it shows evidence of client cooperation.
[ ] **2.** Encourage the client to restrict fluid intake because it leads to accomplishing the goal.
[ ] **3.** Discourage the client from restricting fluid intake because it contributes to constipation.
[ ] **4.** Discourage the client from restricting fluid intake because it potentiates fluid imbalance.

A client with urinary incontinence says to the nurse, "What's the sense in living? I'm just a baby nowadays."

5. Which comment is the best response the nurse can offer?
[ ] **1.** "You're a very nice person."
[ ] **2.** "Cheer up. You can't be serious."
[ ] **3.** "You should expect this at your age."
[ ] **4.** "You're discouraged right now."

Bladder retraining is progressing slower than expected due to the client's mental and physical limitations. The nursing team uses an external catheter at night to prevent skin breakdown.

6. When applying an external catheter to a male client, which action by the nurse is correct?
[ ] **1.** Lubricate the penis before applying the catheter.
[ ] **2.** Measure the length and circumference of the penis.
[ ] **3.** Leave space between the end of the penis and the catheter's drainage end.
[ ] **4.** Retract the foreskin before rolling the catheter sheath over the penis.

7. After inserting an indwelling catheter into a male client, which technique is most appropriate for stabilizing the catheter to avoid damage to the penis?
[ ] **1.** Tape the catheter to the abdomen.
[ ] **2.** Pass the catheter under the client's leg.
[ ] **3.** Fasten the drainage tubing to the bed with a safety pin.
[ ] **4.** Insert the catheter into the tubing of a collecting bag.

Nursing Care of Clients with Infectious and Inflammatory Urologic Disorders

A client with type 1 diabetes mellitus consults a physician regarding urinary problems.

8. When the nurse interviews the client, which symptoms will the client most likely report if a bladder infection has been acquired? Select all that apply.
[ ] **1.** Sharp flank pain
[ ] **2.** Urethral discharge
[ ] **3.** Strong-smelling urine
[ ] **4.** Burning on urination
[ ] **5.** Urgency
[ ] **6.** Frequency

9. Which statements should be included when the nurse instructs a female client about the technique for collecting a clean-catch midstream urine specimen for routine urinalysis? Select all that apply.
[ ] **1.** Clean the urethral area using several circular motions.
[ ] **2.** Void into the plastic liner under the toilet seat.
[ ] **3.** Void a small amount, and then collect a sample of urine.
[ ] **4.** Mix the antiseptic solution with the collected urine specimen.
[ ] **5.** Collect the urine in the nonsterile cup.
[ ] **6.** Drink several caffeinated beverages before collecting the urine.

10. When the nurse reviews the results of the client's urinalysis, which substance in the urine is most suggestive of a bladder infection?
[ ] **1.** Glucose
[ ] **2.** Blood
[ ] **3.** Bilirubin
[ ] **4.** Protein

To relieve the client's symptoms, the physician orders phenazopyridine (Pyridium).

11. It is most appropriate for the nurse to advise the client that taking this medication will have which effect on the urine?
[ ] **1.** The urine will look cloudy.
[ ] **2.** The urine will appear orange.
[ ] **3.** The urine will become scant.
[ ] **4.** The urine will have a strong odor.

12. Which urinary change provides the best evidence that the phenazopyridine (Pyridium) is achieving its intended therapeutic effect?
[ ] **1.** Urinary frequency is decreased.
[ ] **2.** Urinary urgency is decreased.
[ ] **3.** Urinary burning is decreased.
[ ] **4.** Urine output is increased.

A middle-aged client is involved in a motor vehicle accident and will be in traction on bed rest for an extended time.

13. Considering the amount of time the client must remain in bed, why is it imperative for the nurse to monitor for a urinary tract infection?
[ ] **1.** The client will not be able to complete hygiene needs.
[ ] **2.** The client will not be able to fully empty the bladder.
[ ] **3.** The client will not be able to maintain bladder control.
[ ] **4.** The client will not be able to drink sufficient fluids.

Several clients come to the urology clinic with signs and symptoms related to urinary tract infections (UTIs).

14. In evaluating multiple clients with UTIs, the clinic nurse would anticipate which client to be at least risk for developing a UTI?
[ ] 1. A client with urethral mucosa damage
[ ] 2. A client with an altered mental condition
[ ] 3. A client with an altered metabolic state
[ ] 4. An immunocompromised client

15. When a client asks the clinic nurse why women have more bladder infections than men, which answer is most accurate?
[ ] 1. The male urethra is straighter, which facilitates elimination of pathogens.
[ ] 2. The male urethra is lined with a layer of mucous membrane, which traps microorganisms.
[ ] 3. The female urethra is shorter, and pathogens enter the bladder more easily.
[ ] 4. The female urethra has a larger diameter and is more easily contaminated.

16. Which statements made by a diabetic client at the clinic strongly suggest that the client has a urinary tract infection? Select all that apply.
[ ] 1. "I need to urinate frequently."
[ ] 2. "I can't hold my urine."
[ ] 3. "I have a burning sensation when I urinate."
[ ] 4. "I have itching in my perineal area."
[ ] 5. "I pass a large quantity of urine."
[ ] 6. "My urine is foul-smelling."

17. Because the client also has diabetes mellitus, which statement by the nurse best explains why that client is at higher risk for acquiring a bladder infection?
[ ] 1. Glucose in urine supports bacterial growth.
[ ] 2. Diabetes suppresses white blood cell activity.
[ ] 3. Diabetic clients urinate more frequently.
[ ] 4. The urine is more concentrated in diabetic clients.

18. Which recommendations by the nurse are most effective in reducing bacterial growth in a female client's bladder? Select all that apply.
[ ] 1. Drink a large quantity of fluids.
[ ] 2. Change underclothing each day.
[ ] 3. Avoid the use of public restrooms.
[ ] 4. Use only white toilet tissue.
[ ] 5. Urinate after having sexual intercourse.
[ ] 6. Drink fluids that are highly acidic.

19. Which of the following measures performed by the client would offer the best protection against acquiring a urinary tract infection?
[ ] 1. Wiping away from the urinary meatus after bowel elimination
[ ] 2. Performing appropriate hand washing after bowel elimination
[ ] 3. Using a feminine hygiene spray after bowel elimination
[ ] 4. Drying the perineum thoroughly after bowel elimination

20. When teaching a client with cystitis about urinary tract irritants, the nurse correctly identifies which of the following substances as potential irritants to avoid? Select all that apply.
[ ] 1. Alcohol
[ ] 2. Milk
[ ] 3. Tea
[ ] 4. Chocolate
[ ] 5. Coffee
[ ] 6. Pears

21. When the client with cystitis has difficulty visualizing the urinary tract, the nurse shows the client a diagram that includes all the primary structures involved. Identify with an *X* on the diagram the area of inflammation associated with the client's cystitis.

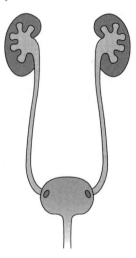

A female paraplegic client is being taught to catheterize herself before being discharged from the rehabilitation unit.

22. When teaching a female client how to catheterize herself, how far into the urethra should the nurse instruct the client to insert the catheter?
[ ] 1. 1″ (2.5 cm)
[ ] 2. 2″ (5 cm)
[ ] 3. 3″ (7.5 cm)
[ ] 4. 4″ (10 cm)

A female client becomes acutely ill with flank pain, fever, and chills. The physician makes a tentative diagnosis of acute pyelonephritis and orders a catheterized urine specimen for culture.

23. When preparing the client for catheterization, how should the nurse position the client?
[ ] **1.** Lithotomy position
[ ] **2.** Recumbent
[ ] **3.** Knee-chest position
[ ] **4.** Prone

24. When the nurse mistakenly inserts the catheter into the client's vagina rather than the urinary meatus, which action is best to take next?
[ ] **1.** Wipe the catheter tip with an alcohol swab.
[ ] **2.** Clean the catheter tip with povidone-iodine solution (Betadine).
[ ] **3.** Discard the catheter and use another sterile one.
[ ] **4.** Withdraw the catheter and insert it in the urethra.

The physician prescribes the combination urinary anti-infective medication trimethoprim and sulfamethoxazole (Bactrim) twice a day for the client who is diagnosed with pyelonephritis.

25. Which nursing instruction is most appropriate for preventing crystal formation in this client's urine?
[ ] **1.** Eat more acidic citrus fruits.
[ ] **2.** Avoid carbonated soft drinks.
[ ] **3.** Drink 3 quarts (3 L) of water daily.
[ ] **4.** Take the medication with food.

The client is scheduled for intravenous pyelography (IVP). The nurse prepares to administer a laxative to the client.

26. What is the primary reason for administering a laxative before the procedure?
[ ] **1.** Emptying the bowel aids in examining the lower GI tract.
[ ] **2.** Emptying the bowel prevents accidental stool incontinence during the X-ray.
[ ] **3.** Emptying the bowel reduces the potential for constipation or impaction.
[ ] **4.** Emptying the bowel improves the ability to visualize the urinary structures.

27. If the client makes the following statements, which information is most important to report to the physician before the client undergoes an intravenous pyelography (IVP)?
[ ] **1.** "The barium they give me to drink causes me to have constipation."
[ ] **2.** "I have a low tolerance for pain during procedures."
[ ] **3.** "I had a reaction when my gallbladder was X-rayed before."
[ ] **4.** "I get claustrophobic when I am put into that big round machine."

A middle-aged client comes to the clinic with vague symptoms of malaise and headache. Even though these symptoms are rather unremarkable, the client is diagnosed with acute glomerulonephritis.

28. Which statements made by the client's spouse most closely correlate with the diagnosis of acute glomerulonephritis? Select all that apply.
[ ] **1.** "My spouse's face looks rather puffy lately."
[ ] **2.** "Recently my spouse has been quite forgetful."
[ ] **3.** "My spouse has been salting food heavily."
[ ] **4.** "It seems that my spouse sleeps quite poorly."
[ ] **5.** "My spouse hasn't been eating very well."
[ ] **6.** "My spouse gets up at night to use the bathroom."

29. When the nurse reviews the client's medical history, which finding most likely precipitated the present illness?
[ ] **1.** Trauma to the lower abdomen
[ ] **2.** An upper respiratory infection
[ ] **3.** Treatment with an antibiotic
[ ] **4.** An allergic reaction to X-ray dye

30. If this client is typical of others with glomerulonephritis, which finding would the nurse expect to observe when conducting a head-to-toe physical assessment?
[ ] **1.** Skin hemorrhages
[ ] **2.** Absence of body hair
[ ] **3.** Flushed appearance
[ ] **4.** Peripheral edema

31. If the physician orders the following laboratory tests, which one is most important for the nurse to monitor when caring for this client?
[ ] **1.** Serum amylase
[ ] **2.** Blood glucose
[ ] **3.** Blood urea nitrogen (BUN)
[ ] **4.** Complete blood count (CBC)

32. Considering the client's diagnosis, which nursing intervention is the priority at this time?
[ ] **1.** Ambulating the client twice daily
[ ] **2.** Instructing the client how to self-catheterize
[ ] **3.** Monitoring the client's weight daily
[ ] **4.** Encouraging the client to increase fluid intake

33. When the client with glomerulonephritis reports having a headache that is rated a 7 on a scale of 0 to 10, with 10 being the most pain, which nursing action should be performed next?
[ ] **1.** Administer a prescribed analgesic.
[ ] **2.** Assess the client's blood pressure.
[ ] **3.** Reduce environmental stimuli.
[ ] **4.** Change the client's position.

The nurse caring for the client with glomerulonephritis is told during the shift report that a 24-hour urine collection for creatinine clearance is to begin at 8 A.M.

34. Which nursing action is most appropriate in relation to collecting the client's urine specimen?
[ ] **1.** Have the client void at 8 A.M., and refrigerate the specimen.
[ ] **2.** Have the client void at 8 A.M., and dispose of the specimen.
[ ] **3.** Have the client void at 8 A.M., and send the specimen to the laboratory.
[ ] **4.** Have the client void at 8 A.M., and place the specimen in a preservative.

The nurse uses a color reagent strip (dipstick) to test a voided urine specimen.

35. If the reagent strip can detect the following substances, which one would the nurse expect to be present in the urine of a client with glomerulonephritis?
[ ] **1.** Glucose
[ ] **2.** Bilirubin
[ ] **3.** Albumin
[ ] **4.** Acetone

36. When the nurse inspects the client's urine specimen, which finding best indicates that the urine contains red blood cells?
[ ] **1.** The urine appears cloudy.
[ ] **2.** The urine appears smoky.
[ ] **3.** The urine appears bright orange.
[ ] **4.** The urine appears dark yellow.

The client is started on a low-sodium diet.

37. Which menu choice is best for the nurse to recommend?
[ ] **1.** Hot dog with potato salad
[ ] **2.** Beef bouillon and crackers
[ ] **3.** Chicken breast on lettuce
[ ] **4.** Cheese pizza with thin crust

The physician prescribes the steroids methylprednisolone (Medrol) and prednisone (Orasone) both on alternate days by oral administration to treat the client's inflammatory process.

38. When the client questions why both drugs are not taken daily, which response by the nurse is best?
[ ] **1.** The medications are too toxic if taken on a daily basis.
[ ] **2.** This alternating schedule maintains adrenal function.
[ ] **3.** Each medication has a prolonged period of action.
[ ] **4.** Most people cannot tolerate the medications' daily side effects.

Nursing Care of Clients with Renal Failure

A client who has chronic glomerulonephritis has deteriorated to the early stages of renal failure.

39. When receiving shift report from the nurse, which of the following information correlates with renal failure?
[ ] **1.** Anemia
[ ] **2.** Hypotension
[ ] **3.** Weight loss
[ ] **4.** Fever

40. If this client's condition is similar to that of others in the oliguric phase of renal failure, the nurse would anticipate the client's urine output to be within what range?
[ ] **1.** 50 to 100 mL/hour
[ ] **2.** 100 to 150 mL/hour
[ ] **3.** 500 to 1,000 mL/day
[ ] **4.** 100 to 500 mL/day

The nursing team meets to address the client's early renal failure in relation to the care plan.

41. Which diagnostic test, considered a sensitive indicator of advanced kidney disease, will need to be closely monitored by the nursing team?
[ ] **1.** Serum creatinine level
[ ] **2.** Serum sodium level
[ ] **3.** Uric acid level
[ ] **4.** Urine specific gravity

42. As the nurse is updating the client's plan of care, which nursing assessment is essential?
[ ] **1.** Monitor body temperature.
[ ] **2.** Measure intake and output.
[ ] **3.** Assess for urine retention.
[ ] **4.** Check the urine for glucose.

The physician orders a fluid challenge of 500 mL of I.V. fluid infused at a rapid rate, followed by the administration of a loop diuretic to sustain or improve renal function.

43. While the fluid is being administered, which nursing assessment is most important?
[ ] **1.** Checking for pedal edema
[ ] **2.** Assessing for rapid weight gain
[ ] **3.** Monitoring specific gravity
[ ] **4.** Auscultating breath sounds

44. Because of the client's impaired urine elimination, which potential skin problem will require additional team planning?
[ ] **1.** Reduced perspiration
[ ] **2.** Extreme oiliness
[ ] **3.** Loss of skin turgor
[ ] **4.** Pronounced itching

The client is placed on a sodium-restricted diet.

45. When the client complains about the bland taste of the food, the nurse appropriately recommends substituting salt with which condiment?
[ ] **1.** Catsup
[ ] **2.** Mustard
[ ] **3.** Soy sauce
[ ] **4.** Lemon juice

46. Which nursing action is most appropriate when the client complains about being thirsty because of the fluid restrictions?
[ ] **1.** Giving the client hard candy to suck
[ ] **2.** Providing the client with ice chips
[ ] **3.** Offering the client an ice cream bar
[ ] **4.** Supplying the client with fresh fruit

When it becomes evident that the client will require long-term hemodialysis, an internal arteriovenous fistula is created.

47. Which nursing assessment is most important to perform regularly when a client has an arteriovenous fistula?
[ ] **1.** Checking the color and temperature of the client's hand
[ ] **2.** Monitoring the client's wrist and finger range of motion
[ ] **3.** Observing the tone and coordination of the client's arm muscles
[ ] **4.** Inspecting the client's forearm skin turgor

48. When performing a physical assessment, which sensation would the nurse expect to detect when palpating the site of the arteriovenous fistula?
[ ] **1.** A pulse
[ ] **2.** A bruit
[ ] **3.** A thrill
[ ] **4.** A click

49. Which nursing intervention is most helpful in assisting the client undergoing hemodialysis to cope with the client's chronic health condition?
[ ] **1.** Giving the client literature to read about renal failure
[ ] **2.** Advising the client's spouse to cook the client's favorite dishes
[ ] **3.** Keeping the client informed of the latest research findings
[ ] **4.** Exploring with the client how this disorder has affected life

The nurse is caring for another client with renal failure who is being treated with peritoneal dialysis.

50. Which assessment before and after peritoneal dialysis is most valuable in evaluating the outcome of treatment?
[ ] **1.** Pulse rate
[ ] **2.** Body weight
[ ] **3.** Abdominal girth
[ ] **4.** Urine output

51. Before peritoneal dialysis begins, the nurse correctly informs the client that the procedure involves the movement of urea and creatinine through the peritoneum by means of which force?
[ ] **1.** Osmosis
[ ] **2.** Diffusion
[ ] **3.** Filtration
[ ] **4.** Gravity

52. Immediately after the dialysate solution has been instilled, which nursing action is correct?
[ ] **1.** Clamping the tubing from the infusion
[ ] **2.** Draining the infused dialysate solution
[ ] **3.** Restricting the client's movement as much as possible
[ ] **4.** Encouraging the client to drink fluids

53. Which of the following findings is the most significant information to report when caring for a client undergoing peritoneal dialysis?
[ ] **1.** Loss of body weight
[ ] **2.** Decreased serum creatinine
[ ] **3.** Elevated body temperature
[ ] **4.** Output that exceeds intake

54. Which finding provides the best evidence that peritoneal dialysis is achieving a therapeutic effect?
[ ] **1.** Urine output increases.
[ ] **2.** Appetite improves.
[ ] **3.** Potassium level falls.
[ ] **4.** Red blood cell count is lower.

55. When the nurse is advising the client about the potential complications associated with peritoneal dialysis, which complication is most important to include?
[ ] **1.** Pulmonary edema
[ ] **2.** Abdominal peritonitis
[ ] **3.** Abdominal hernia
[ ] **4.** Ruptured aorta

A client with renal failure is just informed about being a potential candidate for a kidney transplant.

56. When the client asks about the source of donated kidneys, the nurse correctly identifies which of the following as the preferred donor?
[ ] **1.** A recently deceased human
[ ] **2.** A sibling or living relative
[ ] **3.** An unrelated living human
[ ] **4.** A chimpanzee or other primate

57. Which problem is the nurse's immediate concern after kidney transplant surgery?
[ ] **1.** Hypovolemic shock caused by postoperative bleeding
[ ] **2.** Abdominal distention secondary to delayed peristalsis
[ ] **3.** Postoperative paralytic ileus due to colon manipulation
[ ] **4.** Pneumonia secondary to ineffective breathing patterns

Nursing Care of Clients with Urologic Obstructions

58. Which assessment finding strongly suggests that a client's reduced volume of voided urine is due to an obstructive disorder such as an enlarged prostate gland?
[ ] **1.** The client feels a continued need to void.
[ ] **2.** The client's urine appears dark amber.
[ ] **3.** The client's bladder is below the pubis.
[ ] **4.** The client experiences abdominal cramps.

59. If the physician inserts a suprapubic cystostomy tube to drain the accumulating urine, the nurse should assess the characteristics of urine from a catheter that exits from which location?
[ ] **1.** Urethra
[ ] **2.** Abdomen
[ ] **3.** Ureter
[ ] **4.** Flank

60. Which nursing intervention is essential for evaluating the patency of the suprapubic catheter?
[ ] **1.** Inspecting the client's skin around the insertion site
[ ] **2.** Monitoring the client's urine output every 2 hours
[ ] **3.** Attaching the catheter to a leg bag when the client ambulates
[ ] **4.** Encouraging the client to consume 100 mL of oral fluid hourly

A client comes to the emergency department for relief from severe, stabbing, colicky flank pain. The physician makes a tentative diagnosis of urolithiasis.

61. When the nurse examines the voided urine specimen, which finding is most supportive of the diagnosis of urolithiasis?
[ ] **1.** Cloudy pale urine
[ ] **2.** Blood-tinged urine
[ ] **3.** Light yellow urine
[ ] **4.** Strong-smelling urine

A cystoscopy is scheduled to help diagnose the client's suspected condition.

62. If the client asks the nurse to outline the benefits of the cystoscopy procedure, which ones should the nurse list as positive outcomes? Select all that apply.
[ ] **1.** Involves visual examination of the internal structure of the kidney
[ ] **2.** Helps identify the sources of hematuria, incontinence, and urine retention
[ ] **3.** Allows for collection of tissue samples, cell washings, and urine samples
[ ] **4.** Requires no sedation because it is painless
[ ] **5.** Uses a light source to visualize the internal structure
[ ] **6.** Requires no surgical incision because the scope is introduced into the urethra

63. After the cystoscopy, which urinary symptom can the nurse expect the client to experience?
[ ] **1.** Polyuria
[ ] **2.** Dysuria
[ ] **3.** Anuria
[ ] **4.** Pyuria

64. When the client is definitively diagnosed with urolithiasis, which nursing interventions are most appropriate to add to the care plan? Select all that apply.
[ ] **1.** Restrict fluids to 1,000 mL/day.
[ ] **2.** Maintain the client in Fowler's position.
[ ] **3.** Limit activity to bed rest.
[ ] **4.** Strain all voided urine.
[ ] **5.** Maintain patency of the indwelling catheter.
[ ] **6.** Administer antibiotics per physician order.

65. While the client is awaiting further treatment options, which nursing intervention is appropriate?
[ ] **1.** Increase the client's fluid intake to prevent further stone formation.
[ ] **2.** Interrupt the voiding pattern to strengthen the bladder muscles.
[ ] **3.** Limit the client's voiding to allow for releasing a larger stream of urine.
[ ] **4.** Increase the client's dietary calcium to replace losses to renal calculi.

The client is scheduled for extracorporeal shock wave lithotripsy (ESWL) to pulverize the stone.

66. After the nurse explains the ESWL procedure to the client, which statements provide the best evidence that the client understands the scheduled procedure? Select all that apply.
[ ] **1.** "I'll be placed on a fluid-filled pillow."
[ ] **2.** "Radiation will be focused on my bladder."
[ ] **3.** "A laser beam will be aimed at my kidneys."
[ ] **4.** "I'll experience a tingling sensation."
[ ] **5.** "I cannot eat or drink anything before the test."
[ ] **6.** "I will have general anesthesia for the test."

An older man makes an appointment with a physician concerning urinary symptoms he has been experiencing.

67. When the office nurse obtains the client's history, which statements provides the best indications that the client has benign prostatic hypertrophy (BPH)? Select all that apply.
[ ] **1.** "There is some burning when I urinate."
[ ] **2.** "I wake up each night needing to urinate."
[ ] **3.** "I feel pressure in my back before voiding."
[ ] **4.** "My urine is almost colorless, like water."
[ ] **5.** "My urine stream is really thin and narrow."
[ ] **6.** "I dribble for several minutes after I urinate."

68. To gather more information about symptoms associated with benign prostatic hypertrophy (BPH), which question is most important to ask next?
[ ] 1. "Have you noticed any changes in sexual function?"
[ ] 2. "Have you felt any lumps in your scrotum recently?"
[ ] 3. "Do you have difficulty starting to void?"
[ ] 4. "Do you have problems controlling urination?"

The client with a history of benign prostatic hypertrophy (BPH) tells the nurse that he has been unable to urinate for 18 hours. The physician instructs the nurse to insert a urethral catheter.

69. Which technique is best for helping the nurse insert the tip of the catheter past the enlarged prostate gland?
[ ] 1. Angle the penis in the direction of the toes.
[ ] 2. Massage the tissue below the base of the penis.
[ ] 3. Push the catheter with additional force.
[ ] 4. Grasp the penis firmly within the hand.

70. Which catheter is the best choice to use for a client with BPH?
[ ] 1. A Coudé catheter
[ ] 2. A silicone catheter
[ ] 3. A rubber catheter
[ ] 4. A flexible catheter

The client is scheduled to undergo a transurethral resection of the prostate (TURP).

71. After the TURP, which assessment finding would the nurse expect to observe during the immediate postoperative period?
[ ] 1. Light pink to clear urine
[ ] 2. Mucoid sediments in urine
[ ] 3. Decreased volume of urine
[ ] 4. Grossly bloody urine

The nurse receives orders to provide continuous bladder irrigation (CBI) through a three-way catheter after the client undergoes a transurethral resection of the prostate (TURP).

72. As the nurse instructs the client about CBI, which information should the nurse provide? Select all that apply.
[ ] 1. "You may feel the urge to urinate even though the bladder is empty."
[ ] 2. "Do not to try to urinate around the catheter, because this will cause bladder spasms."
[ ] 3. "You need to limit your fluids to 4 glasses per day."
[ ] 4. "It is normal for the urine to be bloody immediately after surgery."
[ ] 5. "The catheter will be removed in about a week."
[ ] 6. "By the time you are ready to go home, your urine should be pink with a few clots."

Postoperatively, the client tells the nurse that he is having a great deal of discomfort in his bladder area. The physician has written several analgesic drug orders for the client in anticipation of the pain associated with transurethral resection of the prostate (TURP).

73. Before administering an analgesic to the client, which information is most important for the nurse to assess?
[ ] 1. Whether the urine is bloody
[ ] 2. Whether the client has been up walking in the room
[ ] 3. Whether the catheter is draining urine
[ ] 4. Whether the client has been drinking adequate fluids

74. Which medication is most appropriate to administer to the client who is having bladder spasms?
[ ] 1. Aspirin by mouth
[ ] 2. Acetaminophen (Tylenol) by mouth
[ ] 3. Meperidine hydrochloride (Demerol) intramuscularly
[ ] 4. Belladonna and opium (B&O) rectal suppository

A nurse is assigned to care for a client who has undergone a suprapubic prostatectomy. The client has one catheter in the urethra and another in an abdominal incision.

75. When documenting the client's urine output in the medical record, which measurement is correct for the nurse to record?
[ ] 1. Only the output from the urethral catheter
[ ] 2. Only the output from the wound catheter
[ ] 3. The outputs from each catheter separately
[ ] 4. The combined output from both catheters

Several days after the client's procedure, the physician removes the catheter from the abdominal incision.

76. Which nursing intervention is most important to add to the client's care plan after removal of the suprapubic catheter?
[ ] 1. Check the client's urine specific gravity every shift.
[ ] 2. Measure the client's abdominal girth daily.
[ ] 3. Change wet abdominal dressings as needed.
[ ] 4. Perform a credé maneuver every 4 hours.

Nursing Care of Clients with Urologic Tumors

A physician asks the office nurse to schedule a series of examinations and diagnostic tests to determine whether a client has cancer of the prostate gland.

77. To avoid erroneous test results caused by the manipulation of the prostate, the nurse should schedule which diagnostic test before the client's rectal examination?
[ ] 1. Kidneys, ureters, bladder X-ray
[ ] 2. Needle biopsy of the prostate gland
[ ] 3. Prostate specific antigen (PSA) test
[ ] 4. Transrectal ultrasound examination

The client is diagnosed with prostate cancer and undergoes a radical perineal prostatectomy. Postoperatively, the client has an indwelling (Foley) catheter in place.

78. When managing catheter care, which nursing action is most important for promoting wound healing?
[ ] **1.** Avoid tension on the catheter.
[ ] **2.** Encourage oral fluid intake.
[ ] **3.** Clean the urethral meatus daily.
[ ] **4.** Clamp and release the catheter every 2 hours.

The physician prescribes estradiol (Estrace) for the client after the prostatectomy.

79. Which statement by the client provides the best evidence that he understands the potential side effects associated with hormonal therapy? Select all that apply.
[ ] **1.** "My breasts may enlarge."
[ ] **2.** "I may have spontaneous erections."
[ ] **3.** "My sperm count will be higher."
[ ] **4.** "I'll have strong sexual urges."
[ ] **5.** "My voice may become higher."
[ ] **6.** "I may have a rapid weight gain."

A nephrectomy is performed on a client with a kidney tumor.

80. Postoperatively, which assessment finding is most suggestive that the client is hemorrhaging?
[ ] **1.** Acute flank pain
[ ] **2.** Abdominal distention
[ ] **3.** Flushed, warm skin
[ ] **4.** Nausea and vomiting

A nurse is caring for a client with bladder cancer.

81. If this client is typical of others who acquire bladder cancer, which symptoms are most likely to have manifested in the early stage of this disease? Select all that apply.
[ ] **1.** Difficulty voiding
[ ] **2.** Persistent oliguria
[ ] **3.** Painless hematuria
[ ] **4.** Urethral discharge
[ ] **5.** Painful urination
[ ] **6.** Postvoid dribbling

82. When asked about factors that are linked to bladder cancer, the nurse correctly identifies which factors? Select all that apply.
[ ] **1.** Stress incontinence
[ ] **2.** Frequent intercourse
[ ] **3.** Sexual promiscuity
[ ] **4.** Cigarette smoking
[ ] **5.** History of prostate cancer
[ ] **6.** Exposure to asbestos

The physician recommends that the client's bladder cancer be treated conservatively by instilling an antineoplastic drug within the bladder.

83. Following the instillation of the antineoplastic drug, which safety precaution is important for the licensed practical nurse to instruct the nursing assistant to take when disposing of the client's urine?
[ ] **1.** Wear two pairs of latex gloves.
[ ] **2.** Don an air purifying respirator.
[ ] **3.** Avoid wearing clothing with long sleeves.
[ ] **4.** Limit contact time with the client.

Nursing Care of Clients with Urinary Diversions

84. A nurse is assigned to care for a client with a cutaneous ureterostomy. Which of the following images correlates with the client's urinary diversion?

[ ] **1.**

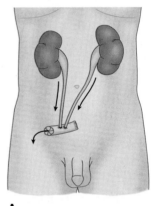

A

[ ] **2.**

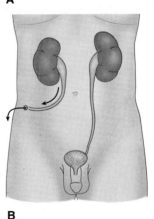

B

[ ] **3.**

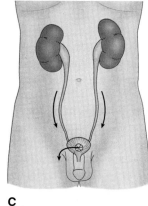

C

[ ] **4.**

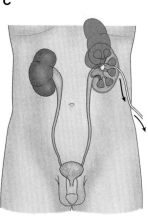

D

A client whose bladder cancer has been unresponsive to treatment will have the bladder surgically removed. An ileal conduit will be created to facilitate urine elimination.

85. When the client asks the nurse to clarify the surgeon's explanation of the procedure, which statement is most accurate?
[ ] **1.** "Your urine will be deposited in your small intestine."
[ ] **2.** "Urine will be eliminated with stool from the rectum."
[ ] **3.** "Urine will drain from an abdominal opening."
[ ] **4.** "Your urine will empty from a special catheter."

The night nurse reports that the preoperative client scheduled for the cystectomy and ileal conduit was awake much of the night and that, when sleeping, the client was restless.

86. Which assessment supports the nurse's assumption that the client's sleep disturbance was most likely due to anxiety?
[ ] **1.** The client's face is pale.
[ ] **2.** Blood pressure is 132/88 mm Hg.
[ ] **3.** Pulse rate is 106 beats/minute at rest.
[ ] **4.** The client requests a midnight snack.

87. To facilitate the client's coping, which statement by the nurse is most therapeutic at this time?
[ ] **1.** "It must be difficult facing this type of surgery."
[ ] **2.** "You have one of the best surgeons at this hospital."
[ ] **3.** "You'll see; everything will turn out okay for you."
[ ] **4.** "Others with your diagnosis have done just fine."

On the morning of surgery, the client tells the nurse, "I don't think I can go through with this surgery. Just the thought of peeing into a bag repulses me."

88. Which response by the nurse is most therapeutic?
[ ] **1.** "Tell me what that means to you."
[ ] **2.** "I know just how you're feeling."
[ ] **3.** "Well, it's not quite as bad as that."
[ ] **4.** "You need to think more positively."

Postoperatively, the client wears an appliance that collects the urine. The client tells the nurse that the skin feels raw and irritated near the stoma.

89. Which nursing action is most appropriate at this time?
[ ] **1.** Increase the client's oral fluids to dilute the urine.
[ ] **2.** Remove the appliance and inspect the skin.
[ ] **3.** Empty the appliance at more frequent intervals.
[ ] **4.** Leave the appliance off for 1 or 2 days.

90. Which postoperative instruction regarding client care is most important for the nurse to relate to the nursing assistant during a shift report?
[ ] **1.** The client independently empties the urine collection device.
[ ] **2.** The client is receiving ostomy care instructions from the enterostomal nurse.
[ ] **3.** The client had a cystectomy and ileal conduit performed three days ago.
[ ] **4.** The client's ileal conduit is patent and draining dark urine.

The nurse also teaches the client how to change the ostomy appliance before being discharged.

91. Which suggestion is most helpful to control leaking urine during the time the appliance is being changed?
[ ] **1.** "When you remove the appliance, let the urine drip into the toilet."
[ ] **2.** "When you remove the appliance, insert a tampon into the stoma."
[ ] **3.** "When you remove the appliance, press a gloved finger over the stoma."
[ ] **4.** "When you remove the appliance, pinch the stoma with two fingers."

Nursing Care of Clients with Culturally Diverse Backgrounds

An elderly Native American male is admitted to the hospital for signs and symptoms related to prostate enlargement. The nurse performs a cultural assessment.

92. If this client shares cultural characteristics of other Native Americans, which findings in the cultural assessment should be included in the client's care plan? Select all that apply.

[ ] **1.** Native Americans may hesitate to share personal information with strangers.
[ ] **2.** Questions regarding health history may be interpreted as prying.
[ ] **3.** Native Americans value listening skills.
[ ] **4.** Touching on the head is considered offensive.
[ ] **5.** Native Americans pattern their lifestyle according to "clock time."
[ ] **6.** Direct eye contact should be used when addressing the client or family.

 Correct Answers, Rationales, and Test Taking Strategies

Nursing Care of Clients with Urinary Incontinence

1. 1. Keeping an incontinence log helps the nurse identify patterns in the frequency of urination. The data are then used to schedule toilet activities to correspond to the filling and emptying patterns demonstrated by the client. Checking the urine's specific gravity, monitoring bladder distention, and weighing incontinence pads are all appropriate assessments when caring for clients having problems with urinary elimination. However, these assessments are not as pertinent to planning a successful bladder-retraining program as identifying urinary elimination patterns.

> **Test Taking Strategy**—*Look at the key words "most important" in reference to the nursing assessment needed before bladder retraining. Recall that it is essential to determine the client's individual pattern of elimination if possible to coordinate retraining efforts. Review information on bladder retraining if you had difficulty answering this question.*
> **Cognitive Level**—*Applying*
> **Client Needs Category**—*Physiological integrity*
> **Client Needs Subcategory**—*Basic care and comfort*

2. 3. The Health Insurance Portability and Accountability Act (HIPAA) is a federal law that protects a client's health information. It ensures that information regarding the client's age; birthdate; Social Security number; address; and past, present, and future medical diagnoses, care, and treatment remains private. By announcing in front of other residents at the nurses' station that the client was incontinent, the patient care technician has violated HIPAA regulations. The Hippocratic Oath is a pledge that physicians take when they enter into practice to do no harm to their patients. The Good Samaritan Act is a law that protects health care providers who provide emergency care and first-aid from any liability should something go wrong. The Emergency Medical Treatment and Liability Act (EMTALA) provides a medical screening if the client comes to the emergency department regardless of the client's ability to pay or insurance status. This law also has strict guidelines regarding transfers to different facilities and treatment that occurs within 250 yards of the facility's main entrance.

> **Test Taking Strategy**—*Analyze to determine what information the question asks for, which is the law that protects the confidentiality of client information. Recall that HIPAA legislation applies to spoken and written health information. Review how HIPAA legislation applies to health care workers if you had difficulty answering this question.*

Cognitive Level—*Applying*
Client Needs Category—*Safe and effective care environment*
Client Needs Subcategory—*Coordinated care*

3. 3. According to the Health Insurance Portability and Accountability Act (HIPAA), health care providers may not disclose any information about the client's medical condition unless the client authorizes them to do so. HIPAA maintains client confidentiality. None of the other choices is appropriate because they reveal information about the client's current condition and treatment.

> *Test Taking Strategy*—*Look at the key words "most appropriate" in reference to a nursing response to a person requesting health information about a client. Recall that HIPAA legislation protects the confidentiality of client information. Review how HIPAA legislation applies to health care workers if you had difficulty answering this question.*
> *Cognitive Level*—*Applying*
> *Client Needs Category*—*Safe and effective care environment*
> *Client Needs Subcategory*—*Coordinated care*

4. 4. The nurse should discourage the client from restricting fluid intake because it can lead to fluid imbalance. In general, maintaining an adequate fluid intake is important because fluids flush toxins and organisms from the body and maintain a state of homeostasis. Restricting fluid leads to more concentrated urine, which is more likely to foster stone formation. Inadequate fluid intake does contribute to constipation, but that is not the main reason for discouraging the client from limiting fluid intake. Although the client is determined to the meet the goal, it is unsafe to encourage a plan to restrict fluid intake.

> *Test Taking Strategy*—*Use the process of elimination to help select the option that identifies the best response to a client's strategy for remaining continent. When discriminating between options, first decide whether the fluid restriction is appropriate in this situation. Options 1 and 2 can be eliminated because supporting the client's intention to restrict fluid is potentially harmful. Option 3 looks like an attractive answer because a client's fluid status does affect the consistency of stool; however, it is not the best answer in this case. Option 4 emerges as the best answer because it identifies the relationship between restricting fluid and the effect it has on fluid balance. Review strategies of bladder retraining if you had difficulty answering this question.*
> *Cognitive Level*—*Applying*
> *Client Needs Category*—*Health promotion and maintenance*
> *Client Needs Subcategory*—*None*

5. 4. Reflecting feelings is a useful therapeutic communication technique that demonstrates empathy. It lets the client know that the nurse has recognized the emotion underlying the spoken words in the verbal statement. Disagreeing with the client may block further communication. Belittling the client's feelings by challenging the seriousness of the statement also interferes with communication. Advising the client to cheer up or to anticipate physical setbacks because of age are inappropriate, nontherapeutic forms of interaction.

> *Test Taking Strategy*—*Use the process of elimination to help select the option that offers the best therapeutic response. Options 1, 2, and 3 can be eliminated because they are examples of nontherapeutic communication techniques involving disagreeing, belittling, and advising. Option 4 emerges as the best answer because it illustrates the therapeutic communication technique called reflecting. Review therapeutic and nontherapeutic communication techniques if you had difficulty answering this question.*
> *Cognitive Level*—*Applying*
> *Client Needs Category*—*Psychosocial integrity*
> *Client Needs Subcategory*—*None*

6. 3. Allowing space between the end of the penis and the drainage end of the catheter helps prevent irritation to the urinary meatus and promotes urine drainage. Lubrication is inappropriate because it would interfere with maintaining the catheter's application. External catheters are similar to latex condoms; they stretch to fit; therefore, measuring the penis is unnecessary. The foreskin of an uncircumcised man is never left in a retracted position because it could have a tourniquet effect and interfere with circulation of blood to the tissue.

> *Test Taking Strategy*—*Analyze to determine what information the question asks for, which is the correct method for applying an external catheter. To reduce the potential for leaking and tissue irritation, it is important to leave a space between the tip of the penis and the proximal end of the drainage tube (option 3). Review the steps in applying an external catheter if you had difficulty answering this question.*
> *Cognitive Level*—*Applying*
> *Client Needs Category*—*Physiological integrity*
> *Client Needs Subcategory*—*Basic care and comfort*

7. 1. Anchoring the indwelling catheter to the abdomen and allowing for slack before taping eliminates pressure and irritation at the penoscrotal angle. Pressure in this area predisposes to fistula formation. The catheter and tubing are passed over a client's leg to prevent obstruction of drainage from body weight. It is appropriate to fasten the drainage tubing to the bed to ensure a straight line from the bed to the collection bag and to insert the catheter into the tubing of the collection bag. However, neither of these nursing actions will prevent damage to the penis and a penoscrotal fistula from forming.

> *Test Taking Strategy*—Look at the key words *"most appropriate"* used in reference to preventing penile injury when stabilizing an indwelling catheter. Recall that tension and torsion on the penis can be eliminated by anchoring the catheter to the abdomen. Review techniques for securing an indwelling catheter in a male if you had difficulty answering this question.
>
> *Cognitive Level*—Applying
> *Client Needs Category*—Physiological integrity
> *Client Needs Subcategory*—Reduction of risk potential

Nursing Care of Clients with Infectious and Inflammatory Urologic Disorders

8. 4, 5, 6. One of the classic symptoms of a urinary tract infection (cystitis) is pain or burning on urination. Other symptoms include urinary frequency and urgency. People who have pyelonephritis more commonly experience flank pain. The client's urine may contain white blood cells, causing it to appear cloudy, but a purulent discharge is not a common complaint. Concentrated urine has a strong odor, but this usually does not occur among those with cystitis. Although the urine may develop an odor depending on bacterial growth and amount of urine retained, clients do not commonly report this finding.

> *Test Taking Strategy*—Analyze to determine what information the question asks for, which is symptoms of a urinary tract infection. Alternative-format *"select all that apply"* questions require considering each option independently to decide its merit in answering the question. Choose options that correlate with signs and symptoms of a bladder infection. Review clinical manifestations associated with cystitis if you had difficulty answering this question.
>
> *Cognitive Level*—Understanding
> *Client Needs Category*—Physiological integrity
> *Client Needs Subcategory*—Physiological adaptation

9. 3. The initial voided stream is discarded and a portion of what follows is collected as the specimen. Women are instructed to clean the urethral area from front to back; men clean the penis using a circular motion. The specimen is collected in a sterile container. The substance used for cleaning is not mixed with the urine specimen. Drinking several caffeinated beverages may stimulate urine formation, but it is not part of instructions related to midstream urine collection.

> *Test Taking Strategy*—Analyze to determine what information the question asks for, which is instructions for collecting a clean-catch urine specimen.

> Alternative-format *"select all that apply"* questions require considering each option independently to decide its merit in answering the question. Choose options that identify correct instructions for collecting a clean-catch midstream urine specimen from a female client. Recall that the method for cleaning the meatus is different in women than in men because of anatomic differences. Review the technique for obtaining a clean-catch midstream urine specimen if you had difficulty answering this question.
>
> *Cognitive Level*—Understanding
> *Client Needs Category*—Physiological integrity
> *Client Needs Subcategory*—Reduction of risk potential

10. 2. Infectious and inflammatory conditions affecting the urinary tract are accompanied by blood and pus in the urine, which may be grossly visible or microscopic. Glucose in the urine may be caused by a metabolic problem such as diabetes mellitus. Liver and gallbladder disorders are evidenced by the presence of bilirubin in the urine. Protein in the urine suggests pathology within the nephrons of the kidneys.

> *Test Taking Strategy*—Look at the key words *"most suggestive"* in reference to a laboratory finding in urine that indicates a bladder infection. Recall that normal urine should not contain any of the substances listed, but blood in the urine may be indicative of a bladder infection. Review normal and abnormal constituents of urine and their significance if you had difficulty answering this question.
>
> *Cognitive Level*—Applying
> *Client Needs Category*—Physiological integrity
> *Client Needs Subcategory*—Physiological adaptation

11. 2. Phenazopyridine (Pyridium) changes the color of the urine to orange. It will not cause the urine to look cloudy, decrease in volume, or smell strong. This drug will also cause staining of the underwear.

> *Test Taking Strategy*—Look at the key words *"most appropriate"* in reference to health teaching about the drug phenazopyridine. Recall that phenazopyridine, a urinary analgesic that soothes the lining of the urinary tract, contains an orange dye. Clients who are unaware of the color change in urine may become distressed by its appearance. Review the recommended health teaching related to drug therapy with phenazopyridine if you had difficulty answering this question.
>
> *Cognitive Level*—Understanding
> *Client Needs Category*—Physiological integrity
> *Client Needs Subcategory*—Pharmacological therapies

12. 3. Phenazopyridine (Pyridium) is a urinary analgesic that rapidly decreases the burning associated with urinary tract infections (UTIs). Reducing discomfort eventually results in less frequent and urgent urination, but these are secondary effects. Emptying the bladder at less frequent intervals may increase the volume eliminated, but this is also a secondary effect of drug therapy.

> *Test Taking Strategy—Use the process of elimination to help select the option that identifies the best evidence of the drug phenazopyridine's effectiveness. Because the drug is classified as a urinary analgesic, option 3 is the best answer because it describes relief from discomfort. Options 1, 2, and 4 describe secondary effects. Review the mechanism of action and use of phenazopyridine for treating the symptoms of a UTI if you had difficulty answering this question.*
> *Cognitive Level—Applying*
> *Client Needs Category—Physiological integrity*
> *Client Needs Subcategory—Pharmacological therapies*

13. 2. The client who must remain on bed rest due to traction has difficulty in fully eliminating urine from the bladder due to the positioning within the bed. This can lead to residual urine in the bladder that prompts bacterial growth. Urinary stagnation can also result in stone formation. Hygiene needs are also important but can be met with regular nursing care. The client should still have bladder control and be able to drink fluids.

> *Test Taking Strategy—Analyze to determine what information the question asks for, which is is the rationale for monitoring a client on prolonged bed rest in a recumbent position for the development of a urinary tract infection (UTI). Recall that stasis of urine secondary to incomplete emptying of the bladder contributes to the potential for a UTI. Review factors that predispose to UTIs if you had difficulty answering this question.*
> *Cognitive Level—Applying*
> *Client Needs Category—Physiological integrity*
> *Client Needs Subcategory—Physiological adaptation*

14. 2. Altered mental states do not necessarily place a client at higher risk for urinary tract infections (UTIs), especially if the client can still attend to personal hygiene. A client is at risk for a UTI if immunocompromised and unable to fight bacteria growth, has suffered trauma to the urethral mucosa, or has an altered metabolic state that could change the composition of the urine.

> *Test Taking Strategy—Use the process of elimination to help select the option that identifies the client who is least likely to develop a UTI. Options 1 and 4 can be eliminated immediately because these conditions place clients at high risk for an infection involving the urinary tract. Although option 3 is somewhat vague because it does not identify a specific metabolic disorder, it can be assumed that anyone with compromised physical health is at risk for infection. When options 1, 3, and 4 are eliminated, option 2 emerges as the best answer. Review factors that*

> predispose to UTIs if you had difficulty answering this question.
> *Cognitive Level—Analyzing*
> *Client Needs Category—Health promotion and maintenance*
> *Client Needs Subcategory—None*

15. 3. Because the female urethra is shorter (about 1½" or nearly 4 cm), pathogens travel to the bladder at a much faster rate than in a man. Also, the female urethra is more easily contaminated with organisms from the rectum and vagina if hygiene is inadequate. Pathogens have to travel farther in the longer male urethra (about 6" [15 cm]). Also, the male urethra is more curved, which tends to act as a barrier to the progression of pathogens toward the bladder. Both male and female urethras are lined with mucous membranes. The diameters of the urethras are similar in both sexes.

> *Test Taking Strategy—Look at the key words "most accurate" in reference to the reason more women than men develop urinary tract infections. Recall the anatomic gender differences in the length of the urethra and the proximity of the urethra to microorganisms that can be transferred there from the rectum. Review factors that contribute to the development of urinary tract infections if you had difficulty answering this question.*
> *Cognitive Level—Applying*
> *Client Needs Category—Health promotion and maintenance*
> *Client Needs Subcategory—None*

16. 1, 3, 6. The client with a urinary tract infection (UTI) typically reports symptoms of urinary frequency, burning on urination, urinary urgency, and concentrated, foul-smelling urine. The client might also report passing a small amount of urine with each frequent voiding. Urinary incontinence and itching in the perineal area are not symptoms of a UTI but should be assessed as well.

> *Test Taking Strategy—Analyze to determine what information the question asks for, which is signs and symptoms of a UTI in a diabetic client. Alternative-format "select all that apply" questions require considering each option independently to decide its merit in answering the question. Choose options that correlate with signs and symptoms of a UTI. Review the manifestations of a UTI if you had difficulty answering this question.*
> *Cognitive Level—Analyzing*
> *Client Needs Category—Physiological integrity*
> *Client Needs Subcategory—Physiological adaptation*

17. 1. Many chronic health states, such as diabetes mellitus, multiple sclerosis, and spinal cord injuries, predispose affected clients to urinary tract infections (UTIs). Glucose in the urine provides a supportive environment for bacterial growth. Diabetes mellitus does not suppress white blood cell activity. Polyuria is a finding in diabetic clients who have not yet been diagnosed. Once diabetic clients are diagnosed and treated, however, they do not void more frequently than nondiabetic clients, nor is their urine more concentrated.

> *Test Taking Strategy—Use the process of elimination to help select the option that is the best explanation for the increased risk for UTIs among those with diabetes mellitus. Option 2 can be eliminated immediately because diabetic clients are not necessarily immunosuppressed. Options 3 and 4 can be eliminated because the increased volume of urine in an untreated or undiagnosed state dilutes the urine; the increased urinary volume then triggers frequent voiding. Both of these factors would tend to reduce colonization of microorganisms. Option 1 remains as the best answer because the presence of glucose in the urine of treated and untreated diabetic clients promotes microbial growth. Review the pathophysiologic factors that contribute to a higher incidence of infections of any type among persons with diabetes mellitus if you had difficulty answering this question.*

Cognitive Level—*Applying*
Client Needs Category—*Physiological integrity*
Client Needs Subcategory—*Physiological adaptation*

18. 1, 5. A large intake of fluids promotes frequent urinary elimination, which causes pathogens to pass out of the bladder with the urine. Decreasing the number of pathogens present in the urinary tract reduces their growth rate. Voiding after intercourse is important to flush the bacteria out of the urethra that may have entered during intercourse. Drinking acidic fluids will not necessarily decrease bacterial growth. Changing underclothing regularly is an appropriate hygiene measure; however, it is not the most effective measure for reducing bacteria in the bladder. Personal hygiene measures are more important than the sanitary condition of restrooms in reducing the incidence of bladder infections. The color of toilet tissue does not contribute to or prevent cystitis.

> *Test Taking Strategy—Analyze to determine what information the question asks for, which is instructions by a nurse to a female client that help reduce bacterial growth in the bladder. Alternative-format "select all that apply" questions require considering each option independently to decide its merit in answering the question. To answer this question, choose options that describe health teaching to reduce the potential for developing a urinary tract infection. Review interventions that are prophylactic for preventing or reducing the incidence of cystitis if you had difficulty answering this question.*

Cognitive Level—*Applying*
Client Needs Category—*Health promotion and maintenance*
Client Needs Subcategory—*None*

19. 1. The most important technique for preventing future urinary tract infections is to eliminate the introduction of organisms from the rectum or vagina through improper wiping. Hand washing after elimination assists in reducing the transmission of pathogens to other body structures, such as the eyes and mouth. However, hand washing is not as effective as correct wiping in reducing the risk of cystitis. The use of chemicals, such as those found in feminine hygiene sprays, should be avoided because they commonly contain irritants or substances to which many people are sensitive. Drying the perineum is a comfort measure that also appropriately eliminates moisture that may facilitate bacterial growth; however, it is not as significant at preventing introduction of pathogens as the manner in which the perineum is wiped.

> *Test Taking Strategy—Use the process of elimination to help select the option that identifies the best strategy for preventing a urinary tract infection. Option 3 can result in skin irritation. Options 2 and 4 are appropriate hygiene measures but are not as effective as proper wiping of the perineum after elimination (option 1). Review how physically wiping the remnants of stool away from the female urethra (and vagina) reduces the transfer of microorganisms to sites where they could facilitate an infection if you had difficulty answering this question.*

Cognitive Level—*Applying*
Client Needs Category—*Health promotion and maintenance*
Client Needs Subcategory—*None*

20. 1, 3, 4, 5. Alcohol, tea, chocolate, and coffee are all urinary irritants. Urinary irritants may exacerbate such conditions as interstitial cystitis. Possible substitutes include apricots, pears, papaya juice, herbal tea, and carob.

> *Test Taking Strategy—Analyze to determine what information the question asks for, which is possible urinary irritants. Alternative-format "select all that apply" questions require considering each option independently to decide its merit in answering the question. Choose substances that potentiate discomfort in a client who is already experiencing urinary frequency. Review dietary substances that promote frequency of urination if you had difficulty answering this question.*

Cognitive Level—*Understanding*
Client Needs Category—*Health promotion and maintenance*
Client Needs Subcategory—*None*

21.

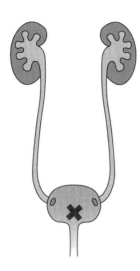

Cystitis is an inflammation of the urinary bladder (indicated by the X). It is usually caused by a bacterial infection.

> *Test Taking Strategy—Analyze to determine what information the question asks for, which is the anatomic structure affected by cystitis. Recall that the prefix cysto- refers to the bladder. Review the gross anatomy of the urinary tract and the location of the bladder if you had difficulty answering this question.*
> *Cognitive Level—Remembering*
> *Client Needs Category—Physiological integrity*
> *Client Needs Subcategory—Physiological adaptation*

22. 3. The nurse should teach the client to catheterize herself by inserting a catheter 3″ (7.5 cm) into the urinary meatus in a downward and backward direction. At approximately 3″, the client should see urine in the tubing.

> *Test Taking Strategy—Analyze to determine what information the question asks for, which is the distance a client should insert a straight catheter during self-catheterization. Recall that the female urethra is approximately 1½″ (4 cm) long, but the catheter must be inserted somewhat farther to ensure that the tip of the catheter is fully within the bladder. Review the technique for straight catheterization if you had difficulty answering this question.*
> *Cognitive Level—Understanding*
> *Client Needs Category—Physiological integrity*
> *Client Needs Subcategory—Reduction of risk potential*

23. 2. Pyelonephritis is a bacterial infection of the kidneys and the renal pelvis and can be acute or chronic. When it is necessary to insert a catheter, the recumbent position is best for most female clients. This position involves placing the client on the back with the knees flexed and the soles of the feet flat on the bed. For women who have arthritis of the hips or another condition that interferes with recumbent positioning, a side-lying position is used as an alternative. The lithotomy position involves supporting the feet in stirrups. It is used when a woman undergoes a pelvic examination. The knee-chest position is used for rectal or lower bowel examinations. The prone position is used when examining the spine and back.

> *Test Taking Strategy—Analyze to determine what information the question asks for, which is the standard position for catheterizing a female. To access the urinary meatus and provide comfort for the client during the catheterization procedure, it is best that the client lies on her back with the knees bent and spread apart. Review images of the positions identified in the options, focusing on the position used for female catheterization, if you had difficulty answering this question.*
> *Cognitive Level—Understanding*
> *Client Needs Category—Physiological integrity*
> *Client Needs Subcategory—Reduction of risk potential*

24. 3. The urinary tract is a sterile environment; therefore, a contaminated catheter should be discarded and a new one obtained before proceeding with the catheterization. Wiping the contaminated catheter with an alcohol swab or cleaning it with povidone-iodine (Betadine) solution will not ensure sterility. If the catheter contaminated from the vagina is reinserted into the urethra, pathogens may be transferred to the urinary tract.

> *Test Taking Strategy—Use the process of elimination to help select the option that is best after mistakenly inserting a catheter intended for urinary insertion in the vagina. Recall that a urinary catheter should remain sterile and the vagina is essentially unsterile. Consequently the catheter is no longer sterile and must be replaced before proceeding further. Review principles of asepsis if you had difficulty answering this question.*
> *Cognitive Level—Applying*
> *Client Needs Category—Safe and effective care environment*
> *Client Needs Subcategory—Safety and infection control*

25. 3. Clients who take sulfonamides such as trimethoprim and sulfamethoxazole (Bactrim) can reduce the risk of developing crystalluria by consuming 3 to 4 quarts (3 to 4 L) of fluid per day. Water is preferred for a diabetic client because it is calorie-free. Sulfonamides are best taken on an empty stomach unless gastric irritation occurs. Carbonated drinks and citrus fruits will not reduce the risk of crystalluria.

> *Test Taking Strategy—Look at the key words "most appropriate" in reference to health teaching that helps a client avoid crystalluria secondary to*

sulfonamide drug therapy. Recall that keeping the urine dilute, which subsequently leads to more frequent urination, reduces the accumulation of a concentrated amount of the drug in the urine. Review the physiologic effects on urinary elimination when fluid intake is increased if you had difficulty answering this question.
***Cognitive Level**—Applying*
***Client Needs Category**—Physiological integrity*
***Client Needs Subcategory**—Pharmacological therapies*

26. **4.** An intravenous pyelogram (IVP) is an X-ray examination of the kidneys, ureters, and urinary bladder that uses contrast material. The client should be instructed not to eat or drink after midnight on the night before the examination and to take a mild laxative (in either pill or liquid form) the evening before the procedure. A laxative is taken to empty the bowel of gas and stool, which, if present, could obstruct the view of the urinary structures during the X-ray. IVP is not used to examine the lower GI tract. Stool incontinence is not generally a problem with IVP. Laxatives are generally given to treat, not prevent, constipation.
> *Test Taking Strategy—Look at the key words "primary reason" as they refer to the rationale for cleansing the bowel before an IVP. Recall that in order to image the urinary structures the radiation must pass through organs in the abdominal cavity such as the large intestine. Anything that increases the density in the large intestine, such as stool, may obscure a crisp image of the kidneys, ureters, and bladder. Review the preparation of a client for an IVP if you had difficulty answering this question.*
***Cognitive Level**—Applying*
***Client Needs Category**—Physiological integrity*
***Client Needs Subcategory**—Reduction of risk potential*

27. **3.** A history of a previous allergic reaction to radiopaque dye indicates the client is at risk for a similar episode. The physician may prescribe a corticosteroid or antihistamine before the test to reduce the potential for an allergic reaction. Other than inserting the I.V. to inject the dye, the procedure is painless; the client lies flat on an X-ray table or is asked to turn to the side as the X-ray tube is adjusted over the client's lower abdomen. In the IVP, iodine dye injected through a vein in the arm collects in the kidneys, ureters, and bladder, giving these areas a bright white and sharply defined appearance on the X-ray images. Barium is not used in this procedure but in those involving upper and lower GI studies.
> *Test Taking Strategy—Look at the key words "most important" in reference to reportable information before an IVP. Recall that an allergic reaction to contrast dye can be life-threatening and needs to be reported before the client undergoes the procedure.*

Review the risks associated with contrast dyes used during diagnostic procedures if you had difficulty answering this question.
***Cognitive Level**—Applying*
***Client Needs Category**—Physiological integrity*
***Client Needs Subcategory**—Reduction of risk potential*

28. **1, 5, 6.** Glomerulonephritis is an inflammatory condition that causes significant kidney damage. More than half of the clients are asymptomatic or have vague symptoms that they feel do not require medical attention. Family members often notice that the face of a person with glomerulonephritis appears pale and puffy. Other symptoms include poor appetite, nocturia, hematuria, ankle edema, and hypertension. Mental status is usually unaffected in the early stages of the disease. Salting food and sleeping poorly are atypical signs of glomerulonephritis.
> *Test Taking Strategy—Analyze to determine what information the question asks for, which is signs and symptoms of acute glomerulonephritis. Alternative-format "select all that apply" questions require considering each option independently to decide its merit in answering the question. Choose options with statements that correlate with signs and symptoms of acute glomerulonephritis. Review information about the clinical manifestations of glomerulonephritis if you had difficulty answering this question.*
***Cognitive Level**—Analyzing*
***Client Needs Category**—Physiological integrity*
***Client Needs Subcategory**—Physiological adaptation*

29. **2.** Although definite evidence linking a streptococcal infection with glomerulonephritis has not been established, many people recall that they experienced an upper respiratory infection or sore throat 2 to 3 weeks before the onset of glomerulonephritis. There is no correlation between acute glomerulonephritis and trauma, antibiotic therapy, or an allergy specific to X-ray dye.
> *Test Taking Strategy—Look at the key words "most likely" in reference to a factor that may have precipitated acute glomerulonephritis. Recall that acute glomerulonephritis is often preceded by an infection such as pharyngitis, caused by beta-hemolytic streptococci. Review etiologic factors associated with acute glomerulonephritis if you had difficulty answering this question.*
***Cognitive Level**—Applying*
***Client Needs Category**—Physiological integrity*
***Client Needs Subcategory**—Physiological adaptation*

30. **4.** A common sign associated with glomerulonephritis is peripheral edema that ranges from slight ankle edema in the evening to generalized fluid retention that may compromise cardiac function. The skin is pale, not flushed. Skin hemorrhages are a common finding in liver disease and blood dyscrasias. The distribution of body hair is not directly related to glomerulonephritis.

> *Test Taking Strategy*—*Analyze to determine what information the question asks for, which is a typical finding when physically assessing a client with acute glomerulonephritis. Recall that because this disorder affects renal function and the ability to excrete excess fluid in urine, the client is likely to present with evidence of fluid retention such as peripheral edema. Review clinical manifestations associated with acute glomerulonephritis if you had difficulty answering this question.*
> *Cognitive Level*—*Applying*
> *Client Needs Category*—*Physiological integrity*
> *Client Needs Subcategory*—*Physiological adaptation*

31. 3. The blood urea nitrogen (BUN) test is primarily used, along with the creatinine level, to evaluate kidney function and to monitor clients with acute or chronic kidney dysfunction or failure. The results of BUN testing indicate how efficiently the glomeruli are removing nitrogen wastes from the blood. An elevation indicates glomerular dysfunction. Serum amylase levels aid in diagnosing and monitoring pancreatitis. A blood glucose test is used for monitoring diabetes mellitus. A complete blood count (CBC) is helpful for baseline information, but it is not as essential in evaluating the course of glomerulonephritis as BUN testing.

> *Test Taking Strategy*—*Look at the key words "most important" in reference to a laboratory test result that is important to monitor when caring for a client with acute glomerulonephritis. Recall that one of the kidneys' functions is to excrete nitrogen wastes. When affected by this disorder, nitrogen wastes accumulate in the blood. Elevations in BUN can lead to seizures if they are not controlled. Review the significance of abnormal BUN levels if you had difficulty answering this question.*
> *Cognitive Level*—*Applying*
> *Client Needs Category*—*Physiological integrity*
> *Client Needs Subcategory*—*Reduction of risk potential*

32. 3. Because glomerulonephritis impairs renal function, monitoring weight on a daily basis is essential for evaluating how much fluid the person is retaining. Ambulation is not usually impaired; however, if the client is hypertensive or has other circulatory complications, activity may be restricted. Many clients with glomerulonephritis are on fluid restriction; therefore, encouraging fluid intake is an inappropriate nursing action. Self-catheterization is not indicated in clients with acute glomerulonephritis.

> *Test Taking Strategy*—*Look at the key word "priority" in reference to the nursing intervention that is most important to perform. Recall that a significant weight gain or loss in a short period is an assessment that generally reflects fluid volume status,*

which is a particular problem of concern when caring for this client. Review nursing interventions when caring for a client with fluid volume excess if you had difficulty answering this question.
> *Cognitive Level*—*Analyzing*
> *Client Needs Category*—*Physiological integrity*
> *Client Needs Subcategory*—*Physiological adaptation*

33. 2. After assessing the severity of the client's pain on the pain scale, it is important for the nurse to assess the client's blood pressure. People with glomerulonephritis are typically hypertensive; hypertension can be accompanied by a headache. Hypertension is also an indication of increased intracranial pressure. If the headache is caused by hypertension, a priority intervention is to reduce the blood pressure and treat the cause. Implementing comfort measures such as reducing environmental stimuli, administering a prescribed analgesic, and changing the client's position are appropriate; however, assessing the client is the nurse's priority in this situation.

> *Test Taking Strategy*—*Analyze to determine what information the question asks for, which is the nursing action that is indicated immediately after the client with acute glomerulonephritis reports a severe headache. Assessing the client's blood pressure helps to confirm or rule out that the headache is a consequence of hypertension secondary to fluid volume excess. If the blood pressure is significantly elevated, the client may need antihypertensive and diuretic medications, more than an analgesic, to prevent complications from occurring. Review the correlation of hypertension with neurologic and cardiac complications if you had difficulty answering this question.*
> *Cognitive Level*—*Analyzing*
> *Client Needs Category*—*Physiological integrity*
> *Client Needs Subcategory*—*Physiological adaptation*

34. 2. Urine that formed before a 24-hour urine collection starts should not be included with the collected urine. Valid results require that the urine collected be produced within the 24-hour period. Properly collected urine is refrigerated in a large container or kept in the container in a basin of ice. After all the urine from the 24-hour period is collected, the entire specimen is sent to the laboratory. The nurse should consult laboratory policy about whether to mix the urine from a 24-hour collection with a preservative or to refrigerate the sample.

> *Test Taking Strategy*—*Look at the key words "most appropriate" in reference to collecting a 24-hour urine specimen. Recall that the client voids at the time the collection begins, but because that urine has been produced earlier, it is discarded. All subsequent voided urine is collected for 24 hours. The test ends with the collection of one last voided urination at the same time the test began the previous day. Review*

the steps in collecting a 24-hour urine specimen if you had difficulty answering this question.
Cognitive Level—Applying
Client Needs Category—Physiological integrity
Client Needs Subcategory—Reduction of risk potential

35. 3. People with glomerulonephritis generally test positive for albuminuria. Albumin is present in the urine due to the increased permeability of the glomerular membrane. Glucose and acetone are expected in the urine of a person with uncontrolled diabetes mellitus. Bilirubin is present in the urine of a person with liver or gallbladder disease.

> *Test Taking Strategy—Analyze to determine what information the question asks for, which is an expected assessment finding when testing the urine of a client with glomerulonephritis using a reagent strip. Recall that when the kidneys are affected by this disorder, it is common to detect proteinuria. Albumin is the smallest of the plasma proteins and is the one most likely to escape glomerular filtration. Review the pathophysiology related to renal disorders if you had difficulty answering this question.*
> *Cognitive Level—Applying*
> *Client Needs Category—Physiological integrity*
> *Client Needs Subcategory—Physiological adaptation*

36. 2. The presence of blood gives a smoky appearance to urine. Cloudy urine suggests the presence of white blood cells. If the urine appears bright orange, the nurse might investigate whether the client has ingested a substance containing a water-soluble dye or has taken a urinary analgesic such as phenazopyridine (Pyridium) for a urinary tract infection (UTI). Concentrated urine is likely to appear dark yellow.

> *Test Taking Strategy—Use the process of elimination to help select the option that identifies the urine characteristic that correlates best with the presence of hematuria. Options 1, 3, and 4, although abnormal, are more indicative of other causative factors. Option 2 is the best choice. Review normal and abnormal characteristics of urine if you had difficulty answering this question.*
> *Cognitive Level—Applying*
> *Client Needs Category—Physiological integrity*
> *Client Needs Subcategory—Physiological adaptation*

37. 3. Chicken breast on lettuce is the menu item that contains the least amount of sodium among the options provided. Processed meats such as hot dogs are highly salted. Bouillon and other canned soups also generally contain a great deal of salt. Dairy products such as cheese are high in sodium. Baked goods, such as crackers and pizza crust, also contain sodium bicarbonate or salt.

> *Test Taking Strategy—Use the process of elimination to help select the menu choice that is lowest in sodium from among the options. Recall that bouil-*

lon, processed meats, and cheese contain hidden salt. Option 3 emerges as the best answer because breast of chicken and lettuce are lower in sodium than the other options. Review the sodium content in the food items listed if you had difficulty answering this question.*
> *Cognitive Level—Applying*
> *Client Needs Category—Health promotion and maintenance*
> *Client Needs Subcategory—None*

38. 2. Steroids are prescribed to treat the inflammatory response caused by the disease process. Alternate-day therapy is used when administering glucocorticoid drugs to prevent adrenal suppression. Alternating oral hormone therapy allows the adrenal cortex to produce natural hormones as the blood level drops the day the hormone replacement is not given. Steroids have many undesirable side effects, but most are tolerable. Steroids can be and are administered on a daily basis when clients require short-term therapy. The duration of action is generally 24 hours.

> *Test Taking Strategy—Use the process of elimination to help select the option that provides the best explanation for alternate-day therapy when administering corticosteroids. Although all drugs can be toxic, option 1 can be eliminated because as long as the client receives a usual dose of corticosteroids and can metabolize and excrete them, toxicity should not develop. Option 3 can be eliminated because the medication's duration of action is not significantly prolonged. Although the side effects of steroid therapy are undesirable, clients can tolerate them. Option 2 emerges as the best answer because daily exogenous sources of steroids can eliminate the adrenal cortex's production of endogenous corticosteroids. Review alternate-day therapy in relation to the administration of corticosteroid drug therapy if you had difficulty answering this question.*
> *Cognitive Level—Applying*
> *Client Needs Category—Physiological integrity*
> *Client Needs Subcategory—Pharmacological therapies*

Nursing Care of Clients with Renal Failure

39. 1. Anemia is common in clients with renal failure. The kidneys produce erythropoietin, which stimulates the production of red blood cells (RBCs). If kidney function is diminished, anemia occurs from the decreased RBC production. Clients with renal failure typically have weight gain, not weight loss, related to fluid retention and hypertension not hypotension. Renal failure does not generally produce a fever.

Test Taking Strategy—*Analyze to determine what information the question asks for, which is a pathophysiologic finding associated with renal failure. Recall that bone marrow requires erythropoietin, which is produced by the kidneys to produce and replace RBCs. If the production of erythropoietin declines, it will lead to anemia. Review the production of erythropoietin and its physiologic role if you had difficulty answering this question.*
Cognitive Level—*Applying*
Client Needs Category—*Physiological integrity*
Client Needs Subcategory—*Physiological adaptation*

40. 4. Normal urine output is between 1,000 and 2,000 mL/day. The first stage of renal failure is generally characterized by oliguria—that is, a urine output of less than 500 mL in 24 hours. The nurse would expect to note a diuretic phase following a period of oliguria or anuria as the client's condition improves.

Test Taking Strategy—*Analyze to determine what information the question asks for, which is urine output that correlates with oliguria. Recall that urine output diminishes significantly in oliguria but does not cease. Review the definition of oliguria if you had difficulty answering this question.*
Cognitive Level—*Applying*
Client Needs Category—*Physiological integrity*
Client Needs Subcategory—*Physiological adaptation*

41. 1. The client's serum creatinine levels should be closely monitored because they are helpful in determining kidney functioning. High serum creatinine levels are commonly noted in conjunction with glomerular damage. Altered levels of serum sodium, uric acid, and blood urea nitrogen may also be seen, but these are not the best indicators of kidney functioning. Specific gravity relates to the concentration of the urine, not kidney function.

Test Taking Strategy—*Analyze to determine what information the question asks for, which is a laboratory test result that, depending on the extent of its abnormal value, provides information about the status of renal function. Recall that creatinine is a nitrogen waste that is excreted by the kidneys; its accumulation in the blood indicates glomerular dysfunction. Review the laboratory tests that are used to diagnose and manage the care of clients with glomerulonephritis if you had difficulty answering this question.*
Cognitive Level—*Applying*
Client Needs Category—*Physiological integrity*
Client Needs Subcategory—*Reduction of risk potential*

42. 2. Measuring intake and output accurately is a priority when planning the care of a client with renal failure. This information aids in evaluating fluid balance and adjusting fluid restrictions. Urine retention is not common in renal failure because the client is not producing

much urine. Generally, a urinary catheter is inserted to aid in monitoring the output of a person in renal failure. The body temperature is monitored to assess for signs of infection or other complications; however, it is not likely to be affected by the primary condition. The nurse would not expect to find glucose in the urine; therefore, checking for evidence with a chemical dipstick or by other means is unnecessary.

Test Taking Strategy—*Use the process of elimination to select the option that identifies an essential nursing assessment when caring for a client with glomerulonephritis. Recall that one of the kidneys' primary functions is the excretion of excess fluid. A decrease or increase in urine excretion indicates how well or poorly the client is responding to treatment. Review the nursing management of a client with chronic glomerulonephritis if you had difficulty answering this question.*
Cognitive Level—*Applying*
Client Needs Category—*Physiological integrity*
Client Needs Subcategory—*Physiological adaptation*

43. 4. It is necessary to assess the client's breath sounds in this situation because administering fluid to someone with oliguria or anuria may lead to heart failure and pulmonary edema. Fluid overload is manifested by pedal edema, but this is not a life-threatening consequence. It is not likely that the nurse will perform frequent weights while the fluids are infusing. Monitoring specific gravity is not a priority during fluid administration. It is assumed that with increased urine output, the concentration of the urine (specific gravity) would decrease.

Test Taking Strategy—*Use the process of elimination to help select the option that identifies the most important assessment when I.V. fluid is infused rapidly. Although options 1, 2, and 3 are assessments that are affected by circulating fluid volume and the kidney's excretion, option 4 is the best answer because it will provide evidence that the rapid infusion may be causing circulatory overload and pulmonary edema, a life-threatening consequence. Review the causes of pulmonary edema and the significance of adventitious lung sounds if you had difficulty answering this question.*
Cognitive Level—*Applying*
Client Needs Category—*Physiological integrity*
Client Needs Subcategory—*Pharmacological therapies*

44. 4. The skin of a client in renal failure becomes dry and intensely itchy due to the excretion and evaporation of nitrogenous wastes through the skin (uremic frost). Skin care involves frequent cleaning with plain, warm water, then patting the skin dry. The client may have increased perspiration due to the excretion process. The skin typically becomes dry, not oily. The nurse may choose to apply a lubricating skin cream or lotion. Edema causes taut, puffy skin, not loss of turgor.

Test Taking Strategy—Analyze to determine what information the question asks for, which is the skin problem characteristically experienced by clients in renal failure. Recall that the skin becomes the organ for excreting nitrogen waste products when the kidneys are not capable of doing so. Review the effects of uremic frost if you had difficulty answering this question.
Cognitive Level—*Applying*
Client Needs Category—*Health promotion and maintenance*
Client Needs Subcategory—*None*

45. 4. Lemon juice is used to enhance the flavor of seafood, fish, eggs, and some vegetables. Other recommended seasonings include fresh herbs, such as parsley, dill, and oregano. Fresh onion is also acceptable. Catsup, prepared mustard, and soy sauce are high in sodium and should be avoided.

Test Taking Strategy—Analyze to determine what information the question asks for, which is an appropriate salt substitute for someone on a sodium-restricted diet. Recall that lemon juice contains 0 mg of sodium, whereas yellow mustard contains 190 mg/tbsp., catsup contains 175 mg/tbsp., and soy sauce contains 914 mg/tbsp. Review the sodium content of various condiments as well as healthier substitutions for seasoning food if you had difficulty answering this question.
Cognitive Level—*Applying*
Client Needs Category—*Physiological integrity*
Client Needs Subcategory—*Basic care and comfort*

46. 1. Hard candy, especially if sour or tart-flavored, increases salivation and reduces the sensation of thirst without increasing fluid intake. Clients in renal failure, unless they are diabetic, are not generally restricted in the amount of carbohydrates they may consume. Ice chips, ice cream, and fresh fruit all contain fluid that must be considered in the fluid restriction. Fruit contains potassium, which is also contraindicated for clients with renal failure.

Test Taking Strategy—Look at the key words "most appropriate" in reference to a nursing action for relieving thirst experienced by a fluid-restricted client with glomerulonephritis. Recall that hard candy does not have any water content, but can stimulate the production of saliva, which could diminish a client's thirst. Review techniques for managing thirst for a client on fluid restrictions if you had difficulty answering this question.
Cognitive Level—*Applying*
Client Needs Category—*Physiological integrity*
Client Needs Subcategory—*Basic care and comfort*

47. 1. An arteriovenous fistula is a surgical procedure connecting an artery and vein located in the forearm.

When dialysis is needed, two venipunctures are performed at either end of the fistula. The color and temperature of the hands are assessed regularly for signs of inadequate circulation. Blood clots may form in the joined vessels and occlude tissue perfusion. Joint range of motion, muscle tone and coordination, and skin turgor are not likely to be affected.

Test Taking Strategy—Look at the key words "most appropriate" in reference to a critical nursing assessment when managing the care of a client with an arteriovenous fistula. Recall that joining these two blood vessels may lead to circulatory complications that are best evidenced by pale color and coldness in the hand used for this measure. Review nursing responsibilities when caring for a client with an arteriovenous fistula if you had difficulty answering this question.
Cognitive Level—*Applying*
Client Needs Category—*Physiological integrity*
Client Needs Subcategory—*Reduction of risk potential*

48. 3. While assessing the arteriovenous fistula, the nurse palpates a thrill, or vibration over the vascular access. The nurse should also expect to hear a bruit—a loud sound caused by turbulent blood flow—at the connection site. Both the thrill (vibration) and bruit (sound) must be present. If they are absent, the nurse should postpone further use of the device and notify the physician. The nurse would not expect to note a pulse or a clicking sound in the assessment.

Test Taking Strategy—Analyze to determine what information the question asks for, which is the expected assessment finding when palpating the skin over the site of the arteriovenous fistula. Recall that arterial blood flowing through the fistula causes turbulence in the blood flow, which creates a vibratory sensation or thrill (option 3). A regular pulse (option 1) or click (option 4) is not consistent with the continuous vibratory sensation. A bruit (option 2) is heard not felt. Review expected physical findings when assessing the site of an arteriovenous fistula created for the purpose of performing hemodialysis if you had difficulty answering this question.
Cognitive Level—*Applying*
Client Needs Category—*Physiological integrity*
Client Needs Subcategory—*Physiological adaptation*

49. 4. Discussing an actual or potential stressor helps to place the event in more realistic perspective. Giving a client an opportunity for discussion empowers the client to confront the issues and acquire support in the process. Having the spouse cook the client's favorite dishes may not be advisable, especially taking into account the sodium, protein, and fluid restrictions. Although the other two options may be explored later, the nurse should focus on the client's feelings about the disorder.

Test Taking Strategy—*Look at the key words "most helpful" in reference to assisting a client cope with a chronic health condition. Recall that assessment is the first step in the nursing process and that verbalizing feelings is therapeutic. Review techniques for improving coping skills if you had difficulty answering this question.*
Cognitive Level—*Applying*
Client Needs Category—*Psychosocial integrity*
Client Needs Subcategory—*None*

50. 2. Peritoneal dialysis is a method of filtering fluid, wastes, and chemicals from the body using the peritoneum, the semipermeable lining of the abdomen. Along with measuring the volume of infused and drained dialysis solution, comparing the client's weight before and after the procedure provides the best objective data for evaluating the outcome of peritoneal dialysis. Most clients requiring peritoneal dialysis do not excrete urine. Typically, the abdominal girth measurements will fluctuate based on the addition or withdrawal of fluids. Pulse rate should not vary and therefore will not affect the outcome of the treatment.

Test Taking Strategy—*Use the process of elimination to help select the option that is the best indication for determining the effectiveness of peritoneal dialysis. Option 4 can be eliminated immediately because a client who requires dialysis would most likely urinate a small amount, if any, between dialysis treatments. Option 1 can be eliminated because a pulse rate may not change very much unless the client experiences significant hypotension. Option 3 has merit because retention or loss of fluid may be reflected in abdominal girth, but it is not the best method for evaluating the effectiveness of peritoneal dialysis. Option 2 emerges as the best answer because there should be an expected weight loss after dialysis due to the change in fluid volume. Review the process of peritoneal dialysis and the physiologic changes associated with it if you had difficulty answering this question.*
Cognitive Level—*Evaluating*
Client Needs Category—*Physiological integrity*
Client Needs Subcategory—*Physiological adaptation*

51. 2. In peritoneal dialysis, the peritoneum serves as a semipermeable membrane. Urea and creatinine, metabolic end products normally excreted by the kidneys, are cleared from the blood by diffusion as the waste products move from an area of higher concentration (the peritoneal blood supply) to an area of lower concentration (the peritoneal cavity). Osmosis, also helpful in the dialysis process, is the movement of water through the semipermeable membrane. Filtration is movement that occurs according to pressure changes. Gravity is the process by which the dialysate is infused.

Test Taking Strategy—*Analyze to determine what information the question asks for, which is the physical*

mechanism by which dialysis removes nitrogen wastes from the blood. Recall that diffusion is a method that transports dissolved substances from higher to lower concentration. Review how fluid and substances dissolved in fluid are transported if you had difficulty answering this question.
Cognitive Level—*Understanding*
Client Needs Category—*Physiological integrity*
Client Needs Subcategory—*Physiological adaptation*

52. 1. The dialysate infusion tubing is clamped, usually for 15 to 45 minutes, to allow osmosis and diffusion to take place between the dialysate and the peritoneum. The peritoneal cavity is then drained after the dwell time. The client is free to ambulate, change positions, or remain in bed during peritoneal dialysis. The amount of activity depends on the client's safety needs. The client may eat and drink during peritoneal dialysis; however, oral fluids continue to be restricted throughout dialysis and for as long as the client is in renal failure.

Test Taking Strategy—*Analyze to determine what information the question asks for, which is the nursing action that is necessary after dialysate has been instilled within the peritoneal cavity. Recall that the dialysate must dwell in the peritoneal cavity for a period of time to optimally facilitate osmosis and diffusion. Clamping the tubing contains the infused solution. Review the process for performing peritoneal dialysis if you had difficulty answering this question.*
Cognitive Level—*Analyzing*
Client Needs Category—*Physiological integrity*
Client Needs Subcategory—*Reduction of risk potential*

53. 3. An elevated temperature is unexpected. Its presence indicates that an infection is occurring, and the nurse should suspect peritonitis. It is expected that a client undergoing peritoneal dialysis will lose weight and have an output that exceeds intake. Clients who require dialysis typically do not have a normal serum creatinine level (1.2 mg/dL).

Test Taking Strategy—*Use the process of elimination to help select the option that identifies an assessment finding that should be reported because it correlates with a potential complication associated with peritoneal dialysis. Options 1, 2, and 4 are findings that are expected or insignificant. Option 3 emerges as the best answer because clients who undergo peritoneal dialysis are susceptible to infection at the site of catheter insertion as well as life-threatening peritonitis. Review complications associated with peritonitis and their clinical manifestations if you had difficulty answering this question.*
Cognitive Level—*Analyzing*
Client Needs Category—*Physiological integrity*
Client Needs Subcategory—*Physiological adaptation*

54. 3. One beneficial effect of dialysis is the lowering of the serum potassium level. A goal of dialysis therapy is to maintain a safe concentration of serum electrolytes. A lower red blood cell count is not a desired effect. Most people with renal failure become anemic because the kidneys' ability to produce erythropoietin is impaired. Blood transfusions or injections of erythropoietin are commonly necessary. Peritoneal dialysis is not expected to improve urine output. Any improvement in renal function is probably due to accompanying therapy or healing at the cellular level. An improved appetite is far too subjective to be used as an indicator of a therapeutic response to peritoneal dialysis.

Test Taking Strategy—Use the process of elimination to help select the option that identifies the best evidence of the therapeutic benefit of peritoneal dialysis. Option 1 can be eliminated immediately because it is unlikely that the client's urine output will improve. Although a client with renal failure is likely to be anorectic, an improvement in appetite (option 2) is not the best evidence of a therapeutic effect. Option 4 can be eliminated because the failed kidneys are not able to manufacture erythropoietin, a function that will be unchanged despite dialysis. Option 3 emerges as the best answer because one of the goals of dialysis is to lower elevated potassium levels. Review expected outcomes of peritoneal dialysis if you had difficulty answering this question.
Cognitive Level—Evaluating
Client Needs Category—Physiological integrity
Client Needs Subcategory—Reduction of risk potential

55. 2. Peritonitis is the most serious and common complication in 60% to 80% of clients on long-term peritoneal dialysis. Pulmonary edema is not a common complication. Although cardiovascular disease commonly occurs due to hypertriglyceridemia, a ruptured aorta is not common. An abdominal hernia is common in clients undergoing long-term peritoneal dialysis because of the continuous increased intra-abdominal pressure; however, a hernia is not as common or as serious as peritonitis.

Test Taking Strategy—Use the process of elimination to help select the option that identifies the complication that is most likely to occur when a client elects to undergo peritoneal dialysis. Options 1 can be eliminated because the dialysate is not infused into the client's circulation. Option 4 can be eliminated because it is unrelated to peritoneal dialysis. Although option 3 is a potential complication, it is not as life-threatening as peritonitis. Review the complications associated with peritoneal dialysis if you had difficulty answering this question.
Cognitive Level—Analyzing
Client Needs Category—Physiological integrity
Client Needs Subcategory—Reduction of risk potential

56. 2. Relatives, especially siblings who were conceived by the same father and mother, prove to be the most compatible genetic matches for clients who receive transplanted organs. Immunosuppressive drugs make it possible to reduce the potential for rejection regardless of the source of human organs. Kidneys from other species are not successfully transplanted.

Test Taking Strategy—Analyze to determine what information the question asks for, which is the best source for a donor kidney. Although all the options, except option 4, are sources of organs for transplantation, a sibling provides the greatest potential for matching the genetic characteristics of an organ recipient. Review organ donor sources if you had difficulty answering this question.
Cognitive Level—Understanding
Client Needs Category—Physiological integrity
Client Needs Subcategory—Reduction of risk potential

57. 1. Because the kidney is a highly vascular organ, hemorrhage and shock are the most immediate complications of renal surgery. Fluid and blood component replacements are often necessary in the immediate postoperative period. Abdominal distention, paralytic ileus, and pneumonia also are potential complications during the postoperative period, but they are not likely to occur immediately after surgery.

Test Taking Strategy—Analyze to determine what information the question asks for, which is the chief nursing concern when caring for a client immediately after renal transplant surgery. Although postoperative complications are low, clients undergoing major surgery involving anastomosis of the donor renal artery and vein to the recipient's iliac artery and vein must be monitored for hemorrhage around the transplanted kidney, peritoneal, and retroperitoneal spaces. Review the postoperative care of a client undergoing renal transplant surgery if you had difficulty answering this question.
Cognitive Level—Analyzing
Client Needs Category—Physiological integrity
Client Needs Subcategory—Reduction of risk potential

Nursing Care of Clients with Urologic Obstructions

58. 1. Subjective data that are associated with obstructive urinary disorders include a persistent feeling of needing to void and dull flank pain. Feeling the urge to void is related to urine accumulating in the bladder secondary to incomplete emptying. A palpable bladder above the pubis is an objective sign that urine is being retained. Dark urine is associated with fluid volume deficit. Abdominal cramping is associated with a problem with the bowel.

Test Taking Strategy—*Analyze to determine what information the question asks for, which is an assessment finding that correlates with a urinary obstruction such as that caused by an enlarged prostate gland. Recall that the prostate gland encircles the male urethra; when enlarged, it interferes with completely emptying the bladder. Review the structures of the urinary system, focusing on the location of the prostate gland in relation to the bladder and urethra, if you had difficulty answering this question.*
Cognitive Level—*Applying*
Client Needs Category—*Physiological integrity*
Client Needs Subcategory—*Physiological adaptation*

59. 2. A cystostomy tube is surgically inserted directly into the bladder through the abdominal wall. A ureterostomy tube is inserted into one of the ureters through a flank incision. A retention catheter, such as a Foley catheter, is inserted through the urethra.

Test Taking Strategy—*Analyze to determine what information the question asks for, which is the location of suprapubic cystostomy tube placement. Recall that the prefix cysto- refers to the bladder and that the bladder is located in the lower abdomen. The word "suprapubic" indicates an area above the pubis. Review the gross anatomy of the urinary system and the terms used in this question if you had difficulty answering this question.*
Cognitive Level—*Applying*
Client Needs Category—*Physiological integrity*
Client Needs Subcategory—*Physiological adaptation*

60. 2. Ensuring that there is adequate urine output from the suprapubic catheter is the best nursing intervention for evaluating patency of the catheter. Inspecting the skin is essential for detecting breakdown or infection. Attaching the catheter to a leg bag promotes the client's ability to move. Encouraging oral intake promotes urine formation, but increased fluid intake is not a measure of catheter patency.

Test Taking Strategy—*Analyze to determine what information the question asks for, which is an essential nursing assessment to determine the patency of a suprapubic catheter. Recall that drainage from this catheter is not controlled by a sphincter muscle; therefore, the nurse can expect that if the catheter is patent, there will be a continuous flow of urine into a collection device. Review techniques for assessing the patency of any type of urinary catheter if you had difficulty answering this question.*
Cognitive Level—*Applying*
Client Needs Category—*Physiological integrity*
Client Needs Subcategory—*Reduction of risk potential*

61. 2. *Urolithiasis* refers to stones that form in the kidneys or urinary tract. Stones are usually made of mineral salts that typically are dissolved in the urine. Stones may be smooth, jagged, or staghorn-shaped. Gross or microscopic hematuria (blood-tinged urine) is more characteristic of trauma from a moving urinary stone than cloudy, light yellow, or strong-smelling urine.

Test Taking Strategy—*Use the process of elimination to help select the option that describes the appearance of urine from a client who is passing a kidney stone. Because stones cause trauma to the urinary tract, blood-tinged urine (option 2) is the best answer. Review the clinical manifestations of urine in relation to urolithiasis if you had difficulty answering this question.*
Cognitive Level—*Applying*
Client Needs Category—*Physiological integrity*
Client Needs Subcategory—*Reduction of risk potential*

62. 2, 3, 5, 6. A cystoscopy is the visual examination of the inside of the bladder, not the kidneys. The cystoscope consists of a lighted tube with a telescopic lens. It is used to help identify the cause of painless hematuria, urinary incontinence, and urine retention. It also helps to evaluate structural and functional changes of the bladder. The cystoscope is introduced through the urethra while the client is under local, spinal, or general anesthesia; no surgical incision is required. Biopsy samples of tissue, cell washing, and a urine sample may be obtained during the procedure.

Test Taking Strategy—*Analyze to determine what information the question asks for, which is the benefits of cystoscopy. Alternative-format "select all that apply" questions require considering each option independently to decide its merit in answering the question. Choose options that identify benefits of performing a cystoscopy. Review the purposes for a cystoscopy if you had difficulty answering this question.*
Cognitive Level—*Applying*
Client Needs Category—*Physiological integrity*
Client Needs Subcategory—*Physiological adaptation*

63. 2. Because of the instrumentation and dilation of the urethra, many clients complain of burning when urinating after a cystoscopy. The nurse can reduce or relieve the discomfort by promoting a liberal fluid intake, providing sitz baths, and administering a prescribed mild analgesic. Polyuria, anuria, and pyuria indicate other complications or conditions affecting the renal system, but these are not directly related to having a cystoscopy.

Test Taking Strategy—*Analyze to determine what information the question asks for, which is the symptom that is most likely to occur after a cystoscopy. Recall that a cystoscope is inserted through the urethra to visualize the interior of the bladder. Consequently, there is likely to be discomfort in the urethra, especially during urination. Review the physical effects that result after a cystoscopic examination if you had difficulty answering this question.*

Cognitive Level—Applying
Client Needs Category—Physiological integrity
Client Needs Subcategory—Reduction of risk potential

64. 4, 6. Urine is strained to assess for evidence that the urinary stone or stones have passed. Antibiotics are administered to treat the cause of a urinary tract infection related to urolithiasis and urinary stasis. Fluids are encouraged rather than restricted. Activity promotes movement of urinary stones. Fowler's position is unlikely to benefit or interfere with the passage of a urinary stone. Indwelling catheters are not used.

Test Taking Strategy—Analyze to determine what information the question asks for, which are appropriate nursing interventions in the care of the client with urolithiasis. Alternative-format "select all that apply" questions require considering each option independently to decide its merit in answering the question. Choose options that identify nursing interventions associated with the care of a client with urolithiasis. Review the nursing care of clients who have developed one or more kidney stones if you had difficulty answering this question.
Cognitive Level—Analyzing
Client Needs Category—Safe and effective care environment
Client Needs Subcategory—Coordinated care

65. 1. Increasing fluid intake helps to move the stone so it may be spontaneously eliminated. The nurse should also encourage the client to increase fluids following stone removal to dilute the urine, prevent further stone production, and flush bacteria from the urinary system. Strengthening the bladder muscles, voiding a larger stream, and increasing calcium in the diet are not related to urolithiasis.

Test Taking Strategy—Analyze to determine what information the question asks for, which is the most important nursing intervention when caring for a client with urolithiasis. Recall that the goal is to promote the expulsion of the stone, which can be done by increasing the client's fluid intake. Review the nursing care of a client with a kidney stone if you had difficulty answering this question.
Cognitive Level—Applying
Client Needs Category—Physiological integrity
Client Needs Subcategory—Reduction of risk potential

66. 1, 5. Extracorporeal shock wave lithotripsy (ESWL) is a procedure that is performed while the client's lower body is submerged in a tank of water or surrounded by a fluid-filled pillow. The client is not allowed to eat or drink anything several hours before the procedure. Ultrasound, not radiation or a laser beam, is the mechanism used to pulverize the stone. Clients are mildly sedated and given preprocedural analgesic medication to reduce the discomfort, which is commonly described as a "blow to the body"

rather than a tingling sensation. It is common for bruises to appear as a consequence of the ultrasonic energy. The procedure generally takes from 45 minutes to 1 hour. Pregnant women should not undergo ESWL.

Test Taking Strategy—Analyze to determine what information the question asks for, which is statements about ESWL that demonstrate that the client understands the procedure. Alternative-format "select all that apply" questions require considering each option independently to decide its merit in answering the question. Choose options that provide statements that are accurate in reference to ESWL. Review the preparation for and performance of ESWL if you had difficulty answering this question.
Cognitive Level—Analyzing
Client Needs Category—Physiological integrity
Client Needs Subcategory—Reduction of risk potential

67. 2, 5, 6. Benign prostatic hypertrophy (BPH) is the enlargement of the prostate. The prostate gland encircles the male urethra like a donut. As the gland enlarges, the client notices that it takes more effort to void, and the urinary stream becomes narrower. Dribbling often occurs. Nocturia, being awakened by a need to urinate, is a common finding among clients with BPH. Burning on urination is more likely a sign of a bladder infection, which could be secondary to BPH. Feeling pressure in the back is more indicative of pathology involving the kidneys. Colorless or very light yellow urine indicates that the urine is dilute. This could be caused by an endocrine disturbance, such as diabetes insipidus, or some other dysfunction affecting renal tubular reabsorption.

Test Taking Strategy—Analyze to determine what information the question asks for, which is signs and symptoms of BPH. Alternative-format "select all that apply" questions require considering each option independently to decide its merit in answering the question. Choose statements made by the client that correspond with signs and symptoms of BPH. Review the clinical manifestations of BPH if you had difficulty answering this question.
Cognitive Level—Analyzing
Client Needs Category—Physiological integrity
Client Needs Subcategory—Physiological adaptation

68. 3. Because of obstruction of the urethra from an enlarging prostate gland, men with benign prostatic hypertrophy (BPH) often describe hesitancy when initiating urination. In other words, they feel the need to urinate but it takes some time before urine is released. The stream of urine is also diminished. BPH usually does not cause sexual dysfunction or incontinence. The prostate gland is not located in the scrotum; it encircles the urethra and can be palpated by rectal examination.

Test Taking Strategy—Use the process of elimination to help select the most important question to ask

after the client describes the signs and symptoms being experienced. Option 1 can be eliminated because BPH does not interfere with erection or ejaculation. Option 2 can be eliminated because prostatic enlargement does not cause alterations in tissues within the scrotum. Option 4 can be eliminated because BPH is more likely to cause urine retention than urinary incontinence. Option 3 emerges as the best answer because an enlarged prostate narrows the lumen of the urethra, and the nurse may wish to determine if the client is experiencing hesitancy. Review the pathophysiology that results from BPH if you had difficulty answering this question.
Cognitive Level—*Analyzing*
Client Needs Category—*Physiological integrity*
Client Needs Subcategory—*Physiological adaptation*

69. 1. Lowering the penis from an upright position to one in which the penis is pointed in the direction of the toes sometimes helps to pass a catheter beyond the narrowing caused by an enlarged prostate gland. The penis is grasped firmly whenever a catheter is inserted. A catheter is never forced if resistance is met during insertion. Massaging the tissue below the base of the penis does not facilitate the catheter's passage past an enlarged prostate gland.

Test Taking Strategy—*Use the process of elimination to help select the option that describes the best technique for inserting a urinary catheter beyond an enlarged prostate gland. Option 3 can be eliminated immediately because using force can cause trauma to tissue and discomfort for the client. Option 2 can be eliminated because it is inappropriate to massage genitourinary structures when attempting to catheterize a client. Although option 4 describes an appropriate technique when catheterizing a male, it does not specifically identify a modification in the procedure when the enlarged prostate interferes with passage of the catheter. Option 1 emerges as the best answer because it alters the anatomic direction through which the catheter must pass. Review the procedure for male catheterization, especially how to deal with factors that affect the ease of catheter insertion, if you had difficulty answering this question.*
Cognitive Level—*Applying*
Client Needs Category—*Physiological integrity*
Client Needs Subcategory—*Reduction of risk potential*

70. 1. A Coudé catheter is used in a client with benign prostatic hypertrophy (BPH) because it has a curved tip that is able to move through the narrowed urethra. An instillable anesthetic lubricant is commonly used to facilitate the procedure. Silicone, rubber, and flexible catheters typically meet the resistance of the prostate gland and cannot be advanced.

Test Taking Strategy—*Use the process of elimination to help select the option that identifies the best choice of catheter to use if a client has BPH. Options 2, 3, and 4 describe flexible catheters that cannot be advanced past the enlarged prostate, leaving option 1 as the best answer. Review the various types of urinary catheters available and the indications for their use if you had difficulty answering this question.*
Cognitive Level—*Analyzing*
Client Needs Category—*Physiological integrity*
Client Needs Subcategory—*Reduction of risk potential*

71. 4. Transurethral resection of the prostate (TURP) is a procedure frequently performed on older men to treat benign prostatic hypertrophy (BPH). Historically it was one of the most common major surgeries performed on men age 65 and older but is rapidly being replaced by laser prostatectomy and other less invasive procedures. Hematuria is generally present for at least 24 hours after a TURP. Vital signs are monitored to evaluate if the volume of blood loss is causing shock. It may take 24 to 48 hours for the urine to become light pink and transparent. After the procedure, the volume of urine is usually within the normal range unless complications, such as hypovolemic shock or obstruction of the catheter, occur. Sediment, if present, is due to the remnants of prostatic tissue; however, the blood that is mixed with the urine initially obscures the nurse's ability to identify the presence of tissue or mucoid debris.

Test Taking Strategy—*Analyze to determine what information the question asks for, which is an assessment finding commonly manifested immediately after a TURP. Although there is no incision, a great deal of blood is lost through the catheter. Review the postoperative nursing care of a client who has undergone a TURP if you had difficulty answering this question.*
Cognitive Level—*Analyzing*
Client Needs Category—*Physiological integrity*
Client Needs Subcategory—*Reduction of risk potential*

72. 1, 2, 4. Bladder irrigation is the process of flushing the bladder to prevent or treat clot formation after a transurethral resection of the prostate (TURP). Bladder irrigation may also be used to instill medications such as antibiotics for treating bladder infections. Bladder irrigation is done over a period of time and runs continuously, instilling normal saline solution hung from an I.V. pole through one lumen of the urinary catheter. The solution flows into the bladder, dilutes the urine and sediment, and drains out the catheter into a gravity drainage bag. Instructing the client that it is normal to feel the urge to urinate even though the bladder is empty is an appropriate nursing action. This is due to feeling the presence of the catheter and balloon. It is also important for the nurse to instruct the client not to try to urinate around the catheter, because this will cause bladder muscles to contract, leading to painful bladder spasms requiring medication. The client also needs to know that it is normal for the urine to be bloody at first. This should clear up gradually and change from bright red, to pink, to dark amber, to clear yellow, usually within 24 hours. The urine will clear faster if the client increases the intake of fluids, so limiting fluid amounts is not an appropriate nursing instruction. The catheter is removed within 24 to 48 hours if complications do not occur. By the time the client is discharged 2 or 3 days after surgery, he should be voiding clear yellow, not pink, urine and no clots should be present.

Test Taking Strategy—Analyze to determine what information the question asks for, which is client teaching after TURP. Alternative-format "select all that apply" questions require considering each option independently to decide its merit in answering the question. Choose options that correspond with accurate client information about the use of a three-way catheter to administer continuous bladder irrigation. Review the use of a three-way catheter and its use, especially as it applies to the postoperative care after a TURP, if you had difficulty answering this question.

Cognitive Level—Analyzing
Client Needs Category—Physiological integrity
Client Needs Subcategory—Reduction of risk potential

73. 3. The nurse should assess whether the catheter is draining well before administering an analgesic for bladder discomfort. Obstruction of the catheter causes bladder spasms. Restoring patency is more appropriate in the case of catheter obstruction than administering an analgesic. Initially, the urine will be bloody with some clot formation; although this is important to note, it is not the cause of the client's bladder spasms. The nurse may need to know about the client's most recent activities, such as walking in the room or drinking fluids, but the patency of the catheter is more important at this time.

Test Taking Strategy—Use the process of elimination to help select the option that identifies the most important information a nurse should assess before administering an analgesic to a client who has undergone a transurethral resection of the prostate (TURP). Although options 1, 2, and 4 describe appropriate data to collect, determining that the catheter is patent (option 3) is the most important fact to confirm or rule out because ensuring that the catheter drains may be the better nursing response. Review care of a client after a TURP if you had difficulty answering this question.

Cognitive Level—Applying
Client Needs Category—Physiological integrity
Client Needs Subcategory—Physiological adaptation

74. 4. Belladonna and opium (B&O) rectal suppositories are considered the most effective drug for relieving bladder spasms after transurethral resection of the pros-

tate (TURP). The belladonna component relaxes smooth muscles in the bladder, and the opium is a centrally acting analgesic. Aspirin is avoided because it increases the tendency to bleed. Meperidine (Demerol) is a synthetic opioid analgesic. Opioids alone do not lessen the spasms but may decrease the pain. Acetaminophen is better for mild pain.

Test Taking Strategy—Look at the key words "most appropriate" in reference to the selection of an analgesic for relieving bladder spasms. Although all of the drugs listed are analgesics, the combination of belladonna with opium in a rectal suppository (option 4) has a unique ability to relieve bladder spasms that cause pain. Review the action and use of B&O suppositories if you had difficulty answering this question.

Cognitive Level—Applying
Client Needs Category—Physiological integrity
Client Needs Subcategory—Pharmacological therapies

75. 3. The best method for recording urine output when a client has more than one catheter is to record the volumes drained from each catheter as separate entries in the medical record. Recording only the output from the urethral catheter or the output from the wound catheter does not provide accurate data on total output. If the two volumes are added and recorded as a single entry, it is difficult to evaluate the status of urine drainage from each catheter.

Test Taking Strategy—Analyze to determine what information the question asks for, which is the correct method for documenting urine output involving two catheters. Recall that it is important to identify urine output separately from each catheter. Review the nursing responsibilities when caring for a client with a suprapubic catheter if you had difficulty answering this question.

Cognitive Level—Applying
Client Needs Category—Physiological integrity
Client Needs Subcategory—Basic care and comfort

76. 3. After a suprapubic catheter is removed, urine may leak from the incisional area and saturate the sterile dressing. A wet dressing provides a wicking action by which microorganisms are attracted in the direction of the impaired tissue. A dressing saturated with urine also leads to skin breakdown. Checking the specific gravity is important only if fluid status is a concern but is not related to removal of the suprapubic catheter. Measuring the client's abdominal girth is an activity related to ascites and cirrhosis of the liver, not the removal of the suprapubic catheter. The Credé maneuver is a technique in which the nurse presses inward and downward over the bladder to increase the abdominal pressure to facilitate bladder emptying. This technique is not needed after removal of the client's suprapubic catheter because the client will either have normal bladder function or the urine will leak out of the catheter insertion site.

Test Taking Strategy—*Use the process of elimination to help select the option that identifies the most important nursing intervention after a suprapubic catheter is removed. Options 2 and 4 can be eliminated because they are unrelated to problems experienced by a client who has a suprapubic prostatectomy. Option 1 may appear to have merit, but the kidneys' ability or inability to concentrate urine is unaffected when the prostate gland is removed. Option 3 emerges as the correct answer because it supports principles of asepsis. Review care of a client after removal of a suprapubic catheter if you had difficulty answering this question.*
Cognitive Level—*Applying*
Client Needs Category—*Physiological integrity*
Client Needs Subcategory—*Reduction of risk potential*

Nursing Care of Clients with Urologic Tumors

77. 3. Prostate specific antigen (PSA) is believed to be a tumor marker for malignancies involving the prostate gland. At this time, the evidence that detecting an increased level improves healthy outcomes is mixed and incomplete. However, clients who are at high risk for prostate cancer or who prefer to have the test performed after being advised of its advantages and disadvantages may be tested. To avoid a falsely elevated finding, the test should be performed before a digital rectal examination or instrumentation around the prostate gland, such as occurs during a cystoscopy. The other examinations and tests are not influenced by physical manipulation of the prostate gland.

Test Taking Strategy—*Analyze to determine what information the question asks for, which is the diagnostic test that should be performed before a digital examination of the prostate gland. The PSA level can be elevated up to 12 days after digital rectal examination or other tests, including cystoscopy. Review the preparation for and significance of a PSA test if you had difficulty answering this question.*
Cognitive Level—*Applying*
Client Needs Category—*Physiological integrity*
Client Needs Subcategory—*Reduction of risk potential*

78. 1. Tension on the catheter may disrupt healing where the bladder and the urethra have been surgically reconnected after removal of the prostate gland and its capsule. Encouraging oral fluids and cleaning the urinary meatus are appropriate postoperative nursing measures, but they are not likely to have as significant an effect on wound healing. Clients who undergo a radical prostatectomy have a high potential for urinary incontinence as a consequence of the surgical procedure. Clamping and releasing the catheter is not likely to promote wound healing.

Test Taking Strategy—*Use the process of elimination to help select the option that correlates with the nursing action that promotes wound healing when providing catheter care after a radical prostatectomy. Option 4 can be eliminated because clamping and releasing the catheter is designed to promote eventual continence, not wound healing. Options 2 and 3 appear to have merit because they promote urinary elimination and prevent an ascending bladder infection, but they are not the best actions for promoting wound healing. Option 1 emerges as the best answer because it avoids traumatizing tissue and delaying wound repair. Review the nursing care of a client after a radical prostatectomy, especially in relation to catheter care, if you had difficulty answering this question.*
Cognitive Level—*Applying*
Client Needs Category—*Physiological integrity*
Client Needs Subcategory—*Reduction of risk potential*

79. 1, 5. Men with advanced prostate cancer are candidates for hormone therapy. Hormone therapy involving estrogens may be prescribed to slow the progression of the malignancy. Men who receive estrogen therapy are prone to developing feminizing characteristics, such as a high voice, breast enlargement, breast tenderness, and testicular atrophy. Hair and fat distribution may also be affected. An alternative approach is to remove both testicles to reduce the production of testosterone. The other effects do not occur as a result of estrogen hormone therapy in males.

Test Taking Strategy—*Analyze to determine what information the question asks for, which is side effects of estrogen therapy for prostate cancer. Alternative-format "select all that apply" questions require considering each option independently to decide its merit in answering the question. Choose options that support correct information about the use of estrogen therapy for clients with prostate cancer. Review the effects of estrogen drug therapy on primary and secondary male sexual characteristics if you had difficulty answering this question.*
Cognitive Level—*Applying*
Client Needs Category—*Physiological integrity*
Client Needs Subcategory—*Pharmacological therapies*

80. 1. The sudden onset of flank pain along with other signs of shock, such as hypotension, restlessness, and tachycardia, is suggestive of hemorrhage. With shock, the skin is generally pale and cool. A distended abdomen is usually caused by the accumulation of intestinal gas. Pain sometimes causes nausea and vomiting, but these signs and symptoms may be due to multiple etiologies.

Test Taking Strategies—*Use the process of elimination to help select the option that identifies the sign or symptom that correlates with hemorrhage in a client who has undergone a nephrectomy. Option 3 can be eliminated immediately because in shock, blood flow is diverted to vital organs rather than the skin, causing the client to appear pale. Option 2 can be eliminated because hemorrhage is more likely to occur in the retroperitoneal area rather than in the abdomen. Option 4 can be eliminated immediately because there could be multiple etiologies for nausea and vomiting, but it is unlikely that hemorrhage is one. Option 1 emerges as the best answer because a nephrectomy is performed through a flank incision and can be accompanied by retroperitoneal discomfort as blood accumulates, causing pressure and pain in the area. Review postoperative complications and their clinical manifestations after a nephrectomy if you had difficulty answering this question.*

Cognitive Level—*Applying*
Client Needs Category—*Physiological integrity*
Client Needs Subcategory—*Reduction of risk potential*

81. 3. The most common symptom of bladder cancer is painless hematuria. Dysuria, if present, is generally due to a concurrent urinary tract infection secondary to obstruction of urine. Oliguria occurs later as the disease becomes more advanced and obstruction occurs. Bladder cancer that has not spread to adjacent pelvic structures is not usually associated with an unusual discharge from any body orifice. Postvoid dribbling and difficulty voiding are associated with an enlarged prostate gland.

Test Taking Strategy—Analyze to determine what information the question asks for, which is early symptoms of bladder cancer. Alternative-format "select all that apply" questions require considering each option independently to decide its merit in answering the question. Choose options that correlate with an early manifestation of bladder cancer; in this case, only one option applies: painless hematuria (option 3). Review the signs and symptoms of bladder cancer focusing on early rather than late signs if you had difficulty answering this question.

Cognitive Level—*Analyzing*
Client Needs Category—*Physiological integrity*
Client Needs Subcategory—*Physiological adaptation*

82. 4, 5. There is a correlation between cigarette smoking, even passive exposure to cigarette smoke, and the development of bladder cancer. Other carcinogenic factors include long-term exposure to chemical solvents and dyes, but exposure to asbestos is related to cancer of the lung, not the bladder. Because of the proximity of the prostate gland to the bladder, clients who have been diagnosed with prostate cancer are at higher risk for cancer of the bladder. Neither stress incontinence nor sexual activities are implicated as a causal agent in bladder cancer.

Test Taking Strategy—Analyze to determine what information the question asks for, which is risk factors for bladder cancer. Alternative-format "select

all that apply" questions require considering each option independently to decide its merit in answering the question. Choose options that identify factors that are believed to contribute to the development of bladder cancer. Review the etiology and contributing factors of bladder cancer if you had difficulty answering this question.

Cognitive Level—*Understanding*
Client Needs Category—*Physiological integrity*
Client Needs Subcategory—*Physiological adaptation*

83. 1. Recommendations for safe handling of toxic chemotherapeutic agents include wearing two pairs of surgical latex gloves, which are less permeable than polyvinyl gloves. A gown with cuffs and a mask or goggles are also worn to prevent direct contact with the drug. An air purifying respirator, also known as an N95 respirator, is used when caring for clients with known or suspected pulmonary tuberculosis or severe acute respiratory syndrome (SARS). The time spent in contact with the client is not considered a safety hazard with chemotherapy, but it is a factor in radiation therapy involving sealed and unsealed implants.

Test Taking Strategy—Analyze to determine what information the question asks for, which is a safety precaution that is required when disposing of urine that contains an antineoplastic medication. Recall that antineoplastic drugs can be absorbed through the skin. Wearing two pair of gloves reduces the potential for skin absorption. Review safety precautions when antineoplastic drugs have been administered if you had difficulty answering this question.

Cognitive Level—*Analyzing*
Client Needs Category—*Safe and effective care environment*
Client Needs Subcategory—*Safety and infection control*

Nursing Care of Clients with Urinary Diversions

84.

2.

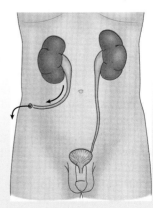

When a cutaneous ureterostomy is created, a ureter is detached from the bladder and brought through the abdominal wall. This type of urinary diversion requires the application of an ostomy appliance that collects urine from the diverted ureter.

Test Taking Strategy—Analyze to determine what information the question asks for, which is the image that depicts a cutaneous ureterostomy. Note that the term cutaneous refers to the skin and ureterostomy indicates that the ureter is brought to the skin, which is illustrated in option 2. Option 1 illustrates an ileal conduit. Option 3 illustrates a vesicotomy. Option 4 is an illustration of a nephrostomy. Review the anatomic changes made with various urinary diversion procedures if you had difficulty answering this question.
Cognitive Level—*Understanding*
Client Needs Category—*Physiological integrity*
Client Needs Subcategory—*Physiological adaptation*

85. 3. An ileal conduit, or ileal loop procedure, involves implanting the ureters into a section of the ileum that has been removed from the small intestine. The section of ileum is fashioned into a stoma that opens onto the abdomen, from which urine will drain. When a ureterosig-moidostomy is performed, the ureters are attached to the sigmoid colon and urine is eliminated with stool by way of the rectum. Currently, there are no procedures in which the ureters are implanted directly into the small intestine. If a Koch pouch, or continent urostomy, is performed, urine is siphoned with a catheter from an internal collection pouch.

Test Taking Strategy—Look at the key words "most accurate" in reference to an explanation about the creation of an ileal conduit. Recall that the word ileal refers to the ileum portion of the small intestine, and the word conduit is used to describe a passageway that, in this case, empties urine through an abdominal opening. Review the anatomic changes that result from an ileal conduit if you had difficulty answering this question.
Cognitive Level—*Analyzing*
Client Needs Category—*Physiological integrity*
Client Needs Subcategory—*Reduction of risk potential*

86. 3. A pulse rate of more than 100 beats/minute in the absence of activity or some accompanying pathology suggests that the sympathetic nervous system is stimulated. The sympathetic nervous system responds when a person is experiencing a real or perceived threat to his or her well-being. Usually a client's face is red or pink when anxious, related to the increase in pulse and blood pressure. Requesting a midnight snack is not a true indicator of anxiety, although some individuals eat when stressed. Because the client is scheduled for surgery, it is likely that the client will be NPO after midnight.

Test Taking Strategy—Look at the key terms "most likely" as they refer to evidence that anxiety is the

etiology for a client's preoperative sleep disturbance. Recall that stimulation of the sympathetic nervous system increases the rate and force of heart contraction as well as many other physiologic changes caused by the fight-or-flight response. Review signs of anxiety and sympathetic nervous system stimulation if you had difficulty answering this question.*
Cognitive Level—*Analyzing*
Client Needs Category—*Psychosocial integrity*
Client Needs Subcategory—*None*

87. 1. Sharing perceptions with the client by stating that it must be difficult shows empathy and allows the client an opportunity to discuss concerns. Telling the client that one of the best surgeons will be doing the procedure does not encourage further verbalization because it is unlikely to stimulate discussion. The cliché that everything will turn out okay offers false reassurance. It also communicates that the nurse is uncomfortable discussing the client's feelings. Saying that others have done just fine minimizes and belittles the uniqueness of the situation from the client's perspective.

Test Taking Strategy—Use the process of elimination to help select the option that provides the most therapeutic statement from the nurse. Option 2 can be eliminated because it is a nontherapeutic communication example of defending. Option 3 can be eliminated because it is impossible to predict the outcome of surgery. Option 4 is an example of a nontherapeutic communication technique known as belittling. Option 1 emerges as the best answer because it promotes verbalization by the client. Review examples of therapeutic and nontherapeutic communication techniques if you had difficulty answering this question.
Cognitive Level—*Applying*
Client Needs Category—*Psychosocial integrity*
Client Needs Subcategory—*None*

88. 1. Encouraging the client to verbalize more and express feelings is an effective therapeutic communication technique. Because it is impossible for a nurse to know how a client is feeling, stating so diminishes the nurse's credibility. The client may lose faith in the ability of the nurse to be truly empathetic. Minimizing the client's despair by saying, "It's not as bad as that," is likely to interfere with any further discussion. Advising the client to think more positively is likely to be interpreted as disapproval of the way the client currently feels.

Test Taking Strategy—Use the process of elimination to help select the option that provides the most therapeutic response to a client who is concerned about the results of the scheduled urologic surgical procedures. Option 2 can be eliminated because it is an example of the nontherapeutic communication technique of agreeing. Option 3 can be eliminated

because it is an example of the nontherapeutic communication technique of disagreeing. Option 4 can be eliminated because it is an example of the nontherapeutic communication technique of giving advice. Option 1 emerges as the most therapeutic statement because it encourages the client to talk about his or her feelings. Review examples of therapeutic and nontherapeutic communication techniques if you had difficulty answering this question.
Cognitive Level—*Applying*
Client Needs Category—*Psychosocial integrity*
Client Needs Subcategory—*None*

89. 2. It is important for the nurse to assess the skin's condition to plan appropriate interventions. If the skin is excoriated, it probably will take more than just diluting the urine or emptying the appliance more frequently to restore skin integrity. It would be impossible to leave the appliance off because urine is released constantly.

Test Taking Strategy—Look at the key words "most appropriate" in reference to the nursing action for addressing the client's discomfort around the stoma. Recall that assessment is the first step in the nursing process. Therefore, inspecting the skin around the stoma should precede any interventions that may follow. Review stomal care if you had difficulty answering this question.
Cognitive Level—*Applying*
Client Needs Category—*Physiological integrity*
Client Needs Subcategory—*Physiological adaptation*

90. 1. The most important information that the nursing assistant needs to know is that which applies to a nursing assistant's scope of practice. A nursing assistant provides clients with personal care including toileting so it is of most importance to know that the client is emptying the urine collection device independently. Information about the client's teaching, the type of surgery the client has undergone, and the character of the urine is not as important.

Test Taking Strategy—Look at the key words "most important" in reference to the postoperative information regarding client care that is pertinent for a nursing assistant to know. Consider how each option affects the direct care that the nursing assistant provides leading to option 1 as the best answer. Review duties assigned to unlicensed assistant personnel (UAPs) if you had difficulty answering this question.
Cognitive Level—*Applying*
Client Needs Category—*Safe and effective care environment*
Client Needs Subcategory—*Coordinated care*

91. 2. Inserting a tampon or gauze square into the stoma momentarily absorbs the urine and keeps the skin dry. Leaning over the toilet puts the client in an awkward position while the appliance is being changed. It gener-

ally takes two hands to manipulate the appliance during its application; therefore, pressing a finger over the stoma or pinching the stoma interferes with the coordination needed.

Test Taking Strategy—Look at the key words "most helpful" in reference to controlling leakage from the ileal conduit stoma. Recall that the skin around the stoma must be dry for the replacement appliance to adhere securely, so absorbing the urine with a tampon (option 2) is the best answer. Review the procedure for changing a urinary stomal appliance if you had difficulty answering this question.
Cognitive Level—*Applying*
Client Needs Category—*Physiological integrity*
Client Needs Subcategory—*Physiological adaptation*

Nursing Care of Clients with Culturally Diverse Backgrounds

92. 1, 2, 3. Performing a cultural assessment for clients with diverse backgrounds provides the nurse with valuable information related to the client's health beliefs, practices, causes of illness, role when ill, and lifestyle choices. These findings should be included in the care plan and communicated from shift to shift. Native Americans are usually private and modest and are reluctant to share much personal information with strangers. This especially includes information related to bowel and bladder function and sexual/reproductive history. The nurse must be cognizant of the need for privacy and should ask questions regarding health history using a patient, nonjudgmental manner. Native Americans value good listening skills because their history is preserved through oral communication. Writing notes when taking a health history should be reserved for after the interview. Native Americans do not pattern their lifestyle after "clock time." "Clock time" refers to time in seconds, minutes, hours, days, months, and years. Asian Americans, (not Native Americans) consider touching on the head offensive. Native Americans view the eyes as a "window to the soul." Native Americans avoid direct eye contact because they view it as disrespectful because it may harm the soul.

Test Taking Strategy—Analyze to determine what information the question asks for, which is cultural characteristics to keep in mind when working with Native American clients. Alternative-format "select all that apply" questions require considering each option independently to decide its merit in answering the question. Choose options that describe cultural characteristics of Native Americans. Review characteristics of clients from various cultures, focusing on those of Native Americans, if you had difficulty answering this question.
Cognitive Level—*Remembering*
Client Needs Category—*Psychosocial integrity*
Client Needs Subcategory—*None*

10 The Nursing Care of Clients with Disorders of the Reproductive System

- Nursing Care of Clients with Breast Disorders
- Nursing Care of Clients with Disturbances in Menstruation
- Nursing Care of Clients with Infectious and Inflammatory Disorders of the Female Reproductive System
- Nursing Care of Clients with Benign and Malignant Disorders of the Uterus and Ovaries
- Nursing Care of Clients with Miscellaneous Disorders of the Female Reproductive System
- Nursing Care of Clients with Inflammatory Disorders of the Male Reproductive System
- Nursing Care of Clients with Structural Disorders of the Male Reproductive System
- Nursing Care of Clients with Benign and Malignant Disorders of the Male Reproductive System
- Nursing Care of Clients with Sexually Transmitted Infections
- Nursing Care of Clients Practicing Family Planning
- Correct Answers, Rationales, and Test Taking Strategies

Directions: *With a pencil, blacken the space in front of the option you have chosen for your correct answer.*

Nursing Care of Clients with Breast Disorders

A 30-year-old woman has an appointment for a routine pelvic examination. She asks the office nurse when she should begin undergoing routine mammography.

1. If the client is asymptomatic and at low risk for breast cancer, the nurse would be correct in advising her to have a baseline mammogram at what age?
[ ] **1.** 35
[ ] **2.** 45
[ ] **3.** 50
[ ] **4.** 55

The nurse asks whether the client currently practices breast self-examination (BSE), then takes the opportunity to show her the proper technique.

2. The client states that she examines her breasts in the shower and while lying down. The nurse recommends that the client should also inspect her breasts from which position?
[ ] **1.** Bending from the waist
[ ] **2.** Standing before a mirror
[ ] **3.** Arching the back
[ ] **4.** Leaning from side-to-side

3. Which breast palpation technique is most correct?
[ ] **1.** Examine the breast while using the heel of the hand.
[ ] **2.** Examine the breast while using the index finger only.
[ ] **3.** Examine the breast while using the index finger and thumb.
[ ] **4.** Examine the breast while using the pads of the fingertips.

4. The nurse correctly informs the client that the breast self-examination (BSE) technique involves palpating each breast moving in small concentric circles, following imaginary spokes in a wheel, or moving in rows from superior to inferior areas of the breast. In addition to the breast tissue, the nurse is also correct to provide nursing instruction on palpating which area?

[ ] **1.** The axillae
[ ] **2.** The sternum
[ ] **3.** The clavicles
[ ] **4.** The ribs

5. If the client chooses to perform breast self-examination (BSE), which statement demonstrates to the nurse the best understanding of when BSE should be performed?

[ ] **1.** "I will perform a BSE on a weekly basis."
[ ] **2.** "I will perform a BSE every 6 months."
[ ] **3.** "I will perform a BSE 1 week before my period begins."
[ ] **4.** "I will perform a BSE 3 to 7 days after my period ends."

A 35-year-old woman makes an appointment with her physician because she has felt several lumps in her right breast. She is scheduled for a mammogram.

6. When the office nurse gives the client instructions on how to prepare for the mammogram, which of the following statements offers accurate information? Select all that apply.

[ ] **1.** "You will need to shave your underarm hair the morning of the test."
[ ] **2.** "Do not wear any underarm deodorant the day of the test."
[ ] **3.** "Wipe each breast with an antiseptic pad before the test."
[ ] **4.** "Do not wear constricting clothing to the test."
[ ] **5.** "Avoid wearing body powder the day of the test."
[ ] **6.** "Refrain from applying lotion to the breasts or axillae."

The nurse collects the woman's health history before the mammogram.

7. Which assessment findings recorded by the nurse indicate high risk factors for developing breast cancer? Select all that apply.

[ ] **1.** The client began menstruating before age 12.
[ ] **2.** The client had three full-term pregnancies.
[ ] **3.** The client has a sister diagnosed with breast cancer.
[ ] **4.** The client has very large breasts.
[ ] **5.** The client has had radiation treatment to the chest.
[ ] **6.** The client has had breast implants.

The radiologist interprets the findings on the mammogram as benign fibrocystic disease.

8. The nurse correctly informs the client that fibrocystic lesions may become larger and more tender at what time?

[ ] **1.** After the menstrual cycle
[ ] **2.** After sexual intercourse
[ ] **3.** Nearer to beginning menopause
[ ] **4.** Just before menstruation

9. Although it has not been conclusively proven, the nurse explains that some women with fibrocystic disease get relief from their symptoms by eliminating which substance from their diet?

[ ] **1.** Alcohol
[ ] **2.** Caffeine
[ ] **3.** Saturated fat
[ ] **4.** Refined sugar

The office manager schedules a mandatory staff meeting for all nursing personnel. As the nurse enters the room, several documents containing the client's name, medical records number, mammogram results, and diagnosis are found unattended on the table.

10. Which nursing actions are appropriate in this situation? Select all that apply.

[ ] **1.** Notify housekeeping to come and dispose of the papers.
[ ] **2.** Toss the papers in the trash.
[ ] **3.** Put the papers into the shredder bin.
[ ] **4.** Try to determine who left the papers unattended.
[ ] **5.** Stack the papers neatly, placing them off to the side.
[ ] **6.** Notify the office manager of the breach in confidentiality.

During a presurgical assessment, a 67-year-old woman tells the nurse that she has felt a lump in her left breast for the past 6 months.

11. If the lump has the following characteristics when the nurse palpates the breast tissue, which characteristic would the nurse identify as most suggestive that the lump may be cancerous?

[ ] **1.** The lump can be easily moved about.
[ ] **2.** The lump is about ½″ (1 cm).
[ ] **3.** The lump is irregularly shaped.
[ ] **4.** The lump is near the areola.

The physician recommends an excisional biopsy followed by an immediate modified radical mastectomy if the biopsy shows malignant cells.

12. If the client tells the nurse that she would prefer to postpone the mastectomy until the biopsy has been more thoroughly examined, which is the most appropriate initial nursing action?

[ ] **1.** Explain that most biopsies are accurate.
[ ] **2.** Advocate for her choice of treatment.
[ ] **3.** Discourage her from opposing the physician.
[ ] **4.** Recommend that she seek a second opinion.

The client's breast tumor is malignant and she undergoes a left modified radical mastectomy.

13. Which nursing interventions are most appropriate to add to the client's immediate postoperative care plan? Select all that apply.

[ ] **1.** Maintain the client in a dorsal recumbent position.
[ ] **2.** Limit oral fluid intake to no more than 2,000 mL/day.
[ ] **3.** Use the right arm when assessing blood pressure.
[ ] **4.** Inspect the incision at least once each shift.
[ ] **5.** Advise the client to avoid sleeping on the affected side.
[ ] **6.** Ask the client to report numbness or tingling in the chest wall.

14. On the basis of the location and extent of this client's surgery, which nursing assessment finding is most indicative of a postoperative complication?

[ ] **1.** Shallow breathing
[ ] **2.** Inadequate nutrition
[ ] **3.** Impaired bowel motility
[ ] **4.** Signs of skin breakdown

15. The physician prescribes tamoxifen (Nolvadex) 10 mg P.O. b.i.d. for a client who underwent a modified radical mastectomy to treat her estrogen-sensitive breast cancer. The drug label indicates that there are 20 mg in each tablet. How many tablets should the nurse administer to the client?

_____

16. Which activity of daily living is most therapeutic for the nurse to recommend for preserving the hospitalized client's muscle strength and joint flexibility in the arm on the operative side?

[ ] **1.** Feeding herself
[ ] **2.** Brushing her hair
[ ] **3.** Writing letters
[ ] **4.** Washing her chest

17. When modifying the postoperative care plan, which nursing measure should the nurse plan to include to prevent swelling of the arm on the client's operative side?

[ ] **1.** Applying an ice pack to the site
[ ] **2.** Applying warm compresses to the site
[ ] **3.** Keeping the arm elevated
[ ] **4.** Ambulating the client frequently

Before the client's discharge, the nurse provides instructions regarding home care.

18. Which instructions should the nurse include in the client's discharge plan? Select all that apply.

[ ] **1.** Continue arm exercises three times per day.
[ ] **2.** Avoid lifting objects weighing more than 15 pounds (6.8 kg).
[ ] **3.** Use gloves while doing yard or house work.
[ ] **4.** Get at least 8 hours of sleep per night.
[ ] **5.** Avoid drinking caffeinated or alcoholic beverages.
[ ] **6.** Postpone getting a prosthesis for at least 6 months.

19. If the client asks for information on special bras and prosthetic devices after her mastectomy, which organization is the best resource to recommend?

[ ] **1.** American Garment Industry
[ ] **2.** American Cancer Society
[ ] **3.** Breast Prosthetics Association
[ ] **4.** Organization for Mammary Cosmetics

20. Before discharging a postmenopausal mastectomy client, which instruction concerning breast self-examination (BSE) is most correct?

[ ] **1.** Examine your remaining breast on awakening from sleep.
[ ] **2.** Examine your remaining breast on the first day of the month.
[ ] **3.** Examine your remaining breast after you finish your shower.
[ ] **4.** Examine your remaining breast before your yearly mammogram.

After the discharge orders have been written, the nurse walks the client down to the car. The client says to the nurse, "I sure hope the cancer hasn't spread. I don't want to have to come back here to have the other breast removed."

21. On the basis of the client's pathology report, the nurse is concerned that the cancer may have already metastasized. Identify with an *X* the area where breast cancer is most likely to metastasize initially.

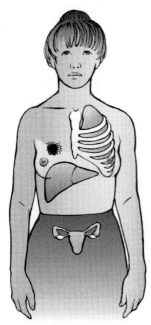

Nursing Care of Clients with Disturbances in Menstruation

22. A nurse has been asked to teach ovulation and menstruation to a class of secondary school students. Place the events listed below in the order in which they occur in the menstrual cycle after menstrual flow ends. Use all the options.

1. Ovum is released.	
2. Progesterone decreases.	
3. Endometrium begins to thicken.	
4. Ovarian follicle matures.	
5. Endometrium is shed.	
6. Corpus luteum forms.	

A nurse obtains a history from a 20-year-old client who says she does not menstruate.

23. Which question is most important for the nurse to ask next?
[ ] **1.** "Have you ever had any menstrual periods?"
[ ] **2.** "Do you have any pubic hair growth?"
[ ] **3.** "Have you ever been sexually attracted to males?"
[ ] **4.** "Are there any siblings with a similar problem?"

A 16-year-old client confides to the school nurse that she has cramps that accompany the onset of menstruation.

24. Besides a mild analgesic such as ibuprofen (Motrin), which therapeutic interventions are most appropriate for the nurse to recommend? Select all that apply.
[ ] **1.** Obtain a prescription for an oral contraceptive.
[ ] **2.** Switch from menstrual pads to tampons.
[ ] **3.** Use local applications of heat.
[ ] **4.** Reduce physical activity.
[ ] **5.** Massage the lower abdomen when experiencing pain.
[ ] **6.** Lie prone while sleeping or napping.

A 34-year-old woman makes an appointment with a physician concerning her pattern of heavy menstrual bleeding. A pelvic examination is scheduled.

25. Which instruction is most appropriate if a Papanicolaou (Pap) smear will be obtained at the time of the pelvic examination?
[ ] **1.** Avoid douching for several days before your appointment.
[ ] **2.** Stop using any and all forms of contraception temporarily.
[ ] **3.** Drink at least 1 quart of liquid an hour before your appointment.
[ ] **4.** Avoid having sexual intercourse for a week before the test.

26. Before taking the client to the room where the pelvic examination will be performed, which nursing action is most appropriate?
[ ] **1.** Ask the client to sign a consent form.
[ ] **2.** Give the client an opportunity to void.
[ ] **3.** Offer the client a mild analgesic.
[ ] **4.** Help the client instill a vaginal lubricant.

27. Which question is most important to ask to ensure valid analysis of the vaginal specimen?
[ ] **1.** "When did you last have sexual intercourse?"
[ ] **2.** "How old were you when you had your first pregnancy?"
[ ] **3.** "What was the date of your last menstrual period?"
[ ] **4.** "Have you ever used oral contraceptives?"

28. The nurse correctly places the client in which position when the physician is ready to perform the pelvic examination?

[ ] **1.** Sims' position
[ ] **2.** Trendelenburg's position
[ ] **3.** Fowler's position
[ ] **4.** Lithotomy position

29. Before the physician performs the vaginal examination, which nursing intervention is most important?

[ ] **1.** Arrange to have a female nurse present during the examination.
[ ] **2.** Instruct the client on the dangers of cervical cancer.
[ ] **3.** Palpate the internal organs to obtain a baseline assessment.
[ ] **4.** Encourage the client to instill a vaginal lubricant.

A 20-year-old college student calls her physician's office and reports to the nurse that she is bleeding vaginally at a time other than her expected menses.

30. If the client reports all of the following data, which factor is most likely contributing to the bleeding?

[ ] **1.** The client has been taking an oral contraceptive for 2 months.
[ ] **2.** The client has just changed employment and is under unusual stress.
[ ] **3.** The client's sexual partner has a sexually transmitted infection.
[ ] **4.** The client has been using a vibrator to elicit sexual arousal.

The physician requests that the client with vaginal bleeding come to the office. When the client arrives, she is accompanied by a female friend. The nurse assigns the client to an examination room, but as the client's friend follows the client into the room, the nurse stops her. The client says to the nurse, "It's OK, we're lesbians."

31. Which action by the nurse is most appropriate?

[ ] **1.** Allow the client's partner to stay in the examination room.
[ ] **2.** Ask the client's friend to remain in the waiting room.
[ ] **3.** Ask the physician to make the decision in this situation.
[ ] **4.** Suggest that the friend wait outside the examination room door.

During the physical and pelvic examination by the physician, the nurse notices that the client has several tattoos on the insides of her thighs and labia and she has nipple and navel piercings.

32. Before the client leaves the office, on which topic should the nurse obtain further information?

[ ] **1.** The name of the person who did the tattoos and piercings
[ ] **2.** Whether the client is practicing safe, protected sex
[ ] **3.** The client's sexual experiences with members of both sexes
[ ] **4.** The names of all of the client's sexual partners

Nursing Care of Clients with Infectious and Inflammatory Disorders of the Female Reproductive System

A 25-year-old woman has repeated vaginal infections. The symptoms suggest that the client has candidiasis caused by the yeastlike microorganism Candida albicans (C. albicans).

33. After *C. albicans* is identified as the causative organism, the nurse would expect the physician to prescribe which treatment?

[ ] **1.** A nonprescription antifungal medication
[ ] **2.** A prescription oral penicillin
[ ] **3.** A prescription broad-spectrum antibiotic
[ ] **4.** A vaginal douche with a vinegar solution

34. Which nursing instruction is best when teaching the client about inserting vaginal medication?

[ ] **1.** Place the applicator just inside the vaginal opening.
[ ] **2.** Insert the applicator while sitting on the toilet.
[ ] **3.** Instill the medication just before retiring for sleep.
[ ] **4.** Put on disposable latex gloves before applying the drug.

35. Which health practice is most appropriate for the nurse to teach this client?

[ ] **1.** Take showers rather than tub baths if possible.
[ ] **2.** Wipe away from the vagina after a bowel movement.
[ ] **3.** Use a lanolin-based soap for genital cleansing.
[ ] **4.** Avoid having sexual intercourse more than once a week.

36. What information provided by the nurse is most appropriate for the client who plans on douching twice a week?

[ ] **1.** Use a concentrated solution of vinegar and water.
[ ] **2.** Avoid frequent douching because it removes helpful microorganisms.
[ ] **3.** Instill no more than 16 oz of irrigant solution with each douching.
[ ] **4.** Discontinue the instillation if cramping occurs.

A 21-year-old client is recovering from acute pelvic inflammatory disease (PID).

37. When assigning a nursing assistant to this client's care, which instruction for disposing of soiled drainage pads is correct?
[ ] **1.** Flush all perineal pads down the toilet.
[ ] **2.** Put the pads in biohazard waste bags.
[ ] **3.** Place the pads in the client's wastebasket.
[ ] **4.** Enclose the soiled pads in a clean paper bag.

38. If the client asks about long-term consequences that are associated with this disorder, the nurse accurately identifies which reproductive sequela?
[ ] **1.** Cancer of the cervix
[ ] **2.** Premature labors
[ ] **3.** Spontaneous abortions
[ ] **4.** Difficulty getting pregnant

A 24-year-old woman is being treated for endometriosis. A laparoscope will be used to remove ectopic tissue.

39. When the client asks where the laparoscope will be inserted, the nurse correctly identifies which structure?
[ ] **1.** Abdomen
[ ] **2.** Vagina
[ ] **3.** Uterine cervix
[ ] **4.** Uterine fundus

40. If the client experiences all of the following signs and symptoms after the laparoscopy, which one can the nurse attribute directly to the endoscopic procedure?
[ ] **1.** Nausea and vomiting
[ ] **2.** Shoulder discomfort
[ ] **3.** Urinary frequency
[ ] **4.** Leg cramps

A 65-year-old woman experiences painful intercourse and is concerned about possible reproductive disease.

41. On the basis of this client's age, which statement by the nurse is the best explanation for the client's discomfort?
[ ] **1.** The pelvic muscles are more sensitive to pressure after menopause.
[ ] **2.** The clitoris is unable to respond to sexual foreplay as women age.
[ ] **3.** The vagina hypertrophies if intercourse is infrequent.
[ ] **4.** The mucus-producing glands decrease with aging.

Nursing Care of Clients with Benign and Malignant Disorders of the Uterus and Ovaries

The physician sees a 42-year-old woman for suspected fibroid tumors (myomas).

42. In addition to pressure in the pelvic region, which sign or symptom is the client most likely to reveal during a nursing history?
[ ] **1.** Heavy menstrual bleeding
[ ] **2.** Light menstrual bleeding
[ ] **3.** Abdominal pain at the time of ovulation
[ ] **4.** Breast tenderness during menstruation

A pelvic ultrasound (sonogram) using a transabdominal approach is scheduled for the client.

43. When preparing the client for the sonogram, which instruction is most important for the nurse to emphasize?
[ ] **1.** Do not void for several hours before the test.
[ ] **2.** Begin fasting at midnight before the test.
[ ] **3.** Take a mild analgesic such as aspirin before the test.
[ ] **4.** Use an antiseptic soap when showering before the test.

After the diagnosis of fibroid tumors is confirmed, the client is scheduled for a dilation and curettage in the ambulatory surgery department.

44. Before the client is discharged, which nursing observation is most important for the nurse to document?
[ ] **1.** The client can eat without nausea.
[ ] **2.** The client can empty her bladder.
[ ] **3.** The client's pelvic pain is relieved.
[ ] **4.** The client's perineal pad has been changed.

A client with an abnormal Pap smear has a colposcopy performed in her physician's office.

45. Before the client leaves the office, the nurse correctly instructs her to report which unusual problem associated with this procedure?
[ ] **1.** Excessive bleeding
[ ] **2.** Inability to void
[ ] **3.** Pressure during bowel elimination
[ ] **4.** Pain in the right lower quadrant

The client is scheduled to undergo electrocauterization after the diagnostic tests confirm that she has an early stage of cervical cancer.

46. After the electrocauterization procedure, which discharge instruction is most appropriate?

[ ] **1.** "Douche in 24 hours to remove debris and blood clots."

[ ] **2.** "Avoid heavy lifting until you have had a follow-up examination."

[ ] **3.** "Remain in bed as much as possible over the next 5 days."

[ ] **4.** "Avoid any sexual activity for 2 months."

The nurse reviews the medical records of several clients looking for risk factors associated with cervical cancer.

47. Which finding in a client profile indicates the highest risk for cervical cancer?

[ ] **1.** Onset of menstruation at age 12 years

[ ] **2.** Spontaneous abortion at age 35 years

[ ] **3.** Human papillomavirus infection at age 28 years

[ ] **4.** Maternal history of breast cancer

A client makes an appointment with her gynecologist because she has been having vaginal bleeding between her regular menstrual periods. On the basis of the client's history and physical examination, the physician suspects cervical cancer and orders further diagnostic tests.

48. To determine the significance of the client's symptomatic bleeding, which questions are most important for the nurse to ask? Select all that apply.

[ ] **1.** "Has your energy level changed remarkably?"

[ ] **2.** "Do you have intercourse more than once a week?"

[ ] **3.** "How many sanitary pads do you use?"

[ ] **4.** "Is the bleeding light or dark red?"

[ ] **5.** "Do you have itching and swelling of the labia?"

[ ] **6.** "Have you lost weight in the past few months?"

Internal radiation therapy is used to treat the client who has been diagnosed with advanced cervical cancer. An applicator containing radioactive material is inserted into the client's vagina.

49. Because the client is receiving this type of radiation therapy, which nursing interventions should the nurse include in the care plan? Select all that apply.

[ ] **1.** Elevate the head of the bed to 90 degrees.

[ ] **2.** Maintain the client on strict bed rest.

[ ] **3.** Place urine and feces in a closed container.

[ ] **4.** Weigh the client daily before breakfast.

[ ] **5.** Stand at a distance and talk with the client from the doorway.

[ ] **6.** Spend as little time as possible with the client.

50. If the nurse finds the radioactive insert in the client's bed, which nursing action is most appropriate?

[ ] **1.** Return it to the nuclear medicine department.

[ ] **2.** Discard it in the infectious waste receptacle.

[ ] **3.** Reinsert it immediately.

[ ] **4.** Place it in a lead container.

51. If the nurse must handle the radioactive implant, which action provides the best protection for the nurse?

[ ] **1.** Putting on sterile vinyl gloves

[ ] **2.** Washing hands before putting on vinyl gloves

[ ] **3.** Using long-handled forceps to handle the implant

[ ] **4.** Enclosing the implant in a glass jar

52. Which staff nurse is best suited to care for a client with a radioactive implant?

[ ] **1.** A male nurse with oncology nursing experience

[ ] **2.** A female nurse who has had a hysterectomy

[ ] **3.** A female nurse who has survived cancer herself

[ ] **4.** A male nurse whose mother died of cancer

A 64-year-old client with uterine cancer is scheduled to undergo an abdominal hysterectomy under general anesthesia. Before the client returns from the postanesthesia care unit, the registered nurse asks the licensed practical nurse to help revise the care plan for the client who has undergone a hysterectomy.

53. Which nursing diagnosis is most appropriate for the nurse to add to the client's care plan at this time?

[ ] **1.** Risk for ineffective airway clearance

[ ] **2.** Risk for imbalanced nutrition

[ ] **3.** Ineffective coping

[ ] **4.** Impaired verbal communication

Postoperative orders include applying antiembolism stockings to the client's legs after the hysterectomy.

54. Which nursing intervention for applying antiembolism stockings is most appropriate to include in the client's care plan?

[ ] **1.** Have the client wear the stockings continuously, but remove and reapply them at least twice a day.

[ ] **2.** Have the client wear the stockings continuously during the day hours, and remove them at night.

[ ] **3.** Have the client wear the stockings only when getting up to ambulate.

[ ] **4.** Have the client wear the stockings only while in bed.

55. The licensed practical nurse (LPN) realizes that the nursing assistant requires further instruction when observing her performing which actions after the client's hysterectomy? Select all that apply.
[ ] 1. Frequently offering the client a variety of oral fluids
[ ] 2. Helping the client ambulate in the hall
[ ] 3. Raising the knee gatch on the hospital bed
[ ] 4. Reporting to the physician that the client's dressing is loose
[ ] 5. Massaging the calves when applying lotion
[ ] 6. Changing the client's perineal pad without using gloves

56. Before surgery a urinary catheter was inserted. Today, the physician orders that the client's catheter can be removed. As the nurse is preparing for catheter removal, which nursing action is performed first?
[ ] 1. Clean the client's labia with soap and water.
[ ] 2. Measure the urine in the drainage bag.
[ ] 3. Remove the fluid from the balloon.
[ ] 4. Disconnect the client's catheter and drainage bag.

The client's bladder is distended after the catheter is removed even though she is urinating approximately 100 mL with each voiding. The physician instructs the nurse to recatheterize the client and measure the residual urine.

57. Which nursing action is most appropriate to carry out the medical order?
[ ] 1. Catheterize the client as soon as possible.
[ ] 2. Catheterize the client after her next voiding.
[ ] 3. Connect the catheter to gravity drainage.
[ ] 4. Use a small-gauge catheter to drain the bladder.

A 59-year-old client with ovarian cancer is receiving antineoplastic chemotherapy after undergoing a total hysterectomy.

58. To accurately determine the dosage of antineoplastic drugs, which information is essential for the nurse to obtain from the client's chart?
[ ] 1. Urine output for the past 24 hours
[ ] 2. Body weight and height
[ ] 3. Date of surgery
[ ] 4. Drug allergies

59. Because many antineoplastic drugs affect bone marrow function, which laboratory test is most important to monitor for client safety?
[ ] 1. Mean cell volume
[ ] 2. Total leukocyte count
[ ] 3. Differential cell count
[ ] 4. Complete blood count

60. The nurse adds the nursing diagnosis of Anxiety related to recent cancer diagnosis as evidenced by inability to complete routine activities. Which client outcome, if met, best reflects improvement in client status?
[ ] 1. The client will maintain personal affairs.
[ ] 2. The client will attend a cancer support group.
[ ] 3. The client will interact with family and friends.
[ ] 4. The client will participate in all health care decisions.

The client experiences almost total hair loss as antineoplastic drug therapy progresses.

61. Which statement is most accurate when discussing hair loss with the client?
[ ] 1. The hair loss is permanent, but attractive wigs are available.
[ ] 2. The hair loss is permanent, but hair transplantation is a possible solution.
[ ] 3. The hair loss is temporary; hair may grow back in several years.
[ ] 4. The hair loss is temporary; hair will regrow after chemotherapy is finished.

Nursing Care of Clients with Miscellaneous Disorders of the Female Reproductive System

The transfer form for a 72-year-old client being admitted to a nursing home indicates that she has a prolapsed uterus.

62. When the nurse does a physical assessment of this client, which technique is best for determining the extent of the prolapse?
[ ] 1. Examine the perineum when the client rolls from side to side.
[ ] 2. Examine the perineum as the client stands and bears down.
[ ] 3. Examine the perineum with the client in a dorsal recumbent position.
[ ] 4. Examine the perineum with a lubricated speculum and flashlight.

A 53-year-old woman becomes symptomatic as a result of a cystocele.

63. During the client's care, when is the most likely time that the nurse can anticipate the client will experience urinary incontinence?
[ ] 1. When she awakens
[ ] 2. As she walks
[ ] 3. During sleep
[ ] 4. Upon sneezing

64. If the cystocele is not severe, which nursing action is best?

[ ] **1.** Recommend wearing absorbent underwear.
[ ] **2.** Show her how to apply an external catheter.
[ ] **3.** Teach her to exercise her perineal muscles.
[ ] **4.** Instruct her to limit her fluid intake.

Because of her persistent symptoms, the client chooses to undergo surgery to correct the cystocele. She is instructed to catheterize herself for approximately 1 week after being discharged.

65. Which outcome best demonstrates that the client is performing self-catheterization appropriately?

[ ] **1.** She empties 50 mL of urine from her bladder each time.
[ ] **2.** She is free of signs of a urinary tract infection.
[ ] **3.** She inserts the catheter for 30 minutes each time.
[ ] **4.** She maintains a urinary record of time and amount.

66. A postmenopausal woman receives a prescription for alendronate (Fosamax). What health teaching information should the nurse provide? Select all that apply.

[ ] **1.** Take the medication with a full glass of water.
[ ] **2.** Refrain from eating for 30 minutes after taking the medication.
[ ] **3.** This medication helps relieve hot flashes and irritability.
[ ] **4.** Take the medication upon awakening.
[ ] **5.** Do not lie down after taking the medication.
[ ] **6.** Take the medication with food or a glass of milk.

Nursing Care of Clients with Inflammatory Disorders of the Male Reproductive System

A physician prescribes an oral antibiotic for a client with prostatitis.

67. Which instruction by the nurse about the client's antibiotic use is a priority?

[ ] **1.** Drink a glass of milk when taking the medication.
[ ] **2.** Report if your urine becomes a lighter color.
[ ] **3.** Take the medication until it is completely gone.
[ ] **4.** Monitor your body temperature on a daily basis.

In addition to a mild analgesic, the physician also recommends that the client use sitz baths as a comfort measure for the prostatitis.

68. Which instruction by the nurse is correct concerning the sitz bath regimen?

[ ] **1.** Use cool tepid water.
[ ] **2.** Soak for 20 minutes.
[ ] **3.** Add mild liquid soap to the water.
[ ] **4.** Massage the scrotum while bathing.

The physician examines a 22-year-old client who has a swollen, painful scrotum. The physician suspects epididymitis and orders a clean-catch urine specimen for a culture and sensitivity test.

69. When the nurse asks the client to repeat the instructions for collecting a clean-catch urine specimen, which statement indicates that the client needs further clarification?

[ ] **1.** "I must clean my penis."
[ ] **2.** "I must collect all the urine."
[ ] **3.** "I must retract the foreskin."
[ ] **4.** "I must use a sterile container."

70. Which suggestion by the nurse will best promote the client's comfort?

[ ] **1.** Using a scrotal support
[ ] **2.** Wearing cotton briefs
[ ] **3.** Buying larger underwear
[ ] **4.** Applying a hot compress

A middle-aged client with inflamed testes is being seen at a local clinic. The physician diagnoses orchitis.

71. When the nurse gathers the client data, which information is most suggestive as the cause of the client's condition?

[ ] **1.** The client has multiple sexual partners.
[ ] **2.** The client is a sexually active homosexual.
[ ] **3.** The client was never immunized for mumps.
[ ] **4.** The client had a previous sports-related scrotal injury.

During a subsequent visit, when the client has recovered from the orchitis, the nurse uses the opportunity to teach him how to perform testicular self-examination.

72. Which statement by the nurse accurately explains the technique for testicular self-examination?

[ ] **1.** Palpate each testicle simultaneously.
[ ] **2.** Roll each testicle between the thumb and fingers.
[ ] **3.** Examine your testicles at least once yearly.
[ ] **4.** Perform the self-examination in a cool room.

Nursing Care of Clients with Structural Disorders of the Male Reproductive System

During a routine sports physical, the nurse notes that a 15-year-old client has an undescended testicle.

73. When the client asks how this condition will affect him sexually, which response by the nurse is most appropriate?

[ ] **1.** "It most likely will have little effect on your masculinity."
[ ] **2.** "It means that you will probably be impotent."
[ ] **3.** "You may notice that your breasts will enlarge later."
[ ] **4.** "Your sex drive will not be like that of other boys."

A 56-year-old client has had difficulty retracting the foreskin over the glans of his penis. He is scheduled for a circumcision.

74. Besides assessing the dressing for signs of bleeding, which other postoperative nursing assessment is a priority after this surgical procedure?
[ ] **1.** Checking the client's deep-breathing efforts
[ ] **2.** Assessing the client's ability to achieve an erection
[ ] **3.** Monitoring the volume of urine output
[ ] **4.** Monitoring the infusion of I.V. antibiotics

A client with a hydrocele has the fluid aspirated from his scrotum. The physician orders a cold application to the area.

75. When carrying out this intervention, which action is most appropriate?
[ ] **1.** Apply ice to the site in a sealed plastic bag.
[ ] **2.** Place a covered ice pack to the scrotum.
[ ] **3.** Position the client on a hypothermia blanket.
[ ] **4.** Seat the client on an ice-filled ring.

Nursing Care of Clients with Benign and Malignant Disorders of the Male Reproductive System

A 65-year-old client makes an appointment for a routine physical examination.

76. When the physician asks the nurse to prepare the client for a prostate examination, which position is preferred?
[ ] **1.** Lithotomy
[ ] **2.** Modified standing
[ ] **3.** Dorsal recumbent
[ ] **4.** Fowler's

77. The nurse provides health teaching to the client about the prostate before the examination. Please place an *X* where the prostate gland is located.

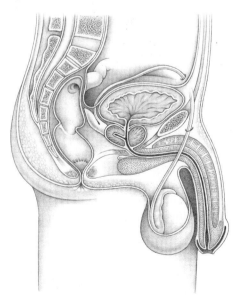

A 72-year-old client with a history of benign prostatic hypertrophy (BPH) phones the nurse at his physician's office, stating that he has not been able to urinate in the past 16 hours.

78. In the early stages of BPH, the nurse expects the physician to monitor the progression of the disease with which diagnostic test?
[ ] **1.** A semiannual prostate-specific antigen (PSA) test
[ ] **2.** An annual cystoscopy
[ ] **3.** A digital rectal examination
[ ] **4.** A retrograde pyelogram

The physician advises the client to go to the emergency department for catheterization.

79. Because an enlarged prostate gland may be the cause for the client's urine retention, place an *X* on the catheter that would be best for the nurse to use in lieu of a Foley retention catheter.

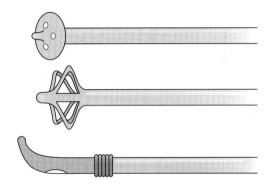

80. During catheterization, at which urine quantity is the nurse most correct to clamp the catheter?
[ ] **1.** 500 mL
[ ] **2.** 1,000 mL
[ ] **3.** 1,500 mL
[ ] **4.** 2,000 mL

The client is scheduled for a sonogram of his prostate.

81. When the nurse provides the client with pretest instructions, which statement is most correct?
[ ] **1.** "You'll need to fast from midnight the night before the test."
[ ] **2.** "You'll need to empty your bladder just before the test begins."
[ ] **3.** "You'll need to consume at least a quart of water an hour before the test."
[ ] **4.** "You'll need to self-administer an enema 1 hour before the test."

The client undergoes a transurethral resection of the prostate (TURP) and is returned to the nursing unit with a three-way catheter for administering intermittent bladder irrigations. Because the physician is concerned about the client's renal status, urine output is calculated every 4 hours.

82. If the nurse instills 1,000 ml of irrigant in the 4-hour time frame, and there is 1,275 ml in the drainage collection bag at the end of the 4 hours, what is the total urine output?

_____

83. When a client with a transurethral resection of the prostate (TURP) complains of bladder discomfort and a feeling of urgency to void, which nursing action is best to take first?
[ ] 1. Check that the urinary drainage catheter is patent.
[ ] 2. Administer a prescribed analgesic as soon as possible.
[ ] 3. Change the client to semi-Fowler's position.
[ ] 4. Get the client out of bed to ambulate for a while.

A 68-year-old client with prostate cancer undergoes a suprapubic prostatectomy. He returns to the nursing unit with an indwelling catheter in his urethra and a cystostomy tube in his abdomen.

84. Which nursing order is most appropriate to add to the client's initial postoperative care plan?
[ ] 1. Connect the cystostomy tube to a leg bag for drainage.
[ ] 2. Secure the cystostomy tube to the client's thigh.
[ ] 3. Ensure that the cystostomy tube is unclamped at all times.
[ ] 4. Clamp the indwelling catheter when the cystostomy tube is irrigated.

85. When providing shift report to the next nurse, which common postoperative complication is most important to discuss?
[ ] 1. Urinary retention
[ ] 2. Flank pain
[ ] 3. Urinary bleeding
[ ] 4. Flatus

A radical inguinal orchiectomy is performed on a 22-year-old client with testicular cancer.

86. Which comment by the client indicates that he has misinterpreted the consequences of his surgery?
[ ] 1. "My beard will continue to grow."
[ ] 2. "My voice will sound higher."
[ ] 3. "My sperm count will be unchanged."
[ ] 4. "My sex drive will be unaffected."

Nursing Care of Clients with Sexually Transmitted Infections

A nurse makes an office appointment for a male teenager who thinks he may have a sexually transmitted infection.

87. To facilitate obtaining truthful information regarding this client's sexual history, which attitude is most important for the nurse to convey?
[ ] 1. Sympathetic
[ ] 2. Nonjudgmental
[ ] 3. Encouraging
[ ] 4. Optimistic

88. When obtaining a sexual history from this client, which question is most important for the nurse to ask?
[ ] 1. "Have you ever had a painless sore on your penis?"
[ ] 2. "Does any sex partner have similar symptoms?"
[ ] 3. "At what age did you first have sexual intercourse?"
[ ] 4. "When did you last have sexual intercourse?"

After obtaining a health and sexual history, the nurse suspects that the client has signs and symptoms of gonorrhea.

89. If the client is typical of others with gonorrhea, which statements made by the client will help to make the diagnosis? Select all that apply.
[ ] 1. "I have burning when I urinate."
[ ] 2. "I have a yellow drainage from my penis."
[ ] 3. "I had sexual intercourse 5 days ago."
[ ] 4. "I have a painless ulceration on my penis."
[ ] 5. "I have little blisters on my penis and scrotum."
[ ] 6. "I have extra skin growing around my penis."

90. The nurse discusses healthy sexual behaviors with the client. Which risk factor predisposes the client to acquiring a sexually transmitted infection?
[ ] 1. Experiencing early puberty
[ ] 2. Finding sex information on the Internet
[ ] 3. Having multiple sex partners
[ ] 4. Receiving limited sex education

91. If a culture is ordered to detect the causative organism, which body substance will the nurse collect?
[ ] 1. Venous blood
[ ] 2. Sterile urine
[ ] 3. Ejaculated semen
[ ] 4. Urethral drainage

92. When collecting a specimen from the client who may have gonorrhea, which nursing action is correct?
[ ] 1. Wearing latex gloves
[ ] 2. Using a disinfectant
[ ] 3. Asking the client to provide the specimen
[ ] 4. Refrigerating the specimen immediately

93. When counseling a female client with a new diagnosis of genital herpes, which statement by the nurse is accurate?
[ ] **1.** "Have a Pap test done at least every 6 months."
[ ] **2.** "Avoid having vaginal intercourse for at least 6 months."
[ ] **3.** "If you take your medicine, you will not infect anyone else."
[ ] **4.** "Your infection provides immunity for any future children."

94. While assessing a male client with tertiary syphilis, which finding is most characteristic of this stage of the disease?
[ ] **1.** Stabbing leg pain
[ ] **2.** Red, raised rash
[ ] **3.** Penile ulcer
[ ] **4.** Patchy hair loss

95. Which comment indicates that the client lacks a clear understanding of syphilis?
[ ] **1.** "I can be cured using antibiotic therapy."
[ ] **2.** "My sex partner should be tested for the disease."
[ ] **3.** "Syphilitic lesions may be present in my partner's vagina."
[ ] **4.** "One infection provides lifelong immunity."

A culture indicates that a client has nonspecific urethritis from Chlamydia trachomatis, a nongonococcal organism. The physician prescribes doxycycline (Vibramycin) 100 mg b.i.d. with a sufficient number of capsules for 7 days of treatment.

96. Which information given by the nurse is most appropriate to provide to the client?
[ ] **1.** Take the medication until the symptoms clear.
[ ] **2.** Refill the prescription if symptoms persist.
[ ] **3.** Take the medication for the full amount of time.
[ ] **4.** Treatment of the infection is likely to be lifelong.

97. Which nursing instruction is best to provide to the client with chlamydia to prevent a recurrence of the infection?
[ ] **1.** Shower or bathe after intercourse.
[ ] **2.** Wash your hands well using an antiseptic soap.
[ ] **3.** Encourage your sexual partners to be tested and treated.
[ ] **4.** Make sure you receive adequate nutrition and fluid intake.

98. Which gynecologic symptom reported by a female client is most suggestive of trichomoniasis?
[ ] **1.** A series of fluid-filled vesicles on the vagina
[ ] **2.** Vaginal drainage that causes intense itching
[ ] **3.** Vaginal drainage that resembles milk curds
[ ] **4.** Tenderness and pressure in the lower abdomen

To prevent infection with the human immunodeficiency virus (HIV), a client says he uses a condom when having intercourse.

99. When managing the care of a client with acquired immunodeficiency syndrome (AIDS), which method best evaluates the effectiveness of zidovudine (AZT) therapy?
[ ] **1.** Assessing the client's vital signs
[ ] **2.** Assessing the client's blood counts
[ ] **3.** Monitoring the client's blood culture reports
[ ] **4.** Monitoring the client's viral load tests

Nursing Care of Clients Practicing Family Planning

A female client receives a 6-month supply of oral contraceptives.

100. Which instruction is appropriate to include when providing the client with oral contraceptive teaching?
[ ] **1.** Take oral contraceptives at the same time each day.
[ ] **2.** Take oral contraceptives on an empty stomach.
[ ] **3.** Take oral contraceptives on the first day of menses.
[ ] **4.** Take oral contraceptives in the morning with food.

101. Which recommendation by the nurse is most appropriate to reduce the risk of blood clots while the client is taking hormonal contraceptives?
[ ] **1.** Stop smoking while taking hormonal contraceptives.
[ ] **2.** Drink a high volume of fluid to dilute the blood.
[ ] **3.** Keep the legs elevated while sitting in a chair.
[ ] **4.** Take a baby aspirin daily at the same time as the oral contraceptive.

A pregnant client is considering a tubal ligation after the birth of her child.

102. Which statement indicates that the client is misinformed?
[ ] **1.** "I will have a small abdominal incision."
[ ] **2.** "This procedure is not easily reversed."
[ ] **3.** "I will no longer menstruate afterward."
[ ] **4.** "Recovery should occur in a brief time."

103. If a female client with an intrauterine device describes the following symptoms, which of them are most likely related to her birth control device? Select all that apply.
[ ] **1.** Breast tenderness
[ ] **2.** Heavy menstrual flow
[ ] **3.** Steady weight gain
[ ] **4.** Chronic acne
[ ] **5.** Periods that last longer than normal
[ ] **6.** Painful menstrual cramping

104. The nurse correctly teaches a couple that immediately after a vasectomy, it is best to continue using an alternative birth control method for which time period?
[ ] **1.** 1 month
[ ] **2.** 6 weeks
[ ] **3.** 12 weeks
[ ] **4.** 6 months

105. When teaching a male client about how to use a condom, which instructions are correct? Select all that apply.
[ ] **1.** "Wait until your penis becomes limp before removing it from the vagina."
[ ] **2.** "You can reuse a condom as long as it is made of silicone."
[ ] **3.** "Leave a small space between the end of the condom and the penis."
[ ] **4.** "Apply spermicide to the penis before applying the condom."
[ ] **5.** "Unroll the condom over an erect penis."
[ ] **6.** "Store condoms in a cool, dry place."

106. The physician prescribes medroxyprogesterone acetate (Depo-Provera) 150 mg I.M. for contraception for a 28-year-old woman. What actions are appropriate when administering this medication? Select all that apply.
[ ] **1.** Confirm that the client is not pregnant.
[ ] **2.** Give the injection deeply into the dorsogluteal site.
[ ] **3.** Schedule administration of the first injection to coincide with the time of ovulation.
[ ] **4.** Inform the client to return every 3 months for another injection.
[ ] **5.** Inform the client to use an additional form of contraception for the first week after an injection.
[ ] **6.** Apply ice to the injection site for 2 to 3 minutes before administering the drug.

A 16-year-old student comes to the local public health department requesting information about birth control. She tells the nurse that she "wants something" so that she does not get pregnant.

107. Which information should be gathered before the nurse can advise the student appropriately regarding methods of birth control? Select all that apply.
[ ] **1.** The adolescent's lifestyle
[ ] **2.** Whether she is currently sexually active
[ ] **3.** Whether she has had a Pap smear in the last year
[ ] **4.** The date of her last menstrual period
[ ] **5.** Where she is currently working

After discussing various birth control methods with the client, the nurse advises her about safe sex practices.

108. Which information regarding safer sex practices should the nurse include in the client's teaching plan? Select all that apply.
[ ] **1.** "Be selective in choosing sexual partners."
[ ] **2.** "Do not share vibrators or other sexual equipment."
[ ] **3.** "Avoid intercourse if you have signs of a sexually transmitted infection."
[ ] **4.** "Urinate after having intercourse."
[ ] **5.** "Store condoms away from excessive heat."
[ ] **6.** "Keep birth control patches in the refrigerator."

The nurse is assigned to discuss family planning and various methods of contraception with a group of women who have expressed an interest in this topic. One participant asks the nurse, "How do oral contraceptives prevent pregnancy?"

109. The nurse correctly explains that the combination oral contraceptives prevent pregnancy by interfering with the sperm reaching the ovum and by which other method?
[ ] **1.** Preventing ovulation
[ ] **2.** Depressing progesterone secretion
[ ] **3.** Depressing formation of the corpus luteum
[ ] **4.** Thickening the uterine lining

Another participant asks the nurse to explain the difference between oral contraceptive packages that have 21 pills and those that have 28 pills.

110. Which statement correctly describes oral contraceptive packages that contain 28 pills?
[ ] **1.** Packages containing 28 pills are biphasic and release a constant amount of estrogen and an increasing amount of progesterone throughout the cycle.
[ ] **2.** Packages containing 28 pills have 7 placebo pills and allow a woman to maintain a routine of taking a pill a day without missing a dose.
[ ] **3.** Packages containing 28 pills have 21 pills that contain estrogen and 7 pills that contain progesterone and are called "combination oral contraceptives."
[ ] **4.** Packages containing 28 pills are prescribed for women who have a 28-day menstrual cycle instead of a 21-day menstrual cycle.

111. Which statement by a participant indicates a need for additional teaching regarding safe and effective use of oral contraceptives?
[ ] **1.** "I need to use an additional form of contraception if I forget to take my pill for days in a row."
[ ] **2.** "Women who have painful menstrual cramping should not take oral contraceptives."
[ ] **3.** "Oral contraceptives should be discontinued 3 to 4 months before I plan to get pregnant."
[ ] **4.** "If I take certain antibiotics at the same time as my oral contraceptives, I could get pregnant."

A participant asks the nurse about the use of the birth control patch that some of her friends have started to use. The nurse explains about the use of the patch and reviews the side effects of this type of birth control.

112. Which side effects should the nurse address in the explanation? Select all that apply.

[ ] **1.** Skin irritation
[ ] **2.** Irregular vaginal bleeding
[ ] **3.** Fluid retention
[ ] **4.** Increased blood pressure
[ ] **5.** Nausea and vomiting
[ ] **6.** Infection

At the family planning class, the nurse describes to the participants the various barrier methods of contraception.

113. Which statement made by a participant indicates the need for additional teaching about barrier methods of contraception?

[ ] **1.** "A diaphragm is refitted or replaced if there is a weight gain or loss of 10 pounds or more."
[ ] **2.** "Use of the intrauterine device is not recommended for women who have never been pregnant."
[ ] **3.** "Toxic shock syndrome is a potential side effect associated with the use of the cervical cap."
[ ] **4.** "Use of the female condom is not recommended for women who are allergic to latex."

One participant states that she is considering using the basal body temperature method of natural family planning and asks the nurse the correct way to use this method.

114. Which statement is correct concerning the proper use of the basal body temperature method of natural family planning?

[ ] **1.** The client should record the pattern of her menstrual cycle for 6 to 8 months before actually using the method.
[ ] **2.** The client should regularly monitor the consistency of vaginal bleeding during menstruation.
[ ] **3.** The client should take her temperature every morning before rising for 6 months before using the method.
[ ] **4.** The client should have her sex partner withdraw his penis from the vagina just before ejaculation.

115. A licensed practical nurse is working at a Women's Health Clinic. Due to a high client volume, the nurse has delegated client instruction on the use of Lo/Ovral birth control pills to the medical assistant. Prior to delegation, which consideration is most important?

[ ] **1.** The medical assistant's moral beliefs
[ ] **2.** Information receptiveness of client
[ ] **3.** Presence of a significant other in the room
[ ] **4.** The medical assistant's medication knowledge

Correct Answers, Rationales, and Test Taking Strategies

Nursing Care of Clients with Breast Disorders

1. 3. Although the American Cancer Society continues to recommend that all women have an initial baseline mammogram beginning at age 40, the U.S. Preventive Services Task Force recently indicated that routine mammograms can be delayed until age 50. The recommendation was based on statistics that indicate the risk for breast cancer between ages 40 and 50 is only 1.4%. Several studies suggest that screening for high-risk women with a family history of breast cancer should begin approximately 10 years before the age of diagnosis of the family member with breast cancer.

> *Test Taking Strategy—Analyze to determine what information the question asks for, which is the age at which routine mammography screening should begin. Recall that there is an ongoing age-related controversy on this subject, with some experts recommending screening should begin at age 40 while others say age 50. Review recommendations by the American Cancer Society and other reputable organizations if you had difficulty answering this question.*

Cognitive Level—*Understanding*
Client Needs Category—*Health promotion and maintenance*
Client Needs Subcategory—*None*

2. 2. Although the American Cancer Society states that monthly breast self-examinations (BSEs) are optional, they are an important way for women to discover early breast changes. When conducting BSE, the client should inspect her breasts during a shower, when lying down, and while standing before a mirror. Ominous signs include a change in the size of one breast, dimpling of the skin, or an altered nipple appearance. A clinical breast examination performed by a physician, nurse, or physician's assistant should be performed every 3 years for women ages 20 to 39 and annually for women once they are age 40.

> *Test Taking Strategy—Analyze to determine what information the question asks for, which is a position, other than standing in the shower and lying down, that is recommended when performing BSE. Recall that looking at the breasts while standing in front of a mirror helps identify significant differences in breast and nipple symmetry and changes in the skin of the breasts. Review the method for performing BSE if you had difficulty answering this question.*

Cognitive Level—*Applying*
Client Needs Category—*Health promotion and maintenance*
Client Needs Subcategory—*None*

3. 4. The pads of the four fingertips are used to feel for breast abnormalities during breast self-examination (BSE). The pads of the fingers are especially sensitive and can note lumps or changes in breast tissue.

> *Test Taking Strategy*—Look at the key words "most correct," and read the descriptions in each option, looking for one that corresponds to the technique that is recommended for palpating breast tissue. Recall that the tips of the fingers are best for identifying characteristics of the tissue beneath the skin. Review the method for performing BSE if you had difficulty answering this question.
> *Cognitive Level*—Applying
> *Client Needs Category*—Health promotion and maintenance
> *Client Needs Subcategory*—None

4. 1. There is more than one method for performing breast self-examination (BSE). The woman may move her fingers in circles, dividing the breast into wedges like the spokes of a wheel, or in rows up and down over the breast, but the method she chooses must be done the same way for each breast. Regardless of the technique chosen, all methods include palpating from the outer margins of the breast into the axillae.

> *Test Taking Strategy*—Analyze to determine what information the question asks for, which is the correct technique for BSE. Consider the anatomy of breast tissue and its lymphatic drainage. Recall that BSE should include the outward margins of the breast (tail of Spence), which is an extension of breast tissue. Review the anatomy of the breast if you had difficulty answering this question.
> *Cognitive Level*—Applying
> *Client Needs Category*—Health promotion and maintenance
> *Client Needs Subcategory*—None

5. 4. Hormonal levels fluctuate each month during the menstrual cycle, which causes changes in the breast tissue. Swelling begins to decrease when the menstrual cycle starts. Premenopausal women should perform breast self-examination (BSE) every month, 3 to 7 days after the period ends. When a client is past menopause, a BSE should be performed on a selected date each month, for example, the first day of the month.

> *Test Taking Strategy*—Use the process of elimination to help select the option that identifies the best time for performing BSE. Options 1 and 2 can be eliminated immediately because BSE need only be performed monthly. Option 3 can be eliminated because breast tissue is more likely to feel tender and lumpy premenstrually. Option 4 remains as the best answer because breast tissue changes would be at their minimum after menstruation and before ovulation. Review BSE standards and the physiology of changes in breast tissue throughout the menstrual cycle if you had difficulty answering this question.

Cognitive Level—Applying
Client Needs Category—Health promotion and maintenance
Client Needs Subcategory—None

6. 2, 5, 6. Underarm deodorant, body powder, lotion, or ointments on the breast can produce artifacts on the mammogram film. The artifacts may be misinterpreted as pathologic findings. The client may wear constricting clothing and a bra before and after the test, but during the mammogram, the clothing is removed from the upper part of the body and a gown is put on. Shaving underarm hair is a cultural choice; it is not a test requirement. Normal hygiene measures are appropriate, but wiping the breasts with an antiseptic before the test is unnecessary.

> *Test Taking Strategy*—Analyze to determine what information the question asks for, which is topics to include when teaching a client preparing for a mammogram. Alternative-format "select all that apply" questions require considering each option independently to decide its merit in answering the question. Choose the options that would promote clear imaging of the breast tissue. Review preparation for a mammographic screening if you had difficulty answering this question.
> *Cognitive Level*—Applying
> *Client Needs Category*—Health promotion and maintenance
> *Client Needs Subcategory*—None

7. 1, 3, 5. Having a close blood relative with breast cancer places the client at high risk for developing this disease. The risk factor increases twofold if the relative is a first-degree female, such as a sister, mother, or daughter. Menstruating before age 12 and not having children are additional predisposing factors. Women who have had radiation therapy to the chest as treatment for cancer (such as Hodgkin's disease or non-Hodgkin's lymphoma) are at significant risk for breast cancer. According to recent research, breast implants are not found to increase the risk of breast cancer, although silicone breast implants can cause scar tissue to form in the breast. Implants make it harder to visualize breast tissue on standard mammograms. The size of the breast is not a risk factor for developing breast cancer.

> *Test Taking Strategy*—Analyze to determine what information the question asks for, which is risk factors for breast cancer. Alternative-format "select all that apply" questions require considering each option independently to decide its merit in answering the question. Choose one or more options that place a person at high risk for developing breast cancer. Review breast cancer risk factors if you had difficulty answering this question.
> *Cognitive Level*—Applying

Client Needs Category—Health promotion and maintenance
Client Needs Subcategory—None

8. 4. Fibrocystic lesions cause more discomfort before menstruation because the lesions are affected by increasing levels of estrogen. Estrogen appears to be a factor because cysts usually disappear after menopause. Many women experience relief of symptoms when menstruation occurs. Symptoms do not commonly increase with aging. Fibrocystic lesions are not affected by sexual activity.

> *Test Taking Strategy—Analyze to determine what information the question asks for, which is the time period when cysts within the breast are likely to become larger and feel tender to the touch. Recall that estrogen rises premenstrually (option 4) and peaks at ovulation to prepare the uterus and breasts for fertilization of an ovum. Review the rise and fall of hormones throughout the menstrual cycle if you had difficulty answering this question.*
> *Cognitive Level—Applying*
> *Client Needs Category—Health promotion and maintenance*
> *Client Needs Subcategory—None*

9. 2. Some women report that eliminating coffee, tea, cola, and chocolate reduces their breast discomfort. Limiting sodium intake, taking a warm bath, or taking an anti-inflammatory such as ibuprofen (Motrin) also helps. Objectively, however, there is no evidence that the fibrocystic lesions become smaller or disappear with any particular diet modification. Consuming a high-fat diet seems to have a relationship to developing breast cancer. Refined sugar and alcohol are not linked to breast disease.

> *Test Taking Strategy—Analyze to determine what information the question asks for, which is a dietary change that may relieve the symptoms of fibrocystic breast disease. Although all four items listed in the options should be consumed in moderation, eliminating caffeine (option 2) has reduced or eliminated the discomfort associated with fibrocystic breast disease for some women. Review information about the management of fibrocystic disease if you had difficulty answering this question.*
> *Cognitive Level—Applying*
> *Client Needs Category—Health promotion and maintenance*
> *Client Needs Subcategory—None*

10. 4, 6. The Health Insurance Portability and Accountability Act (HIPAA) was enacted by Congress in 1996 to protect the client's health information. This includes information such as name, address, Social Security number, phone number, medical records number, diagnosis, admission and discharge dates, and all information from past, present, and future treatments. Leaving this information unattended is considered a major HIPAA violation. The nurse who finds these violations should report them to the office manager, supervisor, or the ethics and compliance officer of that institution. Because the documents are the client's medical records and are legal documents, throwing them away or putting them into the shredder are not appropriate actions. Instead, the nurse should find out who brought the documents to the location of the meeting and remind that person that a HIPAA violation has occurred. Neatly stacking the documents to the side is immaterial at this time because potentially confidentiality has already been violated.

> *Test Taking Strategy—Analyze to determine what information the question asks for, which is the proper action to take in reference to HIPAA regulations. Alternative-format "select all that apply" questions require considering each option independently to decide its merit in answering the question. Choose options that protect the client's confidentiality. Review the HIPAA regulations as they apply to protecting health information from unauthorized access if you had difficulty answering this question.*
> *Cognitive Level—Analyzing*
> *Client Needs Category—Safe effective care environment*
> *Client Needs Subcategory—Coordinated care*

11. 3. Cancerous tumors tend to be irregularly shaped and attached firmly to surrounding tissue. Benign breast tumors tend to have a well-defined border and to be freely movable. Neither the lump's size nor the location can necessarily predict if the lump is benign or malignant. However, cancerous tumors in nulliparous women or those who have not breast-fed infants are more commonly located in the upper outer quadrant of the breast.

> *Test Taking Strategy—Use the process of elimination to help select the option that identifies a characteristic of a cancerous tumor within the breast. Recall that malignant breast tumors feel irregular (option 3), in contrast to their benign counterparts, which feel more like a pellet or marble that can be easily moved about (option 1). Option 2 can be eliminated because the size of the lesion can vary regardless of whether it is benign or malignant. Although a malignant breast tumor can be located anywhere in the breast, nearly half are located in the upper outer quadrant of the breast; less than 20% are located near the nipple, which eliminates option 4. Review the characteristics and locations of malignant breast tumors if you had difficulty answering this question.*
> *Cognitive Level—Applying*
> *Client Needs Category—Physiological integrity*
> *Client Needs Subcategory—Physiological adaptation*

12. 2. Competent adult clients have the right to self-determination once they have all the pertinent information to make a decision. When that occurs, nurses have a duty to facilitate whatever choices the clients make. Discouraging the client from opposing the physician's recommendation promotes passivity. Even if most biopsies are accurate, some are not. Even though a second opinion may eventually prove to be appropriate, the nurse should try to facilitate communication between the client and physician; in most cases, the treatment plan can be modified to suit the client's wishes.

> *Test Taking Strategy—Look at the key words "most appropriate" and "initial nursing action." Recall that a client has the right to make his or her decision about treatment after considering the benefits and risks that are involved. It is the nurse's responsibility to assume the role of client advocate (option 2). Review the right to self-determination if you had difficulty answering this question.*
> *Cognitive Level—Applying*
> *Client Needs Category—Safe and effective care environment*
> *Client Needs Subcategory—Coordinated care*

13. **3, 5, 6.** Because this surgery compromises the client's vascular and lymphatic circulation, blood pressures and any other invasive procedures involving an arm (I.V. sticks, blood draws, injections) are performed on the opposite upper extremity. Postmastectomy clients generally are restricted from turning or sleeping on the affected side initially so that blood and lymph circulation can still occur. A sitting position tends to promote incisional drainage. Numbness and tingling of the chest wall or the inside aspect of the arm should be reported because these findings could indicate neurologic damage. These findings may last for a year or so. Fluids usually are not restricted. It is appropriate to assess the dressing and drainage, but the incisional wound is inspected only at the time of a dressing change, which may take place several days later.

> *Test Taking Strategy—Analyze to determine what information the question asks for, which is the postoperative plan of care for a client who has had a modified radical mastectomy. Alternative-format "select all that apply" questions require considering each option independently to decide its merit in answering the question. Review standard postoperative nursing care of a client after a modified radical mastectomy if you had difficulty answering this question.*
> *Cognitive Level—Applying*
> *Client Needs Category—Physiological integrity*
> *Client Needs Subcategory—Reduction of risk potential*

14. **1.** After a mastectomy, the client's breathing may be compromised due to the thoracic incision and restrictive (pressure) dressing. This type of dressing prevents movement of the chest muscles and therefore reduces lung capacity until the dressing is removed. Having the client take deep breaths and encouraging coughing every 2 hours is critical to prevent such respiratory problems as atelectasis and hypostatic pneumonia. The client should be encouraged to assume her regular diet soon after surgery; therefore, her nutrition should not be compromised. The client should also begin ambulating while decreasing her pain medication, thereby helping to increase bowel motility. Her risk of pressure sores should also decrease when she begins moving.

> *Test Taking Strategy—Look at the key words "most indicative" that are used when asking about an assessment finding that suggests a postoperative complication. Recall that the surgical incision and wound dressing are located in the chest area. Therefore, shallow breathing (option 1) is the best answer. Review potential complications that may occur after a modified radical mastectomy and related nursing assessments to detect them if you had difficulty answering this question.*
> *Cognitive Level—Analyzing*
> *Client Needs Category—Physiological integrity*
> *Client Needs Subcategory—Reduction of risk potential*

15. **0.5 tablet.**
To calculate the drug dosage, use the formula:

$$\frac{\text{Desired dose}}{\text{Dose on hand}} \times \text{Total quantity} = \text{Desired dose}$$

$$\text{In this case, } \frac{10}{20} \times 1 \text{ tablet} = 0.5 \text{ tablet}$$

> *Test Taking Strategy—Analyze to determine what information the question asks for, which requires calculating the number of 20-mg tablets that are necessary to administer 10 mg to the client. Refer to the formula and calculation and review how to calculate oral dosages if you had difficulty answering this question.*
> *Cognitive Level—Understanding*
> *Client Needs Category—Physiological integrity*
> *Client Needs Subcategory—Pharmacological therapies*

16. **2.** Most mastectomy clients tend to avoid raising the arm on the operative side after surgery. If this practice is prolonged, they tend to lose their full range of motion. Using the affected arm for hair brushing requires using muscles that elevate the arm and extend the chest muscles. Although self-feeding, writing, and washing the chest are good activities, they are not as likely to exercise the muscle groups to the same extent as brushing the hair.

> *Test Taking Strategy—Analyze to determine what information the question asks for, which is an activity that will preserve muscle strength and joint flexibility in the arm on the operative side. Recall that in a modified radical mastectomy, the pectoralis major and minor muscles are cut. These muscles, which are attached to the humerus,*

are used to flex and rotate the arm. Based on this knowledge, hair brushing (option 2) is the correct answer because it trains other muscles to maintain arm function. Review postoperative exercises recommended for a client who has had a modified radical mastectomy if you had difficulty answering this question.

Cognitive Level—*Analyzing*
Client Needs Category—*Physiological integrity*
Client Needs Subcategory—*Reduction of risk potential*

17. 3. In postmastectomy clients, the standard practice is to elevate the affected arm on pillows while the client is in bed, to raise the client's arm and exercise the hand muscles, and to support the client's arm in a sling while she is ambulating. Applying ice reduces swelling, and warm compresses dilate blood vessels; however, because this surgery tends to compromise the client's circulation and sensory perception, these two measures are not the most appropriate to use. Frequent ambulation of the client would be contraindicated.

Test Taking Strategy—*Analyze to determine what information the question asks for, which is a nursing measure that will relieve swelling in the client's arm. Recall that blood and lymphatic vessels in the arm are altered when this type of surgery is performed. Gravity (option 3) can be used to support the movement of these two substances by keeping the arm elevated. Review measures to prevent and relieve lymphedema if you had difficulty answering this question.*

Cognitive Level—*Applying*
Client Needs Category—*Physiological integrity*
Client Needs Subcategory—*Reduction of risk potential*

18. 1, 2, 3. Because most mastectomy clients are discharged fairly quickly after surgery, it is imperative that detailed discharge instructions be given to the client and that the client understands them. Arm exercises that are begun postoperatively in the hospital should be continued at home to regain full range of motion, prevent contractures, and promote blood and lymph circulation. The client should avoid lifting or carrying heavy objects weighing more than 15 pounds and should use gloves to prevent injuries that could result in infection. It is important for the client to have assistance when selecting a breast prosthesis, but most women do not postpone getting a prosthetic device and are fitted soon after surgery when healing has occurred. Although getting adequate sleep and avoiding alcohol and caffeine promote a healthy lifestyle, they do not have a bearing on the client's postoperative mastectomy home care.

Test Taking Strategy—*Analyze to determine what information the question asks for, which is appropriate discharge instructions for home care. Alternative-format "select all that apply" questions require*

considering each option independently to decide its merit in answering the question. Focus on the client's safety and rehabilitation when choosing an option. Review precautions the client should take after being discharged if you had difficulty answering this question.

Cognitive Level—*Applying*
Client Needs Category—*Safe and effective care environment*
Client Needs Subcategory—*Coordinated care*

19. 2. The American Cancer Society includes a group of trained volunteers who offer personal support and printed materials for postmastectomy clients in its program called "Reach to Recovery." None of the other associations or organizations listed exists. Some department stores hire individuals who have been certified by the American Board for Certification in Orthotics, Prosthetics & Pedorthics who may assist with fitting postmastectomy clients with an appropriate bra or prosthesis, but these employees may not be located in a commercial department store in a client's area.

Test Taking Strategy—*Use the process of elimination to help select the option that identifies the best resource for information about special bras and prosthetic devices after a mastectomy. Options 1, 3, and 4 can be eliminated because there are no organizations by those names. Option 2 remains as the best answer because the American Cancer Society, which is available to persons in counties throughout the United States, offers comprehensive services, including information about special bras and prosthetics, to mastectomy clients. Review the services that are provided by the American Cancer Society if you had difficulty answering this question.*

Cognitive Level—*Understanding*
Client Needs Category—*Health promotion and maintenance*
Client Needs Subcategory—*None*

20. 2. Clients who have had breast cancer are at risk for cancer in the opposite breast. Therefore, they must be conscientious about performing monthly breast self-examinations (BSEs). Postmenopausal women pick an arbitrary date and perform BSE on that date each month. The time of day is not pertinent. Breasts are examined during a shower, not afterward, when it is easier for the fingers to glide over the breast tissue. BSEs are performed monthly, not once a year.

Test Taking Strategy—*Use the process of elimination to help select the option that provides the most correct information about BSE after menopause. Although BSE is now considered optional, it may be more important to perform as a woman ages when the risk for breast cancer increases. Option 1 can be eliminated because there is no scientific evidence to support an advantage in examining the breast*

on awakening. Option 3 can be eliminated because breast changes may be identified better while showering. Option 4 can be eliminated because performing BSE on a yearly basis is probably not often enough to detect breast changes. Recall that the characteristics of breast tissue are not as susceptible to hormonal changes after menopause; therefore, option 2 is the best answer because it develops a consistent habit for detecting breast changes that may be occurring. Review the recommendation for the pattern for performing BSE after menopause if you had difficulty answering this question.
Cognitive Level—*Applying*
Client Needs Category—*Health promotion and maintenance*
Client Needs Subcategory—*None*

21.

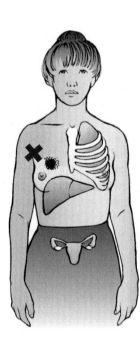

Breast cancer usually spreads first to the axillary lymph nodes, the structures closest to the primary site. Distant metastasis in advanced stages of breast cancer may be found in the bones, liver, lungs, and brain.
Test Taking Strategy—Analyze to determine what information the question asks for, which is the location where breast cancer cells are likely to migrate initially. Recall that when a breast tumor is removed, the surgeon removes various lymph nodes in the axilla to determine if malignant cells are present in that area. Once malignant cells are in lymph nodes, they may travel via lymphatic circulation to other locations in the body. Review common sites of breast metastasis if you had difficulty answering this question.
Cognitive Level—*Applying*
Client Needs Category—*Physiological integrity*
Client Needs Subcategory—*Physiological adaptation*

Nursing Care of Clients with Disturbances in Menstruation

22.

4. Ovarian follicle matures.
3. Endometrium begins to thicken.
1. Ovum is released.
6. Corpus luteum forms.
2. Progesterone decreases.
5. Endometrium is shed.

The ovarian follicle matures when the anterior pituitary gland secretes follicle-stimulating hormone. This is accompanied by an increase in estrogen, which promotes thickening of the endometrium. At about midcycle, the anterior pituitary gland releases luteinizing hormone, which causes the follicle to rupture and release an ovum. The ruptured follicle is transformed into the corpus luteum and secretes progesterone. If fertilization fails to occur, the progesterone level decreases and the endometrium is shed.
Test Taking Strategy—Analyze to determine what information the question asks for, which is the physiologic sequence that occurs during the menstrual cycle. Read each option and place the events in the order in which they occur. Review the processes that occur in the menstrual cycle if you had difficulty answering this question.
Cognitive Level—*Applying*
Client Needs Category—*Health promotion and maintenance*
Client Needs Subcategory—*None*

23. 1. It is important to differentiate between primary amenorrhea, a condition in which a female has never menstruated, and secondary amenorrhea, in which menstruation has occurred but has been absent for more than 3 months. This differentiation can provide important diagnostic information. Although the other questions may be pertinent, they are not as important to know at this time.
Test Taking Strategy—Look at the key words "most important" in reference to a question the nurse should ask when a client reports the absence of menstruation. Recall that it is important to determine if this is a new condition or has been an ongoing problem (option 1). Review the different types of amenorrhea and the characteristics associated with each if you had difficulty answering this question.

Cognitive Level—Applying
Client Needs Category—Health promotion and
  maintenance
Client Needs Subcategory—None

24. **3, 4.** Local applications of heat and mild analgesics are the first line of treatment for minor symptoms of dysmenorrhea, as is reducing strenuous physical activity that could worsen cramping. It would be premature to seek a prescription for an oral contraceptive at this time, although oral contraception is effective in certain cases for relieving dysmenorrhea. There is no correlation between hygiene products and dysmenorrhea. Massaging the lower abdomen may cause further pain due to uterine contractility. Lying on the abdomen in a prone position will not relieve discomfort.

Test Taking Strategy—Analyze to determine what
  information the question asks for, which is thera-
  peutic interventions to relieve dysmenorrhea.
  Alternative-format "select all that apply" questions
  require considering each option independently to
  decide its merit in answering the question. Choose
  options that correlate with measures that can reduce
  discomfort experienced during menstruation. Review
  management of dysmenorrhea if you had difficulty
  answering this question.
Cognitive Level—Applying
Client Needs Category—Health promotion and
  maintenance
Client Needs Subcategory—None

25. **1.** Douching in the days preceding a Pap smear interferes with accurate test results because it removes exfoliated cells. None of the other instructions is necessary when preparing a client for a pelvic examination.

Test Taking Strategy—Look at the key words "most
  appropriate," and apply them to the instructions
  listed. Select the option that identifies accurate
  information. Recall that the purpose for obtain-
  ing a Pap smear is to obtain cervical secretions to
  identify atypical cells that may be cancerous. If the
  client douches (option 1), the diagnostic cells may
  be reduced or eliminated. Review information to tell
  a client when scheduling a Pap smear if you had dif-
  ficulty answering this question.
Cognitive Level—Applying
Client Needs Category—Physiological integrity
Client Needs Subcategory—Reduction of risk potential

26. **2.** If the bladder is empty, pelvic organs are more easily palpated and the client experiences less discomfort. It is inappropriate to instill a vaginal lubricant before the examination. Analgesia is generally unnecessary. No special consent form is required for the examination.

Test Taking Strategy—Apply the key words "most
  appropriate" to the statements listed. Select the

nursing action that should be carried out before a pelvic examination. Recall that a full bladder interferes with the best outcome of a pelvic examination. Review how to prepare a client for a pelvic examination if you had difficulty answering this question.
Cognitive Level—Applying
Client Needs Category—Physiological integrity
Client Needs Subcategory—Reduction of risk potential

27. **3.** The vaginal specimen obtained for a Pap smear test contains exfoliated cells from the uterus. They are examined microscopically to identify precancerous, cancerous, inflammatory, typical, and atypical cells. It is best to document the date of a client's last menstrual period to assist the pathologist in determining if the microscopic cells are appropriate for the current stage in the menstrual cycle. The presence of atypical cells can sometimes be correlated with having the Pap test performed toward the end of menses. Identifying the date of the last menstrual period may eliminate a need for additional testing. Answers to the other questions are immaterial to the results of the Pap smear.

Test Taking Strategy—Apply the key words "most
  important" to each of the four options. Select the
  option that correlates with a question that helps to
  ensure valid vaginal specimen findings. Recall that
  characteristics of the cells may be different depending
  on the changes in the endometrium at different times
  in a woman's menstrual cycle. Therefore, option 3 is
  the best answer. Review information that facilitates a
  valid analysis of a vaginal specimen for a Pap test if
  you had difficulty answering this question.
Cognitive Level—Applying
Client Needs Category—Health promotion and
  maintenance
Client Needs Subcategory—None

28. **4.** A supine lithotomy position is preferred for a pelvic examination. In unusual circumstances, Sims' position may be used. Neither Trendelenburg's nor Fowler's position facilitates access to the vagina.

Test Taking Strategy—Analyze to determine what
  information the question asks for, which is the
  position in which a client should be placed when a
  pelvic examination will be performed. Recall that a
  lithotomy position (option 4) is the usual client posi-
  tion for a pelvic examination because it facilitates
  inserting a vaginal speculum as well as digitally
  palpating the ovaries through the vagina and rectum.
  Review the descriptions of the positions listed if you
  had difficulty answering this question.
Cognitive Level—Understanding
Client Needs Category—Physiological integrity
Client Needs Subcategory—Reduction of risk potential

29. **1.** To reduce the claim of sexual impropriety and to make the client feel more comfortable, an important nursing consideration is to have a female nurse present during the pelvic examination. Instructing on the dangers of cervical cancer is good general information; however, it is not known if the client has cervical cancer. The physician usually completes the internal examination and documents the findings. A vaginal lubricant is not instilled before the examination, although the physician may use a lubricant on the fingers during the internal examination.

> *Test Taking Strategy*—Apply the key words "most important" to each of the four options. Choose the option that identifies the most important nursing intervention from among the choices that are provided. Recall that without a same-gender third party present during the examination (option 1), an examiner of the opposite gender is at risk for allegations of sexual impropriety. Review risk factors for sexual accusations against health care providers and measures to prevent them if you had difficulty answering this question.
> *Cognitive Level*—Applying
> *Client Needs Category*—Safe and effective care environment
> *Client Needs Subcategory*—Coordinated care

30. 1. Breakthrough bleeding or spotting may occur in clients who take oral contraceptives with low dosages of estrogen or progesterone. Stress has been implicated in delaying menses or causing irregularity in a previously regular cycle, but it is uncommon for stress to cause mid-cycle bleeding. Having sexual intercourse with a partner who has a sexually transmitted infection is not smart but is not a common cause of vaginal bleeding. Using a vibrator to elicit sexual arousal typically is not the cause of bleeding or spotting. However, care must be used not to damage genital tissue.

> *Test Taking Strategy*—Look at the key words "most likely," and apply them to the statement in each of the four options. Select the option that is the most probable cause for vaginal bleeding between menses for this client. Recall that a potential side effect of low-dose contraceptives is breakthrough bleeding (option 1). Review the various causes of vaginal bleeding at a time other than menses, focusing on those that may occur in a young client, if you had difficulty answering this question.
> *Cognitive Level*—Analyzing
> *Client Needs Category*—Health promotion and maintenance
> *Client Needs Subcategory*—None

31. 2. Regardless of sexual preference, the client should be provided with privacy when a sensitive medical history is obtained and during a physical/pelvic examination. Confidentiality must also be maintained. Therefore, asking the client's partner to wait outside in the waiting room is most appropriate for this situation.

> *Test Taking Strategy*—Apply the key words "most appropriate" to the choices among the four options. Analyze which nursing response is ethically and legally appropriate for the described situation. Recall that the Health Insurance Portability and Accountability Act (HIPAA) was enacted to protect client health information. Review the requirements of HIPAA legislation as they apply to nurses and other health care workers if you had difficulty answering this question.
> *Cognitive Level*—Applying
> *Client Needs Category*—Safe and effective care environment
> *Client Needs Subcategory*—Coordinated care

32. 2. To promote the client's health, the most appropriate information for the nurse to ask is regarding the practice of protected, safe sex. Although hepatitis B and human immunodeficiency virus can be spread with contaminated tattoo equipment, obtaining the name of the person who tattooed the client and questioning whether the client has sex with men as well as women is not as significant to promoting the client's health as discussing safe sex practices. Obtaining the names of sexual partners is only appropriate if the client has a sexually transmitted infection that could be potentially spread to sex partners.

> *Test Taking Strategy*—Analyze to determine what information the question asks for, which is a topic the nurse should discuss with a client who is sexually active. Recall that many sexually transmitted infections can be prevented by using protected, safe sexual practices (option 2) regardless of whether they involve same- or different-gender partners. Review methods for preventing sexually transmitted infections if you had difficulty answering this question.
> *Cognitive Level*—Analyzing
> *Client Needs Category*—Health promotion and maintenance
> *Client Needs Subcategory*—None

Nursing Care of Clients with Infectious and Inflammatory Disorders of the Female Reproductive System

33. 1. *Candida albicans,* a common cause of vaginitis, is usually treated with an antifungal medication. Several former prescription antifungal drugs are now available without a prescription. Over-the-counter drugs, such as miconazole (Monistat) and clotrimazole (Gyne-Lotrimin), are available in various forms, including vaginal tablets, creams, and suppositories. Oral antibiotics are not used to treat *C. albicans* and, in fact, are frequently the cause of the vaginitis. Irritating vaginal douches are not recommended for treatment.

> *Test Taking Strategy—Analyze to determine what information the question asks for, which is a treatment for C. albicans. Recall that vaginal fungal infections may be treated with over-the-counter medications (option 1), which eliminates options 2 and 3. Although douching with vinegar and water may acidify the vaginal pH, using antifungal medication is more efficient at treating this type of vaginitis. Review the treatment for vaginal infections caused by C. albicans if you had difficulty answering this question.*

Cognitive Level—*Applying*
Client Needs Category—*Physiological integrity*
Client Needs Subcategory—*Pharmacological therapies*

34. 3. Instilling the drug before bedtime aids in retaining the medication within the vagina for a substantial period of time. When this is not possible, the client is instructed to recline for 10 to 30 minutes after insertion. The applicator is inserted approximately 2″ to 4″ (5 to 10 cm) within the vagina. The best position to be in when instilling the drug is reclining in a dorsal recumbent position. Latex gloves are a matter of personal choice when self-administering vaginal medication; however, they are required when instilling the drug into someone else. Good hand washing is important in either case.

> *Test Taking Strategy—Use the process of elimination to help select the option that identifies the best instruction when teaching a client about inserting vaginal medication. Recall that there is no sphincter muscle within the vagina that can help retain topical medication. Therefore, option 3, instilling the medication at a time when it will not leak from the vagina due to gravity, is the best answer. Review the procedure for instilling vaginal medications if you had difficulty answering this question.*

Cognitive Level—*Applying*
Client Needs Category—*Physiological integrity*
Client Needs Subcategory—*Pharmacological therapies*

35. 2. Yeasts are present in the intestinal tract and are introduced into the vagina if stool is wiped across rather than away from the vaginal opening. This is often a common etiologic factor in urinary tract infections as well. Showers versus tub baths are a matter of personal preference as long as the tub is cleaned on a routine basis. Some types of vaginal infections are spread from infected sex partners, but limiting intercourse to once a week is not likely to prevent them. Lanolin soap is no more effective than antiseptic body soaps for reducing microorganism growth.

> *Test Taking Strategy—Apply the key words "most appropriate" to the statements in each option. Select the option that is the best health teaching informa-*

tion to prevent a fungal/yeast infection in the vagina. Recall the close proximity of the vagina to the rectum, where there is an abundance of fungi and yeasts present in stool. Teaching the client to wipe away from the vagina after having a bowel movement (option 2) is a recommended health measure. Review methods for preventing vaginal fungal/yeast infections if you had difficulty answering this question.

Cognitive Level—*Applying*
Client Needs Category—*Health promotion and maintenance*
Client Needs Subcategory—*None*

36. 2. Douching for the purpose of hygiene is unnecessary and can be harmful because it depletes helpful microorganisms that tend to prevent vaginal infections. A vinegar solution alters the pH of the vagina and makes it an inhospitable environment for microbial growth, but it is better to use a dilute solution rather than one that is concentrated. The volume of douche solutions can be more than 16 oz. The solution drains out by gravity when the vaginal capacity is reached. Cramping is not common with douching.

> *Test Taking Strategy—Look at the key words "most appropriate" and apply them when analyzing each of the four options. Select the option that identifies health teaching the nurse should provide to a client who douches frequently. Recall that the vagina is protected by helpful microscopic flora, known as Döderlein bacilli. This species forms a mucosal biofilm that inhibits the growth, adhesion, and spread of pathogenic microorganisms. The colony of Döderlein bacilli can be depleted by frequent douching (option 2), causing the client to be more susceptible to vaginal infections. Review the consequences of frequent douching if you had difficulty answering this question.*

Cognitive Level—*Applying*
Client Needs Category—*Health promotion and maintenance*
Client Needs Subcategory—*None*

37. 2. Pelvic inflammatory disease (PID) refers to infection of the uterus, fallopian tubes, and other reproductive organs. It is a common and serious complication of some sexually transmitted infections (STIs), especially chlamydia and gonorrhea. It is essential to contain any and all infectious drainage from a client with PID within specially marked biohazardous infectious waste bags. Flushing absorbent pads down the toilet could cause plumbing problems. Neither an open wastebasket nor paper bags are sufficient barriers for containing the infectious microorganisms.

> *Test Taking Strategy—Analyze to determine what information the question asks for, which is the best method for disposing of pads that are soiled with*

vaginal drainage. Recall that disposing of materials containing body secretions and potentially infectious drainage should be placed in a biohazard bag (option 2) then subsequently deposited within a covered container in the dirty utility room. Review the procedure for disposing of infectious hazardous waste if you had difficulty answering this question.
Cognitive Level—*Applying*
Client Needs Category—*Safe and effective care environment*
Client Needs Subcategory—*Safety and infection control*

38. 4. Pelvic inflammatory disease (PID) can damage the fallopian tubes and tissues in and near the uterus and ovaries. PID can lead to serious consequences, including ectopic pregnancy, abscess formation, chronic pelvic pain, and infertility. Infertility results from the scarring of fallopian tubes, which subsequently blocks passage for both sperm and ovum. With early and aggressive treatment, the sequelae may be prevented or minimized. Cancer of the cervix, premature labor, and spontaneous abortion are not directly related to a prior incidence of PID.
Test Taking Strategy—*Analyze to determine what information the question asks for, which is a potential reproductive sequela of PID. Recall that this infectious disorder involves an inflammatory process and possible healing with scar tissue. Scar tissue may narrow the lumen of fallopian tubes, leading to infertility (option 4). Review the potential consequences of PID if you had difficulty answering this question.*
Cognitive Level—*Applying*
Client Needs Category—*Physiological integrity*
Client Needs Subcategory—*Physiological adaptation*

39. 1. The endometrium is the inside lining of the uterus. Endometriosis is tissue growth by cells that look and act like endometrial cells. However, these cells grow outside the uterus in other areas, including on or under the ovaries, behind the uterus, or on the tissues that hold the uterus in place. A laparoscope is inserted through the abdominal wall. Once inserted, the instrument is used to visualize the intra-abdominal and pelvic organs, obtain biopsies of tissue, and perform therapeutic procedures.
Test Taking Strategy—*Analyze to determine what information the question asks for, which is the structure into which a laparoscope will be inserted. Recall that a laparoscope is used to visualize intra-abdominal pelvic structures. To do so requires inserting the instrument through the abdomen. Review how laparoscopic procedures are performed if you had difficulty answering this question.*

Cognitive Level—*Understanding*
Client Needs Category—*Physiological integrity*
Client Needs Subcategory—*Reduction of risk potential*

40. 2. Shoulder or abdominal discomfort may be experienced for 1 to 2 days after a laparoscopy. The discomfort is caused by the bolus of carbon dioxide instilled to distend the abdominal cavity. Nausea and leg cramps are unrelated to the laparoscopic procedure. Urinary urgency may occur after removal of the retention catheter used to keep the bladder empty during the laparoscopy, but it is not a direct effect of the procedure.
Test Taking Strategy—*Analyze to determine what information the question asks for, which is a sign or symptom caused by the laparoscopic procedure itself. Recall that gas is instilled within the abdomen to promote visualization. The gas, which is retained, rises to upper levels of the body, potentially causing shoulder or abdominal discomfort (option 2). Review the technique for performing a laparoscopy and signs and symptoms that may be experienced by a client on whom this procedure is performed if you had difficulty answering this question.*
Cognitive Level—*Applying*
Client Needs Category—*Physiological integrity*
Client Needs Subcategory—*Reduction of risk potential*

41. 4. Decreased estrogen production after menopause reduces the potential for vaginal lubrication. A dry vaginal mucous membrane is a common etiologic factor in painful intercourse after menopause. Pelvic muscles usually do not become more pressure sensitive with age. The amount of foreplay, if prolonged, can stimulate the clitoris. The vagina atrophies as a result of age-related changes.
Test Taking Strategy—*Use the process of elimination to help select the option that provides the best reason that an older female experiences discomfort during sexual intercourse. Option 1 can be eliminated immediately because pelvic muscles do not become more pressure-sensitive with age. Option 2 can be eliminated because the clitoris will respond to sexual foreplay, although it requires a longer amount of time to do so. Option 3 can be eliminated because the vagina atrophies in sexually inactive women, but at a marginal level of significance. Option 4 remains as the best answer because a reduction in mucus contributes to sexual discomfort. Review age-related sexual changes among females if you had difficulty answering this question.*
Cognitive Level—*Applying*
Client Needs Category—*Physiological integrity*
Client Needs Subcategory—*Physiological adaptation*

Nursing Care of Clients with Benign and Malignant Disorders of the Uterus and Ovaries

42. 1. Fibroid tumors respond to estrogen stimulation. Heavy menstrual bleeding is a common complaint of clients with myomas. Myomas arise from muscle tissue in the uterus and are usually benign. If pain occurs, it usually accompanies menstruation. Irregular light menses and breast tenderness, if present, are not associated with fibroid tumors.

> *Test Taking Strategy*—*Apply the key words "most likely" to the statements in each option. Select the option that correlates with a sign or symptom that occurs among women who have fibroid tumors. Myomas form on the muscle tissue inside or outside the uterus and respond similarly to the endometrium's response to estrogen levels. This means that when the endometrium is shed during menstruation, the myomas also bleed (option 1) adding to the volume of menstrual blood loss. Review the signs and symptoms caused by fibroid tumors if you had difficulty answering this question.*

Cognitive Level—*Applying*
Client Needs Category—*Physiological integrity*
Client Needs Subcategory—*Physiological adaptation*

43. 1. A full bladder is essential when performing a pelvic sonogram. Clients must consume at least a quart of water 1 hour before the examination and refrain from urinating until the examination is completed. Fasting is unnecessary. The examination is not painful, so an analgesic is unnecessary. No special skin preparation is required before the examination.

> *Test Taking Strategy*—*Apply the key words "most important" to each of the instructions described in the options. Select the option that identifies the most important information to tell a client before having a pelvic ultrasound. Recall that fluid within the bladder intensifies the sound waves, creating a clearer image of pelvic organs. This leads to choosing option 1 as the best answer. Review how a pelvic ultrasound is performed and why avoiding urination before the test can improve the diagnostic outcome if you had difficulty answering this question.*

Cognitive Level—*Applying*
Client Needs Category—*Physiological integrity*
Client Needs Subcategory—*Reduction of risk potential*

44. 2. All the data described are valid facts to document; however, documenting that this client has voided a sufficient amount to empty her bladder is most pertinent to the client's safety after discharge.

> *Test Taking Strategy*—*Look at the key words "most important" in reference to documentation that is essential to record in the medical record before dis-*charging a client who has undergone a dilation and curettage procedure. Recall that discharge criteria after any ambulatory surgery procedure includes that the client's discomfort has been managed, the client has tolerated oral fluids or a light diet, and most of all (option 2), that the client has voided. If the client is discharged without evidence of voiding, the client may need to return to an emergency department later for help to empty the bladder. Review criteria used to evaluate readiness for discharge after ambulatory surgery, focusing on which one is a priority, if you had difficulty answering this question.*

Cognitive Level—*Applying*
Client Needs Category—*Physiological integrity*
Client Needs Subcategory—*Reduction of risk potential*

45. 1. A colposcopy is a diagnostic procedure that is performed if the woman has an abnormal Pap smear. The colposcopy examines the cervix and the tissues of the vagina and vulva by illuminating and magnifying these tissues. It is common to have slight vaginal bleeding after a colposcopy; however, excessive bleeding is unusual and should be reported. None of the other options describes a common problem following colposcopy.

> *Test Taking Strategy*—*Analyze the information that the question asks about a postprocedural problem related to a colposcopy. Recall that a significant amount of vaginal bleeding (option 1) is a cause for concern. Review signs of complications after a colposcopy if you had difficulty answering this question.*

Cognitive Level—*Applying*
Client Needs Category—*Physiological integrity*
Client Needs Subcategory—*Reduction of risk potential*

46. 2. After electrocauterization, the client is told to avoid straining and heavy lifting because these activities may cause bleeding from the cauterized site. The physician usually reexamines the client in 2 to 4 weeks. Absolute bed rest is unnecessary, but the client should rest more than usual. Neither douching nor sexual intercourse is permitted until the physician indicates it is safe to do so, but avoiding sexual intercourse for 2 months is an unusually long time.

> *Test Taking Strategy*—*Apply the key words "most appropriate" to the choices. Select the discharge instruction that ensures the safety and well-being of the client after undergoing electrocauterization. Recall that activities such as heavy lifting that increase intra-abdominal pressure may contribute to excessive bleeding. Review precautions that a client who has undergone electrocauterization should follow until healing occurs if you had difficulty answering this question.*

Cognitive Level—*Analyzing*
Client Needs Category—*Health promotion and maintenance*
Client Needs Subcategory—*None*

47. 3. Like other sexually transmitted infections such as genital herpes, certain strains of human papillomavirus (HPV) are a risk factor for cervical cancer. HPV causes cervical dysplasia (abnormal cells), a precursor of cancer, which validates the necessity for regular Pap tests. Other risk factors include sexual intercourse before age 16, multiple sex partners, and multiple pregnancies. Menstruation beginning at age 12 years is normal. Spontaneous abortion and history of maternal breast cancer are not risk factors for cervical cancer. A vaccination for HPV is available.

Test Taking Strategy—Analyze to determine what information the question asks for, which is identifying the highest risk factor for developing cervical cancer from among the four options. Recall that the HPV virus (option 3), if not destroyed by the immune system, survives and slowly over several years converts cells on the surface of the cervix to cancer. Review the connection between infections with HPV and the development of cervical cancer if you had difficulty answering this question.
Cognitive Level—*Analyzing*
Client Needs Category—*Physiological integrity*
Client Needs Subcategory—*Reduction of risk potential*

48. 1, 3, 6. Cervical cancer is a malignancy involving the cervix (the lower portion of the uterus) or the cervical structures. The early stages of cervical cancer may be completely asymptomatic. Vaginal bleeding occurs in the advanced stages. Identifying the number of sanitary pads used helps quantify the extent of bleeding. Other symptoms of advanced cervical cancer may include anorexia; weight loss due to poor nutrition or as a consequence of the cancer; fatigue due to nutritional deficiencies or chronic vaginal bleeding; pelvic, back, or leg pain; a single swollen leg; and bone fractures. The color of the blood provides a characteristic of the blood loss, but it does not indicate the extent of bleeding. Sexual frequency does not provide clinical data that can be used to make a diagnosis. Itching and swelling of the labia are not related to cervical cancer but to sexually transmitted infectinons.

Test Taking Strategy—Analyze to determine what information the question asks for, which correlates vaginal bleeding and its possible connection to cervical cancer. Alternative-format "select all that apply" questions require considering each option independently to decide its merit in answering the question. Review signs and symptoms of cervical cancer if you had difficulty answering this question.
Cognitive Level—*Analyzing*
Client Needs Category—*Physiological integrity*
Client Needs Subcategory—*Physiological adaptation*

49. 2, 5, 6. There are several methods used to treat cervical cancer depending on the progression of the disease. A hysterectomy may be done in the earlier stages; chemotherapy or radiation therapy or a combination of the two may be used in addition to the hysterectomy in the later stages. Internal radiation therapy is a form of treatment in which a source of radiation is put inside the client's body. Bed rest must be maintained to retain the applicator within the vagina. In fact, the head of the bed should not be raised more than 45 degrees while the radioactive applicator is in place. To provide safety for the nurse and avoid excessive exposure to radiation, the nurse should stand at a distance and talk with the client from the doorway, spending as little time in the room as possible. The client should be instructed about radiation safety precautions before the placement of the implant. Weighing the client is postponed while the radioactive applicator is in place. It is not necessary to contain urine or feces.

Test Taking Strategy—Analyze to determine what information the question asks for, which is the care of a client receiving internal radiation therapy. Alternative-format "select all that apply" questions require considering each option independently to decide its merit in answering the question. Critically appraise each option and select all of the nursing interventions that are appropriate to include in the nursing care plan for this client. Choose options that help to retain the radioactive substance in place as well as protect nursing personnel from accumulating an unsafe level of radiation. Review precautions that should be followed when a client receives internal radiation therapy, especially when a device is implanted vaginally, if you had difficulty answering this question.
Cognitive Level—*Analyzing*
Client Needs Category—*Safe and effective care environment*
Client Needs Subcategory—*Safety and infection control*

50. 4. Displaced radioactive materials are placed in a lead container as soon as they are discovered. The nurse should avoid contact with the radioactive materials if at all possible and should call the radiation safety department or nuclear medicine department. The lead container blocks the transmission of radioactivity. The nuclear medicine department then manages the substance appropriately. Radioactive substances are never discarded. The physician, not the nurse, is responsible for reinserting the implant.

Test Taking Strategy—Apply the key words "most appropriate" to help select an option that identifies a nursing action that should be taken upon finding a displaced radioactive substance. Recall that lead interferes with gamma radiation, making option 4 the correct answer. Review procedures to follow when handling and disposing of radioactive material if you had difficulty answering this question.
Cognitive Level—*Applying*
Client Needs Category—*Safe and effective care environment*
Client Needs Subcategory—*Safety and infection control*

51. 3. Distance is one measure used to reduce exposure to radiation. Therefore, radioactive substances are never held with the hands. A long-handled forceps and lead container should be in the room of a client who has a radioactive implant in a body orifice. Neither washing the hands nor using a glass jar will control exposure to radiation. Rubber gloves rather than vinyl gloves provide better protection, but the radioactive substance should never be touched with the hands.

> *Test Taking Strategy*—*Use the process of elimination to help select the option that identifies the best action that protects the nurse who must retrieve or move a radioactive substance. Always consider measures that reduce exposure to radiation. Eliminate options 1 and 2 as providing little resistance to radiation exposure. Eliminate option 4 because it does not address how the implant was moved to the jar nor does glass act as a barrier to radiation. Option 3 remains as the correct answer because the long-handled forceps are used in lieu of the nurse's hands. Review the radiation exposure protocol if you had difficulty answering this question.*
> *Cognitive Level*—*Applying*
> *Client Needs Category*—*Safe and effective care environment*
> *Client Needs Subcategory*—*Safety and infection control*

52. 2. All the described nurses have strengths that may be helpful to this client. However, because exposure to radiation can affect male and female gametes (sex cells), it is best that a nurse for whom pregnancy is unlikely or a male nurse who has had a vasectomy should care for the client.

> *Test Taking Strategy*—*Use the process of elimination to help select the option that identifies the nurse who is best suited to care for the client with a device delivering internal radiation. Because radiation exposure has the potential for damaging sperm and ova, options 1, 3, and 4 can be eliminated; there is nothing in those options that indicates the reproductive status of the nurses. Option 2 is the best answer because a nurse who has had a hysterectomy is unable to become pregnant with an ovum that has been damaged by radiation. Review the types of cells that are affected by exposure to radiation if you had difficulty answering this question.*
> *Cognitive Level*—*Analyzing*
> *Client Needs Category*—*Safe and effective care environment*
> *Client Needs Subcategory*—*Coordinated care*

53. 1. All clients who receive general anesthesia are prone to respiratory complications. Because a clear airway and breathing are higher priorities than nutrition to maintain immediately postoperatively, Risk for ineffective airway clearance is the most appropriate addition at this time.

It is too early to make the diagnosis *Ineffective coping*. The client should have no difficulty communicating verbally when she returns from the postanesthesia recovery room.

> *Test Taking Strategy*—*Apply the key words "most appropriate" when selecting the nursing diagnosis that pertains to a postoperative client. Regardless of the type of surgery a client has undergone, always consider maintaining a patent airway that is free of secretions (option 1) as a priority nursing diagnosis. Review common postoperative problems that guide the selection of nursing diagnoses and interventions when planning for the client's care if you had difficulty answering this question.*
> *Cognitive Level*—*Applying*
> *Client Needs Category*—*Safe and effective care environment*
> *Client Needs Subcategory*—*Coordinated care*

54. 1. Antiembolism stockings are frequently ordered for postoperative clients and those unable to ambulate to circulate venous blood to the heart. These clients are at high risk for developing a blood clot. Antiembolism stockings are used to reduce stasis of venous blood in the extremities that could cause a thrombus and embolus to occur. Antiembolism stockings should be worn continuously except when removed for assessment and hygiene.

> *Test Taking Strategy*—*Look at the key words "most appropriate," select the option that describes a standard of care involving the use of antiembolism stockings. Recall that pooling of venous blood can occur throughout the client's period of inactivity, which indicates that the stockings should be removed only briefly and then reapplied. Review the policy for applying and removing antiembolism stockings if you had difficulty answering this question.*
> *Cognitive Level*—*Applying*
> *Client Needs Category*—*Physiological integrity*
> *Client Needs Subcategory*—*Basic care and comfort*

55. 3, 4, 5, 6. Clients who have had abdominal surgery are prone to developing blood clots in their lower extremities. Therefore, the knees should not be elevated because doing so promotes stasis of blood flow. In addition, the client's calves should never be massaged. Gloves must be worn when dealing with blood and body fluids. Reporting to the physician that the dressing is loose is a nursing function, not one for the unlicensed assistant. All the other activities are appropriate in the care for a client recovering from a hysterectomy.

> *Test Taking Strategy*—*Analyze to determine what information the question asks for, which are appropriate actions for a nursing assistant to perform for a postoperative hysterectomy client. Alternative-format "select all that apply" questions require considering each option independently to decide its merit in answering the question. Choose the options that indicate an unsafe or*

inappropriate action being performed by the nursing assistant. Review potential complications and the scope of care required when a client has an abdominal hysterectomy if you had difficulty answering this question.
Cognitive Level—Evaluating
Client Needs Category—Safe and effective care environment
Client Needs Subcategory—Coordinated care

56. 3. It is important to deflate the balloon first so that the catheter can be removed from the urethra. Not deflating the balloon can lead to urethral trauma and damage. Cleaning the client's perineum and measuring her urine output are essential actions, but they can be postponed until after the catheter has been removed. It is unnecessary to separate the catheter from the drainage bag. After the bag is emptied, both can be disposed of in an appropriate waste receptacle.
Test Taking Strategy—Look at the key words "most important to perform" and "first" in reference to removing the urinary retention catheter. Recall that the balloon that was inflated with fluid must be emptied first (option 3) to avoid injury to the client. Options 1, 2, and 4 are components of removing the urinary catheter, but they are completed after the catheter is removed. Review the procedure for Foley catheter removal if you had difficulty answering this question.
Cognitive Level—Applying
Client Needs Category—Physiological integrity
Client Needs Subcategory—Basic care and comfort

57. 2. To measure the volume of urine retained in the bladder, it is important to catheterize the client within 10 minutes of voiding. The size of the catheter is relative to the size of the client; however, the size is not pertinent to the purpose of the procedure. The catheter is connected to gravity drainage only if the physician orders a retention catheter based on a certain retained volume.
Test Taking Strategy—Look at the key words "most appropriate" when evaluating the statements in each option. Select the option that describes the correct plan to follow when obtaining and measuring residual urine. By catheterizing the client shortly thereafter (option 2), a decision can be made on whether to replace the catheter, depending on the presence of urine remaining in the bladder and its quantity. The urinary residual should normally measure less than 100 mL. Review the procedure for measuring residual urine if you had difficulty answering this question.
Cognitive Level—Applying
Client Needs Category—Physiological integrity
Client Needs Subcategory—Reduction of risk potential

58. 2. The dosages of many toxic drugs administered to adults, as well as drugs administered to children, are calculated on the basis of the client's body surface area (BSA). BSA is calculated by using both body weight and height. The other options are important to obtain but have no relationship to the dosage of the drug that will be administered.
Test Taking Strategy—Analyze to determine what information the question asks for, which is essential information on which to base the dose of a chemotherapy drug. Recall that many chemotherapy drugs require the client's height and weight (option 2) to calculate a dose based on the individual client's BSA. Review the formula used to calculate BSA and the types of drugs that are prescribed according to BSA if you had difficulty answering this question.
Cognitive Level—Applying
Client Needs Category—Physiological integrity
Client Needs Subcategory—Pharmacological therapies

59. 4. Antineoplastic medications can affect the function of bone marrow, which produces the blood cells. A complete blood count provides information about all the cells that the bone marrow produces. The mean cell volume, total leukocyte count, and differential cell count are all important, but none is as comprehensively informative as a complete blood cell count.
Test Taking Strategy—Apply the key words "most important" when analyzing the choices in the four options to select the laboratory test that is best to monitor for the depletion of bone marrow function. Recall that all blood cells are formed in the bone marrow, making option 4 the best answer because it will determine whether it is safe to continue administering the antineoplastic medication, administer blood or a drug like a colony-stimulating factor to increase blood cell production, or temporarily delay chemotherapy. Review the tests listed and the information they provide if you had difficulty answering this question.
Cognitive Level—Applying
Client Needs Category—Physiological integrity
Client Needs Subcategory—Reduction of risk potential

60. 1. The nurse identifies a priority nursing diagnosis of anxiety evidenced by an inability to manage routine affairs. Clients frequently are overwhelmed with a cancer diagnosis. The best evidence of improvement would be the client's ability to successfully manage personal affairs. Attending support groups, maintaining family/friend relationships and participating in health care decisions are positive actions related to the accepting of the diagnosis.
Test Taking Strategy—Use the process of elimination to help select the option that identifies the best evidence of problem reduction or resolution as it

relates to the nursing diagnostic statement. Review the principles for developing goal statements and expected outcomes if you had difficulty answering this question.
Cognitive Level—*Evaluating*
Client Needs Category—*Safe and effective care environment*
Client Needs Subcategory—*Coordinated care*

61. 4. The hair lost with some antineoplastic drugs returns after chemotherapy is terminated. The return of hair growth varies from client to client, but in all cases it is restored in less than 2 years. However, the new hair growth may be different in color or texture from the past hair type of the individual.
> *Test Taking Strategy—Look at the key words "most accurate," and apply them to the information in the four options. Select the option that correlates with correct information regarding hair loss associated with antineoplastic chemotherapy. Note that there are two pairs of opposite options—two that identify that the hair loss is permanent and two that identify that hair loss is temporary. Decide first if the hair loss is temporary or permanent, which reduces the selection to two remaining options. Option 4 is the best answer because the hair loss is temporary and hair growth resumes after the medication is discontinued. Review the side effects associated with antineoplastic drug therapy, focusing on hair loss and its future outcome, if you had difficulty answering this question.*
Cognitive Level—*Applying*
Client Needs Category—*Physiological integrity*
Client Needs Subcategory—*Pharmacological therapies*

Nursing Care of Clients with Miscellaneous Disorders of the Female Reproductive System

62. 2. A prolapsed uterus is a condition in which the uterus descends or changes position with the surrounding structures in the pelvis. When the supporting structures become stretched or weak, they cannot support the uterus and the uterus falls. Standing and bearing down is the best technique for determining the extent of uterine prolapse. Using this technique, the nurse can evaluate the effect of gravity in relation to the relaxed pelvic muscles. The other assessment techniques are used if the client is unable to stand.
> *Test Taking Strategy—Use the process of elimination to help select the option that describes the best method for assessing the extent of a prolapsed uterus. Note that all of the options describe methods for examining the perineum, but only one method is the best*

choice. Because the prolapse is more obvious when the client stands, option 2 is the best answer. Review techniques for examining a client to determine the extent of uterine prolapse if you had difficulty answering this question.
Cognitive Level—*Applying*
Client Needs Category—*Physiological integrity*
Client Needs Subcategory—*Physiological adaptation*

63. 4. A cystocele occurs when the wall between the bladder and vagina weakens and allows the bladder to fall into the vagina. This condition may cause problems with emptying the bladder. The majority of clients with a cystocele experience stress incontinence. Stress incontinence is manifested by a slight loss of urine when abdominal pressure increases, as with sneezing, coughing, laughing, and lifting heavy objects. Awakening in the morning, walking, and sleeping do not promote stress incontinence.
> *Test Taking Strategy—Look at the key words "most likely," and apply them to the descriptions in the options to determine when a client with a cystocele typically experiences urinary incontinence. Recall that the levator ani muscles elevate the bladder neck and support the urethra. When these become weakened, the urethra is stretched, resulting in leakage of urine, especially when there is an increase in abdominal pressure such as when sneezing (option 4). Review the factors that contribute to urinary incontinence secondary to a cystocele if you had difficulty answering this question.*
Cognitive Level—*Applying*
Client Needs Category—*Physiological integrity*
Client Needs Subcategory—*Physiological adaptation*

64. 3. Perineal exercises, also known as Kegel exercises, strengthen the pubococcygeal muscles, components of the levator ani group of muscles, which help suspend the bladder. Purchasing absorbent underwear is an option if the cystocele is more serious or if the client chooses not to proceed with a surgical repair. Applying an external catheter is an option but not a very effective or popular one. It is inappropriate to limit oral fluid intake as a means of controlling adult incontinence.
> *Test Taking Strategy—Use the process of elimination to help select the option that identifies the best intervention for promoting a client's control over leaking urine. Options 1 and 2 can be eliminated immediately because they are means of collecting urine, not controlling it. Option 4 can be eliminated because an adequate fluid intake is essential for maintaining fluid balance. Option 3 remains as the best answer because strengthening the pubococcygeal muscles by performing Kegel exercises promotes the ability to retain urine within the bladder; it also facilitates reaching orgasm during sexual intercourse. Review*

the function of the pubococcygeal muscles and how they may be strengthened if you had difficulty answering this question.
Cognitive Level—*Applying*
Client Needs Category—*Health promotion and maintenance*
Client Needs Subcategory—*None*

65. **2.** Absence of a urinary tract infection is the best indication that the client is following appropriate aseptic principles when performing self-catheterization. The volume of urine should be more than 50 mL if the bladder is being emptied completely. The catheter should be removed immediately after the bladder is emptied. The frequency of catheterization depends on the client's rate of urine formation and sensation of a need to void. Frequency of catheterization is not an indication of appropriate technique.

> *Test Taking Strategy*—*Use the process of elimination to help select the option that describes the best evidence that a client is performing self-catheterization correctly. Option 1 can be eliminated because self-catheterization should remove more than 50 mL if it is performed when feeling a need to void. Option 3 can be eliminated because the catheter need only remain in place a short amount of time—similar to the amount of time it takes to urinate naturally. Option 4 can be eliminated because keeping a record is not evidence that the procedure is being performed correctly. Option 2 remains as the best answer because if self-catheterization is being performed correctly, the client should be free of a urinary tract infection. Review the expected outcomes for self-catheterization if you had difficulty answering this question.*
Cognitive Level—*Evaluating*
Client Needs Category—*Physiological integrity*
Client Needs Subcategory—*Reduction of risk potential*

66. **1, 2, 4, 5.** Alendronate (Fosamax) may be prescribed to help increase bone mass when bone resorption exceeds bone formation—a condition that occurs among women as they age, especially during the postmenopausal years when estrogen levels decrease significantly. Alendronate may cause esophageal irritation; therefore, measures to promote gastric emptying are encouraged. This includes taking the medication on awakening with 6 to 8 ounces of water (not food or milk) and remaining upright for at least 30 minutes. Alendronate neither relieves hot flashes or irritability nor eases any other discomforts commonly associated with menopause.

> *Test Taking Strategy*—*Analyze to determine what information the question asks for, which is health teaching for a client who will self-administer alendronate (Fosamax). Alternative-format "select all that apply" questions require considering each option independently to decide its merit in answering*

the question. Choose options that contain information a client must know to avoid the risk of side effects. Review health teaching that is appropriate for whomever Fosamax is prescribed if you had difficulty answering this question.
Cognitive Level—*Applying*
Client Needs Category—*Physiological integrity*
Client Needs Subcategory—*Pharmacological therapies*

Nursing Care of Clients with Inflammatory Disorders of the Male Reproductive System

67. **3.** Inadequate treatment leads to the development of a chronic condition. Whenever an antibiotic is prescribed, it is important to stress that the client take all the medication. Taking only a portion of the medication may not be sufficient to destroy the infectious microorganism; it can also contribute to the development of resistant strains. Drinking milk, reporting significant information, and monitoring body temperature may be important in some cases. The latter recommendations are based more on such factors as the side effects of the drug, the condition for which the drug is prescribed, and the client's physical condition.

> *Test Taking Strategy*—*Analyze to determine what information the question asks for, which is information that is a priority when the nurse instructs a client about antibiotic therapy for the treatment of prostatitis. Recall that in order to destroy all the urinary pathogens, the client must take the full amount of the medication for the prescribed amount of time (option 3). Review the factors that contribute to ineffective antibiotic therapy and the potential for developing resistant strains of pathogens if you had difficulty answering this question.*
Cognitive Level—*Applying*
Client Needs Category—*Physiological integrity*
Client Needs Subcategory—*Pharmacological therapies*

68. **2.** The prostate surrounds the urethra and when enlarged can induce discomfort and difficulty passing urine due to a stricture. A sitz bath soothes the area, relieving pain and possible inflammation. It is more effective if it lasts approximately 20 minutes. The water should be about 100°F (37.8°C), which is considered warm, not tepid. Soap is omitted with a sitz bath; the bath's purpose is to apply heat and relieve discomfort, not clean the area. Massaging the scrotum has no direct benefit in relieving the client's symptoms.

> *Test Taking Strategy*—*Analyze to determine what information the question asks for, which is a nursing instruction for using a sitz bath for comfort. Recall that a sitz bath promotes comfort as a result of the warm temperature of the water and the length of time the client's perineum is immersed (option 2).*

Review the purposes for a sitz bath and the manner in which the procedure is performed if you had difficulty answering this question.
Cognitive Level—Applying
Client Needs Category—Physiological integrity
Client Needs Subcategory—Basic care and comfort

69. 2. The epididymis is a tightly coiled tube in the scrotum that is used to transport sperm. An inflammation of this structure is called *epididymitis*. Only a small portion of urine voided in midstream (after the first release of urine is wasted) is collected in a clean-catch specimen. The procedure does require cleaning the penis, retracting the foreskin if the client is uncircumcised, and depositing the urine directly into a sterile container.

Test Taking Strategy—Analyze to determine what information the question asks for, which is an inaccurate client statement about collecting a clean-catch urine specimen. Recall that a urine culture can be performed with as little as 10 to 15 mL of urine. Therefore, the statement in option 2 requires clarification because the amount of urine in a full voiding exceeds that amount. Review the procedure for collecting a clean catch urine specimen if you had difficulty answering this question.
Cognitive Level—Evaluating
Client Needs Category—Physiological integrity
Client Needs Subcategory—Reduction of risk potential

70. 1. Elevating and supporting the scrotum helps to relieve the discomfort of epididymitis. Analgesics are also prescribed. Wearing larger underwear or cotton briefs is a personal choice and does not inherently relieve the client's symptoms. Heat is contraindicated because it can damage sperm.

Test Taking Strategy—Use the process of elimination to help select the option describing the best method for providing comfort for the client with a swollen scrotum. Options 2 and 3 can be eliminated because modifications in underwear are not the best approaches for providing comfort. Option 4 can be eliminated because the term "hot" suggests that the client's scrotal skin may be burned. Option 1 remains as the correct answer because supporting the scrotum reduces scrotal movement, which intensifies pain. Review methods for relieving the scrotal discomfort associated with epididymitis or other conditions such as postvasectomy if you had difficulty answering this question.
Cognitive Level—Applying
Client Needs Category—Physiological integrity
Client Needs Subcategory—Basic care and comfort

71. 3. Orchitis is a painful condition of the testicles involving inflammation, swelling and, frequently, infection. Often it is the result of epididymitis that has spread to the testes. The mumps virus can infect the testes of males who have not been adequately immunized before puberty. A sexually transmitted infection would be likely if the client's testes and epididymis are co-infected, but that is not the case in this situation. Orchitis is not commonly reported in clients who have had sports-related scrotal injuries.

Test Taking Strategy—Look at the key words "most suggestive" in reference to a cause of orchitis. Read the options looking for one that correlates with an etiology for this condition. Recall that the virus that causes mumps can cause orchitis in prepubertal to middle-aged adult males who have not received the mumps immunization. Review the causes of orchitis if you had difficulty answering this question.
Cognitive Level—Applying
Client Needs Category—Physiological integrity
Client Needs Subcategory—Physiological adaptation

72. 2. When performing a testicular self-examination, the client should examine each testicle separately, rolling it between the thumb and fingers. It is easier to palpate the testes when the scrotum is warm, such as during or after a shower. Testicular self-examination should be performed monthly.

Test Taking Strategy—Analyze to determine what information the question asks for, which is how a male should perform testicular self-examination. Recall that the testes lie within the scrotum and that they can be felt when the scrotal tissue is rolled between the thumb and fingers. Review how a testicular self-examination is performed if you had difficulty answering this question.
Cognitive Level—Applying
Client Needs Category—Health promotion and maintenance
Client Needs Subcategory—None

Nursing Care of Clients with Structural Disorders of the Male Reproductive System

73. 1. As long as one testicle is descended, the testicle will most likely produce sufficient testosterone for normal secondary sexual characteristics, adequate sperm for conception, and a healthy sex drive. Impotence, the inability to achieve an erection, is not generally compromised.

Test Taking Strategy—Apply the key words "most appropriate" when considering the statement in each of the four options. Select the option that identifies the effect that having one undescended testicle will have on a male's sexuality. Recall that having one functioning testicle can sustain normal hormone levels for achieving and maintaining secondary sex characteristics and potential fertility (option 1). Review the potential consequences associated with having an undescended testicle if you had difficulty answering this question.

Cognitive Level—Applying
Client Needs Category—Physiological integrity
Client Needs Subcategory—Physiological adaptation

74. 3. The priority nursing assessments after a circumcision include checking the amount of local bleeding and the client's ability to void. Swelling can obstruct the urethra and interfere with urination. Deep breathing is a routine assessment for surgical clients who have received general anesthesia. It would be inappropriate to assess the client's erectile function at this time. I.V. antibiotics are not usually prescribed for this type of surgery.

> *Test Taking Strategy—Analyze to determine what information the question asks for, which is a priority for postoperative nursing assessment after an adult male's circumcision. Based on the surgical procedure, localized swelling around the urethra may interfere with the client's ability to void, which leads to selecting option 3. Review the postoperative nursing management of a client who has had a circumcision if you had difficulty answering this question.*

Cognitive Level—Applying
Client Needs Category—Physiological integrity
Client Needs Subcategory—Reduction of risk potential

75. 2. Whenever a cold or warm device is placed on a client's body, the device is placed within some type of fabric cover. A plastic bag is not an appropriate cover. A hypothermia blanket is too large for the local effect desired. An ice-filled ring would not cover the area sufficiently to produce a local effect.

> *Test Taking Strategy—Apply the key words "most appropriate" and select the option that describes the best method for a cold application to the scrotum. Recall that the scrotum must be protected from an extreme difference in temperature. Enclosing an ice pack within a cover prevents direct contact between the scrotal skin and the cold device. Review principles that apply to applications of heat and cold if you had difficulty answering this question.*

Cognitive Level—Applying
Client Needs Category—Safe and effective care environment
Client Needs Subcategory—Safety and infection control

Nursing Care of Clients with Benign and Malignant Disorders of the Male Reproductive System

76. 2. The best position for assessing the characteristics of the prostate gland is one in which the client leans forward from the waist while standing, bracing his body against the examination table for support. The rectum can be examined with the client in the lithotomy and dorsal recumbent positions, but these are not the preferred positions. A Fowler's position does not facilitate a rectal examination.

> *Test Taking Strategy—Analyze to determine what information the question asks for, which is the preferred position for a prostate examination. Recall that when the prostate is manually examined, the physician inserts a lubricated finger into the rectum, making option 2 the best answer. Visualize the prostate examination procedure, which leads to the correct answer. Knowledge of medical terminology is also helpful in discriminating between options. Review the technique used to do a digital examination of the prostate gland if you had difficulty answering this question.*

Cognitive Level—Applying
Client Needs Category—Health promotion and maintenance
Client Needs Subcategory—None

77.

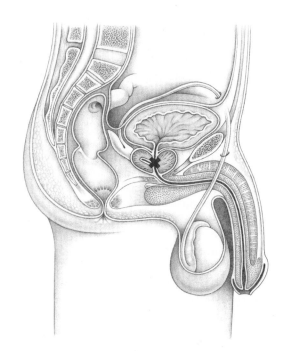

The prostate gland is a walnut-sized structure that surrounds the male urethra just beneath the bladder.

> *Test Taking Strategy—Analyze to determine what information the question asks for, which is the anatomic location of the prostate gland. Recall that when the prostate gland is enlarged, it may obstruct the flow of urine when the client attempts to void. Review the male anatomy if you had difficulty answering this question.*

Cognitive Level—Applying
Client Needs Category—Physiological integrity
Client Needs Subcategory—Physiological adaptation

78. 3. In the early stages of benign prostatic hypertrophy (BPH), the progression of prostatic enlargement is monitored with periodic digital rectal examinations. A prostate-specific antigen (PSA) test is no longer recommended because it has led to unnecessary treatment of prostate cancer in the past. As BPH progresses, the physician may use cystoscopy to determine the extent of the infringement on the urethra and the effects on the bladder. A retrograde pyelogram is a diagnostic test commonly used to provide information about possible damage to the upper urinary tract due to urine retention.

Test Taking Strategy—Analyze to determine what information the question asks for, which is how the progression of BPH is monitored. Recall that a digital rectal examination is the most expedient way to determine the size and shape of the prostate gland. This examination is generally performed during a yearly physical of male clients. Review the manner in which BPH is diagnosed and evaluated if you had difficulty answering this question.
Cognitive Level—Analyzing
Client Needs Category—Physiological integrity
Client Needs Subcategory—Reduction of risk potential

79.

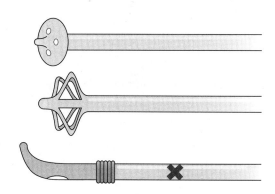

A Coudé catheter is used in lieu of a flexible catheter to overcome urethral obstructions because it has a stiffer and pointed tip. The first catheter in the illustration is a mushroom-shaped de Pezzer catheter and the second is a wing-tipped Malecot catheter; both of these are inserted by a physician and require a stylet.

Test Taking Strategy—Analyze to determine what information the question asks for, which is the most appropriate catheter selection for a client with a urethral obstruction. Relate the differences in the catheters to the difficulties of a urethral obstruction. Recall that Coudé catheters have a unique design that enables them to pass through a small opening. Review urinary catheter styles and function if you had difficulty answering this question.
Cognitive Level—Applying
Client Needs Category—Physiological integrity
Client Needs Subcategory—Reduction of risk potential

80. 2. After draining 700 mL of urine, the client should feel relief. Draining any more than 1,000 mL in a short amount of time can contribute to bladder spasms or loss of bladder tone. More urine can be removed after waiting a period of time. The physician may override this rule of thumb in special circumstances.

Test Taking Strategy—Analyze to determine what information the question asks for, which is the volume of urine that should be removed with a catheter. Recall that the standard of care is to remove no more than 1,000 mL of urine at any one time for whatever reason. Review guidelines for urinary catheterization if you had difficulty answering this question.
Cognitive Level—Understanding
Client Needs Category—Physiological integrity
Client Needs Subcategory—Reduction of risk potential

81. 4. When a prostate sonogram is performed, a rectal probe is inserted. The presence of stool can interfere with imaging the prostate as well as contribute to discomfort. Therefore, it is important to empty the rectum completely. The client may wish to empty his bladder as well, but that is not necessary with this test. The test does not require fasting. Water may be instilled within the sheath surrounding the rectal probe; the client is not required to consume a large volume of water.

Test Taking Strategy—Apply the key words "most correct" when analyzing each of the four options to determine which one is the best answer. Recall that the prostate gland is assessed from the rectal area. Review client preparation before a prostatic sonogram if you had difficulty answering this question.
Cognitive Level—Analyzing
Client Needs Category—Physiological integrity
Client Needs Subcategory—Reduction of risk potential

82. 275 mL.
The irrigation solution is a part of the volume that collects in the drainage bag. Therefore, to find the true urine output, the amount of instilled irrigant is subtracted from the volume in the drainage bag.

Test Taking Strategy—Analyze to determine what information the question asks for, which is the portion of urine contained in the drainage collection bag. Recall that the collection bag has a combination of irrigant and urine. Subtracting the volume of irrigant from the total volume leads to the correct answer. Review principles for calculating intake and output if you had difficulty answering this question.
Cognitive Level—Understanding
Client Needs Category—Physiological integrity
Client Needs Subcategory—Basic care and comfort

83. 1. Obstructions in the drainage catheter are the chief cause of bladder discomfort after transurethral resection of the prostate (TURP). Therefore, the nurse should check for patency of the drainage catheter. A belladonna and opium suppository may be helpful, but this option is not the first course of action. Sitting can increase intra-abdominal pressure and contribute to more bleeding. Ambulating may or may not improve drainage through the catheter, but it is not the first choice of actions.

   Test Taking Strategy—Use the process of elimination to help select the option that identifies the best action to take first when a client who has a catheter feels a need to void. Recall that the bladder should be nearly empty when a retention catheter is in place. Therefore, the first action the nurse should take is to check that the catheter is not obstructed (option 1). Neither option 2 nor option 4 is the first step to take; option 3 can be eliminated because it increases the risk of bleeding. Review factors that may lead to an obstruction in urinary drainage following a TURP if you had difficulty answering this question.
   Cognitive Level—Applying
   Client Needs Category—Physiological integrity
   Client Needs Subcategory—Reduction of risk potential

84. 3. In the immediate postoperative period, all urinary drainage catheters, including the cystostomy tube, are unclamped to facilitate drainage. The suprapubic cystostomy tube is clamped later when bladder retraining is begun. A cystostomy catheter is too short to attach directly to the thigh or a leg bag; it would require a separate drainage tube and urine collection bag.

   Test Taking Strategy—Look at the key words "most appropriate," and apply them when considering the choice in each option. Look for the option that supports the purpose of the cystostomy tube in the immediate postoperative period, which is to provide continuous urinary drainage (option 3). Review the reasons a suprapubic cystostomy tube is inserted and how care of the catheter is managed if you had difficulty answering this question.
   Cognitive Level—Applying
   Client Needs Category—Physiological integrity
   Client Needs Subcategory—Physiological adaptation

85. 3. When caring for a client following a suprapubic prostatectomy, the nurse must assess for the common complication of urinary bleeding. The nurse monitors the color and amount of urine. Urinary retention is not a complication as a catheter drains all urine. Flank pain and flatus are not common complications.

   Test Taking Strategy—Look at the key words "most important," and apply them when analyzing each of the four options describing a common postoperative complication associated with a suprapubic prostatectomy. Look for the option that identifies a common postoperative complication following a suprapubic prostatectomy. Recall that irrigation of the bladder helps to ensure that blood clots do not obstruct the urinary catheter making option 3 bleeding the best answer. Review postoperative complications of a suprapubic prostatectomy if you had difficulty answering this question. Review postoperative care after prostate surgery if you had difficulty answering this question.
   Cognitive Level—Applying
   Client Needs Category—Safe and effective care environment
   Client Needs Subcategory—Coordinated care

86. 3. Orchiectomy is the removal of the testicles when a malignancy occurs. One functioning testis ought to produce enough testosterone to sustain all of a man's secondary sex characteristics and his libido. However, after this surgery, the sperm count is reduced and the motility of the sperm is impaired.

   Test Taking Strategy—Analyze to determine what information the question asks for, which is a statement that indicates the client is mistaken about the consequences of an orchiectomy. Evaluate the options for accuracy. Recall that the remaining testis can produce sufficient sex-related hormones, but the number of sperm that will be produced is altered. Review the sexual consequences of an orchiectomy if you had difficulty answering this question.
   Cognitive Level—Analyzing
   Client Needs Category—Physiological integrity
   Client Needs Subcategory—Physiological adaptation

Nursing Care of Clients with Sexually Transmitted Infections

87. 2. Conveying a nonjudgmental attitude facilitates obtaining truthful information from the person who feels uncomfortable discussing sexual information. Being sympathetic, encouraging, and optimistic are all positive attributes, but none of these is as important as being nonjudgmental.

   Test Taking Strategy—Look at the key words "most important," and apply them to the choices in the options. Look for the attitude that is best for facilitating discussion of information of a sexual nature. Recall that to promote an open dialogue regarding a sensitive topic, it is important to be nonjudgmental (option 2). Review interviewing techniques that are best when collecting sexual information if you had difficulty answering this question.
   Cognitive Level—Applying
   Client Needs Category—Psychosocial integrity
   Client Needs Subcategory—None

88. 2. Asking a person if any sex partner has similar symptoms helps to determine if the cause of the client's symptoms is a sexually transmitted infection. A painless sore is a symptom of syphilis, which is not the most common sexually transmitted infection, but may be asked if the client reports having a lesion on the penis, rectal area, mouth, or nose. The age at which a person first had sexual intercourse is unrelated to the present symptoms. Incubation periods vary among sexually transmitted infections; identifying the most recent date of sexual intercourse will not identify the time at which the infection was transmitted.

> *Test Taking Strategy—The key words are "most important," which indicates that the correct choice is one that represents a priority. Because STIs are infectious, it is most important to determine if there are similar symptoms among the client's sex partner(s), which is option 2. Review information that is important to obtain when obtaining a sexual history, focusing on those that are pertinent to the acquisition of a sexually transmitted infection, if you had difficulty answering this question.*
> *Cognitive Level—Analyzing*
> *Client Needs Category—Physiological integrity*
> *Client Needs Subcategory—Physiological adaptation*

89. 1, 2, 3. Gonorrhea is a common sexually transmitted infection with the highest incidence among 14- to 15-year-olds. It is caused by bacteria, making it easy to treat. The bacteria enter the urethra, vagina, rectum, or throat, depending on the manner of sexual contact. Most females are asymptomatic. Males, if symptomatic, usually experience symptoms 2 to 6 days after exposure and have burning on urination; yellow, white, or green drainage from the penis; and soreness in the scrotum. Painless ulcers (chancres) on the penis are more common with syphilis. Blisters on the penis are common in herpes infections; extra skin (soft, fleshy growths) growing around the penis is common with venereal warts.

> *Test Taking Strategy—Analyze to determine what information the question asks for, which is symptoms of gonorrhea. Alternative-format "select all that apply" questions require considering each option independently to decide its merit in answering the question. Review the signs and symptoms associated with a gonorrheal infection in a male if you had difficulty answering this question.*
> *Cognitive Level—Applying*
> *Client Needs Category—Physiological integrity*
> *Client Needs Subcategory—Physiological adaptation*

90. 3. Intimate sexual contact with one or more sexual partners is the highest risk factor among the options listed for acquiring a sexually transmitted infection. Developing sexually at an early age does not necessarily affect a person's sexual choices. Internet access for children and adolescents can be informative if the site is reputable. Sex education is important, and too little accurate information does predispose individuals to making poor sexual choices. However, it is not as great a risk factor as having multiple sexual partners.

> *Test Taking Strategy—Analyze to determine what information the question asks for, which is a risk factor that predisposes the client to acquiring a sexually transmitted infection. Option 3 is the only option that involves intimate sexual contact; as the number of sex partners increases, so does the potential for acquiring a sexually transmitted infection. Review factors that influence the acquisition of a sexually transmitted infection if you had difficulty answering this question.*
> *Cognitive Level—Applying*
> *Client Needs Category—Health promotion and maintenance*
> *Client Needs Subcategory—None*

91. 4. The most likely substance to be cultured if a client has gonorrhea is urethral drainage. However, the organism might also be cultured from swabs taken from other areas, including the rectum, pharynx, and vagina (in women). The organism causing gonorrhea is not generally found in blood or urine. It is found in semen; however, collection is complicated because producing the specimen requires masturbation and ejaculation.

> *Test Taking Strategy—Analyze to determine what information the question asks for, which is the specimen that should be examined to determine if the client has acquired gonorrhea. Because this is a sexually transmitted infection, a venous blood sample (option 1) and sterile urine from the bladder (option 2) may be eliminated as not specific enough. Discriminate between the remaining two options; the bacteria may be present in each of them, but option 4 is the better choice because urethral drainage is fairly easy to collect. Review diagnostic testing for gonorrhea if you had difficulty answering this question.*
> *Cognitive Level—Applying*
> *Client Needs Category—Physiological integrity*
> *Client Needs Subcategory—Reduction of risk potential*

92. 1. Gloves are worn as a standard precaution when collecting body substances from any client regardless of the tentative diagnosis. The hands should also be washed after glove removal. Using a disinfectant is not appropriate for any specimen collection. As long as gloves are worn, the nurse can touch the client. Cultures for the gonorrhea organism are inoculated onto a culture medium as soon as possible; therefore, refrigeration is undesirable.

> *Test Taking Strategy—Analyze to determine what information the question asks for, which is the correct nursing action when collecting a specimen of urethral drainage. Wearing latex gloves (option 1) is always correct when the hands may be exposed*

to potentially infectious body substances. Latex-free gloves are used if the nurse has a latex allergy. Review standard precautions if you had difficulty answering this question.
Cognitive Level—*Applying*
Client Needs Category—*Safe and effective care environment*
Client Needs Subcategory—*Safety and infection control*

93. 1. Women infected with the herpes simplex virus type 2 are at greater risk for developing cervical cancer. Therefore, frequent Pap smears are necessary. Men infected with the virus are at greater risk for developing prostatic cancer. Clients may have vaginal intercourse, but a condom should be used and all sex partners should be informed of the potential for infection. Drugs may decrease the frequency of outbreaks and reduce the length of time when symptoms are manifested. However, taking medication does not provide protection for others. Spontaneous abortions increase among infected pregnant women. Infants can acquire the herpes virus at the time of vaginal delivery.
Test Taking Strategy—*Analyze to determine what information the question asks for, which is accurate information the nurse should tell a female who has acquired genital herpes. Recall that acquiring a genital herpes infection increases the risk for cervical cancer in a female. Consequently, option 1 is the correct answer because cervical cancer can be identified in an early stage if the client has regular Pap tests. Review the complications associated with an infection of genital herpes in females if you had difficulty answering this question.*
Cognitive Level—*Analyzing*
Client Needs Category—*Health promotion and maintenance*
Client Needs Subcategory—*None*

94. 1. Tertiary syphilis is the final stage in the course of untreated disease. It occurs about 25 to 30 years after the initial infection. In this stage, syphilis presents as a slow, progressive inflammatory disease. One of the manifestations of tertiary syphilis is sharp, stabbing leg pains. The client may also have other organ system damage involving the heart, brain, liver, bones, and eyes. A painless ulcer is a characteristic of primary-stage syphilis. The secondary stage of syphilis is accompanied by a red rash and patchy hair loss.
Test Taking Strategy—*Apply the key words "most characteristic" to the four options and select the option that correlates with a finding that occurs during the tertiary stage of syphilis. Recall that the tertiary stage is the last stage of syphilitic infection, during which a client may develop tabes dorsalis, a degeneration of myelin around peripheral nerves that causes episodic leg pain (option 1), an unsteady gait,*

and loss of coordination and sensation. Review the stages of syphilis and their manifestations, focusing on the pathophysiology of the tertiary stage, if you had difficulty answering this question.
Cognitive Level—*Applying*
Client Needs Category—*Physiological integrity*
Client Needs Subcategory—*Physiological adaptation*

95. 4. There is no lifelong immunity to syphilis. Each new incident is treated with antibiotic therapy. Antibiotic therapy destroys the microorganism and prevents further consequences from the disease. Sex partners are tested and treated if they are infected. Syphilitic lesions can appear on the penis, outside and inside the vagina, around the mouth, and even on the nipple.
Test Taking Strategy—*Analyze to determine what information the question asks for, which is an inaccurate statement. Options 1, 2, and 3 all provide accurate statements about syphilis. Unlike some infectious diseases, acquiring syphilis and being successfully treated does not provide immunity from future infections (option 4). Review the potential for becoming reinfected with syphilis if you had difficulty answering this question.*
Cognitive Level—*Analyzing*
Client Needs Category—*Physiological integrity*
Client Needs Subcategory—*Physiological adaptation*

96. 3. To ensure adequate treatment, the client with a sexually transmitted infection is told to continue taking the prescribed medication for the full amount of time. Symptoms may clear in a short time after initial treatment, but the organisms might not be totally destroyed. The infection may persist without adequate treatment. The need for a refill is at the discretion of the health care professional. Long-term or repeated use of an antibiotic can cause an organism to develop resistance. Aggressive and appropriate short-term treatment is adequate for the present infection. Further treatment is not required unless reinfection occurs.
Test Taking Strategy—*Look at the key words "most appropriate," and select the option that contains accurate information about antibiotic therapy. Recall that organisms can become antibiotic-resistant if the client fails to take the medication for the specified time period (option 3). Review factors that contribute to the development of antibiotic resistant microorganisms if you had difficulty answering this question.*
Cognitive Level—*Applying*
Client Needs Category—*Physiological integrity*
Client Needs Subcategory—*Pharmacological therapies*

97. 3. Although all of the measures listed are important health practices for preventing infections, the most important method for preventing the recurrence of a sexually transmitted infection is to eliminate the infection in other sex partners. Unless this occurs, the pathogenic organism can be retransmitted.

> *Test Taking Strategy*—*Use the process of elimination to help select the option that is best for preventing a recurrence of a chlamydial infection. Focus on an option that relates to the potential for reinfection with a sexually transmitted infection. Options 1, 2, and 4 are important health practices, but they will not eliminate the potential for reinfection. Because Chlamydia is sexually transmitted, infected sexual partner(s) also must be treated to interrupt the cycle of infection and reinfection. Review how an infection with* Chlamydia trachomatis *requires treatment among sexual partners if you had difficulty answering this question.*
> *Cognitive Level*—*Applying*
> *Client Needs Category*—*Health promotion and maintenance*
> *Client Needs Subcategory*—*None*

98. 2. Vaginal pruritus (itching) is a common problem experienced by women infected with *Trichomonas vaginalis*. Other clinical manifestations include yellow-brown malodorous vaginal discharge and thin vaginal secretions. Fluid-filled vesicles are associated with herpetic lesions. Vaginal drainage that seems to contain flecks of milk is characteristic of candidiasis (moniliasis). Women with gonorrhea or chlamydial infections commonly experience abdominal discomfort among other symptoms.

> *Test Taking Strategy*—*The key words are "most suggestive," indicating that the answer reflects a common clinical manifestation of an infection caused by* Trichomonas vaginalis. *Recall that this type of infection causes vaginal itching (option 2) among various other signs and symptoms. Review the signs and symptoms of a* Trichomonas *infection in a female if you had difficulty answering this question.*
> *Cognitive Level*—*Applying*
> *Client Needs Category*—*Physiological integrity*
> *Client Needs Subcategory*—*Physiological adaptation*

99. 4. Viral load tests, which include the p24 antigen and polymerase chain reaction tests, are considered to be the best marker of disease progression in acquired immunodeficiency syndrome (AIDS). They are used to guide drug therapy and follow the progression of the disease. Viral load tests and T4 cell counts are performed every 2 to 3 months once a person tests positive for human immunodeficiency virus (HIV) infection. Blood counts reveal if the cell counts are increasing, decreasing, or staying the same, but they are not as effective as the newer viral load tests. Assessing for changes in vital signs can help signal complications such as infection; however, this is not the best method for monitoring drug effectiveness. Viruses

can only be cultured in living tissue. Consequently, this approach is not used except in research.

> *Test Taking Strategy*—*Use the process of elimination to help select the option that is the best method for evaluating the effectiveness of antiretroviral drug therapy. Once options 1, 2, and 3 are eliminated, option 4 remains as the best answer. Review tests to monitor the progression of HIV infection and the effectiveness of treatment if you had difficulty answering this question.*
> *Cognitive Level*—*Evaluating*
> *Client Needs Category*—*Physiological integrity*
> *Client Needs Subcategory*—*Pharmacological therapies*

Nursing Care of Clients Practicing Family Planning

100. 1. Oral contraceptives should be taken at approximately the same time each day. Dosing begins on the fifth day of menstruation and, depending on the type used, is taken for 20 or 21 days. Some forms of oral contraceptives contain an additional week's worth of placebo tablets so a woman gets into the habit of taking a pill each day.

> *Test Taking Strategy*—*The key word is "appropriate," indicating one option is better than the others in relation to teaching a client about oral contraceptives. Taking the oral contraceptive at the same time each day (option 1) ensures that blood levels rise and fall in a consistent pattern. Developing a pattern for taking medications at the same time also helps avoid missing a dose, which could cause an unwanted pregnancy if it happens over repeated days. Review the pharmacokinetics of medication administration, focusing on the advantage of taking medications at the same time each day; also review actions to take if more than one dose of oral contraceptives is missed consecutively for several days if you had difficulty answering this question.*
> *Cognitive Level*—*Applying*
> *Client Needs Category*—*Physiological integrity*
> *Client Needs Subcategory*—*Pharmacological therapies*

101. 1. Smoking increases the risk of developing blood clots in women who take hormonal contraceptives. Maintaining a high fluid volume and elevating the legs are ways of preventing venous stasis, but they are not directly related to the cause-and-effect nature of this question. Taking a small dose of aspirin may prevent blood clots because of its anticoagulant properties, but before taking aspirin, the client should thoroughly discuss its use with the physician.

> *Test Taking Strategy*—*Look at the key words "most appropriate" and apply them when analyzing each option. Recall that one side effect of oral contraceptives is the formation of thrombi. The risk for this complication is increased in women who smoke*

(option 1). Perhaps the underlying mechanism is that nicotine causes vasoconstriction, which reduces blood flow. Review contraindications for oral contraceptive use if you had difficulty answering this question.
Cognitive Level—*Applying*
Client Needs Category—*Physiological integrity*
Client Needs Subcategory—*Pharmacological therapies*

102. 3. Menstruation continues because the ovarian hormones are circulated in the blood, not through the fallopian tubes. A tubal ligation performed through the abdomen leaves only a small incisional scar. Hospitalization is brief. Although tubal ligations have been reversed, they are still considered a permanent form of contraception.

Test Taking Strategy—Analyze to determine what information the question asks for, which is an inaccurate statement regarding tubal ligation. Recall that the ovaries, which secrete estrogen and progesterone, remain intact and functioning when the fallopian tubes are ligated. Consequently, menstruation will continue because endocrine hormones do not require passage through a duct to achieve their effects (option 3). Review the anatomic changes that occur when a tubal ligation is performed if you had difficulty answering this question.
Cognitive Level—*Applying*
Client Needs Category—*Physiological integrity*
Client Needs Subcategory—*Reduction of risk potential*

103. 2, 5, 6. After an intrauterine device (IUD) is inserted, many women experience menstrual cramps, an increase in blood loss, and longer duration of menstrual periods. These symptoms are related to the plastic or copper, and in some cases, progestin used in the IUD. Breast tenderness, weight gain, and acne are more common with birth control measures that contain estrogen.

Test Taking Strategy—Analyze to determine what information the question asks for, which is symptoms associated with an IUD. Alternative-format "select all that apply" questions require considering each option independently to decide its merit in answering the question. Choose options that correlate with side effects associated with an IUD. Review the mechanisms by which IUDs facilitate contraception and their related side effects if you had difficulty answering this question.
Cognitive Level—*Applying*
Client Needs Category—*Physiological integrity*
Client Needs Subcategory—*Reduction of risk potential*

104. 3. Although a vasectomy is a very reliable method of birth control, having a vasectomy does not ensure sterility immediately. Guidelines typically recommend using an alternative form of birth control for 12 weeks after a vasectomy.

A sperm count should be done to determine if viable sperm are present in sufficient numbers to cause pregnancy before discontinuing alternative birth control measures.

Test Taking Strategy—Analyze to determine what information the question asks for, which is the length of time an alternative birth control measure should be used after a vasectomy to avoid an unwanted pregnancy. Recall that a persistent small number of sperm may remain in ejaculated semen for 3 months, which is the basis for option 3. If any sperm remain after 3 months, they are more likely to be present in low numbers and be nonmotile. Review vasectomy guidelines if you had difficulty answering this question.
Cognitive Level—*Applying*
Client Needs Category—*Health promotion and maintenance*
Client Needs Subcategory—*None*

105. 3, 5, 6. Leaving a space between the tip of the condom and the penis allows an area where the ejaculate can be contained. Condoms are designed for one single use only regardless of what they are made of. A new condom is applied with each new erection. To prevent semen leakage, the condom is grasped as the erect penis is withdrawn from the vagina. Condoms are applied as the penis becomes erect. Condoms should be stored in a cool, dry location to prevent deterioration. Spermicides are not applied directly to the penis, but are often part of the condom's lubricant.

Test Taking Strategy—Analyze to determine what information the question asks for, which is proper condom application and use. Alternative-format "select all that apply" questions require considering each option independently to decide its merit in answering the question. Review the procedure for safe, effective condom use if you had difficulty answering this question.
Cognitive Level—*Applying*
Client Needs Category—*Health promotion and maintenance*
Client Needs Subcategory—*None*

106. 1, 2, 4. Medroxyprogesterone (Depo-Provera) is a form of progesterone that prevents ovulation; changes cervical mucus and the uterine lining, impairing sperm from reaching the uterus; and makes implantation within the uterine wall difficult should fertilization occur. Before administering medroxyprogesterone, the physician should validate that the client is not currently pregnant because the drug can cause birth defects in the fetus. Medroxyprogesterone is administered deeply into the gluteal or deltoid muscle within the first 7 days of the menstrual cycle and thereafter every 3 months. The injection is effective within 24 hours. Because ovulation is unlikely during days 1 through 7 of the menstrual cycle, any additional contraception is unnecessary. There is no reason to apply ice to the injection site before administration.

Test Taking Strategy—Analyze to determine what information the question asks for, which is instructions for the administration of medroxyprogesterone. Alternative-format "select all that apply" questions require considering each option independently to decide its merit in answering the question. Review the pertinent drug information on medroxyprogesterone if you had difficulty answering this question.
Cognitive Level—*Applying*
Client Needs Category—*Physiological integrity*
Client Needs Subcategory—*Pharmacological therapies*

107. **1, 2, 4.** Before advising the client about methods of birth control, the nurse needs to gather more information. Knowing about the client's lifestyle is important because it can provide clues about the need to exclude certain types of birth control. For example, birth control pills may be inadvisable if the client does not like to take pills or cannot remember to take medicine. Also, some forms of birth control are contraindicated if the client is a smoker. The nurse needs to ascertain whether the client is currently sexually active and whether she is practicing safe sex. Both answers can provide additional teaching opportunities regarding the avoidance of pregnancy and sexually transmitted infections. The nurse also needs to explore when the client had her last menstrual period because this will help determine whether she is currently pregnant. Information about the client's last Pap smear and workplace is irrelevant to helping her choose an appropriate birth control method.

Test Taking Strategy—Analyze to determine what information the question asks for, which is baseline information the nurse should obtain before advising a client on methods for birth control. Alternative-format "select all that apply" questions require considering each option independently to decide its merit in answering the question. Choose options that would help in the selection of the best birth control method for a client. Review birth control options if you had difficulty answering this question.
Cognitive Level—*Analyzing*
Client Needs Category—*Health promotion and maintenance*
Client Needs Subcategory—*None*

108. **1, 2, 3, 4, 5.** Safer sex practices (protected sex) are precautions that prevent acquiring a sexually transmitted infection (STI) or giving one to a sex partner. They include being selective in choosing sex partners. Sex with a partner who has had numerous casual encounters with bisexual or same-sex partners or with someone who is an I.V. drug user increases the chance of acquiring a sexually transmitted infection. Sharing vibrators or other sexual equipment can lead to the transfer of infections and should be avoided.

Avoiding intercourse if either partner has signs of a sexually transmitted infection is a safe practice in preventing the spread of infection. Sex partners must always be notified when a sexually transmitted disease has been diagnosed. Urinating after intercourse can help prevent urinary tract infections; it also washes away contaminates on the labia. Storing condoms away from excessive heat helps prevent deterioration of the latex. Storing birth control patches in the refrigerator is inappropriate; they should be kept at room temperature.

Test Taking Strategy—Analyze to determine what information the question asks for, which is recommendations for safer sex practices. Alternative-format "select all that apply" questions require considering each option independently to decide its merit in answering the question. Choose options that avoid risk factors for acquiring a STI and methods that prevent contact with blood or body fluids. Review safe sex practices if you difficulty answering this question.
Cognitive Level—*Applying*
Client Needs Category—*Health promotion and maintenance*
Client Needs Subcategory—*None*

109. **1.** Combination oral contraceptives contain estrogen and progesterone. The estrogen is thought to prevent follicle maturation and thereby prevent ovulation. The progesterone is thought to inhibit thickening of the uterine lining. The other two options do not reflect correct functions of the combination oral contraceptive.

Test Taking Strategy—Analyze to determine what information the question asks for, which is an understanding of how oral contraceptives prevent pregnancy. Review how modifying levels of hormones change menstrual cycle physiology to resemble a pseudo-pregnancy, thus inhibiting ovulation and making the endometrium unsuited for implantation, if you had difficulty answering this question.
Cognitive Level—*Applying*
Client Needs Category—*Physiological integrity*
Client Needs Subcategory—*Pharmacological therapies*

110. **2.** The 28-pill package has 7 placebo pills that allow the woman to maintain a routine of taking the pills daily. This reduces the possibility of the client forgetting to take a pill. The menstrual cycle's length has nothing to do with the number of pills dispensed in the package. Monophasic, biphasic, and triphasic are categories of combination pills that refer to how the estrogen and progesterone are released over the course of the menstrual cycle. All combination oral contraceptives have estrogen and progesterone in each pill.

Test Taking Strategy—Analyze to determine what information the question asks for, which is an explanation for why some contraceptive packages contain

28 tablets rather than 21. Recall that only 21 of the 28 tablets actually contain contraceptive hormones. The remaining 7 are placebos, which supports option 2 as the correct answer. Review information of various combinations of hormones and the manner in which they are packaged by pharmaceutical companies if you had difficulty answering this question.
Cognitive Level—*Applying*
Client Needs Category—*Physiological integrity*
Client Needs Subcategory—*Pharmacological therapies*

111. 2. Oral contraceptives are sometimes prescribed for women who have primary dysmenorrhea because the oral contraceptive is thought to create a better hormonal balance and may help decrease the client's discomfort related to menstrual cramping. All of the other statements are accurate regarding oral contraceptives.

> ***Test Taking Strategy***—*Analyze to determine what information the question asks for, which is a client's statement that is incorrect in relation to safe and effective use of oral contraceptives. Recall that modifying hormones in the menstrual cycle can relieve the monthly discomfort experienced by some women (option 2) and may be a reason other than contraception for which they are prescribed. Review the purposes for which oral contraceptives are prescribed if you had difficulty answering this question.*
> ***Cognitive Level***—*Applying*
> ***Client Needs Category***—*Physiological integrity*
> ***Client Needs Subcategory***—*Pharmacological therapies*

112. 1, 2, 3, 4, 5. Hormonal contraceptives such as the patch are used to prevent pregnancy. The patch transfers hormones through the skin and must stick securely to work properly. The patch is applied once a week for 3 weeks to the abdomen, buttocks, upper outer arm, or upper torso, but not on the breasts. Major side effects include skin irritation or rash at the site of application, irregular vaginal bleeding or spotting (which is temporary), fluid retention that causes edema of the fingers and ankles, a rise in blood pressure (due to fluid retention), and nausea and vomiting. Hepatitis is not a common side effect of the patch. Women with a history of hepatitis, smoking, breast cancer, or liver, gallbladder, kidney, or heart disease should refrain from using the patch. The birth control patch is not known to cause infection.

> ***Test Taking Strategy***—*Analyze to determine what information the question asks for, which is side effects of contraceptive skin patches. Alternative-format "select all that apply" questions require considering each option independently to decide its merit in answering the question. Choose options that correlate with potential side effects involving the application of the patch to the skin as well as the medications within the patch. Review information*

on side effects of contraceptive hormones if you had difficulty answering this question.
Cognitive Level—*Applying*
Client Needs Category—*Physiological integrity*
Client Needs Subcategory—*Pharmacological therapies*

113. 4. The female condom is made of polyurethane, not latex; therefore, the client who has an allergy to latex can use a female condom without experiencing an allergic reaction. All other statements include accurate information about barrier forms of contraception.

> ***Test Taking Strategy***—*Analyze to determine what information the question asks for, which is identifying a client's inaccurate statement about barrier methods of contraception that requires additional teaching. Although the use of a female condom is not as popular as other forms of barrier and nonbarrier methods of contraception, they are available and the nurse should be able to provide information about them. Recall that because individuals may be sensitive to latex, this type of barrier contraceptive is made from nonlatex materials, making option 4 an incorrect statement and the correct answer to the question. Review barrier methods of contraception if you had difficulty answering this question.*
> ***Cognitive Level***—*Applying*
> ***Client Needs Category***—*Health promotion and maintenance*
> ***Client Needs Subcategory***—*None*

114. 3. The client who wishes to use the basal body temperature method of natural family planning should take her temperature every morning before rising for 6 months with a special thermometer. Recording the pattern of the menstrual cycle for 6 to 8 months is used for the rhythm or calendar method of natural family planning. Monitoring the consistency of vaginal bleeding during menses is not a component of natural family planning. Having the male sex partner withdraw his penis from the vagina before ejaculation is called *coitus interruptus* and is not an effective birth control method, because pre-ejaculate fluid produced by Cowper's glands for the purpose of lubricating the vagina may contain sperm.

> ***Test Taking Strategy***—*Use the process of elimination to help select the one option that is correct in relation to using basal body temperature for planning or avoiding a pregnancy. Recall that the term basal means pertaining to the lowest level. Using that information, option 3 can be identified as the best answer because body temperature is lowest on awakening and rises thereafter during the day. Review the basal body temperature method, which may be used for family planning by those who oppose artificial contraceptive methods, if you had difficulty answering this question.*

Cognitive Level—*Applying*
Client Needs Category—*Health promotion and maintenance*
Client Needs Subcategory—*None*

115. 4. The nurse is most correct to consider the 5 rights in the delegation process. The first right is right task where the nurse ensures that the medical assistant has the knowledge base and skill to carry out the delegated assignment. All other options are considerations but not the most important.

Test Taking Strategy—*Analyze to determine what information the question asks for, which is an important consideration prior to delegation. Recall the 5 steps of delegation: right task, right circumstance, to the right person, with the right directions and communication, and right supervision/evaluation. Option 4 can be identified as the best option to meet the steps in delegation. Review applying the steps in delegation if you had difficulty answering this question.*
Cognitive Level—*Analyzing*
Client Needs Category—*Safe and effective care environment*
Client Needs Subcategory—*Coordinated care*

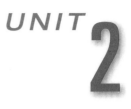

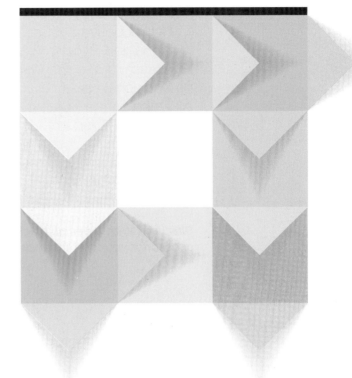

The Nursing Care of the Childbearing Family

UNIT 2

385

TEST

11 The Nursing Care of Clients During the Antepartum Period

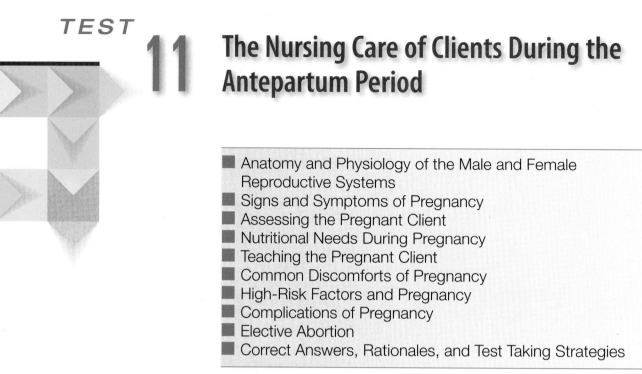

■ Anatomy and Physiology of the Male and Female Reproductive Systems
■ Signs and Symptoms of Pregnancy
■ Assessing the Pregnant Client
■ Nutritional Needs During Pregnancy
■ Teaching the Pregnant Client
■ Common Discomforts of Pregnancy
■ High-Risk Factors and Pregnancy
■ Complications of Pregnancy
■ Elective Abortion
■ Correct Answers, Rationales, and Test Taking Strategies

Directions: *With a pencil, blacken the space in front of the option you have chosen for your correct answer.*

Anatomy and Physiology of the Male and Female Reproductive Systems

A 30-year-old woman and her spouse attend an infertility clinic. They have no children and have had several appointments with the physician regarding their infertility problems. After receiving information about reproduction, the client asks the nurse where fertilization takes place.

1. The nurse correctly explains that fertilization usually takes place in which structure?
[ ] **1.** Fallopian tube
[ ] **2.** Ovary
[ ] **3.** Uterus
[ ] **4.** Vagina

2. When the client asks the nurse about the viability of the ovum after ovulation, the nurse correctly explains that after ovulation, the ovum remains alive for how many hours?
[ ] **1.** 2 hours
[ ] **2.** 24 hours
[ ] **3.** 48 hours
[ ] **4.** 72 hours

3. The client's husband states that he has been diagnosed with a low sperm count. To improve sperm production, the nurse should instruct the client's husband to avoid which activities? Select all that apply.
[ ] **1.** Swimming in chlorinated water
[ ] **2.** Sitting in hot tubs
[ ] **3.** Wearing boxer shorts
[ ] **4.** Wearing colored underwear
[ ] **5.** Smoking cigarettes
[ ] **6.** Refraining from strenuous exercise

The client tells the nurse that despite desperately wanting to have a baby, the client is concerned about a vaginal birth because of small hips.

4. Which response by the nurse is most appropriate when addressing the client's concerns?
[ ] **1.** "Your hips are measured to make an accurate determination of whether or not the baby can be delivered vaginally."
[ ] **2.** "The size of your true pelvis, not the size of your hips, determines whether or not you can deliver a baby vaginally."
[ ] **3.** "It doesn't really matter whether you deliver vaginally or by cesarean birth because the risk for both types of delivery is the same."
[ ] **4.** "The size of the baby's head is the only factor that determines whether the infant can be delivered vaginally."

After discussing various options regarding the correction of their infertility problems, there is a question regarding when the gender of the baby is determined.

5. The nurse accurately explains that the gender of a baby is determined at which point?
[ ] **1.** During maturation of the ovum in the ovaries
[ ] **2.** During maturation of the sperm in the epididymis
[ ] **3.** When the fertilized ovum implants in the uterine lining
[ ] **4.** When the sperm fertilizes the ovum in the fallopian tube

During a discussion regarding menstruation, the client asks the nurse, "Where does the blood flow come from when a woman has her monthly period?"

6. The nurse correctly explains that the bleeding is the result of sloughing of which structure?
[ ] **1.** Endometrium
[ ] **2.** Perimetrium
[ ] **3.** Myometrium
[ ] **4.** Epimetrium

Signs and Symptoms of Pregnancy

A 22-year-old visits the prenatal clinic for the first time. During the health history assessment, the client reveals to the nurse a possibility of being 2 months' pregnant.

7. On the basis of the health history data, how should the nurse record the client's pregnancy status on the prenatal records?
[ ] **1.** Multipara
[ ] **2.** Primipara
[ ] **3.** Primigravida
[ ] **4.** Multigravida

The client informs the nurse that twins "run" in the family. The client asks the nurse why some women have identical twins and others have twins who do not look alike.

8. Which explanation by the nurse correctly describes the occurrence of identical twins?
[ ] **1.** Two separate ova are fertilized by identical sperm.
[ ] **2.** The mother releases two identical ova.
[ ] **3.** One fertilized ovum divides into two identical halves.
[ ] **4.** Two identical ova are fertilized by two identical sperm.

9. If the client reports the following signs and symptoms, which one represents a probable sign of pregnancy?
[ ] **1.** Absence of monthly periods
[ ] **2.** Abdominal enlargement
[ ] **3.** Nausea and vomiting
[ ] **4.** Frequent urination

The physician examines the client and orders a pregnancy test.

10. The nurse correctly sends a requisition and specimen for which laboratory test?
[ ] **1.** Alpha-fetoprotein (AFP)
[ ] **2.** Corticotropin-releasing hormone (CRH)
[ ] **3.** Human chorionic gonadotropin (hCG)
[ ] **4.** Follicle-stimulating hormone (FSH)

The client asks the nurse if an ultrasound could confirm the pregnancy in the second month.

11. Which statement by the nurse regarding an ultrasound is most accurate?
[ ] **1.** "Transvaginal ultrasound is used to diagnose pregnancy as early as 2½ to 3 weeks."
[ ] **2.** "Ultrasounds aren't performed during the first trimester because of the risk to the baby."
[ ] **3.** "An x-ray is just as reliable as an ultrasound and poses less of a risk to the baby."
[ ] **4.** "Ultrasounds aren't used until the uterus ascends out of the pelvis into the abdomen."

The physician informs the client that the pregnancy is confirmed based on the blood test and Chadwick's sign, which was positive during the pelvic examination. After the physician leaves, the client asks the nurse to explain the significance of a positive Chadwick's sign.

12. Which response by the nurse about Chadwick's sign is most accurate?
[ ] **1.** "It's the spontaneous occurrence of intermittent painless contractions that begin early in pregnancy and continue throughout the entire period of gestation."
[ ] **2.** "It's a bluish discoloration of the cervix, vagina, and vulva that occurs as a result of the presence of an increased number of blood vessels."
[ ] **3.** "It's a softening of the cervix that occurs because of an increased amount of blood flowing to the reproductive organs."
[ ] **4.** "It's a dark brown line extending from the umbilicus to the symphysis pubis that occurs as a result of hormonal changes."

When reviewing the client's medical record, the nurse notes that the physician documented the presence of ballottement.

13. On the basis of this finding, the nurse can assume that the client is at least how many months' pregnant?
[ ] **1.** 5 months
[ ] **2.** 6 months
[ ] **3.** 7 months
[ ] **4.** 8 months

The physician also documented that the client had a positive sign of pregnancy.

14. As the nurse is reviewing the physician's documentation, which client finding best represents a positive sign of pregnancy?
[ ] **1.** Palpable fetal outline
[ ] **2.** Blotchy tan facial skin
[ ] **3.** Positive pregnancy test
[ ] **4.** Fetal heartbeat

The client asks the nurse when it will be possible to feel the baby move.

15. In the primigravid client, when is fetal movement typically felt for the first time?
[ ] **1.** Between 10 and 14 weeks' gestation
[ ] **2.** Between 16 and 20 weeks' gestation
[ ] **3.** Between 22 and 26 weeks' gestation
[ ] **4.** Between 28 and 32 weeks' gestation

Assessing the Pregnant Client

A 32-year-old multigravid client visits the prenatal clinic for the first time during this pregnancy and states to the nurse, "I know I'm pregnant; I've already felt the baby move."

16. On the basis of the client's statement, what can the nurse conclude?
[ ] **1.** The client is having twins.
[ ] **2.** The client is between 14 and 18 weeks' gestation.
[ ] **3.** The client is in the first trimester.
[ ] **4.** The client's due date will be difficult to calculate.

During the interview, the client informs the nurse, "I have a son and twin daughters, no abortions, or stillbirths."

17. According to the TPAL method, which of the following accurately records the client's obstetric history?
[ ] **1.** T-III, P-0, A-0, L-III
[ ] **2.** T-III, P-III, A-0, L-0
[ ] **3.** T-III, P-II, A-0, L-II
[ ] **4.** T-II, P-0, A-0, L-III

The client informs the nurse that her last menstrual period began on March 13 and then asks the nurse when the baby is due.

18. Using Nägele's rule, the nurse can assume the client's expected delivery date to be approximately which date?
[ ] **1.** November 13
[ ] **2.** November 23
[ ] **3.** December 3
[ ] **4.** December 20

The physician asks the nurse to prepare the client for a pelvic examination.

19. The nurse correctly assists the client into which position?
[ ] **1.** Lithotomy
[ ] **2.** Prone
[ ] **3.** Sims'
[ ] **4.** Trendelenburg's

20. Before the pelvic examination, which intervention by the nurse is most appropriate?
[ ] **1.** Give the client an enema.
[ ] **2.** Instruct the client to urinate.
[ ] **3.** Shave the client's perineum.
[ ] **4.** Give the client a mild sedative.

21. Which method best promotes client comfort during the pelvic examination?
[ ] **1.** Have the client lift her head off the table.
[ ] **2.** Have the client press her back into the examination table.
[ ] **3.** Have the client tighten her buttocks.
[ ] **4.** Tell the client to let her knees fall outward.

The physician determines that the client is in the 15th week of pregnancy. The client asks if it is too early to hear the baby's heartbeat.

22. How early in a pregnancy can the nurse expect to hear the fetal heartbeat using a Doppler device?
[ ] **1.** 4 to 6 weeks
[ ] **2.** 8 to 10 weeks
[ ] **3.** 12 to 14 weeks
[ ] **4.** 16 to 18 weeks

23. Which action by the nurse best ensures that an accurate fetal heart rate is obtained?
[ ] **1.** Assess the fetal heart rate when the client is lying on her right side.
[ ] **2.** Assess the fetal heart rate when the client reports fetal movement.
[ ] **3.** Assess the fetal heart rate between Braxton Hicks contractions.
[ ] **4.** Assess the maternal pulse and fetal heart rate, and compare the two.

24. Which fetal heart rate must the nurse report immediately to the physician?
[ ] **1.** 100 beats/minute
[ ] **2.** 120 beats/minute
[ ] **3.** 140 beats/minute
[ ] **4.** 160 beats/minute

The client tells the nurse that a cousin's baby was born with spina bifida. The client asks if it is possible to detect the presence of this condition during her pregnancy.

25. Which response by the nurse is most accurate?
[ ] **1.** Fluorescent treponemal antibody absorption (FTA-ABS) test can detect this defect.
[ ] **2.** Hepatitis B surface antigen (HBsAg) test can detect this defect.
[ ] **3.** Maternal serum alpha-fetoprotein (AFP) test can detect this defect.
[ ] **4.** Venereal Disease Research Laboratory (VDRL) test can detect this defect.

Before leaving the clinic, the client asks the nurse about the schedule for the next few perinatal visits.

26. The nurse responds that, for clients with uncomplicated pregnancies, it is usually best to plan monthly visits for the first 28 weeks and then more frequent visits following which schedule?
[ ] **1.** Weekly for the remainder of the pregnancy
[ ] **2.** Every 2 weeks for the remainder of the pregnancy
[ ] **3.** Every 2 weeks up to 36 weeks, then weekly for the last month
[ ] **4.** Weekly up to 36 weeks, then twice weekly for the last month

The client also asks the nurse whether it is safe to continue to exercise routinely throughout the pregnancy.

27. Which nursing instructions concerning exercise during pregnancy are accurate? Select all that apply.
[ ] **1.** Avoid exercising during hot, humid weather.
[ ] **2.** Avoid any jerking, bouncing, or jumping movements.
[ ] **3.** Drink plenty of fluids before and after exercising.
[ ] **4.** Limit strenuous activity to no more than 60 minutes a session.
[ ] **5.** Perform exercises only in the supine position.
[ ] **6.** Limit exercising to once per week.

The client returns for follow-up visits on a regular basis, following the prearranged schedule. According to the most recent examination, the client is estimated to be at 20 weeks' gestation.

28. Where can the nurse expect to palpate the fundus at this time?
[ ] **1.** Just above the symphysis pubis
[ ] **2.** Just below the xiphoid process
[ ] **3.** Near the level of the umbilicus
[ ] **4.** Just below the symphysis pubis

29. When the nurse discusses the tasks to be accomplished during the client's visit at 24 weeks' gestation, which routine test will be performed?
[ ] **1.** Coombs' test
[ ] **2.** Glucose tolerance test
[ ] **3.** Papanicolaou (Pap) smear
[ ] **4.** Rubella titer

The client has progressed to the last month of pregnancy. The physician orders a nonstress test.

30. When planning for this test, which one of the following items should the nurse have available?
[ ] **1.** The emergency crash cart
[ ] **2.** A cardiac monitor
[ ] **3.** I.V. oxytocin (Pitocin)
[ ] **4.** A fetal monitor

A physician recommends amniocentesis for a pregnant woman whose first child has Down syndrome.

31. The nurse advises the client that this test is typically performed at what time during the pregnancy?
[ ] **1.** Just after the pregnancy is confirmed
[ ] **2.** Early in the second trimester
[ ] **3.** In the transition phase of labor
[ ] **4.** Just after the first fetal movements

Nutritional Needs During Pregnancy

During a routine prenatal visit, the physician determines that a client in the fourth month of pregnancy is not eating an appropriate diet and asks whether she has been taking the prenatal vitamins, folic acid, and iron supplements that were previously prescribed. The physician asks the nurse to instruct the client about nutritional needs during pregnancy.

32. Before teaching the client about the nutritional needs during pregnancy, which nursing intervention is most appropriate?
[ ] **1.** Determine if the client needs to gain or lose weight.
[ ] **2.** Assess the client's current eating pattern and preferences.
[ ] **3.** Determine if the client knows how to accurately count calories.
[ ] **4.** Develop a sample menu that includes the required nutrients.

While discussing prepregnancy eating habits with the nurse, the client asks, "What's the normal weight gain during pregnancy?"

33. Which explanation by the nurse accurately identifies the recommended weight gain for a pregnant client who has a normal prepregnancy weight?
[ ] **1.** Less than 15 pounds (<6.8 kg)
[ ] **2.** 15 to 20 pounds (6.8 to 9 kg)
[ ] **3.** 25 to 35 pounds (11.3 to 15.8 kg)
[ ] **4.** No more than 40 pounds (≤18.1 kg)

After interviewing the client, the nurse determines that the client does not have an adequate intake of calcium.

34. The nurse correctly instructs the client to drink how many glasses of milk per day to meet calcium requirements?
[ ] **1.** 1 to 2
[ ] **2.** 3 to 4
[ ] **3.** 5 to 6
[ ] **4.** 7 to 8

The client tells the nurse that it is hard to get the required amount of calcium because of a dislike for milk.

35. Which food provides the best alternative source of calcium?
[ ] **1.** Organ meats
[ ] **2.** White bread
[ ] **3.** Leafy green vegetables
[ ] **4.** Dark turkey meat

The nurse asks whether the client is taking the daily iron supplement. The client states, "I have not been taking the iron routinely because it causes constipation."

36. When providing information about iron supplements, which instruction by the nurse is most appropriate?
[ ] **1.** "Take the supplement with meals."
[ ] **2.** "Be aware that iron can cause abdominal pain."
[ ] **3.** "Make sure you drink plenty of fluids."
[ ] **4.** "You can substitute dietary sources of iron for this medication."

37. To best enhance absorption of the iron supplement, which foods should the nurse recommend the client increase in her diet? Select all that apply.
[ ] **1.** Oranges
[ ] **2.** Cantaloupe
[ ] **3.** Bananas
[ ] **4.** Broccoli
[ ] **5.** Whole milk
[ ] **6.** Carrots

38. What information should the nurse also include about the side effects of iron supplementation?
[ ] **1.** "You may notice that your stools will be black."
[ ] **2.** "Your teeth will become stained."
[ ] **3.** "Vomiting is likely to occur."
[ ] **4.** "You may have diarrhea several times per day."

During the visit, the nurse also asks if the client has been taking the prescribed folic acid.

39. When the client asks why folic acid is important, which response by the nurse is most accurate?
[ ] **1.** "Folic acid helps prevent neural tube defects such as spina bifida."
[ ] **2.** "Folic acid helps build strong bones for your baby."
[ ] **3.** "Folic acid helps your baby become resistant to infections."
[ ] **4.** "Folic acid prevents your baby from becoming anemic."

A 17-year-old primigravid client is seen at the health clinic for the first time. The nurse assesses the teenager's nutritional status and provides nutritional guidance.

40. Which dietary adjustment is most appropriate for a pregnant teenager?
[ ] **1.** Increase caloric intake to 2,500 calories per day.
[ ] **2.** Drink presweetened beverages instead of carbonated ones.
[ ] **3.** Eat foods that are low in carbohydrates and fats.
[ ] **4.** Choose nonspicy, easy to digest foods.

After interviewing the client, the nurse determines that the client lives with her boyfriend and works several hours per week. She frequently skips meals or eats at fast food restaurants. The client drinks beer or wine when with friends and is constantly concerned about weight gain and appearance.

41. How many factors in this scenario place the client at risk for nutritional deficiencies and the need for dietary guidance and counseling?
[ ] **1.** Three
[ ] **2.** Four
[ ] **3.** Five
[ ] **4.** Six

During a subsequent visit, the nurse notes that the client is eating a bag of potato chips and drinking a diet cola. The nurse revises the client's care plan accordingly.

42. Which expected outcome should the nurse include based on the client's eating habits?
[ ] **1.** The client will eat three balanced meals and two snacks daily while pregnant.
[ ] **2.** The client will gain a total of 50 pounds during the pregnancy.
[ ] **3.** The client will take two prenatal vitamins daily.
[ ] **4.** The client will report eating about 2,000 calories per day.

During the visit, the client expresses concern that an increased weight gain over the past month is causing unwanted obesity.

43. Which response by the nurse is most appropriate?
[ ] **1.** "A weight gain of about 10 pounds is recommended during pregnancy."
[ ] **2.** "Your weight gain depends on the amount of food that you eat."
[ ] **3.** "It's normal for adolescent girls to be worried about weight gain."
[ ] **4.** "The average weight gain during pregnancy is between 25 and 35 pounds."

The nurse helps the client compile lists of healthy and unhealthy foods as a guide for the remainder of the pregnancy.

44. Which of the following beverages should be included in the list of unhealthy drinks to avoid? Select all that apply.
[ ] **1.** Alcohol
[ ] **2.** Coffee
[ ] **3.** Tea
[ ] **4.** Cola beverages
[ ] **5.** Sports drinks
[ ] **6.** Orange juice

At a subsequent prenatal visit, the client complains of edema in the lower extremities.

45. After gathering further information about the edema, the nurse advises the client to limit the intake of which substance?
[ ] **1.** Sodium
[ ] **2.** Potassium
[ ] **3.** Vitamin C
[ ] **4.** Magnesium

A nurse conducts a nutrition class at a local public health department for a group of clients who are newly pregnant. During the class, the nurse collects information about each person's nutritional status and assesses the group for nutritional risk factors during pregnancy.

46. Which of the following clients are at risk for nutritional problems during pregnancy? Select all that apply.
[ ] **1.** A 17-year-old primigravid client who works part time
[ ] **2.** A 25-year-old client who weighs 250 pounds (113.4 kg) at conception
[ ] **3.** A 19-year-old client who admits that she smokes cigarettes and drinks alcohol
[ ] **4.** A 30-year-old client who is unemployed and uses food stamps
[ ] **5.** A 25-year-old client whose prepregnancy hemoglobin level is 13 g/100 mL
[ ] **6.** A 30-year-old client who drinks four glasses of milk per day

Teaching the Pregnant Client

A 26-year-old primigravid client visits the obstetrician for the first prenatal visit. The physician confirms that the client is in the ninth week of pregnancy. The nurse and client discuss general health needs during pregnancy.

47. Which client statement regarding bathing indicates a need for additional teaching?
[ ] **1.** "I should avoid taking tub baths if my membranes rupture."
[ ] **2.** "I should avoid taking tub baths during my pregnancy."
[ ] **3.** "I shouldn't sit in a hot tub because the heat could affect my baby."
[ ] **4.** "I should use warm water when I bathe."

The client asks the nurse if sexual intercourse is safe during pregnancy.

48. The nurse correctly explains that sexual intercourse should be avoided at what time?
[ ] **1.** Throughout pregnancy
[ ] **2.** Until the baby is fully developed
[ ] **3.** Once the abdomen starts to enlarge
[ ] **4.** Once the membranes rupture

The client informs the nurse about planning a vacation next month before the pregnancy is too "far along." The client asks if there are any special instructions regarding traveling.

49. Which response by the nurse regarding travel is most appropriate? Select all that apply.
[ ] **1.** "Carry a copy of your medical record with you when traveling."
[ ] **2.** "Refrain from traveling until after the baby is born."
[ ] **3.** "Pack a scale and weigh yourself every day."
[ ] **4.** "Avoid using a seatbelt for extended periods of time."
[ ] **5.** "Eat foods that you are normally accustomed to eating."
[ ] **6.** "If you travel to a foreign country, make sure to get vaccinated."

The client informs the nurse about some spotting during the first week of pregnancy. The client asks if it should be reported to the physician.

50. The nurse documents the information to be shared with the physician, and then instructs that spotting can be normal and the result of which occurrence?
[ ] **1.** The embryo implanting in the lining of the uterus
[ ] **2.** Increased blood circulation to the vaginal area
[ ] **3.** Hormonal changes that occur during pregnancy
[ ] **4.** The cervical opening enlarging and thinning out

At 9 weeks' gestation, the client asks the nurse, "What does my baby look like now?"

51. The nurse explains that between 8 and 12 weeks' gestation, what characteristics have developed?
[ ] **1.** The zygote looks like a lumpy ball.
[ ] **2.** The embryo has a well-defined head.
[ ] **3.** The embryo's sex is distinguishable.
[ ] **4.** The fetus has fully formed arms and legs.

In a discussion regarding fetal development, the nurse informs the client that as growth increases, the amount of amniotic fluid increases. The client asks the nurse to explain the purpose of the amniotic fluid.

52. Which response given by the nurse is most appropriate regarding the purpose of amniotic fluid?
[ ] **1.** It generates fetal antibodies from the mother.
[ ] **2.** It helps protect the fetus from external injury.
[ ] **3.** It provides oxygen for the developing fetus.
[ ] **4.** It helps support the enlarging maternal uterus.

53. In a discussion about hormonal changes, the nurse informs the client that the placenta produces which hormone?
[ ] **1.** Estrogen
[ ] **2.** Testosterone
[ ] **3.** Oxytocin
[ ] **4.** Follicle-stimulating hormone

Common Discomforts of Pregnancy

The nurse conducts a prenatal class on common discomforts of pregnancy. One person attending the class states, "I've been having trouble with constipation."

54. Which responses by the nurse regarding prevention of constipation are most appropriate? Select all that apply.
[ ] **1.** "Resting helps to relieve constipation."
[ ] **2.** "Exercising can help relieve constipation."
[ ] **3.** "A low-fat diet helps to relieve constipation."
[ ] **4.** "Prenatal vitamins help to relieve constipation."
[ ] **5.** "Drink 8 glasses of water per day to add moisture to stool."
[ ] **6.** "Take an over-the-counter laxative to maintain bowel elimination."

Several people attending the prenatal class ask the nurse to discuss the causes of varicose veins and how to relieve the discomfort associated with them.

55. The nurse explains that, in addition to increased blood volume, which other condition causes varicose veins during pregnancy?
[ ] **1.** Impaired venous return
[ ] **2.** Decreased cardiac output
[ ] **3.** Altered center of gravity
[ ] **4.** Impaired kidney function

56. The nurse correctly explains to the group that the discomfort associated with varicose veins is relieved by which activity?
[ ] **1.** Resting with the feet in a dependent position
[ ] **2.** Sitting for periods of time when possible
[ ] **3.** Putting on calf-length, elastic-top hose
[ ] **4.** Moving around after standing in one position

57. When teaching the class about varicose veins, which symptom should the nurse instruct clients to report immediately?
[ ] **1.** The appearance of additional varicose veins
[ ] **2.** Varicose veins that are purple in color
[ ] **3.** Legs that begin to ache and feel heavy
[ ] **4.** Calves that become red, tender, and warm

One of the participants in the prenatal class tells the nurse, "My skin itches so much. What can I do about it?"

58. Which nursing instruction is most appropriate regarding the relief of itchy skin during pregnancy?
[ ] **1.** Take a hot bath daily.
[ ] **2.** Increase fluid intake.
[ ] **3.** Add a daily vitamin C tablet to the diet.
[ ] **4.** Take diphenhydramine (Benadryl) twice per day.

One participant who is in the third trimester says, "I've started to experience shortness of breath and I'm concerned about the baby."

59. Which information about shortness of breath during pregnancy is correct?
[ ] **1.** It is not common during pregnancy and may indicate a blood clot in the lungs.
[ ] **2.** It is probably the result of anxiety about the baby's impending delivery.
[ ] **3.** It is probably caused by the enlarged uterus pressing against the diaphragm.
[ ] **4.** It is probably caused by decreased oxygen secondary to slow venous circulation.

60. Which nursing instruction given to the client complaining about shortness of breath is most appropriate?
[ ] **1.** "Contact your health care provider immediately."
[ ] **2.** "Decrease your activity level to conserve oxygen."
[ ] **3.** "Ask your physician for a mild sedative."
[ ] **4.** "Sleep with your upper body elevated on pillows."

Several participants in the prenatal class complain of frequent urination.

61. The nurse explains to the group that frequent urination during early pregnancy usually subsides at which time?
[ ] **1.** When the placenta is fully developed
[ ] **2.** When fetal kidneys begin to function
[ ] **3.** When the uterus rises into the abdominal cavity
[ ] **4.** When the hormonal balance is reestablished

62. The nurse correctly explains to the group that the most probable cause of frequent urination late in pregnancy is related to what factor?
[ ] 1. Loss of bladder tone in the mother
[ ] 2. The presence of a urinary tract infection
[ ] 3. The enlarging uterus exerting pressure on the bladder
[ ] 4. The growing fetus excreting increased amounts of waste

63. Which statement made by a participant indicates the need for additional teaching regarding management of urinary frequency?
[ ] 1. "Limiting fluid intake will help control this problem."
[ ] 2. "I should report a burning sensation during urination."
[ ] 3. "Urinating before going to bed may help control the problem."
[ ] 4. "Avoiding caffeinated beverages may help control the problem."

One participant who is 5 months' pregnant complains of annoying backaches.

64. Which advice can the nurse give to relieve the client's backache? Select all that apply.
[ ] 1. Avoid clothing that fits tightly around the waist.
[ ] 2. Sleep on a heating pad.
[ ] 3. Take a nonopioid pain reliever regularly.
[ ] 4. Wear low-heeled shoes.
[ ] 5. Carry objects close to your body.
[ ] 6. Squat when picking objects off the floor.

A client in the class reports having intermittent episodes of nausea, especially in the morning. The nurse advises the class about ways to minimize the occurrence of heartburn and nausea.

65. Which statement made by a participant regarding remedies for heartburn and nausea indicates that teaching has been effective?
[ ] 1. "I should eat frequent, small meals."
[ ] 2. "I should take an antacid after eating."
[ ] 3. "I should eat my largest meal in the evening."
[ ] 4. "I should drink extra water with my meals."

66. When one participant asks the nurse what can be done to relieve leg cramps while working, which instruction by the nurse is correct?
[ ] 1. Increase protein intake to five to six servings per day.
[ ] 2. Wear elastic stockings when at work.
[ ] 3. Point the toes frequently toward the head.
[ ] 4. Massage the leg when a cramp occurs.

67. Which response by the nurse is most relevant when another participant talks about having recurrent mood swings?
[ ] 1. "Try to avoid fatigue and decrease your stress."
[ ] 2. "Avoid interactions with people who upset you."
[ ] 3. "You need to be assessed for a possible mood disorder."
[ ] 4. "Are you ambivalent about the pregnancy?"

It is confirmed that a nurse who works in a busy doctor's office is 12 weeks' pregnant. The nurse has been working long hours and is experiencing fatigue.

68. If this nurse is similar to other women experiencing normal pregnancies, which guidelines for pregnant working women should be implemented? Select all that apply.
[ ] 1. Use break and lunch periods for resting.
[ ] 2. Void every 2 hours.
[ ] 3. Eat foods high in carbohydrates.
[ ] 4. Schedule work days close together.
[ ] 5. Refrain from working overtime.
[ ] 6. Get at least 12 hours of sleep per night.

The nurse leads a discussion with the group about distinguishing between danger signs and the common discomforts of pregnancy.

69. The nurse considers prenatal teaching successful when the class correctly identifies which of the following as a danger sign of pregnancy?
[ ] 1. Headache and swelling of the face and fingers
[ ] 2. Constipation and flatulence on a regular basis
[ ] 3. Lower extremity muscle cramping and varicosities
[ ] 4. Large amounts of odorless, colorless vaginal secretions

High-Risk Factors and Pregnancy

A nurse discusses high-risk complications with a group of women at a prenatal clinic.

70. Which client would the nurse identify as being at highest risk for developing complications during pregnancy?
[ ] 1. A 25-year-old gravida I client
[ ] 2. A client with the placenta implanted on the fundus of the uterus
[ ] 3. A client who has nausea and vomiting during the first trimester
[ ] 4. A 35-year-old gravida V client

One participant tells the nurse about drinking a beer every night before going to bed. The participant asks the nurse if occasional alcohol consumption will harm the unborn baby.

71. Which response by the nurse is best?
[ ] 1. "Any alcohol consumption during pregnancy will cause the child to have complications later in life."
[ ] 2. "The minimal safe amount of alcohol consumption during pregnancy has not yet been determined."
[ ] 3. "Alcohol consumption has a harmful effect on the baby only if consumed during the first trimester of pregnancy."
[ ] 4. "Occasional intake of a small amount of alcohol during pregnancy will not adversely affect the unborn baby."

Another participant informs the nurse about smoking about a pack of cigarettes a day.

72. The nurse correctly informs the participants that women who smoke during pregnancy have a greater risk of which problem?
[ ] **1.** Having a premature delivery
[ ] **2.** Having a cesarean birth
[ ] **3.** Having a large, overweight baby
[ ] **4.** Developing a prenatal infection

A 40-year-old participant, a gravida V, para I in the 10th week of pregnancy, tells the nurse of concerns that her age may affect the health of the baby. The participant asks the nurse if there is a test that can identify any genetic disorders that the baby may have.

73. At this point in the client's pregnancy, which test is typically used to detect genetic disorders?
[ ] **1.** Amniocentesis
[ ] **2.** Chorionic villi sampling
[ ] **3.** Rapid plasma reagin
[ ] **4.** Ultrasound

At the clinic, an 18-year-old primigravid client is seen for the first time. The physician determines that the client is 3 months' pregnant and diagnoses chlamydia, a sexually transmitted infection.

74. Which assessment finding best indicates the presence of this condition?
[ ] **1.** Painful blisters on the labia
[ ] **2.** Heavy, grayish white discharge
[ ] **3.** Milky white discharge that smells like fish
[ ] **4.** Thick, white, curdlike vaginal discharge

75. Which statement by the client indicates a need for additional teaching regarding chlamydial infection?
[ ] **1.** "My sex partner(s) will require treatment as well."
[ ] **2.** "I will have to have a cesarean birth to protect my baby."
[ ] **3.** "The physician will treat the infection with an antibiotic."
[ ] **4.** "My Pap smear results may show abnormal cells."

Before leaving the clinic, the nurse teaches the client about danger signs that should be reported immediately to the physician.

76. The nurse correctly instructs the client to contact the physician immediately under which circumstance?
[ ] **1.** When the first fetal movement is felt
[ ] **2.** If the breasts become tender
[ ] **3.** If vaginal bleeding occurs
[ ] **4.** When experiencing frequent urination

A 30-year-old client comes to the clinic reporting episodes of severe nausea and frequent vomiting. The nurse learns that the client has had these symptoms for the past 7 days. The physician determines that the client has hyperemesis gravidarum and is moderately dehydrated. The client is admitted to the hospital.

77. Which of the following should the nurse plan to have available when providing nursing care to this client? Select all that apply.
[ ] **1.** I.V. start kit
[ ] **2.** An intake and output record
[ ] **3.** Oxygen and face mask
[ ] **4.** Cardiac monitor
[ ] **5.** A consent for a blood transfusion
[ ] **6.** A suction machine

Complications of Pregnancy

A nurse on the obstetrics unit cares for several high-risk pregnant clients.

78. Which clients are most likely to be identified as being at high risk for pregnancy complications? Select all that apply.
[ ] **1.** A client who is pregnant for the fifth time
[ ] **2.** A client who has gained 30 pounds (13.6 kg) during the pregnancy
[ ] **3.** A client who has a history of twins in the family
[ ] **4.** A client who has primary hypertensive disease
[ ] **5.** A client who works 40 hours a week in a factory
[ ] **6.** A client who reports spotting in the first trimester

The nurse applies a fetal heart monitor to assess the heart rate of a fetus in the cephalic position.

79. Place an X at the location where the nurse should place the Doppler transducer to auscultate fetal heart tones.

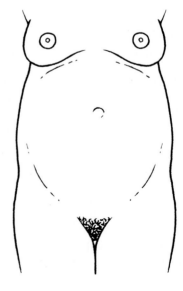

The obstetrician sees a 31-year-old multipara client in the first trimester of pregnancy. When sharing a health history, the client tells the nurse that the last pregnancy ended in a spontaneous abortion because of an incompetent cervix. The client asks the nurse to clarify what is meant by an incompetent cervix.

80. Which statement by the nurse best explains the meaning of an incompetent cervix?
[ ] **1.** The cervix is not large enough for passage of the fetus.
[ ] **2.** The cervix cannot support the weight of the fetus.
[ ] **3.** The cervix has an external opening but not an internal opening.
[ ] **4.** The cervix has an internal opening but not an external opening.

At the end of the first trimester, the physician puts a cerclage in the client's cervix. The client asks the nurse how long the cerclage will remain in place.

81. The nurse correctly explains to the client that the physician will probably leave the cerclage in place until what occurs?
[ ] **1.** The client goes into labor.
[ ] **2.** The client's baby is delivered.
[ ] **3.** The second trimester ends.
[ ] **4.** The client is near term.

A 29-year-old primigravid client is in the 22nd week of pregnancy. The physician determines that the client has pregnancy-induced hypertension (PIH).

82. When assessing a client with a history of pregnancy-induced hypertension (PIH), the nurse should thoroughly explore which finding at each visit?
[ ] **1.** A decrease in urine protein level
[ ] **2.** An increase in urine output
[ ] **3.** A decrease in pulse rate
[ ] **4.** An unexpected weight gain

83. Which assessment finding is most indicative of mild pregnancy-induced hypertension (PIH)?
[ ] **1.** A 15 mm Hg rise in the baseline systolic blood pressure
[ ] **2.** A weight gain of 1 pound per week in the second trimester
[ ] **3.** A +1 protein measured with a urine reagent test strip
[ ] **4.** The presence of frequent ankle edema

The physician decides that the client can manage her pregnancy-induced hypertension (PIH) at home and requests that the nurse provide instructions for home care.

84. Which instruction regarding the home care of pregnancy-induced hypertension (PIH) is most appropriate?
[ ] **1.** Decrease fluid intake.
[ ] **2.** Return for bimonthly checkups.
[ ] **3.** Eat high-protein foods.
[ ] **4.** Limit activity to light housework.

The client's condition worsens and requires admission to the hospital. The physician orders magnesium sulfate.

85. While the client is receiving magnesium sulfate, besides monitoring the client's vital signs, what other nursing assessment is essential to include?
[ ] **1.** Urine for glucose
[ ] **2.** Deep tendon reflexes
[ ] **3.** Stool for blood
[ ] **4.** Pupils for constriction

86. Which medication should the nurse have on hand when the client is receiving magnesium sulfate?
[ ] **1.** Hydralazine (Apresoline)
[ ] **2.** Oxytocin (Pitocin)
[ ] **3.** Methylergonovine (Methergine)
[ ] **4.** Calcium gluconate (Kalcinate)

87. Which assessment finding is the best indication that magnesium sulfate toxicity is developing?
[ ] **1.** Manifesting brisk deep tendon reflexes
[ ] **2.** Taking less than 14 breaths/minute
[ ] **3.** Excreting protein in the urine
[ ] **4.** Having a magnesium level of 5 mg/dL

The nurse frequently assesses the client and finds that the pregnancy-induced hypertension (PIH) has progressed to eclampsia.

88. The nurse notifies the physician immediately when detecting which one of the following assessment findings?
[ ] **1.** Seizures
[ ] **2.** Drowsiness
[ ] **3.** Bradycardia
[ ] **4.** Vomiting

A 28-year-old multipara client is admitted to the hospital for observation during the 10th week of pregnancy. The client has a history of habitual spontaneous abortions.

89. Which findings reported by the client at this time suggest there is a threat of aborting the fetus? Select all that apply.
[ ] **1.** Cold, clammy skin
[ ] **2.** Severe headache
[ ] **3.** Persistent tachycardia
[ ] **4.** Mild irregular uterine cramping
[ ] **5.** Discomfort in the lower back
[ ] **6.** Vaginal bleeding or spotting

The physician examines the client and determines that the cervix is dilated but the fetus and placenta are still in the uterus.

90. Which nursing intervention is most appropriate when a spontaneous abortion is inevitable?
[ ] **1.** Prepare the client for dilation and curettage (D&C).
[ ] **2.** Place the client in Trendelenburg's position.
[ ] **3.** Prepare the client for placement of a purse-string stitch.
[ ] **4.** Place the client in the side-lying position.

The client comments to the nurse, "This is like a recurring nightmare. This same thing happened during my last two pregnancies. I don't want to lose another baby."

91. Which response by the nurse is most appropriate at this time?
[ ] **1.** "I know this is disappointing. Would you like to talk about how you are feeling?"
[ ] **2.** "Be positive. You are young enough to have additional pregnancies."
[ ] **3.** "I know you are scared, but stress will only make the situation worse."
[ ] **4.** "Trust me; everything will work out for the best in the end."

A 22-year-old gravida I, para 0, has insulin-dependent diabetes mellitus and is being seen by the obstetrician for the first time. The client was diagnosed with diabetes at age 6. The diabetes has been well controlled since the initial diagnosis. While waiting to see the physician, the client asks the nurse if the pregnancy will increase the need for insulin.

92. Which explanation by the nurse is correct concerning the client's need for insulin during pregnancy?
[ ] **1.** Insulin requirements will most likely increase.
[ ] **2.** Insulin requirements will most likely decrease.
[ ] **3.** Insulin requirements will most likely fluctuate.
[ ] **4.** Insulin requirements will most likely not change.

The client also asks the nurse what kinds of diabetes-related complications can be expected during pregnancy.

93. The nurse correctly informs the client that diabetics are at risk for developing which condition?
[ ] **1.** Hyperemesis gravidarum
[ ] **2.** Pregnancy-induced hypertension
[ ] **3.** Placenta previa
[ ] **4.** Toxoplasmosis

In the last trimester of pregnancy, the client's diabetes has been well controlled. The client tells the nurse about being excited but also scared that something could be wrong with the baby because of the diabetes.

94. Which response by the nurse is most accurate?
[ ] **1.** "Your baby may be large and may initially need glucose monitoring."
[ ] **2.** "Your baby may be small but otherwise will be healthy."
[ ] **3.** "Your baby will most likely be insulin dependent during adulthood."
[ ] **4.** "Your baby will have difficulty metabolizing simple sugars."

A 21-year-old multigravid client who is 8 months' pregnant is admitted to the obstetric unit for observation. The admission diagnosis is partial placenta previa. The client's partner asks the nurse, "What is placenta previa?"

95. Which response by the nurse provides the best explanation regarding placenta previa?
[ ] **1.** "The placenta is implanted over or close to the internal cervical opening."
[ ] **2.** "The placenta isn't producing the hormones needed to maintain the pregnancy."
[ ] **3.** "The placenta is invaded by polyps that cause premature uterine contractions."
[ ] **4.** "The placenta is producing antibodies that are destroying the baby's red blood cells."

The client's partner verbalizes concern about how placenta previa is treated.

96. The nurse correctly states that the physician is most likely to do which of the following if the client's condition remains stable?
[ ] **1.** Induce labor prematurely.
[ ] **2.** Perform an emergency cesarean birth.
[ ] **3.** Place the client on bed rest until full term.
[ ] **4.** Start the client on ritodrine (Yutopar).

After a short observation period, the client with placenta previa is sent home. One week later, the client reports to the hospital with profuse vaginal bleeding.

97. On the basis of the client's clinical presentation, what information is a priority to obtain at this time? Select all that apply.
[ ] **1.** Height and weight
[ ] **2.** Blood pressure and pulse rate
[ ] **3.** Pregnancy and prior delivery history
[ ] **4.** General health and drug history
[ ] **5.** Urinalysis and beta-streptococcal test results
[ ] **6.** Phone number of the client's obstetrician

A 30-year-old multigravid client who is in the last trimester of pregnancy is diagnosed with abruptio placentae.

98. Which assessment findings are considered predisposing factors for the development of abruptio placentae? Select all that apply.
[ ] **1.** Gestational diabetes
[ ] **2.** Hyperemesis gravidarum
[ ] **3.** Oligohydramnios
[ ] **4.** Pregnancy-induced hypertension
[ ] **5.** History of placenta previa
[ ] **6.** Reports of crack cocaine use

99. Which findings are most indicative of abruptio placentae and should be reported to the physician immediately? Select all that apply.
[ ] **1.** Rigid, boardlike, tender abdomen
[ ] **2.** Severe nausea and vomiting
[ ] **3.** Fetal heart rate of 160 beats/minute
[ ] **4.** Painless vaginal bleeding
[ ] **5.** Dark red vaginal bleeding
[ ] **6.** A seizure lasting several seconds

100. If the client develops a complete abruption, which nursing action is most appropriate?
[ ] **1.** Obtain a written consent for an immediate cesarean birth.
[ ] **2.** Give the client an enema and prepare the abdomen.
[ ] **3.** Place the client in Trendelenburg's position.
[ ] **4.** Prepare the client for a contraction stress test.

A client comes to the clinic in the last month of pregnancy. The client has significant anxiety regarding invasive procedures such as an I.V. line and internal fetal monitoring that may be required during labor and delivery. The doctor, nurses, and client prepare a plan limiting invasive procedures yet maintaining appropriate fetal monitoring and an acceptable pain level for the client.

101. In the labor and delivery suite, the physician orders meperidine (Demerol) 100 mg intramuscularly. The nurse chooses to inject the meperidine via the Z-track (zigzag) method. Which muscle is best for the nurse to select when administering the meperidine to the client?
[ ] **1.** Deltoid
[ ] **2.** Trapezius
[ ] **3.** Gluteus medius
[ ] **4.** Latissimus dorsi

102. Just before inserting the needle into the muscle for a Z-track injection, the nurse appropriately pulls the tissue at the injection site in what direction?
[ ] **1.** Laterally
[ ] **2.** Obliquely
[ ] **3.** Proximally
[ ] **4.** Superiorly

A client, gravida I, para 0, recently immigrated to the United States from Africa and comes to the obstetric (OB) clinic. During the pregnancy history, the client indicates that she believes she is about 12 weeks' pregnant. The client also reports having had rubella (German measles) 2 months ago.

103. Which possible complication should the nurse discuss with the client?
[ ] **1.** Premature labor
[ ] **2.** Fetal abnormalities
[ ] **3.** Severe preeclampsia
[ ] **4.** Hydatidiform mole formation

104. The licensed practical nurse is working in the labor and delivery unit with a registered nurse. The following clients present to the unit. When assessing client needs, to which client will the licensed practical nurse most likely be assigned?
[ ] **1.** A 16-year-old client who is 37 weeks gestation experiencing leg cramps, increased pelvic pressure, and a bloody show.
[ ] **2.** A 22-year-old who is 37 weeks gestation with a passage of clear, odorless fluid from the vagina
[ ] **3.** A 25-year-old who is 38 weeks gestation with the passage of yellow-green fluid from the vagina.
[ ] **4.** A 30-year-old who is 24 weeks gestation having contractions in the abdomen and groin every 5 minutes.

105. Which of the following is most indicative of the presence of hydatidiform mole?
[ ] **1.** A blotchy brown discoloration on the face
[ ] **2.** A positive Chadwick's sign
[ ] **3.** The presence of ballottement
[ ] **4.** A uterus that is larger than expected

106. Which pregnant client should the nurse encourage to undergo hepatitis B testing?
[ ] **1.** A client with a history of cigarette smoking
[ ] **2.** A client who is single and pregnant for the first time
[ ] **3.** A client who emigrated in the past year from Haiti
[ ] **4.** A client who was recently exposed to *Haemophilus influenzae*

Elective Abortion

An 18-year-old primigravid client is considering terminating the pregnancy and wants more information before making a decision. The client asks the nurse, "At what point during pregnancy can a baby live outside the mother?"

107. Which response by the nurse is correct concerning the legal threshold of viability?
[ ] **1.** It is usually estimated to be 36 to 40 weeks.
[ ] **2.** It is usually estimated to be 30 to 35 weeks.
[ ] **3.** It is usually estimated to be 20 to 24 weeks.
[ ] **4.** It is usually estimated to be 10 to 15 weeks.

Correct Answers, Rationales, and Test Taking Strategies

Anatomy and Physiology of the Male and Female Reproductive Systems

1. 1. The ovum is released from the ovary and enters the outer third of the fallopian tube, where the sperm fertilizes it. After fertilization, the fertilized ovum travels through the remainder of the fallopian tube and enters the uterus, where it implants and remains throughout pregnancy.

> *Test Taking Strategy—Analyze to determine what information the question asks for, which is the location of fertilization. Recall that fertilization is different than implantation, and it is important to know the physiologic differences. Recall that the fertilized ovum is implanted in the uterus, thus making the location of fertilization in one of the two fallopian tubes (option 1). Review the fertilization process if you had difficulty answering this question.*
> **Cognitive Level**—*Understanding*
> **Client Needs Category**—*Health promotion and maintenance*
> **Client Needs Subcategory**—*None*

2. 2. The ovum remains viable for 24 hours after being released from the ovary. If fertilization does not occur within this time frame, conception cannot take place.

> *Test Taking Strategy—Analyze to determine what information the question asks for, which is the viability of the ovum after ovulation. Recall that once the ovum is released from the ovary, it must be fertilized with the sperm within 24 hours of being released (option 2) or it will deteriorate. Review the process of ovulation if you had difficulty answering this question.*
> **Cognitive Level**—*Understanding*
> **Client Needs Category**—*Health promotion and maintenance*
> **Client Needs Subcategory**—*None*

3. 2, 5, 6. Because heat can damage or kill sperm, men should avoid hot tubs or taking hot baths if attempting to prevent infertility. Tight-fitting clothing, such as jeans or briefs, may also have the same effect by trapping body heat and elevating the temperature of the testes. Strenuous exercise can also change the temperature of the testes. Testosterone production is changed during strenuous exercise, which may cause a decrease in sperm formation. Smoking is associated with low sperm counts and decreased motility. Swimming does not affect the viability of sperm.

> *Test Taking Strategy—Analyze to determine what information the question asks for, which is techniques for increasing sperm production. Alternative-format "select all that apply" questions require considering each option independently to decide its merit in answering the question. Recall that activities that raise the temperature around the scrotum may decrease the sperm count. Smoking is extremely counterproductive for fertility because it lowers the sperm count by approximately 23% and can damage the nuclei of sperm, causing chromosomal abnormalities. Review factors affecting spermatogenesis and sperm motility if you had difficulty answering this question.*
> **Cognitive Level**—*Applying*
> **Client Needs Category**—*Health promotion and maintenance*
> **Client Needs Subcategory**—*None*

4. 2. The true pelvis is the part of the pelvis that influences the woman's ability to deliver vaginally. The false pelvis, which is formed by the iliac portion of the innominate bone, is what accounts for hip measurements. The fetus must be in an appropriate position and small enough to pass through the true pelvis for a successful vaginal delivery.

> *Test Taking Strategy—Look at the key words "most appropriate" in reference to the nurse's response to the client's concerns about the impact "small hips" will have on a vaginal birth. Recall that the true pelvis consists of the pelvic inlet, pelvic cavity, and pelvic outlet; this is what dictates the bony limits of the birth canal (option 2). Review the prenatal measurements that determine the potential for cephalopelvic disproportion at the time of labor if you had difficulty answering this question.*
> **Cognitive Level**—*Applying*
> **Client Needs Category**—*Health promotion and maintenance*
> **Client Needs Subcategory**—*None*

5. 4. The sex of the baby is determined at fertilization, which occurs in the outer third of the fallopian tube. Each parent contributes one sex chromosome. The mother always contributes an X chromosome. The father contributes an X or a Y chromosome. If a sperm containing an X chromosome fertilizes the ovum, the offspring is a female. If a sperm containing a Y chromosome fertilizes the ovum, the offspring is a male.

> *Test Taking Strategy—Analyze to determine what information the question asks for, which is when sex determination occurs. Recall that a zygote, a fertilized ovum, contains 46 chromosomes, 22 + 1 X chromosome from the mother and 22 + 1 X or Y chromosome from the father. The combination of chromosomes and the resulting gender occur at the time of fertilization (option 4). Review the process of gender determination if you had difficulty answering this question.*
> **Cognitive Level**—*Applying*
> **Client Needs Category**—*Health promotion and maintenance*
> **Client Needs Subcategory**—*None*

6. 1. Vaginal discharge during a woman's monthly period, often called *menstrual flow* or *menses*, consists of endometrial cells sloughed from the thickened uterine lining formed to prepare for pregnancy. When fertilization does not occur, the lining is sloughed. The discharge contains mucus, tissue, and blood. The first day of blood flow is considered the first day of the monthly cycle, which lasts about 28 days. The bleeding continues for 3 to 7 days and may be dark red, bright red, or rust-colored. The perimetrium is the thin outer layer of the uterus. The myometrium is the muscle layer of the uterus. The epimetrium is part of the peritoneum.

> *Test Taking Strategy*—*Analyze to determine what information the question asks for, which is the source of vaginal bleeding during menstruation. Recall that if fertilization does not occur, the resulting decrease in estrogen and progesterone levels causes the endometrium (option 1) to slough, resulting in menstruation. Review the menstrual cycle and hormonal levels that fluctuate during the proliferative, secretory, and menstrual phases if you had difficulty answering this question.*
> *Cognitive Level*—*Understanding*
> *Client Needs Category*—*Health promotion and maintenance*
> *Client Needs Subcategory*—*None*

Signs and Symptoms of Pregnancy

7. 3. Primigravida describes a woman who is pregnant for the first time. Multipara describes a woman who has delivered more than one viable infant. A primipara is a woman who has delivered her first viable infant. Multigravida describes a woman who has been pregnant more than once.

> *Test Taking Strategy*—*Analyze to determine what information the question asks for, which is the term used to describe the obstetric history of a client who is pregnant for the first time. Refer to the terminology used to document a client's obstetric history, which is described in the rationale. Recall that the term gravid refers to being pregnant and the prefix primi-indicates a first pregnancy (option 3). Review terms used to describe an obstetric history if you had difficulty answering this question.*
> *Cognitive Level*—*Understanding*
> *Client Needs Category*—*Health promotion and maintenance*
> *Client Needs Subcategory*—*None*

8. 3. Identical twins result when one fertilized ovum divides into two identical halves that develop into two individuals with the same appearance and same gender. Fraternal twins are the result of two separate ova fertilized by two different sperm at the same time. They may or may not resemble each other and may or may not be of the same gender.

> *Test Taking Strategy*—*Analyze to determine what information the question asks for, which is the physiologic event resulting in the development of identical twins. Recall that monozygotic twins (identical) develop from a single fertilized ovum (option 3) and have the exact same genetics, gender, and physical appearance at birth. Dizygotic twins (fraternal) develop from two separate ova and two separate sperm; they resemble each other, but have different physical characteristics, may be the same or different genders, and look similar to siblings born during other pregnancies. Review the outcome of multifetal pregnancies if you had difficulty answering this question.*
> *Cognitive Level*—*Applying*
> *Client Needs Category*—*Health promotion and maintenance*
> *Client Needs Subcategory*—*None*

9. 2. Abdominal enlargement is considered a probable sign of pregnancy. Amenorrhea (absence of monthly periods), nausea, vomiting, and frequent urination are all considered to be presumptive signs of pregnancy because they can also be indications of conditions other than pregnancy. Positive signs are those that cannot be mistaken for any other condition, such as hearing fetal heart sounds or detecting the presence of the fetus during an ultrasound examination.

> *Test Taking Strategy*—*Use the process of elimination to select the one option that is a probable sign of pregnancy. If unsure, analyze the options. Eliminate options 1, 3, and 4, which occur earliest after conception, but could also be caused by other reasons. Option 2 remains as the correct answer because abdominal enlargement occurs most of the time with a pregnancy but is not totally exclusive to pregnancy. Review the presumptive, probable, and positive signs of pregnancy if you had difficulty answering this question.*
> *Cognitive Level*—*Analyzing*
> *Client Needs Category*—*Health promotion and maintenance*
> *Client Needs Subcategory*—*None*

10. 3. Levels of human chorionic gonadotropin (hCG) rise significantly shortly after implantation of the ovum. Blood and urine testing for hCG is the basis for most pregnancy tests, because hCG can be measured as early as 8 to 11 days after ovulation. The level of hCG doubles every 2 to 3 days and can be used to validate that the pregnancy is continuing and that a miscarriage has not occurred. The alpha-fetoprotein (AFP) test is performed during pregnancy to determine the presence of neural tube defects such as spina bifida. Follicle-stimulating hormone (FSH) is not associated with pregnancy but is related to the maturation of the ovum before ovulation.

> *Test Taking Strategy*—*Analyze to determine what information the question asks for, which is a laboratory test used to confirm pregnancy. Recall that hCG*

is a hormone that is produced by the placenta during pregnancy (option 3). Pregnancy can be confirmed through an examination of the client and a blood test that measures hCG. Review pregnancy testing if you have difficulty answering this question.
Cognitive Level—*Applying*
Client Needs Category—*Health promotion and maintenance*
Client Needs Subcategory—*None*

11. 1. A transvaginal ultrasound can detect pregnancy as early as 2½ to 3 weeks. An abdominal ultrasound can detect pregnancy as early as 5 to 6 weeks, well before the uterus ascends out of the pelvis. The ultrasound has replaced the X-ray as a diagnostic tool for pregnancy, eliminating the risks associated with fetal radiation exposure.
> *Test Taking Strategy*—*Look at the key words "most accurate" when selecting an option that correlates with a statement that is more correct than any of the others regarding the use of an ultrasound to confirm pregnancy. Recall that early in gestation, the uterus is closer to the vagina than to the abdominal wall. The thin transvaginal ultrasound probe can provide a visual image of the fetus (option 1), detect its beating heart, identify structural problems in reproductive organs or the placenta, and provide evidence of more than one fetus. After 18 to 20 weeks of pregnancy, a transabdominal ultrasound is more appropriate. Review use of transvaginal and transabdominal ultrasounds during pregnancy if you had difficulty answering this question.*
Cognitive Level—*Analyzing*
Client Needs Category—*Health promotion and maintenance*
Client Needs Subcategory—*None*

12. 2. Chadwick's sign is a bluish discoloration of the cervix, vagina, and vulva caused by increased vascularization of the reproductive organs. Braxton Hicks contractions are spontaneous intermittent contractions that occur during pregnancy. Goodell's sign is the softening of the cervix, and linea nigra is the dark brown line extending from the umbilicus to the symphysis pubis that appears on the skin of many pregnant women.
> *Test Taking Strategy*—*Look at the key words "most accurate" in reference to the nurse's explanation of the symptom known as Chadwick's sign. Knowledge of the probable signs of pregnancy, such as the bluish discoloration of the reproductive organs known as Chadwick's sign (option 2), facilitates answering this question correctly. Review the description of Chadwick's sign if you had difficulty answering this question.*
Cognitive Level—*Analyzing*
Client Needs Category—*Health promotion and maintenance*
Client Needs Subcategory—*None*

13. 1. Ballottement is observed when the fetus rises (or bounces) in the amniotic fluid, then returns to its normal position after a gentle push or tapping of the lower portion of the uterus by the examiner. Ballottement is usually first observed during the fourth or fifth month of pregnancy.
> *Test Taking Strategy*—*Analyze to determine what information the question asks for, which is the relevance of ballottement to the length of gestation. Recall that ballottement, a term derived from a French word that means "to rise like a ball," is a technique for detecting or examining a floating object, in this case the fetus, in the body. During midpregnancy (option 1), the fetus will rise and quickly rebound to the original position when the cervix is tapped by the examiner's finger. Review the time during pregnancy when ballottement is performed if you had difficulty answering this question.*
Cognitive Level—*Applying*
Client Needs Category—*Health promotion and maintenance*
Client Needs Subcategory—*None*

14. 4. The health care provider's detection of the fetal heartbeat confirms pregnancy. A palpable fetal outline and positive pregnancy test are probable signs of pregnancy but are not conclusive evidence. A blotchy tan discoloration of the face known as *chloasma* is a presumptive sign of pregnancy.
> *Test Taking Strategy*—*Use the process of elimination to select the option that identifies an assessment finding that best represents a positive sign of pregnancy. Options 1, 2, and 3 can be eliminated because they are probable signs of pregnancy, not positive signs. Recall that an actual heartbeat (option 4) is conclusive for pregnancy. Review the positive signs of pregnancy if you had difficulty answering this question.*
Cognitive Level—*Applying*
Client Needs Category—*Health promotion and maintenance*
Client Needs Subcategory—*None*

15. 2. The first fetal movement felt by the mother is referred to as *quickening*. If this is the woman's first pregnancy, quickening is usually experienced between 16 and 20 weeks' gestation.
> *Test Taking Strategy*—*Analyze to determine what information the question asks for, which is the time when fetal movement is first felt in the primigravid client. Recall that fetal movement felt by the mother, known as quickening, is typically felt between 16 and 20 weeks of pregnancy by the primigravid client, which is later than felt by the multigravid client. Review the occurrence of quickening and when it occurs during pregnancy if you had difficulty answering this question.*

Cognitive Level—*Applying*
Client Needs Category—*Health promotion and maintenance*
Client Needs Subcategory—*None*

Assessing the Pregnant Client

16. 2. Quickening, the term attributed to the mother's first feeling of fetal movement, is often described as a fluttering sensation. In a primigravid client, quickening usually occurs in the second trimester, between the 16th and 20th weeks of gestation. In a multipara client, it typically occurs earlier, at about 14 to 18 weeks' gestation. Due dates are calculated based on the first day of the last menstrual period, not on fetal movement. Quickening occurs at about the same time regardless of whether a woman is carrying one or two fetuses.

> *Test Taking Strategy*—*Analyze to determine what information the question asks for, which is the significance of detecting fetal movement reported by the mother on the first prenatal visit. Recall that the multigravid client may feel fetal movement between 14 and 18 weeks of pregnancy (option 2), which is sooner than the primigravid client. Review the stage of pregnancy during which it is likely that a multigravid client will feel first fetal movement if you had difficulty answering this question.*
> *Cognitive Level*—*Applying*
> *Client Needs Category*—*Health promotion and maintenance*
> *Client Needs Subcategory*—*None*

17. 4. TPAL is an acronym used when documenting the client's obstetric history. *T* represents the number of term pregnancies, *P* represents the number of premature infants delivered, *A* represents the number of abortions or miscarriages, and *L* represents the number of living children. The client in this situation has had two term pregnancies, no premature deliveries, no abortions, and has three living children. Therefore, the correct TPAL is T-II, P-0, A-0, L-III.

> *Test Taking Strategy*—*Analyze to determine what information the question asks for, which is the correct interpretation of the TPAL method used to record the client's obstetric history. The client states that she has a son and twin daughters and has had no abortions or stillbirths, making option 4 the correct answer. Review the TPAL method for documenting a client's obstetric history if you had difficulty answering this question.*
> *Cognitive Level*—*Applying*
> *Client Needs Category*—*Health promotion and maintenance*
> *Client Needs Subcategory*—*None*

18. 4. Nägele's rule is one method of determining the estimated date of delivery. When using Nägele's rule, add 7 days to the first day of the last menstrual period (LMP), and count back 3 months. In this situation, the estimated delivery date is December 20.

> *Test Taking Strategy*—*Analyze to determine what information the question asks for, which requires determining a client's expected delivery date using Nägele's rule. Recall that Nägele's rule helps determine a possible date of delivery using a formula based on the first day of the LMP. Using March 13th as the client's first day of the LMP, December 20th (option 4) is the correct answer. Review Nägele's rule if you had difficulty answering this question.*
> *Cognitive Level*—*Applying*
> *Client Needs Category*—*Health promotion and maintenance*
> *Client Needs Subcategory*—*None*

19. 1. When preparing the client for a pelvic examination, the nurse assists her into the lithotomy position. In this position, the client lies on her back with the knees bent and feet resting flat on the table or placed in stirrups. Her buttocks should extend slightly beyond the edge of the examination table. All of the other positions (prone, Sims', and Trendelenburg's) do not accommodate this type of examination.

> *Test Taking Strategy*—*Analyze to determine what information the question asks for, which is the client position used during a pelvic examination. Recall that the lithotomy position (option 1) facilitates an examination of the structures in the female reproductive tract. Review client preparation for a pelvic examination if you had difficulty answering this question.*
> *Cognitive Level*—*Applying*
> *Client Needs Category*—*Health promotion and maintenance*
> *Client Needs Subcategory*—*None*

20. 2. Before the pelvic examination, the client should be encouraged to empty her bladder. This action increases the client's comfort during the examination and facilitates a more accurate assessment of the pelvic structures. It is not necessary nor is it routine for the client to receive an enema, sedative, or shave and prep before having a pelvic examination.

> *Test Taking Strategy*—*Look at the key words "most appropriate" in reference to the nursing intervention that is best before a pelvic examination. Recall the anatomy of the female genitourinary tract and the close proximity of the urinary bladder to the uterus when considering the means to promote comfort during the pelvic examination. Consider that pressure from the pelvic examination may cause additional discomfort during the examination and interfere with assessment*

if the bladder is not emptied (option 2). Review client preparation for a pelvic examination if you had difficulty answering this question.
Cognitive Level—*Applying*
Client Needs Category—*Health promotion and maintenance*
Client Needs Subcategory—*None*

21. 4. The nurse instructs the client to let her knees fall outward and to relax during the examination; this increases the client's comfort level. The client should have a pillow under her head and should not lift her head off the pillow during the examination. Raising the head tightens the abdominal muscles, making the examination more difficult. Having the client press her back into the examination table and tighten her buttocks will not promote relaxation because these actions cause increased tension in the muscles of the perineum.

Test Taking Strategy—*Use the process of elimination to select the option that identifies the best method for promoting the client's comfort during a pelvic examination. Option 4 is the correct answer because relaxing the muscles facilitates a more comfortable examination for the client and increases the ease with which the examiner can assess the client. Review how to prepare a client, pregnant or not, for a pelvic examination if you had difficulty answering this question.*
Cognitive Level—*Applying*
Client Needs Category—*Health promotion and maintenance*
Client Needs Subcategory—*None*

22. 2. With the use of a Doppler device, the examiner can detect fetal heart tones as early as 8 to 10 weeks' gestation. The Doppler bounces harmless sound waves off the fetal heart. When you actually hear the heartbeat over this period depends on the luck of the instrument, position of the uterus, and the mother's body build. The fetal heartbeat is audible with a standard fetoscope between 18 and 20 weeks' gestation.

Test Taking Strategy—*Analyze to determine what information the question asks for, which is when the fetal heartbeat can be detected with a Doppler device. Recall that the embryonic heart starts beating at 22 days after conception or in the 5th week of pregnancy and is able to be detected within the next few weeks (option 2). Review embryonic development and when the heartbeat can initially be heard with an amplifying device such as a Doppler if you had difficulty answering this question.*
Cognitive Level—*Understanding*
Client Needs Category—*Health promotion and maintenance*
Client Needs Subcategory—*None*

23. 4. When auscultating for the fetal heart rate, the nurse may also hear the uterine soufflé (a soft whirling sound produced by the maternal blood moving through the uterine vessels). To differentiate between fetal heart tones and the uterine soufflé, the nurse should count the maternal pulse rate and compare it to the rate obtained when listening for the fetal heart tones. Placing the client on her right side, counting during fetal movement, and counting between Braxton Hicks contractions will not ensure an accurate fetal heart rate.

Test Taking Strategy—*Use the process of elimination to select the option that best ensures an accurate assessment of the fetal heart rate. Option 4 remains as the best answer because differentiating between the maternal pulse rate and the fetal heartbeats ensures an accurate assessment. Review the method for assessing a fetal heart rate if you had difficulty answering this question.*
Cognitive Level—*Applying*
Client Needs Category—*Health promotion and maintenance*
Client Needs Subcategory—*None*

24. 1. The fetal heart rate is normally between 120 and 160 beats/minute. A fetal heart rate less than 120 beats/minute or greater than 160 beats/minute may indicate fetal distress and should be immediately reported.

Test Taking Strategy—*Analyze to determine what information the question asks for, which is a fetal heart rate of significant concern that requires immediate reporting to the physician. Knowledge of the normal fetal heart rate is helpful in answering the question. To narrow the selection, recall that fetal heart rates tend to be rapid. The lowest heart rate, which is 100 beats/minute (option 1), is the correct answer because it is a significantly low heart rate. Review the range of normal fetal heart rates if you had difficulty answering this question.*
Cognitive Level—*Applying*
Client Needs Category—*Physiological integrity*
Client Needs Subcategory—*Physiological adaptation*

25. 3. The maternal serum alpha-fetoprotein (AFP) test is used to screen for neural tube defects such as spina bifida. AFP is a substance made in the liver of an unborn fetus. The amount of AFP in the blood of a pregnant woman can be used to detect neural tube defects, but it can also identify other congenital disorders, such as Down syndrome and abdominal wall defects. This test should be performed between 14 and 16 weeks' gestation. The HBsAg test is used to detect hepatitis B. The VDRL (Venereal Disease Research Laboratory) and FTA-ABS (fluorescent treponemal antibody absorption) tests are used to screen for syphilis.

Test Taking Strategy—*The key words "most accurate" can be used to select the option that correctly identi-*

*fies a test for detecting spina bifida during preg-
nancy. The answer can be narrowed by eliminating
tests that are performed for other obvious reasons.
The prefix feto-, used in fetoprotein, shows some
relationship to the word fetal, which may lead to
selecting option 1 as the correct answer. Review the
purpose for each of the diagnostic tests listed if you
had difficulty answering this question.*
Cognitive Level—*Applying*
Client Needs Category—*Health promotion and
maintenance*
Client Needs Subcategory—*None*

26. 3. A pregnant woman who is experiencing no complications usually visits the health care provider every
4 weeks for the first 28 weeks of pregnancy, then every
2 weeks from 28 to 36 weeks' gestation, and then weekly
from the 37th week to delivery.
Test Taking Strategy—*Use the process of elimination
to select the option that identifies the best plan for
a prenatal visit schedule after 28 weeks. Consider
that the purpose for prenatal visits is to monitor
fetal status and maternal cervical dilation, the
latter of which occurs near the end of gestation.
Analyze the options for a schedule that ends with
weekly examinations. Eliminate options 2 and 4
because they do not end with weekly visits. Discriminate between options 1 and 3. Eliminate option 1;
weekly visits are not scheduled immediately after
28 weeks because there would be no cervical dilation at this point. Review the prenatal schedule of
a normal pregnancy if you had difficulty answering
this question.*
Cognitive Level—*Applying*
Client Needs Category—*Health promotion and
maintenance*
Client Needs Subcategory—*None*

27. 1, 2, 3. Exercise raises body temperature and
speeds the metabolism and heart rate. For these reasons,
exercising during pregnancy should be carefully monitored
so that no harm comes to the mother or baby. The nurse
should advise the client to avoid exercising in hot, humid
weather to ensure that her core body temperature does not
rise and possibly affect the baby. Likewise, she should
avoid any jerking, bouncing, or jumping movements that
could harm the growing fetus. It is important for the client
to drink plenty of fluids before and after exercising to prevent dehydration, which can alter her electrolyte balance
and temperature as well as those of the fetus. She should
also exercise only during the cooler part of the day or in an
air-conditioned environment. Although the client should
be able to tolerate exercising at least three times per week
(not just once weekly), she should limit any strenuous
workouts to no more than 15 minutes per session. Exercises should never be done in the supine position, espe-

cially after the fourth month, to avoid supine hypotension
and insufficient blood flow to the baby.
Test Taking Strategy—*Analyze to determine what information the question asks for, which is components
of client teaching about exercise during pregnancy.
Alternative-format "select all that apply" questions
require considering each option independently to
decide its merit in answering the question. Consider
each option and evaluate the benefits and risks of the
instruction. Review recommendations about exercise
during pregnancy if you had difficulty answering this
question.*
Cognitive Level—*Applying*
Client Needs Category—*Health promotion and
maintenance*
Client Needs Subcategory—*None*

28. 3. At 20 weeks' gestation, the fundus of the uterus
can be palpated near the level of the umbilicus. At
16 weeks' gestation, the fundus is located halfway
between the top of the symphysis pubis and the umbilicus.
Close to term (38 to 40 weeks), the uterus can be palpated
just below the xiphoid process.
Test Taking Strategy—*Analyze to determine what
information the question asks for, which is where
to palpate the fundus at 20 weeks' gestation. The
fundal height is measured from the top of the pubic
bone to the top of the uterus as a reference point for
analyzing maternal progress. Consider the standard
of fundal placement midway through the pregnancy
as at the level of the umbilicus (option 3). Review
standards for fundal height measurement at various
times during gestation if you had difficulty answering this question.*
Cognitive Level—*Applying*
Client Needs Category—*Health promotion and
maintenance*
Client Needs Subcategory—*None*

29. 2. The glucose tolerance test is a routine test performed between 24 and 28 weeks' gestation as a screening
tool for gestational diabetes. A Pap smear and rubella titer
are usually performed at the first prenatal visit. Coombs'
test is not routinely performed during pregnancy; it is used
to determine the possibility of Rh incompatibility between
the mother and fetus or neonate.
Test Taking Strategy—*Analyze to determine what
information the question asks for, which is the test
that is routinely performed at 24 weeks' gestation.
If unsure, consider either the purpose for the test or
actions that will be taken after the test results are
obtained when discriminating among the options.
Option 2 screens for gestational diabetes, requires
additional teaching, and requires diabetic monitoring to avoid complications. The other options do not
have an impact on prenatal care at this stage of the*

pregnancy. Review typical prenatal screening midway during a pregnancy if you had difficulty answering this question.
Cognitive Level—*Applying*
Client Needs Category—*Health promotion and maintenance*
Client Needs Subcategory—*None*

30. 4. To perform the nonstress test, the nurse attaches a fetal monitor to the client's abdomen and monitors the response of the fetal heart rate to fetal movement. The nonstress test is noninvasive and poses little risk to the mother; therefore, an emergency crash cart is not necessary. I.V. oxytocin (Pitocin) may be given for several reasons, including augmentation of labor and control of postpartum hemorrhage. A cardiac monitor is not used during a nonstress test.

> **Test Taking Strategy**—*Analyze to determine what information the question asks for, which is an item the nurse should have available when a nonstress test is performed. A nonstress test is a simple, noninvasive test performed in pregnancies beyond 28 weeks' gestation. Because this test poses no expected complications, options 1, 2, and 3 can be eliminated. A fetal monitor (option 4) should be available to record the data from the test. Review the nonstress test procedure if you had difficulty answering this question.*
> **Cognitive Level**—*Applying*
> **Client Needs Category**—*Health promotion and maintenance*
> **Client Needs Subcategory**—*None*

31. 2. Amniocentesis is an invasive procedure in which a sterile needle is inserted through the uterine wall and a small sample of amniotic fluid is withdrawn and used for analysis. This test is usually performed early in the second trimester to rule out congenital abnormalities, such as Down syndrome or spinal cord defects. It may also be used during the third trimester to assess fetal lung maturity, postmaturity of the fetus, or fetal death. An amniocentesis is usually performed after the 14th week of gestation, when there is sufficient fluid to sample.

> **Test Taking Strategy**—*Analyze to determine what information the question asks for, which is when an amniocentesis is typically performed. When analyzing the options, consider factors that would make the amniocentesis procedure unsafe for the fetus or provide inaccurate results. Note that options 1 and 4 are early in the pregnancy, making it difficult to withdraw sufficient amniotic fluid; thus, both can be eliminated. Next consider options 2 and 3 as midway in the pregnancy and during labor. Eliminate option 3 because delivery is close at hand, which makes option 2 the correct answer. Review the protocol for performing an amniocentesis if you had difficulty answering this question.*

Cognitive Level—*Applying*
Client Needs Category—*Health promotion and maintenance*
Client Needs Subcategory—*None*

Nutritional Needs During Pregnancy

32. 2. The client's current eating pattern and preferences should be assessed before a teaching plan can be formulated and implemented. Once this information is obtained, the nurse can show the client what foods to add or delete to ensure a balanced, nutritious diet. The nurse should include the client in the planning process to ensure her cooperation with the choices made and to advise her on calorie recommendations, nutritional requirements, and food equivalencies (such as 1 cup of milk equaling 10 mg of calcium). After initiating this teaching, the nurse can work with the client to develop sample menus to meet her nutritional needs during the pregnancy. Regardless of her prepregnancy weight, a pregnant client should gain sufficient weight to meet the needs of the baby.

> **Test Taking Strategy**—*Note the key words "most appropriate," which indicate that one option is better than the others. Recall that when instructing clients, assessment is the first step before providing information. Option 2 is the only option that addresses this priority. Review principles of teaching, especially as they relate to nutritional needs during pregnancy, if you had difficulty answering this question.*
> **Cognitive Level**—*Applying*
> **Client Needs Category**—*Health promotion and maintenance*
> **Client Needs Subcategory**—*None*

33. 3. The weight gain recommended during pregnancy is individualized, and the client's prepregnancy weight must be taken into consideration. Being small for gestational age is associated with detrimental outcomes for infants, but not mothers. Being large for gestational age predisposes to harmful consequences for both infants and mothers. The guidelines for weight gain for the client with a normal prepregnancy weight is between 25 and 35 pounds (11.3 and 15.9 kg). A weight gain of 28 to 40 pounds (12.7 to 18.1 kg) is generally recommended for a client who is underweight. Clients who are moderately overweight can gain between 15 and 25 pounds (6.8 and 11.3 kg). Clients who are very overweight (obese) can gain approximately 11 to 20 pounds (4. 9 to 9 kg).

> **Test Taking Strategy**—*Analyze the information the question asks, which is the recommended weight gain during pregnancy for a woman whose prepregnancy weight is normal for height. If unsure, eliminate the extremes (options 1 and 4) as too little or*

too much weight gain. Discriminate between options 2 and 3. Recall that weight gain during pregnancy results from weight of the baby, placenta, amniotic fluid, breast tissue, blood supply, additional fat stores, and increase in uterine size. Considering all of the sources that contribute to the total weight leads to selecting option 3 as the correct answer. Review weight gain during pregnancy if you had difficulty answering this question.
Cognitive Level—*Applying*
Client Needs Category—*Health promotion and maintenance*
Client Needs Subcategory—*None*

34. 2. During pregnancy, the recommended intake of milk is 3 to 4 servings (3 to 4 cups) daily. Milk is an excellent source of calcium and protein, both of which are essential for the proper development of strong bones, healthy teeth, healthy nerves and muscles, and normal blood clotting for the client and her fetus. Calcium is also present in prenatal vitamins.
Test Taking Strategy—Analyze to determine what information the question asks for, which is the daily recommended servings of milk during pregnancy. Recall that 3 servings a day from the dairy group is a typical recommendation on the food pyramid. Increasing to 4 servings per day (option 2) provides additional calcium and allows for the fetus to obtain calcium without depleting it from the mother. Review nutritional needs during pregnancy, especially for milk and calcium, if you had difficulty answering this question.
Cognitive Level—*Applying*
Client Needs Category—*Health promotion and maintenance*
Client Needs Subcategory—*None*

35. 3. Of the foods listed, leafy green vegetables, such as broccoli, Brussels sprouts, collards, kale, and Swiss chard, contain the highest amount of highly absorbable calcium from among the nondairy sources. Eating four slices of bread provides 31% of the daily need for calcium. One cup of turkey provides 4% of the daily requirement for calcium, and organ meats such as liver and heart provide even less.
Test Taking Strategy—Use the process of elimination to select the option that identifies the best source of calcium other than milk and dairy products. Knowledge of nutrients in foods is helpful in answering the question. If unsure, recall that green leafy vegetables (option 3) are high in a variety of dietary nutrients. Review calcium-rich foods if you had difficulty answering this question.
Cognitive Level—*Applying*
Client Needs Category—*Health promotion and maintenance*
Client Needs Subcategory—*None*

36. 3. A client receiving iron supplements may complain of constipation or an upset stomach. The nurse should encourage the client to increase fiber and fluids to help prevent or control this problem. Iron requirements double during pregnancy, and the demand for iron usually exceeds the amount that can be provided from dietary sources. Therefore, if the physician orders an iron supplement, the client should not attempt to substitute dietary sources of iron for the prescribed iron supplement. Iron supplements are best absorbed when taken between meals, on an empty stomach. Iron usually does not cause abdominal pain unless it is associated with constipation.
Test Taking Strategy—Note the key words "most appropriate" when selecting an option regarding an iron supplement and constipation. Immediately eliminate option 4 because it would be difficult to obtain sufficient iron from the usual servings of food to equal that in an iron supplement. Option 1 can be eliminated because it reduces the amount of iron that can be absorbed. Eliminate option 2 because it provides knowledge but is not helpful for eliminating constipation. Option 3 is correct because increasing fluid intake moistens stool, making it easier to eliminate. Review methods for relieving constipation if you had difficulty answering this question.
Cognitive Level—*Applying*
Client Needs Category—*Physiological integrity*
Client Needs Subcategory—*Pharmacological therapies*

37. 1, 2, 4. Increasing the client's daily amounts of ascorbic acid (vitamin C) will enhance the absorption of iron. Vitamin C is found in citrus foods, such as oranges, grapefruit, lemons, and limes. It is also found in other fruits, such as kiwi, strawberries, and cantaloupe, and in vegetables such as broccoli and Brussels sprouts. Vitamin C is not found in bananas, milk, or carrots.
Test Taking Strategy—Analyze to determine what information the question asks for, which is foods that increase the absorption of an iron supplement. Alternative-format "select all that apply" questions require considering each option independently to decide its merit in answering the question. Review the link between ascorbic acid (vitamin C) and foods that are high in that vitamin, as well as the absorption of iron, if you had difficulty answering this question.
Cognitive Level—*Applying*
Client Needs Category—*Physiological integrity*
Client Needs Subcategory—*Pharmacological therapies*

38. 1. Because the client's iron requirements will increase during pregnancy, constipation may become a problem. The nurse should advise the client that her stools may become greenish black, hard, and dry and offer instructions on how to prevent constipation. Diarrhea is not a side effect of iron supplements and vomiting is unlikely to occur, although gastric upset is possible. The teeth are not likely to become stained unless the iron preparation is in liquid form. Most prenatal iron supplements, however, come in tablet form.

> *Test Taking Strategy—Analyze to determine what information the question asks for, which is information to include in client teaching about the side effects of iron supplements. Link the common side effects to nursing instructions. Recall that iron that is not absorbed is eliminated in the stool, causing it to appear black. Option 1 correlates with a common side effect about which instruction is needed. Review the side effects of iron administration if you had difficulty answering this question.*
> **Cognitive Level**—*Applying*
> **Client Needs Category**—*Physiological integrity*
> **Client Needs Subcategory**—*Pharmacological therapies*

39. 1. Folic acid, a B vitamin, is thought to prevent neural tube defects. Neural tube defects occur in embryonic development when the spinal column fails to close. In general, good sources of folic acid and B vitamins include eggs, beans, whole grains, and dark, leafy green vegetables. The recommended amount of folic acid for pregnant women is 0.4 mg/day. Calcium is needed for fetal bone formation. Vitamin A helps build fetal resistance to infection. Iron is needed to build the fetus' hemoglobin and blood supply.

> *Test Taking Strategy—Note the key words "most accurate," and the option that includes a correct statement that identifies the reason folic acid is especially important during pregnancy. Recall that folic acid plays a crucial role in preventing a congenital defect such as spina bifida (option 1). Review the benefits of folic acid before and during pregnancy if you had difficulty answering this question.*
> **Cognitive Level**—*Analyzing*
> **Client Needs Category**—*Health promotion and maintenance*
> **Client Needs Subcategory**—*None*

40. 1. To meet the pregnant teenager's energy needs, a diet of 2,500 calories per day is necessary. Adequate nutrition is a problem for pregnant teens because of their own growth coupled with the demands of pregnancy. Pregnant teenagers are often deficient in calcium, iron, folic acid, and calories. In their search for independence and identity, pregnant adolescents often refuse to eat foods suggested by their parents; instead, they eat fast food and snack on junk food that is not highly nutritious throughout the day. Eating centers on social gatherings and peer pressure. Presweetened beverages contain sugar and empty calories, so substituting them in place of soft drinks is not appropriate. Milk is a better choice. Carbohydrates and fats are needed every day to meet the teenager's energy needs. Limiting them does not ensure adequate nutrition. Diges-

tion is not affected in the pregnant teenager, so limiting spicy foods is a personal choice.

> *Test Taking Strategy—Analyze to determine what information the question asks for regarding nutrition and the pregnant teenager. Note the words "dietary adjustment," indicating a needed dietary change. Consider the personal growth of a pregnant teenager and that of the developing fetus, which increase caloric and nutritional needs (option 1). Review the nutritional needs of pregnant adolescents if you had difficulty answering this question.*
> **Cognitive Level**—*Applying*
> **Client Needs Category**—*Health promotion and maintenance*
> **Client Needs Subcategory**—*None*

41. 2. Adolescent girls frequently exhibit poor food choices and irregular eating habits due to their active schedules and busy lifestyles. Risk factors related to poor nutritional intake include frequently omitting meals, eating fast food, and consuming alcoholic beverages during a pregnancy, as well as being concerned about body weight and appearance, which may lead to limiting consumption of food. Fast food, which is easily accessible, is high in fat and sodium and low in nutrition. Adolescent girls are usually social and spend large amounts of time with peers, but living with a boyfriend is not necessarily a risk factor for nutritional deficiencies.

> *Test Taking Strategy—Analyze to determine what information the question asks for, which is to quantify the issues in the client's current history that are a dietary concern. Scrutinize the scenario to identify facts that could affect the nutrition of the pregnant teenager. Be careful not to include other areas of concern such as social or economic information when answering the question; as a result, four factors (option 2) can be identified. Review how the lifestyle of an adolescent affects nutritional needs during pregnancy if you had difficulty answering this question.*
> **Cognitive Level**—*Analyzing*
> **Client Needs Category**—*Health promotion and maintenance*
> **Client Needs Subcategory**—*None*

42. 1. An acceptable expected outcome for a pregnant adolescent client is that she will eat three balanced meals and two nutritious snacks each day. Normal weight gain during pregnancy is between 25 and 35 pounds (11.3 and 15.9 kg). Therefore, a total weight gain of 50 pounds (22.7 kg) is an inappropriate outcome. Only one prenatal vitamin is required per day. Normal caloric intake should increase to about 2,300 to 2,500 calories during pregnancy to support fetal growth.

> *Test Taking Strategy—Analyze to determine what information the question asks for, which is an expected outcome in light of the client's current dietary habits. Eliminate option 2 because a nurse would not*

set an outcome that is beyond acceptable standards. Eliminate option 3 because prenatal vitamins are a medication, and the nurse does not adjust prescription medication. Eliminate option 4 because focusing on calories, rather than eating nutritious food, is not better than option 1, a goal that will ensure nutrition and provide the best outcome for the pregnant adolescent. Review nutritional goals when a client has a less than nutritious dietary intake during pregnancy if you had difficulty answering this question.
Cognitive Level—*Analyzing*
Client Needs Category—*Safe and effective care environment*
Client Needs Subcategory—*Coordinated care*

43. 4. The average recommended weight gain during pregnancy is between 25 and 35 pounds (11.3 and 15.9 kg). Therefore, a weight gain of 10 pounds (4.5 kg) is inadequate to maintain fetal growth. Although weight gain is affected by food intake, this is not the most appropriate response. The nurse needs to point out the normalcy of gaining weight during pregnancy. Likewise, even though it may be normal for adolescents to be concerned about body image and appearances, pregnant adolescents need to be counseled and carefully monitored to ensure they gain adequate weight.
> **Test Taking Strategy**—*The key words are "most appropriate," indicating that one answer is best. Recall that option 4 provides factual information for the adolescent to compare her status with that which has been scientifically established. Review standards for weight gain during pregnancy if you had difficulty answering this question.*
Cognitive Level—*Applying*
Client Needs Category—*Health promotion and maintenance*
Client Needs Subcategory—*None*

44. 1, 2, 3, 4, 5. Alcohol should be avoided during pregnancy because of the numerous documented psychophysiologic effects it has on the developing fetus. Coffee, tea, and cola beverages contain caffeine, a central nervous system stimulant that increases the heart rate of both the mother and fetus. Sports drinks such as Gatorade should be limited because the effects on the fetus are not yet known. Orange juice is recommended because it is a good source of vitamin C, an essential vitamin that also helps with iron absorption.
> **Test Taking Strategy**—*Analyze to determine what information the question asks for regarding unhealthy drinks to avoid. Alternative-format "select all that apply" questions require considering each option independently to decide its merit in answering the question. In evaluating each option, consider the nutritional value and effect on the pregnant adolescent. Review drink choices that provide little nutritional value, especially during pregnancy, if you had difficulty answering this question.*

Cognitive Level—*Applying*
Client Needs Category—*Health promotion and maintenance*
Client Needs Subcategory—*None*

45. 1. Edema is affected by sodium retention. Therefore, omitting or limiting salt from the diet will help alleviate lower extremity edema. Some edema is normal during the latter stages of pregnancy. However, a client with edema of the hands and face may have pregnancy-induced hypertension, a serious complication. Vitamin C, magnesium, and potassium are not associated with fluid retention and edema.
> **Test Taking Strategy**—*Analyze to determine what information the question asks for, which is the substance the nurse should advise the client with edema to limit. Recall that sodium (option 1) causes retention of body fluid, and limiting table salt and foods that are high in sodium could relieve the client's current edema. The nurse should provide the client with examples of food items to avoid or eat sparingly. Review the correlation of sodium and fluid retention if you had difficulty answering this question.*
Cognitive Level—*Applying*
Client Needs Category—*Health promotion and maintenance*
Client Needs Subcategory—*None*

46. 1, 2, 3, 4. Because of their rapid growth and development, there are a number of nutritional concerns for pregnant adolescents related to their need for additional calories and increased levels of vitamins and minerals. Women who are overweight or underweight at the time of conception are at risk for nutritional deficits based on their prepregnancy eating patterns. Women who consume alcohol or smoke cigarettes during pregnancy are robbing their bodies and their growing fetuses of valuable nutritional intake; they are also placing their fetus at risk for fetal alcohol syndrome. Those with a low income are at risk for nutritional problems because they may not have the financial resources to eat well-balanced meals or buy prenatal vitamins. Women who have a prepregnancy hemoglobin level of 13 g/100 mL are within normal limits and are not at risk for nutritional problems such as anemia. Drinking four glasses of milk is the recommended daily requirement for pregnant women.
> **Test Taking Strategy**—*Analyze to determine what information the question asks for, which requires identifying pregnant clients at risk for nutritional problems. Alternative-format "select all that apply" questions require considering each option independently to decide its merit in answering the question. Refer to the rationale for the reasons the identified options contain information that impacts client nutrition. Review nutritional requirements as they relate to various situations during pregnancy if you had difficulty answering this question.*

Cognitive Level—Evaluating
Client Needs Category—Health promotion and
maintenance
Client Needs Subcategory—None

Teaching the Pregnant Client

47. 2. Daily tub baths or showers are recommended
for the client during pregnancy because women usually
perspire more heavily and have a heavier vaginal discharge
at this time. However, tub baths during the latter part of
pregnancy increase the risk for falls because the protruding abdomen shifts the client's center of gravity. Safety
mats, handgrips, and other safety precautions are recommended to prevent falls. Hot tubs and hot water used for
bathing should be avoided because an elevated maternal
core body temperature can produce harmful effects on the
fetus. Warm water is acceptable for bathing or showering.
Once the membranes rupture, tub baths should be avoided
because of the increased risk of developing an infection.

> *Test Taking Strategy*—Analyze to determine what
> information the question asks for, which is an
> incorrect client statement that indicates a need for
> additional teaching. Narrow the selection by elimi-
> nating any correct statements regarding bathing.
> Because option 2 does not qualify when a tub bath
> may be inappropriate, but rather indicates that tub
> baths in general should be avoided, it is a statement
> that requires clarification. Review health teaching
> regarding bathing during pregnancy if you had dif-
> ficulty answering this question.
> *Cognitive Level*—Applying
> *Client Needs Category*—Physiological integrity
> *Client Needs Subcategory*—Basic care and comfort

48. 4. If the client has a healthy pregnancy, no restrictions are placed on sexual intercourse. However, sexual
intercourse is contraindicated if the client experiences
vaginal bleeding, if the physician has diagnosed placenta
previa, or if the membranes have ruptured. Also, a client with a history of premature labor should be cautioned
about the danger of premature labor when experiencing
orgasms after 32 weeks' gestation.

> *Test Taking Strategy*—Analyze to determine what
> information the question asks for, which is the
> time during pregnancy when sexual intercourse
> should be avoided. Recall that sexual intercourse
> throughout pregnancy is a personal decision as
> long as the client does not feel uncomfortable,
> but it should be avoided if the membranes have
> ruptured (option 4) or if atypical vaginal
> drainage such as blood is present. Review
> precautions related to sexual intercourse during
> pregnancy if you had difficulty answering this
> question.

Cognitive Level—Applying
Client Needs Category—Health promotion and
maintenance
Client Needs Subcategory—None

49. 1, 4. Travel restrictions during pregnancy are
indicated only when the client is unhealthy or experiencing complications. The optimal time for travel is
during the second trimester of pregnancy, when the
client is typically most comfortable. The client should
be encouraged to carry a copy of her medical record
whenever traveling. Wearing a seatbelt is the law in
most states, but the pregnant woman should avoid wearing it for extended periods of time. When traveling,
the pregnant woman should avoid sitting for prolonged
periods and should walk every couple of hours to avoid
complications related to venous stasis. It is permissible for pregnant women to eat different foods during
travel. Typically, vaccinations are not given to pregnant
women because of the risk to the developing fetus.
Daily weights are not necessary when at home or during
traveling.

> *Test Taking Strategy*—Analyze to determine what
> information the question asks for regarding trave-
> ling during pregnancy. Alternative-format "select
> all that apply" questions require considering each
> option independently to decide its merit in answer-
> ing the question. To narrow the selection, consider
> physiological changes in the body and normal
> guidelines for pregnancy that impact travel during
> a normal pregnancy. Review travel restrictions dur-
> ing pregnancy if you had difficulty answering this
> question.
> *Cognitive Level*—Analyzing
> *Client Needs Category*—Health promotion and
> maintenance
> *Client Needs Subcategory*—None

50. 1. Once fertilized, the ovum travels through the
fallopian tube to the uterus, where it will be implanted,
usually within 7 days. At the time of implantation there
may be a small amount of bleeding similar to menstrual
spotting. Such spotting is unrelated to increased circulation to the vagina or to hormonal changes. Dilation and
effacement (enlargement and thinning of the cervix) occur
during labor; they are not associated with spotting during
the early stages of pregnancy.

> *Test Taking Strategy*—Analyze to determine what
> information the question asks for, which is the cause
> of spotting during the first week of pregnancy. Recall
> that spotting may coincide with implantation (option
> 1), which occurs between 6 and 10 days after ferti-
> lization when the zygote attaches to the lining of the
> uterus. However, if spotting or bleeding is accompa-
> nied by cramping, the physician could be consulted
> because it may indicate a miscarriage. Review the

significance of spotting during the early first trimester if you had difficulty answering this question.
Cognitive Level—*Applying*
Client Needs Category—*Health promotion and maintenance*
Client Needs Subcategory—*None*

51. 4. By the eighth week of gestation, the embryo has developed enough to be called a fetus. The fetal stage of development, which lasts from the 8th week until term (40 weeks), mostly involves growth and maturation of structures begun during the embryonic stage. At 8 weeks, the extremities are developed; by the 12th week, the fetus not only has arms and legs, but also has fingers and toes. A *zygote* is the term used to identify the newly formed cell that develops when the sperm penetrates the ovum and fertilization occurs. During this stage, which lasts from fertilization to implantation in the uterus (usually 3 to 4 days), the zygote cell divides and grows, resembling a lumpy ball. During the embryonic stage, which marks the time from implantation to about 8 weeks' gestation, the body begins forming and the gender becomes distinguishable.

Test Taking Strategy—Analyze to determine what information the question asks for, which is characteristics of the fetus late in the first trimester. Knowledge of fetal development is helpful in answering the question. Recall that a full fetal skeleton (option 4) is developed by the 12th week of pregnancy; the feet measure almost a half inch, and fingernails and toenails are present. Review fetal development if you had difficulty answering this question.
Cognitive Level—*Applying*
Client Needs Category—*Health promotion and maintenance*
Client Needs Subcategory—*None*

52. 2. The amniotic fluid primarily serves as a medium to protect the fetus. It allows the fetus to move while keeping the fetal environment at a constant temperature. It also prevents the amnion from adhering to the fetus. It helps to maintain a consistent temperature within the uterine environment. The amniotic fluid does not provide the fetus with antibodies or oxygen. The broad and round ligaments support the uterus.

Test Taking Strategy—Note the key words "most appropriate," which indicates one answer is better than any of the others. Select the option that accurately identifies the purpose of amniotic fluid. Recall that the amniotic fluid that surrounds the fetus simply provides a buoyant environment that cushions it from blows or jarring movements to the maternal abdomen (option 2). Review the purpose of amniotic fluid if you had difficulty answering this question.
Cognitive Level—*Applying*
Client Needs Category—*Health promotion and maintenance*
Client Needs Subcategory—*None*

53. 1. During pregnancy, the placenta is considered a temporary endocrine gland. It secretes estrogen as well as progesterone and human chorionic gonadotropin. Testosterone is a male hormone. Oxytocin, a hormone secreted by the posterior pituitary gland, is normally released near the time of delivery to begin and maintain uterine contractions during labor. It is also administered in some cases to augment labor and prevent postpartal hemorrhage. Oxytocin also causes the release of breast milk. Follicle-stimulating hormone is excreted by the anterior pituitary gland before pregnancy and matures the follicle in the ovary before ovulation.

Test Taking Strategy—Analyze to determine what information the question asks for, which is the hormone that the placenta secretes. If you are unsure, eliminate option 2 because it is a male hormone. Next, eliminate options 3 and 4 because they are pituitary hormones. Option 1, which remains after eliminating the other choices, is the correct answer. Review hormonal regulation during pregnancy if you had difficulty with this question.
Cognitive Level—*Understanding*
Client Needs Category—*Health promotion and maintenance*
Client Needs Subcategory—*None*

54. 2, 5. Constipation may occur because of hormonal changes, increased uterine size, and decreased peristalsis later in pregnancy. Exercise, not rest, may assist with the control or relief of this discomfort. Also, a diet containing fresh fruit and vegetables, whole grains, and increased fluids will assist with controlling or relieving constipation. In addition, increasing fluids will help prevent constipation. Prenatal vitamins will not relieve constipation and may even contribute to it if each tablet contains minerals such as iron. A low-fat diet is not associated with constipation or its relief. Over-the-counter laxatives and other medications that stimulate bowel elimination are contraindicated unless prescribed by the physician. This includes enemas, use of mineral oil, and suppositories.

Test Taking Strategy—Analyze to determine what information the question asks for, which is prevention of constipation during pregnancy. Alternative-format "select all that apply" questions require considering each option independently to decide its merit in answering the question. Choose options that provide information about maintaining normal bowel elimination. Review ways of preventing constipation if you had difficulty answering this question.
Cognitive Level—*Applying*
Client Needs Category—*Health promotion and maintenance*
Client Needs Subcategory—*None*

55. **1.** During pregnancy, the client may develop varicose veins, especially in the lower extremities and rectal area (hemorrhoids). Varicose veins occur during pregnancy primarily because of impaired venous return, which is caused by the pressure of the enlarged uterus on venous circulation and the increased blood volume normally associated with pregnancy. Decreased cardiac output and changes in the body's center of gravity are not associated with the occurrence of varicose veins. Kidney function is not normally impaired during pregnancy.

Test Taking Strategy—Analyze to determine what information the question asks for, which is the cause of varicose veins during pregnancy. Note that the stem of the question identifies increased blood volume as one component that contributes to varicose veins during pregnancy. Recall that venous blood must move against gravity in the lower areas of the body as it travels toward the heart and that an enlarging fetus may impede return circulation (option 1). Review factors that contribute to the development or worsening of varicose veins during pregnancy if you had difficulty answering this question.
Cognitive Level—*Applying*
Client Needs Category—*Health promotion and maintenance*
Client Needs Subcategory—*None*

56. **4.** It is recommended that pregnant women with varicose veins move around after standing for extended time periods. This prevents stasis of blood in the lower extremities. Clients with varicose veins should be instructed to rest with their feet elevated, not in a dependent position. They should avoid wearing garters or knee-length or calf-length elastic-top hose because of the risk of impaired circulation.

Test Taking Strategy—Analyze to determine what information the question asks for, which is an action that relieves the discomfort associated with varicose veins. Recall that muscle contraction is the means by which venous blood moves toward the heart. Moving about (option 4) supports this physiological process, whereas the other options contribute to the accumulation and stagnation of venous blood. Review causes and prevention of varicose veins if you had difficulty answering this question.
Cognitive Level—*Applying*
Client Needs Category—*Health promotion and maintenance*
Client Needs Subcategory—*None*

57. **4.** A client with varicose veins whose calves are red, tender, or warm to the touch should report this finding immediately because it could signal thrombophlebitis, a more serious problem. The presence of additional varicose veins is not a condition that needs immediate attention from the physician but should be addressed at the next routine visit. Varicose veins are normally purple in color. The client with varicose veins may complain of her legs feeling achy, tired, and heavy.

Test Taking Strategy—After analyzing to determine what information the question seeks, note the word "immediately," indicating a serious complication related to varicose veins. Recall that impaired venous circulation predisposes to the formation of thrombi, the symptoms of which are described in option 4. The other options describe the expected appearance and symptoms of varicose veins not accompanied by thrombosis. Review complications of varicose veins if you had difficulty answering this question.
Cognitive Level—*Applying*
Client Needs Category—*Physiological integrity*
Client Needs Subcategory—*Reduction of risk potential*

58. **2.** Itching of the skin is a common and annoying discomfort of pregnancy. It may occur during pregnancy because the enlarging uterus causes the abdominal skin to stretch. Drying agents, such as soaps and alcohol, as well as hot baths, may also increase itching. Increasing fluid intake may improve skin elasticity and decrease the occurrence of itching. There is no correlation between vitamin C intake and decreased itching. Benadryl is used for itching, but it is contraindicated for use during pregnancy because of the risk of fetal damage.

Test Taking Strategy—Note the key words "most appropriate," which indicate that one option is better than the others. Select the option that identifies the best information for relieving itchy skin during pregnancy. Recall that increasing fluid intake (option 2) contributes to a greater volume of water in all the cells and tissues of the body and would relieve dry skin due to its hydrating effect. The remaining options lack therapeutic benefit because they either contribute to skin dryness or are ineffective or contraindicated during pregnancy. Review skin care techniques for relieving dry skin during pregnancy if you had difficulty answering this question.
Cognitive Level—*Applying*
Client Needs Category—*Physiological integrity*
Client Needs Subcategory—*Basic care and comfort*

59. **3.** The uterus rising in the abdomen exerts pressure on the diaphragm, thereby decreasing the client's lung capacity and causing her to feel short of breath. This problem is common during the third trimester of pregnancy and is considered normal. Shortness of breath during the third trimester is not related to anxiety about the impending delivery, nor is it associated with a decreased oxygen supply secondary to slow venous circulation or clots in the lungs.

Test Taking Strategy—*Use the process of elimination to select the option that identifies correct information about shortness of breath that occurs during the third trimester of pregnancy. Option 1 can be eliminated because shortness of breath is commonly experienced and is unlikely due to a pulmonary embolism. Eliminate option 2 because anxiety is a consequence of sensing a threat to one's well-being, which is unlikely in the course of a normal pregnancy. Eliminate option 4 because despite factors that affect venous circulation, it is not generally the reason a pregnant woman develops shortness of breath when nearing a delivery date. Option 3 is the correct answer because it offers a physiological rationale for compromised breathing. Review how breathing may be affected during the late stage of pregnancy and its cause if you had difficulty answering this question.*
Cognitive Level—*Analyzing*
Client Needs Category—*Health promotion and maintenance*
Client Needs Subcategory—*None*

60. 4. Elevating the upper body on pillows while resting may help to relieve shortness of breath. Maintaining an erect posture when sitting or standing may also help to relieve this problem by increasing oxygen intake. It is unnecessary for the client to notify the physician immediately, but the physician should be made aware of any difficulty in breathing to rule out the presence of a serious problem. A mild sedative is not indicated for clients who exhibit shortness of breath. Decreasing activity may reduce the shortness of breath, but only temporarily.
Test Taking Strategy—*Note the key words "most appropriate," indicating that more than one option may have some hint of accuracy, but one option is best. Option 1 may be a valid answer, but because the client's symptom does not suggest a life-threatening condition, it is not the best answer. Although decreasing activity (option 2) may relieve breathlessness due to cardiopulmonary disorders, activity is not the underlying cause of the client's shortness of breath. A sedative (option 3) may relieve anxiety and promote rest, but this type of medication is not likely to be prescribed during pregnancy. Elevating the upper body on pillows (option 4) is a basic nursing measure that helps to relieve the pressure of the enlarged uterus on the thoracic cavity. This option requires no pharmacologic therapy and limited lifestyle change, making it the most appropriate early intervention. Review methods for relieving shortness of breath during the late stage of pregnancy if you had difficulty answering this question.*
Cognitive Level—*Applying*
Client Needs Category—*Physiological integrity*
Client Needs Subcategory—*Basic care and comfort*

61. 3. Frequent urination is common early in pregnancy because the enlarging uterus causes pressure on the urinary bladder. When the uterus rises into the abdominal cavity, urinary frequency subsides. Placental maturity, fetal kidney function, and hormonal balance are not usually causes of urinary frequency during early pregnancy.
Test Taking Strategy—*Analyze to determine what information the question asks for, which is the time when frequent urination during early pregnancy is likely to subside. Urination is increased during pregnancy because the maternal blood volume increases and requires greater fluid elimination through increased urination. Although this is a continuing factor during pregnancy, many women get some relief as the uterus expands in the direction of the abdominal cavity (option 3) and there is less secondary pressure on the bladder itself. However, urinary frequency is likely to become bothersome again in the last trimester when the room for expansion is limited and the mass of the uterus presses on the bladder once again. Review the cause and relief of common discomforts of pregnancy if you had difficulty answering this question.*
Cognitive Level—*Applying*
Client Needs Category—*Health promotion and maintenance*
Client Needs Subcategory—*None*

62. 3. Frequent urination is common in late pregnancy because the enlarged uterus descends into the pelvis, causing pressure on the urinary bladder. Frequency is unrelated to increased fetal waste. A urinary tract infection could cause frequency, but this is not the most probable cause late in pregnancy. A urinary tract infection is likely to cause additional symptoms, such as burning and painful urination. During the late stages of pregnancy, loss of bladder tone resulting in urinary frequency does not commonly occur.
Test Taking Strategy—*Analyze to determine what information the question asks for, which is a factor later in pregnancy that contributes to frequent urination. Option 4 directly relates to the enlarging uterus (a changing factor of pregnancy) and pressure on the bladder causing the frequent urination. Review factors that contribute to increased urination during pregnancy if you had difficulty answering this question.*
Cognitive Level—*Applying*
Client Needs Category—*Health promotion and maintenance*
Client Needs Subcategory—*None*

63. 1. Although limiting fluid intake before going to bed at night may help to manage nighttime urinary frequency, the patient should be advised to maintain adequate intake during the day to help prevent dehydration. Reducing the intake of high-caffeine fluids and voiding before going to bed are both acceptable means of controlling urinary frequency. The client should also be taught to recognize and report signs of a urinary tract infection.

Test Taking Strategy—Analyze to determine what information the question asks for, which requires selecting an incorrect or unsafe statement that indicates a need for additional teaching. Evaluate the options, eliminating the correct statements and identifying the incorrect one. The statement regarding limiting fluids (option 1) requires more teaching because fluid volume, which is increased during pregnancy, must be compensated by having a liberal fluid intake. Review the potential problem that may develop if a pregnant woman limits fluid intake if you had difficulty answering this question.
Cognitive Level—*Analyzing*
Client Needs Category—*Health promotion and maintenance*
Client Needs Subcategory—*None*

64. **4, 5, 6.** Wearing low-heeled shoes helps maintain the back in a more proper alignment and may relieve backaches associated with pregnancy. In addition, carrying objects close to the body and squatting when picking objects up from the floor will prevent back strain and consequently, backaches. A firm mattress may also help to relieve backaches by providing increased support to the lower back. Sleeping on a heating pad is likely to cause burns and may increase the maternal core temperature, which could harm the fetus. Regular use of pain relievers is contraindicated during pregnancy. Tight-fitting clothes do not usually cause backaches in pregnancy.

Test Taking Strategy—Analyze to determine what information the question asks for regarding measures to relieve backaches during pregnancy. Alternative-format "select all that apply" questions require considering each option independently to decide its merit in answering the question. Choose options that include factors that contribute to backaches during pregnancy and nursing instructions that can provide relief. Options 2 and 3 are unsafe or contraindicated and should be eliminated for those reasons. Review methods that are safe and therapeutic for relieving backaches during pregnancy if you had difficulty answering this question.
Cognitive Level—*Applying*
Client Needs Category—*Physiological integrity*
Client Needs Subcategory—*Basic care and comfort*

65. **1.** Nausea and heartburn, which are common discomforts during pregnancy, are believed to occur because of hormonal changes, decreased gastric motility, and displacement of the stomach and duodenum by the enlarging uterus. Eating frequent small meals, avoiding liquids during meals, and avoiding lying down after meals can prevent or limit nausea and heartburn.

Antacid preparations may relieve these discomforts, but they should be taken only under a physician's direction because they can affect iron absorption, cause fluid and electrolyte imbalance, and cause additional constipation. Eating the largest meal at night will add to heartburn, not help prevent it.

Test Taking Strategy—Analyze to determine what information the question asks for, which is a statement that indicates effective teaching regarding a method for relieving nausea during pregnancy. Recall that eating small meals frequently (option 1) will meet a client's caloric and nutritional needs without distending the stomach. Review methods for relieving symptoms of nausea during pregnancy if you had difficulty answering this question.
Cognitive Level—*Evaluating*
Client Needs Category—*Physiological integrity*
Client Needs Subcategory—*Basic care and comfort*

66. **3.** Decreased calcium levels and normal tension on muscles and tendons cause leg cramps during pregnancy. Pointing the toes toward the head (rather than the floor) may help to relieve leg cramps. Increasing milk rather than recommending generic protein intake will increase calcium levels. The client should be instructed not to massage her legs because of the danger of dislodging clots. Wearing support stockings will help prevent varicosities, not muscle cramps.

Test Taking Strategy—Use the process of elimination to select the correct nursing response to the client's question about a measure to relieve leg cramps. Although ingesting sufficient calcium may prevent muscle spasms, recall that stretching the muscle will temporarily terminate the cramp if one develops. Review the relationship between calcium and muscle cramps and the technique for relieving a leg cramp once it occurs if you had difficulty answering this question.
Cognitive Level—*Applying*
Client Needs Category—*Physiological integrity*
Client Needs Subcategory—*Basic care and comfort*

67. **1.** Mood swings are common during pregnancy and are related to the hormonal and psychological changes that accompany pregnancy. Mood changes are often unpredictable and can cause tension with the client's partner and within the family. Fatigue and stress decrease normal coping defenses and may cause or contribute to unpredictable behavior. The nurse should advise the client to avoid becoming fatigued and stressed and to get plenty of sleep. Mood swings produce erratic behavior; a situation that may appear acceptable one minute may be unacceptable the next. Therefore, it is unrealistic to advise the client to avoid interactions as a means of controlling her mood. Suggesting that the client be assessed for a mood disorder suggests prematurely that emotional instability is pathologic in this case. Asking the client if she has discussed mood swings with her physician and stating concern about her emotional lability implies that there is something abnormal or wrong with the client; therefore, these responses are inappropriate.

> *Test Taking Strategy—Note the key words "most relevant," which indicate that one option is better than the others when responding to information about mood swings during pregnancy. Evaluate each option for its therapeutic benefit. Recall that stress is a crucial factor in mood swings, which is exacerbated by fatigue (option 1) and the hormonal and psychological changes occurring during pregnancy. Review suggestions that may help a client maintain emotional stability during pregnancy if you had difficulty answering this question.*
> *Cognitive Level—Analyzing*
> *Client Needs Category—Psychosocial integrity*
> *Client Needs Subcategory—None*

68. 1, 2, 5. Pregnant women who work should use breaks and lunch periods to rest. (This means that breaks and lunch periods must be taken.) Elevating the feet and legs on a chair during breaks and at lunch will help with fatigue, edema, backaches, and varicosities. To avoid urinary tract infections, the pregnant working woman should void every 2 hours or so. Avoiding excessive overtime will help with fatigue, and spacing work schedules out will also allow rest during days off. The pregnant working woman should get extra rest on her days off and on the weekends and may require extra sleep at night, but requiring 12 hours of sleep per night may not be feasible. Eating foods high in carbohydrates is not appropriate and will lead to weight gain. A well-balanced diet is important while working and when at home.

> *Test Taking Strategy—Analyze to determine what information the question asks for, which is measures to take regarding working and pregnancy. Alternative-format "select all that apply" questions require considering each option independently to decide its merit in answering the question. When evaluating each option, consider the physical effects of pregnancy and methods that can maintain or promote health and well-being. Research how employers must adapt the environment and working conditions to accommodate for the needs of pregnant employees if you had difficulty answering this question.*
> *Cognitive Level—Analyzing*
> *Client Needs Category—Health promotion and maintenance*
> *Client Needs Subcategory—None*

69. 1. The nurse is responsible for teaching pregnant clients about signs and symptoms of potentially serious problems or complications associated with pregnancy or

delivery. Headache and swelling of the face and fingers are signs of pregnancy-induced hypertension and need to be reported immediately. Constipation, flatulence, muscle cramping, varicosities, and an increase in colorless, odorless vaginal secretions are all uncomfortable during pregnancy; however, they are not generally considered causes for alarm.

> *Test Taking Strategy—Analyze to determine what information the question asks for, which is evidence of a danger sign during pregnancy. Consider the implications of each option and their significance. Recall that pregnancy-induced hypertension, a complication that can affect the well-being of the mother and fetus, is accompanied by headaches and peripheral edema (option 1). Review the signs and symptoms of pregnancy-induced hypertension as well as its implications if you had difficulty answering this question.*
> *Cognitive Level—Applying*
> *Client Needs Category—Physiological integrity*
> *Client Needs Subcategory—Reduction of risk potential*

High-Risk Factors and Pregnancy

70. 4. A client who is older than age 35 or younger than age 18 is considered at the highest risk for complications during pregnancy. A client who has had more than four pregnancies is also considered at risk for complications. A 25-year-old client experiencing her first pregnancy is not typically at an increased risk for complications. Nausea and vomiting are common in the first trimester, and placental attachment to the fundus is normal.

> *Test Taking Strategy—Use the process of elimination to select the option that identifies the client who is at highest risk for complications during pregnancy. Consider that more than one client profile may be a person who is predisposed to risks, but one is at higher risk than the others. Note that options 1, 2, and 3 are normal or low-risk factors and can be immediately eliminated. Recall the criteria used to classify high-risk pregnancies, which include age and number of previous pregnancies (option 4) as a basis for evaluation. Review the factors that contribute to a high-risk pregnancy if you had difficulty answering this question.*
> *Cognitive Level—Analyzing*
> *Client Needs Category—Physiological integrity*
> *Client Needs Subcategory—Physiological adaptation*

71. 2. There is no known safe amount of alcohol that can be consumed by the mother during pregnancy. The effects of a mother's occasional alcohol consumption on the fetus are unknown. Because the fetus is unable to eliminate the by-products of maternal alcohol consumption, which can lead to vitamin deficiencies and neurologic damage, the pregnant woman is encouraged to stop drinking all alcoholic beverages during pregnancy. Harmful effects of alcoholism can occur throughout pregnancy, not just in the first trimester. Pregnant women with alcohol abuse problems are referred to rehabilitation programs.

> *Test Taking Strategy—Use the process of elimination to select the option that identifies the best response to the client's question concerning the fetal effect of alcohol consumption during pregnancy. Although the responses in options 1, 3, and 4 are potentially good responses, the information is without substantial scientific validation. Option 2 is the best answer because standards of care prescribed by most reputable authorities of obstetrics advise pregnant women to abstain from drinking alcohol. Review the potential adverse effects from alcohol consumption during pregnancy if you had difficulty answering this question.*

Cognitive Level—Analyzing
Client Needs Category—Health promotion and maintenance
Client Needs Subcategory—None

72. 1. A woman who smokes during pregnancy increases the risk of complications for herself and her unborn child. Smoking constricts the blood vessels; during pregnancy, it is linked to premature births, low-birth-weight infants (not overweight ones), spontaneous abortions, and delayed mental and physical development of the child. In addition, there is a higher incidence of sudden infant death syndrome among infants who are exposed to second-hand smoke after birth. There is no known association between cigarette smoking and prenatal infections or increased incidence of cesarean births.

> *Test Taking Strategy—Analyze to determine what information the question asks for, which is a consequence that may occur from smoking during pregnancy. Consider the effects of inhaling nicotine, carbon monoxide, and tar on the fetus. These chemicals can lessen the amount of oxygen that gets to the fetus and, in turn, can cause premature births and low-birthweight infants (option 1). Review how smoking affects the fetus and newborn if you had difficulty answering this question.*

Cognitive Level—Applying
Client Needs Category—Health promotion and maintenance
Client Needs Subcategory—None

73. 2. Chorionic villi sampling (CVS) involves removal of a small portion of placental tissue by inserting a plastic tube through the cervix or using a transabdominal needle. Ultrasound images assist in guiding the placement of the sampling tube. CVS is the preferred procedure for the client because it can be done as early as 8 to 11 weeks' gestation. An additional advantage of CVS is that the results, which can identify fetal DNA and chromosomes that may be abnormal, are obtained within 1 to 7 days of the procedure. Amniocentesis cannot be performed until the client is between 14 and 20 weeks'

gestation, and the results usually are not available for 1½ to 4 weeks. Ultrasound can detect some congenital anomalies, but it is more useful as an adjunct to other tests such as amniocentesis. The rapid plasma reagin test is designed to screen for syphilis and does not detect genetic defects in the fetus.

> *Test Taking Strategy—Analyze the information the question asks which requires identifying a test to detect genetic disorders specifically for this time of gestation. Knowledge of diagnostic testing of the mother and fetus is helpful in successfully answering the question. Option 2 is the only option that directly relates to the defined situation. Review the purpose and timeline for performing CVS if you had difficulty answering this question.*

Cognitive Level—Analyzing
Client Needs Category—Physiological integrity
Client Needs Subcategory—Reduction of risk potential

74. 2. Chlamydia is a sexually transmitted infection caused by the bacterium *Chlamydia trachomatis*. A female client with this infection usually presents with a heavy, grayish white discharge and a complaint of intense itching. Pain during urination and intercourse also occurs. Diagnosis is made by culture of the organism. Painful blisters are associated with herpes simplex type 2 virus infection. A white, curdlike vaginal discharge is associated with candidiasis (yeast infection), and a milky discharge that smells like fish is characteristic of bacterial vaginosis.

> *Test Taking Strategy—Use the process of elimination to select the option that provides the best evidence of a chlamydial infection. After eliminating the incorrect options, Option 2 remains as the best answer. Review the symptoms caused by Chlamydia trachomatis if you had difficulty answering this question.*

Cognitive Level—Applying
Client Needs Category—Physiological integrity
Client Needs Subcategory—Physiological adaptation

75. 2. Chlamydia is the most common sexually transmitted infection in the United States, and all pregnant women should be tested as soon as antepartum visits begin. The pregnant woman with a chlamydial infection requires further teaching if she states that she will need to deliver her baby by cesarean birth. This procedure is unnecessary because antibiotics can eradicate the infection before labor and delivery. Azithromycin (Zithromax) given orally in a single dose is the drug of choice for pregnant clients, whereas either tetracycline or doxycycline is used for nonpregnant clients (tetracycline is harmful to the fetus). Sex partners of the client with *Chlamydia trachomatis* infection should be treated because this is a sexually transmitted infection, meaning that if infected sex partners are untreated, reinfection can occur. Also, males who are infected can develop urethritis, epididymitis, and orchitis. Newborns of untreated mothers are at risk for pneumonia and conjunctivitis. Atypical cells may show up on the Pap smear results.

> *Test Taking Strategy—Analyze to determine what information the question asks for, which is an incorrect statement that indicates a need for additional teaching regarding chlamydial infection. Knowledge of sexually transmitted infections, chlamydia in particular, and their effects on delivery, the fetus, the newborn, and sexual partners is essential in answering the question. Recall that treatment of a chlamydial infection is relatively simple and effective and does not necessitate a cesarean delivery (option 2). Review the significance of a chlamydial infection during pregnancy and delivery if you had difficulty answering this question.*
>
> *Cognitive Level—Applying*
> *Client Needs Category—Physiological integrity*
> *Client Needs Subcategory—Reduction of risk potential*

76. 3. Bleeding from the vagina may indicate a complication of pregnancy, such as abruptio placentae, spontaneous abortion, or placenta previa. This problem must be brought to the physician's attention immediately. Breast tenderness, fetal movement, and frequent urination are usually normal occurrences during pregnancy and can be discussed with the physician during a routine visit.

> *Test Taking Strategy—Analyze to determine what information the question asks for, which is a serious concern that warrants contacting the physician immediately. Evaluate each option for symptoms that correlate with a complication of pregnancy. Bleeding any time during pregnancy indicates a potentially serious condition (option 3) that should be evaluated as soon as it develops. Review the significance of bleeding during pregnancy if you had difficulty answering this question.*
>
> *Cognitive Level—Applying*
> *Client Needs Category—Physiological integrity*
> *Client Needs Subcategory—Reduction of risk potential*

77. 1, 2. Hyperemesis gravidarum is a serious condition characterized by persistent vomiting. It can result in dehydration and electrolyte imbalances. Severe cases of hyperemesis gravidarum require hospitalization for I.V. therapy to correct the dehydration and electrolyte imbalances. Because of frequent vomiting, it is imperative that the nurse record the amount and frequency of emesis. Therefore, an intake and output record is important when providing care for this client. The other choices listed may be ordered for various other reasons but are not routinely used in the care of the client hospitalized for hyperemesis gravidarum.

> *Test Taking Strategy—Analyze to determine what information the question asks for regarding care of a client with hyperemesis gravidarum who is dehydrated. Alternative-format "select all that apply" questions require considering each option independently to decide its merit in answering the question. Evaluate the*

options with reference to the primary problems, which are nausea, vomiting, and dehydration. Review the nursing care of a client with hyperemesis gravidarum if you had difficulty answering this question.

> *Cognitive Level—Analyzing*
> *Client Needs Category—Physiological integrity*
> *Client Needs Subcategory—Physiological adaptation*

Complications of Pregnancy

78. 1, 4. Pregnant clients with a preexisting disease such as hypertensive disease have an increased risk of developing complications during pregnancy. Pregnant clients who have had more than four pregnancies are also considered to be at increased risk for complications. A family history of twins does not increase the client's risk of complications. Normal weight gain during pregnancy is between 25 and 35 pounds (11.3 and 15.9 kg). Women who work 40 hours a week in a factory or elsewhere are not necessarily at high risk. Spotting is relatively normal in the first trimester as the fertilized egg attaches to the uterine wall.

> *Test Taking Strategy—Analyze to determine what information the question asks for regarding clients who meet the criteria for a high-risk pregnancy. Alternative-format "select all that apply" questions require considering each option independently to decide its merit in answering the question. Evaluate each option, identifying if the condition fits high-risk pregnancy criteria, which place the mother or fetus at risk for obstetric complications. Review criteria for a high-risk pregnancy if you had difficulty answering this question.*
>
> *Cognitive Level—Analyzing*
> *Client Needs Category—Physiological integrity*
> *Client Needs Subcategory—Reduction of risk potential*

79.

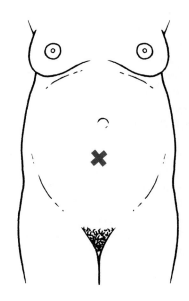

The cephalic position is the term used to indicate that the fetus's head lies in the direction of the mother's cervix. When the fetus is in this position, fetal heart tones are best auscultated midway between the mother's symphysis pubis and umbilicus.

> *Test Taking Strategy—Analyze to determine what information the question asks for regarding the best location for placing a transducer on the maternal abdomen to auscultate fetal heart tones of a fetus in the cephalic position. Consider the relation of the fetal head to its feet with the best location for obtaining heart tones being between the two. Review fetal presentation and positioning if you had difficulty answering this question.*
> **Cognitive Level**—*Analyzing*
> **Client Needs Category**—*Health promotion and maintenance*
> **Client Needs Subcategory**—*None*

80. 2. The cervix is the lower portion of the uterus that dilates and thins during labor. An incompetent cervix dilates prematurely because it is unable to support the weight of the growing fetus. This complication occurs without labor, is painless, and usually occurs during the second trimester of pregnancy. If untreated, an incompetent cervix may result in a spontaneous abortion or premature birth if the baby is viable. None of the remaining options describes this complication.

> *Test Taking Strategy—Use the process of elimination to select the option that identifies the best meaning for an incompetent cervix. Consider the definition of the word incompetent to be "inadequate." Option 1 can be eliminated because rather than being an insufficient size for the fetus to pass through, the cervix is too weak to stay closed. Options 3 and 4 can be eliminated because the external os and internal os, the openings at opposite ends of the cervix, are both present. Thus, option 2 remains as the correct answer because when the cervix opens prematurely, the fetus is in jeopardy of being expelled while still underdeveloped. Review the pathophysiology of an incompetent cervix if you had difficulty answering this question.*
> **Cognitive Level**—*Understanding*
> **Client Needs Category**—*Health promotion and maintenance*
> **Client Needs Subcategory**—*None*

81. 4. The treatment of choice for a client with an incompetent cervix who is not experiencing labor contractions is the placement of a purse-string suture (cerclage) in the cervix to close the cervical opening. The suture is left in place until the client is near term, when the client may go into labor spontaneously or be a candidate for a cesarean birth. The cerclage must be removed before delivery. Removing the cerclage at the end of the second trimester is too early and may precipitate preterm labor and delivery.

> *Test Taking Strategy—Analyze to determine what information the question asks for regarding the length of time the cerclage will remain in place. Recall that the purpose for the cerclage is to keep the cervix closed and prevent premature labor and delivery. The best timeframe for removing the cerclage is near the client's expected date of delivery before labor has begun (option 4). Review the purpose for a cerclage and the duration of its use if you had difficulty answering this question.*
> **Cognitive Level**—*Applying*
> **Client Needs Category**—*Physiological integrity*
> **Client Needs Subcategory**—*Reduction of risk potential*

82. 4. The nurse should suspect pregnancy-induced hypertension (PIH) when a client has any unexpected weight gain. Other signs include proteinuria, decreased urine output, and a rise in blood pressure (over 140/90 mm Hg).

> *Test Taking Strategy—Analyze to determine what information the question asks for, which is a finding that is of greatest concern when assessing a client with PIH. Consider the physiology of PIH and recall that an unexpected weight gain (option 4) correlates with fluid retention and an elevation in blood pressure. Review the assessment findings for PIH if you had difficulty answering this question.*
> **Cognitive Level**—*Applying*
> **Client Needs Category**—*Physiological integrity*
> **Client Needs Subcategory**—*Physiological adaptation*

83. 3. Clients experiencing mild pregnancy-induced hypertension (PIH) will have proteinuria, with a +1 or +2 measurement using a urine reagent test strip. Other findings include a 30 mm Hg rise in the baseline systolic blood pressure or a 15 mm Hg rise in the baseline diastolic blood pressure, and a weight gain of 2 or more pounds (0.9 kg) per week during the second trimester. Edema may be present, but it is usually noted in the face and hands. Ankle edema may be present during pregnancy for reasons other than PIH.

> *Test Taking Strategy—Note the key words "most indicative," indicating one option is better than any of the others in describing an indication of PIH that is mild in nature. Recall that proteinuria (option 3) accompanies PIH, whereas the assessment findings in the other options are either unrelated to PIH or normal. Review the clinical manifestations of PIH if you had difficulty answering this question.*
> **Cognitive Level**—*Analyzing*
> **Client Needs Category**—*Physiological integrity*
> **Client Needs Subcategory**—*Reduction of risk potential*

84. 3. The care of the client with mild pregnancy-induced hypertension (PIH) can usually be managed at home; however, it is important for the client to return to the physician on a weekly basis. The client also needs to eat a diet high in protein and ensure that she is consuming adequate fluids because of protein loss during urination. She should also be instructed to remain on bed rest. The nurse should teach the client about danger signs, such as seizures, that must be reported to the physician immediately.

Test Taking Strategy—*Note the key words "most appropriate" used in the stem of the question. These words indicate that one option is better than any of the others. Select the option that provides accurate information about how the client with PIH should proceed with home care. Even though this client's PIH is considered mild, it is nevertheless dangerous. The client must be advised that weekly follow-up appointments with the physician are imperative. Review how the client's prognosis is evaluated when managing PIH at home if you had difficulty answering this question.*

Cognitive Level—*Applying*
Client Needs Category—*Physiological integrity*
Client Needs Subcategory—*Reduction of risk potential*

85. 2. Magnesium sulfate is the drug of choice for seizure prophylaxis in women who have severe pregnancy-induced hypertension (PIH). Magnesium sulfate prevents calcium ion transport, dilates cerebral blood vessels, and prevents platelet aggregation. In addition to assessing the vital signs, the nurse should check the client's deep tendon reflexes, urine output, fetal heart tones, oxygen saturation, respiratory rate, and serum magnesium blood level. Close monitoring of these findings is necessary to detect the presence of or potential for magnesium toxicity. Glucose in the urine, blood in the stool, and constricted pupils are unrelated to magnesium toxicity.

Test Taking Strategy—*Analyze to determine what information the question asks for, which is an assessment finding that is essential to monitor when a client receives magnesium sulfate for PIH. Magnesium toxicity is manifested by a loss of patellar tendon reflexes (option 2), an assessment that must be checked every 4 hours during administration of magnesium sulfate. Review assessments that must be monitored to detect magnesium toxicity if you had difficulty answering this question.*

Cognitive Level—*Applying*
Client Needs Category—*Physiological integrity*
Client Needs Subcategory—*Pharmacological therapies*

86. 4. The antidote for magnesium toxicity is a 10% solution of calcium gluconate (Kalcinate). Recall that magnesium sulfate prevents calcium ion transport. For a muscle to contract, calcium ions must enter calcium channels on the membrane of motor neurons. If magnesium sulfate inhibits the flow of calcium ions, contraction of muscles—including the diaphragm, which is necessary for breathing—is impaired. Calcium gluconate is usually given I.V. and is injected over 3 or more minutes to prevent the occurrence of ventricular fibrillation. Hydralazine (Apresoline) is an antihypertensive; methylergonovine (Methergine) is usually given to control postpartum bleeding; and oxytocin (Pitocin) is used to augment labor and to control postpartum bleeding.

Test Taking Strategy—*Analyze to determine what information the question asks for, which is the medication to have on hand when administering magnesium sulfate. If skeletal muscle contraction becomes significantly impaired while administering magnesium sulfate, this life-threatening consequence can be reversed with calcium gluconate (option 4), which should be available before initiating the infusion of magnesium sulfate. Review the manifestations of magnesium toxicity and the antidote for managing it if you had difficulty answering this question.*

Cognitive Level—*Applying*
Client Needs Category—*Physiological integrity*
Client Needs Subcategory—*Pharmacological therapies*

87. 2. A respiratory rate of less than 14 breaths/minute is associated with magnesium toxicity. Additional indications of magnesium toxicity include diminished deep tendon reflexes, urine output of less than 100 mL in 4 hours, signs of fetal distress, and a magnesium serum level above 10 mg/dL. If any of these occur, magnesium sulfate should be discontinued and the physician notified immediately.

Test Taking Strategy—*Use the process of elimination to select the option that identifies the best indication that magnesium sulfate toxicity is developing. Eliminate options 1 and 4 because these are assessment findings that are essentially normal. Although finding protein in the urine is abnormal, it can be eliminated because it is a manifestation of PIH rather than magnesium toxicity. Option 2 remains as the correct answer because an inhibition of calcium due to magnesium toxicity interferes with skeletal muscle contraction, which includes contraction of the diaphragm. Review signs of magnesium toxicity if you had difficulty answering this question.*

Cognitive Level—*Analyzing*
Client Needs Category—*Physiological integrity*
Client Needs Subcategory—*Pharmacological therapies*

88. 1. The client with pregnancy-induced hypertension (PIH) is said to have developed eclampsia if she begins to have seizures. Severe headache, abdominal pain, muscle hyperirritability, apprehension, and twitching often precede seizures associated with eclampsia. The other signs and symptoms listed are not manifestations of eclampsia.

Test Taking Strategy—*Analyze to determine what information the question asks for, which is the assessment finding that must be reported immediately because it indicates that PIH has progressed to eclampsia. Knowledge of eclampsia is essential in successfully answering the question. If unsure, consider the rationale for administering magnesium sulfate, which is to prevent seizures. Recall that the onset of seizures (option 1) due to cerebral edema indicates the development of eclampsia. Eclampsia can lead to a comatose state and maternal as well as fetal mortality. Review the clinical manifestations of eclampsia if you had difficulty answering this question.*
Cognitive Level—*Applying*
Client Needs Category—*Physiological integrity*
Client Needs Subcategory—*Physiological adaptation*

89. **4, 5, 6.** Vaginal bleeding, abdominal cramping, and backaches are typical symptoms that clients report with the occurrence of a threatened abortion. These signs and symptoms may resolve without losing the fetus, but the opposite may occur as well. Severe headaches and persistent tachycardia are not normal and should be reported to the health care provider, but someone experiencing a spontaneous abortion does not usually manifest these symptoms. Cold, clammy skin also is not associated with spontaneous abortion.

Test Taking Strategy—*Analyze to determine what information the question asks for, which is signs that suggest an impending spontaneous abortion. Alternative-format "select all that apply" questions require considering each option independently to decide its merit in answering the question. If unsure, consider that the symptoms of labor are similar to those when a spontaneous abortion is threatened. Review signs of a threatened abortion, which also is referred to as a spontaneous abortion, if you had difficulty answering this question.*
Cognitive Level—*Analyzing*
Client Needs Category—*Physiological integrity*
Client Needs Subcategory—*Reduction of risk potential*

90. **1.** When the cervix is dilated but the fetus and placenta remain in the uterus, spontaneous abortion is inevitable and the client will more than likely require a dilation and curettage (D&C) to remove the remaining products of conception. The client should be prepared physically and emotionally for the procedure. The other options are not usually included in the care of the client experiencing an inevitable spontaneous abortion.

Test Taking Strategy—*Note the key words "most appropriate," which indicates that one answer is better than the others. Recall that the word "inevitable" means that the client's condition has progressed to the point that there is no hope for the pregnancy*

continuing. Nursing interventions are adjusted from measures to save the pregnancy to care of the mother. Option 1 is the correct answer because the products of conception must be removed, generally with a D&C. Review the nursing interventions that are performed when managing the care of a mother when an abortion is inevitable if you had difficulty answering this question.*
Cognitive Level—*Applying*
Client Needs Category—*Physiological integrity*
Client Needs Subcategory—*Physiological adaptation*

91. **1.** An inevitable abortion means that there is no hope of saving the fetus. The nurse must provide much-needed emotional support. The client and family members are encouraged to verbalize their feelings to facilitate their abilities to cope with the situation. Telling the client that there are opportunities for additional pregnancies in the future disregards the significance of the mother's present loss. Suggesting that the client avoid stress does not facilitate expression of her feelings and hinders her ability to cope with the situation. Telling the client that things will work out for the best does not acknowledge the justifiable sorrow that the client is experiencing. It also does not show much-needed emotional support.

Test Taking Strategy—*Analyze to determine what information the question asks for, which is the most therapeutic response to a client experiencing a spontaneous abortion. Option 1 is the best answer because encouraging a client to verbalize her feelings openly while the nurse actively listens relieves some of the emotional distress the client is feeling. Review therapeutic communication techniques when a client experiences a loss and is grieving if you had difficulty answering this question.*
Cognitive Level—*Applying*
Client Needs Category—*Psychosocial integrity*
Client Needs Subcategory—*None*

92. **3.** The insulin requirement for the pregnant diabetic client will fluctuate during pregnancy. During implantation, progesterone levels raise, counteracting the effect of insulin and causing a temporary increased need. After the 5th and 6th weeks of pregnancy, the need for insulin decreases because the mother is transporting increased amounts of glucose to the growing fetus. Later in pregnancy, the need for insulin usually increases because of the increasing amounts of the hormones estrogen and progesterone, which cause insulin resistance in the client. During the postpartum period, the hormone levels are lower, thereby decreasing the requirements for insulin.

Test Taking Strategy—*Use the process of elimination to identify the insulin level during pregnancy. It is incorrect to indicate that insulin requirements will be consistently increased, decreased, or stay the same. In fact, the requirements fluctuate (option 3) with the*

changes in reproductive hormone levels. Review how insulin requirements change during pregnancy if you had difficulty answering this question.
Cognitive Level—*Applying*
Client Needs Category—*Physiological integrity*
Client Needs Subcategory—*Pharmacological therapies*

93. 2. A pregnant client who has diabetes is predisposed to higher risks for complications than nondiabetic clients. The pregnant diabetic client has an increased risk of developing pregnancy-induced hypertension (PIH), especially if vascular changes secondary to diabetes have already developed. Some other complications that may occur secondary to diabetes include infection due to elevated blood glucose levels that support pathogenic growth; hydramnios, an increase in the volume of amniotic fluid, thought to be caused by increased urination by the fetus in utero from fetal hyperglycemia; dystocia, difficult labor, due to a large-birthweight infant; possible birth trauma related to the large size of the fetus; and postpartum hemorrhage. Hyperemesis gravidarum, placenta previa, and toxoplasmosis are not associated with diabetes during pregnancy.

> *Test Taking Strategy*—*Analyze to determine what information the question asks for, which is regarding complications during pregnancy secondary to diabetes. Obesity and vascular changes that are often components of diabetes increase the risk for developing PIH (option 2). PIH is a potential problem even for those with gestational diabetes, a condition in which a woman who has never been diagnosed with diabetes develops impaired glucose tolerance during pregnancy but which resolves following delivery. Review diabetic complications during pregnancy if you had difficulty answering this question.*
Cognitive Level—*Applying*
Client Needs Category—*Physiological integrity*
Client Needs Subcategory—*Physiological adaptation*

94. 1. The pregnant diabetic client is at greatest risk for having a baby that is larger than average in both size and weight. During pregnancy, the fetus stores glycogen from the mother's elevated blood glucose. After birth, the infant's supply of insulin metabolizes the glucose, predisposing the infant to hypoglycemia. Because hypoglycemia is a complication, the baby will require frequent blood glucose testing for the first several hours. Other fetal effects of diabetes include congenital deformities, prematurity, and respiratory distress syndrome. However, a client whose diabetes is well controlled during pregnancy rarely experiences the other fetal effects listed here.

> *Test Taking Strategy*—*Apply the key words "most accurate" when considering the choice in each option. Select the option that is validated by evidence-based information. Recall that infants born to diabetic mothers generally have higher birth weights and*

require temporary monitoring of blood glucose because their blood glucose level falls precipitously when separated from the maternal source of glucose. Review the effect of diabetes on a newborn infant if you had difficulty answering this question.
Cognitive Level—*Applying*
Client Needs Category—*Physiological integrity*
Client Needs Subcategory—*Physiological adaptation*

95. 1. Placenta previa is a condition in which the placenta is abnormally placed and partially or totally covers the cervix because it is implanted low in the uterus. It is the most common cause of painless bleeding during the third trimester of pregnancy. The bleeding is due to a separation of the placenta from the uterus in the area that is near or covers the cervical os. The separation occurs when the cervix stretches and thins before delivery. Severe bleeding can cause anemia in the mother, but the gravest danger of placenta previa is to the infant, who may experience respiratory distress syndrome after birth due to premature delivery. Placenta previa is unrelated to the development of polyps, hormonal deficiencies, or antibody production.

> *Test Taking Strategy*—*Use the process of elimination to select the option that identifies the best explanation for placenta previa. Options 2 and 4 can be eliminated because placenta previa does not involve a deficit of placental hormones or antibodies against fetal red blood cells. Option 3 can be eliminated because uterine polyps, known as fibroids, do not invade the placenta. Option 1 remains as the correct answer because it describes a malplacement of the placenta that makes it subject to bleeding before the beginning of labor. Review the description of placenta previa and its etiology if you had difficulty answering the question.*
Cognitive Level—*Understanding*
Client Needs Category—*Physiological integrity*
Client Needs Subcategory—*Physiological adaptation*

96. 3. The preferred course of treatment is to maintain the pregnancy as close to term as possible. If the client is stable, the physician usually orders bed rest and continuous client observation. With marginal or partial placenta previa, vaginal birth is possible. Uncontrolled hemorrhaging, fetal distress, or complete placenta previa requires immediate delivery of the baby, usually by cesarean birth. Ritodrine (Yutopar) is indicated for premature labor; however, this medication is not routinely used for clients with placenta previa.

> *Test Taking Strategy*—*Note the key words "most likely" in reference to the course of action the physician may take after detecting placenta previa. Recall that as long as the placenta remains attached, the fetus will survive. Recall that supporting the pregnancy as long as possible (option 3) eliminates*

the need to induce labor prematurely, inhibit the progress of labor, or perform an emergency cesarean section if hemorrhage occurs. Review how placenta previa is managed in the absence of a life-threatening situation if you had difficulty answering this question.
Cognitive Level—*Applying*
Client Needs Category—*Physiological integrity*
Client Needs Subcategory—*Physiological adaptation*

97. **2, 6.** The client with placenta previa is at risk for shock due to hemorrhaging. Therefore, a baseline blood pressure measurement and a pulse rate should be obtained so that those involved in the client's care can evaluate further changes. Significant findings must also be reported to the physician immediately because this is a condition that is a medical emergency. When a client is admitted to the hospital, the client's height and weight as well as her obstetric, general health, and drug histories are obtained. In this situation, obtaining the client's blood pressure and pulse takes priority over admittance information. The urinalysis and beta-streptococcal laboratory results are not priorities at this point.

> *Test Taking Strategy—Analyze to determine what information the question asks for, which is regarding priority information when the client with placenta previa is experiencing profuse vaginal bleeding. Alternative-format "select all that apply" questions require considering each option independently to decide its merit in answering the question. Review information that is essential to obtain when it appears that placenta previa is now complete if you had difficulty answering this question.*
> **Cognitive Level**—*Analyzing*
> **Client Needs Category**—*Physiological integrity*
> **Client Needs Subcategory**—*Physiological adaptation*

98. **4, 5, 6.** Abruptio placentae is a separation of the placenta from its site of implantation. It differs from placenta previa in that the client experiences painful bleeding rather than painless bleeding. The bleeding is accompanied by uterine contractions and fetal distress. The client with pregnancy-induced hypertension is at risk for developing abruptio placentae. Other factors associated with the occurrence of abruptio placentae include essential hypertension, previous history of placenta previa, dietary deficiencies, trauma to the abdomen, multiparity, and a history of alcohol or cocaine abuse, the latter of which may be responsible for vasospasm of uterine blood vessels. Gestational diabetes, hyperemesis gravidarum, and oligohydramnios are not associated with abruptio placentae.

> *Test Taking Strategy—Analyze to determine what information the question asks for regarding predisposing factors associated with abruptio placentae. Alternative-format "select all that apply" questions require considering each option independently to*

decide its merit in answering the question. Select options that have an effect on a client's vasculature. Review conditions that place pregnant clients at risk for developing abruptio placentae if you had difficulty answering this question.
Cognitive Level—*Analyzing*
Client Needs Category—*Physiological integrity*
Client Needs Subcategory—*Physiological adaptation*

99. **1, 5.** The bleeding associated with abruptio placentae may be obvious or concealed. A rigid, boardlike abdomen is commonly observed in clients with concealed hemorrhaging. Other signs and symptoms of abruptio placentae include severe abdominal pain, dark red vaginal bleeding, maternal shock, and fetal distress with a heart rate less than 100 beats/minute. Severe nausea and vomiting, painless vaginal bleeding, and seizures are not manifestations of abruptio placentae.

> *Test Taking Strategy—Analyze to determine what information the question asks for regarding the findings most indicative of abruptio placentae that must be reported immediately. Alternative-format "select all that apply" questions require considering each option independently to decide its merit in answering the question. Review assessment findings associated with abruptio placentae if you had difficulty answering this question.*
> **Cognitive Level**—*Analyzing*
> **Client Needs Category**—*Physiological integrity*
> **Client Needs Subcategory**—*Physiological adaptation*

100. **1.** Abruptio placentae requires an emergency cesarean birth because without an intact, functioning placenta, the fetus will not receive adequate oxygenation or nutrients to survive. Written consent should be obtained immediately from the client or a family member. A client with vaginal bleeding is not given an enema. A client with a complete abruption is not usually placed in Trendelenburg's position (where the feet are higher than the head) because of the pooling of blood in the uterus. A contraction stress test is inappropriate for a client with any type of abruption.

> *Test Taking Strategy—Note the key words "most appropriate," indicating that one answer is better than the others. Consider which option identifies a nursing action that is most important to perform when a client is hemorrhaging and the fetus is in jeopardy of hypoxemia. Recall that abruptio placentae is an obstetric emergency, requiring a cesarean section to preserve the lives of the fetus and mother. Emergency surgery necessitates that the nurse obtain written consent for the procedure to proceed. Review nursing care of a client with an abruption of the placenta if you had difficulty answering this question.*
> **Cognitive Level**—*Applying*
> **Client Needs Category**—*Physiological integrity*
> **Client Needs Subcategory**—*Physiological adaptation*

101. 3. Any I.M. injection can be administered using the Z-track method, but there are certain medications for which this method is mandatory. Z-track injections are given deeply into a large muscle. The ventrogluteal site, which includes the gluteus medius and gluteus minimus muscles, is the preferred site for administering an injection by the Z-track technique. The deltoid muscle is used for I.M. injections; however, it is a smaller muscle in comparison to other I.M. injection sites and cannot accommodate large amounts of medication. Neither the trapezius muscle (located in the back and the shoulder) nor the latissimus dorsi (the widest muscle in the back) is used for the injections.

Test Taking Strategy—Use the process of elimination to select the option that identifies the proper site to administer an I.M. injection using the Z-track technique. The gluteus medius muscle (option 3) is the correct answer because it is sufficiently large enough to insert a needle deeply within the muscle. Review the sites for a Z-track technique if you had difficulty answering this question.
Cognitive Level—Applying
Client Needs Category—Safe and effective care environment
Client Needs Subcategory—Safety and infection control

102. 1. Using the Z-track technique allows the nurse to deposit a medication deeply into the muscle so that the tissue will self-seal, thereby keeping the medication from leaking into the subcutaneous tissues. It also reduces pain during the injection. It is especially important to use this method when injecting medication that irritates or stains tissue, such as iron preparations, and medications that require absorption over a long period of time, such as those the pharmaceutical company advocates be given as a depot injection. When giving a medication by Z-track technique, the nurse pulls the tissue laterally (to the side) about 1″ to 1½″ until it is taut, holds the tissue in position during the actual injection, releasing it only after the needle is withdrawn. It is inappropriate to pull the tissue superiorly, proximally, or obliquely when using this technique.

Test Taking Strategy—Analyze to determine what information the question asks for, which is the direction in which the tissue is pulled when preparing to administer an I.M. injection using the Z-track technique. Visualize the letter Z or the term "zig-zag" for which the injection technique is named. Recall that the nondominant hand displaces the tissue laterally before the injection. Review the Z-track injection technique if you had difficulty with this question.
Cognitive Level—Applying
Client Needs Category—Safe and effective care environment
Client Needs Subcategory—Safety and infection control

103. 2. Exposure to rubella (German measles) during the first trimester of pregnancy increases the risk of the fetus developing congenital rubella syndrome. Major manifestations of this congenital condition include blindness, deafness, heart defects, mental retardation, cleft lip, and cleft palate. Premature labor, severe preeclampsia, and hydatidiform moles are not associated with rubella exposure.

Test Taking Strategy—Analyze to determine what information the question asks for, which is a complication from a possible rubella infection. Although rubella does not cause symptoms as severe as rubeola, rubella that occurs during pregnancy is dangerous to a fetus because it causes many congenital defects (option 2). Review the impact of rubella during the first trimester of pregnancy if you had difficulty answering this question.
Cognitive Level—Applying
Client Needs Category—Health promotion and maintenance
Client Needs Subcategory—None

104. 2. The LPN is co-assigned duties with the registered nurse. The LPN is best assigned routine intrapartum clients. The best assignment is the 22-year-old who is close to term pregnancy. The other options are clients experiencing potential complications.

Test Taking Strategy—Use the process of elimination to identify the client best suited to the LPN scope of practice. Analyze the four client options to determine those which would need advanced assessment skills. Note the routine labor and delivery client with no immediate complications which leads to the correct answer. Review the signs and symptoms of labor if you had difficulty answering this question.
Cognitive Level—Evaluating
Client Needs Category—Safe and effective care environment
Client Needs Subcategory—Coordinated care

105. 4. A hydatidiform mole is a mass of tissue that forms within the uterus as the result of a genetic error during the fertilization process, when a nonviable, fertilized egg implants in the uterus. A grapelike mass composed of numerous clear vesicles develops as the tissue deteriorates. A malignancy called *choriocarcinoma* may develop from a hydatidiform mole. A hydatidiform mole is suspected when there is abnormally rapid uterine growth resulting in a uterus that is larger than expected for the woman's gestational dates. This condition is also suspected when fetal heart tones and fetal movement are not detected, when there is excessive or persistent nausea and vomiting, and when pregnancy-induced hypertension develops before 20 to 24 weeks' gestation. Vaginal bleeding may be continuous or intermittent, and the human chorionic gonadotropin level is greatly elevated. A blotchy brown discoloration to the face (chloasma) is not associated with this condition. A positive Chadwick's sign refers to the purple coloring of the vulva and vagina early in pregnancy; this is a normal finding. Ballottement is a normal indication of pregnancy occurring between the 16th and 20th weeks of gestation; it is elicited when the examiner taps the uterus and the fetus floats to the top of the uterus, then back down.

> ***Test Taking Strategy**—Note the key words "most indicative" in reference to a characteristic finding of a hydatidiform mole. Consider that the hydatidiform mole is a mass or growth that forms in the uterus at the beginning of pregnancy. The growth may be made of placental tissue and atypical fetal or even malignant cells. The only option that correlates with a growth within the uterus is option 4. Review manifestations of a hydatidiform mole and its etiology if you had difficulty answering this question.*
> ***Cognitive Level**—Applying*
> ***Client Needs Category**—Physiological integrity*
> ***Client Needs Subcategory**—Reduction of risk potential*

106. 3. The U.S. Centers for Disease Control and Prevention recommends that pregnant women who are at risk for hepatitis B virus (HBV) be tested during pregnancy. High-risk groups include women of Asian, Pacific Island, Alaskan Eskimo, and Haitian descent; recipients of repeated blood transfusions; I.V. drug users or partners of I.V. drug users; women who have been exposed to HBV; and women who have multiple sex partners. HBV infection is not linked to clients who smoke, who are single and pregnant for the first time, or who have been exposed to *Haemophilus influenzae*.

> ***Test Taking Strategy**—Analyze to determine what information the question asks for, which is the pregnant client the nurse should encourage to undergo testing for HBV. Recall that HBV is transmitted through contact with blood or body fluids of an infected person, similarly to human immunodeficiency virus (HIV). Note that emigrating from a poverty-stricken country with poor health care, such as Haiti, places a pregnant client at high risk for HBV (option 3). Review the pregnant populations that are at high risk for being infected with HBV if you had difficulty answering this question.*
> ***Cognitive Level**—Applying*
> ***Client Needs Category**—Health promotion and maintenance*
> ***Client Needs Subcategory**—None*

Elective Abortion

107. 3. During the first trimester of pregnancy, a woman has the right to have an abortion without legal restraints. During the second trimester, states can regulate the conditions under which an abortion is performed but cannot prohibit abortion. After viability, which according to legal guidelines is considered after 22 weeks' gestation, the state may, and usually does, prohibit abortion except in a situation that is perceived as a threat to the life or health of the pregnant woman.

> ***Test Taking Strategy**—Analyze to determine what information the question asks for regarding the legal threshold of fetal viability. Viability refers to the fetus's ability to survive outside the uterus, which depends on its stage of embryonic development. If unsure, divide a pregnancy into trimesters and recall that a common timeframe for viability is just before 6 months (option 3). Review the most current literature on the threshold of viability and the maximum stage of pregnancy during which an elective legal abortion may be performed if you had difficulty answering this question.*
> ***Cognitive Level**—Applying*
> ***Client Needs Category**—Health promotion and maintenance*
> ***Client Needs Subcategory**—None*

12 The Nursing Care of Intrapartum, Postpartum, and Newborn Clients

- ■ Admission of the Client to a Labor and Delivery Facility
- ■ Nursing Care of Clients During the First Stage of Labor
- ■ Nursing Care of Clients During the Second Stage of Labor
- ■ Nursing Care of Clients During the Third Stage of Labor
- ■ Nursing Care of Clients During the Fourth Stage of Labor
- ■ Nursing Care of Clients Having a Cesarean Birth
- ■ Nursing Care of Clients Having an Emergency Delivery
- ■ Nursing Care of Clients Having a Stillborn Baby
- ■ Nursing Care of Clients During the Postpartum Period
- ■ Nursing Care of the Newborn Client
- ■ Nursing Care of Newborns with Complications
- ■ Correct Answers, Rationales, and Test Taking Strategies

Directions: With a pencil, blacken the space in front of the option you have chosen for your correct answer.

Admission of the Client to a Labor and Delivery Facility

A 25-year-old primigravid client in the last trimester of pregnancy calls the physician's office and tells the nurse, "I think I'm in labor."

1. Which findings warrant instructing the client to notify the physician and report to the hospital's labor and delivery unit immediately? Select all that apply.
[ ] **1.** The client is having contractions every 5 minutes.
[ ] **2.** The client feels a burst of energy.
[ ] **3.** The client experiences a sudden gush of fluid from her vagina.
[ ] **4.** The client experiences urinary frequency.
[ ] **5.** The client notices blood-tinged mucus from her vagina.
[ ] **6.** The client reports that she has felt the baby "drop."

The client arrives at the hospital and is admitted to the labor, delivery, recovery, and postpartum (LDRP) unit. The nurse obtains the client's health and pregnancy history.

2. As the nurse collects the client's history, which question has the lowest priority?
[ ] **1.** "When did you last eat?"
[ ] **2.** "Have you ever had an enema?"
[ ] **3.** "When did your contractions start?"
[ ] **4.** "When is your baby due?"

The client informs the nurse about a previous admission to the unit 3 days ago with "false labor."

3. Which statement made by the client indicates a characteristic of Braxton Hicks contractions?
[ ] **1.** "The contractions are less strong when I walk."
[ ] **2.** "The contractions are regular and I can time them."
[ ] **3.** "The contractions get stronger no matter what I am doing."
[ ] **4.** "The contractions start in my lower back."

During the admission process, the nurse obtains the client's vital signs.

4. When is the most appropriate time to take the client's blood pressure?
[ ] **1.** After a contraction before the next one begins
[ ] **2.** At the end of a contraction before it is complete
[ ] **3.** At the onset of the contraction before its peak intensity
[ ] **4.** Midway in the contraction when it is at its greatest intensity

The nurse palpates the uterus to measure the fundal height of a pregnant woman at 40 weeks' gestation.

5. Identify with an *X* the area on the abdomen where the nurse should feel the uterine fundus.

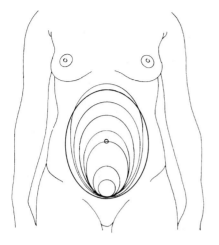

Nursing Care of Clients During the First Stage of Labor

A 30-year-old primigravid client is admitted to the labor, delivery, recovery, and postpartum (LDRP) unit of a local hospital. The physician plans to perform a vaginal examination to determine the status of labor.

6. How can the nurse best prepare to assist with the vaginal examination?
[ ] **1.** By having sterile gloves available for the examiner
[ ] **2.** By placing the client in the left side-lying position
[ ] **3.** By instructing the client to halt breathing during the exam
[ ] **4.** By giving the client an enema before the exam

After the vaginal examination, the physician indicates that the client is in the latent phase of the first stage of labor. A progress note is written in the client's admission records.

7. When the nurse reviews the client's admission records, which assessment finding is the most reliable indicator that the client is in true labor?
[ ] **1.** Contractions are regular and increasing in duration and intensity.
[ ] **2.** Contractions radiate from the lower back to the lower abdomen.
[ ] **3.** Bloody show is present.
[ ] **4.** The cervix is dilating.

8. During the latent phase, which findings can the nurse expect to notice when assessing the client? Select all that apply.
[ ] **1.** Contractions occurring every 10 to 15 minutes
[ ] **2.** Fetal heart rate of 120 to 160 beats/minute
[ ] **3.** Bulging perineum
[ ] **4.** Early decelerations
[ ] **5.** Irritable mood in the client
[ ] **6.** Client report, "I feel my bowels may move."

9. Which of the following nursing instructions are appropriate to make to the client during the latent phase of labor? Select all that apply.
[ ] **1.** "As long as your membranes are intact, you may walk around the unit."
[ ] **2.** "You may have clear liquids or ice chips as needed."
[ ] **3.** "Pant when you experience a contraction."
[ ] **4.** "Avoid bathing until after the delivery."
[ ] **5.** "Put on your call light when you feel a contraction coming on."
[ ] **6.** "You may have pain medication when your contractions are 2 minutes apart."

10. During the latent phase of the first stage of labor, how often should the nurse plan to assess the fetal heart rate?
[ ] **1.** Every 5 to 15 minutes
[ ] **2.** Every 15 to 30 minutes
[ ] **3.** Every 30 to 60 minutes
[ ] **4.** Every 60 to 90 minutes

The primigravid client tells the nurse, "I plan to have an epidural for pain management," and asks the nurse, "When can I expect to receive it?"

11. An epidural is best performed when the client is how many centimeters dilated?
[ ] **1.** 3 to 4
[ ] **2.** 5 to 6
[ ] **3.** 7 to 8
[ ] **4.** 9 to 10

The registered nurse performs a vaginal examination of the client. The nurse determines that the labor is progressing and the cervix is dilated 6 cm.

12. When assessing the frequency and duration of the client's contractions during this phase of labor, the nurse expects to find that the contractions are occurring every 3 to 5 minutes and lasting up to how many seconds?
[ ] **1.** 30
[ ] **2.** 40
[ ] **3.** 60
[ ] **4.** 90

Labor has progressed, and the client enters the transition phase of the first stage of labor.

13. Which assessment finding can the nurse expect to observe during this phase?
[ ] **1.** Cervix dilated to 10 cm
[ ] **2.** Crowning of the presenting part
[ ] **3.** Increased bloody show
[ ] **4.** Contractions lasting up to 60 seconds

14. Which nursing action is best for meeting the client's needs during the transition phase?
[ ] **1.** Encouraging the client to ambulate
[ ] **2.** Praising the client frequently
[ ] **3.** Instructing the client to push with each contraction
[ ] **4.** Massaging the client's back between contractions

A 29-year-old multiparous client who has had an uneventful, healthy pregnancy is admitted to the hospital. The physician informs the client that the active phase of the first stage of labor is in progress. The records also show that the full-term baby is in the left occipitoposterior (LOP) position.

15. When the fetus is in the LOP position, which nursing intervention is most appropriate?
[ ] **1.** Assisting the client to the knee-chest position to relieve back pain
[ ] **2.** Placing the client in Trendelenburg's position to prevent cord prolapse
[ ] **3.** Assisting with preparation of equipment for a precipitous delivery
[ ] **4.** Having the client void frequently to minimize displacement of the uterus

16. To prevent distention of the client's bladder during the active phase of labor, which nursing intervention is most appropriate?
[ ] **1.** Instructing the client to limit fluid intake
[ ] **2.** Decreasing the rate of the I.V. infusion
[ ] **3.** Offering solid foods instead of liquids
[ ] **4.** Encouraging the client to void every 2 hours

17. The nurse places an eternal fetal monitor on the client and observes this monitoring strip:

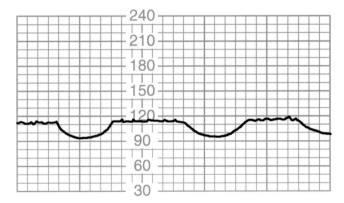

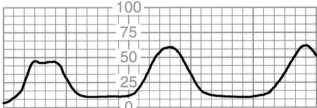

After analyzing the monitoring strip, into which of the following positions should the nurse assist the client?
[ ] **1.** Left lateral
[ ] **2.** Right lateral
[ ] **3.** Supine
[ ] **4.** Prone

18. To correctly assess the duration of a contraction, the nurse counts the time between which intervals?
[ ] **1.** The beginning of one contraction and the end of the same contraction
[ ] **2.** The end of one contraction and the beginning of the next contraction
[ ] **3.** The beginning of one contraction and the end of the next contraction
[ ] **4.** The beginning of one contraction and the beginning of the next contraction

19. Which method represents the most accurate technique to use when assessing the client's contractions?
[ ] **1.** Place the hand over the fundus of the uterus, which is located just above the umbilicus.
[ ] **2.** Place the hand over the inferior portion of the uterus, which is located just above the umbilicus.
[ ] **3.** Place the hand over the fundus of the uterus, which is located midway between the umbilicus and the symphysis pubis.
[ ] **4.** Place the hand over the inferior portion of the uterus, which is located midway between the umbilicus and the symphysis pubis.

The client tells the nurse, "I think my membranes have ruptured." The nurse performs a nitrazine test and confirms that the membranes have ruptured.

20. Which test result indicates that the membranes have ruptured?
[ ] **1.** The test strip turns blue.
[ ] **2.** The test strip turns yellow.
[ ] **3.** The test strip turns red.
[ ] **4.** The test strip turns green.

21. Which actions should the nurse perform immediately after the membranes are ruptured? Select all that apply.
[ ] **1.** Check the client's pulse.
[ ] **2.** Insert an indwelling catheter.
[ ] **3.** Perform a vaginal examination.
[ ] **4.** Check the fetal heart rate.
[ ] **5.** Inspect the fluid for meconium.
[ ] **6.** Prepare the room for imminent delivery.

22. After the membranes have ruptured, how often should the nurse take the client's temperature?
[ ] **1.** Every hour
[ ] **2.** Every 2 hours
[ ] **3.** Every 3 hours
[ ] **4.** Every 4 hours

Because the nitrazine test results indicate that the membranes have ruptured, the physician orders internal electronic fetal monitoring. The client asks the nurse, "Is there any danger of this procedure causing harm to my baby?"

23. Which response by the nurse provides the best explanation of the procedure and potential risks, if any, associated with internal electronic fetal monitoring?
[ ] **1.** "The procedure requires attachment of a small spiral electrode to the fetal scalp and poses a slight risk of soft-tissue injury and infection."
[ ] **2.** "The procedure requires insertion of a soft, water-filled catheter into the uterus and poses no risk of injury to you or your baby."
[ ] **3.** "The procedure requires placement of an ultrasound transducer over your abdomen and poses no risk to you or your baby."
[ ] **4.** "The procedure requires application of a suction cup to the fetal scalp and poses a slight risk for the development of a hematoma."

24. Which assessment finding is most indicative of fetal distress?
[ ] **1.** Fetal heart rate of 140 beats/minute
[ ] **2.** Presence of fetal heart rate accelerations
[ ] **3.** Presence of green amniotic fluid
[ ] **4.** Increased amount of bloody show

The client continues in active labor and tells the nurse, "I haven't had anything to eat for 24 hours. Can I have something to eat now?"

25. Which response by the nurse is the best explanation for why solid food is not given at this time?
[ ] **1.** "It may alter the absorption of regional anesthetics."
[ ] **2.** "It may alter the duration and frequency of contractions."
[ ] **3.** "It may cause fetal distress."
[ ] **4.** "It may cause nausea and vomiting."

After a sterile vaginal examination is performed, the client tells the nurse, "I overheard the physician say that the baby is in the vertex position. What does that mean?"

26. Which response by the nurse provides the best explanation regarding vertex positioning?
[ ] **1.** "The head is entering the birth canal first."
[ ] **2.** "The feet are entering the birth canal first."
[ ] **3.** "The buttocks are entering the birth canal first."
[ ] **4.** "The shoulder is entering the birth canal first."

27. During evaluation of the client's contractions during the active phase of the first stage of labor, when is it important for the nurse to notify the physician?
[ ] **1.** When the contractions occur every 3 to 5 minutes
[ ] **2.** When the contractions last longer than 45 seconds
[ ] **3.** When the uterus relaxes between contractions
[ ] **4.** When the fetal heart rate drops after the acme of a contraction

The nurse is caring for a client in preterm labor. The physician writes an order for terbutaline sulfate (Brethine).

28. The nurse should carefully monitor the client for which adverse reactions to terbutaline sulfate? Select all that apply.
[ ] **1.** Anxiety
[ ] **2.** Tremors
[ ] **3.** Nervousness
[ ] **4.** Hypoglycemia
[ ] **5.** Oliguria
[ ] **6.** Rash

29. When is it necessary for the nurse to withhold the terbutaline sulfate (Brethine) and notify the physician?
[ ] **1.** When the electronic monitor reveals that the client is having mild contractions
[ ] **2.** When the cervix is dilated 4 cm or greater or is effaced 50% or more
[ ] **3.** When the electronic monitor reveals the presence of fetal heart rate variability
[ ] **4.** When the client states that the contractions are milder and occurring less frequently

Nursing Care of Clients During the Second Stage of Labor

The nurse cares for a 30-year-old multiparous client who is in the transition phase of the first stage of labor.

30. Which assessment finding is the best indication that the client has entered the second stage of labor?
[ ] **1.** The perineum is bulging.
[ ] **2.** Contractions are lasting 30 to 60 seconds.
[ ] **3.** The cervix is dilated to 8 cm.
[ ] **4.** The client becomes agitated with her spouse.

31. When should the nurse begin preparing this client for delivery?
[ ] **1.** When the client is about 7 cm dilated
[ ] **2.** When the fetal head begins to crown
[ ] **3.** When the physician or midwife arrives
[ ] **4.** When the client is completely dilated

The client tells the nurse, "I feel like I need to push."

32. Which action should the nurse take first?
[ ] **1.** Instruct the client to push with the next contraction.
[ ] **2.** Place the client in a semi-Fowler's position.
[ ] **3.** Check that the client's cervix is fully dilated.
[ ] **4.** Advise taking a cleansing breath before pushing.

The client complains of pain and asks the nurse, "Can I have some more Stadol?"

33. The nurse correctly explains that butorphanol tartrate (Stadol) is not given at this time because opioid analgesics during this stage of labor may have which effect?
[ ] **1.** Decrease the effectiveness of the contractions
[ ] **2.** Cause the uterus to rupture
[ ] **3.** Result in respiratory depression in the newborn
[ ] **4.** Cause increased fetal activity

The obstetrician arrives for delivery and requests that the client be prepared for epidural anesthesia.

34. The nurse is aware that, the epidural anesthetic will take how long to become effective?

[ ] **1.** Immediately
[ ] **2.** In 10 to 20 minutes
[ ] **3.** In 30 to 40 minutes
[ ] **4.** In approximately 1 hour

35. For which complication should the nurse assess the client immediately after the administration of the epidural anesthetic?

[ ] **1.** Maternal hypotension
[ ] **2.** Fetal tachycardia
[ ] **3.** Spinal headache
[ ] **4.** Lower extremity paralysis

36. Which modification to the client's care plan is required after the client has undergone the epidural?

[ ] **1.** Oxygen is administered to prevent hypoxia.
[ ] **2.** The nurse instructs the client when to push.
[ ] **3.** Oxytocin (Pitocin) is administered to augment labor.
[ ] **4.** The client is catheterized to prevent incontinence.

37. Which sequence should the nurse follow when cleaning the client's perineum in preparation for delivery of the baby?

[ ] **1.** Pubic bone to lower abdomen, both inner thighs, right and left labia, vagina to anus
[ ] **2.** Vagina to anus, right and left labia, both inner thighs, pubic bone to lower abdomen
[ ] **3.** Both inner thighs, right and left labia, vagina to anus, pubic bone to lower abdomen
[ ] **4.** Left and right labia, vagina to anus, both inner thighs, pubic bone to lower abdomen

The physician informs the client that she needs to have an episiotomy. The client begins to cry and asks the nurse, "Why do I have to have an episiotomy?"

38. Which response by the nurse best explains the need for an episiotomy?

[ ] **1.** "An episiotomy is necessary to prevent uterine rupture."
[ ] **2.** "An episiotomy is necessary to prevent postpartum infection."
[ ] **3.** "An episiotomy is necessary to prevent perineal laceration."
[ ] **4.** "An episiotomy is necessary to prevent rectal trauma."

Nursing Care of Clients During the Third Stage of Labor

A 31-year-old client has just delivered a healthy baby girl. While waiting for the expulsion of the placenta, the nurse's attention is focused on caring for the newborn.

39. Which one of the following items should the nurse have available to meet the infant's priority need immediately after delivery?

[ ] **1.** Cord clamp
[ ] **2.** Warm blanket
[ ] **3.** Bulb syringe
[ ] **4.** Oxygen supply

The newborn is assigned an Apgar score of 7 at 5 minutes.

40. The nurse understands that the newborn is in what condition based on the Apgar score?

[ ] **1.** Severely distressed
[ ] **2.** Moderately distressed
[ ] **3.** Stable but requiring close monitoring
[ ] **4.** Vigorous with no signs of distress

41. What should the nurse do initially to facilitate mother-infant attachment and prevent the newborn from developing distress?

[ ] **1.** Give the newborn to the mother immediately after initial care is given in the delivery room.
[ ] **2.** Immediately dry the newborn, and then place the infant skin-to-skin on the mother's abdomen.
[ ] **3.** Place the newborn in a radiant warmer for 5 minutes, then wrap the newborn and give the infant to the mother.
[ ] **4.** Place the newborn in the radiant warmer, and position the warmer so the mother can see the infant.

The nurse tells the father that the infant will receive an injection of vitamin K (AquaMEPHYTON) and erythromycin (Ilotycin) eye ointment.

42. When preparing to administer vitamin K (AquaMEPHYTON) to the infant, the nurse chooses which site for injection? Place an *X* on the appropriate site:

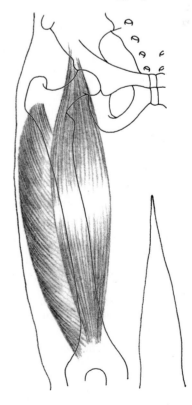

43. When the infant's father asks what the purpose of vitamin K is, the nurse correctly explains that vitamin K (AquaMEPHYTON) is given for what reason?
[ ] 1. To stimulate respirations
[ ] 2. To promote peristalsis
[ ] 3. To decrease the risk for hemorrhage
[ ] 4. To increase calcium absorption

The infant's father also wants to know about the ointment that is being placed in the baby's eyes.

44. The nurse explains to the father that erythromycin (Ilotycin) is given to protect the infant from neonatal blindness, which can occur if the infant develops an eye infection caused by which organisms?
[ ] 1. Gonococcal and chlamydial organisms
[ ] 2. Gonococcal and streptococcal organisms
[ ] 3. Gonococcal organisms and *Candida albicans*
[ ] 4. Gonococcal organisms and *Pneumocystis carinii*

The nursing assistant weighs the newborn.

45. Which action indicates a need for additional teaching regarding accurate and safe assessment of the newborn's weight?
[ ] 1. The nursing assistant undresses the newborn before obtaining the weight.
[ ] 2. The nursing assistant places a diaper or paper barrier on the scale before balancing it.
[ ] 3. The nursing assistant keeps one hand over the newborn while obtaining the weight.
[ ] 4. The nursing assistant cleans the scale with an antiseptic before using it.

46. Which intervention is most important for the nurse to implement before transporting the newborn from the delivery area to the nursery?
[ ] 1. Placing matching identification bracelets on mother and baby
[ ] 2. Administering prophylactic eye medication
[ ] 3. Giving I.M. vitamin K (AquaMEPHYTON)
[ ] 4. Obtaining a blood sample for phenylketonuria (PKU) testing

The nurse observes the client for signs of impending delivery of the placenta.

47. To facilitate delivery of the placenta, what should the nurse instruct the client to do?
[ ] 1. Turn on the right or left side.
[ ] 2. Breathe slowly and deeply.
[ ] 3. Tighten and relax the perineum intermittently.
[ ] 4. Push when feeling a contraction occurring.

48. Which nursing observation suggests an impending separation of the placenta from the uterine lining?
[ ] 1. Bulging perineum
[ ] 2. Shortening of the umbilical cord
[ ] 3. Rise of the fundus in the abdomen
[ ] 4. Decreased vaginal discharge

Nursing Care of Clients During the Fourth Stage of Labor

Just after the delivery of the placenta, the client complains of uncontrollable shaking and of being cold.

49. Which actions by the nurse are most appropriate at this time? Select all that apply.
[ ] 1. Explain that the shaking is normal.
[ ] 2. Place a warmed blanket over the client.
[ ] 3. Suggest the client try to ignore the shaking.
[ ] 4. Notify the physician or nurse-midwife.
[ ] 5. Take the client's temperature.
[ ] 6. Provide a warm beverage.

After the placenta is delivered, the physician sutures the episiotomy and instructs the nurse to add oxytocin (Pitocin) to the client's I.V. fluids. The client asks the nurse, "Why do I need this drug?"

50. The nurse explains that oxytocin (Pitocin) is given after delivery of the baby and placenta for which purpose?
[ ] 1. To increase the blood pressure
[ ] 2. To prevent the uterus from inverting
[ ] 3. To decrease the likelihood of hemorrhage
[ ] 4. To prevent rupture of the uterus

51. When performing postpartal checks just after delivery, which assessment findings should the nurse report immediately? Select all that apply.
[ ] 1. A pulse rate between 120 and 130 beats/minute
[ ] 2. Presence of dark red, fleshy-smelling lochia
[ ] 3. Saturation of one perineal pad per hour
[ ] 4. A systolic blood pressure less than 90 mm Hg
[ ] 5. A respiratory rate of 24 breaths/minute
[ ] 6. Cool, clammy skin

Nursing Care of Clients Having a Cesarean Birth

A 26-year-old gravida I client is admitted to the hospital in active labor. During the physician's examination, it is determined that the client has cephalopelvic disproportion. A cesarean birth using epidural anesthesia is scheduled. The physician orders the insertion of an indwelling urinary catheter before surgery. The client asks the nurse, "Why do I need a urinary catheter?"

52. Which response by the nurse regarding the placement of the indwelling catheter is most accurate?
[ ] 1. "It prevents the development of postpartum hemorrhaging."
[ ] 2. "It keeps the bladder empty during the surgical procedure."
[ ] 3. "It's used as a landmark for the physician during surgery."
[ ] 4. "It's inserted to provide a safe way of collecting urine specimens."

The client asks the nurse if she will feel any pain while the surgery is performed.

53. Which response by the nurse regarding the client's pain is most appropriate?
[ ] **1.** "You may experience pressure, but you will not feel any pain during the procedure."
[ ] **2.** "You may experience a brief sting when the first incision is made."
[ ] **3.** "You won't remember anything about the procedure because you will be asleep."
[ ] **4.** "You won't feel any pain once the anesthesia takes effect."

The client's husband asks the nurse if he can remain with his wife during the cesarean birth.

54. Which statement by the nurse is most appropriate in response to the husband's request?
[ ] **1.** "Only your wife and surgical personnel are allowed in the operating room to maintain a sterile environment."
[ ] **2.** "You can join your wife in the operating room only after the baby has been delivered and your wife and baby are stable."
[ ] **3.** "You can join your wife in the operating room after you change into the appropriate attire."
[ ] **4.** "You can join your wife at the time of transfer to the recovery area and the effects of the anesthesia have worn off."

The client is transferred to the operating room. The physician plans to perform a lower-segment transverse incision and requests that the nurse perform the surgical skin preparation.

55. Which method of cleansing the abdomen is most appropriate?
[ ] **1.** The nurse cleanses the entire abdomen beginning at the level of the nipple line.
[ ] **2.** The nurse cleanses the entire abdomen beginning at the top of the uterine fundus.
[ ] **3.** The nurse cleanses the entire abdomen beginning at the level of the umbilicus.
[ ] **4.** The nurse cleanses the entire abdomen beginning 6″ (15 cm) above the mons pubis.

The cesarean birth is performed without complications. About 1½ hours after surgery, the client is transferred in stable condition to the postpartum unit. The abdominal dressing is dry and intact, the indwelling catheter is patent and draining clear yellow urine, and I.V. fluids are infusing at the prescribed rate. The client also has a continuous infusion of epidural morphine sulfate.

56. While the client is receiving an epidural of morphine sulfate, the nurse closely monitors the client for which adverse reaction?
[ ] **1.** Urinary incontinence
[ ] **2.** Pupil dilation
[ ] **3.** Respiratory depression
[ ] **4.** Elevated blood pressure

57. Which medication should the nurse plan to have readily available while the client is receiving an epidural of morphine sulfate?
[ ] **1.** Buprenorphine hydrochloride (Buprenex)
[ ] **2.** Calcium gluconate (Calsan)
[ ] **3.** Atropine sulfate (Atropair)
[ ] **4.** Naloxone hydrochloride (Narcan)

Twenty-four hours after surgery, the physician writes orders to discontinue the morphine epidural, I.V. therapy, and indwelling catheter and to administer the combination drug oxycodone and acetaminophen (Percocet) 2 tabs P.O. every 3 to 4 hours p.r.n. for pain. The physician also removes the abdominal dressing and says the client may shower and ambulate as tolerated.

58. Which assessment finding is the best indication that an infection is present in the abdominal incision line?
[ ] **1.** The client states that the incision line feels numb.
[ ] **2.** The client's oral temperature is 99°F (37.2°C).
[ ] **3.** The incision line is approximated.
[ ] **4.** The incision line is red and swollen.

The day after surgery, the client complains of abdominal pain and bloating. The nurse notes that the client's abdomen is distended.

59. Which intervention should the nurse perform initially to relieve the client's discomfort?
[ ] **1.** Assist the client to ambulate in the hall.
[ ] **2.** Insert a rectal tube to monitor bowel function.
[ ] **3.** Administer the prescribed pain medication.
[ ] **4.** Instruct the client to use a straw when drinking fluids.

The client tells the nurse, "I'm disappointed that it was necessary to have a delivery by cesarean section," then asks the nurse, "If I have another baby, will I have to have another cesarean?"

60. Which response by the nurse is most accurate regarding a vaginal birth after a cesarean birth (VBAC)?
[ ] **1.** "It may be possible to have a VBAC if the previous cesarean was done with other than a vertical incision."
[ ] **2.** "A vaginal birth is not recommended after a cesarean birth because of the danger of uterine rupture."
[ ] **3.** "A vaginal birth is just as painful as a cesarean birth because an episiotomy has to be performed."
[ ] **4.** "A VBAC may be possible if there is no history of medical conditions that prohibit it."

Nursing Care of Clients Having an Emergency Delivery

A 25-year-old primigravid client is in the active phase of the first stage of labor when her membranes rupture. The nurse notes a decrease in the fetal heart rate on the electronic monitor. Upon inspection of the perineum, the nurse observes that the umbilical cord is protruding through the vagina.

61. Which action is most appropriate for the nurse to take initially?
[ ] **1.** Turn the client on the left side.
[ ] **2.** Notify the physician of the findings.
[ ] **3.** Place the client in Trendelenburg's position.
[ ] **4.** Prepare a sterile field for delivery of the baby.

A 32-year-old client with a history of precipitous labor is admitted to the hospital. She states that contractions are occurring every 2 to 3 minutes. When observing the client's perineum, the nurse notes that the baby's head is crowning. The nurse is alone with the client and unable to obtain assistance.

62. At this point, what is most appropriate for the nurse to do after putting on sterile gloves?
[ ] **1.** Gently place one hand on the crowning head, and allow the head to emerge slowly between contractions.
[ ] **2.** Push back firmly on the head, and place pressure on the vaginal meatus until the physician arrives.
[ ] **3.** Place a sterile towel over the perineal area, and have the client bring the legs close together.
[ ] **4.** Slide a finger into the vagina, and enlarge its exit while delivering the head during a contraction.

Nursing Care of Clients Having a Stillborn Baby

A 26-year-old primigravid client at 40 weeks' gestation is admitted to the hospital after contacting the physician about not having felt the baby move for 24 hours. The nurse is unable to detect a fetal heartbeat using the external fetal monitor. The physician examines the client and determines that there has been intrauterine fetal demise (the fetus is dead). An infusion of oxytocin (Pitocin) is ordered for induction of labor. The client is crying and tells the nurse, "This can't be true. You must have made a mistake."

63. Which nursing intervention is most appropriate at this time?
[ ] **1.** Recheck the fetal heart tones with the electronic external fetal monitor so that the client can listen.
[ ] **2.** Express sorrow about the client's loss and encourage the client to express feelings.
[ ] **3.** Redirect the client's attention to the laboring process and the correct use of breathing techniques.
[ ] **4.** Explain that the baby probably would have been born with severe long-term health problems.

The baby is delivered stillborn. After the client is stabilized, she is transferred to a private room on a wing adjacent to the labor, delivery, recovery, and postpartum (LDRP) unit. The client's husband is present. The client asks the nurse about seeing the baby.

64. Which action is most appropriate for the nurse to take at this time?
[ ] **1.** Substitute a memory packet with a picture of the baby and footprints.
[ ] **2.** Bring the infant and allow the couple to view the baby privately.
[ ] **3.** Suggest postponing the viewing until seeing the hospital chaplain.
[ ] **4.** Bring the infant, but do not allow the parents to hold or touch the infant.

Nursing Care of Clients During the Postpartum Period

65. Which finding would the nurse consider abnormal for the postpartum client who delivered within the past 24 hours?
[ ] **1.** The client has passed a couple of nickel-sized clots.
[ ] **2.** The client has calf pain when a foot is dorsiflexed.
[ ] **3.** The client has abdominal cramping while breast-feeding.
[ ] **4.** The client's vaginal discharge is dark red.

66. Which of the following clients is at highest risk for developing postpartum hemorrhage? Select all that apply.
[ ] **1.** A client with placenta previa
[ ] **2.** A client who just delivered triplets
[ ] **3.** A client who delivered her sixth baby
[ ] **4.** A client whose fetus had late decelerations
[ ] **5.** A client with a history of primary hypertension
[ ] **6.** A client who had a precipitious delivery

67. To prevent hemorrhage, when should the nurse massage the fundus during the postpartum period?
[ ] **1.** When the fundus is firm and hard
[ ] **2.** When the fundus is at the umbilicus
[ ] **3.** When the amount of lochia decreases
[ ] **4.** When the fundus is soft and boggy

68. The nurse correctly massages the fundus by placing one hand on the fundus and the other hand where?
[ ] **1.** Just above the symphysis pubis
[ ] **2.** To the right side of the abdomen
[ ] **3.** Just below the xiphoid process
[ ] **4.** To the left side of the abdomen

A 33-year-old client delivered a healthy infant vaginally 6 hours ago. During the delivery, the physician performed a right mediolateral episiotomy. Although in stable condition, the client experiences incisional discomfort.

69. On the illustration below, identify with an *X* the area where the incision would have been made:

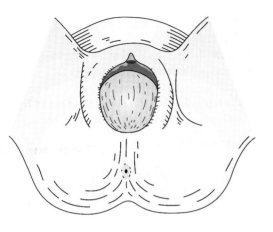

70. How should the nurse position the client when assessing the perineum after an episiotomy?
[ ] **1.** Prone
[ ] **2.** Supine
[ ] **3.** Sims' position
[ ] **4.** Lithotomy position

71. Which nursing intervention is most appropriate for initially relieving discomfort associated with an episiotomy?
[ ] **1.** Sitz bath
[ ] **2.** Ice pack
[ ] **3.** Heat lamp
[ ] **4.** Topical cortisone

72. Which assessment finding by the nurse is the best indication that a perineal hematoma is present?
[ ] **1.** The client complains of a feeling of fullness in the vagina.
[ ] **2.** Lochia rubra is heavy and foul-smelling.
[ ] **3.** There is separation and purulent drainage from the episiotomy.
[ ] **4.** The client complains of severe pain in the perineal area.

During the initial assessment, the nurse notes that the client's fundus is firm and left of midline.

73. What nursing action is warranted at this time?
[ ] **1.** Massage the uterus vigorously.
[ ] **2.** Have the client empty her bladder.
[ ] **3.** Reassess the client in 4 hours.
[ ] **4.** No action is presently required.

The nursing assistant helps the client with perineal hygiene.

74. Which observation by the nurse indicates that the nursing assistant needs additional instruction?
[ ] **1.** The nursing assistant applies the peripad from back to front.
[ ] **2.** The nursing assistant wears gloves while providing perineal care.
[ ] **3.** The nursing assistant fills the peri bottle with warm tap water.
[ ] **4.** The nursing assistant places the sitz bath on the toilet.

The client tells the nurse about feeling the urge to urinate but being unsuccessful.

75. Which nursing action is most appropriate to implement initially?
[ ] **1.** Catheterize the client with a straight catheter.
[ ] **2.** Assist the client with ambulation.
[ ] **3.** Have the client drink more fluids.
[ ] **4.** Assist the client with a warm sitz bath.

When reviewing the client's medical records, the nurse notes that the client's rubella titer is low (less than 1:10) and is scheduled to receive the rubella vaccine before discharge.

76. Before giving the vaccine, the nurse should determine if the client is allergic to which medication?
[ ] **1.** Neomycin sulfate (Mycifradin)
[ ] **2.** Erythromycin estolate (Ilosone)
[ ] **3.** Tetracycline (Panmycin)
[ ] **4.** Doxycycline (Vibramycin)

77. When administering Rho(D) immune globulin (RhoGAM) to an Rh-negative mother who has delivered an Rh-positive infant, what is the maximum length of time the nurse has to give the medication?
[ ] **1.** 48 hours after delivery
[ ] **2.** 72 hours after delivery
[ ] **3.** At the 6-week postpartum checkup
[ ] **4.** Within the first 24 hours of delivery

78. Which finding by the nurse is most suggestive of cystitis in the postpartum client?
[ ] **1.** Boggy uterus displaced to the right of the abdominal midline
[ ] **2.** Complaint of increased thirst and voiding large amounts of urine
[ ] **3.** Urine retention and swelling of the lower extremities
[ ] **4.** Complaint of painful urination and presence of blood in the urine

Twenty-four hours after the client delivers her baby, the obstetrician writes discharge orders. The nurse reviews home care instructions with the client in anticipation of discharge.

79. After the nurse instructs the client about ways to avoid constipation, which statement made by the client indicates a need for additional teaching?
[ ] **1.** "I should drink at least 2 to 3 quarts of fluid daily."
[ ] **2.** "I will need to take a stool softener every other day."
[ ] **3.** "I should include raw fruits and vegetables in my diet."
[ ] **4.** "I will need to continue taking daily walks."

80. The nurse correctly instructs the client to notify the health care provider if what occurs?
[ ] **1.** The client experiences difficulty urinating.
[ ] **2.** The lochia becomes creamy yellow after the first postpartum week.
[ ] **3.** The client experiences unexplained feelings of tearfulness and sadness.
[ ] **4.** The client's breasts become slightly firm after 48 hours.

The client informs the nurse about plans to continue breast-feeding after being discharged and asks what should be done about breast engorgement if it occurs at home.

81. Which nursing instruction is most appropriate regarding breast engorgement?
[ ] **1.** "Pump your breasts between breast-feedings."
[ ] **2.** "Limit your fluid intake for 24 hours."
[ ] **3.** "Feed your baby every 2 to 3 hours."
[ ] **4.** "Apply ice packs to your full breasts."

82. Which instruction should the nurse plan to include in the discharge teaching plan for the client who is at risk for developing mastitis?
[ ] **1.** Wear a breast binder between breast-feedings.
[ ] **2.** Apply petroleum jelly to the nipples before breast-feeding.
[ ] **3.** Clean the nipples with soap and water after breast-feeding.
[ ] **4.** Wash both hands before handling the breasts.

The client asks the nurse how long after discharge should sexual intercourse be delayed.

83. The best nursing response is that sexual intercourse may be resumed at which time?
[ ] **1.** As soon as the lochia has ceased and the perineum is healed
[ ] **2.** As soon as an acceptable birth control method is selected
[ ] **3.** After the postpartum checkup in 4 to 6 weeks
[ ] **4.** After the uterus has returned to its normal position

84. When the client tells the nurse, "I'm nervous about going home with the new baby," which nursing action is most appropriate?
[ ] **1.** Suggest that the client ask the physician to postpone discharge.
[ ] **2.** Tell the client that this is a normal feeling that will go away in time.
[ ] **3.** Make sure the client has written instructions on infant care before discharge.
[ ] **4.** Provide the facility's telephone number with encouragement to call as needed.

The client is readmitted to the hospital on the fifth postpartum day with a tentative diagnosis of puerperal infection.

85. If this client is typical of other women with a puerperal infection, which assessment findings are most characteristic? Select all that apply.
[ ] **1.** Pulse rate over 100 beats/minute
[ ] **2.** Complaint of abdominal tenderness
[ ] **3.** A decrease in the size of the uterus
[ ] **4.** Presence of lochia serosa
[ ] **5.** Hematoma on the perineum
[ ] **6.** Continuous trickle of blood from the vagina

Nursing Care of the Newborn Client

Two hours after a female newborn is delivered at 39 weeks' gestation, the newborn is admitted to the well-baby nursery. The nurse performs a newborn physical assessment and observes normal variations to the skin.

86. Which skin variations are considered normal and require no further intervention? Select all that apply.
[ ] **1.** Mongolian spot
[ ] **2.** Milia
[ ] **3.** Epstein's pearls
[ ] **4.** Erythema toxicum
[ ] **5.** Molding
[ ] **6.** Cephalhematoma

87. When the nurse documents the following newborn profile information on the flow sheet, which data require notifying the pediatrician immediately? Select all that apply.
[ ] **1.** Head circumference of 20″ (50.8 cm)
[ ] **2.** Chest circumference of 13″ (33 cm)
[ ] **3.** Length of 19½″ (49.5 cm)
[ ] **4.** Heart rate of 100 beats/minute
[ ] **5.** Weight of 11 pounds (5 kg)
[ ] **6.** Abdominal circumference of 11½″ (29.2 cm)

The nurse proceeds with the assessment, observing the newborn's reflexes.

88. Which reflexes would the nurse expect to find in a newborn of this gestational age? Select all that apply.

[ ] **1.** Rooting reflex
[ ] **2.** Moro reflex
[ ] **3.** Tonic neck reflex
[ ] **4.** Extrusion reflex
[ ] **5.** Barlow reflex
[ ] **6.** Ortolani reflex

The length and weight are recorded on the newborn's name card. The weight has been documented in kilograms, and the nurse must convert the weight into pounds.

89. If the newborn weighs 3.5 kg, what is the weight in pounds?

_____

After the newborn's temperature has stabilized, the nurse gives the first bath.

90. Which findings noted by the nurse bathing the newborn should be reported immediately? Select all that apply.

[ ] **1.** The hands and feet are bluish in color.
[ ] **2.** The pulse rate is 140 beats/minute.
[ ] **3.** The skin has a yellowish discoloration.
[ ] **4.** The labia are slightly swollen.
[ ] **5.** There is nasal flaring.
[ ] **6.** Substernal and intercostal retractions are noted.

After the bath is completed, the nurse rechecks the newborn's axillary temperature and records it as 97°F (36.1°C).

91. Which nursing intervention is most appropriate at this time?

[ ] **1.** Dress and wrap the newborn in a blanket, place in an open crib, and recheck the temperature every 4 to 8 hours.
[ ] **2.** Place the newborn on a preheated radiant warmer, and gradually rewarm over a period of 2 or more hours.
[ ] **3.** Dress the newborn, wrap in double blankets, place in an open crib, and recheck the temperature in 30 to 60 minutes.
[ ] **4.** Place the newborn on a preheated radiant warmer, and rewarm over a period of 15 to 30 minutes.

Four hours after admission to the nursery, the newborn's condition is stable and there are no signs of distress. The newborn is taken to the mother's room for a visit.

92. When the nurse begins gathering data for a discussion about methods to keep the baby safe while in the hospital, which information should be included in the teaching plan? Select all that apply.

[ ] **1.** Identification bands must be kept on the newborn at all times.
[ ] **2.** When the client is showering, the crib should be placed outside the bathroom door.

[ ] **3.** Hospital staff assigned to the obstetric (OB) department should check the baby's name bands when entering the room.
[ ] **4.** Hospital staff assigned to the OB department must wear a visible, valid hospital ID.
[ ] **5.** The newborn can sleep in bed with the mother.
[ ] **6.** Visitors coming to the hospital must wash their hands before holding or caring for the infant.

93. Which of the following observations by the nurse indicate that an appropriate mother-infant bond is occurring? Select all that apply.

[ ] **1.** The mother holds her baby away from her body.
[ ] **2.** The mother makes eye contact with her baby.
[ ] **3.** The mother talks or sings to her baby.
[ ] **4.** The mother discusses the baby's physical attributes.
[ ] **5.** The mother becomes upset because the baby has spit up.
[ ] **6.** The mother repeatedly asks the nurse if the baby is going to live.

The nurse instructs the mother about initial breast-feeding. The client says to the nurse, "My breasts are small. Will I be able to breast-feed my baby?"

94. Which response by the nurse is most appropriate?

[ ] **1.** "The size of your breasts does not affect your ability to breast-feed."
[ ] **2.** "You should attempt to breast-feed and give supplemental formula."
[ ] **3.** "Bottle-feeding is just as nutritious as breast-feeding."
[ ] **4.** "You can do exercises to increase the size of your breasts."

The client thinks it is best to give the baby formula until breast milk comes in. She tells the nurse, "I started to breast-feed my first child, but changed to bottle-feeding because the baby lost lots of weight before being discharged from the hospital."

95. Which response by the nurse is most appropriate regarding neonatal weight loss?

[ ] **1.** "It's normal for both bottle-fed and breast-fed infants to lose up to 10% of their birth weight during the first few days after birth."
[ ] **2.** "If your baby begins bottle-feeding, the infant won't be successful breast-feeding because of a preference for the bottle nipple."
[ ] **3.** "A baby is more prone to lose weight with bottle-feeding than breast-feeding because formula is more difficult to digest."
[ ] **4.** "Until the baby is ready to begin breast-feeding, you should pump your breasts to promote the let-down reflex."

96. The nurse also explains that during the first few days after the newborn's birth, the client's breasts will secrete colostrum, which is beneficial to the baby because it contains which substance?

[ ] **1.** Estrogen, which will prevent the newborn from developing breakthrough bleeding

[ ] **2.** Antibodies, which provide protection against certain types of infections

[ ] **3.** Predigested fats, which increase the newborn's ability to absorb fat-soluble vitamins

[ ] **4.** Digestive enzymes, which increase the newborn's ability to absorb nutrients

The nurse gives the mother verbal instructions about how to breast-feed correctly. The nurse then remains in the room to assist the mother.

97. Which action by the client indicates a need for additional teaching regarding proper breast-feeding technique?

[ ] **1.** The mother uses the thumb of the free hand to gently press the breast away from the baby's nose.

[ ] **2.** The mother gently strokes the baby's lips with the nipple when ready to breast-feed.

[ ] **3.** The mother places a breast shield over the nipple before placing the nipple in the baby's mouth.

[ ] **4.** The mother gently pulls down on the baby's chin before removing the nipple from the baby's mouth.

Before leaving the newborn with the parents, the nurse hands the mother a bulb syringe and provides instructions on its use.

98. Which statement made by the client indicates a need for additional teaching regarding proper use of the bulb syringe?

[ ] **1.** The mother states that the baby's mouth should be suctioned before the nose is suctioned.

[ ] **2.** The mother states that the bulb syringe should be compressed before it is placed in the baby's mouth or nose.

[ ] **3.** The mother states that, when suctioning the mouth, the bulb syringe should not touch the back of the baby's throat.

[ ] **4.** The mother states that the bulb syringe should remain compressed until it is removed from the baby's nose or mouth.

The newborn's father asks about positioning the baby in the crib after being fed.

99. The nurse correctly explains that it is best to place the newborn in which position in the crib after feeding?

[ ] **1.** Right side-lying

[ ] **2.** Left side-lying

[ ] **3.** Prone

[ ] **4.** Supine

The client asks the nurse, "How will I know that my baby is getting enough to eat?"

100. Which nursing explanation is suggestive that a breastfed newborn's nutritional needs are not being adequately met?

[ ] **1.** The infant awakens during the night for a feeding.

[ ] **2.** The infant has fewer than six wet diapers per day.

[ ] **3.** The infant has loose, pale-yellow stools.

[ ] **4.** The infant is breastfed every 2 to 3 hours.

The client tells the nurse about plans to continue breast-feeding after returning to work and to pump both breasts when unable to breast-feed. The client asks the nurse, "How long can I store pumped breast milk?"

101. The nurse correctly responds that breast milk can be safely stored in the refrigerator for how long after pumping?

[ ] **1.** Up to 8 hours

[ ] **2.** 2 to 3 days

[ ] **3.** 5 to 8 days

[ ] **4.** Up to 2 weeks

A postterm male newborn in no apparent distress is admitted to the nursery after an uneventful planned cesarean birth.

102. During an initial assessment, the nurse would expect to note which finding that is characteristic of a postterm newborn?

[ ] **1.** Few sole creases

[ ] **2.** Flat, shapeless ears

[ ] **3.** Legs in a froglike position

[ ] **4.** Dry, cracked, peeling skin

103. Which assessment finding would the nurse consider abnormal for this newborn?

[ ] **1.** A scrotal sac that has numerous rugae

[ ] **2.** An umbilical cord that has one vein and one artery

[ ] **3.** Minimal vernix caseosa with remnants in skin creases

[ ] **4.** Bluish discoloration of the hands and feet

104. Which assessment finding would the nurse consider most indicative of congenital hip dysplasia in a newborn?

[ ] **1.** Asymmetry of the gluteal skin folds

[ ] **2.** Limited adduction of the affected hip

[ ] **3.** No spontaneous movement of the affected leg

[ ] **4.** Exaggerated curvature of the lumbar spine

Six hours after admission to the nursery, the newborn is taken to the mother for the first feeding. The mother wants to bottle-feed the newborn. The nurse reviews basic principles of bottle-feeding with the mother.

105. When the nurse observes the mother, which action by the mother is incorrect, indicating that the mother needs a review of the technique for bottle-feeding the infant?
[ ] **1.** The mother places the nipple of the bottle on top of the baby's tongue.
[ ] **2.** During feeding, the mother places the baby in the supine position.
[ ] **3.** The mother burps the baby after the baby takes each ounce of formula.
[ ] **4.** The mother places the baby in the right side-lying position after feeding.

The mother asks the nurse why it is important to keep the bottle nipple full of formula.

106. Holding the bottle so that the nipple is always full of formula helps prevent which consequence in the newborn?
[ ] **1.** Damaging the gums
[ ] **2.** Getting tired while feeding
[ ] **3.** Gulping the formula
[ ] **4.** Swallowing air when sucking

The mother tells the nurse of a plan to use concentrated liquid infant formula at home. The nurse gathers information about formula preparations and reviews this with the parents.

107. Which statement made by the mother indicates a need for additional teaching?
[ ] **1.** "I can wash the formula bottles in a dishwasher."
[ ] **2.** "I should use warm tap water to dilute the concentrate."
[ ] **3.** "The formula should be used immediately after it is prepared."
[ ] **4.** "The lid of the can of formula must be wiped before it is opened."

The infant's total bilirubin level is 11 mg/dL. The physician orders conventional phototherapy using lights suspended above the infant rather than a biliblanket that is placed directly on the skin.

108. When providing care for a newborn receiving phototherapy, which nursing intervention is most appropriate?
[ ] **1.** Cover the infant's eyes when providing treatment.
[ ] **2.** Dress the infant in a diaper and lightweight nightshirt.
[ ] **3.** Apply a cream with a sun protection factor (SPF) of 15.
[ ] **4.** Place a nonreflective pad on the surface of the bassinette.

After 2 days of therapy, the newborn's total bilirubin level decreases to 9 mg/dL and phototherapy is discontinued. The pediatrician prepares for a circumcision using the Plastibell technique.

109. After the circumcision, which nursing action is most appropriate?
[ ] **1.** Maintain a petroleum gauze dressing over the penis.
[ ] **2.** Monitor vital signs every 15 minutes for the first hour.
[ ] **3.** Observe the penis frequently for swelling and bleeding.
[ ] **4.** Place the infant in a prone position after the circumcision is completed.

The pediatrician writes orders for the newborn to be discharged if no complications occur within 4 hours of the circumcision. Before discharge, the nurse reviews home care of the circumcision.

110. Which statement by the parents indicates that teaching has been effective?
[ ] **1.** "We'll notify the pediatrician if we see any drainage from the baby's penis."
[ ] **2.** "We'll clean the baby's penis three times a day with alcohol."
[ ] **3.** "We'll remove the Plastibell ring in 1 week if it has not fallen off by then."
[ ] **4.** "We'll apply petroleum jelly to the baby's penis with each diaper change."

Before discharge, the nurse prepares to perform a phenylketonuria (PKU) test.

111. Which information is most important for the nurse to obtain before performing the PKU test?
[ ] **1.** Whether the newborn has been feeding for at least 2 to 3 days
[ ] **2.** Whether the newborn was large for gestational age at birth
[ ] **3.** Whether the mother had gestational diabetes during the pregnancy
[ ] **4.** Whether there is a family history of mental retardation

112. Which area of the infant's foot should the nurse puncture to obtain the phenylketonuria (PKU) test? Place an X on the appropriate area on the photo:

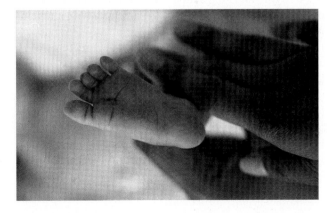

113. When obtaining the blood specimen for the phenylketonuria (PKU) test, which action by the nurse is incorrect?

[ ] 1. The nurse warms the site for the puncture for 5 to 10 minutes.
[ ] 2. The nurse applies pressure to obtain a large drop of blood.
[ ] 3. The nurse fills each circle on the collection card completely.
[ ] 4. The nurse closes the card while the circles of blood are wet.

A nurse educator teaches the staff about how to prevent infant abduction from the hospital. A drill is conducted to test the staff's knowledge.

114. Which actions by the hospital staff indicate that they have a good understanding of what to do in case an infant is abducted from the nursery? Select all that apply.

[ ] 1. Question any person carrying a box or bag.
[ ] 2. Call the Federal Bureau of Investigation (FBI) immediately.
[ ] 3. Report suspicious persons to security STAT.
[ ] 4. Search closets and stairwells where a baby can be hidden.
[ ] 5. Thoroughly question all visitors in the hospital.
[ ] 6. Ask the mother why the baby was left unattended.

Nursing Care of Newborns with Complications

A 38-year-old multiparous client gave birth a day ago to a full-term newborn with a myelomeningocele.

115. Which assessment finding is the best indication that the client is grieving over the loss of a "perfect" baby?

[ ] 1. The client has not selected a name for the baby.
[ ] 2. The client visits the nursery frequently but only stays for a few minutes.
[ ] 3. The client asks the physician to postpone discharge from the hospital.
[ ] 4. The client leaves the nursery when the baby receives treatments.

116. Which nursing action is best for facilitating the client's acceptance and care of the newborn with a myelomeningocele?

[ ] 1. Show the client "before" and "after" pictures of other infants born with myelomeningocele.
[ ] 2. Feed, hold, and change the newborn in the client's presence.
[ ] 3. Explain to the client that surgery will most probably eliminate the defect and its consequences.
[ ] 4. Assure the client that social agencies will most likely assume responsibility for full care of the newborn.

An infant who is born at 27 weeks' gestation is taken to the neonatal intensive care unit (NICU) at a nearby hospital in respiratory distress.

117. Which nursing intervention is essential for preventing retinopathy of prematurity (ROP) in the preterm newborn?

[ ] 1. Monitor the oxygen concentration level.
[ ] 2. Monitor the bilirubin level.
[ ] 3. Check the hemoglobin level.
[ ] 4. Check the pupil response.

After the newborn's respiratory condition stabilizes and the infant is weaned from the ventilator, the neonatologist writes an order to begin feedings.

118. When feeding the preterm newborn, which method is most appropriate?

[ ] 1. Feed the infant every hour around the clock.
[ ] 2. Give the infant no more than 3 to 4 ounces per feeding.
[ ] 3. Feed the infant with a nasogastric tube.
[ ] 4. Give the infant glucose solution for the first month.

The parents of a preterm newborn ask the nurse why their baby is being monitored for signs of infection.

119. The nurse correctly explains that preterm newborns are at risk for developing infections primarily for which reason?

[ ] 1. Their fragile skin may tear.
[ ] 2. They lack maternal antibody protection.
[ ] 3. They are exposed to numerous bacterial organisms.
[ ] 4. They need to undergo many invasive procedures.

120. Which nursing action is best to ensure that the thermoregulation needs of the preterm newborn are being met?

[ ] 1. The newborn is wrapped in a cotton blanket.
[ ] 2. The nursery is maintained at 75°F (23.9°C).
[ ] 3. The newborn is in an isolette or radiant warmer.
[ ] 4. The crib is located away from sources of drafts.

A gravida II, para I client in the 38th week of pregnancy comes to the emergency department in active labor. An Rh-positive newborn is delivered with congenital hemolytic disease caused by Rh incompatibility.

121. Which assessment finding is most indicative of the presence of Rh incompatibility?

[ ] 1. A slow and irregular respiratory rate
[ ] 2. Absence of newborn reflexes
[ ] 3. Limited movement in the lower extremities
[ ] 4. Jaundice within 24 to 36 hours of birth

A direct Coombs' test is ordered to confirm the diagnosis of hemolytic disease.

122. The nurse should be prepared to assist with the collection of a blood specimen from which source?
[ ] **1.** The newborn's father
[ ] **2.** The newborn's mother
[ ] **3.** The newborn's sibling
[ ] **4.** The newborn's umbilical cord

A newborn is delivered at 32 weeks' gestation to a gravida I, para I client with human immunodeficiency virus (HIV) infection.

123. When providing care for this newborn, the nurse should follow which precautions?
[ ] **1.** Standard precautions
[ ] **2.** Airborne precautions
[ ] **3.** Droplet precautions
[ ] **4.** Contact precautions

The mother asks the nurse when the baby will be tested for HIV, and how long it usually takes before HIV-positive babies develop acquired immunodeficiency syndrome (AIDS).

124. Which statement by the nurse about HIV testing is most appropriate?
[ ] **1.** "Your baby won't be tested because babies of HIV-positive mothers are already HIV-positive."
[ ] **2.** "Your baby will be tested within 24 hours for HIV antibodies to facilitate early treatment."
[ ] **3.** "Your baby won't be tested for HIV antibodies until age 3 months."
[ ] **4.** "Your baby will be tested for HIV antibodies yearly until test results are positive."

125. It would be correct for the nurse to explain that most untreated infants who contract HIV in utero typically develop AIDS symptoms at which age?
[ ] **1.** By age 4 weeks
[ ] **2.** By age 2 to 6 months
[ ] **3.** By age 6 to 12 months
[ ] **4.** By age 1 to 2 years

The client asks the nurse about breast-feeding the baby.

126. Which explanation by the nurse is most appropriate regarding breast-feeding this newborn?
[ ] **1.** "It's OK to breast-feed the baby if the anti-HIV test results are positive."
[ ] **2.** "It's OK to breast-feed the baby as long as he is symptom-free."
[ ] **3.** "You can't breast-feed the baby because you are HIV-positive."
[ ] **4.** "You can't breast-feed the baby if you have developed symptoms of AIDS."

The father of a toddler brings the child to the hospital to see the newborn sibling. The toddler acts out and throws the newborn's pacifier onto the floor. The parents are embarassed about their toddler's behavior.

127. Which parental advice regarding sibling rivalry is most appropriate at this time?
[ ] **1.** After going home, each parent should spend time with the toddler doing activities the toddler enjoys.
[ ] **2.** The toddler should be sent to a grandparent's home for the first week until a routine can be established with the newborn.
[ ] **3.** Set firm limits on the toddler's behavior providing appropriate discipline and punishment.
[ ] **4.** Keep the toddler and the newborn separated for the first few days until the toddler can adjust to the new sibling.

128. A nurse is caring for 5 clients in the newborn nursery. A new obstetric licensed practical nurse (LPN) informs the charge nurse that documentation on his/her assignment will not be completed at the end of the shift. Which statement by the LPN mentor is best?
[ ] **1.** "I will assist you in your documentation to get you finished in time."
[ ] **2.** "Why do you not have it done? We will reduce your patient load next time."
[ ] **3.** "I will grant you overtime to complete your documentation."
[ ] **4.** "By not having your documentation done, it will be on your personal record."

Correct Answers, Rationales, and Test Taking Strategies

Admission of the Client to a Labor and Delivery Facility

1. **1, 3.** The client should come to the hospital or health care facility when contractions are 5 minutes apart. A sudden gush of fluid from the vagina indicates that the membranes have ruptured. Once the membranes rupture, there is an increased risk for intrauterine infection and umbilical cord prolapse if the fetal head has not engaged. A sudden burst of energy, also known as the *nesting instinct*, is a preliminary sign of approaching labor and may occur a few days before the beginning of labor; it does not require reporting to the health care facility. Urinary frequency may occur as the fetus settles into the pelvic outlet. The primigravid client may experience urinary frequency as early as 2 to 3 weeks before the beginning of labor. Having the baby descend into the pelvis may occur several weeks before delivery and is not a sign of labor. Blood-tinged mucus is also known as *bloody show* and may be the start of labor as the cervix dilates and effaces, but it may be several hours or a day or two before labor begins. Therefore, it is too early to take the steps of notifying the physician and reporting to the labor and delivery unit.

Test Taking Strategy—Analyze to determine what information the question asks for regarding the initiation of true labor. Alternative-format "select all that apply" questions require considering each option independently to decide its merit in answering the question. Consider that true labor includes regular contractions intended to push the fetus down the birth canal. The contractions are accompanied by pelvic pressure and pain. False labor, including Braxton Hicks contractions, occur irregularly and do not progress. Choose options that correlate with signs and symptoms of true labor or indications of potential complications of labor. Compare and contrast signs and symptoms of true labor if you had difficulty answering this question.
Cognitive Level—Applying
Client Needs Category—Health promotion and maintenance
Client Needs Subcategory—None

2. **2.** When admitting a client in labor, the information that is least important is whether she has ever had an enema. Not every client requires an enema, so the best time to ask about this is shortly before administering one. It is more pertinent to ask whether the client's membranes have ruptured, when her contractions started, and when she last ate. The timing of the last meal is especially important in case the client requires anesthesia for delivery.

Test Taking Strategy—Use the process of elimination to select the option that does not correlate with essential information needed on admission to the labor, delivery, recovery, and postpartum unit. Options 1, 3, and 4 are of higher priority than option 2. Recall that determining if the client has ever had an enema is of lowest priority and contingent upon whether the client will require an enema before delivery. Review the standard information that is routinely collected when a client arrives on the obstetric unit if you had difficulty answering this question.
Cognitive Level—Analyzing
Client Needs Category—Health promotion and maintenance
Client Needs Subcategory—None

3. **1.** Braxton Hicks contractions are irregular, painless contractions that occur intermittently (in some cases, every 10 to 20 minutes). They tend to disappear with walking and sleeping and become more uncomfortable closer to delivery. Because of their irregularity, Braxton Hicks contractions cannot be timed, and they do not increase in frequency or intensity. These contractions begin and remain in the abdomen, whereas true labor contractions begin in the lower back and progress to the abdomen. The main difference between true labor and false labor contractions, however, is that Braxton Hicks contractions do not dilate the cervix.

Test Taking Strategy—Analyze to determine what information the question asks for, which is evidence of a manifestation of Braxton Hicks contractions. Recall that Braxton Hicks contractions, which may occur throughout a pregnancy, may be misinterpreted as the onset of labor, especially when they occur late in the third trimester. Movement (option 1) and changing positions tends to relieve any associated discomfort. Review the differences between Braxton Hicks contractions and the contractions experienced just before delivery if you had difficulty answering this question.
Cognitive Level—Applying
Client Needs Category—Health promotion and maintenance
Client Needs Subcategory—None

4. **1.** Blood pressure begins to rise several seconds before a contraction begins and returns to resting level when the contraction subsides. To obtain the most accurate blood pressure reading, it should be assessed between contractions. Taking the blood pressure when the contraction is over minimizes the possibility of obtaining an inaccurate measurement. Some believe that in addition to taking the blood pressure between contractions, the client should be in a left lateral position to relieve compression on the inferior vena cava, which can alter the blood pressure as well.

Test Taking Strategy—Note the key words "most appropriate" in reference to the best time to obtain

the blood pressure of a client who is in labor. Recall how the size of the uterus, uterine contractions, and the client's position affect the circulation of arterial blood. Review the physiological changes that affect blood flow and blood pressure during labor if you had difficulty answering this question.
Cognitive Level—*Applying*
Client Needs Category—*Health promotion and maintenance*
Client Needs Subcategory—*None*

5.

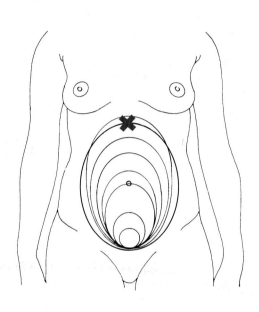

Uterine height is measured from the top of the maternal symphysis pubis to the top of the uterine fundus. By the 36th week, the uterine fundus should touch the xiphoid process. About 2 weeks before term (the 38th week), the fetal head settles into the pelvis to prepare for birth and the uterus returns to its height at 36 weeks.
Test Taking Strategy—Analyze to determine what information the question asks for regarding the location of the uterine fundus at 40 weeks. Recall that fundal height is related to gestational age and fetal position. Because the client is at 40 weeks' gestation, the X should be at the top of the abdomen under the xiphoid process. Review how uterine height is measured if you had difficulty answering this question.
Cognitive Level—Applying
Client Needs Category—Health promotion and maintenance
Client Needs Subcategory—None

Nursing Care of Clients During the First Stage of Labor

6. 1. When performing a vaginal examination, the examiner wears a pair of sterile gloves to avoid the introduction of bacteria and the risk of infection. The client should be assisted to the supine (not side-lying) position and assisted to use breathing techniques (breathing slowly through an open mouth) to help her relax. An enema is not usually part of client preparation for a vaginal examination.
Test Taking Strategy—Use the process of elimination to help select the option that identifies the best method the nurse can use to prepare the client for a vaginal examination. Options 2, 3 and 4 are not part of a vaginal examination and therefore can be eliminated. Option 1 remains as the correct answer because wearing sterile gloves is an aseptic practice that prevents transmitting pathogens to tissues that have an abundant supply of blood. Review the steps for preparing a client in labor for a vaginal examination if you had difficulty answering this question.
Cognitive Level—*Applying*
Client Needs Category—*Safe and effective care environment*
Client Needs Subcategory—*Safety and infection control*

7. 4. Dilation and effacement of the cervix are the only definite, reliable indicators of true labor. Regular, progressing contractions and the presence of bloody show are also signs of labor, but they are not considered as reliable as dilation.
Test Taking Strategy—Note the key words "most reliable," which indicates that the sign in more than one option may be present during labor, although one option identifies the best sign of true labor. Recall that options 2, 3, and 4 may occur in both true and false labor, but option 1 occurs only in true labor and therefore is the best answer. Compare and contrast true labor and false labor if you had difficulty answering this question.
Cognitive Level—*Analyzing*
Client Needs Category—*Health promotion and maintenance*
Client Needs Subcategory—*None*

8. 1, 2. The latent phase is the beginning of the first stage of labor. During the latent phase, also known as the early phase, the normal fetal heart rate ranges from 120 to 160 beats/minute. During the latent phase of the first stage of labor, contractions occur every 5 to 30 minutes. The perineum does not begin to bulge until the transition phase of the first stage of labor, and early decelerations usually occur late in labor as a result of head compression. Irritability is a sign exhibited during the transition stage, and feeling the need to have a bowel movement is common as the client feels the need to push in the late stage of labor.
Test Taking Strategy—Analyze to determine what information the question asks for, which is signs and symptoms of the latent (early) phase of labor, often occurring at home or upon hospital admission. Alternative-format "select all that apply" questions require considering each option independently to decide its merit in answering the question. Choose

options that correlate with the signs and symptoms of the latent (early) phase of labor. Review the stages and phases of labor if you had difficulty answering this question.
Cognitive Level—*Applying*
Client Needs Category—*Health promotion and maintenance*
Client Needs Subcategory—*None*

9. 1, 2. If the client's membranes are intact and contractions are not very frequent or intense, the client may be allowed to ambulate and take a warm shower or Jacuzzi bath. During the latent phase of the first stage of labor, the client is encouraged to drink clear liquids or moisten the lips/mouth with ice chips. The client usually uses a panting breathing pattern during the transition phase of the first stage of labor. The client's contractions are monitored; therefore, the nurse will know when the contraction begins and ends. In the latent phase of labor, contractions are far apart. Pain medication is generally unnecessary during the latent phase of labor.

> *Test Taking Strategy*—*Analyze to determine what information the question asks for, which is appropriate instructions for the nurse to give the client in the latent phase of labor. Alternative-format "select all that apply" questions require considering each option independently to decide its merit in answering the question. Choose all the options that correlate with the nursing interventions for the client in the latent phase of labor. Recall that this phase may last 4 to 6 hours, amniotic membranes may be intact, and clear liquids are offered to prevent dehydration. Review the nursing care of the woman in the latent phase of labor if you had difficulty answering this question.*

Cognitive Level—*Applying*
Client Needs Category—*Health promotion and maintenance*
Client Needs Subcategory—*None*

10. 3. According to the Association of Women's Health, Obstetric and Neonatal Nurses (AWHOONN) guidelines, the fetal heart rate is assessed every 15 to 30 minutes during the active phase of the first stage of labor, every 30 to 60 minutes during the latent phase of the first stage of labor, and every 5 to 15 minutes during the second stage of labor.

> *Test Taking Strategy*—*Analyze to determine what information the question asks for, which is the frequency of fetal heart rate assessment during the active phase of labor. Recall that the need to assess the fetal heart rate increases in frequency as labor progresses; the norm during the active stage of labor would be every 15 minutes (option 3). However, the frequency of the assessment should not be rigidly set because it can vary depending on maternal and fetal risk factors. Review fetal heart rate assessment during labor if you had difficulty answering this question.*

Cognitive Level—*Applying*
Client Needs Category—*Health promotion and maintenance*
Client Needs Subcategory—*None*

11. 2. Epidural anesthesia can be administered at any time, but it is usually administered to a primigravid client at 5 to 6 cm dilation. If the client is multigravid, an epidural is generally given at 3 to 4 cm dilation.

> *Test Taking Strategy*—*Use the process of elimination to help select the option that correctly identifies when epidural anesthesia is administered to a primigravid client. Option 1 can be eliminated because the primigravid client's progression through labor is typically slower, and administration of the epidural anesthesia when the cervix is only dilated 3 to 4 cm may prolong labor. Options 3 and 4 can be eliminated because administration of an epidural anesthesia during the transition stage of labor (cervical dilation 7–10 cm) does not provide therapeutic pain management when contraction frequency, duration and intensity have increased. Option 2 remains as the best answer because an epidural is administered when active labor is progressing as evidenced by a dilation of 5 to 6 cm. Review regional analgesics and anesthetics if you had difficulty answering this question.*

Cognitive Level—*Applying*
Client Needs Category—*Physiological integrity*
Client Needs Subcategory—*Pharmacological therapies*

12. 3. Contractions during the active phase of labor usually occur every 3 to 5 minutes and last between 45 and 60 seconds. Contractions last up to 30 seconds during the latent phase of the first stage of labor. They can last up to 90 seconds during the transition phase of the first stage of labor as well as during the second stage of labor.

> *Test Taking Strategy*—*Analyze to determine what information the question asks for, which is the duration of contractions during the active phase of labor. Recall that during this phase of labor, contractions that previously only lasted 20 or 30 seconds now occur more frequently and have a longer duration (option 3), but they do not usually last 90 seconds until the transition phase. Review contraction frequency, duration, and intensity during the latent, active, and transition phases of labor if you had difficulty answering this question.*

Cognitive Level—*Applying*
Client Needs Category—*Health promotion and maintenance*
Client Needs Subcategory—*None*

13. 3. During the transition phase of the first stage of labor, which ends when the cervix is completely dilated, the client usually has an increase in bloody show and the contractions last up to 90 seconds. Crowning of the pre-senting part does not occur until the cervix is completely dilated (10 cm), during the second stage of labor.

> *Test Taking Strategy—Analyze to determine what infor-mation the question asks for, which is an assessment finding that correlates with the transition phase of labor. Recall that this phase is noted as the labor progresses and approaches delivery. At this time there is a marked increase in the bloody show due to rupture of capillary blood vessels in the cervix and lower uterus (option 3). Review the assessment find-ings of the client in the latent, active, and transition phases of the first stage of labor if you had difficulty answering this question.*

Cognitive Level—*Applying*
Client Needs Category—*Health promotion and maintenance*
Client Needs Subcategory—*None*

14. 2. During the transition phase of the first stage of labor, the client is at risk for losing control because of intense discomfort, fatigue, and the frequency and length of the contractions. Praising the client's efforts frequently at this time can help her to maintain control of the situa-tion. During the transition phase of labor, the membranes usually rupture if they have not already done so, and the client may receive an opioid analgesic or regional anes-thetic; therefore, ambulation is not usually recommended. The client should not push until the cervix is completely dilated, which occurs during the second stage of labor. Application of sacral pressure can relieve back discomfort. Some women have a low tolerance to touch during this phase of labor; therefore, every client should be assessed individually to determine her preference.

> *Test Taking Strategy—Use the process of elimination to select the option that identifies the best nursing action for meeting the needs of a client during the transition phase of the first stage of labor. Option 2 emerges as the best answer because the client has difficulty coping with the increasing discomfort and benefits from words of encouragement from the nurse to persevere as labor progresses. Review the nurs-ing care of the woman in labor if you had difficulty answering this question.*

Cognitive Level—*Applying*
Client Needs Category—*Health promotion and maintenance*
Client Needs Subcategory—*None*

15. 1. When the fetus presents in the posterior instead of the anterior position, the client experiences back discomfort and there is a danger of maternal laceration if the fetus does not rotate before delivery. The posterior position usually prolongs labor, so preparing for a pre-cipitous delivery is not necessary. The client should be assisted to a more comfortable position. The knee-chest

position is commonly recommended because it relieves discomfort associated with the posterior presentation of the head and facilitates rotation of the head. Trendelen-burg's position does not assist with rotation of the head to the anterior position. During this phase, the client should avoid lying on her back to avoid compression of the vena cava by the uterus. The uterus usually is not dis-placed with a posterior presentation, so having the client void is inappropriate.

> *Test Taking Strategy—Note the use of the key words "most appropriate," indicating that one option is better than the others for facilitating normal progression through the active phase of labor when the fetus presents in the posterior position. Recall that the anterior position is the most favorable for normal labor. When the occiput faces the posterior section of the woman's pelvis, a longer "back labor" birth process is anticipated. Option 1 emerges as the best answer because the knee-chest position helps relieve back pressure and pain. Review fetal presen-tation and position during labor if you had difficulty answering this question.*

Cognitive Level—*Applying*
Client Needs Category—*Physiological integrity*
Client Needs Subcategory—*Basic care and comfort*

16. 4. The client should be encouraged to void every 2 hours to minimize bladder distention, which may prolong labor. The client should be encouraged to drink clear liquids at frequent intervals to prevent dehydration. The I.V. infusion rate is not decreased unless ordered by the physician. Maintaining the prescribed I.V. infusion rate also prevents dehydration. No solid foods are given during labor because peristalsis is slowed during this time, and nausea and vomiting can occur.

> *Test Taking Strategy—Consider the key words "most appropriate" when analyzing the four options and select the option that identifies the nursing interven-tion that will best prevent bladder distention during the active phase of labor. Option 4 prevents bladder distention by promoting frequent emptying of the bladder. Review nursing interventions for preventing bladder distention for the client in active labor if you had difficulty answering this question.*

Cognitive Level—*Applying*
Client Needs Category—*Physiological integrity*
Client Needs Subcategory—*Reduction of risk potential*

17. 1. This fetal heart rate monitoring strip shows late decelerations, which indicates insufficient uteroplacental circulation, which can lead to fetal hypoxia and acidosis if the underlying cause is not corrected. The client should be assisted to her left side to increase placental perfusion and decrease the frequency of contractions. The right lateral, supine, and prone positions do not increase placental perfusion.

Test Taking Strategy—Analyze the fetal heart rate monitoring strip to determine if it is normal or abnormal and in which position to place the laboring client. Remember that the fetal heart rate pattern should mirror uterine contractions; if it does not, an abnormality is present. Based on that premise, the abnormality, which is decelerations, can be relieved if the nurse places the client in a left lateral position to improve placental perfusion. Review nursing management of a client whose fetal heart rate monitoring strip shows late decelerations if you had difficulty with this question.
Cognitive Level—Analyzing
Client Needs Category—Physiological integrity
Client Needs Subcategory—Reduction of risk potential

18. 1. The *contraction duration* is defined as the time interval between the beginning of a contraction and the end of the same contraction. The time interval between the end of one contraction and the beginning of the next contraction is called the *relaxation period*. The time interval between the beginning of one contraction and the end of the next contraction is insignificant when assessing the client's labor pattern and is not generally measured. The time interval between the beginning of one contraction and the beginning of the next contraction is defined as the *frequency of the contractions.*
Test Taking Strategy—Analyze to determine what information the question asks for, which is the correct method for assessing the duration of contractions. Recall that the duration of a contraction is measured from the beginning of one contraction until the same contraction ends (option 1). Review the characteristics of a contraction, which include the duration, frequency, interval, and intensity, if you had difficulty answering this question.
Cognitive Level—Applying
Client Needs Category—Health promotion and maintenance
Client Needs Subcategory—None

19. 1. The nurse should palpate the fundus of the uterus, which is usually located just above the umbilicus in the full-term client. The fundus is palpated because muscular contractions are strongest and easiest to assess at this location.
Test Taking Strategy—Use the process of elimination to help select the option that provides a description of the method to use for accurately assessing a client's contractions. Recall that contractions can be assessed by palpation or by continuous external fetal monitoring. The correct technique for contraction assessment using palpation is to place the entire hand lightly on the abdomen above the umbilicus (option 1) and note the tightening of the fundus as the myometrium contracts in a downward direction.

Options 2 and 4 can therefore be eliminated. Also recall that fundal height increases approximately 1 cm per week of pregnancy; therefore, a full-term client's fundus would be above the umbilicus, eliminating option 3. Review contraction assessment if you had difficulty answering this question.
Cognitive Level—Applying
Client Needs Category—Health promotion and maintenance
Client Needs Subcategory—None

20. 1. When there is a question about whether the membranes have ruptured, a nitrazine test may be performed. The nitrazine test involves placing a drop or two of fluid onto a paper strip prepared with nitrazine dye. A chemical reaction occurs and the strip changes color based on the pH of the fluid being tested. Amniotic fluid turns the nitrazine test strip blue because amniotic fluid is alkaline. The nitrazine test remains yellow when exposed to vaginal secretions and urine, which are usually acidic. Red and green are not colors associated with nitrazine testing.
Test Taking Strategy—Analyze to determine what information the question asks for, which is the nitrazine test result that indicates the amniotic membranes have ruptured. Recall that the difference in pH determines whether fluid assessed with nitrazine test paper is amniotic fluid, urine, or vaginal secretions. The pH of amniotic fluid is between 7 and 7.5, which is alkaline. The pH of urine is around 5.5, and the pH of vaginal secretions is 4.5 to 5.5, both of which are acidic. The reagent used on the nitrazine paper turns blue in an alkaline environment and yellow in an acidic environment. Review the procedure for a nitrazine test if you had difficulty answering this question.
Cognitive Level—Applying
Client Needs Category—Physiological integrity
Client Needs Subcategory—Reduction of risk potential

21. 4, 5. The fetal heart rate should be checked immediately after the membranes rupture. A drop in the fetal heart rate may indicate umbilical cord prolapse. Prolapse of the umbilical cord may occur because of the sudden gush of fluid from the vagina, especially if the presenting part is not engaged. Inspecting the fluid for meconium is important because meconium-stained amniotic fluid indicates fetal distress. Rupture of the membranes can happen at any time before or during labor. Therefore, preparing for imminent delivery may be premature. The client's pulse is not affected by the rupturing of the membranes. The registered nurse usually performs vaginal examinations, and an indwelling catheter is not usually indicated when the membranes rupture.
Test Taking Strategy—Analyze to determine what information the question asks for, which is nursing actions that should be performed immediately after

the membranes rupture. Alternative-format "select all that apply" questions require considering each option independently to decide its merit in answering the question. Choose options that correlate with the nursing actions necessary to detect risks to the infant (options 4 and 5) when the membranes rupture. Review assessments that should be performed after rupture of membranes if you had difficulty answering this question.
Cognitive Level—Analyzing
Client Needs Category—Physiological integrity
Client Needs Subcategory—Reduction of risk potential

22. 1. The client's temperature should be assessed every hour after the membranes rupture because of the increased risk of infection. The temperature is assessed every 4 hours if the membranes are intact.

> *Test Taking Strategy—Analyze to determine what information the question asks for, which is the frequency of temperature assessment after rupture of the membranes. Recall that once the amniotic membranes have ruptured, the barrier of protection against invading microorganisms is eliminated. Temperature elevation is an early sign of infection and must be evaluated every hour (option 1). Review nursing care of the client after rupture of membranes if you had difficulty answering this question.*
> *Cognitive Level—Applying*
> *Client Needs Category—Safe and effective care environment*
> *Client Needs Subcategory—Safety and infection control*

23. 1. Internal electronic fetal monitoring requires the application of an electrode to the fetal scalp. Infection and soft-tissue injury can occur with the use of internal electronic fetal monitoring, but both are rare. A soft, water-filled catheter is inserted into the uterus for internal electronic monitoring of uterine contractions. A transducer is applied to the mother's abdomen when external electronic monitoring is used. A suction cup is applied to the fetal scalp when a vacuum extraction is being performed to assist with delivery of the fetal head.

> *Test Taking Strategy—Use the process of elimination to identify the option that provides an accurate explanation of internal electronic fetal monitoring and potential risks involved in its use. Recall that placing an electrode on the infant's scalp provides a route for the entry of pathogens and trauma from the scalp-implanted electrode (option 1). Review the advantages and disadvantages of internal electronic fetal monitoring if you had difficulty answering this question.*
> *Cognitive Level—Applying*
> *Client Needs Category—Health promotion and maintenance*
> *Client Needs Subcategory—None*

24. 3. The presence of green amniotic fluid indicates that the fetus has passed a meconium stool in utero. Passage of meconium in utero when the fetus is presenting in the vertex position is an indication of fetal distress and should be reported immediately. To avoid meconium aspiration, the mouth, nose, and throat should be suctioned before the delivery of the baby. The normal range for the fetal heart rate is 120 to 140 beats/minute, which suggests a well-oxygenated fetus. It is normal for the fetal heart rate to accelerate. An increase in bloody show is normal and indicates that the second stage of labor is imminent.

> *Test Taking Strategy—Look at the key words "most indicative" in reference to evidence of fetal distress. Recall that normal amniotic fluid is colorless; green amniotic fluid indicates fetal distress (option 3). Review signs and symptoms of fetal distress after rupture of membranes if you had difficulty answering this question.*
> *Cognitive Level—Analyzing*
> *Client Needs Category—Physiological integrity*
> *Client Needs Subcategory—Physiological adaptation*

25. 4. Although there is a trend toward more liberal food policies, the argument for avoiding solid food during active labor is that it may cause nausea and vomiting. The potential problem arises because gastric emptying is delayed during labor and there is decreased tone of the lower esophageal sphincter, both of which predispose to food passively entering the pharynx and lungs, causing aspiration. Eating solid food is not known to alter the absorption of regional anesthetics or to alter the duration and frequency of uterine contractions; it also does not cause fetal distress.

> *Test Taking Strategy—Use the process of elimination to select the option that identifies the best explanation for why eating solid food during active labor is contraindicated. Options 1, 2, and 3 can be eliminated because there is no scientific evidence that eating food during labor results in the negative outcomes referred to in those options. Option 4 remains as the best answer because physiologic changes may cause nausea and vomiting. Review the effects of labor on GI physiology if you had difficulty answering this question.*
> *Cognitive Level—Applying*
> *Client Needs Category—Health promotion and maintenance*
> *Client Needs Subcategory—None*

26. 1. When the fetus presents in the vertex position, the head descends into the birth canal first. If the feet or buttocks enter the birth canal first, the presentation is considered a *breech*. A shoulder presentation is when the shoulder enters the birth canal first. Both breech and shoulder presentations are considered malpresentations and make delivery more difficult. Often these types of presentations result in a cesarean section.

> *Test Taking Strategy—Use the process of elimination to help select the option that correctly explains the term vertex position from among the options provided. Options 2, 3, and 4 can be eliminated because they describe atypical positions that involve the presentation of body parts other than the head and complicate delivery. Recall that the vertex presentation is one in which the fetal head is the presenting part (option 1), making it the most favorable cephalic presentation because the smallest possible diameter enters the pelvis. Review fetal presentation and position during labor if you had difficulty answering this question.*
> **Cognitive Level**—Understanding
> **Client Needs Category**—Health promotion and maintenance
> **Client Needs Subcategory**—None

27. 4. A drop in the fetal heart rate after the contraction acme is defined as a *late deceleration*. The fetal heart requires a significant amount of oxygen; slowing of the heart rate is an ominous sign of fetal hypoxia that should be reported immediately. The other options describe processes that normally occur during the active phase of the first stage of labor.

> *Test Taking Strategy—Analyze to determine what information the question asks for, which is a finding about which the physician should be notified when it occurs in the active phase of the first stage of labor. Recall that a drop in fetal heart rate after the peak of contraction indicates a decrease in blood flow to the infant (option 4). If late decelerations are repetitive and do not respond to remediation, a cesarean section is indicated to rescue the compromised fetus. Review late decelerations and their significance if you had difficulty answering this question.*
> **Cognitive Level**—Analyzing
> **Client Needs Category**—Physiological integrity
> **Client Needs Subcategory**—Physiological adaptation

28. 1, 2, 3. Drugs such as terbutaline sulfate (Brethine) are used to slow or prevent uterine contractions occurring before 34 weeks' gestation. It is used as a tocolytic for interrupting preterm labor, although it has not been approved by the U.S. Food and Drug Administration for that use. Terbutaline provides short-term prolongation of the pregnancy, thereby increasing time to administer other drugs that can promote fetal maturity or to transfer the pregnant client to a facility that is equipped to handle premature births. Adverse reactions to terbutaline sulfate include anxiety, tremors, nervousness, headache,

hypertension, palpitations, hypokalemia, pulmonary edema, and restlessness. Hypoglycemia, oliguria, and a rash are not common adverse reactions to terbutaline sulfate.

> *Test Taking Strategy—Analyze to determine what information the question asks for, which is signs of adverse reactions to terbutaline. Alternative-format "select all that apply" questions require considering each option independently to decide its merit in answering the question. Choose all the options that correlate with adverse reactions associated with the administration of terbutaline sulfate. Recall that terbutaline sulfate is a sympathomimetic, meaning its actions are similar to those of the sympathetic nervous system. Review the actions of tocolytics and terbutaline in particular if you had difficulty answering this question.*
> **Cognitive Level**—Applying
> **Client Needs Category**—Physiological integrity
> **Client Needs Subcategory**—Pharmacological therapies

29. 2. Tocolytic agents such as terbutaline sulfate (Brethine) should be withheld if the client's cervix is dilated 4 cm or more or is effaced 50% or more. Tocolytic agents should also be withheld when the client is hemorrhaging or has severe pregnancy-induced hypertension, or when fetal distress is evident. The presence of mild contractions indicates that the client continues to be in preterm labor, so it would be appropriate to give the client the tocolytic medication. Fetal heart rate variability is of no consequence as long as it does not differ more than 10 to 15 beats over any 1 minute. The client's perception that contractions are occurring less frequently is not substantial enough to withhold the medication; more objective data are necessary.

> *Test Taking Strategy—Analyze to determine what information the question asks for, which is the indication for withholding the administration of terbutaline and notifying the physician. Terbutaline relaxes bronchial, vascular, and uterine smooth muscle; the latter inhibits preterm contractions. However, its administration should be withheld when the client has reached active labor, evidenced by cervical dilation and effacement (option 2). Inhibiting uterine contractions during active labor could lead to prolonging labor by suppressing contractions that are strong enough to deliver the fetus. Review indications that make it medically necessary to withhold the administration of terbutaline if you had difficulty answering this question.*
> **Cognitive Level**—Analyzing
> **Client Needs Category**—Physiological integrity
> **Client Needs Subcategory**—Pharmacological therapies

Nursing Care of Clients During the Second Stage of Labor

30. 1. The second stage of labor begins when the cervix is fully dilated to 10 cm and ends when the baby is delivered. The perineum usually begins to bulge and the presenting part begins to crown during the second stage of labor. The contractions usually last for 60 to 90 seconds, and the cervix is completely dilated (10 cm). During transition, when the cervix is dilating from 7 to 10 cm, the client is likely to become agitated, and irritable, often times losing control.

> *Test Taking Strategy*—*Use the process of elimination to select the option that identifies the evidence that accurately indicates that the client is in the second stage of labor. Options 2, 3, and 4 can be eliminated because they are characteristics of the first stage of labor. Recall that the second stage of labor, the stage during which the fetus is delivered, is preceded by bulging of the perineum. Review the clinical manifestations that occur in the stages of labor, focusing on those that correlate with the second stage of labor, if you had difficulty answering this question.*
> *Cognitive Level*—*Applying*
> *Client Needs Category*—*Health promotion and maintenance*
> *Client Needs Subcategory*—*None*

31. 1. Preparation for delivery for a multiparous client should begin when she is 6 to 7 cm dilated. Preparation for a primiparous client is usually delayed until the client is completely dilated (10 cm) because it generally takes longer to achieve full dilation with a woman's first delivery. The arrival time of the physician or midwife varies and usually is not used as an indicator for when to begin preparing for delivery.

> *Test Taking Strategy*—*Analyze to determine what information the question asks for, which is the finding that indicates delivery is imminent. Recall that the multiparous client has given birth to more than one child, and her progression through the first and second stages of labor is generally expected to be quicker. Delaying preparation of the client until the events described in options 2, 3, and 4 may result in a precipitous birth rather than one occurring in the delivery room. Review the differences between when a primiparous and multiparous client should be prepared for delivery if you had difficulty answering this question.*
> *Cognitive Level*—*Applying*
> *Client Needs Category*—*Health promotion and maintenance*
> *Client Needs Subcategory*—*None*

32. 3. A vaginal examination should be performed to determine whether the cervix is 10 cm dilated and 100% effaced before the client begins to push. This precaution prevents edema or lacerations to the cervix that would prevent further dilation, prolong labor, and possibly require delivery by cesarean birth. The other options are appropriate if the nurse has already determined that the client is fully dilated.

> *Test Taking Strategy*—*Look at the key word "first," which indicates that one action described is a priority that should be completed before any of the others when the client feels the need to push. Recall that until the cervix is fully dilated (option 4), the client may experience fatigue or cervical or vaginal trauma. Review the nursing care of a client in the second stage of labor if you had difficulty answering this question.*
> *Cognitive Level*—*Applying*
> *Client Needs Category*—*Health promotion and maintenance*
> *Client Needs Subcategory*—*None*

33. 3. If an opioid analgesic such as butorphanol tartrate (Stadol) is given too late during labor, the medication can cross the placental barrier and may be present after the newborn is delivered, resulting in respiratory depression. Conversely, giving an opioid analgesic too early in labor may interfere with labor progression and decrease the contractions' effectiveness. Administration of an opioid analgesic is not associated with uterine rupture or increased fetal activity.

> *Test Taking Strategy*—*Analyze to determine what information the question asks for, which is the reason an opioid narcotic is not warranted during the second stage of labor. Consider the actions and side effects of opioid narcotics on the mother and fetus. Recall that the infant's breathing may be impaired due to placental distribution of the recently administered drug. Review the effects of narcotics on the fetus before delivery if you had difficulty answering this question.*
> *Cognitive Level*—*Applying*
> *Client Needs Category*—*Physiological integrity*
> *Client Needs Subcategory*—*Pharmacological therapies*

34. 1. An epidural block is a type of local (regional) anesthetic delivered through a catheter placed in the space between the dura mater and the surface of the spinal cord. Epidural anesthesia provides pain relief during labor and delivery by numbing and paralyzing muscles below the ribcage. Epidural anesthesia also is useful for clients who have preexisting conditions, such as heart disease, pulmonary disease, or diabetes. An epidural usually takes effect immediately and reaches its maximum potency within 3 to 5 minutes of administration. However, the procedure for placing the catheter requires additional time.

Test Taking Strategy—Analyze to determine what information the question asks for, which is the length of time required for the onset of analgesia with an epidural anesthetic. Recall that after a local anesthetic is injected to reduce discomfort during the insertion of the catheter, the anesthetic agent eliminates sensation. Review regional analgesics and anesthetics if you had difficulty answering this question.
Cognitive Level—*Applying*
Client Needs Category—*Physiological integrity*
Client Needs Subcategory—*Pharmacological therapies*

35. 1. During the period immediately after administering an epidural anesthetic, the client's blood pressure should be assessed and evaluated for the presence of hypotension. A drop in blood pressure occasionally occurs secondary to sympathetic blockade and may decrease the oxygen supply to the fetus, which is manifested by fetal bradycardia (not tachycardia). Paralysis of the lower extremities is an expected result. The client may experience a spinal headache within 24 to 72 hours of the procedure, but not immediately. Ensuring that the client is well hydrated (usually through I.V. infusion) before, during, and after the procedure minimizes both maternal hypotension and spinal headache.

Test Taking Strategy—Analyze to determine what information the question asks for, which is a complication that may occur immediately after the administration of an epidural block and for which the nurse must monitor. Recall that sympathetic blockade causes vasodilation, which decreases cardiac output, resulting in maternal hypotension (option 1) and compromised fetal oxygenation. The degree of hypotension depends on the level of anesthesia and the position of the client. Review regional analgesics and anesthetics if you had difficulty answering this question.
Cognitive Level—*Applying*
Client Needs Category—*Physiological integrity*
Client Needs Subcategory—*Pharmacological therapies*

36. 2. The client to whom an epidural anesthesia has been administered is instructed when to push because she is unable to feel contractions. Oxygen is not routinely required unless complications arise. The client is not usually catheterized after this type of anesthesia, and the epidural is usually given late in labor (second stage) or for cesarean birth; therefore, it usually does not slow the progress of labor, which would require the use of oxytocin (Pitocin).

Test Taking Strategy—Analyze to determine what information the question asks for, which is the nursing management of the client who has received an epidural block. Recall that an epidural block elicits both analgesic and anesthetic effects, which interferes with the client's ability to feel uterine contractions. Consequently, the nurse manually palpates the client's abdomen and indicates when

the client should push when a contraction occurs. Review the effects of an epidural anesthetic administered during labor if you had difficulty answering this question.*
Cognitive Level—*Applying*
Client Needs Category—*Physiological integrity*
Client Needs Subcategory—*Pharmacological therapies*

37. 1. When cleaning the perineum in preparation for delivery, the nurse should use the technique that poses the least possibility of infection and increases visibility of the area. The usual procedure of cleaning the area is as follows: pubic bone to lower abdomen, the inner thighs (both), the right and left labia, and the vagina to the anus. The vagina is always the last area cleaned.

Test Taking Strategy—Analyze to determine what information the question asks for, which is the sequence used to prepare the perineum for delivery. Recall that secretions and dried blood are removed to prevent contamination of the urethral and vaginal areas following medically aseptic principles (option 1). Review the technique for performing a perineal scrub as well as the principles of asepsis if you had difficulty answering this question.
Cognitive Level—*Applying*
Client Needs Category—*Safe and effective care environment*
Client Needs Subcategory—*Safety and infection control*

38. 3. An episiotomy is an incision made into the perineum tissue to enlarge the vaginal opening. It is usually performed to prevent lacerations within the vagina and, in extreme cases, lacerations in the rectum. An episiotomy also diminishes the possibility of prolonged pressure on the fetal head and speeds the delivery process. Episiotomies are not associated with uterine rupture or postpartum infection. Although an episiotomy may prevent rectal trauma, that is not the primary reason for which it is done.

Test Taking Strategy—Use the process of elimination to select the option that identifies the best reason for performing an episiotomy. Option 1 can be eliminated because the episiotomy in the perineum between the vagina and anus is not prophylactic for uterine rupture. Option 2 can be eliminated because a postpartum infection is a consequence of pathogens that invade local tissue. Option 4 can be eliminated because a rectal tear occurs less often than a vaginal tear, making option 3 a better answer. Recall that an episiotomy is performed to control the location and extent of vaginal enlargement as well as create a cleanly incised margin of tissue that will heal more efficiently than one that is torn irregularly (option 3). Review the purposes for performing an episiotomy and the problems associated with a vaginal and rectal laceration if you had difficulty answering this question.

Cognitive Level—*Applying*
Client Needs Category—*Health promotion and maintenance*
Client Needs Subcategory—*None*

Nursing Care of Clients During the Third Stage of Labor

39. 3. The priority need of the newborn immediately after delivery is establishment of a patent airway. This is best accomplished by suctioning the newborn's nose and mouth with a bulb syringe after the head is delivered but before complete delivery of the body. Oxygen is not given before the airway is cleared; it is only administered if needed. Applying the cord clamp and warming the newborn do not take priority over establishment and maintenance of respirations.

Test Taking Strategy—*Analyze to determine what information the question asks for, which is an item that should be available to meet the newborn infant's priority need. Recall that breathing is a priority need that depends on ensuring a patent airway; having a bulb syringe (option 3) available to remove fluid from the infant's nose and oral pharynx helps to meet that need by providing a tool to keep the airway clear. Review nursing care of the newborn immediately after delivery if you had difficulty answering this question.*
Cognitive Level—*Applying*
Client Needs Category—*Health promotion and maintenance*
Client Needs Subcategory—*None*

40. 4. The Apgar scoring system is a tool used to assess the infant at 1 minute of age and at 5 minutes. It assesses heart rate, respiratory effort, muscle tone, reflexes, and color. The maximum score an infant can achieve is 10 (2 points for each of the five categories). An Apgar score of 7 to 10 is considered good and does not require any intervention. A score between 4 and 6 indicates moderate distress, in which case the newborn requires close monitoring and possible intervention with oxygen. A score between 0 and 3 is considered poor and indicates a definite need for resuscitation efforts and medical intervention.

Test Taking Strategy—*Analyze to determine what information the question asks for regarding interpretation of an Apgar score. Recall that an Apgar score of 7 at 5 minutes after birth indicates an expected assessment finding in a newborn and no signs of distress. If unsure, recall that 10 is the highest score obtained and 0 is the lowest. Review the Apgar scoring system if you had difficulty answering this question.*
Cognitive Level—*Applying*
Client Needs Category—*Health promotion and maintenance*
Client Needs Subcategory—*None*

41. 2. The newborn is dried first to prevent heat loss secondary to evaporation, placed on the mother's abdomen in skin-to-skin contact, and then covered with a warmed blanket. The mother's abdomen is usually warm, so direct newborn-mother contact does not pose a danger of heat loss. The other options either interfere with maintaining the newborn's warmth or do not promote mother-infant attachment.

Test Taking Strategy—*Note the key word "initially" in reference to the nursing action that should be performed first to facilitate mother-infant bonding and, at the same time, promote physiologic stability of the newborn. Consider the option that meets both objectives. Review newborn physiologic changes after birth and mother-infant bonding if you had difficulty answering this question.*
Cognitive Level—*Applying*
Client Needs Category—*Health promotion and maintenance*
Client Needs Subcategory—*None*

42.

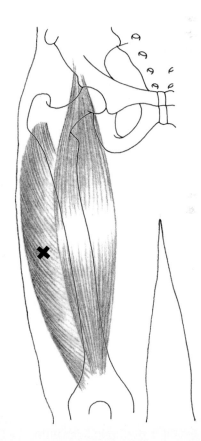

The preferred site for I.M. injections in a newborn and children up to age 3 years is the vastus lateralis muscle. This site is located on the outside aspect of the thigh between the greater trochanter and the knee. The ventrogluteal muscle and the gluteus maximus muscles are not used in newborns because of the risk of sciatic nerve damage. The deltoid muscle should not be used until a child is 3 years old. The rectus femoris muscle on the anterior

thigh is not a recommended site for a newborn because what appears to be a bulky muscle is predominantly subcutaneous fat. In addition, there is a neurovascular bundle beneath the site.

Test Taking Strategy—Analyze to determine what information the question asks for, which is the injection site for administering vitamin K (AquaMEPHYTON) to an infant. Recall that the vastus lateralis muscle is an ideal and recommended I.M. injection site because it has few nerves and blood vessels, will hold a reasonable amount of injected volume, and is the largest muscle mass in this age group. Review administering parenteral medications to the newborn if you had difficulty answering this question.

Cognitive Level—*Applying*
Client Needs Category—*Safe and effective care environment*
Client Needs Subcategory—*Safety and infection control*

43. 3. Bacteria normally found in the intestines synthesize vitamin K. The newborn is given vitamin K (AquaMEPHYTON) at birth because the intestines of the newborn are sterile and the infant cannot synthesize vitamin K. Vitamin K is needed for the formation of prothrombin and other clotting factors that help prevent bleeding. Vitamin K does not stimulate respirations, promote peristalsis, or increase calcium absorption.

Test Taking Strategy—Analyze to determine what information the question asks for, which is the rationale for administering vitamin K to a newborn. Recall that newborns need vitamin K to assist in blood clotting, and the intestinal flora necessary to naturally produce vitamin K are absent. One single dose is administered, usually within 1 hour of birth. Review indications for vitamin K administration to the newborn if you had difficulty answering this question.

Cognitive Level—*Understanding*
Client Needs Category—*Physiological integrity*
Client Needs Subcategory—*Pharmacological therapies*

44. 1. Neonatal blindness can occur as a result of eye infections caused by gonococcal and chlamydial organisms. Erythromycin (Ilotycin) ophthalmic ointment is used prophylactically in the newborn to prevent blindness that may result from exposure to these organisms during passage through the mother's birth canal. *Candida albicans* causes yeast infections, and *Pneumocystis carinii* is associated with acquired immunodeficiency syndrome.

Test Taking Strategy—Analyze to determine what information the question asks for, which is the pathogens that, if left untreated, may cause neonatal blindness. Recall that chlamydial infections are the most common sexually transmitted infection and

that those caused by Neisseria gonorrhoeae *rank second. These organisms are sensitive to erythromycin; therefore, all newborns are given prophylactic erythromycin ophthalmic ointment generally within an hour of being born. Review indications for administering erythromycin ophthalmic ointment in the newborn if you had difficulty answering this question.*

Cognitive Level—*Applying*
Client Needs Category—*Physiological integrity*
Client Needs Subcategory—*Pharmacological therapies*

45. 3. The nursing assistant or nurse should keep one hand over the newborn while weighing it. Keeping a hand on the newborn will affect the weight's accuracy. Undressing the newborn before the weight is obtained, placing a diaper or paper barrier on the scale before balancing it, and cleaning the scale with an antiseptic before and after use are all correct techniques to implement when weighing a newborn.

Test Taking Strategy—Analyze to determine what information the question asks for, which is a technique for weighing an infant that indicates a need for additional teaching. Option 3 is the best answer because the infant's weight will be inaccurate if the measurement includes weight from a source other than the infant which in this case is the technician's hand. Review the technique for weighing a newborn if you had difficulty answering this question.

Cognitive Level—*Applying*
Client Needs Category—*Safe and effective care environment*
Client Needs Subcategory—*Safety and infection control*

46. 1. To prevent the risk of the mother receiving the wrong baby, matching identification bracelets should be placed on both the newborn and mother before the newborn leaves the delivery area. Eye prophylaxis and administration of vitamin K (AquaMEPHYTON) are usually delayed to facilitate early bonding between the mother and baby but are completed in the delivery room or in the nursery. Phenylketonuria (PKU) testing should be performed when the baby has begun to eat.

Test Taking Strategy—Use the process of elimination to select the option that identifies the most important nursing intervention before the newborn leaves the delivery area. Eliminate options 2 and 3 as they may be performed in the delivery room or the nursery. Option 4 can be eliminated because it is performed after the infant's first feeding. Option 1 remains as the correct answer because care must be taken that infants and mothers are not mismatched. Review nursing care of the newborn

after delivery if you had difficulty answering this question.
Cognitive Level—*Applying*
Client Needs Category—*Safe and effective care environment*
Client Needs Subcategory—*Safety and infection control*

47. 4. The placenta is delivered after it has separated from the wall of the uterus. This is usually accomplished by having the client bear down. In some cases, the attending health care provider may manually express the placenta. Breathing slowly and deeply, assuming a side-lying position, and tightening and relaxing the perineum will not facilitate delivery of the placenta.
Test Taking Strategy—Analyze to determine what information the question asks for, which is the action that facilitates the delivery of the placenta. Recall that during the third stage of labor, uterine contractions shear the placenta from its site of attachment. Pushing while experiencing the contraction facilitates expulsion of the placenta (option 4). Review the nursing interventions during the fourth stage of labor if you had difficulty answering this question.
Cognitive Level—*Applying*
Client Needs Category—*Health promotion and maintenance*
Client Needs Subcategory—*None*

48. 3. A rise of the fundus in the abdomen, lengthening of the umbilical cord, and a sudden gush of blood from the vagina are signs of impending delivery of the placenta. The perineum does not bulge with delivery of the placenta.
Test Taking Strategy—Analyze to determine what information the question asks for, which is a finding that suggests placental separation. Recall that when the placenta separates, the uterine fundus moves in an upward direction (option 3). It becomes firmer and more globular in shape after placental detachment. Review the characteristics of the third stage of labor if you had difficulty answering this question.
Cognitive Level—*Applying*
Client Needs Category—*Health promotion and maintenance*
Client Needs Subcategory—*None*

Nursing Care of Clients During the Fourth Stage of Labor

49. 1, 2. The client's needs are best met by placing a warmed blanket over her. The nurse can also explain that the shaking is a normal response due to sudden physiological changes and fluid shifts; however, this will not relieve her shaking and coldness. Suggesting that the client try not to think about the shaking will not resolve the underlying cause; therefore, this does not adequately address the client's complaint. Notifying the physician is unnecessary because this is a normal physiological process. Because the shaking and feelings of being cold are related to fluid shifts and sudden physiological changes, taking the client's temperature is not necessary. Providing a warm drink may provide warmth but will not control the shaking. Therefore, it is not an immediate action.
Test Taking Strategy—Note the key words "most appropriate," which indicate a need to discriminate among the options, looking for answers that are more pertinent than others. Alternative-format "select all that apply" questions require considering each option independently to decide its merit in answering the question. Choose options that are specific for the uncontrollable shaking and feeling of cold that is experienced by the client. Review signs and symptoms that the client may develop in the fourth stage of labor if you had difficulty answering this question.
Cognitive Level—*Applying*
Client Needs Category—*Physiological integrity*
Client Needs Subcategory—*Basic care and comfort*

50. 3. Oxytocin is a natural hormone released by the posterior pituitary gland. Massaging the fundus, breastfeeding the infant, and nipple stimulation can supplement its release after delivery, but its biosynthesized form can be administered as a medication. When oxytocin (Pitocin) is administered prophylactically after delivery of the placenta, it is classified as a uterotonic medication because it causes the uterus to contract, which decreases the risk for postpartum hemorrhage. The client's blood pressure should be monitored closely because hypertension is a side effect of this medication. Also, uterine rupture may occur with the administration of oxytocin if hyperstimulation of the uterus secondary to a toxic dose of the medication occurs. Administering oxytocin will not prevent the uterus from inverting. When palpating the uterus, the nurse commonly supports it just above the symphysis pubis to prevent the uterus from inverting.
Test Taking Strategy—Analyze to determine what information the question asks for, which is the rationale for administering oxytocin (Pitocin) during the fourth stage of labor. Recall that firm contraction of the uterus kept at the consistency of a tightened thigh muscle with supplemental oxytocin prevents excessive blood loss (option 3) after the infant is delivered. Review the action of oxytocin if you had difficulty answering this question.
Cognitive Level—*Applying*
Client Needs Category—*Physiological integrity*
Client Needs Subcategory—*Pharmacological therapies*

51. **1, 4, 6.** A systolic blood pressure of 100 mm Hg or less should be reported because it could indicate that the client is hemorrhaging. Signs of hypovolemic shock occur when about 400 to 500 mL of blood have been lost. Besides a drop in blood pressure, other signs of shock related to hemorrhage include increased pulse rate, increased respiratory rate, cold and clammy skin, decreased urine output, and dizziness. The normal pulse rate is slightly lower during the fourth stage of labor than during previous stages because of decreased cardiac strain. The pulse rate can range between 40 and 80 beats/minute and still be considered normal. During the fourth stage of labor, the lochia is usually dark red with a fleshy, not foul, odor. The client may saturate one perineal pad within 1 hour. Also, it is common for clients to exhibit a slightly elevated temperature (up to 100.4°F [38°C]) just after delivery.

> *Test Taking Strategy—Analyze to determine what information the question asks for, which is signs of complications after delivery. Alternative-format "select all that apply" questions require considering each option independently to decide its merit in answering the question. Choose options that correlate with abnormal postpartum assessment findings that are noted immediately after delivery. Review physiological changes and indications of complications occurring in the fourth stage of labor if you had difficulty answering this question.*
> *Cognitive Level—Analyzing*
> *Client Needs Category—Physiological integrity*
> *Client Needs Subcategory—Reduction of risk potential*

Nursing Care of Clients Having a Cesarean Birth

52. **2.** The client is catheterized before abdominal surgery to prevent bladder trauma that may occur if the bladder becomes distended during surgery. Such catheterization is not performed to reduce postpartum hemorrhage, provide a landmark for the physician, or provide a safe way of collecting urine specimens.

> *Test Taking Strategy—Note the key words "most accurate," indicating that one option is more correct than the others. Select the option that provides accurate client education in reference to why a urinary catheter is inserted before a cesarean delivery. Recall the close proximity of the urinary bladder to the uterus, which relates to the need to keep the bladder empty and out of harm's way during the cesarean delivery. Review preoperative nursing care of the client undergoing a cesarean birth if you had difficulty answering this question.*
> *Cognitive Level—Analyzing*
> *Client Needs Category—Safe and effective care environment*
> *Client Needs Subcategory—Safety and infection control*

53. **1.** When a cesarean birth is performed using epidural anesthesia, the client may feel pressure but does not experience pain or stinging because the nerve roots (source of pain) are blocked. Clients are not asleep when this type of anesthesia is used.

> *Test Taking Strategy—Note the use of the key words "most appropriate," indicating that one answer is better than the others. Select the option that provides the best explanation regarding the expected effects of an epidural anesthesia. Recall that during epidural anesthesia, the client is awake and aware of the surroundings. Consider that the client does not experience pain but will comment on pressure (option 1), especially at the time of delivery. Review the use of regional anesthesia during cesarean birth if you had difficulty answering this question.*
> *Cognitive Level—Applying*
> *Client Needs Category—Physiological integrity*
> *Client Needs Subcategory—Pharmacological therapies*

54. **3.** The client's husband (or partner or coach, who is sometimes referred to as a *doula*) is usually allowed in the operating room during the cesarean birth. However, because of the sterile environment, whoever is observing the birth must change into the appropriate surgical attire and perform hand hygiene at the scrub sink before entering into the delivery area when the cesarean section is ready to begin. Then the person is usually seated near the client's head.

> *Test Taking Strategy—Apply the key words "most appropriate" when discriminating among the options. Select one option that is better than any of the others in reference to the husband's request to be present during the cesarean birth. Recall that persons designated by the birthing mother may be present, but to maintain an aseptic and safe environment, surgical standards must be followed (option 3). Review standards that apply to the presence of laypersons within an operating room if you had difficulty answering this question.*
> *Cognitive Level—Applying*
> *Client Needs Category—Safe and effective care environment*
> *Client Needs Subcategory—Safety and infection control*

55. **1.** According to the World Health Organization, women who have cesarean sections are five times more likely to develop a postpartum infection than women who have vaginal births. The majority of surgical site infections are caused by microorganisms on the client's own skin. Therefore, extensive skin preparation is required. Before a cesarean birth, the nurse follows the standard abdominal-perineal skin preparation. The area prepared begins at the nipple line and extends vertically to the perineal area and then horizontally from one side of the abdomen to the other side of the abdomen.

Test Taking Strategy—*Look at the key words "most appropriate" in reference to the technique for completing the surgical skin preparation of the client scheduled for a lower-segment transverse incision. Recall that the entire abdomen is prepared both vertically and horizontally (option 1) to achieve a reduction in skin bacterial counts. Review surgical skin preparations for cesarean deliveries if you had difficulty answering this question.*
Cognitive Level—*Applying*
Client Needs Category—*Safe and effective care environment*
Client Needs Subcategory—*Safety and infection control*

56. 3. When morphine is administered via the epidural route, it produces a long duration of pain relief. However, an ongoing risk is that severe respiratory depression may occur because of the slow circulation of cerebrospinal fluid to the brain. The client should be monitored closely for respiratory depression, evidenced by a slow respiratory rate and unusual drowsiness or sleepiness, when receiving morphine by the epidural route. The client may also experience urine retention, pinpoint pupils, and circulatory collapse.
Test Taking Strategy—*Analyze to determine what information the question asks for, which is an adverse effect from the administration of epidural morphine sulfate. Recall that morphine sulfate is an opioid narcotic and has a greater potential for causing central respiratory depression (option 3) when given by the epidural route. Review adverse effects of morphine sulfate, especially when given intrathecally (within the spinal canal), if you had difficulty answering this question.*
Cognitive Level—*Applying*
Client Needs Category—*Physiological integrity*
Client Needs Subcategory—*Pharmacological therapies*

57. 4. An opioid antagonist such as naloxone hydrochloride (Narcan) should be readily available in case respiratory depression occurs. If naloxone is used, the nurse should monitor the client for the onset of extreme pain because naloxone reverses both the analgesic and side effects of opioids. The medications identified in the other options are not required when the client is receiving epidural morphine sulfate.
Test Taking Strategy—*Analyze to determine what information the question asks for, which is the medication that should be readily available for use in an emergency situation that requires quick action. Recall that naloxone (option 4) is the antidote for managing the side effects of morphine sulfate or an overdose of morphine sulfate. Review the life-threatening effects of opioid narcotics, antidotes used, and epidural administration of opioids if you had difficulty answering this question.*

Cognitive Level—*Applying*
Client Needs Category—*Physiological integrity*
Client Needs Subcategory—*Pharmacological therapies*

58. 4. Redness and swelling around the incision usually indicate the presence of an infection. Other signs of infection include an elevated temperature (100.4°F [38°C] or greater orally) 2 to 3 days after delivery, severe pain, and incisional drainage. It is normal for the incision line to feel numb for several months after a cesarean birth.
Test Taking Strategy—*Use the process of elimination to select the option that identifies the best indication of an incisional infection. Recall the acronym REEDA (Redness, Edema, Ecchymosis, Drainage, and Approximation) which highlights the signs of infection. Redness and swelling (option 4) are indications that the incision is infected. Review signs of a wound infection if you had difficulty answering this question.*
Cognitive Level—*Applying*
Client Needs Category—*Physiological integrity*
Client Needs Subcategory—*Physiological adaptation*

59. 1. Ambulation improves intestinal motility and may relieve intestinal gas. Other interventions include a diet low in gas-forming foods, small enemas, and antiflatulence medications, which can be used to reduce abdominal discomfort experienced by the client who has had a cesarean birth. Pain medications, such as meperidine hydrochloride (Demerol) and morphine sulfate, can contribute to the abdominal discomfort instead of relieving it because they slow peristalsis. Rectal tubes are invasive and should only be used as a last resort after evaluating the outcome of other methods for relieving intestinal gas. Drinking from a straw is discouraged because it causes the client to swallow more air, which further aggravates the problem.
Test Taking Strategy—*Note the key word "initially," which indicates the answer is an action that should be performed before any of the others to relieve abdominal pain and bloating 1 day after cesarean delivery. Consider strategies that would assist in eliminating gas from the intestinal system, either by the rectal or oral route. Recall that a rectal tube, which ordinarily may be helpful, is not the best choice initially because of the close proximity of the bowel and its organisms to the vagina and uterus, which has been incised. Review postoperative nursing care of the client undergoing a cesarean delivery if you had difficulty answering this question.*
Cognitive Level—*Applying*
Client Needs Category—*Physiological integrity*
Client Needs Subcategory—*Basic care and comfort*

60. 1. Vaginal birth after a cesarean birth (VBAC) is possible if the client has had a previous low transverse incision and wishes to attempt to have a vaginal birth.

Although the client must have no history of medical conditions that prohibit a vaginal birth, that is not the major factor in qualifying for VBAC. The reason it was believed that "once a cesarean section, always a cesarean section" was based on the fear that the uterus would rupture if there was a subsequent vaginal delivery. That fear was based on the earlier technique of performing vertical incisions. Currently the uterus ruptures in only 1% of VBACs.

Test Taking Strategy—Look at the key words "most accurate" in reference to the potential for a VBAC. More than 80% of women who have had a previous cesarean section are now able to have a vaginal delivery. Recall that there is a high success rate for VBAC (option 1) as a result of the recent type of incision performed for the initial cesarean section. Review the indications and contraindications of VBAC if you had difficulty answering this question.
Cognitive Level—Applying
Client Needs Category—Health promotion and maintenance
Client Needs Subcategory—None

Nursing Care of Clients Having an Emergency Delivery

61. 3. If the nurse observes prolapse of the umbilical cord, the client should be placed in Trendelenburg's position or knee-chest position. Both positions help to relieve the pressure of the presenting part on the umbilical cord. The nurse may also attempt to lift the presenting part off the cord with a gloved finger or hand until the physician or midwife arrives. Oxygen is usually administered, but the client is not positioned on the left side. The newborn is usually delivered by cesarean birth; however, preparation of the delivery area and notification of the physician do not take priority over relieving the cord compression.

Test Taking Strategy—The key words are "most appropriate" and "initially," meaning there is one priority nursing action at the current time that should be performed before any of the others when the umbilical cord protrudes from the vagina during the active phase of labor. Recall that immediate relief of compression on the umbilical vessels is necessary to maintain oxygenation of the fetus. This is initially accomplished by placing the client in Trendelenburg's position (option 3) or knee-chest position. Review management of the client experiencing umbilical cord compression if you have difficulty answering this question.
Cognitive Level—Applying
Client Needs Category—Physiological integrity
Client Needs Subcategory—Reduction of risk potential

62. 1. When birth is imminent and no help is available, the nurse should gently control the delivery of the head, allow it to emerge, and deliver the newborn between

contractions. The nurse should not hold back the baby's head to prevent birth or attempt to enter or enlarge the vaginal opening.

Test Taking Strategy—Look at the key words "most appropriate" in reference to an action that is best when the infant's head is crowning and the nurse is alone. Recall that contractions occurring every 2 to 3 minutes and crowning are characteristics of the second stage of labor and indicate imminent birth. Rather than forestall the birth, which could result in life-threatening consequences for the infant, the nurse should facilitate the natural birthing process (option 1). Review the nursing care of the client experiencing a precipitous birth if you had difficulty answering this question.
Cognitive Level—Applying
Client Needs Category—Physiological integrity
Client Needs Subcategory—Reduction of risk potential

Nursing Care of Clients Having a Stillborn Baby

63. 2. The nurse should encourage the client to express her feelings, including sorrow over her baby's loss. These actions allow the client to sort through her feelings and facilitate the establishment of a trusting relationship between the client and nurse. The fetal heart rate should be checked only once by an experienced nurse; any rechecking may give the client false hope, which is inappropriate. Redirecting the client's attention to the laboring process does not allow the client the opportunity to sort through her feelings. Explaining that the baby probably would have been born with severe long-term health problems is not necessarily an accurate statement and also does nothing to ease the client's sorrow.

Test Taking Strategy—Look at the key words "most appropriate" in reference to the nursing care of the primigravid client whose fetus has died in utero. Choose the option that facilitates a therapeutic outcome. Recall that it is always therapeutic to acknowledge the client's loss and facilitate the grieving process by listening to the client express feelings about the death of the infant (option 2). Review therapeutic communication and the stages of grief if you had difficulty answering this question.
Cognitive Level—Applying
Client Needs Category—Psychosocial integrity
Client Needs Subcategory—None

64. 2. Allowing the parents to visit with their baby affords them an opportunity to say their last goodbyes and helps them accept the infant's death. The infant is bathed and diapered, and the parents are allowed to hold and touch the infant. Although a memory packet may also be presented, it does not substitute for an actual visit if the parents desire one. Postponing the visit may interfere with the grieving process.

Test Taking Strategy—Apply the key words "most appropriate" when analyzing the choices in the four options. Select the option that describes the nursing action that is best for promoting a therapeutic outcome for the grieving parents. Recall that seeing and holding the stillborn infant (option 2) dispels any preconceived fears about the condition of the infant, confirms the reality of the loss, yet allows the parents to bond and form memories about the identity of the infant for whom they will always be parents. Review the nursing care of the family who has experienced a stillbirth if you had difficulty answering this question.
Cognitive Level—Analyzing
Client Needs Category—Psychosocial integrity
Client Needs Subcategory—None

Nursing Care of Clients During the Postpartum Period

65. 2. Calf pain when the foot is dorsiflexed is a manifestation of thrombophlebitis. This response is also called a *positive Homans' sign*. Thrombophlebitis, the inflammation of the lining of a blood vessel with clot formation, can involve superficial or deep veins. Clients at risk for developing thrombophlebitis include obese women, those with varicose veins, multiparas, and those older than age 30. It is normal for the client to pass a couple of nickel-sized clots during the first 24 hours after delivery. The client may experience abdominal cramping similar to contraction pain during labor; these contractions, which accompany the involution of the uterus, can be caused by the release of oxytocin when the client is breast-feeding and are more common in multiparous clients. The vaginal discharge is normally dark red during this time.
Test Taking Strategy—Analyze to determine what information the question asks for, which is an abnormal assessment finding in the client who delivered within the past 24 hours. Recall that the physiologic changes occurring postpartum include increased clotting factors, which predispose the postpartum patient to develop thrombosis evidenced by calf pain (option 2). Review postpartum physiological changes and signs of complications if you had difficulty answering this question.
Cognitive Level—Applying
Client Needs Category—Physiological integrity
Client Needs Subcategory—Physiological adaptation

66. 1, 2, 3, 6. Postpartum hemorrhage is a serious, life-threatening condition that can occur within the first 24 hours and up to the first 6 weeks postpartum. The nurse must observe the client closely during the first 24 hours and recognize those clients who are at greatest risk for hemorrhaging. These clients include those who had placenta previa or abruptio placentae, clients who have just delivered multiple infants, clients with high parity, and

those who have had a precipitious (rapid) delivery. Other clients who are at risk for postpartum hemorrhage include those who have had a difficult or prolonged delivery, hydramnios, induction of labor using oxytocin (Pitocin), and a forceps delivery. The presence of late decelerations of the fetal heart rate is not a risk factor for maternal postpartum hemorrhage, nor is primary hypertension.
Test Taking Strategy—Analyze to determine what information the question asks for, which is risk factors for postpartum hemorrhage. Alternative-format "select all that apply" questions require considering each option independently to decide its merit in answering the question. Choose options that correlate with conditions that predispose a client to developing postpartum hemorrhage. Review early and late postpartum hemorrhage and contributing factors if you had difficulty answering this question.
Cognitive Level—Analyzing
Client Needs Category—Physiological integrity
Client Needs Subcategory—Reduction of risk potential

67. 4. Normally, the fundus is firm, hard, and located at, or just below, the level of the umbilicus. Thereafter, it decreases in size each day. Involution eventually returns the uterus to its prepregnant state or a near similar size. A soft and boggy fundus and an increase in lochia are characteristics of uterine bleeding. The first step in controlling uterine bleeding is massaging the fundus, but if bleeding is not reduced, the condition should also be reported to the physician. An oxytocic medication may be indicated to further stimulate uterine contraction.
Test Taking Strategy—Analyze to determine what information the question asks for, which is when fundal massage is indicated during the postpartum period. Recall that bleeding from large uterine blood vessels at the site where the placenta was located is controlled by compression of the contracted uterine muscle. A contracted fundus feels firm, but one that is atonic (relaxed) feels boggy (option 4), predisposing the client to hemorrhage. Massaging the fundus stimulates the uterine muscle to contract. Review characteristics of an atonic fundus and indications for fundal massage if you had difficulty answering this question.
Cognitive Level—Applying
Client Needs Category—Physiological integrity
Client Needs Subcategory—Reduction of risk potential

68. 1. Placing one hand on the fundus of the uterus and the other hand just above the symphysis pubis stabilizes the fundus and prevents the uterus from becoming inverted. The hand placement in the other options will not prevent the uterus from inverting.
Test Taking Strategy—Analyze to determine what information the question asks for regarding correct hand placement during fundal massage. Recall that the hand at the top of the fundus performs the massage while the hand positioned above the symphysis

pubis holds the fundus in place (option 1). Review the technique for fundal massage if you had difficulty answering this question.
Cognitive Level—*Applying*
Client Needs Category—*Health promotion and maintenance*
Client Needs Subcategory—*None*

69.

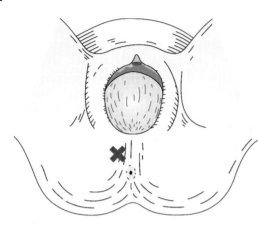

An episiotomy is a surgical enlargement of the vaginal opening that allows easier delivery of the fetus and prevents tearing of the perineum. The incision in a right mediolateral episiotomy begins at the vaginal opening in the midline and then is directed toward the right buttocks at a 45-degree angle. Its main advantage over a midline episiotomy is that it is less likely to extend or tear into the anal sphincter and rectum. However, it is more difficult to repair and the client experiences more discomfort afterward.
   Test Taking Strategy—*Analyze to determine what information the question asks for, which is the location of a right lateral episiotomy. Use the anatomic terms to determine the location of the perineal incision. Note that the right buttock of the client is on the left in the diagram, coinciding with a traditional anatomic position. Review the location of episiotomy sites if you had difficulty answering this question.*
Cognitive Level—*Applying*
Client Needs Category—*Health promotion and maintenance*
Client Needs Subcategory—*None*

70. 3. An episiotomy is the surgical incision made by the physician to avoid perineal tears during delivery. When assessing the perineum of the client who received an episiotomy, the nurse should assist the client to the left side-lying position with the right leg flexed at the knee (Sims' position). The upper buttock is lifted to expose the anus and perineum. This technique allows the best visualization of the perineal area. The positions identified in the other options do not allow for maximal visualization of this area.
   Test Taking Strategy—*Analyze to determine what information the question asks for, which is the client*

position that facilitates assessment of an episiotomy incision. Recall that the episiotomy incision is performed on the obstetrical perineum, which lies between the vaginal opening and the anus. The best position to view this area is the Sims' position (option 3). Review postpartum assessments if you had difficulty answering this question.
Cognitive Level—*Applying*
Client Needs Category—*Health promotion and maintenance*
Client Needs Subcategory—*None*

71. 2. An episiotomy is a surgical incision into the perineum to widen the vaginal opening. If the client has an episiotomy, ice is applied to the perineum initially to reduce the swelling and subsequently decrease the discomfort that may occur from swelling. Sitz baths, heat lamp treatments, and topical cortisone are usually ordered for use after the fourth stage of labor.
   Test Taking Strategy—*Note the key words "most appropriate" and "initially" in reference to the nursing intervention for relieving discomfort associated with an episiotomy repair. For this question, more than one choice may relieve discomfort, but one option is better than the others. Consider measures such as cleanliness, improving circulation, decreasing swelling, and the timeframe since the episiotomy to discriminate among the options. Decide between heat and cold options. Due to the timeframe, an ice pack (option 2) is the most appropriate selection. Review nursing care of the postpartum client if you had difficulty answering questions.*
Cognitive Level—*Analyzing*
Client Needs Category—*Physiological integrity*
Client Needs Subcategory—*Basic care and comfort*

72. 4. A hematoma is the collection of blood in tissue that occurs when a vessel ruptures. A client who develops a perineal hematoma usually complains of a great deal of pain in the perineal area, especially when sutures were needed to repair the episiotomy. The condition should be reported promptly. A hematoma is not associated with a feeling of fullness in the vagina, the presence of heavy and foul-smelling lochia rubra, or separation and purulent drainage from an episiotomy.
   Test Taking Strategy—*Use the process of elimination to help select the option that provides the best indication of the presence of a perineal hematoma. Eliminate options 1, 2, and 3 because they are not characteristic of a hematoma. Recall that the client with a hematoma of the reproductive tract experiences severe, unrelenting pain that analgesics do not relieve (option 4). Review signs and symptoms of complications after delivery if you had difficulty answering this question.*

Cognitive Level—Applying
Client Needs Category—Physiological integrity
Client Needs Subcategory—Reduction of risk potential

73. 2. The fundus of the uterus should feel firm like a grapefruit and in midline when it is palpated after delivery of the infant and placenta. If the fundus deviates to either side, the nurse should suspect that it is caused by a full bladder. Massaging the uterus is unnecessary because the fundus is firm. Waiting to check the client again in 4 hours allows the bladder to fill with an even greater volume of urine. Action should be taken as soon as the nurse notes the fundal deviation.

> *Test Taking Strategy*—Analyze to determine what information the question asks for, which is the action that is appropriate on finding that the fundus deviates from midline. Recall that a full bladder may cause postpartum hemorrhage because it interferes with the uterus contracting appropriately. Having the client empty her bladder (option 2) and then rechecking the fundus is the best nursing action. Review assessment findings of the fundus in the initial postpartum period if you had difficulty with this question.

Cognitive Level—Applying
Client Needs Category—Health promotion and maintenance
Client Needs Subcategory—None

74. 1. The peripad is always applied and removed from front to back to avoid contamination of the perineum. Peripads are changed frequently during the first few days because blood harbors microorganisms that can lead to infection. The nursing assistant should perform hand hygiene before and after helping with perineal care and should wear gloves for the procedure. A peri bottle, if used, should be filled with warm water. A sitz bath is placed on the toilet under the seat and connected to a bag of warm water which soothes the perineal area.

> *Test Taking Strategy*—Analyze to determine what information the question asks for, which is an action in the course of providing perineal hygiene that indicates the nursing assistant requires additional instruction. Evaluate the options for one that is incorrect. Recall the principles of asepsis in which cleaning takes place from clean to dirty areas to reduce the transfer of microorganisms into tissues where healing and avoiding an infection are imperative. Review how to perform perineal care and principles of asepsis if you had difficulty answering this question.

Cognitive Level—Applying
Client Needs Category—Safe and effective care environment
Client Needs Subcategory—Safety and infection control

75. 4. Clients typically have an increase in urine output within the first 24 hours of delivery and void frequently during that time. If an ambulatory client cannot void, the nurse may try giving a warm sitz bath or having the client shower to help her void. If these techniques are unsuccessful, the client should be catheterized with a straight catheter to avoid bladder complications. If the client has to be catheterized more than once, the health care provider may order the insertion of an indwelling catheter. Having the client drink more fluid usually makes the situation worse because it increases the bladder distention.

> *Test Taking Strategy*—The key words are "most appropriate" and "initially," suggesting that the nursing action at the current time may be different from one that may be necessary later or may be utilized if the initial measure is unsuccessful. Recall that initial nursing measures to promote complete emptying of the bladder should use the least invasive means possible, such as assisting with a sitz bath. Review nursing care of the postpartum client and techniques for promoting urination if you had difficulty answering this question.

Cognitive Level—Applying
Client Needs Category—Physiological integrity
Client Needs Subcategory—Basic care and comfort

76. 1. Vaccines may contain small amounts of other components, and it is the nurse's responsibility to be aware of such components to identify potential allergic reactions. The client should be asked if she is allergic to neomycin sulfate (Mycifradin) because the rubella vaccine contains neomycin. It is unnecessary to ask the client if she is allergic to any of the other medications listed because the rubella vaccine does not contain those drugs.

> *Test Taking Strategy*—Analyze to determine what information the question asks for, which is an aspect of the client's allergy history that relates to a component of the rubella vaccine. Recall that neomycin sulfate an additive used to prevent contamination of the vaccine. Anyone who is extremely sensitive to this antibiotic should not be given the rubella vaccine (option 1). Pregnant women should wait to get the vaccine until after they have given birth and avoid getting pregnant for 4 weeks after it has been administered. Review nursing considerations, patient teaching, indications, and contraindications of rubella vaccine administration if you had difficulty answering this question.

Cognitive Level—Applying
Client Needs Category—Health promotion and maintenance
Client Needs Subcategory—Pharmacological therapies

77. 2. Rho(D) immune globulin (RhoGAM) is an injectable immune globulin given to Rh-negative mothers whose fetus is Rh-positive. During the postpartum period, Rho(D) immune globulin should be administered within 72 hours of delivery of the newborn. If it is not administered within this timeframe, the mother is at increased risk for developing antibodies that can cause hemolytic disease in infants who are Rh-positive in the future.

Test Taking Strategy—Analyze to determine what information the question asks for, which is the timeframe during which Rho(D) immune globulin (RhoGAM) can be administered after delivery. Recall that an Rh-negative mother who delivers an Rh-positive infant can produce antibodies within 72 hours to fetal cells that enter the maternal bloodstream after the placenta separates. Administering the immune globulin before those critical 72 hours pass blocks maternal sensitization and antibody production (option 2). Review indications for administering Rho(D) immune globulin if you had difficulty answering this question.
Cognitive Level—*Applying*
Client Needs Category—*Physiological integrity*
Client Needs Subcategory—*Pharmacological therapies*

78. 4. Dysuria (painful urination) and hematuria (blood in the urine) are clinical manifestations of a urinary tract infection (cystitis). A boggy, displaced uterus is usually associated with bladder distention. Urine retention and swelling of the lower extremities are associated with kidney or circulatory problems. Increased thirst (polydipsia) and voiding large amounts of urine (polyuria) are common symptoms of diabetes mellitus.

Test Taking Strategy—Look at the key words "most suggestive" in reference to signs and symptoms of cystitis in the postpartum client. The key words indicate that one option provides a more accurate description than any of the others. Recall that signs and symptoms of cystitis in any client—not just one who is postpartum—include dysuria and hematuria (option 4). Review the manifestations of cystitis if you had difficulty answering this question.
Cognitive Level—*Applying*
Client Needs Category—*Physiological integrity*
Client Needs Subcategory—*Physiological adaptation*

79. 2. Stool softeners should be used only when the client has difficulty passing stools. Drinking at least 2 to 3 quarts of fluids daily, including raw fruits and vegetables in the diet, and taking daily walks are effective ways of preventing constipation.

Test Taking Strategy—Analyze to determine what information the question asks for, which is an incorrect statement by the client that indicates that the client needs additional teaching about methods for avoiding constipation. Identify the option that provides a statement that reflects a misconception by the client. Although a stool softener may eventually promote eliminating moist stool with less effort, medication should be reserved until nonpharmacologic methods prove ineffective. Therefore, option 2 is a statement that warrants additional teaching. Review methods

to facilitate normal bowed elimination if you had difficulty answering this question.
Cognitive Level—*Applying*
Client Needs Category—*Health promotion and maintenance*
Client Needs Subcategory—*None*

80. 1. Normal bladder function usually returns within a few days of delivery. Therefore, the client should notify the health care provider of any difficulty with urination, including burning on urination and the inability to void. These are considered danger signs and may indicate infection or some other complication. Creamy or yellow lochia, *lochia alba*, may be evident at the end of the second or beginning of the third week after delivery. It is composed of white blood cells, remnants of cells, mucus, fat, and other substances that are considered normal as long as it is not accompanied by a foul odor. Changes in lochia color, tearfulness, and breast engorgement are all considered normal findings during the postpartum period.

Test Taking Strategy—Analyze to determine what information the question asks for, which is a symptom that would necessitate notification of the health care provider after the client returns home. Evaluate each option for a symptom that indicates a postpartum complication or deviation in the normal recovery process. Recall that an inability to void (option 1) is significantly abnormal. Review manifestations of postpartum complications if you had difficulty answering this question.
Cognitive Level—*Applying*
Client Needs Category—*Health promotion and maintenance*
Client Needs Subcategory—*None*

81. 3. The best method for alleviating breast engorgement is to breast-feed the newborn frequently. Pumping the breast usually increases the milk supply and further aggravates engorgement. Limiting fluid intake and applying cold compresses or ice packs will suppress lactation and interfere with the production of an adequate amount of milk for feeding. The client can try applying warmth to the breast area instead or wearing a support bra.

Test Taking Strategy—Note the key words "most appropriate" in reference to a suggestion for relieving breast engorgement. Note that one answer is better than the others, some of which may contain accurate information but are not the best answer. Recall that the term engorgement means that the breasts are full of breast milk; nursing the infant (option 3) reduces the volume within the breast. Note that stasis of milk within the breast may lead to mastitis. Review methods for managing breast engorgement if you had difficulty answering this question.
Cognitive Level—*Applying*

Client Needs Category—Health promotion and maintenance
Client Needs Subcategory—None

82. 4. Mastitis is an infection of the breast tissue usually caused by *Staphylococcus aureus*. This infection usually occurs in the second or third postpartum week and is more frequent in primigravidas. To prevent contamination and inflammation of the breast (mastitis), it is important for the client to wash her hands thoroughly or use a hand sanitizer before handling her breasts. A client who is breast-feeding should not wear a breast binder, which may suppress milk production. The nipples should not be cleaned with soap because soap contributes to drying and cracking of the nipples, thereby causing a route for bacteria to enter the breast. Petroleum jelly also should not be applied to the nipples.

> *Test Taking Strategy—Analyze to determine what information the question asks for, which is information that will help the client prevent mastitis. Recall that hand hygiene is the best method for preventing infections (option 4). Review principles of asepsis in relation to interrupting the transmission of microorganisms if you had difficulty answering this question.*
> *Cognitive Level—Applying*
> *Client Needs Category—Safe and effective care environment*
> *Client Needs Subcategory—Safety and infection control*

83. 1. The client may resume sexual intercourse when the perineum is healed and the lochia has ceased. This generally occurs by the third postpartum week, which may be before the postpartum checkup. It is unnecessary to wait for complete involution of the uterus before having sexual intercourse. Also, the client should decide about whether or not to use birth control before resuming intercourse, especially if she wants to avoid becoming pregnant so soon. Ovulation and the potential for becoming pregnant may occur around 6 weeks after delivery. However, the choice of an appropriate method of birth control is not necessarily the most significant factor to consider when deciding when to resume sexual relations. Menses may occur by 9 weeks in a woman who does not breast-feed and around 30 to 36 weeks in one who is lactating. Breast-feeding and the absence of menstruation do not eliminate the potential for ovulation, which was once believed to be true.

> *Test Taking Strategy—Use the process of elimination to select the option that provides the best answer to the client's question about resuming sexual intercourse. Although many postpartum clients experience a low interest in sexual activity for a variety of reasons such as pain from an episiotomy, fatigue, or the presence of lochia, most couples resume sexual intercourse by the third week postpartum (option 1).*

Review sexuality and fertility after delivery of an infant if you had difficulty answering this question.
Cognitive Level—Applying
Client Needs Category—Health promotion and maintenance
Client Needs Subcategory—None

84. 4. The client who feels nervous about going home with a new baby will benefit most from knowing that she can contact the health care facility after her discharge if she has questions. Some facilities also make follow-up phone calls to check on the new mother. The client will probably have the same nervous feeling at the time of the rescheduled discharge if the discharge is postponed, so this action will only relieve the nervousness temporarily. Nervousness is not usually an acceptable reason for postponing the client's discharge. The nurse should acknowledge that the client's feelings are normal and provide her with written instructions on infant care, but these actions alone probably will not alleviate her nervousness.

> *Test Taking Strategy—Note the key words "most appropriate," indicating that one response is better than the others. Providing a means of contacting nursing personnel after discharge (option 4) provides not only a source for reinforcing information on infant care, but also maternal support and reassurance, which written information does not. Review methods for continuity of care after a postpartum discharge if you had difficulty answering this question.*
> *Cognitive Level—Applying*
> *Client Needs Category—Psychosocial integrity*
> *Client Needs Subcategory—None*

85. 1, 2. A puerperal infection is an infection that most often occurs at the unhealed site of placental attachment. It can occur any time during the postpartum period. An elevated temperature, tachycardia over 100 beats/minute, abdominal tenderness, foul-smelling lochia, an abnormally large uterus, and chills are all manifestations of a puerperal infection. When infection is present, the pulse usually increases. The presence of lochia serosa on the fifth postpartum day is considered within normal limits. A continuous trickle of blood is a sign of postpartum hemorrhage, not a puerperal infection. A hematoma is the result of trauma to a blood vessel and is not a sign of a puerperal infection.

> *Test Taking Strategy—Analyze to determine what information the question asks for, which is the most characteristic assessment findings of a puerperal infection. Alternative-format "select all that apply" questions require considering each option independently to decide its merit in answering the question. Choose options that correlate with an infection rather than options that describe normal findings or those associated with complications that are unrelated to the question. Review the signs and symptoms*

of puerperal infection if you had difficulty answering this question.

Cognitive Level—*Applying*
Client Needs Category—*Physiological integrity*
Client Needs Subcategory—*Physiological adaptation*

Nursing Care of the Newborn Client

86. 1, 2, 4. A Mongolian spot is bluish gray pigmentation found on the sacrum, buttocks, or scrotum of children of Asian, southern European, and African American descent. This pigmentation fades by school age and is considered a normal variation of the skin. Milia are pinpoint papules on the nose and cheek that are filled with sebaceous material. They disappear after a couple of weeks and are also considered a normal variation of the skin. Epstein's pearls are small, hard, shiny white specks on the gums and hard palate, not on the skin. They disappear a few days after birth and are of no significance. Erythema toxicum, commonly called newborn rash, is found on the cheeks. It disappears by the third day and is a normal variation of the skin. Molding refers to the shape the newborn's head assumes and retains as it molds to the cervix during delivery. Although a normal finding (especially in primiparous women), it is not associated with the skin. A cephalhematoma is a collection of blood between the periosteum and skull bones that occurs about 1 day after delivery. Although a fairly common finding in newborns, cephalhematoma is not a normal variation of the skin.

> *Test Taking Strategy*—*Analyze to determine what information the question asks for, which is normal skin conditions of the newborn. Alternative-format "select all that apply" questions require considering each option independently to decide its merit in answering the question. Review normal newborn skin variations if you had difficulty answering this question.*

Cognitive Level—*Applying*
Client Needs Category—*Health promotion and maintenance*
Client Needs Subcategory—*None*

87. 1, 4, 5. The normal head circumference of a term newborn is 13″ to 14½″ (34 to 35 cm). Therefore, a head circumference of 20″ (50 cm) is quite large and should be reported immediately because it may be an indication of hydrocephalus resulting from a neural tube disorder. The heart rate of a normal newborn is between 140 and 160 beats/minute; consequently, a heart rate of 100 beats/minute indicates bradycardia and requires immediate attention. A weight of 11 pounds (5 kg) is also considered abnormal and requires immediate notification. A newborn's weight is generally between 5 and 10 pounds (2.5 and 4.7 kg); any weight above this range may be caused by gestational diabetes. Because newborns of

diabetic mothers are generally larger, these newborns are prone to low blood glucose levels and require frequent glucose level monitoring.

A chest circumference of 13″ (33 cm) is within the normal range of 12½″ to 14″ (31.8 to 35.6 cm) for a newborn. Also, a length of 19½″ (50 cm) is within the normal range of 19″ to 21″ (48 to 53 cm). Generally, the chest and abdominal circumferences should be similar in measurement. An abdominal circumference of 11½″ (30 cm) is within normal range for a term newborn.

> *Test Taking Strategy*—*Analyze to determine what information the question asks for regarding abnormal newborn data. Alternative-format "select all that apply" questions require considering each option independently to decide its merit in answering the question. Choose all options that correlate with abnormal, rather than normal, physical assessment findings of the newborn for a correct answer. Review normal ranges for physical assessment findings of the newborn if you had difficulty answering this question.*

Cognitive Level—*Applying*
Client Needs Category—*Physiological integrity*
Client Needs Subcategory—*Reduction of risk potential*

88. 1, 2, 3, 4. The nurse should expect to find the rooting, Moro, tonic neck, and extrusion reflexes in a normal newborn. The rooting reflex serves to help the newborn find food. It is manifested when stroking the newborn's cheek or mouth causes him to turn his head toward the same direction. The rooting reflex disappears at about 2 months, when the infant's eyesight improves. The Moro reflex, also called the *startle reflex*, is a protective mechanism that fades by the fourth to fifth month, when the infant can roll away from danger. The tonic neck reflex is described as a fencing position: When the newborn lies supine, the head is usually turned to the side, and the arm and leg on the same side are extended while the arm and leg on the opposite side are contracted. The tonic neck reflex does not appear to have a particular function, as the other reflexes do. The extrusion reflex is a protective mechanism that prevents the infant from swallowing inedible substances. It is manifested by protrusion of the tongue when any substance is placed on its tip (the infant appears to spit out the substance). This reflex usually fades at about 4 months, at which time solid foods are usually introduced. Barlow and Ortolani are not reflexes. The terms are associated with the assessment of congenital hip dislocation.

> *Test Taking Strategy*—*Analyze to determine what information the question asks for regarding normal reflexes in the full-term newborn. Alternative-format "select all that apply" questions require considering each option independently to decide its merit in answering the question. Review newborn reflexes if you had difficulty answering this question.*

Cognitive Level—Applying
Client Needs Category—Health promotion and maintenance
Client Needs Subcategory—None

89. 7.7 pounds (or 7 pounds, 11 ounces).
Remember that 1 kg = 2.2 pounds. To convert, multiply 3.5 kg by 2.2 pounds = 7.7 pounds.

Test Taking Strategy—Analyze to determine what information the question asks for, which involves converting the infant's weight in kilograms to its equivalent in pounds and ounces. Recall that a weight in kilograms is less than in pounds. Review conversion equivalents if you had difficulty answering this question.
Cognitive Level—Applying
Client Needs Category—Health promotion and maintenance
Client Needs Subcategory—None

90. 3, 5, 6. Yellow skin discoloration within 24 hours of the newborn's birth indicates physiologic jaundice. This finding should be reported immediately so that the health care provider can order the appropriate treatment. Nasal flaring and substernal and intercostal retractions are signs of respiratory distress and should be reported immediately. Respiratory distress may occur as a result of cold stress; therefore, if these findings are seen, the nurse should stop bathing the baby. Bluish discoloration of the hands and feet, a pulse rate of 140 beats/minute, and slightly swollen labia are all normal findings in a female newborn.

Test Taking Strategy—Analyze to determine what information the question asks for, which is assessment findings that must be reported "immediately." Alternative-format "select all that apply" questions require considering each option independently to decide its merit in answering the question. Choose options that correlate with abnormalities in the newborn. Review expected physical characteristics of the newborn and signs that warrant concern if you had difficulty answering this question.
Cognitive Level—Applying
Client Needs Category—Physiological integrity
Client Needs Subcategory—Physiological adaptation

91. 2. The axillary temperature of a normal newborn ranges from 97.7°F to 98.6°F (36.5°C to 37°C). Any lower temperature is associated with hypothermia. The hypothermic newborn should be placed on a prewarmed radiant warmer and rewarmed gradually over a period of approximately 2 hours. Warming the newborn too rapidly can result in apnea and acidosis. When the temperature is within the acceptable range, the newborn can be dressed, wrapped in a blanket, and placed in an open crib; the temperature should be rechecked again in 4 to 8 hours.

Test Taking Strategy—Use the key terms "most appropriate" to select the option that is better than

the others based on an evaluation of the infant's temperature. Recall that the newborn's temperature is below normal and indicates that warming measures are necessary. Consider nursing actions, such as skin-to-skin contact with the mother, applying a knitted cap, and placing the newborn in a radiant warmer until body temperature increases. Review the acceptable range in newborn temperature and methods for warming the infant if you had difficulty answering this question.*
Cognitive Level—Applying
Client Needs Category—Physiological integrity
Client Needs Subcategory—Reduction of risk potential

92. 1, 3, 4, 6. Newborn safety is a major focus in the hospital. Therefore, addressing this issue with the parents is the prudent thing to do. The nurse should instruct the parents to look at their baby's ID band during each visit because these bracelets are prone to falling off and becoming lost when dressing and undressing the newborn. The mother (and, in some cases, the father or significant other) should also wear an ID bracelet throughout her stay. Hospital personnel should check the name bracelets of both the mother and baby on entering the room. Because only authorized hospital personnel should be allowed in the mother's room, the nurse should instruct the mother to look for a valid hospital ID on anyone entering the room. To prevent infections, visitors who come to see the mother and baby should be instructed to wash their hands or use an alcohol-based hand sanitizer before holding or caring for the infant. In addition, the mother should be instructed to wash her hands before attending to the baby's needs. The mother is instructed to never leave the baby unattended when showering or leaving the room and ask that the baby be taken back to the nursery.

After delivery, most mothers are extremely tired. Having the newborn sleep in bed with the mother is not considered safe practice. Mothers should also be advised not to breast-feed or bottle-feed their babies in bed during the night after returning home.

Test Taking Strategy—Analyze to determine what information the question asks for regarding newborn safety in the hospital. Alternative-format "select all that apply" questions require considering each option independently to decide its merit in answering the question. Choose options that correlate with safe care and protection of the newborn. Review safety principles that apply to the newborn if you had difficulty answering this question.
Cognitive Level—Applying
Client Needs Category—Safe and effective care environment
Client Needs Subcategory—Safety and infection control

93. 2, 3, 4. Mother-infant bonding is usually a natural occurrence after delivery. To adequately assess bonding, the nurse should observe the mother's interactions with the baby and listen to what she is saying. The nurse should also assess the mother's nonverbal cues, such as how she looks at the baby during the first few hours after birth and while breast-feeding. The mother should be touching the baby and making good eye contact. Talking or singing to the baby and discussing the baby's physical attributes are also good signs of mother-infant bonding. To facilitate bonding, the mother should hold her baby close to her (not far away). Becoming upset because the baby spits up should alert the nurse that further observation is warranted. Repeatedly asking if the baby is going to live indicates an unwillingness to invest in the bonding process.

Test Taking Strategy—Analyze to determine what information the question asks for, which is maternal actions that indicate mother–infant bonding. Alternative-format "select all that apply" questions require considering each option independently to decide its merit in answering the question. Select all the options that correlate with maternal actions that indicate mother-infant bonding. Review characteristics of mother-infant bonding and nursing care to promote emotional attachment if you had difficulty answering this question.
***Cognitive Level—**Applying*
***Client Needs Category—**Psychosocial integrity*
***Client Needs Subcategory—**None*

94. 1. Each breast consists of lobules that house the milk-secreting cells. The size of the breast is determined by the amount of adipose tissue, not the milk-secreting cells. Therefore, breast size has nothing to do with a woman's ability to breast-feed.

Test Taking Strategy—Apply the key words "most appropriate" when analyzing the options. Note that one response to the client's question about breast size and the ability to breast-feed is better than the others. Recall that the structures that produce breast milk are normally present regardless of the breast's physical size (option 1). Review the process of lactation if you had difficulty answering this question.
***Cognitive Level—**Applying*
***Client Needs Category—**Health promotion and maintenance*
***Client Needs Subcategory—**None*

95. 1. During the first few days after delivery, all newborns normally lose up to 10% of their birth weight, but gain approximately 4 to 7 ounces (113 to 198) per week in the first month after birth. It is not necessarily true that a newborn who bottle-feeds first will not successfully breast-feed because of a preference for a bottle nipple. The nurse should advise the client that it is preferable to breast-feed rather than pump the breast because the infant's sucking stimulates production of an adequate amount of milk to meet the newborn's needs. Also, breast-fed newborns benefit from the colostrum initially present in breast milk.

Test Taking Strategy—Note the key words "most appropriate," indicating one option is a better choice than the others. Some options may be true depending on unique situations and personal experiences, but the best answer is option 1 because it offers the mother factual information that applies to the weight pattern of almost all newborns. Review growth and weight patterns during the neonatal period if you had difficulty answering this question.
***Cognitive Level—**Analyzing*
***Client Needs Category—**Health promotion and maintenance*
***Client Needs Subcategory—**None*

96. 2. Newborns have very small digestive systems, and colostrum delivers its components in a very concentrated low-volume form. Colostrum is a thin, yellowish fluid that contains maternal antibodies known as immunoglobulins as well as other highly nutritional and protective substances. The maternal antibodies found in colostrum prevent infection and provide passive immunity for the newborn. Also, colostrum has a laxative effect and helps the newborn expel the thick meconium normally present in the intestinal tract at birth. Colostrum does not contain estrogen, predigested fats, or digestive enzymes.

Test Taking Strategy—Analyze to determine what information the question asks for regarding the beneficial substance contained in colostrum. Recall that colostrum contains maternal antibodies (option 2) that are not present in commercial formula. Review the components in colostrum if you had difficulty answering this question.
***Cognitive Level—**Applying*
***Client Needs Category—**Health promotion and maintenance*
***Client Needs Subcategory—**None*

97. 3. A breast or nipple shield is not routinely used for breast-feeding. A breast shield is worn when the nipple is flat or inverted, occasionally when the nipple is sore and cracked, or when a premature infant cannot latch on to the maternal nipple. Because the infant has to rely on suction alone to transfer milk, nipple shields can drastically reduce milk production, milk intake, and possibly cause slow or inadequate weight gain. The other options identify correct breast-feeding techniques.

Test Taking Strategy—Analyze to determine what information the question asks for, which is an action by the new mother in reference to breast-feeding that indicates the mother needs additional teaching. Read the options carefully because the correct answer must correlate with an incorrect action. Because a breast shield is unnecessary in most circumstances, a client who routinely incorporates its use requires more information. Review principles for promoting successful breastfeeding if you had difficulty answering this question.

Cognitive Level—*Applying*
Client Needs Category—*Health promotion and maintenance*
Client Needs Subcategory—*None*

98. 4. When suctioning the newborn with a bulb syringe, the bulb should be compressed before it is placed in the nose or mouth, and then decompressed once it is inserted so that mucus can be aspirated. The mouth should be suctioned before the nose to prevent aspiration during the gag response. Also, the back of the throat should not be touched when suctioning the mouth because the gag reflex may be stimulated.

> *Test Taking Strategy*—*Analyze to determine what information the question asks for, which is an indication that the mother requires additional teaching regarding the use of a bulb syringe. Select the option that describes an incorrect statement concerning the technique for removing secretions from the infant's nose and mouth. Recall that secretions cannot be removed if the bulb syringe remains compressed (option 4). Review how to clear an infant's nose and mouth of secretions using a bulb syringe if you had difficulty answering this question.*
> *Cognitive Level*—*Applying*
> *Client Needs Category*—*Health promotion and maintenance*
> *Client Needs Subcategory*—*None*

99. 4. The newborn should be placed supine (on the back) when positioned in the crib. If swaddled, the infant's head must be exposed and the practice discontinued when the infant is able to roll over. Placing a newborn or infant in the prone position (on the stomach) is associated with sudden infant death syndrome (SIDS). Pillows, comforters, bumper pads, and soft toys should be avoided until the infant is at least 8 months old. The side-lying position may prevent aspiration, but does not facilitate gastric emptying, and an active infant could roll onto his or her stomach.

> *Test Taking Strategy*—*Use the process of elimination to select the option that identifies the best position to place an infant when putting the infant in a crib. Recall that the American Academy of Pediatrics and the American Public Health Association advise that newborns be placed in a supine position when in a crib. Review the recommended position for a sleeping infant if you had difficulty answering this question.*
> *Cognitive Level*—*Applying*
> *Client Needs Category*—*Health promotion and maintenance*
> *Client Needs Subcategory*—*None*

100. 2. A newborn whose nutritional needs are not being met is at risk for developing dehydration. One indication of dehydration in a newborn is having fewer than six wet diapers per day. It is normal for a breast-fed newborn to have loose, pale-yellow stools, sometimes after each feeding, to awaken during the night for a feeding, and to feed every 2 to 3 hours.

> *Test Taking Strategy*—*Analyze to determine what information the question asks for, which is evidence that a newborn is not receiving adequate nutrition from breast-feeding. Evaluate each option for characteristics that are typical among newborns. Recall that fluid volume is regulated primarily by urine excretion. Hence, if the intake of breast milk is low, the number of wet diapers will decrease (option 2). Review methods for evaluating the adequacy of nourishment in an infant who is breastfed if you had difficulty answering this question.*
> *Cognitive Level*—*Analyzing*
> *Client Needs Category*—*Health promotion and maintenance*
> *Client Needs Subcategory*—*None*

101. 3. Breast milk should be refrigerated immediately after being pumped; it should not be allowed to sit at room temperature. Refrigerated breast milk can be stored for up to 5 days, according to the American Academy of Pediatrics and the Centers for Disease Control and Prevention. La Leche League International says that breast milk stored in the refrigerator is best used within 72 hours but will remain acceptable for up to 8 days. The breast milk should be stored in clear hard plastic bottles, glass containers with tight-fitting lids, or in breast milk bags (not disposable bottle liners) that are marked with the date. After collection, the breast milk should be placed in the back of the main body of the refrigerator to reduce the potential for warming when the door is opened. Breast milk can be stored in a freezer (one with separate refrigerator and freezer doors) for up to 3 months or in a deep-freezer for up to 12 months. However, the antibodies in frozen breast milk are not as well preserved as those in refrigerated breast milk.

> *Test Taking Strategy*—*Analyze to determine what information the question asks for, which is proper storage guidelines for breast milk. Recall that breast milk that has been properly refrigerated can be safely used up to 8 days after its collection (option 3). Review protocols for storing refrigerated breast milk if you had difficulty answering this question.*
> *Cognitive Level*—*Understanding*
> *Client Needs Category*—*Health promotion and maintenance*
> *Client Needs Subcategory*—*None*

102. 4. Postterm newborns (delivered at 41 weeks' gestation or more) are at risk for such complications as meconium aspiration if the pregnancy is allowed to progress longer than 42 weeks. Usually, labor needs to be induced.

Postterm newborns are usually lighter in weight because of placental insufficiency and have dry, cracked, leathery skin. They also lack vernix and have longer than normal fingernails. Premature babies tend to have flat, shapeless ears; legs in a froglike position; and few sole creases.

> *Test Taking Strategy*—*Analyze to determine what information the question asks for, which is a characteristic of a postterm newborn that differs from one that is preterm or full term. Recall that infants born after remaining in the womb for longer than 41 weeks have little remaining vernix caseosa, a substance rich in sebum. Consequently, the skin is dry, cracked, wrinkled, peeling, and whiter than a newborn at or near full term. Review the characteristics of infants born after a prolonged pregnancy if you had difficulty answering this question.*
> *Cognitive Level*—*Applying*
> *Client Needs Category*—*Health promotion and maintenance*
> *Client Needs Subcategory*—*None*

103. 2. The umbilical cord normally has two arteries and one vein. The presence of one single umbilical artery (SUA) may occur because one artery stops growing or the embryonic umbilical artery does not divide properly. The anomaly occurs in 1 of 100 newborns and is not exclusive or predominantly seen among postterm infants. Having an SUA is associated with congenital anomalies, particularly kidney defects. However, although SUA is one of the most common umbilical abnormalities, half to two thirds of infants with SUA are born healthy with no chromosomal or congenital abnormalities. Normal findings in a postterm infant include a pendulous scrotum with numerous rugae, minimal vernix caseosa with remnants in body creases, and bluish discoloration of the hands and feet (acrocyanosis).

> *Test Taking Strategy*—*Analyze to determine what information the question asks for, which is an abnormal assessment finding in the newborn. Recall that having a single umbilical artery (option 2) may be associated with other physical defects and should prompt the nurse to examine the newborn for evidence of other abnormalities. Review the anatomy of normal umbilical blood vessels and the significance if there are fewer vessels than the expected norm if you had difficulty answering this question.*
> *Cognitive Level*—*Applying*
> *Client Needs Category*—*Health promotion and maintenance*
> *Client Needs Subcategory*—*None*

104. 1. Congenital hip dysplasia is a defect that occurs when the head of the femur is not located securely within the acetabulum or rides on its rim. Asymmetry of the gluteal skin folds, limited abduction of the affected hip, apparent shortening of the femur, and a clicking sound heard when abducting the hips are signs of congenital hip dys-

plasia. Early identification and treatment are essential for preventing a chronic deformity. To correct the deformity, the hip needs to be maintained in a position of flexion and abduction for 3 to 4 months. Absence of spontaneous leg movement may be associated with other musculoskeletal disorders but usually is not seen in a newborn with congenital hip dysplasia. An exaggerated curvature of the lumbar spine (lordosis) is unrelated to congenital hip dysplasia.

> *Test Taking Strategy*—*Note the key words are "most indicative" when analyzing the options, looking for one that describes an assessment finding of a newborn with congenital hip dysplasia. Recall that one of the characteristic signs of this defect is that the folds of the buttocks are not symmetrical (option 1), with more creases being on the side of the dysplastic hip. Review the signs of congenital hip dysplasia if you had difficulty answering this question.*
> *Cognitive Level*—*Applying*
> *Client Needs Category*—*Physiological integrity*
> *Client Needs Subcategory*—*Physiological adaptation*

105. 2. The newborn should be positioned semi-upright rather than in the supine position during feeding. Infants seem to bottle-feed best when held close and at a 45-degree angle, which keeps air bubbles from being swallowed. A supine position increases the risk for aspiration and the possibility for the infant to develop otitis media if milk enters the eustachian tubes. The techniques stated in the other options are correct for bottle-feeding the newborn.

> *Test Taking Strategy*—*Analyze to determine what information the question asks for, which is an incorrect bottle-feeding technique that is potentially unsafe. Recall that some women prefer to position the infant on a feeding pillow or wedge that facilitates elevating the infant's body while being fed to avoid a supine position (option 2). Review principles for bottle-feeding if you had difficulty answering this question.*
> *Cognitive Level*—*Applying*
> *Client Needs Category*—*Health promotion and maintenance*
> *Client Needs Subcategory*—*None*

106. 4. Positioning the bottle so that the nipple remains full of formula throughout the feeding prevents the baby from swallowing air. Keeping the nipple full of formula does not affect the infant's gums, nor will it cause the infant to gulp formula; gulping is generally due to nipple holes that are too large. This technique also does not appear to prevent the infant from getting tired while feeding.

> *Test Taking Strategy*—*Analyze to determine what information the question asks for regarding the consequence of not keeping the nipple on the bottle filled with formula. Recall that having air in the nipple means that the newborn is ingesting air as well as formula. Swallowing air (option 4) from a partially filled nipple can lead to the infant experiencing gas pains, especially*

if burping is not effective or sufficient to expel the air orally. Review techniques for bottle-feeding an infant if you had difficulty answering this question.
Cognitive Level—*Applying*
Client Needs Category—*Health promotion and maintenance*
Client Needs Subcategory—*None*

107. **3.** Prepared formula can be refrigerated for up to 48 hours. However, any formula remaining in the bottle when the newborn has finished feeding should be discarded. Bottles can be washed in a dishwasher or with hot, soapy water or warm tap water. If the water source is questionable, tap water should be boiled first. Also, the lid of the can of formula concentrate should be wiped before being opened to prevent transferring microorganisms to the contents of the can.

> **Test Taking Strategy**—*Analyze to determine what information the question asks for, which is an incorrect statement regarding formula preparation that demonstrates a need for additional teaching. Consider that appropriate teaching about bottle-feeding addresses equipment such as the bottles as well as formula preparation. Recall that like breast milk, a supply of reconstituted commercial formula can be stored for a period of time, making option 3 an incorrect statement. Consult information about how commercial formula should be prepared and stored if you had difficulty answering this question.*
Cognitive Level—*Applying*
Client Needs Category—*Health promotion and maintenance*
Client Needs Subcategory—*None*

108. **1.** Phototherapy is a noninvasive method for treating hyperbilirubinemia that involves exposing the infant's skin to fluorescent light or bulbs in the blue-light spectrum. Phototherapy alters the structure of bilirubin to a soluble form that is easier to excrete. The nurse should apply protective eyeshields to prevent retinopathy from exposure to ultraviolet lights used in the treatment. The infant should be naked except for a diaper. Applying a topical SPF15 cream defeats the purpose of phototherapy. Reflective—not nonreflective—material, such as white linen, is used to cover the inside of the bassinet. The nurse should monitor the newborn's temperature frequently, assessing for hypothermia (from being unclothed) and hyperthermia (because of exposure to the light source). The infant's position should be changed frequently to ensure exposure of all body surfaces to the ultraviolet light.

> **Test Taking Strategy**—*The key words "most appropriate" may indicate that more than one option may have some valid information, but one answer is better than the others. Consider the nature of phototherapy and its inherent risks to the infant. Protecting the infant's eyes (option 1) is a priority. Review nurs-*

ing responsibilities when managing the care of an infant undergoing phototherapy if you had difficulty answering this question.
Cognitive Level—*Applying*
Client Needs Category—*Physiological integrity*
Client Needs Subcategory—*Reduction of risk potential*

109. **3.** After circumcision, the newborn's penis should be frequently assessed for signs of swelling and bleeding, the most common complications associated with the circumcision procedure. If penile swelling occurs, the urinary meatus may be occluded, affecting urine output. Therefore, monitoring urine elimination is an appropriate nursing intervention. Petroleum gauze dressings are not required when a Plastibell is in place. In most cases, it is unnecessary to check the vital signs more frequently unless there are complications such as hemorrhage. Bacteriostatic ointments may be applied if a Gomco circumcision has been performed; otherwise, the health care provider should be consulted for further instructions when an infection is suspected. Placing the newborn on his abdomen is inappropriate because the nurse cannot assess the amount of bleeding if it occurs; also, newborns should not be positioned this way because of the risk of sudden infant death syndrome.

> **Test Taking Strategy**—*The key words "most appropriate" may indicate that more than one option contains information with some validity, but one option is better than the others. Recall that bleeding and swelling (option 3) are likely to occur after the foreskin of the penis is removed. Review the nursing care of an infant after a circumcision if you had difficulty answering this question.*
Cognitive Level—*Applying*
Client Needs Category—*Physiological integrity*
Client Needs Subcategory—*Reduction of risk potential*

110. **1.** The physician should be notified if there is any drainage from the penis, if there are any blood spots larger than the size of a quarter, if the infant is not voiding, and if the Plastibell ring has not fallen off in 7 days. The Plastibell ring should not be removed manually. The penis should be gently cleaned with soap and water. It is unnecessary to apply petroleum jelly to the penis if a Plastibell ring is in place.

> **Test Taking Strategy**—*Analyze to determine what information the question asks for, which is evidence that the nursing instructions on the care of the circumcised infant have been effective. Recall that penile skin and tissue have been impaired, creating a potential for infection. Therefore, consulting the pediatrician if unusual penile drainage is observed (option 1) indicates that the parents have understood the teaching the nurse has provided concerning a potential complication. Review home care of an infant after a circumcision if you had difficulty answering this question.*

Cognitive Level—*Applying*
Client Needs Category—*Health promotion and maintenance*
Client Needs Subcategory—*None*

111. 1. A phenylketonuria (PKU) test is done to check whether a newborn lacks an enzyme needed to metabolize phenylalanine, an essential amino acid that is needed for normal brain function. Mental retardation occurs if the condition is untreated. The newborn should be drinking breast milk or formula for at least 2 to 3 days before a phenylketonuria (PKU) test is performed. If the newborn has not been receiving nutrition for the prescribed time, the result may be inaccurate. Newborns discharged before this time should have the test performed within the prescribed amount of time in an outpatient setting, such as the pediatrician's office or a clinic. The data identified in the remaining options are not needed when performing the PKU test.

> *Test Taking Strategy*—*Note the key words "most important" in reference to information that is essential to obtain before the PKU screening test. Phenylalanine is present in milk and other protein food sources. If there has been an insufficient intake of milk (option 1), the test will be unable to detect an accumulation of phenylalanine in the infant's blood and will be of no benefit in diagnosing the genetic disorder at this time. Review guidelines for performing a PKU screening test on a newborn if you had difficulty answering this question.*
> *Cognitive Level*—*Applying*
> *Client Needs Category*—*Physiological integrity*
> *Client Needs Subcategory*—*Reduction of risk potential*

112.

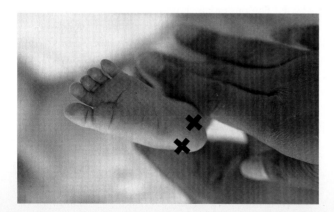

A sample of capillary blood from a newborn is obtained by performing a heelstick. The area that is punctured is located on the lateral aspect of the baby's heel on either the left or right side.

> *Test Taking Strategy*—*Analyze to determine what information the question asks for, which is the location for obtaining a sample of blood for a PKU screening*

test. The anatomic location where the heel is punctured is an area of least sensitivity for the infant. Review the procedure for obtaining a specimen of blood with a heelstick on a newborn if you had difficulty answering this question.
> *Cognitive Level*—*Applying*
> *Client Needs Category*—*Physiological integrity*
> *Client Needs Subcategory*—*Reduction of risk potential*

113. 4. The blood that has been applied within the circles on the test collection card must dry at room temperature, out of heat and direct light for 3 to 4 hours, before closing the specimen card. The nurse is correct to warm the heel, apply pressure to the heel once it has been punctured to obtain a large drop of blood, and completely fill the circle with blood on the collection card when performing the phenylketonuria (PKU) test.

> *Test Taking Strategy*—*Analyze to determine what information the question asks for, which is an incorrect nursing action when performing a PKU screening test. Recall that closing the collection card before the drops of blood have completely dried may alter the test results. Review the procedure for obtaining a specimen of capillary blood for a PKU screening test if you had difficulty answering this question.*
> *Cognitive Level*—*Applying*
> *Client Needs Category*—*Physiological integrity*
> *Client Needs Subcategory*—*Reduction of risk potential*

114. 1, 3, 4. Safety of all patients is a priority for hospital employees. If an infant is abducted from the nursery, each hospital employee should be observant of persons carrying boxes or bags where an infant may be hidden. Making a thorough search of areas such as closets, stairwells, laundry bins, and other places where an infant may be hidden is also appropriate. It is always prudent to report suspicious persons to security. Calling in the Federal Bureau of Investigation (FBI) before a thorough search is made is not timely. Typically local law enforcement is called before notifying the FBI. Questioning every visitor in the building is time-consuming and will take away valuable opportunity needed to search for the missing infant. Questioning the mother about why she left the child unattended is accusatory, and this line of questioning will not help locate the missing baby.

> *Test Taking Strategy*—*Analyze to determine what information the question asks for, which is priority actions to take if an infant is abducted from a hospital nursery. Alternative-format "select all that apply" questions require considering each option independently to decide its merit in answering the question. Choose options that prevent an infant's abduction. Review procedures that ensure the safety of infants in a newborn nursery if you had difficulty answering this question.*

Cognitive Level—Applying
Client Needs Category—Safe and effective care
  environment
Client Needs Subcategory—Safety and infection control

Nursing Care of Newborns with Complications

115. 1. A client who is experiencing grief may delay naming her newborn, may be reluctant to visit the baby in the nursery, or may focus on equipment and treatments rather than the baby when visiting. Asking the physician to postpone her discharge from the hospital is not a sign of anticipatory grieving; instead, this request is often made because the client does not want to leave the newborn.

> *Test Taking Strategy—Use the process of elimination to select the option that identifies the best indication that a mother is disappointed with having given birth to a child with physical abnormalities. Option 2 can be eliminated because a grieving mother may distance herself from the infant rather than visiting frequently. Option 3 can be eliminated because postponing discharge may be a way of indicating a fear of being ultimately responsible for the infant's care. Option 4 can be eliminated because the mother may be fearful or stressed when the infant is undergoing procedures. Although all of the options describe behaviors that are atypical for most new mothers, Option 1 is the most pathological because not giving the child a name indicates that the mother has not fully accepted the reality of the infant's identity and is avoiding a personal relationship with the infant who is less than ideal. Review maternal reactions to an infant born with disabilities if you had difficulty answering this question.*

Cognitive Level—Analyzing
Client Needs Category—Psychosocial integrity
Client Needs Subcategory—None

116. 2. A myelomeningocele is a neural tube defect that occurs during the embryonic development of the nervous system, when the spinal column fails to cover the spinal cord. This defect is evident by the presence of the meninges and spinal cord protruding outside the vertebral column. Because of the exposure of the meninges, meningitis is a realistic complication. Motor and sensory functions are affected beyond the point of the defect, resulting in paralysis of the lower extremities and loss of bowel and bladder function. Hydrocephalus and clubfoot are common findings in conjunction with this defect. To facilitate acceptance and care of the newborn with this defect, the nurse should act as a role model by demonstrating the proper way to feed, hold, and change the newborn. This will encourage the parents to interact with their baby and promote early bonding. Although surgery will result in closure of the defect, it may not correct the neurologic

deficit that accompanies this condition. Showing the parents "before" and "after" surgery pictures is usually more effective when the surgical intervention results in correction of the deformity or disorder; however, this is not the case with myelomeningocele. Social agencies usually do not take custody or assume care of an infant unless there is due cause, such as neglect or abuse.

> *Test Taking Strategy—Use the process of elimination to select the best nursing action for promoting the mother's acceptance and care of the infant with a myelomeningocele. Recall that by demonstrating nurturing care of the infant (option 2) the nurse is modeling behaviors that hopefully the mother will imitate. Review the desired outcome of the nurse acting as a role model for a new mother if you had difficulty answering this question.*

Cognitive Level—Applying
Client Needs Category—Psychosocial integrity
Client Needs Subcategory—None

117. 1. Retinopathy of prematurity (ROP) is abnormal blood vessel development in the retina of the eye. When oxygen is given in high concentrations to a premature newborn in respiratory distress, the newborn becomes especially vulnerable to developing blindness due to hemorrhage of blood vessels in the eyes followed by retinal detachment. Therefore, frequent monitoring of the oxygen concentration is necessary to ensure that excessive amounts are not given. Assessment of the bilirubin level, hemoglobin level, and pupillary response will not assist the nurse in preventing ROP.

> *Test Taking Strategy—The key word is "essential," indicating that the statement in one option is a priority for preventing the development of ROP. Recall that excessive oxygen levels used to treat premature babies can stimulate abnormal growth of blood vessels in the retina. If oxygen concentrations within the isolette are closely monitored (option 1), the condition may not develop. Review ROP if you had difficulty answering this question.*

Cognitive Level—Applying
Client Needs Category—Safe and effective care
  environment
Client Needs Subcategory—Safety and infection
  control

118. 3. Preterm newborns may have weak or absent sucking and swallowing reflexes. These infants may require nasogastric formula or breast milk feeding, or feedings of parenteral fluids (total parenteral nutrition [TPN] and lipids) by an umbilical catheter or peripheral vein. The normal interval between formula or breast milk feedings is 2 to 3 hours. The amount fed depends on the infant's weight, but it may be as little as 1 to 5 mL for each feeding. If glucose is tolerated, the physician may order a formula similar to that fed to normal-sized newborns.

Test Taking Strategy—*Apply the key words "most appropriate" to the statements in each option. Select the option that identifies the best method for feeding a preterm infant. Recall that an infant born before 35 weeks' gestation lacks the ability to coordinate sucking, swallowing, and breathing making oral feeding potentially unsafe. Gavage feeding (option 3) also causes less fatigue, allowing the infant to conserve energy and gain weight. Review the challenges involved in providing nutrition for a preterm infant's growth and development if you had difficulty answering this question.*
Cognitive Level—*Applying*
Client Needs Category—*Health promotion and maintenance*
Client Needs Subcategory—*None*

119. 2. The primary reason that a preterm newborn is at risk for developing infections is the lack of maternal antibodies normally supplied during the third trimester of pregnancy and the newborn's inability to produce antibodies independently. Care is taken to prevent exposure to bacterial and viral infections; procedures are done using strict asepsis. The preterm newborn does have fragile skin, but appropriate measures are taken to prevent skin breakdown.
Test Taking Strategy—*Analyze to determine what information the question asks for regarding the primary risk factor that predisposes the preterm infant to acquiring an infection. Recall that a preterm infant is exposed to life support systems involving ventilators and various types of catheters, which compromise an already poorly developed immune system (option 2). Review risk factors that affect low-birthweight infants.*
Cognitive Level—*Applying*
Client Needs Category—*Physiological integrity*
Client Needs Subcategory—*Physiological adaptation*

120. 3. The preterm newborn is kept in an isolette or radiant warmer because of the increased risk of cold stress due to the immaturity of the brain's temperature-regulating centers, the absence of subcutaneous fat, and the large surface area of the newborn's head. The other actions are appropriate to maintain thermoregulation in a full-term newborn but are inadequate for the preterm newborn's special needs.
Test Taking Strategy—*Use the process of elimination to select the option that identifies the best method for preventing the preterm infant from a lower than desired body temperature. Options 1, 2, and 4 are appropriate for infants who are born at term but are not the best choice for preterm infants. Option 3 is the best answer because an isolette or radiant warmer provides a direct source of heat to the infant. Review nursing care of a preterm infant,*

especially in relation to preventing low body temperature, if you had difficulty answering this question.
Cognitive Level—*Applying*
Client Needs Category—*Physiological integrity*
Client Needs Subcategory—*Physiological adaptation*

121. 4. Congenital hemolytic disease of the newborn is also known as *erythroblastosis fetalis*. Erythroblastosis fetalis results from Rh incompatibility between a Rh-positive neonate and an Rh-negative mother who was previously sensitized by carrying an Rh-positive infant and never received Rho(D) immune globulin (RhoGAM). Jaundice within 24 to 36 hours of birth indicates erythroblastosis fetalis. Physiological jaundice, which occurs in some newborns, is seen 3 to 4 days after birth. Alterations in the respiratory rate, newborn reflexes, and movement of extremities are not usual manifestations associated with Rh incompatibility.
Test Taking Strategy—*The key words "most indicative" indicate that one option is best for describing a key characteristic of an infant who is born with erythroblastosis fetalis. Recall that the neonate's red blood cells (RBCs) are extensively destroyed during fetal development. To compensate, the fetus's bone marrow makes more and more immature RBCs (erythroblasts). The destroyed RBCs elevate bilirubin, causing jaundice (option 4). Review the etiology and clinical manifestations of erythroblastosis fetalis if you had difficulty answering this question.*
Cognitive Level—*Applying*
Client Needs Category—*Physiological integrity*
Client Needs Subcategory—*Physiological adaptation*

122. 4. The direct Coombs' test requires a sample of the newborn's blood. The usual procedure is to obtain a specimen from the umbilical cord after the newborn is delivered and the cord is cut. An indirect Coombs' test is performed using a specimen of maternal blood. Paternal blood and sibling blood are not used for a direct or indirect Coombs' test.
Test Taking Strategy—*Analyze to determine what information the question asks for, which is the source of the blood specimen for performing a direct Coombs' test. Recall that if Rh-positive sensitization was suspected during the prenatal period, an indirect Coombs' test on maternal blood would be done to confirm a previous exposure to Rh antigens. Without prior testing, a direct Coombs' test can be performed postnatally on umbilical cord blood (option 4). A positive test result confirms the diagnosis. Review the indications for performing a direct and indirect Coombs' test and the significance of the test results if you had difficulty answering this question.*

Cognitive Level—*Understanding*
Client Needs Category—*Physiological integrity*
Client Needs Subcategory—*Reduction of risk potential*

123. 1. When the human immunodeficiency virus (HIV) infection status of any client is unknown, which includes a newborn with an HIV-positive mother, standard precautions are implemented. Standard precautions were developed by the U.S. Centers for Disease Control and Prevention in an effort to reduce the risk of transmitting bloodborne and body fluid pathogens when the infectious status of a person is unknown. Generally, if the HIV-positive status of the mother is known prenatally, antiretroviral therapy is begun before delivery to significantly reduce mother-to-neonate transmission. In the absence of prophylactic treatment, the neonate is tested for HIV within the first 24 hours after birth. The mother may not breast-feed the infant while awaiting the infant's test results. The infant will be given a non-nucleoside reverse transcriptase inhibitor (NNRTI), such as nevirapine (Viramune), or a nucleoside reverse transcriptase inhibitor (NRTI), such as zidovudine (Retrovir), within 48 to 72 hours of being born. Depending on the outcome of the test, the infant will be monitored and treated by a pediatric infectious disease specialist, pediatrician, or primary care physician. The other forms of isolation are not necessary unless additional protection is needed for a specific disorder.

> *Test Taking Strategy*—*Analyze to determine what information the question asks for regarding infection control precautions that are indicated when caring for an infant born to an HIV-positive mother. Recall that when the infectious status of a client, even a newborn, is unknown, standard precautions are always used (option 1). Review the categories of infection control precautions and indications for implementing each type if you had difficulty answering this question.*
> *Cognitive Level*—*Applying*
> *Client Needs Category*—*Safe and effective care environment*
> *Client Needs Subcategory*—*Safety and infection control*

124. 2. In almost all cases of acquired immunodeficiency syndrome (AIDS) in infants and children, the disease was acquired through maternal transmission at the time of pregnancy or shortly thereafter. Infants of HIV-positive mothers are tested within 24 hours of birth on other than cord blood. The preferred test is an HIV DNA polymerase chain reaction (PCR) test, which detects the genetic material in HIV, also known as the *viral load*. The test is repeated when the infant is 1 to 2 months old, and again at age 4 to 6 months. If the tests remain negative throughout the timetable for testing, the likelihood is greater than 95% that the infant has not acquired HIV.

> *Test Taking Strategy*—*Note the key words "most appropriate," and select the option that identifies the earliest timeframe for detecting the infant's HIV status (option 2). Recall that HIV antibody testing with an enzyme-linked immunosorbent assay (ELISA) or Western blot test is not as useful as an HIV DNA PCR test in the early neonatal period because the infant's blood almost always contains HIV antibodies if the mother is infected even if the infant is not. Review laboratory monitoring of the neonate for HIV if you had difficulty answering this question.*
> *Cognitive Level*—*Applying*
> *Client Needs Category*—*Physiological integrity*
> *Client Needs Subcategory*—*Physiological adaptation*

125. 4. Infants who are human immunodeficiency virus (HIV)–positive are typically asymptomatic at birth. About 20% develop symptoms suggestive of acquired immunodeficiency syndrome (AIDS) by age 1 to 2 years. The remaining 80% remain symptom-free until around age 3 years or even later. The first signs of HIV infection in children include slowed growth and development, recurring diarrhea, lung infections, or fungal infections within the mouth. During the first 15 months of life, it is not unusual for HIV-infected children who have been untreated to have at least one episode of *Pneumocystis* pneumonia.

> *Test Taking Strategy*—*Analyze to determine what information the question asks for, which is the age at which most untreated infants infected with HIV become symptomatic. Recall that symptoms develop as the immune system deteriorates. Most untreated HIV-positive infants will have health issues and recurrent infections by their first birthday (option 4), but some will continue to remain symptom-free into the toddler years. Review the disease progression of HIV if you had difficulty with this question.*
> *Cognitive Level*—*Applying*
> *Client Needs Category*—*Physiological integrity*
> *Client Needs Subcategory*—*Physiological adaptation*

126. 3. Human immunodeficiency virus (HIV) can be transmitted through breast milk; therefore, HIV-positive mothers in the United States are instructed not to breast-feed their newborns because of the possibility of transmitting the disease. Commercial formulas are substituted because they are easily available, affordable, and safe. However, there is a dilemma for mothers who live in underdeveloped countries and are advised to substitute formula for breast milk. Because the water may be unsafe, infants may be exposed to life-threatening conditions other than HIV. Reconstituting formula with water that is unsanitary or diluting it to such an extent that it results in malnutrition is just as potentially lethal as transmitting HIV through breast-feeding.

> *Test Taking Strategy*—*Note the key words "most appropriate," and analyze the options, looking for*

one that is factual in reference to whether the HIV-positive mother can breast-feed the infant. Recall that the virus is transmitted through breast milk, and the infant may become infected through this mode (option 3). Review HIV transmission precautions, especially as they apply to an HIV-positive mother and breast-feeding, if you had difficulty answering this question.
Cognitive Level—*Applying*
Client Needs Category—*Health promotion and maintenance*
Client Needs Subcategory—*None*

127. 1. Toddlers have a difficult time accepting and adjusting to new siblings in the family. They often lose control, regress, and act out. Toddlers also have a difficult time sharing parental love. By having each parent spend time with the toddler, the toddler will adjust more quickly to the new sibling. The parents may also want to include the toddler in basic care of the newborn such as assisting with feeding, bathing, and diaper changing. Sending the child away reinforces the idea that the newborn is more important than the toddler, which may lead to resentment on the part of the toddler. The parents should expect that the toddler will be acting out and lose control at times. They should praise appropriate behavior and ignore regressive behavior. Instead of disciplining the toddler for loss of control, the parents should provide the toddler with simple commands and explanations that will help the child regain and maintain control. Separating the siblings for the first few days will not foster sibling bonding.
> **Test Taking Strategy**—*The key words are "most appropriate" and "at this time" in reference to managing*

the toddler's behavior. Recall that the acting out displayed by the toddler provides attention even if it is for unacceptable behavior. However, by giving the child attention at other times (option 1), especially when the child is behaving well, the toddler may act out less and less. Review therapeutic parenting techniques in response to sibling rivalry and acting out if you had difficulty answering this question.
Cognitive Level—*Applying*
Client Needs Category—*Psychosocial integrity*
Client Needs Subcategory—*None*

128. 3. The LPN mentor is correct to identify that documentation of a client assignment must be completed by the nurse assigned, even if that means that overtime is required. A standard of care is that the nurse who performs the care documents the care provided. Neither scolding the nurse nor stating that this will be noted in a personal record is helpful in completing the required documentation. Mentoring the new nurse on time management can be completed at a later time.
> **Test Taking Strategy**—*Use the process of elimination to determine the best statement by the LPN mentor. Recall nursing standards regarding nursing documentation which includes documentation completed by the nurse completing care, and if it is not documented, it was not done. Documentation is essential as an important step in nursing care. Review the standards of nursing documentation if you had difficulty answering this question.*
Cognitive Level—*Analyzing*
Client Needs Category—*Safe and effective care environment*
Client Needs Subcategory—*Coordinated care*

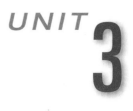

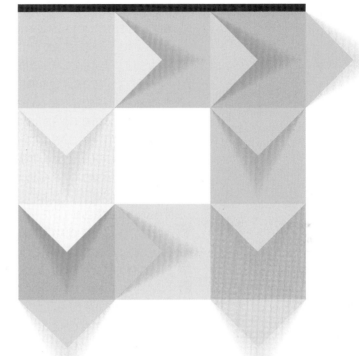

The Nursing Care of Children

13 The Nursing Care of Infants, Toddlers, and Preschool Children

Directions: With a pencil, blacken the space in front of the option you have chosen for your correct answer.

Normal Growth and Development of Infants, Toddlers, and Preschool Children

The nurse in a well-baby clinic assesses the growth and development of healthy infants and toddlers and uses that information as a basis for teaching.

1. Which assessment finding would the nurse document as normal development for a 3-month-old?
[ ] **1.** Able to hold a bottle
[ ] **2.** Able to lift head and shoulders
[ ] **3.** Able to roll from back to abdomen
[ ] **4.** Able to sit with support

2. After a routine immunization for measles, mumps, and rubella (MMR), which one of the following should the nurse instruct the parents of a 15-month-old child to report?
[ ] **1.** Fever that occurs within 7 to 10 days of the immunization
[ ] **2.** Rash that appears 2 to 4 days after the immunization
[ ] **3.** Crying for more than 3 hours, even after comfort measures are taken
[ ] **4.** Soreness, redness, and swelling at the injection site

3. During a home health visit to a family with a 20-month-old child, the nurse would expect to discuss childhood safety issues with the parent when noticing which finding?
[ ] **1.** Electrical outlets are covered.
[ ] **2.** The child is eating a raw carrot stick.
[ ] **3.** Furniture has rounded edges.
[ ] **4.** The child is building a tower with large blocks.

4. The nurse is caring for a 2-year-old diagnosed with Kawasaki's disease. When assessing the toddler's pulse, which site is most appropriate?
[ ] **1.** Apical
[ ] **2.** Brachial
[ ] **3.** Carotid
[ ] **4.** Radial

5. The nurse is caring for an Asian infant brought to the emergency department after a motor vehicle accident. When a cluster of family members are present, to whom should the nurse direct questions regarding the infant's health history?
[ ] **1.** The father
[ ] **2.** The mother
[ ] **3.** The entire family
[ ] **4.** The parents together

The nurse provides instructions about the proper administration of oral medications in liquid form to the parents of an infant.

6. The nurse assumes the parents understand the medication instructions when they make which statement?
[ ] **1.** "We'll add the medication to the bottle of formula."
[ ] **2.** "We should pinch the baby's nose when we're giving the medicine."
[ ] **3.** "We'll use a rubber-tipped medicine dropper to give the medicine."
[ ] **4.** "We should give the medicine while the baby is lying down."

7. Which assessment technique used by the nurse is most accurate for counting the respirations of an infant during a well-child checkup?
[ ] **1.** Count the respirations for 10 seconds and multiply by 6.
[ ] **2.** Count the respirations for 15 seconds and multiply by 4.
[ ] **3.** Count the respirations for 30 seconds and multiply by 2.
[ ] **4.** Count the respirations for 60 seconds or 1 full minute.

8. Which statement by a toddler's parent to the nurse suggests the need for further teaching about signs of readiness for toilet-training?
[ ] **1.** "I won't start toilet-training my child until age 18 months because sphincter control isn't usually accomplished before then."
[ ] **2.** "I should begin bladder training before bowel training."
[ ] **3.** "I'll wait until my child can communicate the need to go to the bathroom."
[ ] **4.** "I should wait to begin toilet-training until my child can independently remove underwear."

9. Which is the best advice a nurse can give parents who are helping a 3-year-old child overcome the rivalry created by the birth of a sibling?
[ ] **1.** Enroll the child in a full-day preschool program with friends.
[ ] **2.** Arrange for the child to have visits with grandparents.
[ ] **3.** Find ways that the child can assist with the infant's care.
[ ] **4.** Invite other similarly aged children to play with the child.

10. Which teaching aid provided by the nurse is developmentally appropriate for a preschooler who is about to have a bone marrow puncture?
[ ] **1.** Dolls or puppets
[ ] **2.** Pamphlets or booklets
[ ] **3.** Colored diagrams
[ ] **4.** Commercial videotapes

11. Which action by parents of a 16-month-old toddler indicates to the nurse that they understand how to best minimize separation anxiety during their child's hospitalization?
[ ] **1.** The parents bring the child's favorite toy to the hospital.
[ ] **2.** The parents explain all procedures to the child.
[ ] **3.** The parents remain with the child during the hospital stay.
[ ] **4.** The parents bring the siblings to visit the child.

12. The nurse instructs the parents of a 6-month-old child about the introduction of solid foods into the child's diet. Which response given by the parents indicates the need for further nursing instruction?
[ ] **1.** "We will begin with cereal made for infants that is fortified with iron."
[ ] **2.** "We will not breast-feed or bottle-feed until after solid food has been given."
[ ] **3.** "We will introduce one food at a time at an interval of every 4 to 5 days."
[ ] **4.** "We will postpone giving solid food if our baby pushes it out of the mouth with the tongue."

13. Which developmental finding of an 18-month-old would the nurse bring to the physician's attention for further assessment?
[ ] **1.** The 18-month-old has a vocabulary of about six words.
[ ] **2.** The 18-month-old uses a spoon when eating meals.
[ ] **3.** The 18-month-old walks with additional support from others.
[ ] **4.** The 18-month-old shows readiness for toilet training.

14. Which observation by the nurse indicates that the parents of a toddler need additional teaching regarding household safety?

[ ] **1.** Household cleaners are in their original containers.
[ ] **2.** Medicines are stored on a high shelf out of the child's reach.
[ ] **3.** The hot water heater thermostat is set at 120°F (48.8°C).
[ ] **4.** The number for the poison control center is posted by the telephone.

15. If the parent of a 4-year-old child tells the nurse about concerns that the child frequently talks about a make-believe playmate, which response by the nurse is best?

[ ] **1.** "This type of behavior is normal for a preschooler."
[ ] **2.** "Can you identify any stressors that may be causing this regression?"
[ ] **3.** "You may need a referral to see a child psychologist."
[ ] **4.** "Give a time-out when this behavior occurs."

A young, first-time parent expresses concern regarding normal physical growth and development. The parent states, "I'm unsure when I need to childproof my home."

16. Prioritize the parent's actions for keeping the infant safe in relation to the normal progression of physical development. Sequence the list from birth through the infant's first year of life. Use all the options.

1. Cover the electrical outlets.	
2. Have straps on the changing table.	
3. Turn pot handles inward when cooking.	
4. Remove stuffed animals with small pieces from the child's grasp.	
5. Lower crib mattresses.	
6. Maintain water temperature under 120°F (48.8°C).	

Nursing Care of an Infant with Myelomeningocele

An infant is born with a myelomeningocele high in the spinal column.

17. Which nursing action is most important for the nurse to include during the preoperative period?

[ ] **1.** Keep the diaper area clean to prevent contamination of the myelomeningocele.
[ ] **2.** Position the infant so that there is no pressure on the myelomeningocele.
[ ] **3.** Keep the infant's myelomeningocele clean by washing it with antiseptic soap.
[ ] **4.** Encourage the parents to cuddle and hold the infant to promote bonding.

A surgical repair of the myelomeningocele is successfully completed.

18. Unless the physician orders otherwise, in which position should the nurse place the infant during the postoperative period?

[ ] **1.** Supine
[ ] **2.** Prone
[ ] **3.** Right or left side-lying
[ ] **4.** Whichever position is most comfortable for the infant

19. In planning the infant's home care, which of the following orthopedic considerations is essential for the nurse to include to diminish musculoskeletal problems?

[ ] **1.** Instruct the parents on range-of-motion exercises to reduce joint contractures.
[ ] **2.** Arrange for specialized assistive devices within the home setting.
[ ] **3.** Place the infant in a position so all extremities are unrestricted.
[ ] **4.** Use lotions and ointments to massage large muscle groups twice daily.

20. What should the nurse plan to teach the parents as the child gets older to prepare them for managing their child's urinary incontinence at home?

[ ] **1.** How to care for a retention catheter
[ ] **2.** How to insert a straight catheter
[ ] **3.** How to reapply a ureterostomy appliance
[ ] **4.** How to attach an external catheter

The infant also has talipes equinovarus (clubfoot) and developmental dysplasia of the hip (DDH).

21. What is the priority nursing intervention to prevent contractures of the infant's lower extremities?
[ ] **1.** Massage the lower extremities.
[ ] **2.** Reposition the infant frequently.
[ ] **3.** Place sheepskin under the bony prominences.
[ ] **4.** Perform range-of-motion exercises.

Nursing Care of an Infant with Hydrocephalus

A 1-week-old infant who was born with hydrocephalus is scheduled for surgery.

22. Which assessment finding for an infant with hydrocephalus is most characteristic of the disorder?
[ ] **1.** Increased head size
[ ] **2.** Paralysis of the lower extremities
[ ] **3.** Absence of the sucking reflex
[ ] **4.** Marked depression of the anterior fontanel

The parents ask the nurse to explain why their baby has hydrocephalus.

23. The nurse correctly explains which of the following as the common cause of hydrocephalus?
[ ] **1.** Absence of the dura mater
[ ] **2.** Blockage of cerebrospinal fluid (CSF) circulation
[ ] **3.** Increased CSF in the subarachnoid space
[ ] **4.** Occlusion in the cerebral arteries

24. After feeding the infant with hydrocephalus, in which position should the infant be placed?
[ ] **1.** Sitting
[ ] **2.** Supine
[ ] **3.** Prone
[ ] **4.** Side-lying

25. Which measure is most appropriate for the nurse to use to reduce the potential for a pressure ulcer developing on the head of an infant with hydrocephalus?
[ ] **1.** Place a sheepskin under the infant's head.
[ ] **2.** Massage the circumference of the infant's skull.
[ ] **3.** Support the infant's head on two pillows.
[ ] **4.** Apply a padded helmet to the infant's head.

26. If a ventriculoperitoneal (V/P) shunt is placed on the right side of the infant's head, which postoperative position is most appropriate for the nurse to use?
[ ] **1.** The right side, to increase absorption of cerebrospinal fluid
[ ] **2.** The abdomen, to prevent obstruction in the shunt catheter
[ ] **3.** The left side, to avoid pressure on the operative site
[ ] **4.** The back, to promote ventricular drainage

27. Postoperatively, which sign is the best indication that the infant is developing increased intracranial pressure?
[ ] **1.** Depression of the fontanel
[ ] **2.** Decreased pulse and respiratory rates
[ ] **3.** Change in frequency of bowel movements
[ ] **4.** Sudden increase in weight

28. Postoperatively, which nursing action is most appropriate if the nurse observes that the infant's anterior fontanel is sunken?
[ ] **1.** Document the finding and take no further action.
[ ] **2.** Place the infant in the supine position.
[ ] **3.** Elevate the infant's head.
[ ] **4.** Notify the charge nurse or physician immediately.

Nursing Care of an Infant with Cleft Lip

The nurse is caring for a newborn infant with a cleft lip.

29. During the initial data collection process in the nursery, the nurse palpates the roof of the newborn's mouth to assess for which finding?
[ ] **1.** The infant's ability to suck
[ ] **2.** The presence of a gag reflex
[ ] **3.** An opening in the palate
[ ] **4.** Position of the uvula

30. When taking the newborn to the parents for the first visit, which action is the nurse's priority?
[ ] **1.** Teaching the parents how to feed the infant
[ ] **2.** Demonstrating open acceptance of the infant
[ ] **3.** Discussing the plans for surgical repair of the defect
[ ] **4.** Showing the parents how to use a bulb syringe

31. Which observation by the nurse indicates that the parents understand how to minimize the risk of aspiration?
[ ] **1.** They burp the newborn frequently during feedings.
[ ] **2.** They position the newborn prone for feedings.
[ ] **3.** They feed the newborn formula thickened with rice cereal.
[ ] **4.** They feed the newborn only glucose water until after surgical repair of the defect.

32. Before surgery, which utensil is best for the nurse to use when feeding the infant with a cleft lip that extends from the lip into the gum line?
[ ] **1.** Gavage tube
[ ] **2.** Bulb syringe
[ ] **3.** Nipple with enlarged hole
[ ] **4.** Nipple that is extra firm

33. Which restraint is best for the nurse to use for a child who has had a cleft lip repair?
[ ] **1.** Papoose board
[ ] **2.** Leg restraints
[ ] **3.** Elbow restraints
[ ] **4.** Posey belt or jacket

34. When developing a care plan for a child who has undergone surgery to correct a cleft lip, how frequently should the nurse plan to remove and reapply the restraints?
[ ] **1.** Daily
[ ] **2.** Every 8 hours
[ ] **3.** Every 4 hours
[ ] **4.** Every 2 hours

Nursing Care of an Infant with Pyloric Stenosis

The nurse is caring for a 3-week-old infant who has been admitted to the hospital for surgical correction of pyloric stenosis.

35. Which assessment finding is most significant during the data collection process?
[ ] **1.** The infant is eager to suck.
[ ] **2.** The anterior fontanel is flat.
[ ] **3.** The gastric peristaltic waves are visible.
[ ] **4.** The mucous membranes are dry.

The physician orders an I.V. infusion of dextrose 2.5% in normal saline solution.

36. Which information regarding infant I.V. therapy is correct?
[ ] **1.** The I.V. catheter will be sutured to the scalp.
[ ] **2.** A buretrol will be added to the infusion tubing.
[ ] **3.** The infant may be restless during I.V. therapy.
[ ] **4.** The area around the I.V. site will swell slightly.

37. After surgical correction of the defect, in which position should the nurse instruct the parents to place the infant after feeding?
[ ] **1.** On the abdomen
[ ] **2.** On the side
[ ] **3.** On the back
[ ] **4.** In a comfortable position

Nursing Care of an Infant with Bilateral Clubfoot

A 1-week-old infant with bilateral talipes equinovarus (bilateral clubfoot) is being seen at the pediatrician's office.

38. Which of the following information gathered by the nurse in the infant's birth history is most indicative of a true clubfoot condition?
[ ] **1.** The infant was born in the breech position.
[ ] **2.** The heels were drawn in and the feet turned inward.
[ ] **3.** The feet could not be corrected to a neutral position.
[ ] **4.** The bilateral defect was present at birth.

After nonsurgical treatment failed to correct the infant's defect, bilateral leg casts are applied.

39. When the parent asks why the ends of the cast have adhesive "petals," how should the nurse respond?
[ ] **1.** "The adhesive petals ensure that nothing is placed between the cast and the skin."
[ ] **2.** "The adhesive petals allow air circulation between the cast and the skin."
[ ] **3.** "The adhesive petals prevent the plaster of the cast from irritating the skin."
[ ] **4.** "The adhesive petals allow for stronger bonding of the plaster cast materials."

40. Which finding noted by the nurse is the best indication that the infant is experiencing a neurovascular complication?
[ ] **1.** The infant cries 4 hours after the last feeding.
[ ] **2.** The infant's toes are wiggling.
[ ] **3.** The infant's toes are pale and cold.
[ ] **4.** The infant's pulse is 110 beats/minute.

41. Which nursing action will minimize swelling of the infant's feet?
[ ] **1.** Elevate the legs and feet on a pillow.
[ ] **2.** Place the infant in the prone position.
[ ] **3.** Petal the edges of the cast.
[ ] **4.** Apply ice packs over the cast.

42. The nurse correctly informs the infant's parents that initially the casts will be changed how frequently?
[ ] **1.** Every 3 to 7 days
[ ] **2.** Every 1 to 2 weeks
[ ] **3.** On a monthly basis
[ ] **4.** Every other month

At age 8 weeks, an infant is seen in the pediatrician's office for a routine cast change. The nurse uses this opportunity to teach the parents ways to promote normal growth and development.

43. Which age-appropriate developmental instruction can the nurse recommend to the parents during this visit?
[ ] **1.** Encourage the infant to crawl about in the crib.
[ ] **2.** Play peek-a-boo with the infant's favorite blanket.
[ ] **3.** Motivate the infant to reach for cuddly toys.
[ ] **4.** Place a brightly colored mobile over the crib.

The parents tell the nurse that they can barely feel the soft spot in the back of the infant's head and ask whether this is normal.

44. Which statement by the nurse is most correct?
[ ] **1.** "Barely feeling the soft spot is normal because the posterior fontanel usually closes between 2 and 3 months."
[ ] **2.** "Barely feeling the soft spot is abnormal because the posterior fontanel usually closes between 9 and 18 months."
[ ] **3.** "Barely feeling the soft spot is abnormal because the posterior fontanel usually remains open longer in children."
[ ] **4.** "Barely feeling the soft spot is normal because the posterior fontanel usually closes earlier in children with congenital skeletal defects."

Nursing Care of a Child with Otitis Media

A 6-month-old infant is examined by the physician and found to have otitis media.

45. Which nursing observation best indicates the presence of ear pain in an infant?
[ ] **1.** The infant refuses to suck a bottle.
[ ] **2.** The infant pulls on one ear.
[ ] **3.** The infant's temperature is elevated.
[ ] **4.** There is drainage from the infant's ear.

The pediatrician prescribes Amoxicillin 125 mg P.O. every 12 hours for 10 days. The office nurse gives the first dose to the infant.

46. When preparing to give medications, which action by the nurse best ensures that the prescribed dose of medication is a safe dose for the infant?
[ ] **1.** Reading the physician's orders carefully
[ ] **2.** Checking the weight/dose range in a drug reference
[ ] **3.** Determining the infant's medication allergies
[ ] **4.** Reading the medication label carefully

47. When explaining the prescribed antibiotic treatment to the parents, which instruction should the nurse emphasize?
[ ] **1.** "Use a side-lying position after giving the antibiotic."
[ ] **2.** "Give the antibiotic with feedings."
[ ] **3.** "Store the antibiotic at room temperature."
[ ] **4.** "Give the antibiotic for the full 10 days."

48. The physician orders Pediazole 6 mL P.O. every 8 hours for a child with an ear infection. The child weighs 38 lb (17.2 kg). Pediazole contains erythromycin ethylsuccinate 200 mg and sulfisoxazole acetyl 600 mg in a 5 mL suspension. How many milligrams of erythromycin will the child receive in a 24-hour period?

Nursing Care of a Child with a Congenital Heart Defect

A 2-week-old infant with a diagnosis of coarctation of the aorta is being cared for in the high-risk nursery.

49. Which of the following admission data is the best indication that the infant has coarctation of the aorta?
[ ] **1.** Generalized cyanosis, especially when the infant cries
[ ] **2.** Clubbing of the fingers and toes
[ ] **3.** Bounding brachial pulses and weak femoral pulses
[ ] **4.** Rapid and irregular apical heartbeat

50. The nurse correctly advises the parents that the optimal time for surgical correction is when?
[ ] **1.** As soon as the child's condition stabilizes
[ ] **2.** When the child is 6 months old
[ ] **3.** Before the child is 2 years old
[ ] **4.** When the child is between ages 2 and 4

The infant receives digoxin (Lanoxin) while in the nursery.

51. Which nursing intervention is most important to perform before giving digoxin (Lanoxin)?
[ ] **1.** Check the apical pulse for 1 minute.
[ ] **2.** Position the infant with the head slightly elevated.
[ ] **3.** Check the expiration date on the medication label.
[ ] **4.** Monitor the infant's urine output.

52. The nurse can best facilitate a reduction of the infant's heart workload by which method?
[ ] **1.** Limiting the amount of holding and cuddling by the infant's parents
[ ] **2.** Organizing nursing care so that the infant has longer rest periods
[ ] **3.** Feeding only by the nasogastric route
[ ] **4.** Keeping the infant mildly sedated at all times

The nurse provides discharge instructions regarding medication administration.

53. Which statement by the parents indicates a need for additional teaching from the nurse about administering digoxin (Lanoxin) at home?
[ ] **1.** "If we miss giving a dose, we should give the next dose at the regularly scheduled time."
[ ] **2.** "We need to check the baby's apical pulse before giving each dose of the medication."
[ ] **3.** "We should mix each dose of the medication in a small amount of formula."
[ ] **4.** "We should never increase or decrease the dose except if ordered by the doctor."

Nursing Care of a Child with an Infectious Disease

A 7-month-old infant with chickenpox is seen in the emergency department. The infant is admitted to the hospital because of moderate dehydration. An I.V. infusion is begun.

54. Which transmission-based precautions category assigned by the nurse following hospital policy is most appropriate for a child with chickenpox in the early stage of infection?
[ ] **1.** Airborne precautions
[ ] **2.** Droplet precautions
[ ] **3.** Contact precautions
[ ] **4.** Standard precautions

55. Which nursing action is correct when implementing the prescribed transmission-based precaution?
[ ] **1.** A supply of clean masks is placed in the infant's room.
[ ] **2.** Specimens are sent to the laboratory in a zip-closure biohazard bag.
[ ] **3.** The infant is assigned to a semiprivate room.
[ ] **4.** A glass thermometer is used and wiped with alcohol after use.

56. The nurse assesses the child who has been admitted for chickenpox. After obtaining all of the following data, which is most important to report to the charge nurse?
[ ] **1.** The child sleeps for short intervals during the day.
[ ] **2.** There is an increase in the frequency and amount of urine.
[ ] **3.** The child occasionally cries when disturbed by noise.
[ ] **4.** There is an increase in the I.V. infusion drip rate.

57. A child weighing 18 pounds is receiving maintenance I.V. fluids. Using the standard formula of 100 mL/kg/day for the first 10 kg of body weight, 50 mL/kg/day for the next 10 kg of body weight, then 20 mL/kg/day for each kilogram above 20 kg of body weight, what would be the daily I.V. fluid volume for this child?

Nursing Care of a Child with Human Immunodeficiency Virus Infection

A 2-month-old infant with human immunodeficiency virus (HIV) infection is discharged from the hospital. At age 4 months, the infant is seen in the physician's office for a routine checkup.

58. Which of the following assessment data documented by the nurse is considered a high-risk factor for developing acquired immunodeficiency syndrome (AIDS)?
[ ] **1.** The infant has pinpoint white spots on the nose.
[ ] **2.** The parent states that the infant has had thrush twice.
[ ] **3.** The infant's respirations have an irregular pattern.
[ ] **4.** The mother states that the infant wets six diapers per day.

59. While developing a care plan for a 2-year-old child with perinatally acquired human immunodeficiency virus (HIV) infection, which assessment findings would indicate that the child has clinical signs of acquired immunodeficiency syndrome (AIDS)? Select all that apply.
[ ] **1.** History of bacterial infections
[ ] **2.** Herpes simplex lesions around the mouth
[ ] **3.** White patches in the mouth area
[ ] **4.** Lung consolidation on a chest X-ray
[ ] **5.** Limited muscle tone
[ ] **6.** Increased blood pressure

Nursing Care of a Child with Atopic Dermatitis

A 2-year-old child in the clinic is diagnosed with atopic dermatitis. The parent asks what caused the child's skin condition and why the physician had many questions about the home environment.

60. The nurse is correct in correlating which factor as a probable cause of this child's atopic dermatitis?
[ ] **1.** Poor nutrition
[ ] **2.** Premature birth
[ ] **3.** Allergic reaction
[ ] **4.** Hormonal imbalance

61. Which disease symptom is the nurse most likely to focus on when providing the parent with preventive care measures?
[ ] **1.** Nausea
[ ] **2.** Ecchymoses
[ ] **3.** Itching
[ ] **4.** Drowsiness

The physician prescribes hydrocortisone ointment (Cortaid) for the child's skin lesions and instructs the parent to give colloid baths.

62. On a subsequent visit, which outcome demonstrates that the ointment has been effective?
[ ] **1.** The child's skin is no longer weeping.
[ ] **2.** There is no further spread of the skin lesions.
[ ] **3.** The skin inflammation has decreased.
[ ] **4.** The child's white blood cell count is increased.

63. When instructing the mother on how to give a colloid bath, the nurse correctly explains that a typical colloid bath consists of tepid water and which additive?
[ ] **1.** Cornstarch
[ ] **2.** Mineral oil
[ ] **3.** Liquid glycerin soap
[ ] **4.** Iodized salt

Nursing Care of a Toddler with Sickle Cell Crisis

An acutely ill 21-month-old child is admitted to the hospital with vaso-occlusive sickle cell crisis. The child has a 6-year-old sibling who also has sickle cell disease.

64. When admitting the child, which nursing assessment is an initial priority?
[ ] 1. Assessing for pain
[ ] 2. Assessing for dehydration
[ ] 3. Assessing for hemorrhage
[ ] 4. Assessing for bradycardia

65. Which nursing action can the nurse anticipate will be involved in this child's care?
[ ] 1. Administering an I.V. transfusion of plasma
[ ] 2. Initiating measures to decrease the hemoglobin level
[ ] 3. Beginning an administration of large doses of iron
[ ] 4. Promoting measures to rehydrate the child

The nurse is informed that one parent has sickle cell trait and the other parent has sickle cell disease.

66. Which statement indicates that the parent understands how sickle cell disease is transmitted?
[ ] 1. "All of our children will have sickle cell disease."
[ ] 2. "With each pregnancy, there is a 50% chance that the baby will be born with sickle cell disease."
[ ] 3. "If I conceive again, our baby will be born with sickle cell trait."
[ ] 4. "With each pregnancy, there is a 75% chance that the baby will be born with sickle cell disease."

67. Which instructions provided by the nurse are essential for preventing further sickle cell crises? Select all that apply.
[ ] 1. Obtain plenty of rest.
[ ] 2. Drink plenty of fluids.
[ ] 3. Use routine pain medication.
[ ] 4. Complete a full course of antibiotics.
[ ] 5. Use proper hand washing techniques.
[ ] 6. Avoid crowds.

Nursing Care of a Toddler with Cystic Fibrosis

An 18-month-old toddler with a diagnosis of cystic fibrosis is admitted to the hospital because of increasing respiratory difficulty and repeated respiratory infections.

68. When the nurse reads the child's health history, what documented information is typical for a child with cystic fibrosis? Select all that apply.
[ ] 1. The child sleeps for brief periods of time.
[ ] 2. The child has gained a lot of weight.
[ ] 3. The child tastes salty when kissed.
[ ] 4. The child has poor head control.
[ ] 5. The child has periods of breathing difficulties.
[ ] 6. The child lags in achieving developmental milestones.

69. Which assessment finding does the nurse anticipate in the child with cystic fibrosis?
[ ] 1. Poor appetite
[ ] 2. Excessive perspiration
[ ] 3. Low urine output
[ ] 4. Bulky, foul-smelling stools

70. Which is the priority nursing goal when managing the care of the child with cystic fibrosis?
[ ] 1. The child will consume appropriate nutrients to meet body needs.
[ ] 2. The child will maintain an effective breathing pattern.
[ ] 3. The child will consume an adequate amount of fluids to meet body needs.
[ ] 4. The child will demonstrate a decreased level of anxiety.

The physician prescribes an Albuterol inhaler 2 puffs every 3 to 4 hours and a flutter mucus clearing device for the child.

71. The nurse determines that this type of therapy is successful if which one of the following is accomplished?
[ ] 1. There is decreased mucus in the stools.
[ ] 2. The serum sodium level decreases.
[ ] 3. The breathing pattern improves.
[ ] 4. Excess fat is excreted from the body.

After collecting additional data, the nurse determines that modifying the child's diet may be therapeutic.

72. Which one of the following modifications would be best for the nurse to recommend?
[ ] 1. Increasing dietary fat intake
[ ] 2. Decreasing protein in the diet
[ ] 3. Limiting the use of salt
[ ] 4. Adding more calories to the diet

The parents ask the nurse whether the physician can prescribe a larger dosage of pancrelipase (Pancrease) given twice daily instead of the current dosage, which is given with each meal.

73. The nurse correctly explains that Pancrease must be given with meals for which reason?
[ ] 1. To prevent gastrointestinal upset
[ ] 2. To increase nutrient absorption
[ ] 3. To prevent salt depletion
[ ] 4. To increase the child's desire to eat

74. The nurse further explains that it is necessary to increase the child's fluid intake for which reason?
[ ] 1. To prevent kidney failure
[ ] 2. To increase cardiac function
[ ] 3. To reduce pain and discomfort
[ ] 4. To liquefy lung secretions

75. The parental identification of which option below confirms an understanding of what the child should most avoid in order to reduce the potential for life-threatening complications?

[ ] **1.** Exposure to airborne pollen
[ ] **2.** Exposure to respiratory pathogens
[ ] **3.** Exposure to pet dander
[ ] **4.** Exposure to bright sunlight

Nursing Care of a Toddler with Asthma

The physician sees a 3-year-old toddler with allergic (extrinsic) asthma triggered by an upper respiratory tract infection.

76. If the nurse collects all the following data, which assessment finding is the best indication that the child is having an acute asthma attack?

[ ] **1.** Presence of expiratory wheezing
[ ] **2.** Respiratory rate between 20 and 30 breaths/ minute
[ ] **3.** Thoracic breathing pattern
[ ] **4.** Clear, watery nasal drainage

77. Which nursing action is most appropriate for relieving the child's respiratory distress?

[ ] **1.** Provide oxygen at 2 L per nasal cannula.
[ ] **2.** Position a steam vaporizer at the bedside.
[ ] **3.** Give antibiotics as ordered.
[ ] **4.** Place the child in semi-Fowler's position.

The child responds to treatment and is scheduled to be discharged. The physician has prescribed breathing exercises for the child.

78. Which nursing intervention best facilitates the child's performance of breathing exercises?

[ ] **1.** Promise to give the child a treat after the exercises.
[ ] **2.** Have the parents assist the child with the exercises.
[ ] **3.** Demonstrate the exercise, and then have the child do the exercise.
[ ] **4.** Instruct the parents to have the child blow bubbles.

79. Which nursing instruction is most appropriate to include during discharge teaching?

[ ] **1.** Instruct the parents to give breathing treatments every 2 hours.
[ ] **2.** Instruct the parents to eliminate vegetables from the child's diet.
[ ] **3.** Instruct the parents to limit the child's fluid intake.
[ ] **4.** Instruct the parents to remove area rugs from the home.

Nursing Care of a Toddler Who Has Swallowed a Toxic Substance

The parent of a 15-month-old toddler calls the physician's office and reports that the child swallowed a lye-based cleaner.

80. Which initial instruction by the nurse is most appropriate to give to the parent?

[ ] **1.** Begin cardiopulmonary resuscitation on the child immediately.
[ ] **2.** Induce vomiting with syrup of ipecac immediately.
[ ] **3.** Give the child water to drink to dilute the substance.
[ ] **4.** Take the child and substance to the nearest emergency department.

The child is taken to the emergency department. After examination, the physician decides to admit the child for further observation.

81. If the nurse documents all the following data on admission, which finding is the best indication that the child needs to be monitored with a pulse oximeter?

[ ] **1.** Substernal and intercostal retractions
[ ] **2.** Red, swollen lips
[ ] **3.** Thin, clear mucus drooling from lips
[ ] **4.** Pulse rate of 105 beats/minute

82. In addition to monitoring the child with a pulse oximeter, which intervention would the nurse expect to perform?

[ ] **1.** Administering gastric lavage
[ ] **2.** Implementing pain-relief measures
[ ] **3.** Maintaining the child on nothing-by-mouth status
[ ] **4.** Performing neurovascular checks

83. Which statement by the parent is the best indication he or she understands how to prevent the child from ingesting poisonous substances in the future?

[ ] **1.** "I'll remove all toxic substances from my home."
[ ] **2.** "I won't ever let my child out of my sight again."
[ ] **3.** "I'll place all toxic substances out of my child's reach."
[ ] **4.** "I'll keep all toxic substances in a locked cabinet."

Nursing Care of a Toddler with Croup

A 2½-year-old toddler is seen in the pediatrician's office because of coughing and difficulty breathing, which began the previous night. The physician makes a diagnosis of laryngotracheobronchitis (croup).

84. When the parents ask how croup occurs, the nurse correctly informs them about which etiology of the disorder?

[ ] **1.** Croup is primarily caused by various viruses.
[ ] **2.** Croup occurs in children with chronic asthma.
[ ] **3.** Croup is another name for whooping cough.
[ ] **4.** Croup is a complication of underdeveloped lungs.

85. Which common characteristic of croup would the nurse expect to document in the child's chart?
[ ] **1.** Moist cough
[ ] **2.** Barky cough
[ ] **3.** Muffled cough
[ ] **4.** Wheezy cough

86. Which recommendation by the nurse commonly relieves the symptoms caused by croup?
[ ] **1.** Providing central heating throughout the house
[ ] **2.** Maintaining an air-conditioned environment
[ ] **3.** Placing a cool-mist humidifier in the child's room
[ ] **4.** Ensuring that the child's room is dust-free

87. The nurse acts correctly by instructing the parents to contact the physician immediately if the child develops which one of the following, which suggests a worsening of the child's condition?
[ ] **1.** Fluctuating fever
[ ] **2.** Intense anxiety
[ ] **3.** Persistent coughing
[ ] **4.** Frequent napping

88. Which statement by the parents indicates a need for further teaching?
[ ] **1.** "Our child may have recurrent episodes of croup for one or two more nights."
[ ] **2.** "We'll give our child aspirin for a temperature greater than 101°F (38.3°C)."
[ ] **3.** "We'll place a cool-mist humidifier at the head of our child's bed."
[ ] **4.** "We'll offer our child small sips of clear liquids at frequent intervals."

The child develops acute respiratory distress during the night and is taken to the hospital's emergency department. The physician admits the child for further treatment.

89. Which medication can the nurse expect the child with croup to receive?
[ ] **1.** Ampicillin (Omnipen)
[ ] **2.** Ferrous sulfate (Feosol)
[ ] **3.** Metoclopramide (Reglan)
[ ] **4.** Racemic epinephrine (Vaponefrin)

90. Which beverage should the nurse avoid when offering liquids to a child with croup?
[ ] **1.** Ginger ale
[ ] **2.** Apple juice
[ ] **3.** Whole milk
[ ] **4.** Cold water

Nursing Care of a Toddler with Pneumonia

A 2½-year-old toddler is admitted to the hospital with a diagnosis of pneumococcal pneumonia. On admission, the child has an intermittent, productive cough. The parents report that the child has been lethargic and anorexic for several days.

91. In addition to the above manifestations, the nurse would expect to find which manifestation of the disease process?
[ ] **1.** Clubbing of the fingers
[ ] **2.** Synchronized chest movement
[ ] **3.** Slow pulse rate
[ ] **4.** Rapid and shallow respirations

92. When providing care for the child with pneumonia, which nursing assessment data is most appropriate for determining the child's hydration status?
[ ] **1.** Urine output
[ ] **2.** Urine pH
[ ] **3.** Blood pressure
[ ] **4.** Respiratory rate

93. Before beginning antibiotic therapy, which of the following diagnostic test findings would the nurse check?
[ ] **1.** Electrolyte panel
[ ] **2.** Pulse oximeter
[ ] **3.** Chest X-ray
[ ] **4.** Sputum culture

94. Which medication can the nurse expect to give to the child with pneumonia who has a productive, moist cough?
[ ] **1.** Antibiotic
[ ] **2.** Bronchodilator
[ ] **3.** Expectorant
[ ] **4.** Cough suppressant

The physician leaves orders to give the child a sponge bath for a temperature of 103°F (39.4°C) or more rectally.

95. When the parents ask to participate, which nursing instruction regarding the sponge bath is essential for the parents to know?
[ ] **1.** The sponge bath should be given for at least 1 hour.
[ ] **2.** The water temperature of the bath should be cool.
[ ] **3.** The bath should be discontinued if the child begins to shiver.
[ ] **4.** The bath should be given until the temperature is below 101°F (38.3°C).

96. A child with pneumonia is ordered cephalexin monohydrate (Keflex) 0.5 g P.O. every 8 hours. The pharmacy dispenses 500 mg per teaspoon. How many milliliters should the nurse administer?

After 3 days of treatment, the child's condition improves significantly. The physician writes discharge orders that include instructions for home care. The parents speak some English, but their primary language is Spanish.

97. Which action is best to ensure that the parents understand the discharge instructions?
[ ] **1.** Give the parents a copy of the instructions written in Spanish.
[ ] **2.** Have an interpreter present when instructions are given.
[ ] **3.** Have the physician give the instructions.
[ ] **4.** Instruct the parents to call if questions arise when they get home.

Nursing Care of a Preschooler with Seizure Disorder

A 4½-year-old preschooler is admitted to the hospital with a tentative diagnosis of tonic-clonic seizures.

98. Of the following history findings reported by the parents, which information given to the nurse best indicates that the child had a tonic-clonic seizure?
[ ] **1.** The child had a high fever.
[ ] **2.** The child has begun wetting the bed.
[ ] **3.** The child suddenly dropped to the floor.
[ ] **4.** The child's whole body was jerking.

99. Which nursing action is most appropriate when preparing the hospital room for the child's admission?
[ ] **1.** Padding the side rails on the bed
[ ] **2.** Keeping phenobarbital at the bedside
[ ] **3.** Placing the bed in Trendelenburg's position
[ ] **4.** Posting a "Seizure Precautions" sign on the child's door

100. Which equipment is least important for the nurse to have at this child's bedside?
[ ] **1.** Suction equipment
[ ] **2.** Oral airway
[ ] **3.** Oxygen sources
[ ] **4.** Cool-mist humidifier

The child has a tonic-clonic seizure while the nurse is at the bedside.

101. Which action should the nurse take first?
[ ] **1.** Calling for assistance
[ ] **2.** Placing the child in a side-lying position
[ ] **3.** Inserting a padded tongue blade in the child's mouth
[ ] **4.** Administering oxygen

The physician prescribes phenytoin (Dilantin). After several days on the medication, the child has no further seizure activity. The physician writes discharge orders, which include administering Dilantin at home.

102. During the discharge process, which long-term adverse effect of phenytoin (Dilantin) should the nurse include in the instructions to the parents?
[ ] **1.** Poor appetite
[ ] **2.** Urinary incontinence
[ ] **3.** Painful joints
[ ] **4.** Gum overgrowth

103. Which statement by the parents indicates a correct understanding of the care and prognosis of their child who has a seizure disorder?
[ ] **1.** "We'll restrict activities to those that are sedentary."
[ ] **2.** "We'll avoid restraining our child during a seizure."
[ ] **3.** "Our child will become developmentally disabled."
[ ] **4.** "We're aware that our child should no longer attend preschool."

104. Which is the most characteristic statement that reflects a preschooler's preconceived idea as to why he or she acquired a health-related problem?
[ ] **1.** "I have seizures because I am unlucky."
[ ] **2.** "I have seizures because I've been bad."
[ ] **3.** "I have seizures because I'm a sickly child."
[ ] **4.** "I have seizures because I don't eat right."

Nursing Care of a Preschooler with Leukemia

A 5-year-old Hispanic American child suspected of having leukemia is admitted to the hospital for diagnosis and treatment.

105. The nurse correctly explains to the parents that the most accurate way to confirm a diagnosis of leukemia is which test?
[ ] **1.** Complete blood count (CBC)
[ ] **2.** Spinal fluid examination
[ ] **3.** Bone marrow aspiration
[ ] **4.** X-ray of long bones

Tests confirm that the child has acute lymphoblastic leukemia (ALL). Induction therapy is begun. The child is started on vincristine sulfate, prednisone, and asparaginase (Elspar). The physician also places the child under protective isolation precautions.

106. Which instructions should the nurse give to those visiting a child on protective isolation? Select all that apply.
[ ] **1.** Only washable toys are allowed into the child's room.
[ ] **2.** Children younger than age 12 are restricted from the room.
[ ] **3.** Fresh fruit that cannot be peeled is prohibited in the room.
[ ] **4.** Only immediate family members may visit in the room.
[ ] **5.** Avoid visiting if there is evidence of cold or flu symptoms.
[ ] **6.** Use an alcohol-based hand rub when entering and leaving the room.

107. Which route of temperature assessment is contraindicated for a child with leukemia?
[ ] **1.** Axillary
[ ] **2.** Oral
[ ] **3.** Rectal
[ ] **4.** Tympanic

108. In the case of an allergic reaction, which medication should the nurse have on hand when asparaginase (Elspar) is given?
[ ] **1.** Epinephrine (Adrenalin)
[ ] **2.** Calcium gluconate
[ ] **3.** Sodium bicarbonate
[ ] **4.** Furosemide (Lasix)

The child receives a transfusion of packed red blood cells.

109. Which of the following is an indication the child may be experiencing a transfusion reaction? Select all that apply.
[ ] **1.** The child is thirsty.
[ ] **2.** The child feels chilled.
[ ] **3.** The child feels tired.
[ ] **4.** The child feels hungry.
[ ] **5.** The child experiences itching.
[ ] **6.** The child feels nauseous.

110. Which is the most appropriate initial nursing action if the child experiences a transfusion reaction?
[ ] **1.** Administer oxygen, and be prepared to start cardiopulmonary resuscitation.
[ ] **2.** Check the child's temperature, and give acetaminophen (Tylenol).
[ ] **3.** Stop the transfusion, and keep the I.V. line open with normal saline solution.
[ ] **4.** Notify the charge nurse, and return the blood to the blood bank for testing.

The child asks the nurse, "Am I going to die?"

111. What is the most appropriate response by the nurse?
[ ] **1.** "Are you feeling especially bad today? Tell me more about how you feel."
[ ] **2.** "You shouldn't worry about things like that. You are only a child."
[ ] **3.** "We are all going to die some day. Usually we die when we get old."
[ ] **4.** "Let's talk about something else. What is your favorite television program?"

The nurse is aware of the parents' strong Christian religious beliefs.

112. Which of the following statements would the nurse most anticipate from the parents of the child regarding disease progression?
[ ] **1.** Energy can be restored by means of acupuncture.
[ ] **2.** We pray to God and light candles asking for healing.
[ ] **3.** Our child's illness is a punishment for our sins.
[ ] **4.** We need to balance the yin and yang for healing.

113. Which statement by a parent of the child indicates a need for additional teaching about the child's condition?
[ ] **1.** "My child should continue all immunizations as scheduled."
[ ] **2.** "My child should avoid high-contact play activities."
[ ] **3.** "My child should eat small but frequent high-protein meals."
[ ] **4.** "My child shouldn't be around individuals with infections."

Nursing Care of a Preschooler with Strabismus

A 4-year-old child is to be admitted to an ambulatory surgical center for the correction of strabismus (crossed eyes). The day before the surgery, the child and parents go to the surgical center for preoperative teaching.

114. Which preoperative instruction is most important for the nurse to give the parents in preparation for the surgical procedure?
[ ] **1.** Clean the child's eyelid with an antiseptic at bedtime.
[ ] **2.** Trim the child's eyebrow in the mornings.
[ ] **3.** Withhold food and fluids from the child after midnight.
[ ] **4.** Give the child a dose of acetaminophen (Tylenol) at bedtime.

The child asks if the surgery will "hurt."

115. Which response by the nurse to the child is most appropriate?
[ ] **1.** "Don't think about that now."
[ ] **2.** "No, you won't feel any pain."
[ ] **3.** "I don't know. Ask the physician."
[ ] **4.** "Your eye may be sore after surgery."

116. Which type of game is the best preparation of the child for the postoperative period?
[ ] **1.** Tic-Tac-Toe on a large piece of paper
[ ] **2.** Pretending the child is a pirate with a patch
[ ] **3.** Hide-and-seek within the hospital room
[ ] **4.** Peek-a-boo with a member of the hospital staff

The child is admitted the following morning and undergoes surgery.

117. Which statement by the parents indicates a need for additional teaching?
[ ] **1.** "Our child can be up and about after the anesthesia wears off."
[ ] **2.** "Our child can have a regular diet after nausea has ceased."
[ ] **3.** "Our child cannot play with toys for at least 4 weeks."
[ ] **4.** "The restraints can be removed when we are holding our child."

Nursing Care of a Preschooler Having a Tonsillectomy and Adenoidectomy

A 5-year-old child who is scheduled for a tonsillectomy and adenoidectomy arrives in the outpatient department the morning of surgery. The nurse admitting the child assesses the vital signs.

118. Which assessment finding should be reported immediately to the charge nurse or physician?
[ ] **1.** Blood pressure of 96/60 mm Hg
[ ] **2.** Temperature of 101°F (38.3°C)
[ ] **3.** Respiratory rate of 20 breaths/minute
[ ] **4.** Pulse rate of 110 beats/minute

After surgery, the physician writes orders for pain medication and diet as the child prepares to be discharged from the outpatient care department.

119. Which food is most appropriate for the nurse to advise the parents to offer the child after surgery?
[ ] **1.** Orange juice
[ ] **2.** Apple juice
[ ] **3.** Ice cream
[ ] **4.** Cream of chicken soup

120. If the nurse observes all of the following behaviors, which one is a concern in the immediate postoperative period?
[ ] **1.** The ice collar is removed from the child's neck.
[ ] **2.** The child sucks liquids through a straw.
[ ] **3.** The parents left the room to get coffee.
[ ] **4.** The child uses a tissue to wipe blood from the lips.

121. If the nurse collects all of the following data, which observation indicates that the child may have postoperative complications?
[ ] **1.** Small amount of dark red emesis
[ ] **2.** Respiratory rate of 30 breaths/minute
[ ] **3.** Complaint of throat pain
[ ] **4.** Frequent swallowing

122. Which instruction is most appropriate to give to the parents during discharge teaching?
[ ] **1.** The child should be kept quiet for a few days after discharge.
[ ] **2.** The child's fluid intake should be limited for the next 48 hours.
[ ] **3.** The child should be given aspirin for discomfort and fever.
[ ] **4.** The child should resume a regular diet after nausea subsides.

123. The pediatric licensed practical nurse is called to the emergency department to care for a 3-year-old critically-ill child in which the staff is having difficulty obtaining an intravenous line. When leading the team, which nursing suggestion provides the best chance of initiating medication quickly into the child?
[ ] **1.** Use a ventrogluteal intramuscular site
[ ] **2.** Obtain a liquid dose for oral administration
[ ] **3.** Place the child under anesthesia to insert an intravenous line
[ ] **4.** Use the femur for an intraosseous site

Correct Answers, Rationales, and Test Taking Strategies

Normal Growth and Development of Infants, Toddlers, and Preschool Children

1. 2. When in the prone position, a 3-month-old infant should be able to raise the head and shoulders 45 to 90 degrees. The other developmental skills are accomplished later in infancy. Sitting with support and rolling from the abdomen to the back occur at approximately 5 months. Holding a bottle occurs when the infant is about 4½ months old.

Test Taking Strategy—Analyze to determine what information the question asks for, which is a normal developmental milestone for a 3-month-old infant. Remember that normal development occurs cephalocaudal (head to toe) and proximal to distal (from middle to outside). Review infant growth and development if you had difficulty answering this question.
Cognitive Level—Applying
Client Needs Category—Health promotion and maintenance
Client Needs Subcategory—None

2. 3. Crying for long periods of time, even after comfort measures have been used, is unusual and should be reported to the health care provider. The other signs and symptoms mentioned are usual side effects of the measles-mumps-rubella (MMR) immunization, which is given at 15 months, and do not require notifying the health care provider.

Test Taking Strategy—Analyze to determine what information the question asks for, which is an atypical response after MMR immunization that should be reported to the physician. Remember that inconsolable crying is not normal and the cause needs to be investigated. Review expected symptoms, which are generally minor, after an MMR immunization.
Cognitive Level—Applying
Client Needs Category—Health promotion and maintenance
Client Needs Subcategory—None

3. 2. A raw carrot should not be given to the toddler unless it is shredded because it (as well as nuts, raisins, and popcorn) may be a choking hazard. All the other findings observed by the nurse demonstrate that the parents understand the toddler's safety needs.

Test Taking Strategy—Use the process of elimination to identify the option that best describes a safety issue relative to a 20-month-old child. Options 1, 3, and 4, which include covering electrical outlets, ensuring that furniture corners are rounded, and providing large blocks for play, can be eliminated because

these are measures that promote the child's safety. Option 2 remains as a safety concern because the molars, which are needed for chewing, have not yet erupted in a child of this age. If the child bites large pieces of carrot or swallows the pieces whole, they may obstruct the airway or be aspirated into the lungs. Review factors that contribute to accidents and injuries in this age group if you had difficulty answering this question.
Cognitive Level—Analyzing
Client Needs Category—Safe and effective care environment
Client Needs Subcategory—Safety and infection critical

4. 1. The child's diagnosis is irrelevant; the apical site is preferred when assessing the pulse of a child younger than age 5. A satisfactory radial pulse cannot be obtained until the child is 2 years old, and even then the child may be so uncooperative that the assessment is invalid. The carotid site is not routinely used when assessing children; however, it is the preferred site when performing child cardiopulmonary resuscitation (CPR). The brachial site is not routinely used when assessing children, but it is the preferred site when performing infant CPR.

Test Taking Strategy—Use the process of elimination to select the option identifying the best location for assessing the pulse on a 2-year-old child. Option 1 is the best answer because the apical pulse is easier to locate; it is also easier to obtain on a child age 2 who is unable to cooperate with the other methods. Review the preferred sites for assessing the pulse in infants and toddlers if you had difficulty answering this question.
Cognitive Level—Applying
Client Needs Category—Health promotion and maintenance
Client Needs Subcategory—None

5. 1. The cultural heritage structure of Asian families is hierarchical. Therefore, the oldest male is usually the authority figure and makes the decision for the child. In this case, it would be the father providing health information not the mother, entire family unit, or parental unit. Other cultural characteristics include that the family is reluctant to have others provide physical care for the child, family values are important, and the parents may be reluctant to be honest and forthright regarding their feelings.

Test Taking Strategy—Analyze to determine what information the question asks for, which is the person to question when obtaining health information from Asian family members. Recall that in an Asian culture, males—in this case, the father—are the figures of authority in the family structure. Review the hierarchical family structure among Asian cultures if you had difficulty answering this question.
Cognitive Level—Applying
Client Needs Category—Psychosocial integrity
Client Needs Subcategory—None

6. 3. The correct way to give liquid medication to an infant is to position the infant upright and slowly administer the medication using a rubber-tipped medicine dropper. The medication may also be given through the nipple from a bottle. However, oral medications should not be added to the infant's formula; there is no guarantee that all of the medication will be administered if the infant does not drink all of the formula. Pinching the infant's nose is inappropriate; when the infant inhales through the mouth, it may cause the infant to aspirate the medication. Using the supine position may also cause the child to aspirate the medication or may allow the medication to leak from the side of the mouth.

Test Taking Strategy—Analyze to determine what information the question asks for, which is evidence that the parents understand an appropriate technique for administering liquid medication to an infant. Option 3 is the best answer because a medicine dropper can be easily placed in an infant's mouth without spilling portions of the liquid if the child struggles in the process of its administration. Review equipment used for pediatric oral medication administration if you had difficulty answering this question.
Cognitive Level—*Analyzing*
Client Needs Category—*Health promotion and maintenance*
Client Needs Subcategory—*None*

7. 4. An infant's respiratory rate is generally counted for 1 full minute because of normal irregularities. When assessing an older child, respirations may be counted for 30 seconds and then multiplied by 2.

Test Taking Strategy—Use the process of elimination to select the option that best describes how to count an infant's respiratory rate. Options 1, 2, and 3 can be eliminated because the lengths of assessment time are too brief to accommodate for an infant's irregular breathing patterns. Review the recommended amount of time for assessing infant respirations, which normally range from 30 to 60 breaths/minute, if you had difficulty answering this question.
Cognitive Level—*Applying*
Client Needs Category—*Health promotion and maintenance*
Client Needs Subcategory—*None*

8. 2. Bowel control is usually easier to accomplish than bladder control and is usually achieved first. All the other statements indicate the child's readiness to toilet-train.

Test Taking Strategy—Analyze to determine what information the question asks for, which is signs of readiness for toilet-training in a toddler. Read the question carefully, because it involves choosing an option that reflects a parent's incorrect statement. Option 2 is the best answer because bowel control is easier to accomplish due to the fact that toddlers usually have one to three stools per day, they occur at somewhat predictable times, and they are

accompanied by behaviors that suggest bowel elimination is about to occur. Review the age at which a child is physically able to voluntarily control urine elimination, which is about age 2 to 3 years, when higher levels of the central nervous system develop, if you had difficulty answering this question.*
Cognitive Level—*Analyzing*
Client Needs Category—*Health promotion and maintenance*
Client Needs Subcategory—*None*

9. 3. Finding age-related tasks that involve nurturing and responsibility tends to promote a feeling that the child's contributions are valued and appreciated. Sending the child to a preschool program or arranging visits with grandparents may further reinforce feelings of abandonment. Although playing with same-age children promotes socialization skills, it does not relieve sibling rivalry.

Test Taking Strategy—Use the process of elimination to identify the option that identifies the best advice for managing sibling rivalry. Option 3 remains as the best answer, because participating in the care of a new baby fosters acceptance and a sense of worth in the older child. Although some sibling rivalry is normal, review resources that discuss techniques for relieving sibling rivalry that may be considered more than ordinary if you had difficulty answering this question.
Cognitive Level—*Applying*
Client Needs Category—*Psychosocial integrity*
Client Needs Subcategory—*None*

10. 1. Using dolls or puppets as a teaching aid is the most appropriate strategy for a preschooler's cognitive ability. Other strategies include motivating the child with some form of reward. Pamphlets and diagrams are too abstract for the cognitive level of children age 3, 4, or 5 years. The use of a videotape might be confused as a form of entertainment rather than personal instruction.

Test Taking Strategy—Analyze to determine what information the question asks for, which is a developmentally appropriate teaching aid for use with a preschool child. Option 1 is the best answer because at a preschooler's cognitive level, dolls or puppets can be easily substituted for applications that involve learning new information. Review age-related differences among learners, especially pedagogic learners, if you had difficulty answering this question.
Cognitive Level—*Analyzing*
Client Needs Category—*Psychosocial integrity*
Client Needs Subcategory—*None*

11. 3. The most effective means for minimizing separation anxiety is having a parent remain with the child during hospitalization. A 16-month-old child has difficulty grasping the fact that parents are coming back after leaving, which leads to crying and other troubling behaviors. A familiar toy may help the child deal with the separation, but it is not as effective as a parent actually being there. Likewise, a sibling visit is not a substitute for the parents' presence; it may or may not assist with minimizing separation anxiety, depending on the child's relationship with the siblings. Explaining the procedure to the child will not decrease separation anxiety.

> *Test Taking Strategy—Use the process of elimination to select the option that identifies the best method for minimizing separation anxiety experienced by a hospitalized child. Recall that separation anxiety is normal in this age-group regardless of whether the child is hospitalized or not. Option 3 is the best answer because, in this case, remaining with the child in an unfamiliar environment provides emotional support and stability. Review references that indicate the age at which a child begins to understand that a parent who leaves will return, which is typically between 19 and 24 months, if you had difficulty answering this question.*
> *Cognitive Level—Applying*
> *Client Needs Category—Psychosocial integrity*
> *Client Needs Subcategory—None*

12. 2. When solid foods are introduced too early, antibodies are produced, predisposing the infant to food allergies. It may be necessary to breast-feed or bottle-feed a hungry infant before giving solid food to relieve his or her hunger and promote receptiveness to the new experience. Introducing one food at a time makes it easier to identify food intolerances and allergies. If solid foods are offered too early, infants normally push food out of their mouths when spoon-fed because of the extrusion reflex, a protective mechanism seen in infants up to age 6 months. Because the throat muscles and tongue are not developed enough to swallow solids until about age 6 months, solid foods are usually spit out. It is roughly around age 6 months that the baby will be able to use the tongue to transfer food from the front to the back of the mouth and then to swallow. Cereals should be the first solid food introduced because they are least likely to cause food allergies, are easy to digest, and contain added iron. By age 6 months, the child will need additional iron because the iron stores that are present at birth are diminished

> *Test Taking Strategy—Analyze to determine what information the question asks for, which is the need to include additional teaching for parents who wish to introduce solid foods to their 6-month-old child. Recall that a slow introduction of solid food (option 3) helps to evaluate the infant's digestive and immunologic responses. Review guidelines for introducing solid food and the basis for those guidelines if you had difficulty answering this question.*
> *Cognitive Level—Analyzing*
> *Client Needs Category—Health promotion and maintenance*
> *Client Needs Subcategory—None*

13. 3. An 18-month-old child should be able to walk without support. Infants on average begin taking steps around age 12 months, and most are walking well by 18 months, although there can be differences. The other findings are normal and should have been accomplished by a toddler of this age.

> *Test Taking Strategy—Analyze to determine what information the question asks for, which is an abnormal assessment finding when examining an 18-month-old child. Read the options carefully because it requires looking for a motor skill that deviates from that expected for a child of this age. Review discussions of the age range when walking commences and is mastered if you had difficulty answering this question.*
> *Cognitive Level—Applying*
> *Client Needs Category—Health promotion and maintenance*
> *Client Needs Subcategory—None*

14. 2. Medicine and other toxic substances should be kept in a locked cabinet. Merely keeping such substances out of reach is inadequate; the child might be able to climb higher than anticipated. The other observations are correct safety measures.

> *Test Taking Strategy—Analyze to determine what information the question asks for, which is a statement that identifies a safety concern and need for parental health teaching when raising a toddler. Recall that toddlers are very active and curious, and can climb to reach objects even if they are on a high shelf. Review the developmental characteristics of toddlers and potential risks for accidents and injuries in this age group if you had difficulty answering this question.*
> *Cognitive Level—Applying*
> *Client Needs Category—Health promotion and maintenance*
> *Client Needs Subcategory—None*

15. 1. It is developmentally normal for a 4-year-old child to talk to an imaginary playmate. Imaginary friends often appear between ages 3 and 6 because fantasy and pretending are common at this age-group's cognitive level. Imaginary friends may meet needs for companionship or comfort, filling a void for loneliness. Parents should respect and accept the imaginary friend, who is real to the child, and avoid discouraging or belittling the child's belief. Preschoolers usually abandon imaginary playmates when they begin to interact more with children their own age. Because the behavior is not pathologic, it would be inappropriate to look for unusual stressors, recommend the services of a child psychologist, or invoke a disciplinary time-out period.

> *Test Taking Strategy—Use the process of elimination to select the option that identifies the best response to a parent's concern about a preschooler's belief in an imaginary playmate. Recall that preschoolers have a*

vivid imagination, and having an imaginary play-mate is not unusual for a child of this age. Review factors that distinguish the normalcy of imaginary friends from those that suggest pathology if you had difficulty answering this question.
Cognitive level—*Analyzing*
Client Needs Category—*Health promotion and maintenance*
Client Needs Subcategory—*None*

16.

6. Maintain water temperatures under 120°F (48.8°C).
2. Have straps on the changing table.
4. Remove stuffed animals with small pieces from the child's grasp.
1. Cover the electrical outlets.
3. Turn pot handles inward when cooking.
5. Lower crib mattress.

Water temperatures should be set under 120°F to ensure that the fragile skin of the newborn is protected. Because of the child's placement on top of tables, straps should be placed on the changing table. Parents should not leave the child unattended. Stuffed animals with small pieces should be removed from the child's environment to avoid the child's accidental ingestion or inhalation. When the child begins to crawl, electrical outlet plugs should be included in childproofing the home. As the child begins to pull up from the floor, pot handles should be turned inward so as not to have hot objects spilled. As the child becomes tall enough to extend over crib rails, the crib mattress should be lowered.

Test Taking Strategy—Analyze to determine what information the question asks for, which is prioritizing safety measures from birth through age 12 months. Recall that at birth the infant is totally helpless, then begins to roll over, develops prehension for grasping objects, learns by mouthing objects, crawls, pulls himself or herself to a standing position, and stands alone. Review normal progression of growth and development during the first year of life if you had difficulty answering this question.
Cognitive Level—*Analyzing*
Client Needs Category—*Health promotion and maintenance*
Client Needs Subcategory—*None*

Nursing Care of an Infant with Myelomeningocele

17. **2.** A myelomeningocele is described as a congenital neural tube defect involving the protrusion of an external sac containing part of the spinal cord and its meninges. This is also called *spina bifida*. Hydrocephalus and mental retardation are also frequent findings. The most important nursing measure would be to avoid pressure on and prevent injury to the sac. This is important because a break in the sac could lead to serious infection. Washing the area would not be appropriate because of the danger of injury to the sac. Preventing skin breakdown is important but not as important as preventing injury to the sac. The normal care of the diaper area is maintained because the sac is high in the spinal column. Parents are encouraged to bond with the infant using touch and eye contact. Cuddling and holding the infant could potentially cause trauma to the sac.

Test Taking Strategy—Use the process of elimination to select the option that identifies the most important nursing measure when caring for an infant with a myelomeningocele preoperatively. Recall that the protruding sac must be protected until it is surgically repaired (option 2). Option 1 can be eliminated because this client's myelomeningocele is described in the stem as being located higher. Eliminate options 3 and 4 because those actions would cause trauma to the sac. Review illustrations of a myelomeningocele as well as discussions of how to manage the care of an infant with this congenital defect if you had difficulty answering this question.
Cognitive Level—*Analyzing*
Client Needs Category—*Physiological integrity*
Client Needs Subcategory—*Reduction of risk potential*

18. **2.** The prone position (lying on the abdomen) is used after surgical repair of a myelomeningocele. This position is maintained until the operative site heals. To prevent infection, it is important to keep the operative site clean and free of pressure. Infants undergoing this procedure should not be placed supine (on the back) or on their side, because these positions may put stress on the operative site. The most comfortable position may not be the most appropriate position for care of the surgical site.

Test Taking Strategy—Analyze to determine what information the question asks for, which is the best postoperative position for an infant after repair of a myelomeningocele. Recall that the surgical incision is located in the midback; therefore, positioning on the stomach (option 2) is recommended. Review the postoperative nursing care after myelomeningocele repair if you had difficulty answering this question.
Cognitive Level—*Applying*
Client Needs Category—*Physiological integrity*
Client Needs Subcategory—*Physiological adaptation*

19. 1. In planning the infant's home care, an essential orthopedic consideration would include instructing the parents on range-of-motion (ROM) exercises to reduce joint contractures. Completing ROM exercises proactively promotes improved function. Arranging for specialized assistive devices, allowing the infant to move all extremities, and using lotions and ointments to massage large muscle groups may be appropriate but not as essential as the parents completing ROM exercises.

Test Taking Strategy—Analyze to determine what information the question asks for, which is home care to reduce musculoskeletal problems for a child with a myelomeningocele repair. Recall that despite the surgical repair, the infant cannot move his or her legs. Therefore, teaching the parents how to do ROM exercises on the infant's legs (option 1) is essential for maintaining muscle tone and joint mobility. Review the musculoskeletal deficits associated with a myelomeningocele and measures that can prevent or reduce additional problems if you had difficulty answering this question.
Cognitive Level—Applying
Client Needs Category—Physiological integrity
Client Needs Subcategory—Reduction of risk potential

20. 2. Urinary and bowel control problems occur in children with spina bifida and myelomeningocele. Because intermittent catheterization is required in most cases, the parents should be instructed on how to insert a straight catheter using a clean technique. During the early school years, the child will also be taught how to perform this procedure. The child with a myelomeningocele usually does not require a retention catheter or ureterostomy.

Test Taking Strategy—Analyze to determine what information the question asks for, which is instruction the parents will need to manage their child's urinary incontinence. Recall that diapers can be used during infancy, but straight catheterization will become necessary after the child gets older. Review the most common method for controlling urinary incontinence in an older child who has a repaired myelomeningocele if you had difficulty answering this question.
Cognitive Level—Applying
Client Needs Category—Physiological integrity
Client Needs Subcategory—Basic care and comfort

21. 4. Infants with spina bifida and a myelomeningocele commonly have clubfoot and congenital hip dysplasia. Because the defect typically causes a loss of motion in the lower extremities, range-of-motion (ROM) exercises are most effective in preventing contractures. Although massaging the lower extremities, repositioning the infant, and placing sheepskin under the bony prominences are good nursing interventions, they will not prevent contractures.

Test Taking Strategy—Analyze to determine what information the question asks for, which is the priority

nursing intervention for preventing contractures in a child who has clubfoot and a hip dysplasia. Recall that contractures are a consequence of shortened muscles and lengthening of those in opposition. Unless exercised, the joint becomes fixed. ROM exercises (option 4) that are performed frequently and consistently help to prevent or reduce the potential for developing contractures. Review methods for preventing contractures if you had difficulty answering this question.*
Cognitive Level—Applying
Client Needs Category—Physiological integrity
Client Needs Subcategory—Reduction of risk potential

Nursing Care of an Infant with Hydrocephalus

22. 1. In an infant, hydrocephalus (commonly called water on the brain) is a neurologic problem related to an accumulation of cerebrospinal fluid (CSF) around the brain and spinal cord caused by a blockage within the path in which it circulates. The buildup of fluid around the brain puts pressure on the child's brain, causing damage to the brain and surrounding structures. An increase in head size is the most prominent characteristic of hydrocephalus. Because of the accumulation of fluid, the child's sutures in the skull separate as the head grows. The fontanels usually bulge. Some hydrocephalic infants also have spina bifida with a myelomeningocele and may have lower-extremity paralysis, but this neurologic deficit is not a prominent symptom of hydrocephalus. The presence or absence of the sucking reflex also is not considered a prominent sign.

Test Taking Strategy—Use the process of elimination to identify the option that describes the most characteristic assessment finding when examining an infant with hydrocephalus. Recalling that the prefix hydro- refers to water and -cephalus is derived from the word meaning head, option 1 becomes the obvious answer. Review the physical manifestations associated with hydrocephalus if you had difficulty answering this question.
Cognitive Level—Applying
Client Needs Category—Physiological integrity
Client Needs Subcategory—Physiological adaptation

23. 2. The cause of hydrocephalus in most infants is a blockage (obstruction) that prevents proper circulation of cerebrospinal fluid (CSF). This is known as noncommunicating congenital hydrocephalus. Absence of the dura mater, increased CSF in the subarachnoid space, and blockage of the cerebral arteries are not known to cause hydrocephalus.

Test Taking Strategy—Analyze to determine what information the question asks for, which is the most common cause of hydrocephalus in infants. Option 2 is the best answer because in infants, hydrocephalus

usually develops when there is a narrowing of the aqueduct of Sylvius, a small passage between the third and fourth ventricles in the brain, which interferes with the circulation of CSF. Review the manner in which CSF is formed and circulates, and compare that with information about the etiology of hydrocephalus, if you had difficulty answering this question.
Cognitive Level—*Applying*
Client Needs Category—*Physiological integrity*
Client Needs Subcategory—*Physiological adaptation*

24. 4. The side-lying position is the preferred way to place an infant with hydrocephalus after feeding. Because such infants are at risk for vomiting as a result of increased intracranial pressure, placing them on their side allows vomitus to easily escape, decreasing the chance of aspiration. The positions identified in the remaining options may result in aspiration.
Test Taking Strategy—*Analyze to determine what information the question asks for, which is the position in which a child with hydrocephalus should be placed after feeding. Recall that this child may not be able to change his or her head position because of its enlarged size. A side-lying (lateral) position (option 4) reduces the potential for regurgitated liquid entering the airway. Stomach contents are more likely to be expelled onto the surface, supporting the infant in a side-lying position. Review the anatomic consequences of an enlarged head and the physics that apply to a side-lying position in relation to preventing aspiration, if you had difficulty answering this question.*
Cognitive Level—*Applying*
Client Needs Category—*Physiological integrity*
Client Needs Subcategory—*Reduction of risk potential*

25. 1. The head and ears of an infant with hydrocephalus are especially prone to the development of pressure ulcers. The primary reason for using a sheepskin in this situation is to help relieve pressure on the head and ears. The infant's position should also be changed frequently to prevent complications due to inactivity. The other options are incorrect because they will not relieve pressure on the infant's head.
Test Taking Strategy—*Look at the key words "most appropriate" used in reference to a nursing measure for reducing the risk of a pressure ulcer developing on the infant's head. Recall that sheepskin (option 1) or some other pressure-relieving device promotes the maintenance of capillary blood flow that will keep tissue perfused and intact. Review methods for preventing pressure ulcers if you had difficulty answering this question.*
Cognitive Level—*Applying*
Client Needs Category—*Physiological integrity*
Client Needs Subcategory—*Basic care and comfort*

26. 3. The purpose of a ventriculoperitoneal (V/P) shunt is to drain the excess fluid from the brain and thereby release intracranial pressure. The position of choice after inserting a V/P shunt is on the side opposite the site of the surgical incision. This position prevents damage to the shunt valve. The infant described in this question should be placed on the left side postoperatively because the surgical site of entry was on the right side of the head.
Test Taking Strategy—*Look at the key words "most appropriate" in reference to postoperative positioning after a shunt insertion on the right side. Recall that a burr hole is made to place the shunt in the ventricle and internal tubing is tunneled behind the right ear to the peritoneal cavity. Therefore, placing the child on the unaffected left side is an appropriate nursing action. Review postoperative care of an infant having a shunt inserted, especially in relation to the preferred body position, if you had difficulty answering this question.*
Cognitive Level—*Applying*
Client Needs Category—*Physiological integrity*
Client Needs Subcategory—*Reduction of risk potential*

27. 2. A child with hydrocephalus has increased intracranial pressure due to the accumulation of cerebrospinal fluid, which should be relieved after the placement of a shunt. If the child develops signs and symptoms of increased intracranial pressure postoperatively, the nurse can assume that there is a problem with fluid draining through the shunt. Signs of increased intracranial pressure in an infant include bulging or tense fontanels, decreased pulse and respiratory rates, irritability, and vomiting. Seizures may also be evident. Changes in weight and bowel elimination are not common indicators of increased intracranial pressure.
Test Taking Strategy—*Use the process of elimination to identify the option that best describes a sign of increased intracranial pressure. Remember that if fluid increases due to a malfunction of the shunt, pressure on the brain stem, which includes the pons and medulla, can cause an alteration in vital signs such as pulse and respiratory rates (option 2). Review the signs associated with increased intracranial pressure if you had difficulty answering this question.*
Cognitive Level—*Analyzing*
Client Needs Category—*Physiological integrity*
Client Needs Subcategory—*Physiological adaptation*

28. 2. Sunken fontanels, especially the anterior fontanel, which is the largest one in the skull, are a sign of dehydration. The finding in an infant with a ventriculoperitoneal (V/P) shunt may indicate that more than the desired amount of cerebrospinal fluid (CSF) has drained through the shunt. On detecting the depressed anterior fontanel, the most appropriate action is to keep the infant flat in a supine position. This position limits a further decrease in intracranial pressure. If the fontanel is bulging, the head would be elevated. It would be appropriate to notify the charge nurse or physician after positioning the infant.

> *Test Taking Strategy—Look at the key words "most appropriate" in reference to a nursing action after finding that the postoperative infant with a V/P shunt has a sunken anterior fontanel. Keeping the child supine (option 2) counteracts the effect of gravity and decreases the volume of CSF leaving the ventricles. Review the significance of sunken fontanels, especially in relation to a child with a V/P shunt, if you had difficulty answering this question.*
> *Cognitive Level—Applying*
> *Client Needs Category—Physiological integrity*
> *Client Needs Subcategory—Physiological adaptation*

Nursing Care of an Infant with Cleft Lip

29. 3. A cleft lip is a congenital birth defect in which the lip or palate does not correctly form during gestation. The nurse assesses the newborn on admission to the nursery, looking for obvious signs of physical anomalies, such as cleft lip and cleft palate. A cleft lip is easily identified during inspection due to the obvious appearance of the lip. However, a cleft palate is a fissure in the midline of the palate and therefore requires palpating the roof of the mouth. The nurse does not palpate the roof of the mouth to elicit the gag reflex, assess the infant's sucking ability, or determine the position of the uvula.

> *Test Taking Strategy—Analyze to determine what information the question asks for, which is the rationale for palpating inside the mouth of a newborn with a cleft lip. A cleft palate occurs in about 50% of those born with a cleft lip, especially bilateral cleft lip. To confirm or rule out that a cleft palate exists, the nurse must palpate the roof of the newborn's mouth (option 3). Review the assessment technique for identifying a cleft palate if you had difficulty answering this question.*
> *Cognitive Level—Applying*
> *Client Needs Category—Physiological integrity*
> *Client Needs Subcategory—Physiological adaptation*

30. 2. One of the nurse's primary considerations when caring for an infant with a cleft lip is dealing with the parents' reaction to the child's appearance. The nurse can facilitate parental adjustment by demonstrating acceptance of the child, encouraging the parents to express their feelings, and acknowledging the appropriateness of their feelings. Discussions about the infant's special needs, including feeding, surgical repair, and use of the bulb syringe, are important; however, the parents must first begin to adjust to their child's appearance before they can deal with other issues.

> *Test Taking Strategy—Use the process of elimination to help select the option that identifies the nursing priority when bringing the newborn with a cleft lip to the parents. Recall that the nurse can model behavior for the parents. Showing acceptance (option 2) can influence a similar attitude on the part of the parents. Options 1, 3, and 4 are not the priorities at this time. Review techniques for promoting acceptance of a special needs infant by parents if you had difficulty answering this question.*
> *Cognitive Level—Analyzing*
> *Client Needs Category—Psychosocial integrity*
> *Client Needs Subcategory—None*

31. 1. Infants with cleft lip swallow more air than usual; therefore, they should be burped frequently to decrease the chance of vomiting and subsequent aspiration. Lying horizontal with the face down in the prone position should be avoided because this position makes feeding difficult and the risk for aspiration is high. An infant scheduled for cleft lip repair is fed regular formula or breast milk before surgery.

> *Test Taking Strategy—Analyze to determine what information the question asks for, which is evidence that the parents understand how to reduce the risk of aspiration in the newborn with a cleft lip. Recall that because of the oral defect, the infant swallows a great deal of air, which increases the risk for vomiting. Burping the infant frequently (option 1) relieves gastric pressure and reduces the risk for vomiting and aspiration. Review techniques for feeding an infant with a cleft lip or cleft palate if you had difficulty answering this question.*
> *Cognitive Level—Applying*
> *Client Needs Category—Physiological integrity*
> *Client Needs Subcategory—Reduction of risk potential*

32. 3. Although breast-feeding is possible, of the four options, a bottle with a nipple that has an enlarged hole is the best method of feeding the infant with a cleft lip that extends into the gum line. The enlarged hole provides a freer flow of formula or breast milk. A hole can be created in a standard nipple by making a cross-cut in the tip, or commercial nipples such as those for premature infants may be purchased. Using a bottle with a firm nipple makes the infant work harder to obtain nourishment. A bulb syringe with a tube that extends from the tip is appropriate for an infant who has a cleft palate rather than cleft lip. Gavage feeding is not usually necessary because of the options available for oral feeding and support from the nurse.

> *Test Taking Strategy—Analyze to determine what information the question asks for, which is the utensil that is best for feeding an infant with a cleft lip. Various utensils are available for feeding the infant, depending on the size of the cleft, but using a nipple with an enlarged hole (option 3) helps deliver sufficient formula or breast milk for weight gain when the infant's*

ability to suck and swallow is compromised. Review methods for feeding an infant with a cleft lip versus those for an infant with both a cleft lip and palate if you had difficulty answering this question.
Cognitive Level—*Applying*
Client Needs Category—*Physiological integrity*
Client Needs Subcategory—*Basic care and comfort*

33. 3. Elbow restraints allow movement of the arms but prevent the infant from touching the face. A papoose board or a mummy restraint prevents movement of the entire body; these forms of restraint are not usually necessary for this type of surgery. A Posey belt or jacket will not prevent a child from touching the face; such devices are used to keep a client in bed or in a wheelchair. Leg restraints are not used because the infant cannot use the legs to injure the surgical site.

Test Taking Strategy—Use the process of elimination to identify the option that describes the best type of restraint to use for a child who has had a cleft lip repair. Recall that the goal is to keep the infant's hands away from the face so that the surgical repair is not altered without totally restricting the infant's movement. The goal can be accomplished by using elbow restraints (option 3). Review the method for applying elbow restraints and their effect on movement if you had difficulty answering this question.
Cognitive Level—*Applying*
Client Needs Category—*Safe and effective care environment*
Client Needs Subcategory—*Safety and infection control*

34. 4. Unless the physician orders otherwise, most restraints are removed and reapplied at least every 2 hours to check skin integrity and maintain adequate circulation and movement. The child is monitored when restraints are removed. Checking the restraints daily every 4 or 8 hours prevents adequate assessment and movement of the extremity.

Test Taking Strategy—Analyze to determine what information the question asks for, which is the frequency with which the infant's restraint should be removed. Recall that restraints of any type should be removed every 2 hours (option 4) to avoid circulatory and neurologic injury. Recall the purpose and frequency for removing and reapplying restraints if you had difficulty answering this question.
Cognitive Level—*Applying*
Client Needs Category—*Safe and effective care environment*
Client Needs Subcategory—*Safety and infection control*

Nursing Care of an Infant with Pyloric Stenosis

35. 4. The pylorus is the sphincter, also called a valve, located between the stomach and the duodenum of the small intestine. In the case of pyloric stenosis, the sphincter

is narrow, impairing passage of stomach contents into the small intestine. Projectile vomiting is the first sign of the problem; the vomiting without sufficient nutrition leads to dehydration. Dry mucous membranes are an indication of dehydration. The infant must be rehydrated and electrolytes must be within normal limits before undergoing surgery. The anterior fontanel is normally flat. Hunger and visible gastric peristaltic waves are present with pyloric stenosis, but they are less significant because they do not indicate the same health risk as dehydration.

Test Taking Strategy—Look at the key words "most significant" in reference to the assessment findings listed. Dehydration (option 4) is a more significant finding than the other three assessment findings. Review the consequences of pyloric stenosis if you had difficulty answering this question.
Cognitive Level—*Applying*
Client Needs Category—*Physiological integrity*
Client Needs Subcategory—*Physiological adaptation*

36. 2. A buretrol is added to the infusion tubing to ensure that a large volume of intravenous fluid does not inadvertently infuse into the client. Typically, 1 to 2 hours worth of fluid is held within the buretrol to be infused. The I.V. catheter is not sutured to the scalp. Most often, tape secures the site. Restlessness and swelling are unusual findings which need to be reported immediately as they may indicate infiltration.

Test Taking Strategy—Analyze to determine what information the question asks for, which is an accurate statement about I.V. fluid administration to an infant with pyloric stenosis. Recall that oral nutrition results in vomiting, which necessitates administering I.V. therapy utilizing a buretrol (option 2). Review methods for maintaining nutrition and hydration for infants with pyloric stenosis if you had difficulty answering this question.
Cognitive Level—*Applying*
Client Needs Category—*Physiological integrity*
Client Needs Subcategory—*Physiological adaptation*

37. 2. After feeding, the infant should be placed on the right side or in an infant seat. These positions aid in emptying the stomach and preventing aspiration. The left side does not facilitate gastric emptying. The prone position is not recommended because of its association with the occurrence of sudden infant death syndrome. Placing the infant on his or her back creates a greater risk for aspiration of stomach contents. The most comfortable position may not necessarily be the best choice for this infant, given the nature of the infant's condition.

Test Taking Strategy—Analyze to determine what information the question asks for, which is the position that is used after feeding the infant with a repaired pyloric sphincter. Recall that the pyloric sphincter is between the stomach and small intestine within a right-sided curve. Placing the infant on the right side

(option 2) facilitates the movement of chyme into the intestinal tract. Review the anatomy of the stomach and small intestine, focusing on the location of the pyloric sphincter, if you had difficulty answering this question.
Cognitive Level—*Applying*
Client Needs Category—*Physiological integrity*
Client Needs Subcategory—*Physiological adaptation*

Nursing Care of an Infant with Bilateral Clubfoot

38. 3. True clubfoot is fixed and cannot be corrected to a neutral or natural position. An infant should be evaluated carefully because the feet may appear to be clubbed at birth but are actually the result of fetal positioning in utero. One or both feet may be involved. In both the infant with true clubfoot and the infant with false clubfoot, the heels may be drawn in and the feet turned inward. Not all infants who are born breech develop clubfoot.

> *Test Taking Strategy—Analyze to determine what information the question asks for, which is the data that indicates true clubbing of the infant's feet. Recall that true clubbing of the feet requires surgical intervention because they will not assume a neutral position (option 3), whereas false clubbing can be corrected with exercise, splints, casts, continuous passive motion machines, and orthopedic shoes. Review the characteristics of true clubbed feet if you had difficulty answering this question.*
Cognitive Level—*Applying*
Client Needs Category—*Physiological integrity*
Client Needs Subcategory—*Physiological adaptation*

39. 3. Adhesive petals are placed around the cast edges to prevent the plaster from irritating the skin. The material is smooth and is placed on the opening at the top of the cast and around the toes. Such petaling is not used to keep materials from getting between the cast and the skin or to keep air circulating between the skin and the cast. It is also not intended or needed to make the cast stronger.

> *Test Taking Strategy—Analyze to determine what information the question asks for, which is the reason for using adhesive petals around the edge of the infant's casts. Recall that the purpose of the petals is to prevent skin breakdown due to cast irritation (option 3). Review nursing care of a client with a cast, focusing specifically on methods for preventing skin breakdown, if you had difficulty answering this question.*
Cognitive Level—*Applying*
Client Needs Category—*Physiological integrity*
Client Needs Subcategory—*Reduction of risk potential*

40. 3. Pale, cold extremities are signs of impaired circulation caused by the pressure of the cast. This problem

must be reported immediately. Crying four hours after the last feeding is normal because the infant is likely to be hungry, but unexplained crying may indicate pain or discomfort. Wiggling the toes is a sign that the nervous system has not been compromised by application of a cast. A pulse rate of 110 beats/minute is normal.

> *Test Taking Strategy—Use the process of elimination to select the option that describes the best indication of a neurovascular complication manifested by the infant with bilateral leg casts. Recall that pink, warm toes would indicate adequate circulation; the opposite would be true for impaired circulation (option 3). Options 1, 2, and 4 represent normal findings in an infant. Review the care of a client in a cast, focusing on indications of neurovascular complications, if you had difficulty answering this question.*
Cognitive Level—*Applying*
Client Needs Category—*Physiological integrity*
Client Needs Subcategory—*Reduction of risk potential*

41. 1. After a cast is applied to the lower extremities, the extremities are elevated on pillows to improve circulation and prevent swelling. The infant's position is usually changed every 2 hours to promote even drying. Petaling the edges is performed to prevent skin breakdown. Ice packs are not used to decrease swelling associated with casting.

> *Test Taking Strategy—Analyze to determine what information the question asks for, which is an action that will minimize swelling of the child's feet after a cast is applied. Recall that elevating the extremities (option 1), regardless of the cause, reduces swelling by promoting venous circulation from the extremities. Review techniques for relieving edema in lower extremities if you had difficulty answering this question.*
Cognitive Level—*Applying*
Client Needs Category—*Physiological integrity*
Client Needs Subcategory—*Basic care and comfort*

42. 1. The purpose of casting is to gradually correct the defect without causing trauma; therefore, the casts are changed every few days initially, then every 1 to 2 weeks. Correction is usually achieved in approximately 6 to 8 weeks.

> *Test Taking Strategy—Analyze to determine what information the question asks for, which is the timeline for changing the infant's casts in the early stages of correcting the abnormal foot position. Recall that the casts will be initially removed and reapplied as often as weekly (option 1) to gradually stretch tendons to achieve an externally rotated foot position. Review the use of casts when correcting a clubfoot deformity if you had difficulty answering this question.*
Cognitive Level—*Applying*
Client Needs Category—*Physiological integrity*
Client Needs Subcategory—*Physiological adaptation*

43. 4. An infant develops the ability to look at surroundings during the first month of life. By age 2 months, the infant can follow an object with both eyes; therefore, a mobile is an appropriate amusement for a child of this age. By age 4 months, the infant typically can reach for objects. By age 7 to 9 months, the infant usually can crawl and play peek-a-boo. It would be inappropriate, however, to encourage an infant in a cast to crawl.

> *Test Taking Strategy—Analyze to determine what information the question asks for, which is an age-appropriate activity that the nurse can suggest to the parents of an 8-week-old infant. Recall that eye coordination is developing at this time, making option 4, stimulating the infant with a colorful mobile, an age-appropriate activity. Review activities that promote normal growth and development for an infant who is 2 months old if you had difficulty answering this question.*
> ***Cognitive Level—****Applying*
> ***Client Needs Category—****Health promotion and maintenance*
> ***Client Needs Subcategory—****None*

44. 1. A fontanel is a space covered by tough membranes between the bones of an infant's cranium. The posterior fontanel closes quite soon after birth, between age 2 and 3 months, in comparison to the anterior fontanel, which remains open until about age 2 years.

> *Test Taking Strategy—Use the process of elimination to select the option that describes an accurate response to the parents' question about the infant's posterior fontanel. Options 2 and 3 can be eliminated because it is not abnormal to barely feel the posterior fontanel at age 2 months. Option 4 can be eliminated because the posterior fontanel does not close earlier in children with skeletal defects. Option 1 is the remaining and best answer because it is normal to barely feel the posterior fontanel at age 2 months. Review the age at which the fontanels close if you had difficulty answering this question.*
> ***Cognitive Level—****Applying*
> ***Client Needs Category—****Health promotion and maintenance*
> ***Client Needs Subcategory—****None*

Nursing Care of a Child with Otitis Media

45. 2. Otitis media is an infection in the middle ear, which is connected to the pharynx by the eustachian tube. It is usually a sequela of an upper respiratory infection during which time the eustachian tube swells, allowing fluid to become trapped. The fluid provides an environment in which bacteria grow. The infected fluid creates pressure in the confined space, leading to intense pain. An infant

or young child with otitis media typically pulls at or rubs the affected ear in response to the pain. Although the other options may be present with otitis media, they are not caused by or related to the pain.

> *Test Taking Strategy—Analyze to determine what information the question asks for, which is the best indicator that an infant is experiencing pain due to otitis media. Recall that an infant cannot verbalize the location of the discomfort, but pulling at the ear (option 2) is a nonverbal sign of ear pain. Review the signs and symptoms of otitis media, especially in relation to clinical manifestations exhibited by an infant, if you had difficulty answering this question.*
> ***Cognitive Level—****Applying*
> ***Client Needs Category—****Physiological integrity*
> ***Client Needs Subcategory—****Physiological adaptation*

46. 2. Although the physician prescribes the amount of medication to be given, the nurse is responsible for determining whether the prescribed dose is within the recommended safe dosage range. The most reliable method of determining the recommended safe dosage range requires calculating the child's dose based on weight. The other options are important steps in medication administration but do not relate specifically to determining the safe dose.

> *Test Taking Strategy—Use the process of elimination to select the option that identifies the best method for ensuring that an infant's dose of medication is accurate. Option 1 can be eliminated because a physician may have written an incorrect dosage in the order. Option 2 can be eliminated because checking for an allergy is unrelated to determining an accurate dosage. Option 4 has some merit because a pharmaceutical company's label may provide the recommended pediatric dose base on weight, but this may not be true for medications such as those repackaged by a pharmacist. Checking a drug reference and calculating the dose based on the recommendation for the weight of the child (option 2) is the best answer. Review how to calculate medication dosages for pediatric clients if you had difficulty answering this question.*
> ***Cognitive Level—****Applying*
> ***Client Needs Category—****Physiological integrity*
> ***Client Needs Subcategory—****Pharmacological therapies*

47. 4. The nurse should instruct the parents to complete the full course of antibiotics even though the infant's condition may improve after 2 to 3 days of treatment. Failure to complete the full course of antibiotics may lead to recurrent infection and other associated complications. Whether the antibiotic is given with food and how the antibiotic is stored varies, depending on the specific antibiotic. Placing the infant on the side after giving an antibiotic is not usually required unless the medication was instilled by eardrop. In this case, the infant is receiving an oral antibiotic.

Test Taking Strategy—*Analyze to determine what information the question asks for, which is information that should be emphasized when teaching parents who will administer medication to the infant. Recall that treating an infection effectively requires complying with the full prescribed drug regimen (option 4). Review the causes of drug resistant pathogens especially as it relates to undertreating infections if you had difficulty answering this question.*
Cognitive Level—*Applying*
Client Needs Category—*Physiological integrity*
Client Needs Subcategory—*Pharmacological therapies*

48. **1. 720 mg.**
Erythromycin is supplied as 200 mg/5 mL or 40 mg/mL. A 6-mL volume provides 240 mg every 8 hours. Multiplied by three 8-hour periods in 24 hours, the child receives 720 mg/day.
Test Taking Strategy—*Analyze to determine what information the question asks for, which relates to calculating a total daily drug dosage. In this case, the child's weight is not necessary for solving the problem. Review the processes for calculating drug dosages if you had difficulty answering this question.*
Cognitive Level—*Applying*
Client Needs Category—*Physiological integrity*
Client Needs Subcategory—*Pharmacological therapies*

Nursing Care of a Child with a Congenital Heart Defect

49. **3.** A coarctation of the aorta is a congenital defect in which the aorta is narrowed. This makes the heart work harder to pump oxygenated blood through the small pathway to the rest of the body. In the child with coarctation of the aorta, the pulses are typically bounding in the upper extremities and weak in the lower extremities. Also, the blood pressure is higher in the upper extremities than in the lower extremities. This happens because of the narrowing of the aorta that occurs with coarctation. The other choices may develop at some point, but they may also be associated with other defects.
Test Taking Strategy—*Use the process of elimination to help select the option identifying the best indication of coarctation of the aorta. Option 1 can be eliminated because cyanosis is not generally associated with coarctation of the aorta. Option 2 can be eliminated because clubbed fingers are the result of long-standing cardiopulmonary disorders. Option 4 can be eliminated because this disorder does not cause arrhythmias, but it does cause alterations in the amplitude of the pulse at various peripheral pulse sites as described in option 3, which is the best answer. Review the pathophysiology associated with coarctation of the aorta, focusing especially on the*

comparative findings in peripheral pulses, if you had difficulty answering this question.
Cognitive Level—*Analyzing*
Client Needs Category—*Physiological integrity*
Client Needs Subcategory—*Physiological adaptation*

50. **3.** Initially, the infant with coarctation of the aorta may be given prostaglandin E to dilate the narrowed aorta. However, the corrective treatment is surgical repair, which is usually performed before the child is 2 years old. If the correction is not performed, life-threatening complications may develop.
Test Taking Strategy—*Analyze to determine what information the question asks for, which is the optimum time for surgically correcting coarctation of the aorta. Depending on the severity of the infant's symptoms, surgical repair may be delayed to determine if other noninvasive treatment options and medications, such as those for managing congestive heart failure, improve the infant's quality of life. If surgery is needed, it is usually performed before the infant is 2 years old (option 3). Review the treatment of clients with coarctation of the aorta if you had difficulty answering this question.*
Cognitive Level—*Applying*
Client Needs Category—*Physiological integrity*
Client Needs Subcategory—*Physiological adaptation*

51. **1.** The nurse should check the infant's apical pulse for 1 full minute before giving digoxin (Lanoxin). If the pulse is slower than the normal lower limit, the nurse should withhold the medication and notify the physician. When giving any medication, not just digoxin, an infant's head should be slightly elevated. The nurse should always check the expiration date before giving any medication to a client. The infant's kidney function should be adequate because medications are primarily excreted by the kidneys; however, these factors are not unique to digoxin.
Test Taking Strategy—*Look at the key words "most important," which implies a priority in this case when administering digoxin. Recall that digoxin is a cardiac glycoside that slows the heart rate and increases the force of the heart's contraction. Therefore, option 1, counting the heart rate for a full minute, determines if the heart rate is sufficient so that the infant will not be endangered. Review the action of cardiac glycosides and the nursing responsibilities when administering this category of drugs if you had difficulty answering this question.*
Cognitive Level—*Applying*
Client Needs Category—*Physiological integrity*
Client Needs Subcategory—*Pharmacological therapies*

52. **2.** Organizing nursing care to allow for longer rest periods decreases the infant's energy demands, thereby decreasing the workload of the heart. The nurse should encourage the parents to hold and cuddle their infant. A nasogastric route is used only if the infant has a poor suck reflex or the feedings take too long, which increases the energy expenditure. The infant would not be routinely sedated.

> *Test Taking Strategy—Use the process of elimination to help select the option that identifies the best method for reducing the heart's workload. Option 1 can be eliminated immediately because holding and cuddling promotes bonding between parents and the infant and meets the infant's psychosocial needs. Option 3 can be eliminated because regardless of the manner in which the infant is fed, the same amount of energy is needed for digestive processes. Option 4 seems to have merit, but sedating the infant is an extreme measure for reducing cardiac activity. Option 2 remains as the best answer because rest slows the heart rate and decreases oxygenation needs. Review how metabolic energy equivalents (METs) increase with various forms of activity if you had difficulty answering this question.*
>
> *Cognitive Level—Applying*
> *Client Needs Category—Physiological integrity*
> *Client Needs Subcategory—Reduction of risk potential*

53. 3. Digoxin (Lanoxin) should not be mixed in the infant's formula or food. Administering medication this way does not ensure that the child will receive the full dose, especially if all of the food is not ingested. All the other statements are correct and indicate that the parents understood the nurse's instructions.

> *Test Taking Strategy—Analyze to determine what information the question asks for, which is an incorrect statement related to the home administration of digoxin that requires further clarification by the nurse. Recall that mixing the medication with formula (option 3) is incorrect because the child may not get the full dose. Review methods for administering oral medications to infants if you had difficulty answering this question.*
>
> *Cognitive Level—Analyzing*
> *Client Needs Category—Health promotion and maintenance*
> *Client Needs Subcategory—None*

Nursing Care of a Child with an Infectious Disease

54. 1. Although standard precautions are used in the care of all clients, airborne precautions are added for clients who have illnesses that are transmitted by airborne droplet nuclei, such as chickenpox during the early stage of infection. Droplet precautions are initiated when a client is known or suspected to have illnesses transmitted by large-particle droplets. Contact precautions are initiated for clients when direct contact or contact with client items may spread the disease.

> *Test Taking Strategy—Look at the key terms "most appropriate" used in reference to the transmission-based precaution for preventing the spread of chickenpox in its early stage to other vulnerable clients in the hospital. Recall that chickenpox (varicella) is a virus that requires airborne precautions in the early stage of transmission and contact precautions later when weeping vesicles are present. Review each category of transmission-based precautions and examples of infectious diseases for which they are used if you had difficulty answering this question.*
>
> *Cognitive Level—Applying*
> *Client Needs Category—Safe and effective care environment*
> *Client Needs Subcategory—Safety and infection control*

55. 2. Specimens are placed in a zip-closure biohazard bag before being sent to the laboratory. The zip-closure prevents contamination of the environment during transportation. The infant is in airborne precautions; therefore, masks and personal protective equipment are placed *outside the room* because the room environment is considered contaminated. The infant is placed in a private room to prevent the potential spread of chickenpox to other clients. A disposable thermometer is placed in the room and then disposed of or sent for proper cleaning upon discharge.

> *Test Taking Strategy—Analyze to determine what information the question asks for, which is a correct action to prevent the transmission of infectious agents. Recall that infection control policies include safely securing a laboratory specimen in a zip-lock bag (option 2) before transporting it to the laboratory. Review common infection control practices if you had difficulty answering this question.*
>
> *Cognitive Level—Applying*
> *Client Needs Category—Safe and effective care environment*
> *Client Needs Subcategory—Safety and infection control*

56. 4. It is important to monitor the infusion rate carefully to prevent circulatory overload. Therefore, any increase in the rate should be reported immediately to the charge nurse. Normal behaviors for a child include voiding frequently, sleeping, and crying when disturbed by noise.

> *Test Taking Strategy—Use the process of elimination to select the option that identifies data that is most important to report. Remember that children are more vulnerable to circulatory overload than adults. Therefore, option 4 is the best answer because it facilitates preventing or reducing life-threatening complications associated with excess fluid volume. Review the causes of circulatory overload and its consequences if you had difficulty answering this question.*
>
> *Cognitive Level—Applying*
> *Client Needs Category—Physiological integrity*
> *Client Needs Subcategory—Reduction of risk potential*

57. **820 mL.**

The formula to calculate the daily rate of pediatric mainte-nance I.V. fluids is:

100 mL/kg/day for the first 10 kg of body weight
50 mL/kg/day for the next 10 kg of body weight
20 mL/kg/day for each kilogram above 20 kg of body weight

First, the nurse must convert the pounds (lb) to kilograms (kg); therefore, 18 lb divided by 2.2 equals 8.2 kg.

100 mL/kg/day multiplied by 8.2 kg = 820 mL

> *Test Taking Strategy—Analyze to determine what infor-mation the question asks for, which requires calcu-lating the safe fluid volume intake based on criteria provided in the stem. Review dosage calculations if you had difficulty answering this question.*
> *Cognitive Level—Applying*
> *Client Needs Category—Physiological integrity*
> *Client Needs Subcategory—Basic care and comfort*

Nursing Care of a Child with Human Immunodeficiency Virus Infection

58. **2.** Infants who are human immunodeficiency virus (HIV)-positive and develop acquired immunodeficiency syndrome (AIDS) often present with thrush, mouth sores, and severe diaper rashes. In some cases, such children also develop bacterial infections and *Pneumocystis carinii* pneumonia. The other options are examples of normal infant behaviors or characteristics.

> *Test Taking Strategy—Analyze to determine what infor-mation the question asks for, which is data suggesting that an HIV infection has progressed to AIDS. Recall that AIDS is a disease that interferes with a person's ability to resist infections that others with normal immune systems survive or suppress. Therefore, having had thrush (option 2), an opportunistic infec-tion, suggests that the infant's disease has destroyed sufficient T-cell lymphocytes to cause an increased susceptibility to pathogens. Review evidence that suggests a change from HIV-positive status to AIDS if you had difficulty answering this question.*
> *Cognitive Level—Applying*
> *Client Needs Category—Physiological integrity*
> *Client Needs Subcategory—Physiological adaptation*

59. **1, 2, 3, 4, 5.** The Centers for Disease Control and Prevention (CDC) developed a classification system to describe the spectrum of human immunodeficiency virus (HIV) disease in children (AIDS-defining conditions). The system indicates the severity of clinical signs or symptoms and the degree of immunosuppression. A history of bacte-rial infections, herpes simplex disease, oral and pulmonary candidiasis (white patches in the mouth area and larynx), *Pneumocystis carinii* or lymphoid interstitial pneumo-nia (consolidation areas on a chest X-ray), and wasting

syndrome (limited muscle tone) all indicate a moderate status for AIDS-defining conditions. An increase in blood pressure may be associated with a disease process but is not closely linked to an AIDS-defining condition.

> *Test Taking Strategy—Analyze to determine what infor-mation the question asks for, which is AIDS-defining conditions. Alternative-format "select all that apply" questions require considering each option indepen-dently to decide its merit in answering the question. Choose the options that best correlate with the signs and symptoms of AIDS in children. Review the AIDS-Defining Conditions identified by the CDC if you had difficulty answering this question.*
> *Cognitive Level—Understanding*
> *Client Needs Category—Physiological integrity*
> *Client Needs Subcategory—Physiological adaptation*

Nursing Care of a Child with Atopic Dermatitis

60. **3.** It is thought that atopic dermatitis (infantile eczema) is caused, at least in part, by an allergic reaction to an irritant, which is why the physician asked about the home environment. The chronic inflammation of the skin causes it to be dry, itchy, and flaky. Hereditary factors may also play a role. Poor nutrition, premature birth, and hormonal imbalances are not associated with the develop-ment of atopic dermatitis.

> *Test Taking Strategy—Analyze to determine what infor-mation the question asks for, which is a factor that contributes to the signs and symptoms associated with atopic dermatitis. Recall that the word derma-titis indicates a skin condition that has an inflamma-tory component, which is compatible with an allergic response (option 3). Review the description of the disorder and its potential causes if you had difficulty answering this question.*
> *Cognitive Level—Applying*
> *Client Needs Category—Health promotion and maintenance*
> *Client Needs Subcategory—None*

61. **3.** An infant with atopic dermatitis experiences severe itching of the skin lesions. The nurse must provide the parents with itch-relief measures to prevent the child from scratching and introducing microorganisms into the lesions, which will cause a secondary infection to develop. Nausea, ecchymosis, and drowsiness are not usual symp-toms of atopic dermatitis.

> *Test Taking Strategy—Analyze to determine what information the question asks for, which is a symptom that may respond to preventive care to avoid potential complications. Recall that itching (option 3) leads to scratching, and scratching leads to skin abrasions, increasing the risk for infection.*

Review the signs and symptoms of atopic dermatitis, focusing on one that has the potential for causing complications, if you had difficulty answering this question.
Cognitive Level—*Applying*
Client Needs Category—*Health promotion and maintenance*
Client Needs Subcategory—*None*

62. 3. Hydrocortisone (Cortaid) is an anti-inflammatory drug. It helps reduce inflammation and its symptoms, such as swelling, redness, heat, and discomfort. This medication does not influence the weeping of lesions, spread of the disease, or white blood cell count.

> **Test Taking Strategy**—*Analyze to determine what information the question asks for, which is evidence that the application of hydrocortisone cream is having a beneficial effect. Because hydrocortisone is an anti-inflammatory agent, option 3 is the best answer. Review the uses for topical applications of hydrocortisone if you had difficulty answering this question.*
> **Cognitive Level**—*Evaluating*
> **Client Needs Category**—*Physiological integrity*
> **Client Needs Subcategory**—*Pharmacological therapies*

63. 1. Colloid baths have been found effective for their soothing effects on the irritated and itching skin of a child with atopic dermatitis. The most commonly used type of colloid bath preparation is cornstarch added to tepid water. Other colloid bath preparations include cooked oatmeal and commercial bath preparations. Mineral oil, liquid glycerin soap, and salt are not components of a colloid bath.

> **Test Taking Strategy**—*Analyze to determine what information the question asks for, which is the additive that is typically used when administering a colloid bath. Recall that when mixed with water, a colloid produces a gelatinous or mucinous solution. The tiny particles in cornstarch (option 1), which do not completely dissolve, float in the water, creating a thick liquid that coats the surface of skin and causes a soothing effect. Review therapeutic uses for administering a colloid bath and the substances that are commonly used if you had difficulty answering this question.*
> **Cognitive Level**—*Understanding*
> **Client Needs Category**—*Health promotion and maintenance*
> **Client Needs Subcategory**—*None*

Nursing Care of a Toddler with Sickle Cell Crisis

64. 1. The sickle-shaped cells tend to clump together in vessels and obstruct normal blood flow. A thrombus may form and cause death of tissue because of poor blood circulation. Severe pain in the affected body part is the characteristic symptom when tissue is denied normal blood circulation. Bradycardia and hemorrhage are not usually associated with sickle cell crisis. Although dehydration may lead to a potential sickle cell crisis, this is not the initial nursing priority.

> **Test Taking Strategy**—*Analyze to determine what information the question asks for, which is the initial priority for a child experiencing a sickle cell crisis. Recall that tissue ischemia from clustered sickled cells creates severe pain (option 1). Once the pain is managed, the nurse can address other aspects of client care, such as increasing circulating fluid volume. Review the pathophysiology of sickle cell diseases, focusing on the symptoms associated in a crisis, if you had difficulty answering this question.*
> **Cognitive Level**—*Applying*
> **Client Needs Category**—*Physiological integrity*
> **Client Needs Subcategory**—*Physiological adaptation*

65. 4. The child with sickle cell crisis is prone to dehydration, which contributes to creating a cluster of sickled cells. The child is encouraged to drink fluids. It is helpful to offer the child appealing fluids, such as juices, popsicles, and gelatins. It may be necessary during the acute stage to rehydrate the child with I.V. fluids. Whole-blood transfusions may be given to increase hemoglobin levels. Iron is of no value in the treatment of this blood disorder.

> **Test Taking Strategy**—*Analyze to determine what information the question asks for, which is a component of nursing care that is specific for a child experiencing a sickle cell crisis. Recall that hydrating the client may help to improve the flow of blood through the area where the sickled cells have collected. Review the manner in which a sickle cell crisis is managed if you had difficulty answering this question.*
> **Cognitive Level**—*Applying*
> **Client Needs Category**—*Physiological integrity*
> **Client Needs Subcategory**—*Physiological adaptation*

66. 2. Sickle cell disease occurs when the child inherits the trait from both parents. If one parent has the disease and one parent has the trait, then all offspring will have at least the trait. Furthermore, there is a 50% chance that the offspring will have sickle cell disease. Information about the probability of offspring having sickle cell disease or trait can be given only in terms of each conception. The only instance in which it is possible to predict that all offspring will definitely have the disease is when both parents are known to have sickle cell disease.

> **Test Taking Strategy**—*Analyze to determine what information the question asks for, which is evidence that a parent understands how sickle cell disease is acquired. Recall that sickle cell disease is acquired through autosomal recessive genetic inheritance.*

Option 2 accurately reflects the etiology. Review how sickle cell anemia is acquired and transmitted to a fetus if you had difficulty answering this question.
Cognitive Level—*Understanding*
Client Needs Category—*Health promotion and maintenance*
Client Needs Subcategory—*None*

67. 1, 2, 4, 5, 6. Because infection contributes to many sickle cell crises and death, the nurse needs to stress the importance of measures to reduce infection. Obtaining plenty of rest, using proper hand-washing techniques, and avoiding crowds, especially during cold and flu season, are all important measures. Some individuals are placed on antibiotic therapy prophylactically. It is important to finish the full course of antibiotic therapy. Maintaining good hydration is an important step in preventing cell sickling. Using pain medication is not typical in preventing a sickle cell crisis.

> *Test Taking Strategy*—*Analyze to determine what information the question asks for, which is measures to take to avoid sickle cell crises. Alternative-format "select all that apply" questions require considering each option independently to decide its merit in answering the question. Choose the options that are essential nursing instructions for avoiding sickle cell crises in the future. Review prophylaxis of sickle cell crises if you had difficulty answering this question.*
Cognitive Level—*Applying*
Client Needs Category—*Health promotion and maintenance*
Client Needs Subcategory—*None*

Nursing Care of a Toddler with Cystic Fibrosis

68. 3, 5, 6. Cystic fibrosis is a genetic disease that causes thick, sticky mucus to accumulate in the lungs and digestive tract. It is a chronic disease causing numerous complications. In many cases, the parents of a child with cystic fibrosis report that their child tastes salty when kissed. This is because the child's perspiration, tears, and saliva contain abnormally high concentrations of salt. Consequently, sweat analysis is an important diagnostic tool when children are examined for cystic fibrosis. Because of the excessive mucus within the lungs in this disorder, children often have bouts of impaired breathing and coughing. Children with cystic fibrosis may be in lower percentiles for growth and development compared to children of a similar age. These children are typically underweight. Disturbed sleep patterns, weight gain, and poor head control, if they occur, are findings associated with other disorders.

> *Test Taking Strategy*—*Analyze to determine what information the question asks for, which is findings associated with cystic fibrosis. Alternative-format "select all that apply" questions require considering each option independently to decide its merit in*

answering the question. Choose the options that best correlate with the signs and symptoms of cystic fibrosis. Review the signs and symptoms of cystic fibrosis if you had difficulty answering this question.
Cognitive level—*Applying*
Client Needs Category—*Physiological integrity*
Client Needs Subcategory—*Physiological adaptation*

69. 4. Typically, the stools of a child with cystic fibrosis are large, sticky, and foul-smelling. The condition is due to diminished or absent flow of pancreatic enzymes, which leads to faulty absorption of dietary fat and fat-soluble vitamins. Besides the unpleasant odor, the stool tends to float and appear a lighter color than normal stools. Other signs and symptoms of cystic fibrosis include malnutrition despite a hearty appetite, chronic coughing, and a distended abdomen. Children with cystic fibrosis usually eat very well but fail to gain weight. Typically, they do not perspire excessively or have a low urine output.

> *Test Taking Strategy*—*Analyze to determine what information the question asks for, which is an assessment finding common among children with cystic fibrosis. Recall that children with cystic fibrosis have bulky, foul-smelling stools because they excrete undigested fat in their stools. Review the pathophysiology of cystic fibrosis and apply the information to the signs and symptoms of the disease process if you had difficulty answering this question.*
Cognitive Level—*Applying*
Client Needs Category—*Physiological integrity*
Client Needs Subcategory—*Physiological adaptation*

70. 2. The cause of death in children with cystic fibrosis is most often related to respiratory or cardiac failure; therefore, the priority goal would be maintenance of an effective breathing pattern. All the other goals are appropriate for the child with cystic fibrosis, but maintaining respiratory function is the priority.

> *Test Taking Strategy*—*Analyze to determine what information the question asks for, which is a nursing goal when managing the care of a child with cystic fibrosis. Recall that the leading cause of death in children diagnosed with this disease is respiratory failure. Therefore, formulating a goal to maintain effective breathing (option 2) is a priority. Review the potentially life-threatening symptoms of cystic fibrosis if you had difficulty answering this question.*
Cognitive Level—*Analyzing*
Client Needs Category—*Safe and effective care environment*
Client Needs Subcategory—*Coordinated care*

71. 3. The air passages of the lungs of persons with cystic fibrosis become clogged with mucus, thereby decreasing the amount of oxygen reaching the lungs. A bronchodilator increases the diameter of the bronchi, thereby allowing more air to enter the lungs so breathing is improved. A flutter mucus clearing device vibrates the airways to loosen mucus; increases endobronchial pressure, which helps to keep the airway open as mucus is moved upward within the respiratory passages; and increases expiratory airflow, facilitating expectoration of mucous secretions. Characteristics of the stool, serum sodium levels, and fat excretion by the body are not affected by bronchodilators or a flutter mucus clearing device.

Test Taking Strategy—Analyze to determine what information the question asks for, which is evidence that the treatment measures have achieved a desired outcome. Option 3 is the best answer because these treatment measures, whether used for a child or an adult, are targeted at improving the ability to breathe. Review the mechanism of action of a flutter mucus clearing device if you had difficulty answering this question.
Cognitive Level—Evaluating
Client Needs Category—Physiological integrity
Client Needs Subcategory—Pharmacological therapies

72. 4. A child with cystic fibrosis may need 1½ to 2 times the normal caloric intake to meet caloric needs. The diet should be high in protein and carbohydrates. Dietary fat should not be excessive, but rather balanced with pancreatic enzyme replacement. Salt need not be restricted; rather, the child may require an increase in salt intake during summer months, when excessive sweating may occur.

Test Taking Strategy—Use the process of elimination to help select the option that identifies a therapeutic dietary modification that will be best for the child with cystic fibrosis. Option 2 can be eliminated because protein is necessary for cellular growth and repair. Option 1 can be eliminated because increasing dietary fat is counterproductive for a child who lacks pancreatic enzymes with which to digest it. Although it is healthy for everyone to decrease salt consumption, option 3 can be eliminated because it is not as therapeutic as option 4, which will facilitate weight gain. Review dietary nutrients that are important for promoting weight gain when a client is underweight if you had difficulty answering this question.
Cognitive Level—Applying
Client Needs Category—Physiological integrity
Client Needs Subcategory—Physiological adaptation

73. 2. Commercially prepared pancreatic enzymes should be given with meals and snacks to facilitate nutrient absorption. Pancreatic enzyme preparations have no relationship to the child's appetite, prevention of salt depletion, or prevention of gastric upset.

Test Taking Strategy—Analyze to determine what information the question asks for, which is the correct explanation for administering pancrelipase with the child's meals. Note that pancreatic enzymes

must be given when food is eaten because a person with cystic fibrosis requires the enzyme to digest and absorb nutrients. Review the function of pancreatic enzymes and relate it to an appropriate time for administering a replacement if you had difficulty answering this question.
Cognitive Level—Applying
Client Needs Category—Physiological integrity
Client Needs Subcategory—Pharmacological therapies

74. 4. In children with cystic fibrosis, sodium and chloride become trapped in the cells of the lining of the lungs. The salt draws liquids from the airways and causes the mucus in the airways to become thick and sticky. Maintaining adequate fluid intake will help liquefy secretions in the airways, which ultimately helps improve breathing. The goal of increased fluid intake for the child with cystic fibrosis is not to prevent kidney failure, improve cardiac function, or reduce pain and discomfort.

Test Taking Strategy—Analyze to determine what information the question asks for, which is the reason for recommending a liberal intake of oral fluids in a child with cystic fibrosis. Recall that the child has thick, mucoid pulmonary secretions and that increasing fluid intake will thin those secretions (option 4), facilitating easier expectoration. Review measures for thinning viscid respiratory secretions if you had difficulty answering this question.
Cognitive Level—Applying
Client Needs Category—Physiological integrity
Client Needs Subcategory—Reduction of risk potential

75. 2. Children with cystic fibrosis are very susceptible to infections, especially infections of the respiratory tract. Protecting a child with cystic fibrosis from exposure to persons who may currently have a respiratory infection can be a life-saving measure. Immunization against childhood diseases is highly recommended, especially against diseases that may place the respiratory tract at risk. Airborne pollen and pet dander are usually avoided when the child has a history of respiratory symptoms secondary to environmental allergies. Avoiding exposure to bright sunlight is not necessarily important unless this poses the risk of excessive sweating, which could result in excessive sodium loss. However, protecting the child against respiratory infections takes priority over preventing exposure to bright sunlight.

Test Taking Strategy—Use the process of elimination to identify the option that indicates the exposure most important to avoid when a child has cystic fibrosis. Recall that this child is extremely susceptible to life-threatening problems if a respiratory infection compounds the respiratory symptoms caused by the disorder. Review the potential consequences of each exposure on a child with cystic fibrosis if you had difficulty answering this question.

Cognitive Level—*Applying*
Client Needs Category—*Physiological integrity*
Client Needs Subcategory—*Physiological adaptation*

Nursing Care of a Toddler with Asthma

76. 1. Wheezing and a dry, hacking cough are major manifestations of an acute asthma attack. The normal respiratory rate for a 3-year-old child is 20 to 30 breaths/ minute. Children also begin to assume a thoracic breathing pattern around this age. Clear, watery nasal drainage is usually seen in upper respiratory tract disorders, not acute asthma attacks.

Test Taking Strategy—*Use the process of elimination to help select the option that identifies the assessment finding that provides the best indication that a child is experiencing an acute attack of asthma. Recall that wheezing breath sounds (option 1) occur during an asthma attack because the airways swell and narrow. Options 2 and 3 can be eliminated because they are normal findings. Option 4 can be eliminated because this is a symptom of an upper respiratory disorder rather than asthma. Review the signs and symptoms experienced by a person having an acute asthma attack if you had difficulty answering this question.*
Cognitive Level—*Applying*
Client Needs Category—*Physiological integrity*
Client Needs Subcategory—*Physiological adaptation*

77. 4. The most effective method of relieving acute respiratory distress is to place the client in semi-Fowler's position. An older child may be more comfortable leaning forward on a pillow on an over-bed table. Applying oxygen may also be helpful in reducing oxygen demand. Cool-mist humidifiers, not steam vaporizers, may be used as well. Antibiotics will not relieve the acute respiratory distress. Distracting the child with age-appropriate toys is not an effective strategy when the child is experiencing acute distress.

Test Taking Strategy—*Look at the key words "most appropriate," which are used in reference to a nursing action that relieves respiratory distress. Recall that sitting upright (option 4) lowers abdominal organs away from the diaphragm, allowing a larger exchange of gases. Review the anatomic and physiologic changes that occur when a semi-Fowler's position is assumed if you had difficulty answering this question.*
Cognitive Level—*Analyzing*
Client Needs Category—*Physiological integrity*
Client Needs Subcategory—*Physiological adaptation*

78. 4. If breathing exercises are incorporated into play activities such as blowing bubbles, the child is more likely to enjoy them and may practice the exercises more. This

is a creative teaching strategy. Promises of treats, parental assistance with the exercise, demonstrations, and return demonstrations are not likely to be as effective as incorporating exercises into play activities.

Test Taking Strategy—*Use the process of elimination to identify the option that identifies a nursing intervention that is best for facilitating the performance of breathing exercises. Recall that blowing bubbles (option 4) is an age-appropriate activity that a 3-year-old is likely to enjoy and that imitates the actions used to perform breathing exercises. Although options 1, 2, and 3 are methods for motivating or teaching the child, they are not as appealing to the child as blowing bubbles. Review age-appropriate play activities that are similar to performing breathing exercises if you had difficulty answering this question.*
Cognitive Level—*Applying*
Client Needs Category—*Health promotion and maintenance*
Client Needs Subcategory—*None*

79. 4. When a client has asthma due to an allergy to one or more environmental factors, general control of the environment is necessary to reduce chances of future asthma attacks. Removing area rugs helps to eliminate a potential allergen and control the environment. The physician orders breathing treatments every 2 hours in the acute stage of the disease process. A generous fluid intake is recommended because fluid is lost through sweating and an increased respiratory rate. A well-balanced diet is necessary, especially for a growing child. Asthma cannot be cured, but it can often be controlled.

Test Taking Strategy—*Look at the key words "most appropriate" used in reference to parental discharge instructions. Recall that asthma attacks are generally triggered by exposure to an allergen. Because area rugs harbor dust, dust mites, and pet dander (if there is a pet in the house), it is best to remove them (option 4) and substitute hardwood floors. Review how the home environment can be modified to reduce exposure to allergens if you had difficulty answering this question.*
Cognitive Level—*Applying*
Client Needs Category—*Health promotion and maintenance*
Client Needs Subcategory—*None*

Nursing Care of a Toddler Who Has Swallowed a Toxic Substance

80. 3. Parents should be instructed to notify medical professionals at the physician's office or Poison Control Center immediately when a poison is ingested. When a caustic substance is ingested, water or milk should be given to dilute the substance. Vomiting should not be induced because the substance may cause additional injury when regurgitated. There is also a danger of respiratory complications secondary to aspiration of vomitus. It is important to address life-threatening concerns immediately before taking the child to the emergency department. Cardiopulmonary resuscitation may or may not be necessary, depending on the specific injury incurred.

Test Taking Strategy—Look at the key words "most appropriate," which should lead to an option that describes the best recommendation for an incident involving the ingestion of a lye-based cleaner. Recall that lye is a highly alkaline substance that burns tissue as it is swallowed, contraindicating the induction of vomiting. Diluting the cleaner by ingesting water (option 3) is the most appropriate action from among those listed. Review poison control measures for the ingestion of caustic substances if you had difficulty answering this question.
Cognitive level—Applying
Client Needs Category—Physiological integrity
Client Needs Subcategory—Physiological adaptation

81. 1. Substernal and intercostal retractions indicate that the child is experiencing respiratory distress. This child's oxygen saturation level should be monitored to assist in determining the need for additional therapy to relieve or minimize respiratory distress. The child may manifest all the other symptoms, but they do not indicate respiratory distress.

Test Taking Strategy—Use the process of elimination to select the option that identifies the best indication that the child should be assessed with a pulse oximeter. Recall that a pulse oximeter is used to measure the oxygen saturation in arterial blood, a level that may be affected by chemical burns in the pharynx and esophagus. Although red, swollen lips and drooling from the lips may be evident, options 2 and 3 can be eliminated because they are not the most serious indication for using a pulse oximeter. A pulse rate of 105 beats/minute is within a normal range for a toddler, eliminating option 4. Option 1 remains as the best answer because accessory muscles are used when there is respiratory distress. Review the signs and symptoms of respiratory distress, which is the basis for using a pulse oximeter to assess the client, if you had difficulty answering this question.
Cognitive Level—Applying
Client Needs Category—Physiological integrity
Client Needs Subcategory—Reduction of risk potential

82. 2. The child may experience pain related to burns on the lips and in the mouth from the lye-based substance. Gastric lavage is not performed when caustic substances have been ingested; however, a gastrostomy may be necessary with severe damage. The child is given liquids by mouth as tolerated. Neurovascular checks are not usually required.

Test Taking Strategy—Analyze to determine what information the question asks for, which is a nursing intervention that the nurse should perform when caring for the child who swallowed a cleaning substance containing lye. Recall that the mouth and lips will be burned, making pain management (option 2) a necessity. Review the consequences of ingesting a caustic chemical if you had difficulty answering this question.
Cognitive Level—Applying
Client Needs Category—Physiological integrity
Client Needs Subcategory—Physiological adaptation

83. 4. All poisonous substances should be placed in locked compartments or cabinets. Children are often capable of climbing and reaching areas higher than anticipated. It would be unrealistic to remove all poisonous substances from the home or to keep a constant eye on the child.

Test Taking Strategy—Use the process of elimination to identify the option that provides a statement that describes the best method for the safekeeping of toxic substances. Recall that keeping toxic substances confined in a locked area (option 4) reduces the potential that the child will gain access to them. Review safety measures that are appropriate in a household with a toddler if you had difficulty answering this question.
Cognitive Level—Applying
Client Needs Category—Safe and effective care environment
Client Needs Subcategory—Safety and infection control

Nursing Care of a Toddler with Croup

84. 1. Croup, also known as *laryngotracheobronchitis*, is a respiratory condition that has a rapid onset. It is usually triggered by a viral infection that affects the upper respiratory tract. The most common viruses that cause croup are parainfluenza virus, adenovirus, and respiratory syncytial virus (RSV). The infection leads to pharyngeal and vocal cord edema, which interferes with breathing and produces a "barking" cough, stridor, and hoarseness. Pertussis is another name for whooping cough, an infectious disease for which most infants have been immunized. It also causes a cough, but the cough is followed by a "whooping" sound created by a high-pitched intake of air. Whooping cough does not have a rapid onset like croup. Croup is not associated with inadequate lung development, and it can occur in toddlers with or without a history of asthma.

Test Taking Strategy—Analyze the information the question asks which is the etiology that causes the symptoms associated with croup. Recall that the suffix -itis indicates an inflammation, which is the result, in this case, of a viral infection. Review the causes of croup and the course of the disease if you had difficulty answering this question.
Cognitive Level—Understanding
Client Needs Category—Physiological integrity
Client Needs Subcategory—Physiological adaptation

85. 2. The child with croup has a cough that sounds hoarse, much like a loud, barking, metallic sound. The cough is usually dry rather than moist, loud, and muffled. *Wheezing* is a term used to describe breath sounds, not cough characteristics.

> **Test Taking Strategy**—*Analyze to determine what information the question asks for, which is the characteristics of the cough caused by croup. Recall that the cough that develops with croup has been described as sounding like a barking seal. Review words that are used to describe the cough associated with croup if you had difficulty answering this question.*
> **Cognitive Level**—*Applying*
> **Client Needs Category**—*Physiological integrity*
> **Client Needs Subcategory**—*Physiological adaptation*

86. 3. To help reduce laryngeal edema, the child with croup should breathe air that is high in humidity. A mist tent, a cool-mist vaporizer, or placing the child in the bathroom while hot water fills the area with steam may be used for this purpose. A dust-free environment is required for children who are allergic to dust. Central heating and air conditioning do not provide relief for children with croup.

> **Test Taking Strategy**—*Analyze the information the question asks, which is a nursing recommendation that helps relieve symptoms caused by croup. Recall that humidified air (option 3) soothes the respiratory mucosa. It also helps reduce laryngeal edema and the frequency of coughing episodes. Review treatment measures for croup if you had difficulty answering this question.*
> **Cognitive Level**—*Applying*
> **Client Needs Category**—*Physiological integrity*
> **Client Needs Subcategory**—*Reduction of risk potential*

87. 2. Intense anxiety is a sign that the child senses a worsening of respiratory distress and feels helpless to relieve the symptoms that are being experienced. When noting the change in the child's reaction, the physician should be contacted immediately because there may be more serious involvement of the trachea and bronchial tree. A fluctuation in the child's fever, persistent coughing, and frequent napping are not considered signs the child's condition is becoming worse.

> **Test Taking Strategy**—*Analyze to determine what information the question asks for, which is a sign of a worsening of the child's croup and respiratory distress. Recall that anxiety (option 2) occurs in response to feeling a threat to one's safety and well-being. Review the complications of croup and factors that trigger anxiety if you had difficulty answering this question.*
> **Cognitive Level**—*Applying*
> **Client Needs Category**—*Physiological integrity*
> **Client Needs Subcategory**—*Physiological adaptation*

88. 2. Aspirin, a salicylate, is contraindicated in young children with a fever, flulike symptoms, or chickenpox. Its use has been associated with Reye's syndrome, a potentially fatal condition that results in multisystem organ failure, especially liver and brain injury. All of the other options reflect a correct understanding of croup and appropriate measures to treat it.

> **Test Taking Strategy**—*Analyze to determine what information the question asks for, which is a parental statement that indicates a need for additional teaching. Read the question carefully because it requires identifying incorrect information. Recall that aspirin is not given to children to relieve a fever (option 2) because it is associated with a risk of developing Reye's syndrome. Review the contraindication for administering aspirin to children if you had difficulty answering this question.*
> **Cognitive Level**—*Applying*
> **Client Needs Category**—*Health promotion and maintenance*
> **Client Needs Subcategory**—*None*

89. 4. The physician may order racemic epinephrine (Vaponefrin) through a nebulizer. This drug is used for its topical vasoconstrictive effect, which will reduce laryngeal edema and produce relaxation of bronchial smooth muscle, resulting in bronchodilation. Racemic epinephrine works within 10 minutes, but wears off in approximately 2 hours, at which time the nurse should assess the child to determine if symptoms of respiratory distress are developing again. Because a virus is the usual cause of croup, antibiotics such as ampicillin are not typically used. The other two medications also are not routinely given to children with croup.

> **Test Taking Strategy**—*Analyze to determine what information the question asks for, which is the drug of choice for relieving acute respiratory distress caused by croup. Recall that racemic epinephrine (option 4) produces a rapid short-acting response, resulting in the relief of respiratory distress. Review the actions of the drugs listed, focusing on which one is used for respiratory emergencies, if you had difficulty answering this question.*
> **Cognitive Level**—*Applying*
> **Client Needs Category**—*Physiological integrity*
> **Client Needs Subcategory**—*Pharmacological therapies*

90. 3. Whole milk should be temporarily avoided because the butter fat in whole milk relaxes the esophageal sphincter and increases gastric acidity, predisposing to gastric reflux, which may contribute to coughing. Coughing occurs because the *arytenoids*, the ends of the folds in the vocal cords that are attached near the esophageal sphincter, become irritated from the reflux of acidic secretions from the stomach. Many food items besides milk cause coughing from gastric reflux. Clear liquids, such as ginger ale, popsicles, apple juice, and gelatin, are permitted because they help to liquefy secretions and allow easier expectoration.

Test Taking Strategy—Analyze to determine what information the question asks for, which is a beverage that should be temporarily withheld when providing oral fluids to the child with croup. Look at the options, and note that three are clear liquids, whereas milk is not. Review fluids to avoid in order to relieve a cough, especially one caused by gastric reflux, if you had difficulty answering this question.
Cognitive Level—Remembering
Client Needs Category—Physiological integrity
Client Needs Subcategory—Reduction of risk potential

Nursing Care of a Toddler with Pneumonia

91. 4. The respiratory pattern in children with pneumonia is usually rapid and shallow. The rapid respiratory rate is the body's way of compensating for decreased ventilation in the lungs. The pulse is usually elevated in the child with pneumonia. Clubbing of the fingers is seen in chronic illnesses associated with a chronic lack of oxygen. Synchronized breathing is characteristic of a normal breathing pattern.

Test Taking Strategy—Analyze to determine what information the question asks for, which is the clinical presentation the nurse should expect in a child with pneumonia. Recall that pneumonia is a respiratory infection and logically it affects ventilation. Rapid breathing (option 4) is a homeostatic mechanism to compensate for decreased oxygenation; respirations also increase from the increased metabolic rate caused by a fever. Review the signs and symptoms of pneumonia, especially the effects on breathing, if you had difficulty answering this question.
Cognitive Level—Applying
Client Needs Category—Physiological integrity
Client Needs Subcategory—Physiological adaptation

92. 1. Recording the child's urine output will assist in determining fluid needs. Fluid loss commonly occurs because of the high fever, vomiting, and increased respiratory rate associated with pneumonia. Such loss results in a decreased amount of urine, which is usually dark in color with a high specific gravity. To ensure that fluid needs are met, the nurse should monitor the child's fluid intake as well. The pH of the urine will indicate whether the urine is acidic or alkalotic; it will not indicate hydration status. A child may have a normal blood pressure yet still be dehydrated. A drop in blood pressure occurs with circulatory collapse, which is a late sign of dehydration. An increased respiratory rate may result in an increased insensible fluid loss, which indicates a risk of dehydration, but this does not indicate the child's hydration status.

Test Taking Strategy—Look at the key words "most appropriate" used in reference to a method for determining the fluid status of a child recovering from pneumonia. Remember that in order to have fluid balance, intake should approximate equal output. Therefore, monitoring urine output is the most appropriate nursing intervention, making option 1 the best answer. Review assessment methods for determining a client's fluid status if you had difficulty answering this question.
Cognitive Level—Applying
Client Needs Category—Physiological integrity
Client Needs Subcategory—Physiological adaptation

93. 4. Before the implementation of antibiotic therapy, typically a sputum culture is needed to identify the causative bacteria. Obtaining a sputum specimen from a child as young as the one in the scenario (2½ years old) may be difficult, however. If the sputum specimen is not available, the physician may elect to start antibiotics based on clinical presentation and provide close monitoring for improvement or worsening of symptoms. Electrolyte levels, pulse oximeter readings, and a chest X-ray can provide appropriate data; however, these data are not as essential in determining antibiotic therapy.

Test Taking Strategy—Analyze to determine what information the question asks for, which is a diagnostic test finding the nurse should check before beginning antibiotic drug therapy. Recall that there are many categories of antibiotics, each of which is administered to combat specific types of infectious agents identified on a culture (option 4). Review the purpose for each of the tests listed, focusing on which one correlates with the administration of an antibiotic, if you had difficulty answering this question.
Cognitive Level—Applying
Client Needs Category—Physiological integrity
Client Needs Subcategory—Reduction of risk potential

94. 3. Expectorants help to loosen secretions so that the client can expectorate mucus that has accumulated in the airways. A moist cough indicates secretions in the airway need to be removed. A cough suppressant would prevent the child from coughing, resulting in retained secretions. Cough suppressants are generally used to relieve a dry cough that causes fatigue and sleeplessness. An antibiotic may relieve the cough by eliminating the cause of the infection, but they are not given primarily to manage a cough. Bronchodilators are used to relax smooth muscles in the airways to promote the ease of breathing.

Test Taking Strategy—Analyze to determine what information the question asks for, which is a drug category given to relieve a productive moist cough. Although all of the drugs listed may be helpful in various ways, an expectorant (option 3) is used to facilitate raising sputum from lower airways. Review

the uses for the drug categories listed if you had difficulty answering this question.
Cognitive Level—Applying
Client Needs Category—Physiological integrity
Client Needs Subcategory—Pharmacological therapies

95. 3. If the child is observed shivering, the bath should be stopped immediately because shivering will further increase the core body temperature. The bath should not be given for more than 30 minutes. Tepid water is used for the bath. The child's temperature should drop, but not below 101°F (38.3°C).

Test Taking Strategy—Use the process of elimination to help select the option that identifies essential information the parents should know about administering a sponge bath to relieve the child's fever. Option 3 remains as the best answer because shivering generates heat, which is contrary to the desired goal of fever reduction. Review physiologic mechanisms that raise body temperature, specifically the effect produced by shivering, if you had difficulty answering this question.
Cognitive Level—Applying
Client Needs Category—Physiological integrity
Client Needs Subcategory—Reduction of risk potential

96. 5 mL.
Conversion equivalents are as follows:

$$1 \text{ g} = 1,000 \text{ mg}$$
$$1 \text{ tsp} = 5 \text{ mL}$$
$$0.5 \text{ g} = 0.5 \text{ g} \times 1,000 \text{ mg} = 500 \text{ mg}$$

5 mL would fulfill the physician's order.

Test Taking Strategy—Analyze to determine what information the question asks for, which involves calculating the correct dosage of medication when there are different measurements in the physician's order and on the medication label. Review conversion equivalents between household and metric measurements if you had difficulty answering this question.
Cognitive Level—Applying
Client Needs Category—Physiological integrity
Client Needs Subcategory—Pharmacological therapies

97. 2. Having an interpreter present when instructions are given allows the nurse to give clear instructions with rationales as well as to validate the parents' understanding of those instructions. Full communication between the two parties can be used. Providing a copy of the instructions in Spanish should be used as reinforcement, but it does not guarantee that the parents understand the instructions; therefore, comprehension is not assessed. Having the physician give the instructions is unnecessary unless the physician speaks Spanish. The parents should be encouraged to call if questions arise after discharge, but the nurse must ensure that they have a basic understanding of the instructions before they leave.

Test Taking Strategy—Use the process of elimination to help select the option that identifies the best action for ensuring that the parents who speak English as a second language understand the discharge instructions. Recall that using an interpreter (option 2) provides the best assurance that the parents understand the instructions and can ask questions after the information has been processed. Options 1, 3, and 4 all have some merit, but none is the best answer. Review methods for communicating with clients from another culture, particularly the advantage of using a qualified—or even certified—interpreter, if you had difficulty answering this question.
Cognitive Level—Applying
Client Needs Category—Safe and effective care environment
Client Needs Subcategory—Coordinated care

Nursing Care of a Preschooler with a Seizure Disorder

98. 4. Tonic-clonic seizures, formerly known as *grand mal seizures*, are one of several types of seizures. Tonic-clonic seizures are considered an example of a generalized seizure because they involve the entire brain. In the tonic phase of the seizure, consciousness is lost and the body becomes rigid. In the clonic phase, there is generalized involuntary body movement that alternates between muscle contraction and relaxation. A child may have seizures associated with fever, but not all children who have a fever have seizures. The child could also drop to the floor with other disorders, such as muscle weakness and unconsciousness. The child may wet the bed after a seizure has ceased, but bedwetting could occur for other reasons.

Test Taking Strategy—Use the process of elimination to help select the option that describes the best indication that the child is having a tonic-clonic type of generalized seizure. Recall that when a tonic-clonic seizure occurs, the entire body appears to have repetitive jerking movements (option 4). Review how seizures are classified and the characteristics of each type if you had difficulty answering this question.
Cognitive Level—Applying
Client Needs Category—Physiological integrity
Client Needs Subcategory—Physiological adaptation

99. 1. The priority nursing action for a child experiencing a generalized seizure is protection from injury. Padding the side rails is one means of protecting the child. Phenobarbital may be given to a child who has tonic-clonic seizures, but the medication is not kept in the child's room. Placing a child in Trendelenburg position is not routinely used in caring for the child with tonic-clonic seizures. Posting a sign on the child's door stating that "Seizure Precautions" are in place is a violation of Health Insurance Portability and Accountability Act (HIPAA) requirements and is a breach of confidentiality.

Test Taking Strategy—Look at the key words "most appropriate," indicating that one answer is better than all the others. This question requires selecting an action that is a component of the standard care for a client who is prone to seizures. Recall that safety is a priority when caring for a child who has seizures, making option 1 the best answer. Review nursing actions that are carried out when a client is prone to having seizures if you had difficulty answering this question.
Cognitive Level—*Applying*
Client Needs Category—*Safe and effective care environment*
Client Needs Subcategory—*Safety and infection control*

100. 4. It is unnecessary to have a cool-mist humidifier at the bedside of a child subject to seizure activity. Suction equipment may be required to remove mucus from the child's mouth. An oral airway and oxygen may be needed in the case of respiratory arrest, which can occur with generalized seizures.
Test Taking Strategy—Look at the key words "least important." Read the options carefully to facilitate selecting one that identifies an item that is basically unrelated to the care of a client prone to seizures. Options 2, 3, and 4 are items appropriate to place at the child's bedside, but option 4, a cool-mist humidifier, has no meaningful reason to be there unless the client has a respiratory problem. If you had difficulty answering this question correctly, review the equipment that may be needed when caring for a client who has a seizure.
Cognitive Level—*Analyzing*
Client Needs Category—*Physiological integrity*
Client Needs Subcategory—*Reduction of risk potential*

101. 2. Placing the child in the side-lying position establishes a patent airway and prevents aspiration of saliva. Inserting a padded tongue blade is no longer recommended because injury to the mouth and teeth may occur. The nurse should be prepared to administer oxygen after the seizure, if required. The nurse should implement necessary measures to minimize injury to the child before calling for assistance.
Test Taking Strategy—Analyze to determine what information the question asks for, which is a nursing action that should be performed first in a sequence of actions when responding to a client having a seizure. Recall that ensuring a client's safety is always a priority, making option 2 the best answer because it reduces the risk of aspirating oral secretions or vomitus. After doing so, calling for assistance is a good second choice followed by administering oxygen when the seizure ends. Review interventions that are performed when caring for a client during a seizure if you had difficulty answering this question.

Cognitive Level—*Analyzing*
Client Needs Category—*Physiological integrity*
Client Needs Subcategory—*Physiological adaptation*

102. 4. Prolonged use of phenytoin (Dilantin) tends to cause an overgrowth of gum tissues. Poor appetite, urinary incontinence, and painful joints are not associated with the use of this medication.
Test Taking Strategy—Analyze to determine what information the question asks for, which is an adverse effect the nurse should inform the parents about in relation to the long-term administration of phenytoin. Recall that phenytoin is known to cause gingival hyperplasia (option 4), which increases the risk for periodontal disease and tooth decay. Review the side effects associated with phenytoin, focusing on its long-term effects, if you had difficulty answering this question.
Cognitive Level—*Applying*
Client Needs Category—*Physiological integrity*
Client Needs Subcategory—*Pharmacological therapies*

103. 2. The child should not be restrained during seizure activity because this may injure rather than protect the child. The parents should be encouraged to maintain as normal a lifestyle as possible for the child, continue their child's enrollment in preschool, and encourage participation in the child's areas of interest. Developmental disability does not always occur with a seizure disorder.
Test Taking Strategy—Analyze to determine what information the question asks for, which is a correct understanding of the care and prognosis of the child with a seizure disorder. Of all the options, option 2 is the best answer because avoiding physical restraint during a seizure reduces the risk for injury. Review myths that are associated with seizure disorders and how to prevent injuries during a seizure if you had difficulty answering this question.
Cognitive Level—*Analyzing*
Client Needs Category—*Health promotion and maintenance*
Client Needs Subcategory—*None*

104. 2. A preschool child often thinks that illness or painful treatments are a punishment for having done something bad, a concept Piaget, a developmental psychologist, labeled as *immanent justice*. It is important to explain to the child that the seizure activity is not a punishment. Piaget's theory has been challenged recently by researchers who believe preschoolers ascribe to the germ theory as the cause of all diseases. Regardless of which theory is believed, the nurse must always be honest with the child, explaining that health problems happen to people who are good as well as bad and from many causes, not just "germs." It is unusual for a preschooler to attribute his or her health status to luck, eating patterns, or previous health history.

Test Taking Strategy—*Analyze to determine what information the question asks for, which is a statement that reflects a common preconceived idea among preschoolers as to the reason for a health-related disorder. Recall that preschoolers feel that illness is a consequence of having done something for which they are being punished (option 2). Review the manner in which preschoolers commonly view a serious change in their health status, as well as Piaget's observation of immanent justice, if you had difficulty answering this question.*

Cognitive Level—*Applying*

Client Needs Category—*Health promotion and maintenance*

Client Needs Subcategory—*None*

Nursing Care of a Preschooler with Leukemia

105. 3. Bone marrow aspiration is commonly used to confirm a diagnosis of leukemia. The bone marrow of the child with leukemia is characterized as being hypercellular, lacking fat globules, and containing blast cells (immature white cells). The complete blood count (CBC) and spinal fluid examinations are part of the battery of tests a client may undergo when leukemia is suspected, but they do not confirm the diagnosis. An X-ray of the long bones also does not confirm the diagnosis.

Test Taking Strategy—*Use the process of elimination to select the option that identifies the best test for diagnosing leukemia. Recall that a hematologist, a physician who is an expert at diagnosing blood disorders, examines the bone marrow (option 3) to determine whether the blood cells are normal and present in appropriate numbers. The presence of abnormal cells or an atypical number of cells is characteristic of specific cancers such as leukemia. Review the tests used to diagnose leukemia if you had difficulty answering this question.*

Cognitive Level—*Applying*

Client Needs Category—*Physiological integrity*

Client Needs Subcategory—*Physiological adaptation*

106. 3, 5, 6. Protective isolation, also known as neutropenic precautions, is used for clients who have low white blood cell counts and who are immunocompromised. Fresh fruits that cannot be peeled should not be taken into the child's room because they may harbor organisms that can cause life-threatening illnesses in someone with leukemia. The risk of contracting a life-threatening illness is increased because of the child's compromised immune system. Therefore, visitors who have a cold or flu symptoms should not be allowed to visit until they become asymptomatic. Visitors should adhere strictly to hand hygiene protocols like using an alcohol-based lotion when

entering the child's room and when leaving it. Allowing only washable toys is appropriate for a child with a contagious disease who is in isolation to prevent the spread of infection to other individuals. However, in this case, the child's disease is not contagious; also, the child is more likely to contract an infection than spread one to someone else. Visitation requirements vary by facility. Generally, family members, including children younger than age 12, are permitted to visit as long as they do not have any type of active infectious disease.

Test Taking Strategy—*Analyze to determine what information the question asks for, which is steps to take to prevent infection in a child in protective isolation. Alternative-format "select all that apply" questions require considering each option independently to decide its merit in answering the question. Choose one or more options that correlate best with methods for reducing the risk for acquiring infectious disorders. Review neutropenic precautions if you had difficulty answering this question.*

Cognitive Level—*Applying*

Client Needs Category—*Safe and effective care environment*

Client Needs Subcategory—*Safety and infection control*

107. 3. Because of the child's immunosuppressed state, the nurse should avoid taking rectal temperatures. This route increases the child's risk of developing a perirectal abscess, which can lead to a life-threatening complication. Temperature taken by the axillary, oral, or tympanic route is appropriate for the child with leukemia.

Test Taking Strategy—*Analyze to determine what information the question asks for, which is a method for assessing body temperature that is contraindicated when caring for a client with leukemia. Recall that the rectal area (option 3) harbors many bacteria, and an injury in this area from a thermometer probe could cause an infectious process. Review how leukemia increases susceptibility to infection if you had difficulty answering this question.*

Cognitive Level—*Applying*

Client Needs Category—*Physiological integrity*

Client Needs Subcategory—*Reduction of risk potential*

108. 1. Asparaginase (Elspar) is a cell cycle-nonspecific chemotherapeutic medication given in combination with other drugs to clients with leukemia to destroy cancerous white blood cells. Frequent allergic reactions have occurred in clients receiving asparaginase treatment. Epinephrine (Adrenalin) and oxygen should be on hand when giving asparaginase (Elspar) because of the increased risk of an anaphylactic reaction. The other medications are not required.

Test Taking Strategy—*Analyze to determine what information the question asks for, which is a drug that*

should be available if an allergic reaction occurs. Recall that epinephrine (option 1) is a drug used in emergencies to raise blood pressure associated with shock and relieve bronchoconstriction caused by an acute allergic reaction. Review the side effects of asparaginase and how an allergic reaction would be managed if you had difficulty answering this question.
Cognitive Level—*Applying*
Client Needs Category—*Physiological integrity*
Client Needs Subcategory—*Pharmacological therapies*

109. 2, 5. Signs of a transfusion reaction include feeling cold and having chills, fever, and a rapid pulse rate. The child may also complain of itching and low back pain. If the child experiences chilliness very early in a blood transfusion, it may be the result of the cold transfused blood entering the body. Nevertheless, the nurse should suspect a transfusion reaction until proved otherwise. Complaints of hunger, thirst, tiredness, and nausea are not common indicators of a blood transfusion reaction.
Test Taking Strategy—*Analyze to determine what information the question asks for, which is signs of a transfusion reaction. Alternative-format "select all that apply" questions require considering each option independently to decide its merit in answering the question. Choose one or more options that correlate with a sign or symptom of a blood transfusion reaction. Review clinical manifestations of transfusion reactions if you had difficulty answering this question.*
Cognitive Level—*Applying*
Client Needs Category—*Physiological integrity*
Client Needs Subcategory—*Reduction of risk potential*

110. 3. If a client is having a reaction to blood, the nurse should first clamp the tubing from the unit of blood to stop the infusion, then administer normal saline solution to maintain I.V. access. The temperature is taken, and acetaminophen (Tylenol) may be given if ordered and necessary. The charge nurse should be notified but not before the infusion is stopped.
Test Taking Strategy—*Look at the key words "most appropriate," which should lead to an option that identifies the initial nursing action when a transfusion reaction occurs. Recall that the infusing blood is the cause of the reaction. Therefore, preventing any more blood from entering the client's circulation (option 3) is the best answer. Review nursing responsibilities when responding to a transfusion reaction, particularly the action that should be performed first, if you had difficulty answering this question.*
Cognitive Level—*Analyzing*
Client Needs Category—*Physiological integrity*
Client Needs Subcategory—*Physiological adaptation*

111. 1. Preschoolers have a limited ability to grasp complex concepts such as death and dying. "Am I going to die?" is a question that can be answered in different ways. However, the nurse's response should encourage the child to ventilate feelings about dying. The nurse should avoid responses that would either make the child feel guilty or discourage the child from talking about anxieties experienced. Also, the nurse's response should not reinforce feelings of denial and unrealistic perceptions of the child's prognosis. When dealing with children, it is important to answer questions honestly based on the child's level of understanding and development.
Test Taking Strategy—*Look at the key words "most appropriate," which should lead to an option that identifies a therapeutic response to the child's question about dying. Recall that it is always therapeutic to provide the client with an opportunity to discuss his or her thoughts and feelings (option 1). Review principles of therapeutic and nontherapeutic communication and examples of each if you had difficulty answering this question.*
Cognitive Level—*Applying*
Client Needs Category—*Psychosocial integrity*
Client Needs Subcategory—*None*

112. 2. In the Hispanic-American culture, most would identify themselves as Christians. Saying prayers and lighting candles are common Christian practices. Although some Christians may believe that illness is a punishment for sins, it is not the dominant belief. Japanese culture believes that energy is restored by acupuncture. Chinese culture believes in the balance of yin and yang.
Test Taking Strategy—*Use the process of elimination to identify the option that best describes a common cultural practice among Hispanics when a family member has a life-threatening illness. Recall that in cultures in which Christianity is practiced, it is common to seek God's intercession for a specific request through prayer and lighting candles (option 2). Review religious practices for seeking relief for a serious health-related issue in Christian cultures if you had difficulty answering this question.*
Cognitive Level—*Applying*
Client Needs Category—*Psychosocial integrity*
Client Needs Subcategory—*None*

113. 1. Children with leukemia should postpone live-virus vaccines for 6 to 12 months after chemotherapy has been discontinued and after blood count levels are within normal ranges. Five vaccines (measles, mumps, rubella, polio, and varicella) are live-virus vaccines. All the other statements by the parents are consistent with the recommended treatment plan.
Test Taking Strategy—*Analyze to determine what information the question asks for, which is a statement*

that implies that a parent has incorrect information that requires clarification. Read the options carefully to ensure selecting a statement that is wrong. Recall that a child who is immunosuppressed is temporarily susceptible to infection from live-virus vaccines, making option 1 the best answer. Review common childhood immunizations that contain live viruses and review the reason leukemic clients should postpone receiving them until their cancer is in remission if you had difficulty answering this question.
Cognitive Level—*Applying*
Client Needs Category—*Health promotion and maintenance*
Client Needs Subcategory—*None*

Nursing Care of a Preschooler with Strabismus

114. 3. Foods and fluids are generally withheld for 6 to 12 hours before surgery to reduce the risk of aspirating vomitus when the client is under anesthesia or recovering from anesthesia. Preparation of the eyelids is usually carried out in the clinical setting. Trimming an eyebrow is not necessary for this type of surgery. There is no basis for administering acetaminophen (Tylenol) preoperatively before this child's eye surgery.
Test Taking Strategy—Use the process of elimination to help select the option that identifies the most important preoperative instruction to provide parents of a child scheduled for eye surgery. Option 1 can be eliminated because the parents do not perform this action. Options 2 and 4 can be eliminated because they are unnecessary. Recall that maintaining an empty stomach reduces the potential for perioperative complications. Review the typical preoperative preparation before eye surgery if you had difficulty answering this question.
Cognitive Level—*Applying*
Client Needs Category—*Physiological integrity*
Client Needs Subcategory—*Reduction of risk potential*

115. 4. Some soreness may occur after this type of eye surgery. The child's question should not be ignored or minimized and deserves an honest response. Any responses or explanations should be developmentally appropriate.
Test Taking Strategy—Look at the key words "most appropriate" used in reference to a nursing response to a child who is concerned about the potential for experiencing discomfort after undergoing eye surgery. Recall that children feel betrayed by less than truthful responses to a valid question or by having

their question dismissed. Understanding this concept leads to selecting option 4 as the best answer. Review examples of therapeutic and nontherapeutic communication techniques if you had difficulty answering this question.
Cognitive Level—*Applying*
Client Needs Category—*Psychosocial integrity*
Client Needs Subcategory—*None*

116. 2. Pretending the child is a pirate affords an opportunity to wear an eye patch, thereby restricting the child's vision and giving the child a perception of the postoperative experience. Done in a nonthreatening manner, this game will decrease the child's anxiety during the postoperative period. The other games do not relate to preparation of the child's postoperative needs.
Test Taking Strategy—Use the process of elimination to identify the option that provides the best game for preparing the child for the postoperative period after eye surgery. Option 4 can be eliminated immediately because playing peek-a-boo is not compatible with this child's age. Although the child may enjoy playing tic-tac-toe and hide-and-seek, neither of these activities prepares the child as much as pretending to play pirate (option 2) with an eye patch. Review the postoperative care after ophthalmic surgery, which often includes covering the operative eye with a dressing and Fox aluminum shield or black vinyl eye patch with an elastic strap, if you had difficulty answering this question.
Cognitive Level—*Applying*
Client Needs Category—*Psychosocial integrity*
Client Needs Subcategory—*None*

117. 3. Unless both eyes are bandaged, there is no reason why the child cannot play with toys while under an adult's supervision. In most cases, the child can resume a regular diet and activity as soon as nausea has ceased and the anesthesia has worn off. Restraints are removed while the child is under adult supervision.
Test Taking Strategy—Analyze to determine what information the question asks for, which is incorrect information that requires clarification. Read the options carefully to find the inaccurate statement. Recall that playing with toys occupies a great deal of the day's activity for children of this age and restricting it for 4 weeks because one eye is patched is inconsiderate as well as unnecessary. Review postoperative home care after surgery to correct strabismus if you had difficulty answering this question.
Cognitive Level—*Analyzing*
Client Needs Category—*Health promotion and maintenance*
Client Needs Subcategory—*None*

Nursing Care of a Preschooler Having a Tonsillectomy and Adenoidectomy

118. 2. It is important to promptly report an elevated temperature of a preoperative client along with any other signs of infection, such as a sore throat, cough, or excessive nasal discharge. Surgery will be canceled if the child has an infection. The other vital signs listed are normal for a child of this age.

> *Test Taking Strategy—Analyze to determine what information the question asks for, which is an assessment finding that causes concern in a child who will undergo a tonsillectomy. Recall that a fever of 101°F suggests a current infectious process that could jeopardize the child's safety if the planned surgery occurs. Review factors that contraindicate surgical procedures if you had difficulty answering this question.*
> *Cognitive Level—Applying*
> *Client Needs Category—Physiological integrity*
> *Client Needs Subcategory—Reduction of risk potential*

119. 2. Clear liquids include clear broth, gelatin, synthetic juices, water, and ice chips. Natural juices, such as orange juice, are irritating to the throat and are not clear. When a full liquid diet can be tolerated, such foods as ice cream, puddings, creamed soups, and custards can be added to the menu.

> *Test Taking Strategy—Look at the key words "most appropriate," which are used when asking for a food choice in the immediate postoperative period. Recall that clear liquids, especially those that are cool, are generally the first food items allowed after surgery. Apple juice (option 2) is the only option listed that correlates with a clear liquid. Review the postoperative diet after a tonsillectomy and adenoidectomy if you had difficulty answering this question.*
> *Cognitive Level—Applying*
> *Client Needs Category—Physiological integrity*
> *Client Needs Subcategory—Basic care and comfort*

120. 2. The child should not be allowed to drink from a straw because sucking can dislodge clots and sutures and lead to hemorrhage. An ice collar is typically applied to promote comfort; however, it may be removed if the child is more comfortable without one. It is permissible for the child whose throat is sore, making swallowing difficult, to use a tissue for wiping bloody oral secretions. It is preferable for the parents to stay with the child postoperatively, but it is not mandatory if they choose to leave.

> *Test Taking Strategy—Analyze to determine what information the question asks for, which is an action that is of concern for the child in the immediate postoperative period after a tonsillectomy. A sucking action*

(option 2) is contraindicated because it increases the potential for bleeding or hemorrhage from the surgical site. Review activities that are contraindicated after a tonsillectomy until healing occurs if you had difficulty answering this question.
> *Cognitive Level—Applying*
> *Client Needs Category—Physiological integrity*
> *Client Needs Subcategory—Physiological adaptation*

121. 4. Signs of excessive bleeding after a tonsillectomy include frequent swallowing (which may be due to blood trickling down the back of the throat), a rapid pulse rate, restlessness, and vomiting bright red blood. Vomiting dark (old) blood is expected and should not cause concern unless there is a large amount of emesis. Throat pain is a common postoperative finding. A respiratory rate of 30 breaths/minute is within the normal range for a 5-year-old child.

> *Test Taking Strategy—Analyze to determine what information the question asks for, which is a sign associated with a postoperative complication after a tonsillectomy. Recall that bleeding and hemorrhage are high on the list of potential complications, and that the site of bleeding is in the oropharynx. Although inspecting the tonsillar fossa for oozing blood is a definitive assessment, frequent swallowing (option 4) is one sign that blood is accumulating rather than being expectorated. Vomiting often follows after swallowing blood. Review signs of post-tonsillectomy hemorrhage if you had difficulty answering this question.*
> *Cognitive Leve—Applying*
> *Client Needs Category—Physiological integrity*
> *Client Needs Subcategory—Physiological adaptation*

122. 1. It is recommended to keep a child quiet for a few days after a tonsillectomy to discourage bleeding at the operative site. Fluids and soft foods can be taken as desired, but a regular diet is not usually recommended for several days because certain foods may cause irritation and bleeding of the operative site. Aspirin is contraindicated for a child of this age because its use has been associated with Reye syndrome. Aspirin may also affect the blood's ability to clot and therefore increases bleeding tendencies.

> *Test Taking Strategy—Look at the key words "most appropriate," used to refer to teaching that should be included during discharge instructions for a child who is recovering from a tonsillectomy and adenoidectomy. Recall that activity increases heart rate and blood pressure, which can contribute to bleeding postoperatively. Keeping the child quiet for a few days (option 1) is the best answer. Options 2, 3, and 4 contain inaccurate and even unsafe instructions. Review recommendations for postdischarge care while*

a child recovers from a tonsillectomy and adenoidectomy if you had difficulty answering this question.
Cognitive Level—*Applying*
Client Needs Category—*Health promotion and maintenance*
Client Needs Subcategory—*None*

123. 4. The pediatric licensed practical nurse is most correct to suggest that the critically-ill 3-year-old have emergency medication administered by the intraosseous route in the femur. The intraosseous route is the best choice during emergency situations when the intravenous route is unable to be obtained. Intraosseous administration is equally rapid in delivering systemic medications and more rapid than the oral and intramuscular route.

In an emergency situation, waiting for the child to be anesthetized delays treatment.
Test Taking Strategy—*Look at the key words "critically-ill" and "initiating medication quickly" in reference to the fastest route for medication action. Analyze each option considering route of administration. Recall that the intraosseous route is similar to the intravenous route and the route of choice if an intravenous line is unable to be obtained in an emergency. Review medication routes of administration if you had difficulty answering this question.*
Cognitive Level—*Analyzing*
Client Needs Category—*Physiological integrity*
Client Needs Subcategory—*Physiological adaptation*

14 The Nursing Care of School-Age Children and Adolescents

Directions: *With a pencil, blacken the space in front of the option you have chosen for your correct answer.*

Nursing Care of a Child with Rheumatic Fever

A 7-year-old child is admitted to the hospital with possible rheumatic fever.

1. If the parents report all the following history findings to the nurse, which one is most closely correlated with an increased risk of rheumatic fever?

[ ] **1.** The child was exposed to measles within the past 4 weeks.
[ ] **2.** The child had a severe sore throat within the past 2 weeks.
[ ] **3.** The child is lethargic and no longer interested in schoolwork.
[ ] **4.** The child received a bump on the head while playing.

2. Which finding documented by the nurse is most indicative of a client with rheumatic fever?

[ ] **1.** Slow, irregular heartbeat
[ ] **2.** Blotchy, diffuse erythema
[ ] **3.** Decreased antistreptolysin O titer (ASO titer)
[ ] **4.** Generalized migrating joint tenderness

The child is placed on bed rest and started on penicillin V (Pen-Vee-K) and aspirin.

3. Which diversional activity suggested by the nurse is most appropriate for the child during the acute phase of rheumatic fever?

[ ] **1.** Playing with action figures
[ ] **2.** Playing video games
[ ] **3.** Reading an adventure story
[ ] **4.** Pounding wooden pegs with a mallet

4. The nurse would expect to withhold penicillin V (Pen-Vee-K) and notify the physician if the child had a previous allergic reaction to a medication from which drug group?
[ ] **1.** Aminoglycosides
[ ] **2.** Cephalosporins
[ ] **3.** Macrolides
[ ] **4.** Sulfonamides

The parents ask why the child is receiving aspirin instead of acetaminophen (Tylenol) and are worried about their child getting Reye's syndrome.

5. Which response by the nurse best explains why aspirin is preferred to acetaminophen (Tylenol) in the treatment of rheumatic fever?
[ ] **1.** "Aspirin controls fever better."
[ ] **2.** "Aspirin prevents infections."
[ ] **3.** "Aspirin relieves joint inflammation."
[ ] **4.** "Aspirin prevents cardiac enlargement."

The parents question how their child got rheumatic fever and ask if the child can get it again. The nurse teaches the parents the disease process and potential consequences in the future.

6. Which statement by the parents best indicates that the nurse's teaching has been effective?
[ ] **1.** "We'll give our child the penicillin for the full 10 days."
[ ] **2.** "We will keep our child at home until fully recovered."
[ ] **3.** "We will make sure that our child stays out of the sun while being treated."
[ ] **4.** "We'll notify the physician if our child has a sore throat."

7. If the child develops shortness of breath when ambulating to the bathroom in the hospital, which intervention should the nurse add to the care plan?
[ ] **1.** Have the child use a bedside commode for elimination.
[ ] **2.** Administer oxygen after the child uses the bathroom.
[ ] **3.** Instruct the child to call for assistance when ambulating to the bathroom.
[ ] **4.** Provide a walker for the child to use when ambulating to the bathroom.

Nursing Care of a Child with Diabetes Mellitus

A 9-year-old child is admitted to the hospital with a tentative diagnosis of type 1 (insulin-dependent) diabetes mellitus. The parents state that the child has been complaining of feeling sick for several days. The physician states that the child has signs and symptoms of diabetic ketoacidosis.

8. Which findings by the nurse best indicate that the child is experiencing diabetic ketoacidosis? Select all that apply.
[ ] **1.** Blood glucose level of 120 mg/dL
[ ] **2.** Fruity-smelling breath
[ ] **3.** Pale-colored face
[ ] **4.** Excessive perspiration
[ ] **5.** Deep, rapid breathing
[ ] **6.** Dry, flushed skin

9. Which of the following is a priority for the nurse to assess when testing the child's urine?
[ ] **1.** Blood in the urine
[ ] **2.** Bilirubin in the urine
[ ] **3.** Ketones in the urine
[ ] **4.** White blood cells in the urine

10. The physician orders I.V. insulin, and the registered nurse (RN) prepares to give it. The licensed practical nurse (LPN) is assisting the RN with the unstable client. Which of the following types of insulin should the LPN anticipate that the physician will order?
[ ] **1.** Regular insulin (Humulin R)
[ ] **2.** Isophane insulin suspension (Humulin N)
[ ] **3.** Insulin glargine (Lantus)
[ ] **4.** Insulin aspart (NovoLog)

After further tests, the diagnosis of type 1 diabetes mellitus is confirmed. The child's condition improves and blood glucose readings range between 100 and 128 mg/dL. The physician writes orders to discontinue the I.V. infusion and to begin subcutaneous Humulin R and NPH (isophane insulin suspension) insulin therapy. The physician also orders a dietary consultation.

11. When is the correct time for the nurse to administer the child's morning dose of a combination regular and NPH insulin?
[ ] **1.** 30 minutes before breakfast is served
[ ] **2.** 15 minutes before breakfast is served
[ ] **3.** 30 minutes after breakfast is served
[ ] **4.** 15 minutes after breakfast is served

12. Which client symptoms documented by the nurse best indicate that the child is having a hypoglycemic reaction? Select all that apply.
[ ] **1.** The child complains of being thirsty.
[ ] **2.** The child's breathing is labored and prolonged.
[ ] **3.** The child's urine tests positive for glucose.
[ ] **4.** The child complains of feeling shaky.
[ ] **5.** The child reports feeling light-headed.
[ ] **6.** The child states his or her heart is racing.

13. Which of the following is the priority nursing action if the child develops symptoms of hypoglycemia?
[ ] **1.** Give the child orange juice or milk to drink.
[ ] **2.** Give the child 10% glucose I.V.
[ ] **3.** Notify the physician immediately.
[ ] **4.** Administer a second dose of insulin.

The child's parents ask the nurse why the child cannot receive the insulin in the form of a pill.

14. Which response by the nurse best explains why insulin must be given subcutaneously?
[ ] **1.** "The oral form of insulin can lead to the worsening of diabetic symptoms."
[ ] **2.** "Insulin is destroyed by digestive enzymes when given by mouth."
[ ] **3.** "Insulin causes vomiting and dehydration when given by mouth."
[ ] **4.** "The oral form of insulin isn't effective in treating children with diabetes."

The child has completely recovered from ketoacidosis and is receiving regular insulin (Humulin R) and isophane insulin suspension (Humulin NPH) subcutaneously. The blood glucose levels have stabilized, and the physician requests that diabetic home care teaching be started.

15. The nurse correctly instructs the child and parents that insulin injection sites should be rotated from one anatomic injection site to another for which reason?
[ ] **1.** To slow the absorption of insulin from the subcutaneous tissue
[ ] **2.** To prevent accumulation of insulin in the subcutaneous tissue
[ ] **3.** To decrease the duration of action of the insulin
[ ] **4.** To prevent lipodystrophy of subcutaneous tissue

16. Which statement by the child indicates to the nurse that diabetic teaching has been effective?
[ ] **1.** "If I eat more food, I won't need as much insulin."
[ ] **2.** "If I'm more active, I won't need as much insulin."
[ ] **3.** "If I get an infection, I won't need as much insulin."
[ ] **4.** "If I get real upset, I won't need as much insulin."

The parents state that their child is very active in sports and likes to swim, play basketball, and soccer. The parents ask the nurse if the child will be able to continue these activities.

17. Which is the best response by the nurse?
[ ] **1.** "You should redirect your child to participate in activities that require less energy."
[ ] **2.** "You should encourage swimming because it lowers the metabolism, but discourage playing basketball or soccer."
[ ] **3.** "You should allow your child to continue these activities, but athletic staff should be aware of possible diabetic complications."
[ ] **4.** "You should permit your child to play basketball and soccer, but swimming will increase the insulin needs."

18. In addition to routine blood glucose assessments, if the child is athletic and very competitive, the nurse should recommend checking the child's blood glucose level how often?
[ ] **1.** After participating in athletics
[ ] **2.** Before participating in athletics
[ ] **3.** Every 4 hours throughout the day
[ ] **4.** When a hypoglycemic reaction occurs

19. The nurse is caring for a diabetic child whose 11 A.M. blood glucose monitoring check is 269 mg/dL. The physician orders the following coverage schedule:
  150 to 200 mg/dL—2 units of Humulin R
  201 to 250 mg/dL—4 units of Humulin R
  251 to 300 mg/dL—6 units of Humulin R
  301 to 350 mg/dL—8 units of Humulin R
  351 to 399 mg/dL—10 units of Humulin R
  Over 400 mg/dL—Call the physician
Draw a line at the calibrated mark on the syringe identifying the amount of insulin that should be drawn into the syringe.

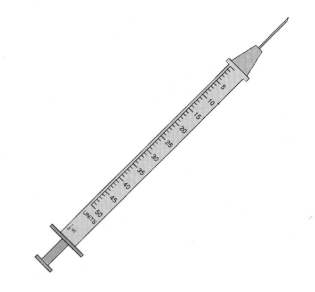

The diabetic child begins using an insulin pump. A diabetes nurse educator has been consulted to assist with insulin pump education and regulation.

20. Which statement by a diabetic child indicates a need for additional instructions on how to use an insulin pump?
[ ] **1.** "I like the insulin pump because I can wear it under my clothes without anyone noticing I have it on."
[ ] **2.** "I like the insulin pump because I only have to change the needle site every 24 to 48 hours."
[ ] **3.** "I like the insulin pump because when I need extra insulin, all I have to do is push a button on the pump."
[ ] **4.** "I like the insulin pump because I don't have to check my blood glucose level; the pump checks the level for me."

Nursing Care of a Child with Partial-Thickness and Full-Thickness Burns

An 8-year-old child is hospitalized for treatment of extensive partial-thickness and full-thickness burns on the face, neck, anterior chest, and left arm as a result of a house fire.

21. Which clinical manifestation of the client's full-thickness burns would the nurse detect during an assessment?
[ ] 1. Moderate level of pain due to exposed nerve endings
[ ] 2. Edema formation throughout the area of the burn
[ ] 3. The appearance of blister formation throughout the area of the burn
[ ] 4. Noted tissue destruction extending to the subcutaneous layer

22. The nurse should plan to keep which equipment or supplies in the burned child's room in case an emergency arises?
[ ] 1. An extra supply of sterile dressing
[ ] 2. An endotracheal tube and oxygen supply
[ ] 3. Equipment to administer pain medication
[ ] 4. Additional bags of I.V. fluid

23. Which nursing interventions are essential to restore the child's fluid and electrolyte balance during the emergent phase of burn care and treatment? Select all that apply.
[ ] 1. Initiate the administration of I.V. fluids.
[ ] 2. Track the child's vital signs.
[ ] 3. Give the child sips of water.
[ ] 4. Encourage the child to consume protein-rich feedings.
[ ] 5. Monitor the child's urine output.
[ ] 6. Assemble equipment for a small-gauge venous catheter.

24. During early postburn care of the child, it is essential for the nurse to closely monitor which of the following?
[ ] 1. Unburned skin
[ ] 2. Bowel elimination
[ ] 3. I.V. fluid therapy
[ ] 4. Pupillary response to light

The physician admits the child to the pediatric intensive care unit (PICU) for close assessment and nursing care.

25. Which of the following assessment findings would alert the nurse that the child may be exhibiting early signs of sepsis?
[ ] 1. Increased level of pain
[ ] 2. Disorientation
[ ] 3. Decreased urine output
[ ] 4. Jitteriness

26. The physician orders an I.V. opioid analgesic. Which finding by the nurse would best indicate that the I.V. opioid analgesic is effective?
[ ] 1. The respiratory rate is within normal limits.
[ ] 2. The child's pain level remains stable.
[ ] 3. The child is watching television.
[ ] 4. The urine output is 30 mL/hour.

27. Because the burned child is confined to bed, the nurse assesses for footdrop. Which nursing action best prevents the development of footdrop?
[ ] 1. Apply braces to the feet and ankles.
[ ] 2. Keep the child in the side-lying position.
[ ] 3. Keep sheets tucked in at the foot of the bed.
[ ] 4. Rest the child's feet against a footboard.

28. Which finding documented by the nurse is most indicative of the presence of a Curling's ulcer in the burned child?
[ ] 1. Absence of bowel sounds
[ ] 2. A positive Hemoccult test
[ ] 3. An elevated hematocrit
[ ] 4. A distended abdomen

After the burned child's condition stabilizes, the child is placed on a high-protein diet.

29. If the following snacks are available, which one is best to meet the child's need for protein?
[ ] 1. Strawberry milkshake
[ ] 2. Apple sprinkled with cinnamon
[ ] 3. Cubes of flavored gelatin
[ ] 4. Warmed beef broth

30. Which diversional activity is best for meeting the burned child's developmental needs?
[ ] 1. Reading the newspaper
[ ] 2. Coloring simple designs
[ ] 3. Playing with an action figure
[ ] 4. Playing a solitary card game

Nursing Care of a Child with Juvenile Rheumatoid Arthritis

A 10-year-old child who has juvenile rheumatoid arthritis (JRA) is seen in the joint disorders specialty clinic 2 weeks after an acute episode of the disorder. The nurse discusses home care with the child and parents.

31. Which statement by the child indicates teaching about the use of ibuprofen (Motrin) has been effective?
[ ] 1. "I should take Motrin every day to control my joint inflammation."
[ ] 2. "I should take Motrin when my temperature is 101°F (38.3°C) or higher."
[ ] 3. "I should take Motrin only when I'm having muscle spasms."
[ ] 4. "I should take Motrin every day to thin my blood."

32. The parents of the child with juvenile rheumatoid arthritis (JRA) ask the nurse why the child cannot have aspirin. The parents further explain that they have heard that aspirin is used in the elderly for arthritis aches and pains. The nurse correctly explains that children with JRA are given different medications than adults with arthritis and explains that the toxic effects of aspirin include which manifestations?
[ ] **1.** Constipation, weight gain, and fluid retention
[ ] **2.** Ringing in the ears, nausea, and vomiting
[ ] **3.** Anorexia, weight loss, and double vision
[ ] **4.** Headache, dry mouth, and dental cavities

33. Which activity is most appropriate for the child with juvenile rheumatoid arthritis?
[ ] **1.** Skipping rope
[ ] **2.** Softball
[ ] **3.** Gymnastics
[ ] **4.** Swimming

34. Which statement by the parents indicates they understand the home care instructions given by the nurse?
[ ] **1.** "We've made arrangements for a homebound teacher."
[ ] **2.** "We'll put ice packs on our child's joints during episodes of inflammation."
[ ] **3.** "We'll serve meals that prevent excess weight gain."
[ ] **4.** "We'll keep our child in bed most of the time."

35. The nurse advises the parents that, to detect possible complications of juvenile rheumatoid arthritis, the child will require which periodic evaluation?
[ ] **1.** Chest X-rays
[ ] **2.** Dental examinations
[ ] **3.** Hearing examinations
[ ] **4.** Eye examinations

Nursing Care of a Child with an Injury

A nurse in a rural community clinic provides nursing care and age-appropriate instruction for pediatric clients with minor injuries. Throughout the day, children with a variety of injuries come in for medical care.

36. Which nursing instruction concerning ice applications is appropriate to give the parents of a 12-year-old child with a sprained ankle?
[ ] **1.** "Ice can be applied and left on until the swelling is gone."
[ ] **2.** "Ice can be applied but must be removed every 30 minutes to 1 hour to check the ankle."
[ ] **3.** "Ice should not be used for treating sprains; heat should be used instead."
[ ] **4.** "There is no danger associated with the application of ice."

37. Which nursing action is most appropriate when caring for a school-age child who is experiencing a nosebleed?
[ ] **1.** Tilt the child's head backward, and apply an ice pack to the nose.
[ ] **2.** Position the child's head forward while gently pinching the nostrils.
[ ] **3.** Pack the affected nostril with a small amount of clean cotton.
[ ] **4.** Clean the affected nostril, and instill saline nose drops.

38. When a 10-year-old child falls from a bicycle and loses a permanent incisor tooth, which advice can the nurse provide the parents before they take the child to see a dentist?
[ ] **1.** Submerge the tooth in milk.
[ ] **2.** Place the tooth in a plastic bag.
[ ] **3.** Wrap the tooth in a clean cloth.
[ ] **4.** Clean the tooth with alcohol.

39. Which intervention is most appropriate initially for an 8-year-old child who selects the fourth face on the Wong-Baker FACES Pain Rating Scale?

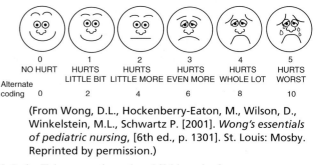

(From Wong, D.L., Hockenberry-Eaton, M., Wilson, D., Winkelstein, M.L., Schwartz P. [2001]. *Wong's essentials of pediatric nursing*, [6th ed., p. 1301]. St. Louis: Mosby. Reprinted by permission.)

[ ] **1.** Take no action; the child is pain-free.
[ ] **2.** Provide diversional activities to relieve the child's pain.
[ ] **3.** Document findings, and recheck the child later.
[ ] **4.** Give the prescribed analgesic to relieve the pain.

Nursing Care of a Child with a Head Injury

A 9-year-old child is admitted to the hospital for observation after falling off a bicycle. The parents state that the child's head hit the pavement during the fall.

40. If the nurse collects the following data, which assessment finding best indicates the presence of increased intracranial pressure?
[ ] **1.** Rapid bilateral pupillary response to light
[ ] **2.** Tympanic temperature of 97.9°F (36.6°C)
[ ] **3.** Blood pressure of 150/90 mm Hg
[ ] **4.** Deep tendon reflexes +2

41. Which assessment finding should the nurse report immediately to the charge nurse or physician?
[ ] 1. Clear, watery nasal drainage
[ ] 2. Glasgow Coma Scale score of 15
[ ] 3. Child does not know the time of day
[ ] 4. Apical pulse of 80 beats/minute

The child is monitored overnight, and no complications are observed. The physician discharges the client in the morning. Before they leave the clinic, the child and parents meet with the nurse to review safety needs.

42. Which statement by the child indicates a need for further teaching about bicycle safety?
[ ] 1. "I'll wear my helmet whenever I ride my bicycle."
[ ] 2. "I'll ride my bicycle in the opposite direction of traffic flow."
[ ] 3. "I'll stop at all intersections and look both ways before proceeding."
[ ] 4. "I won't ride my bicycle after dark on the street."

Another child is being assessed in the emergency department after a blow to the head. The physician determines that the child may be discharged home. The nurse provides discharge instructions to the client and parents.

43. Which instruction is essential to give the parents before discharge?
[ ] 1. Return the child for a follow-up visit in 3 to 5 days.
[ ] 2. Give the child nothing by mouth for the next 12 hours.
[ ] 3. Check the child's pupillary response every 4 hours.
[ ] 4. Awaken the child every 4 hours during the first night.

Nursing Care of a Child with a Brain Tumor

An 11-year-old child is admitted to the hospital with complaints of headaches, dizziness, and vomiting.

44. Which information reported by the parents indicates a high risk for the presence of a brain tumor?
[ ] 1. The child vomits when first getting out of bed.
[ ] 2. The child frequently complains of nausea.
[ ] 3. The child forgets where homework is placed.
[ ] 4. The child's head tilts toward the side when sleeping.

45. If the physician orders a magnetic resonance imaging (MRI) study for the child with a brain tumor, which statement by the nurse would best prepare the child for the diagnostic test?
[ ] 1. "MRI machines differ with some being tunnel-like and others open."
[ ] 2. "A slight headache may occur when the dye is injected into the vein."
[ ] 3. "You'll be given medicine that will make you sleep during the test."
[ ] 4. "You'll have little electrodes placed on your head with a special gel."

The results of the magnetic resonance imaging (MRI) study show that the child has a brain tumor, and the child is taken immediately to surgery. A craniotomy is performed, and the tumor is partially removed. When the child returns from surgery, the nurse observes a moderate amount of clear drainage on the head dressing.

46. Which nursing action is most appropriate at this time?
[ ] 1. Recognize that the fluid is cerebrospinal fluid (CSF) and remove the dressing, observing for the source of the leakage.
[ ] 2. Recognize that the fluid is CSF and call the chaplain because death of the child is imminent.
[ ] 3. Recognize that the fluid is CSF and notify the operating room because additional surgery will be necessary.
[ ] 4. Recognize that the fluid is CSF and reinforce the dressing until the physician can change it.

The child's parents express their feelings of helplessness and anxiety to the nurse after learning about their child's diagnosis.

47. Which statement by the nurse would best help the parents cope with their feelings?
[ ] 1. "Perhaps you'd feel better if you visited your child for shorter periods of time."
[ ] 2. "Don't worry. You're doing a great job, and everything will work out for the best."
[ ] 3. "This is painful for you. Let's identify things you can do to help make your child feel good."
[ ] 4. "It's sad that you feel helpless. What do you usually do to take your mind off your worries?"

The oncologist visits and writes orders for the child to begin chemotherapy.

48. Which nursing action would best help the child to cope with the effects of the chemotherapy?
[ ] 1. Serve the child a well-balanced meal before beginning the chemotherapy.
[ ] 2. Give the child an antiemetic before beginning the chemotherapy.
[ ] 3. Encourage the child to get plenty of rest before beginning the chemotherapy.
[ ] 4. Give the child pain medication before beginning the chemotherapy.

The physician orders an I.V. to maintain fluid replacement for this child.

49. If the child weighs 30 kg, what is the hourly flow rate in milliliters? Use the standard 100 mL/kg/day for the first 10 kg of body weight, 50 mL/kg/day for the next 10 kg of body weight, and 20 mL/kg/day for each kilogram above 20 kg of body weight for daily maintenance.

After losing hair from the chemotherapy treatments, the child cries and says, "Everybody is going to laugh at me. I never want to go to school again!"

50. Which nursing action best facilitates the child's reestablishment of friendships with peers?

[ ] **1.** Encourage the child to make friends with children who have cancer.

[ ] **2.** Tell the child that real friends do not care how you look on the outside.

[ ] **3.** Encourage the child's friends to visit while the child is still in the hospital.

[ ] **4.** Tell the child that the appearance changes are temporary and not that bad.

The physician orders a lumbar puncture for a 3-year-old child suspected of having meningitis.

51. How should the nurse position a child who is about to undergo a lumbar puncture?

[ ] **1.** Prone position

[ ] **2.** Trendelenburg's position

[ ] **3.** Supine position

[ ] **4.** Side-lying position

Nursing Care of a Child in Traction

A 9-year-old is admitted to the pediatric unit with a fractured right femur. The child is in skeletal traction.

52. Which nursing interventions should be included in the care plan of a child in skeletal traction? Select all that apply.

[ ] **1.** Maintain the child in the prone position.

[ ] **2.** Clean the pin site every 8 hours.

[ ] **3.** Perform range-of-motion exercises on each leg.

[ ] **4.** Release weights on the traction every 2 hours.

[ ] **5.** Monitor client for signs of cloudy urine.

[ ] **6.** Cover protruding tips of pins with protective materials.

53. Because of the length of time the client must remain in skeletal traction, the nurse correctly assesses for evidence of skin breakdown in which area?

[ ] **1.** Over the child's calves

[ ] **2.** Over the child's scapulae

[ ] **3.** On the child's knees

[ ] **4.** On the child's buttocks

54. Which assessment finding should the nurse report immediately to the physician or charge nurse?

[ ] **1.** The pin protrudes through the skin on both sides.

[ ] **2.** The foot of the bed is elevated on blocks.

[ ] **3.** The weights of the traction are hanging freely.

[ ] **4.** A traction rope is out of the pulley groove.

55. Which intervention is best to prevent complications associated with traction and immobility?

[ ] **1.** Offer the child fluids on a frequent basis.

[ ] **2.** Assist the child to select low-fiber foods.

[ ] **3.** Assist the child with right leg exercises daily.

[ ] **4.** Reposition the child onto the side every 2 hours.

56. Which assessment finding may indicate a serious neurovascular problem that should be reported immediately to the charge nurse or physician?

[ ] **1.** The pulse is palpable in the right foot.

[ ] **2.** The toes of both feet are cool to the touch.

[ ] **3.** The child is unable to wiggle the toes of the right foot.

[ ] **4.** The capillary refill in the toes of the right foot is 2 seconds.

Nursing Care of a Child with a Kidney Disorder

A 7-year-old child is brought to the pediatrician's office when the parent notes that the child is voiding dark-colored urine. The child is being evaluated for acute glomerular nephritis.

57. Which finding best indicates that a school-age child has acute glomerular nephritis?

[ ] **1.** Periorbital edema

[ ] **2.** Excessive urination

[ ] **3.** Increased appetite

[ ] **4.** Low blood pressure

A school-age child is examined by the pediatrician and diagnosed with nephrotic syndrome. The parents are concerned due to the generalized edema throughout the child's body.

58. Which nursing actions are most appropriate to include in the care plan of a child with nephrotic syndrome? Select all that apply.

[ ] **1.** Restricting the intake of protein

[ ] **2.** Weighing the child daily

[ ] **3.** Completing range-of-motion exercises

[ ] **4.** Measuring abdominal circumference

[ ] **5.** Collecting a 24-hour urine specimen

[ ] **6.** Monitoring blood urea nitrogen (BUN) and creatinine levels

A 12-year-old child is diagnosed with renal tubular dysfunction. Blood chemistry results reveal a potassium level of 2.5 mEq/L.

59. Which finding by the nurse strongly indicates that a child is experiencing hypokalemia?

[ ] **1.** Full, bounding pulses

[ ] **2.** Muscle weakness

[ ] **3.** Elevated blood pressure

[ ] **4.** Hyperactive bowel sounds

A mother notes that her child's clothes do not fit around the waist due to a lump in the abdomen. After evaluation, the child is diagnosed with Wilms' tumor.

60. Which nursing action should be avoided when giving care to a child diagnosed with Wilms' tumor?
[ ] **1.** Palpating the child's abdomen
[ ] **2.** Collecting a catheterized urine sample
[ ] **3.** Assessing pupillary reflex with a penlight
[ ] **4.** Eliciting a patellar reflex with a reflex hammer

Nursing Care of a Child with a Blood Disorder

A child is brought to the public health office for a routine checkup.

61. Which of the following findings during a routine wellness checkup best indicates that a child has iron deficiency anemia?
[ ] **1.** Weight gain and hypertension
[ ] **2.** Nervousness and diarrhea
[ ] **3.** Nausea and vomiting
[ ] **4.** Pallor and listlessness

The nurse is providing discharge instructions to the parents of a client recently diagnosed with hemophilia.

62. The nurse correctly advises the parents to avoid administering medications containing which ingredient to their child who has hemophilia?
[ ] **1.** Aspirin
[ ] **2.** Caffeine
[ ] **3.** Barbiturates
[ ] **4.** Antacids

Nursing Care of a Child with a Communicable Disease

A public health nurse is presenting information on communicable diseases at the local health fair. After the presentation, as individuals are picking up brochures with specific information of interest, many ask questions of the nurse.

63. Which statement by the parent of a school-age child with tinea capitis indicates that the nurse's teaching was effective?
[ ] **1.** "I'll comb my child's hair with a fine-tooth comb dipped in vinegar to remove the nits."
[ ] **2.** "I'll give the griseofulvin (Grisactin) with whole milk to increase absorption of the medication."
[ ] **3.** "I'll give the medication for the full 2 weeks to prevent spreading of the lesions."
[ ] **4.** "I'll apply the medication to my child's scalp three times a day until the lesions are gone."

One family asks if there is any literature on pinworms. They state that a relative had them and they are wondering if their son does as well.

64. Which finding would the nurse most expect the parents to report if their child is suspected of having pinworms?
[ ] **1.** Increased flatulence
[ ] **2.** Abdominal pain
[ ] **3.** Anal itching
[ ] **4.** Bulky, greasy stools

Two parents express frustration because their child has frequent outbreaks of impetigo. The nurse assesses their knowledge of the disease process.

65. Which statement by a parent indicates a need for additional teaching?
[ ] **1.** "I can give oral antihistamines to decrease the inflammation and itching."
[ ] **2.** "Antibiotic treatment isn't necessary because the infection is self-limited."
[ ] **3.** "I'll be sure to trim my child's nails to prevent scratching of the lesions."
[ ] **4.** "I'll take the necessary precautions to prevent my child from spreading the infection to others."

Nursing Care of a Child with a Nutritional Deficiency

Orphans from another country are brought to the United States for adoption. After a complete physical examination, the children are found to be in generally good health but thin, and several of the children are diagnosed with rickets.

66. When developing a care plan for a child with rickets, the nurse appropriately includes providing nutritional sources of which vitamin?
[ ] **1.** Vitamin A
[ ] **2.** Vitamin B$_{12}$
[ ] **3.** Vitamin C
[ ] **4.** Vitamin D

The school nurse identifies a 7-year-old child who does not like to drink milk as possibly being deficient in calcium.

67. Which of the following foods provide excellent sources of calcium for this school-age child? Select all that apply.
[ ] **1.** A serving of broccoli
[ ] **2.** Blueberry yogurt
[ ] **3.** Chocolate ice cream
[ ] **4.** A serving of chicken
[ ] **5.** Cheese and crackers
[ ] **6.** A medium-sized apple

Before the beginning of the new school year, a school nurse teaches the elementary school faculty about peanut allergies.

68. Which of the following signs and symptoms should be included in the nurse's presentation? Select all that apply.
[ ] **1.** Hives with redness and swelling
[ ] **2.** Itching or tingling in or around the mouth and throat
[ ] **3.** Digestive problems such as diarrhea and vomiting
[ ] **4.** Runny or stuffy nose
[ ] **5.** Red, watery eyes
[ ] **6.** Swelling of the hands and fingers

69. The school nurse is asked about foods that should be avoided if a student has a peanut allergy. Which foods should be avoided? Select all that apply.
[ ] **1.** Cookies and pastries
[ ] **2.** Ice cream and frozen desserts
[ ] **3.** Energy bars
[ ] **4.** Cereals and granola
[ ] **5.** Yogurt and sour cream
[ ] **6.** Cheeseburger and cola

Nursing Care of a Child with a Musculoskeletal Disability

A pediatric nurse is providing guidance to parents whose child was recently diagnosed with cerebral palsy.

70. When discussing cerebral palsy with the parents of a newly diagnosed child, which information is correct?
[ ] **1.** Cerebral palsy is a nonprogressive disease caused by damage to the brain.
[ ] **2.** Brain surgery commonly helps or even cures children with cerebral palsy.
[ ] **3.** Physical therapy is of little value to a child with cerebral palsy.
[ ] **4.** Cerebral palsy is the result of injury to the sensory areas of the brain.

A child is brought to the pediatrician's office for a follow-up visit because the child has fallen behind in developmental milestones. The parents state, "My child's muscles don't seem to be as strong as they once were and he needs more rest." After genetic testing, an electromyelogram, and muscle biopsy, the child is diagnosed with Duchenne's muscular dystrophy.

71. If the parents of a child with Duchenne's muscular dystrophy are having a difficult time accepting the diagnosis, which nursing action is most beneficial to the family?
[ ] **1.** Recommend that the parents place the child in a long-term health care facility.
[ ] **2.** Recommend that the parents contact the local social welfare agency.
[ ] **3.** Recommend that the parents talk with other parents who have children with muscular dystrophy.
[ ] **4.** Recommend that the parents read as much literature as possible about treatment of muscular dystrophy.

Nursing Care of an Adolescent with Appendicitis

A 15-year-old is seen in the emergency department with an elevated temperature and complaint of generalized abdominal pain. The physician suspects appendicitis, and the teenager is admitted for observation and possible appendectomy.

72. If the nurse documents all the following data, which finding should be reported immediately?
[ ] **1.** Refusal to eat
[ ] **2.** Complaint of nausea
[ ] **3.** Absent bowel sounds
[ ] **4.** Temperature of 101°F (38.3°C) orally

73. During preoperative preparation, which nursing action is most appropriate?
[ ] **1.** Give analgesics.
[ ] **2.** Give nothing by mouth (NPO).
[ ] **3.** Give an enema.
[ ] **4.** Apply heat to the abdomen.

Surgery is performed, and the appendix is removed intact. The client is returned to the pediatric unit with an I.V. infusion in progress and an abdominal dressing in place. The physician has written orders to continue the I.V. infusion at a rate of 1,000 mL over 8 hours.

74. The nurse would be correct to set the infusion pump for which hourly rate?
[ ] **1.** 50 mL
[ ] **2.** 75 mL
[ ] **3.** 100 mL
[ ] **4.** 125 mL

75. For the teenager recovering from an appendectomy, which nursing measure is most appropriate to prevent respiratory complications during the postoperative period?
[ ] **1.** Give a bronchodilator by inhalation.
[ ] **2.** Administer oxygen by nasal cannula.
[ ] **3.** Give the child a corticosteroid.
[ ] **4.** Have the child use an incentive spirometer.

The physician visits on the second postoperative day and writes an order to ambulate the client three times a day. The nurse enters the client's room and begins to assist with ambulation. The teenager begins to cry and states, "I'm scared."

76. Which statement by the nurse is most therapeutic in addressing the teen's behavior?
[ ] **1.** "There's nothing to be scared of. This won't hurt."
[ ] **2.** "The stitches are strong. They won't come out."
[ ] **3.** "I know you're scared, but you must be brave."
[ ] **4.** "Let's do this later, when you're better prepared."

The parents ask when their child who is recovering from an appendectomy will be able to return to school.

77. The nurse advises the parents that, in most cases, children who have had an appendectomy usually return to school within what time frame?

[ ] **1.** 5 days
[ ] **2.** 2 weeks
[ ] **3.** 4 weeks
[ ] **4.** 6 weeks

Nursing Care of an Adolescent with Dysmenorrhea

A parent brings a 16-year-old girl to the pediatric clinic because of recurrent complaints of pain and discomfort during her menstrual cycle. The physician diagnoses primary dysmenorrhea and recommends the use of ibuprofen (Advil) for the pain and discomfort. The physician also asks the nurse to discuss other measures that can be taken to reduce the client's pain and discomfort.

78. Which suggestion by the nurse would be most helpful in relieving the teenager's menstrual pain and discomfort?

[ ] **1.** "Stay in bed until cramping is relieved, increase your fluid intake, and eat a low-fat diet."
[ ] **2.** "Drink plenty of cold liquids, add extra salt to your diet, and take a nap in the afternoon."
[ ] **3.** "Apply ice packs to the abdomen, eat a high-calorie diet, and have your largest meal at noon."
[ ] **4.** "Get at least 8 hours of sleep, eat a well-balanced diet, and apply heat to your abdomen."

79. Which of the following is given highest priority by the nurse when caring for an adolescent with dysmenorrhea?

[ ] **1.** The effects of dysmenorrhea disrupt the client's ability to participate in gym class.
[ ] **2.** The effects of dysmenorrhea interfere with the client attending social functions.
[ ] **3.** The effects of dysmenorrhea require multiple physician appointments.
[ ] **4.** The effects of dysmenorrhea interrupt family relationships.

The adolescent is upset about outbreaks of acne on her face, back, and shoulders before her menstrual cycle. The adolescent is started on systemic and topical medications to treat the acne.

80. Which statement by an adolescent with acne indicates that additional teaching about taking tetracycline hydrochloride (Panmycin) is needed?

[ ] **1.** "I'll take the medication with a full glass of water."
[ ] **2.** "I won't take any antacids with this medication."
[ ] **3.** "I'll take this medication with food."
[ ] **4.** "I'll avoid sun exposure while taking this medication."

Nursing Care of an Adolescent Who Is Engaging in Risk-Taking Behaviors

The parents of a 14-year-old adolescent call the pediatrician because they have discovered boxes of pseudoephedrine in the teenager's room and suspect involvement in producing methamphetamine as well as abuse of the substance.

81. Which information about methamphetamine use is most accurate and important for the parents to know?

[ ] **1.** Methamphetamines are tried by most adolescents and cause no harm.
[ ] **2.** Methamphetamines are known to lead to addiction.
[ ] **3.** Methamphetamines are a central nervous system depressant.
[ ] **4.** Methamphetamines are harmful only if taken intravenously.

82. Which symptom reported by the parents is the best indicator of methamphetamine abuse by the adolescent?

[ ] **1.** Watery eyes
[ ] **2.** Drowsiness
[ ] **3.** Excessive nasal drainage
[ ] **4.** Marked nervousness

The parents ask the nurse, "What's wrong with our child? Why has this happened?" The parents tell the nurse that the child associates with a gang that is known for getting into trouble and abusing drugs.

83. The nurse correctly explains that, during adolescence, being with a peer group and mimicking peer behaviors is part of the process of achieving which developmental task?

[ ] **1.** Identity
[ ] **2.** Intimacy
[ ] **3.** Integrity
[ ] **4.** Idealism

The parents ask the nurse whether they should force their child to enter a drug treatment program.

84. Which response by the nurse would be most helpful in this situation?

[ ] **1.** "You should attempt to discuss the dangers of drug abuse with your child before deciding that treatment is necessary."
[ ] **2.** "It will be necessary to get a court order before you can force your child to enter a drug treatment program."
[ ] **3.** "The success of the drug treatment program will depend on your child's desire to become drug-free."
[ ] **4.** "It's best that you force your child into the treatment program because otherwise participation probably will not occur."

While the adolescent is talking with the physician, the nurse reviews the child's immunization records and discovers that the last immunization received was at 6 years of age.

85. The nurse advises the parents that the child is due to receive which of the following immunization boosters?
[ ] **1.** *Haemophilus influenzae* type b (Hib)
[ ] **2.** Polio (IPV)
[ ] **3.** Smallpox
[ ] **4.** Tetanus

A 16-year-old approaches the school nurse for information on getting a tattoo.

86. What information regarding the dangers of tattooing should the nurse provide for this client? Select all that apply.
[ ] **1.** Tattooing can lead to skin cancer.
[ ] **2.** There can be an allergic reaction to the tattoo ink.
[ ] **3.** Tattooing can result in skin infections.
[ ] **4.** There is a risk for contracting hepatitis B and human immunodeficiency virus (HIV) if dirty needles are used in tattooing.
[ ] **5.** Tattooing can cause spontaneous abortions in pregnant women.
[ ] **6.** Tattooing can result in heart and lung conditions.

Nursing Care of an Adolescent with a Sexually Transmitted Infection

A 16-year-old girl has been exposed to gonorrhea and visits the clinic for diagnosis and treatment.

87. When preparing the adolescent for the examination, the nurse correctly explains that a specimen should be collected and sent to the laboratory. Which specimen should the nurse collect?
[ ] **1.** Blood sample
[ ] **2.** Urine sample
[ ] **3.** Vaginal smear
[ ] **4.** Biopsy of the cervix

The physician confirms the diagnosis of gonorrhea and informs the client that she also has Chlamydia trachomatis infection, another sexually transmitted infection. The physician orders an I.M. injection of ceftriaxone (Rocephin) to treat the gonorrhea and a prescription for oral doxycycline (Vibramycin) to treat the chlamydia.

88. Which instruction is most appropriate to give to the client regarding doxycycline?
[ ] **1.** "The medication normally causes a dark orange discoloration of urine."
[ ] **2.** "Take the medication 1 hour before or 2 hours after a meal."
[ ] **3.** "Don't drink water for at least 30 minutes after taking the medication."
[ ] **4.** "Report any symptoms of GI upset to the health care provider."

Before leaving the clinic, the client asks the nurse, "When can I be certain that I'm no longer infectious?"

89. The nurse correctly advises the client that she is still considered infectious until which time?
[ ] **1.** She no longer has foul-smelling vaginal discharge.
[ ] **2.** She no longer experiences discomfort during her menstrual periods.
[ ] **3.** She has a negative culture after being off antibiotics for at least 7 days.
[ ] **4.** She has taken the prescribed doses of ceftriaxone (Rocephin) for 1 day.

A 17-year-old adolescent is seen in the sexually transmitted infections specialty clinic and is diagnosed with genital herpes (herpes simplex type 2).

90. Which of the following best illustrates the type of lesions manifested in genital herpes?

[ ] **1.**
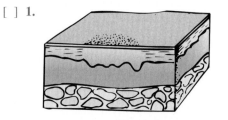

[ ] **2.**
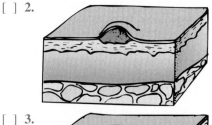

[ ] **3.**
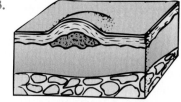

[ ] **4.**
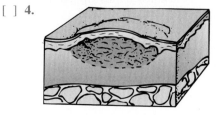

91. Which statement by the client indicates a need for additional teaching about genital herpes?

[ ] **1.** "Males who have genital herpes need a yearly prostate-specific antigen (PSA) test."

[ ] **2.** "Females who have genital herpes need a Papanicolaou (Pap) test every 6 months."

[ ] **3.** "Genital herpes is closely associated with the occurrence of sterility."

[ ] **4.** "Genital herpes is closely associated with Hodgkin's disease."

Oral and topical forms of acyclovir (Zovirax) are prescribed for the client.

92. Which medication instruction provided by the nurse is most accurate?

[ ] **1.** "Taking your acyclovir as prescribed will prevent the recurrence of lesions."

[ ] **2.** "Your sex partners also need to be treated for 10 days with oral acyclovir."

[ ] **3.** "Use a glove to apply topical acyclovir."

[ ] **4.** "Take the oral acyclovir even when the disease is in remission."

The nurse discusses the sexual transmission of herpes with the client.

93. Which statement by the client indicates that teaching has been effective?

[ ] **1.** "My partner should use a condom when lesions are present to prevent transmission."

[ ] **2.** "I should douche after intercourse to prevent becoming infected."

[ ] **3.** "I should apply acyclovir to lesions before intercourse to prevent transmission."

[ ] **4.** "I should avoid sexual contact, especially when lesions or symptoms are present."

The client notices a pamphlet about acquired immunodeficiency syndrome (AIDS) while waiting for the physician in the examination room and asks the nurse, "What are the symptoms of AIDS?"

94. The nurse informs the client that acquired immunodeficiency syndrome (AIDS) is commonly associated with which symptoms?

[ ] **1.** Increased appetite and chills during the night

[ ] **2.** Tachycardia, dyspnea, and constipation

[ ] **3.** Fatigue, fever, and persistent yeast infections

[ ] **4.** Weight gain, peripheral edema, and jaundice

The adolescent client also asks the nurse if human immunodeficiency virus (HIV) infection can be contracted from a sex partner who has no symptoms of acquired immunodeficiency syndrome (AIDS).

95. Which response by the nurse provides the best clarification about the disease process?

[ ] **1.** "If you're afraid of getting HIV, you'll be safer if you avoid having sex with past sex partners."

[ ] **2.** "An HIV-positive individual may not develop symptoms of AIDS for years."

[ ] **3.** "HIV can only be transmitted when symptoms of AIDS are present."

[ ] **4.** "The medication prescribed for AIDS also protects against HIV infection."

Several months later the adolescent client returns to the clinic and is diagnosed with acquired immunodeficiency syndrome (AIDS). The client reports having oral lesions that interfere with eating.

96. Which diet is most appropriate for an adolescent with thrush and a herpes simplex infection of the oral cavity secondary to acquired immunodeficiency syndrome (AIDS)?

[ ] **1.** High-calorie, bland diet

[ ] **2.** Soft, low-protein diet

[ ] **3.** Low-residue, low-fat diet

[ ] **4.** High-residue, low-cholesterol diet

After being diagnosed with a sexually transmitted infection, a 16-year-old client asks the nurse about safe sex practices.

97. If the client asks the nurse for instructions on safe condom use, which information needs to be stressed?

[ ] **1.** Condoms should be stored in a warm, dry place to prevent damage.

[ ] **2.** Condoms are generally lubricated with mineral oil or petroleum jelly.

[ ] **3.** A condom should be applied before the penis becomes erect.

[ ] **4.** During application, a ½″ space should be left at the end of the condom.

The client also tells the nurse that he is concerned about developing testicular cancer because his father died of it.

98. When teaching an adolescent male client about testicular self-examination, which instruction should the nurse include?

[ ] **1.** "Do the examination after a warm bath or shower."

[ ] **2.** "Report any difference in the size of your testicles to the physician."

[ ] **3.** "Malignant lumps are usually located on the front side of the testicles."

[ ] **4.** "Both testicles should be examined simultaneously to detect differences."

Nursing Care of an Adolescent with Scoliosis

A 14-year-old girl is referred for further evaluation after the school nurse discovers lateral spinal curvature during routine scoliosis screening.

99. Which of the following statements made by the adolescent best supports the nurse's suspicion of scoliosis?
[ ] 1. "My friends are getting taller faster than I am."
[ ] 2. "One of my sleeves is always shorter than the other."
[ ] 3. "I have a difficult time sleeping on my side at night."
[ ] 4. "I always roll crooked when I am doing a somersault."

100. The orthopedic physician orders a series of X-rays to confirm scoliosis. Which question is most important for the nurse to ask the adolescent girl in preparation for X-rays?
[ ] 1. "Is there any possibility that you're pregnant?"
[ ] 2. "Have you eaten anything in the past 24 hours?"
[ ] 3. "Have you taken any medications in the past 24 hours?"
[ ] 4. "Are you allergic to iodine or shellfish?"

A diagnosis of structural scoliosis is confirmed, and the physician determines that the adolescent has a 35-degree curvature. The parents ask the nurse if treatment is really necessary.

101. Which explanation by the nurse is most accurate?
[ ] 1. "Your child's condition, which involves a 35-degree curvature, may improve without treatment."
[ ] 2. "Your child may develop problems with bladder control without treatment."
[ ] 3. "Your child may develop problems with bowel control without treatment."
[ ] 4. "Your child may develop breathing problems without treatment."

The child is fitted for a Milwaukee brace. The adolescent asks if the brace has to be worn when at school.

102. The nurse correctly advises the adolescent that the brace has to be worn during which time period?
[ ] 1. At all times except when bathing
[ ] 2. At least 8 hours each day
[ ] 3. At night while sleeping
[ ] 4. At all times, without exception

103. Which nursing action would best promote the adolescent's compliance with wearing the brace?
[ ] 1. Advising the parents to keep a constant watch on their daughter to make sure she wears her brace
[ ] 2. Suggesting that the parents help their daughter find stylish clothing that will hide the brace
[ ] 3. Telling the parents that it might be best to arrange for a homebound teacher during treatment
[ ] 4. Telling the adolescent that the problem will only get worse if she does not wear her brace

Dosage Calculations for Children and Adolescents

104. The physician orders cefaclor (Ceclor) 125 mg P.O. If the Ceclor suspension is available in 250 mg/5 mL, how many milliliters should the nurse give the pediatric client?

_____

105. The nurse is caring for a 52-pound child with an elevated temperature. If the recommended dosage of acetaminophen (Tylenol) for children is 10 to 15 mg/kg P.O. every 4 to 6 hours, what is the highest single dose of acetaminophen that would be safe for this child?

_____

Correct Answers, Rationales, and Test Taking Strategies

Nursing Care of a Child with Rheumatic Fever

1. 2. Rheumatic fever is an inflammatory disease that affects school-age children and can cause damage to heart valves. The exact cause of rheumatic fever is not clearly understood. However, evidence suggests that rheumatic fever is associated with a recent bacterial infection caused by group A β-hemolytic streptococci. These microorganisms cause some, but not all, sore throats; therefore, of the symptoms reported, a sore throat is most closely correlated with rheumatic fever and should be brought to the physician's attention. Rheumatic fever usually occurs 2½ to 3 weeks after the occurrence of a sore throat. Measles is caused by a viral infection, not streptococci. A bump on the head and a disinterest in schoolwork probably are not related to rheumatic fever but should be recorded in the health history.

Test Taking Strategy—Analyze to determine what information the question asks for, which is a suspected etiology for rheumatic fever. Recall that the symptoms of rheumatic fever typically follow untreated pharyngitis caused by β-hemolytic streptococci. Review possible causes of rheumatic fever if you had difficulty answering this question.
Cognitive Level—Applying
Client Needs Category—Physiological integrity
Client Needs Subcategory—Physiological adaptation

2. 4. Migrating joint pain is a major manifestation of rheumatic fever. The antistreptolysin (ASO) titer and the pulse rate are usually elevated with this disease. The child may also have erythema marginatum, which is a distinctive rash found on the trunk and extremities.

Test Taking Strategy—Look for key words "most indicative finding" in reference to a clinical finding associated with rheumatic fever. Recall that polyarthritis is the most common presenting complaint in the majority of clients with rheumatic fever. Review signs and symptoms of rheumatic fever if you had difficulty answering this question.
Cognitive Level—Applying
Client Needs Category—Physiological integrity
Client Needs Subcategory—Physiological adaptation

3. 3. Because the heart valves can be involved, it is prudent for the nurse to keep the oxygen demands and the metabolic needs of the heart decreased. This involves keeping the child in bed and quiet. Reading an adventure story would be the most appropriate activity for the child during the acute phase of the illness. The child will need both physical and emotional rest; therefore, quiet,

age-appropriate activities are recommended to prevent overexertion as well as the boredom and emotional upset that may occur if the child is not permitted any activity. Preschoolers usually enjoy playing with action figures; also, this activity may cause excitement, which will increase energy consumption. Video games may also cause too much excitement. Toy mallets and wooden pegs are more appropriate for a toddler.

Test Taking Strategy—Look for key words "most appropriate" in reference to diversional activity for a child with rheumatic fever. Recall that reading is a sedentary diversional activity as long as the book is at the child's level or if someone reads the story to the child. Review age-appropriate activities for a school-age child who requires bed rest if you had difficulty answering this question.
Cognitive Level—Applying
Client Needs Category—Health promotion and maintenance
Client Needs Subcategory—None

4. 2. There is a slight cross-sensitivity between medications in the penicillin group and those in the cephalosporin group. Therefore, the nurse should exercise caution and notify the charge nurse or physician before giving the medication. There is no cross-sensitivity between penicillin and the other medication categories listed.

Test Taking Strategy—Analyze to determine what information the question asks for, which is a drug category with a cross-sensitivity with penicillin. Review these categories of antimicrobials for precautions when administering if you had difficulty answering this question.
Cognitive Level—Applying
Client Needs Category—Physiological integrity
Client Needs Subcategory—Pharmacological therapies

5. 3. Reye's syndrome is a disease that causes multisystem organ failure and can be fatal. It is associated with aspirin use, but also is associated with viral infections. Despite the risk of Reye's syndrome, aspirin is given instead of acetaminophen because it not only controls fever, but also relieves joint inflammation, which is a major manifestation of rheumatic fever. Aspirin is not necessarily more effective in reducing fever than acetaminophen, and it does not prevent infection or cardiac enlargement.

Test Taking Strategy—Analyze to determine what information the question asks for, which is a rationale for the use of aspirin to manage the symptoms of rheumatic fever. Recall that aspirin has an anti-inflammatory action in addition to being an analgesic and antipyretic medication. Review the therapeutic uses for aspirin in comparison to acetaminophen if you had difficulty answering this question.
Cognitive Level—Applying
Client Needs Category—Physiological integrity
Client Needs Subcategory—Pharmacological therapies

6. 4. A child who has had rheumatic fever may develop the disease again. Although streptococci do not cause all sore throats, the child would be at risk for a recurrence of the disease if the child develops a sore throat. Therefore, any sign of a sore throat should be reported promptly to facilitate immediate diagnosis and treatment. Antibiotics (in this case, penicillin) should be taken for the prescribed course unless otherwise indicated by the physician, but this would not affect future consequences. Keeping the child home is not an incorrect answer because the child should be fully recovered before returning to the school setting; however, it is not the best evidence for a future consequence of the disease.

Test Taking Strategy—Analyze to determine what information the question asks for, which requires evidence of effective teaching for avoiding potential consequences in the future. Recall that a previous case of rheumatic fever does not confer immunity. Therefore, if the child develops pharyngitis, the physician should be contacted and subsequently treated if it is caused by β-hemolytic streptococci. Review the potential for a recurrence of rheumatic fever if you had difficulty answering this question.
Cognitive Level—Analyzing
Client Needs Category—Health promotion and maintenance
Client Needs Subcategory—None

7. 1. The use of a bedside commode is an appropriate alternative to reduce the heart's workload. Shortness of breath indicates that the heart is unable to adapt to the demands required during ambulation. Giving oxygen after elimination or having the child continue to ambulate, even with the assistance of the nurse or a walker, is not likely to prevent or reduce the heart's effort in response to activity.

Test Taking Strategy—Analyze to determine what information the question asks for, which is an intervention that limits cardiopulmonary symptoms brought on by ambulation. Recall that use of a bedside commode limits the demands for cardiopulmonary function. Review interventions for preventing or reducing dyspnea when it occurs in relation to ambulating to the bathroom if you had difficulty answering this question.
Cognitive Level—Applying
Client Needs Category—Physiological integrity
Client Needs Subcategory—Physiological adaptation

Nursing Care of a Child with Diabetes Mellitus

8. 2, 5, 6. Diabetic ketoacidosis is a complication of diabetes that occurs when the body's cells use fat for cellular metabolism because it cannot use sugar (glucose) as a fuel source; the body has no insulin or not enough insulin. By-products of fat metabolism, called *ketones*, accumulate in the body. Fruity-smelling breath is a manifestation of diabetic ketoacidosis, as are deep, rapid breathing and dry,

flushed skin. Other signs and symptoms include hyperglycemia, nausea and vomiting, and abdominal pain. Excessive perspiration and pallor are signs of hypoglycemia. A blood glucose reading of 120 mg/dL is within the normal range.

Test Taking Strategy—Analyze to determine what information the question asks for, which is signs and symptoms of diabetic ketoacidosis. Alternative-format "select all that apply" questions require considering each option independently to decide its merit in answering the question. Review complications of diabetes mellitus, especially those that are associated with ketoacidosis that are different from hypoglycemia, if you had difficulty answering this question.
Cognitive Level—Applying
Client Needs Category—Physiological integrity
Client Needs Subcategory—Physiological adaptation

9. 3. A client experiencing diabetic ketoacidosis will have glucose and ketones in the urine. Blood, white blood cells, and bilirubin are not usually present in ketoacidosis.

Test Taking Strategy—Analyze to determine what information the question asks for, which is the identification of a substance that may be found in the urine of a client with uncontrolled diabetes mellitus. Recall that finding ketones in the urine indicates that the body is breaking down stored fat as a substitute source of energy and excreting a fat metabolite in the urine. Review assessment data that relate to a client with diabetes mellitus as well as complications of diabetes if you had difficulty answering this question.
Cognitive Level—Applying
Client Needs Category—Physiological integrity
Client Needs Subcategory—Physiological adaptation

10. 1. Regular insulin (Humulin R) is the only type of insulin given intravenously. Regular insulin can also be given subcutaneously as can insulin zinc suspension (Humulin L), insulin zinc suspension, extended (Humulin U), and isophane insulin suspension (Humulin N).

Test Taking Strategy—Analyze to determine what information the question asks for, which requires identifying a type of insulin that can be administered intravenously. Recall that regular insulin can be given subcutaneously as well as intravenously. Review types of insulins and how they are administered if you had difficulty answering this question.
Cognitive Level—Applying
Client Needs Category—Physiological integrity
Client Needs Subcategory—Pharmacological therapies

11. 1. Regular insulin (Humulin R) is given 30 minutes before a meal because the onset of action is 30 minutes to 1 hour. Isophane insulin suspension (NPH) is an intermediate-acting insulin that has a later peak and duration. Giving the insulin within a shorter period might result in inadequate coverage because the insulin will not have had a chance to take effect. Giving the insulin after eating will not provide coverage for the food already consumed.

Test Taking Strategy—Analyze to determine what information the question asks for, which is an appropriate time for administering a morning dose of insulin. Recall that regular insulin is a short-acting type of insulin and should be given ½ hour before its onset of action. Review the peak, onset, and duration of each insulin type if you had difficulty answering this question.

Cognitive Level—Applying
Client Needs Category—Physiological integrity
Client Needs Subcategory—Pharmacological therapies

12. **4, 5, 6.** Shakiness is a common sign of hypoglycemia. Other symptoms of hypoglycemia include dizziness or light-headedness, erratic heart rate or tachycardia, sweating, tremors, weakness, and hunger. The remaining options are signs and symptoms of hyperglycemia.

Test Taking Strategy—Analyze to determine what information the question asks for, which is signs and symptoms of hypoglycemia. Alternative-format "select all that apply" questions require considering each option independently to decide its merit in answering the question. Choose options that correlate with the signs and symptoms of hypoglycemia. Review complications of diabetes mellitus, especially those associated with a low blood sugar level, if you had difficulty answering this question.

Cognitive Level—Understanding
Client Needs Category—Physiological integrity
Client Needs Subcategory—Physiological adaptation

13. **1.** Hypoglycemia must be corrected immediately. If the child is awake and able to swallow, the nurse should offer a concentrated source of sugar such as orange juice. In addition, milk supplies the child with lactose or milk sugar, as well as a good source of protein and fat to aid in decreased absorption. I.V. administration of glucose is reserved for those who have a change in level of consciousness and are unable to swallow. Insulin would not be given because the child already has too much insulin. The physician should be notified after the problem is corrected or if the child's condition worsens.

Test Taking Strategy—Analyze to determine what information the question asks for, which is the nursing action that should be done before all other options in response to a client's low blood sugar. Recall that restoring the blood sugar to within normal range is a priority. Normal capillary blood glucose level is 90 to 130 mg/dL before meals and less than 180 mg/dL 1 to 2 hours after meals. Review the nursing care and management of hypoglycemia if you had difficulty answering this question.

Cognitive Level—Applying
Client Needs Category—Physiological integrity
Client Needs Subcategory—Physiological adaptation

14. **2.** Persons with type 1 diabetes mellitus require insulin to control the disease. The hormone insulin cannot be given by mouth because digestive enzymes would destroy the insulin before it reaches the site of action. Also, the child is not a candidate for oral hypoglycemic agents because the pancreas has to be capable of producing some insulin for the child to benefit from the oral hypoglycemics; this is not the case with a child with type 1 diabetes mellitus.

Test Taking Strategy—Analyze to determine what information the question asks for, which is the reason insulin is administered subcutaneously. Because it would be broken down by digestive enzymes, insulin is not given orally, eliminating options 1, 3, and 4. Review the effect of GI secretions on a protein substance, in this case insulin, if you had difficulty answering this question.

Cognitive Level—Applying
Client Needs Category—Physiological integrity
Client Needs Subcategory—Pharmacological therapies

15. **4.** If insulin sites are not rotated following a planned rotation schedule, atrophy (lipodystrophy) of subcutaneous fat may occur. Lipodystrophy can interfere with insulin absorption if insulin is given in areas affected by this problem. Rotating the injection sites does not slow the absorption, prevent accumulation, or decrease the duration of insulin.

Test Taking Strategy—Analyze to determine what information the question asks for, which is a rationale for rotating insulin injection sites. Recall that using the same site repeatedly damages tissue and eventually reduces drug absorption. Review principles for insulin administration if you had difficulty answering this question.

Cognitive Level—Applying
Client Needs Category—Health promotion and maintenance
Client Needs Subcategory—None

16. **2.** Activity requires glucose for energy. Therefore, increasing activity uses up glucose and, consequently, the body requires less-than-usual amounts of insulin. Eating too much, having an infection, and experiencing emotional stress are situations in which a diabetic patient tends to require more, not less, insulin.

Test Taking Strategy—Analyze to determine what information the question asks for, which is evidence that the client has an accurate understanding of the factors that affect the maintenance of blood sugar within a controlled range. Recall that glucose is the body's primary source for quick energy. Review factors such as dietary intake, activity, illness, fever, and stress and the manner in which they affect blood sugar levels if you had difficulty answering this question.

Cognitive Level—Analyzing
Client Needs Category—Health promotion and maintenance
Client Needs Subcategory—None

17. 3. The diabetic child can participate in normal activities. However, certain precautions are necessary to promote safety. For example, the parents should ensure that the child goes swimming with an adult or responsible person who knows that the child is diabetic. The child can participate in activities requiring increased energy expenditure, such as basketball and soccer, as long as the activity is taken into consideration when planning the child's meals and insulin requirements. Generally, the child should consume a snack before engaging in the activity or have a simple form of glucose on hand in case a hypoglycemic reaction should occur.

> *Test Taking Strategy—Analyze to determine what information the question asks for, which is the most accurate information about the relationship between various activities and diabetes. Recall that participating in sports activities is not contraindicated by having diabetes as long as there are individuals present who can identify and respond to emergencies. Review factors such as dietary intake and activity and the manner in which they affect blood sugar levels if you had difficulty answering this question.*
> *Cognitive Level—Analyzing*
> *Client Needs Category—Health promotion and maintenance*
> *Client Needs Subcategory—None*

18. 2. It is important for the newly diagnosed diabetic athlete to check a blood glucose level before participating in exercises or athletics. If the blood glucose level is high, additional glucagon, growth hormone, and catecholamines may be released. This causes the liver to release more glucose, resulting in a higher blood glucose level. If the child's blood glucose level is within the normal range or lower, exercise may lower it. Some individuals are instructed to eat a carbohydrate snack before engaging in exercise to prevent unexpected hypoglycemia.

> *Test Taking Strategy—Analyze to determine what information the question asks for, which is an appropriate time for assessing blood sugar for a very active diabetic client. Although checking the blood sugar after being active has merit, it is best to know a baseline before the activity begins. Review how activity affects blood sugar levels if you had difficulty answering this question.*
> *Cognitive Level—Applying*
> *Client Needs Category—Physiological integrity*
> *Client Needs Subcategory—Physiological adaptation*

19.

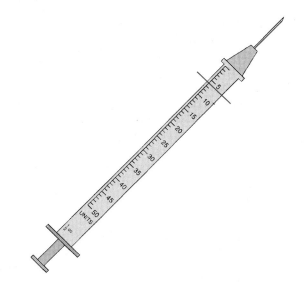

The child's blood glucose level is 269 mg/dL, thus falling within the 6-unit range (251 to 300 mg/dL) specified by the physician. Therefore, the nurse would administer 6 units of Humulin R insulin.

> *Test Taking Strategy—Look for key words, such as a blood sugar level of 269 mg/dL. Correlate the information with the coverage schedule for insulin administration, and identify the appropriate mark on the displayed insulin syringe, which is calibrated in 1-unit increments. Review types of syringes, especially insulin syringes, and their use in administering parenteral medications if you had difficulty answering this question.*
> *Cognitive Level—Applying*
> *Client Needs Category—Physiological integrity*
> *Client Needs Subcategory—Pharmacological therapies*

20. 4. The child will need to continue to monitor blood glucose levels because the insulin pump only delivers the insulin; it does not monitor the blood glucose level. The other options indicate the child correctly understands how to use an insulin pump.

> *Test Taking Strategy—Analyze to determine what information the question asks for, which is evidence that the client has incorrectly understood instructions that relate to an insulin pump. Recall that an insulin pump delivers a dose of insulin according to the client's metabolic needs. Review the use of and advantages of an insulin pump if you had difficulty answering this question.*
> *Cognitive Level—Analyzing*
> *Client Needs Category—Physiological integrity*
> *Client Needs Subcategory—Physiological adaptation*

Nursing Care of a Child with Partial- and Full-Thickness Burns

21. 4. A burn is classified according to the depth of tissue destruction. Burns may be superficial partial-thickness injuries, deep partial-thickness injuries, or full-thickness injuries. A full-thickness burn involves total destruction of the epidermis, dermis, and underlying tissues. The wound color ranges widely from white to red, brown, or black. The burned area is painless because nerve fibers are destroyed. Edema may be present.

> *Test Taking Strategy—Analyze to determine what information the question asks for, which is a manifestation of a full-thickness burn. Recall that a full-thickness burn includes damage to the epidermis, dermis, and subcutaneous tissue. Review depths of burn injuries and their characteristics if you had difficulty answering this question.*
> *Cognitive Level—Applying*
> *Client Needs Category—Physiological integrity*
> *Client Needs Subcategory—Physiological adaptation*

22. 2. It is important for the nurse to remain alert for the possibility of respiratory distress from a blocked airway after burns to the head, face, neck, and chest. Therefore, it is imperative to keep an endotracheal tube and oxygen supply on hand in the burned client's room. An oral airway should also be readily available. The other devices and equipment mentioned are not appropriate for treating an emergency arising from respiratory distress.

> *Test Taking Strategy—Analyze to determine what information the question asks for, which is an item that is essential for managing an emergency that is likely to occur during the care of a client with burns. Remember the principle of maintaining the airway and breathing when managing an emergency. Review complications associated with burn injuries if you had difficulty answering this question.*
> *Cognitive Level—Applying*
> *Client Needs Category—Physiological integrity*
> *Client Needs Subcategory—Physiological adaptation*

23. 1, 2, 5. The emergent phase marks the first 24 to 48 hours after a burn injury. During this time, the primary emphasis is on the treatment of burn shock, specifically restoring the child's fluid and electrolyte balance. Careful tracking of vital signs, urine output, and I.V. infusion is essential. Large-bore I.V. catheters are used whenever possible because of the potential need for rapid infusions or blood products. The child would receive nothing by mouth during the emergent phase because of the risk of a paralytic ileus.

> *Test Taking Strategy—Analyze to determine what information the question asks for, which is steps to take to restore fluid balance in the burn patient. Alternative-*

> *format "select all that apply" questions require considering each option independently to decide its merit in answering the question. Choose options that correlate with interventions for restoring fluid and electrolyte imbalance in the early stages of burn management. Review the phases of burn management, fluid resuscitation measures, and potential GI complications as they apply to a client with burns if you had difficulty answering this question.*
> *Cognitive Level—Applying*
> *Client Needs Category—Physiological integrity*
> *Client Needs Subcategory—Physiological adaptation*

24. 3. A burn victim is placed on I.V. fluid therapy during the first 24 hours to restore fluid and electrolyte balance and to maintain perfusion of vital organs. During I.V. fluid therapy, the child is at risk for fluid overload; therefore, the nurse must closely monitor the I.V. infusion. Monitoring skin integrity and bowel elimination is a regular, ongoing assessment consideration. Checking pupillary response to light is part of a neurologic assessment; this would typically be done if the child's neurologic status was compromised.

> *Test Taking Strategy—Analyze to determine what information the question asks for, which is the data that are essential to monitor in early burn care. Based on Maslow's hierarchy, restoring fluid and electrolyte balance is the most important physiologic need at this time. Review the nursing management of a client with burns if you had difficulty answering this question.*
> *Cognitive Level—Analyzing*
> *Client Needs Category—Physiological integrity*
> *Client Needs Subcategory—Physiological adaptation*

25. 2. Because the skin's integrity is compromised and fluids are out of balance in clients with burns, sepsis is a major concern. During a nursing assessment, disorientation is one of the first signs of sepsis. Any time there is a change in mental status, the nurse should document the abnormal finding. A spiking fever and diminished bowel sounds are also noted at this time. Pain is common after burns and is not an early indicator of sepsis. Renal output and jitteriness are closely assessed but are not early indicators of sepsis.

> *Test Taking Strategy—Analyze to determine what information the question asks for, which is an early sign of sepsis. Recall that sepsis is often accompanied by an acute alteration in mental status. Review the signs and symptoms associated with sepsis if you had difficulty answering this question.*
> *Cognitive Level—Applying*
> *Client Needs Category—Physiological integrity*
> *Client Needs Subcategory—Physiological adaptation*

26. 3. Because severe burns produce considerable pain, an opioid analgesic is commonly used as part of treatment. If the child no longer complains of pain, rates the pain as 0 to 2 on a pain scale (in which 0 represents no pain and 10, the worst pain imaginable), or is able to concentrate on another activity such as watching television, the pain medication is considered effective. Respiratory depression and urine retention are adverse effects of these drugs.

> **Test Taking Strategy**—*Analyze to determine what information the question asks for, which is a sign of opioid analgesic effectiveness. Recall that once acute pain is relieved, performing activities of daily living becomes possible. Review pain assessment techniques and evidence of expected outcomes of adequately managed pain if you had difficulty answering this question.*
> **Cognitive Level**—*Analyzing*
> **Client Needs Category**—*Physiological integrity*
> **Client Needs Subcategory**—*Pharmacological therapies*

27. 4. Footdrop describes the inability to dorsiflex the foot due to weakness or paralysis of the muscles that lift the foot. A footboard is an effective device that the nurse can use to help support the feet in a functional position. Braces cannot be used without a physician's order. Keeping the child in a side-lying position will not prevent footdrop; this problem can only be prevented when the feet are supported in an anatomic position. The top sheet should fit loosely over the feet to assist with preventing footdrop.

> **Test Taking Strategy**—*Analyze to determine what information the question asks for, which is a nursing technique for preventing footdrop. Recall that footdrop results from shortening of the calf muscles and lengthening of the opposing muscles on the anterior leg. By keeping the feet in a position of dorsiflexion, footdrop can be prevented. Review complications of immobility, especially footdrop, and nursing measures for preventing their occurrence if you had difficulty answering this question.*
> **Cognitive Level**—*Applying*
> **Client Needs Category**—*Physiological integrity*
> **Client Needs Subcategory**—*Basic care and comfort*

28. 2. Stress ulcers, also called *Curling's ulcers*, commonly occur in the stomach or duodenum as a complication of burns. Curling's ulcers can be fatal for burned children as a result of perforation and hemorrhage of the bowel secondary to sloughing of the gastric mucosa. If the ulcer bleeds, the client will have blood in the stool, which is detected by a positive Hemoccult test and black, tarry stools. The other findings are not usual manifestations of Curling's ulcers.

> **Test Taking Strategy**—*Analyze to determine what information the question asks for, which is a manifestation of Curling's ulcer. Recall that an ulcer of any type is often accompanied by bleeding. Blood that is incorporated within stool will produce a positive*

finding on a Hemoccult test (option 2). Review the signs and symptoms of ulcers, which would include Curling's ulcer, and data for detecting this condition if you had difficulty answering this question.
> **Cognitive Level**—*Applying*
> **Client Needs Category**—*Physiological integrity*
> **Client Needs Subcategory**—*Physiological adaptation*

29. 1. The child requires a diet rich in protein to help rebuild body tissues destroyed by the burns. A milkshake is a good source of protein. Protein is the only nutrient that can build or repair tissues. Apples, broth, and gelatin contain little or no protein.

> **Test Taking Strategy**—*Analyze to determine what information the question asks for, which is the best source of dietary protein from among the provided options. Recall that a serving of milk contained in a milkshake is higher in protein than apples, gelatin, or broth. Review foods that are high in protein if you had difficulty answering this question.*
> **Cognitive Level**—*Applying*
> **Client Needs Category**—*Physiological integrity*
> **Client Needs Subcategory**—*Basic care and comfort*

30. 3. Of the diversional activities described in this item, an 8-year-old is likely to enjoy playing with an action figure. Television may also provide diversion. Playing a solitary game of cards, reading the newspaper, or coloring a simple design probably would not appeal to a child of this age.

> **Test Taking Strategy**—*Use the process of elimination to help select the option that identifies a diversional activity that is appropriate for the developmental needs of an 8-year-old. Options 1 and 4 can be eliminated because they are not likely to hold a school-age child's interest. Option 2 can be eliminated because the child of this age is capable of coloring a design that has detail. Option 3 emerges as the best answer because school-age children are imaginative and enjoy activities that combine fantasy and reality. Review activities that are appropriate for a young school-age client if you had difficulty answering this question.*
> **Cognitive Level**—*Applying*
> **Client Needs Category**—*Health promotion and maintenance*
> **Client Needs Subcategory**—*None*

Nursing Care of a Child with Juvenile Rheumatoid Arthritis

31. 1. The cause of juvenile rheumatoid arthritis (JRA) is not known, but it is thought to be an autoimmune disorder that results in joint pain and swelling. The primary reason for using ibuprofen (Motrin) in the treatment of JRA is the drug's ability to reduce inflammation in the joints, which relieves pain, swelling, and joint stiffness.

Although ibuprofen also lowers the body temperature, this is not the foremost reason for using this drug. Muscle spasms are not prevented by the administration of ibuprofen (Motrin). Ibuprofen (Motrin) is not an anticoagulant.

> *Test Taking Strategy—Analyze to determine what information the question asks for, which is evidence of effective teaching about self-administration of an anti-inflammatory drug. Recall that joint inflammation is a problem for those affected by JRA. Review the use and administration of a nonsteroidal anti-inflammatory drug like ibuprofen in the management of symptoms caused by JRA if you had difficulty answering this question.*
> *Cognitive Level—Applying*
> *Client Needs Category—Physiological integrity*
> *Client Needs Subcategory—Pharmacological therapies*

32. 2. Side effects of aspirin are the same as symptoms of aspirin toxicity, which include tinnitus (ringing in the ears), nausea, vomiting, difficulty hearing, lassitude, dizziness, oliguria, hyperpnea, and mental confusion. The signs and symptoms identified in the other options are not usual manifestations of aspirin toxicity.

> *Test Taking Strategy—Use the process of elimination to identify the option that best describes symptoms of salicylate (aspirin) toxicity. Review the signs and symptoms of salicylate overdose if you had difficulty answering this question.*
> *Cognitive Level—Applying*
> *Client Needs Category—Physiological integrity*
> *Client Needs Subcategory—Pharmacological therapies*

33. 4. Children with juvenile rheumatoid arthritis (JRA) should stay active and keep their muscles strong. Acceptable activities for these children include walking, bicycling, and swimming. Children should learn to warm up before exercising. Of the four activities listed, swimming would most likely be the safest form of exercise for a child with JRA because it causes the least trauma to the affected joints.

> *Test Taking Strategy—Look at the key words "most appropriate" used in reference to an activity for a child affected by JRA. Recall that a child with this diagnosis would benefit from an activity that reduces stress on inflamed joints. Review activities that are appropriate for a client with a chronic joint disorder if you had difficulty answering this question.*
> *Cognitive Level—Applying*
> *Client Needs Category—Health promotion and maintenance*
> *Client Needs Subcategory—None*

34. 3. This child needs to avoid gaining excessive weight because extra weight places additional stress on the joints. Serving well-balanced meals is an effective way to ensure that the child receives enough of the right nutrients to promote growth while keeping the weight in check. After the acute phase, the child should be encouraged to lead as normal a life as possible, which includes going to school and participating in age-appropriate activities. Heat, not cold, should be applied to joints to treat inflammation.

> *Test Taking Strategy—Use the process of elimination to identify the option that accurately describes parental understanding of home care of the child with JRA. Options 1 and 4 can be eliminated because home-schooling and confinement to bed are not indicated for a child with JRA. Option 2 can be eliminated because heat rather than ice is more therapeutic for discomfort associated with inflammation. Option 3 emerges as the best answer because weight gain puts additional stress on joints that are already painful. Review the long-term management of a child with a chronic disease such as one affecting the joints if you had difficulty answering this question.*
> *Cognitive Level—Analyzing*
> *Client Needs Category—Health promotion and maintenance*
> *Client Needs Subcategory—None*

35. 4. Uveitis, an inflammatory disorder of the eye, is a complication of juvenile rheumatoid arthritis (JRA) that can occur without any noticeable symptoms. Therefore, children with JRA should have regular eye examinations. Chest X-rays, dental checkups, and routine hearing examinations are not recommended any more frequently than for a child without JRA.

> *Test Taking Strategy—Analyze to determine what information the question asks for, which is a test used to detect a complication of JRA. Recall that those affected by JRA are at risk for inflammatory eye disease, which can result in functional blindness. Review the complications of JRA and methods for monitoring them if you had difficulty answering this question.*
> *Cognitive Level—Applying*
> *Client Needs Category—Health promotion and maintenance*
> *Client Needs Subcategory—None*

Nursing Care of a Child with an Injury

36. 2. When the foot twists, rolls, or turns beyond its normal limits, injury occurs to the tendon, ligaments, and soft tissue and is considered an ankle sprain. An ice bag can be used safely as long as it is removed every 30 minutes to 1 hour to check the skin and allow the area to return to normal. Continuous application of cold results in vasoconstriction, which, if allowed to continue, could result in impaired blood supply to the affected part and possible gangrene.

> *Test Taking Strategy—Analyze to determine what information the question asks for, which is appropriate*

(and accurate) home teaching for managing a sprained ankle. Recall the acronym RICE (rest, ice, compression, and elevation), which applies to first-aid after a musculoskeletal injury. Review the principles that apply to using cold applications if you had difficulty answering this question.
Cognitive Level—*Applying*
Client Needs Category—*Physiological integrity*
Client Needs Subcategory—*Reduction of risk potential*

37. 2. A child experiencing a nosebleed should be placed in a sitting position with the head tilted forward while the nostrils are gently compressed between the thumb and forefinger. Tilting the head backward may lead to nausea, vomiting, and aspiration. Applying ice may or may not help stop the bleeding. If bleeding does not stop, the nose should be packed with a small piece of gauze that is preferably impregnated with petroleum jelly or a solution such as aqueous epinephrine (1:1,000).
Test Taking Strategy—*Use the process of elimination to select the best option for managing a nosebleed. Eliminate option 1, because tilting the head back may lead to nausea and vomiting. Eliminate options 3 and 4 because these are not the best actions to take. Review epistaxis and its management if you had difficulty answering this question.*
Cognitive Level—*Understanding*
Client Needs Category—*Physiological integrity*
Client Needs Subcategory—*Reduction of risk potential*

38. 1. Temporarily placing the tooth in a liquid such as milk preserves the tooth for re-implantation if the client and tooth are brought to the dentist within 30 minutes of tooth loss. Alcohol and exposure to air can damage the root and reduce the potential success of re-implantation. Option 2 places the tooth in a plastic bag allowing the tooth exposed to air even though it is in plastic. Option 1 allows the tooth to be placed in a liquid to preserve the tooth for re-implantation if the client is brought to the dentist within 30 minutes of tooth loss. Review managing trauma to dentition if you had difficulty answering this question.
Test Taking Strategy—*Use the process of elimination to identify the best approach for keeping a displaced tooth viable before treatment by a dentist. Options 2 and 3 can be eliminated because the tooth is exposed to air. Option 4 can be eliminated because keeping the tooth in alcohol does not ensure preservation of the tooth. Option 2 emerges as the best answer because keeping the tooth in milk resembles the components of salivary liquid. Review managing trauma to dentition if you had difficulty answering this question.*
Cognitive Level—*Applying*
Client Needs Category—*Physiological integrity*
Client Needs Subcategory—*Physiological adaptation*

39. 4. The fourth face on the Wong-Baker FACES Pain Rating Scale indicates that the child is experiencing a lot of pain; therefore, the child should be medicated with the prescribed analgesic. Diversional activities can be used with analgesics to increase their effectiveness or alone when the child has mild pain. Documenting the child's pain and rechecking later do not relieve or change the pain that the child is currently experiencing.
Test Taking Strategy—*Analyze to determine what information the question asks for, which is an appropriate nursing action based on a pediatric pain assessment tool. Recall that Face 4 on the Wong-Baker FACES Pain Rating Scale indicates that the child "hurts even more." It is the equivalent of a numerical score of 6, indicating the need for analgesic medication. Review the Wong-Baker FACES Pain Rating Scale and techniques for relieving pain that correlate with a variety of assessment scores if you had difficulty answering this question.*
Cognitive Level—*Applying*
Client Needs Category—*Physiological integrity*
Client Needs Subcategory—*Pharmacological therapies*

Nursing Care of a Child with a Head Injury

40. 3. The classic signs of increased intracranial pressure are a change in the level of consciousness, a rise in blood pressure, an increase in body temperature, a decrease in the pulse rate, and a widening pulse pressure. Brisk pupillary response to light, tympanic temperature of 97.9°F (36.6°C), and +2 deep tendon reflexes are indicative of normal central nervous system function.
Test Taking Strategy—*Use the process of elimination to identify the best option that correlates with a manifestation of increased intracranial pressure. Options 1, 2, and 4 can be eliminated because they are normal findings. Recall Cushing's triad, which includes a rising systolic blood pressure (option 3) and occurs late in the development of increased intracranial pressure. Review signs and symptoms of increased intracranial pressure if you had difficulty answering this question.*
Cognitive Level—*Analyzing*
Client Needs Category—*Physiological integrity*
Client Needs Subcategory—*Physiological adaptation*

41. 1. Cerebrospinal fluid is commonly seen leaking from the nose of the child who has sustained a basilar skull fracture. The presence of this finding should be reported immediately because this is the most serious type of skull fracture. A child who has had a head injury may have lost consciousness and may not know the time of day. A Glasgow Coma Scale score of 15 and an apical pulse of 80 beats/minute are within the normal ranges.

Test Taking Strategy—*Look at the key word "immediately," which indicates urgency and a priority for reporting to the charge nurse or physician. Use Maslow's hierarchy to identify a condition that threatens a physiologic need. Although disorientation to time could be pathologic, it is a common abnormality when assessing orientation. The greater threat to the client's well-being is the evidence of leaking cerebrospinal fluid. Review manifestations of head trauma if you had difficulty answering this question.*
Cognitive Level—*Analyzing*
Client Needs Category—*Physiological integrity*
Client Needs Subcategory—*Physiological adaptation*

42. 2. When riding a bicycle, the child should travel in the same direction as the flow of traffic. The other options are correct safety measures that should be followed when riding a bicycle.
Test Taking Strategy—*Use the process of elimination to identify the option that is inaccurate in relation to bicycle safety. Options 1, 3, and 4 can be eliminated because they are appropriate safety precautions. Option 2 requires further teaching because it is incorrect information. Review pedestrian and bicycle safety if you had difficulty answering this question.*
Cognitive Level—*Analyzing*
Client Needs Category—*Safe and effective care environment*
Client Needs Subcategory—*Safety and infection control*

43. 4. The person sustaining a head injury should be observed for signs of intracranial bleeding, which can occur after even a mild or slight head injury. Because signs of bleeding are most likely to occur in the first 24 hours, the parents are instructed to awaken the child every 4 hours during the first night to check for an altered level of consciousness. Examples of changes requiring prompt notification of the health care provider include slurred speech, headache, visual problems, or difficulty arousing the child from sleep.
Test Taking Strategy—*Use the process of elimination to select the discharge instruction that is essential to provide to parents of a child who sustains a closed head injury. Option 3 can be eliminated because it is unrealistic to instruct parents to assess pupil reactions. Option 2 can be eliminated because it is not critical that the child be kept in a fasting state. Option 1 has merit, but it is not the most essential information to provide before discharging the client. Option 4 emerges as the best answer because it indicates a neurologic deterioration caused by the child's injury. Review the signs and symptoms of rising intracranial pressure from a subdural or epidural hemorrhage if you had difficulty answering this question.*
Cognitive Level—*Applying*
Client Needs Category—*Physiological integrity*
Client Needs Subcategory—*Reduction of risk potential*

Nursing Care of a Child with a Brain Tumor

44. 1. The signs and symptoms of a brain tumor usually occur as a result of increased intracranial pressure. Vomiting, especially early in the morning, is one sign in the child with a brain tumor. Nausea is not a common symptom. The child may not want to go to school and that should be documented, but this is not considered a risk factor for the presence of a brain tumor. Tilting the head to one side while sleeping does not correspond with a diagnosis of a brain tumor.
Test Taking Strategy—*Use the process of elimination to select the option that correlates most with a sign or symptom of a brain tumor. Vomiting in the morning (option 1) is a sign of increased intracranial pressure, which points to a brain tumor. Review the manifestations of a brain tumor if you had difficulty answering this question.*
Cognitive Level—*Applying*
Client Needs Category—*Physiological integrity*
Client Needs Subcategory—*Physiological adaptation*

45. 1. The child undergoing magnetic resonance imaging (MRI) will generally be placed in a tunnel-like scanner, which is more commonly available than open scanners. Sedation is used only if the client is restless or claustrophobic. Electrodes are not placed on the child's head, and headaches do not usually occur during this procedure.
Test Taking Strategy—*Use the process of elimination to select the option that most accurately describes the preparation of a client for an MRI. Option 2 can be eliminated because a headache is not a component of dye injection. Option 4 can be eliminated because it correlates with information for someone undergoing an EEG. Option 3 may be an attractive answer, but it can be eliminated because a hypnotic is not given; a sedative that still preserves a conscious state may be administered. Review neurologic diagnostic tests and related client preparation if you had difficulty answering this question.*
Cognitive Level—*Analyzing*
Client Needs Category—*Physiological integrity*
Client Needs Subcategory—*Reduction of risk potential*

46. 4. The head dressing of a child who has undergone a craniotomy may become damp from cerebrospinal fluid (CSF) drainage. The nurse should reinforce the dressing until the physician can change it. The child will require further intervention to prevent the possibility of an infection at the operative site; however, complications may occur if the dressing is changed or removed. Notifying the chaplain is not appropriate unless the child is exhibiting other signs of impending death. Draining of CSF is not an indication of death. Notifying the operating room of the possibility of additional surgery is premature and may not be needed. This should certainly not be done until after the physician has evaluated the child.

> *Test Taking Strategy*—*Look at the key words "most appropriate" and "at this time" in reference to the standard of care for a dressing that becomes moist in the immediate postoperative period. Recall that a wet dressing acts as a wick, pulling microorganisms from the surface toward the incisional area and tissues that lie beneath. Review principles that relate to wound care if you had difficulty answering this question.*
> *Cognitive Level*—*Analyzing*
> *Client Needs Category*—*Physiological integrity*
> *Client Needs Subcategory*—*Reduction of risk potential*

47. 3. The nurse should encourage the parents to express their feelings without being judged by the nurse. The parents need to know that the feelings they are experiencing are normal. Besides listening, the nurse can suggest ways in which the parents can cope with their feelings. Suggesting that the parents identify things they can do to make the child feel good will assist them in coping with their feelings of helplessness.

> *Test Taking Strategy*—*Use the process of elimination to help select the response that can best help parents cope with their feelings of helplessness. Options 1, 2, and 4 contain elements that are nontherapeutic. Option 3, on the other hand, demonstrates empathy and changes the parent's focus from helplessness to being helpful. Review therapeutic and nontherapeutic communication techniques and methods that promote coping strategies if you had difficulty answering this question.*
> *Cognitive Level*—*Analyzing*
> *Client Needs Category*—*Psychosocial integrity*
> *Client Needs Subcategory*—*None*

48. 2. Most chemotherapeutic agents cause some degree of nausea and vomiting. To lessen or prevent this side effect, the nurse should give a prescribed antiemetic before administering the chemotherapeutic agent. The child should always consume well-balanced meals, but serving the child a meal before chemotherapy may cause increased nausea and vomiting. The child should get plenty of rest whether receiving chemotherapy or not. Administration of pain medication is not usually indicated before beginning chemotherapy.

> *Test Taking Strategy*—*Use the process of elimination to select the option that describes the best method for managing a common side effect of chemotherapy medications. Option 4 can be eliminated because pain is not a common experience associated with chemotherapy. Options 1 and 3 are healthy recommendations, but option 2 is the best answer because it provides a means of preventing nausea and vomiting, which some clients who receive chemotherapy experience. Review the side effects associated with chemotherapy and nursing measures to manage or minimize them if you had difficulty answering this question.*

> *Cognitive Level*—*Applying*
> *Client Needs Category*—*Physiological integrity*
> *Client Needs Subcategory*—*Reduction of risk potential*

49. 71 mL. To find the answer, use this formula as a guide:

100 mL/kg/day for the first 10 kg of body weight
50 mL/kg/day for the next 10 kg of body weight
20 mL/kg/day for each kilogram above 20 kg of body

Calculate:

$$100 \text{ mL/kg/day} \times 10 \text{ kg} = 1{,}000 \text{ mL/day}$$
(for the first 10 kg)
$$50 \text{ mL/kg/day} \times 10 \text{ kg} = 500 \text{ mL/day}$$
(for the next 10 kg)
$$20 \text{ mL/kg/day} \times 10 \text{ kg} = 200 \text{ mL/day}$$
(for the remaining 10 kg)

Total the amounts:

$$1{,}000 \text{ mL/day} + 500 \text{ mL/day} + 200 \text{ mL/day} = 1{,}700 \text{ mL/day}$$

To find the hourly rate, divide by 24:

$$1{,}700 \text{ mL} \div 24 \text{ hr} = 70.9 \text{ or } 71 \text{ mL}$$

> *Test Taking Strategy*—*Look for key information needed to calculate the answer to this problem. They include the child's weight and fluid volume per kilogram. Review mathematical processes for calculating I.V. fluid volume if you had difficulty answering this question.*
> *Cognitive Level*—*Applying*
> *Client Needs Category*—*Physiological integrity*
> *Client Needs Subcategory*—*Pharmacological therapies*

50. 3. The nurse should encourage early and consistent visits from the child's friends to promote support and acceptance of the condition and enable the child to deal with the reactions of friends. Although any changes in appearance resulting from treatment are usually temporary, such changes can be very distressing to a child and the nurse should not minimize the child's feelings.

> *Test Taking Strategy*—*Use the process of elimination to select the option that describes the best nursing suggestion for maintaining social relationships between a sick child and school peers. Option 1 can be eliminated because relationships with children who have cancer will not re-establish former friendships. Although option 2 appears attractive, it can be eliminated because it may be difficult for the child to accept. Option 4 can be eliminated because the meaningfulness of being bald is significant to the child. Option 3 emerges as the best answer because it promotes the continuation of former friendships throughout the child's treatment. Review methods for promoting socialization and acceptance among school-age children if you had difficulty answering this question.*
> *Cognitive Level*—*Applying*
> *Client Needs Category*—*Psychosocial integrity*
> *Client Needs Subcategory*—*None*

51. 4. The side-lying position with knees drawn up is the position of choice when a lumbar puncture is performed. This position widens the space between the vertebrae, thereby aiding with insertion of the needle. The supine and Trendelenburg positions are not suitable for this procedure because they do not allow exposure of the lumbar region. The prone position does not facilitate widening of intervertebral spaces; thus, this also is not used.

> *Test Taking Strategy—Analyze to determine what information the question asks for, which is the proper positioning for a lumbar puncture. Eliminate options 1, 2, and 3 because they do not allow access to the invertebral spaces for performance of the puncture. Review nursing actions during a lumbar puncture if you had difficulty answering this question.*
> *Cognitive Level—Applying*
> *Client Needs Category—Physiological integrity*
> *Client Needs Subcategory—Reduction of risk potential*

Nursing Care of a Child in Traction

52. 2, 5, 6. Skeletal traction is used most frequently in the treatment of fractures of the femur, tibia, humerus, and cervical spine. The traction is applied directly to the bone by use of a metal pin, rod, or wire inserted into or through the bone. The pin, rod, or wire is then attached to the traction apparatus. Because of risk of injury to the client and to caregivers, it is prudent to cover the protruding pins, rods, or wires with corks or other materials to protect caregivers from becoming injured. Because of the added risk of infection with skeletal traction, the pin site should be monitored for signs of infection and routinely cleaned. In addition, the nurse should monitor the client for signs and symptoms of a urinary tract infection (UTI), which could be the result of urinary stasis from incomplete voiding. Cloudy or foul-smelling urine, as well as feelings of urgency, burning, and pressure, are all indications of a UTI. The child should be placed in the supine position (not prone). Range-of-motion exercises cannot be performed on the right leg because of the traction, and the weights should not be released.

> *Test Taking Strategy—Analyze to determine what information the question asks for, which is actions to take when providing nursing care to a client in skeletal traction. Alternative-format "select all that apply" questions require considering each option independently to decide its merit in answering the question. Choose options that support principles for nursing care of a client in skeletal traction. Review skeletal traction and related nursing interventions if you had difficulty answering this question.*
> *Cognitive Level—Applying*
> *Client Needs Category—Physiological integrity*
> *Client Needs Subcategory—Basic care and comfort*

53. 2. Pressure areas and skin breakdown are most likely to develop first over bony prominences, such as the heels, elbows, sacrum, ankles, and scapulae.

> *Test Taking Strategy—Analyze to determine what information the question asks for, which is the most likely location of pressure sore development in a client in skeletal traction applied to the leg. Recall that a client in skeletal leg traction is in a supine position, which causes pressure on the scapulae. Review common locations and causes of pressure sore development if you had difficulty answering this question.*
> *Cognitive Level—Applying*
> *Client Needs Category—Physiological integrity*
> *Client Needs Subcategory—Basic care and comfort*

54. 4. A traction rope that has slipped out of a pulley should be replaced in the pulley groove. The physician or registered nurse skilled in orthopedic care should perform this action.

> *Test Taking Strategy—Look at the key word "immediately," which indicates a priority assessment finding that requires reporting. Recall that ropes that are not positioned within the pulley interfere with the therapeutic effect of treatment. Review the principles involved in caring for a client in traction if you had difficulty answering this question.*
> *Cognitive Level—Applying*
> *Client Needs Category—Physiological integrity*
> *Client Needs Subcategory—Basic care and comfort*

55. 1. A high fluid intake and a diet high in fiber are recommended to prevent constipation and other complications of immobilization, such as kidney stones and urinary tract infections. The right leg, which is in traction, is kept immobile. Turning the client is not routinely performed.

> *Test Taking Strategy—Use the process of elimination to select the option that describes a nursing measure for preventing a common complication among pediatric clients who are in traction. Option 1 is the best answer because an immobilized client may not be able to drink independently due to being confined. Confinement also interferes with normal bowel function. Options 2, 3, and 4 are inappropriate nursing measures for this client. Review the principles involved in caring for a client in traction if you had difficulty answering this question.*
> *Cognitive Level—Applying*
> *Client Needs Category—Physiological integrity*
> *Client Needs Subcategory—Basic care and comfort*

56. 3. The child should be able to move the toes freely; an inability to do so may indicate an alteration in neurovascular status. If the toes on both feet are cool, it is probably due to the environmental temperature rather than neurovascular impairment. The other parameters indicate intact neurovascular function.

Test Taking Strategy—Analyze to determine what information the question asks for, which is an immediate reportable finding that indicates a neurovascular problem. The word "immediately" indicates a threat to the client's safety if unresolved. Although option 2 has merit, because the coolness is present bilaterally, it is not as significant a finding as option 3. Review methods for assessing neurovascular status and the implications of abnormalities if you had difficulty answering this question.
Cognitive Level—*Applying*
Client Needs Category—*Physiological integrity*
Client Needs Subcategory—*Physiological adaptation*

Nursing Care of a Child with a Kidney Disorder

57. 1. Glomerular nephritis is an inflammation of the glomeruli, which are the kidneys' filtering mechanisms. Glomerular nephritis is more common in boys than girls, and occurs in toddlers and school-age children who have had recent streptococcal infections (primarily strep throat). Acute glomerular nephritis (AGN) is a disease characterized by the sudden appearance of generalized edema, periorbital edema that is worse in the morning, hematuria, proteinuria, decreased urination, anorexia, and hypertension.

Test Taking Strategy—Use the process of elimination to select the option that best correlates with the signs and symptoms of AGN. Options 2 and 4 can be immediately eliminated. Option 4 is not a common manifestation; in fact, anorexia is generally the rule. Review the signs and symptoms of AGN if you had difficulty answering this question.
Cognitive Level—*Applying*
Client Needs Category—*Physiological integrity*
Client Needs Subcategory—*Physiological adaptation*

58. 2, 4, 5, 6. Nephrotic syndrome is caused by damage to the glomeruli and results in a large amount of protein being excreted in the urine, which in turn results in hypoalbuminemia, hyperlipidemia, and generalized edema. The child with nephrotic syndrome should be weighed daily to monitor the amount of edema present. The abdominal circumference is also measured. Abdominal circumference measurements are indicated because of the large amounts of generalized edema, including fluid trapped in the peritoneal cavity (called *ascites*). Collecting a 24-hour urine specimen will provide more accurate accounts of the protein in the urine than can be identified by using a chemical dipstick to assess the urine. Monitoring blood urea nitrogen and creatinine is essential for assessing the proper functioning of the kidneys and the effectiveness of the treatment. The child is able to maintain range of motion and independently perform activities of daily living. A high-protein, low-sodium diet is commonly required as part of the treatment plan.

Test Taking Strategy—Analyze to determine what information the question asks for, which is the nursing actions to take for a client with nephrotic syndrome. Alternative-format "select all that apply" questions require considering each option independently to decide its merit in answering the question. Choose options that describe the nursing care of a client with nephrotic syndrome. Review the renal pathophysiology associated with nephrotic syndrome and related nursing care if you had difficulty answering this question.
Cognitive Level—*Applying*
Client Needs Category—*Physiological integrity*
Client Needs Subcategory—*Physiological adaptation*

59. 2. Weak pulse, hypotension, muscular weakness, diminished reflexes, loss of peristalsis, and cardiac arrest are signs and symptoms of hypokalemia.

Test Taking Strategy—Analyze to determine what information the question asks for, which involves identifying a manifestation of hypokalemia. Options 1, 3, and 4 can be eliminated because they are not signs and symptoms associated with hypokalemia. Review electrolyte imbalances, specifically hypokalemia, and their effects if you had difficulty answering this question.
Cognitive Level—*Analyzing*
Client Needs Category—*Physiological integrity*
Client Needs Subcategory—*Physiological adaptation*

60. 1. A Wilms' tumor is a congenital, cancerous tumor of the kidney. Feeling, touching, or handling the client's abdomen may result in rupture of the renal capsule and the spread of cancerous tumor cells. Collecting a urine specimen, assessing the pupils, or eliciting a patellar reflex will not exert pressure on the renal capsule.

Test Taking Strategy—Use the process of elimination to select the option that describes an inappropriate or unsafe nursing action when caring for a child with Wilms' tumor. Options 2, 3, and 4 are safe and appropriate nursing activities. Option 1 describes an action that is contraindicated because it exerts pressure on the renal capsule. Review Wilms' tumor and methods for avoiding complications if you had difficulty answering this question.
Cognitive Level—*Applying*
Client Needs Category—*Physiological integrity*
Client Needs Subcategory—*Reduction of risk potential*

Nursing Care of a Child with a Blood Disorder

61. 4. Pallor, listlessness, and irritability are observable signs of iron deficiency anemia. The child's history may also reveal anorexia, weight loss, and a decrease in normal activity.

Test Taking Strategy—*Use the process of elimination to select the option that describes an assessment finding common among clients with anemia regardless of its cause. Options 1, 2, and 3 can be eliminated because they are not among the signs and symptoms of anemia. Review the function of hemoglobin and red blood cells in maintaining cellular oxygenation and how physiology is affected when there are insufficient amounts of either substance if you had difficulty answering this question.*
Cognitive Level—*Understanding*
Client Needs Category—*Physiological integrity*
Client Needs Subcategory—*Physiological adaptation*

62. 1. Salicylates prolong bleeding time by interfering with the blood's ability to clot. Acetylsalicylic acid (aspirin), a salicylate, is contraindicated for anyone with a bleeding disorder because it is usually extremely difficult to stop the bleeding. A child who receives aspirin could bleed to death from even a relatively small lesion. Although caffeine, barbiturates, and antacids are not contraindicated for those with hemophilia, they are not routinely given.

Test Taking Strategy—*Analyze to determine what information the question asks for, which is a drug that may cause further complications for a client who has hemophilia. Recall that a side effect of salicylates is a potential for frank or occult blood loss. Review the actions and side effects of the substances listed if you had difficulty answering this question.*
Cognitive Level—*Applying*
Client Needs Category—*Physiological integrity*
Client Needs Subcategory—*Pharmacological therapies*

Nursing Care of a Child with a Communicable Disease

63. 2. Tinea capitis is a superficial fungal infection usually found on the scalp. The preferred treatment for tinea capitis (ringworm) is oral griseofulvin (Grisactin) for a minimum of 6 weeks. It is recommended that the medication be taken with milk or ice cream to increase its absorption. Nits are found in pediculosis capitis (lice infestation), not tinea capitis. Topical medications alone are ineffective in the treatment of tinea capitis.

Test Taking Strategy—*Analyze to determine what information the question asks for, which is a statement that describes effective teaching about tinea capitis. Recall that ringworm is treated systemically rather than topically. Review tinea capitis and the nursing implications when administering griseofulvin if you had difficulty answering this question.*
Cognitive Level—*Analyzing*
Client Needs Category—*Health promotion and maintenance*
Client Needs Subcategory—*None*

64. 3. Pinworms are small, white worms that live in the intestines. Pinworm infestations are common in young children, easily transmitted from child to child, and easily treated. The most common manifestation of pinworms is anal itching as the female worms exit from the intestine and lay eggs around the anus. Increased flatulence, abdominal pain, and bulky, greasy stools are not usual findings.

Test Taking Strategy—*Use the process of elimination to select the option that most accurately describes a common finding among those with pinworms. Review pinworm infestation and its signs and symptoms if you had difficulty answering this question.*
Cognitive Level—*Analyzing*
Client Needs Category—*Physiological integrity*
Client Needs Subcategory—*Physiological adaptation*

65. 2. Impetigo is a contagious disorder caused by a streptococcal or staphylococcal skin infection. Both systemic and topical antibiotics are usually prescribed. The lesions are itchy, therefore necessitating the need for short nails, and oral antihistamines are sometimes ordered to decrease the inflammation and itching. It is easily spread from child to child.

Test Taking Strategy—*Use the process of elimination to select an option that indicates incorrect parental recall of information. Options 1, 3, and 4 can be eliminated because they represent inaccurate statements. Review the dermatologic disorder of impetigo, how it is managed, and how a client can be reinfected or transmit it to others if you had difficulty answering this question.*
Cognitive Level—*Analyzing*
Client Needs Category—*Safe and effective care environment*
Client Needs Subcategory—*Safety and infection control*

Nursing Care of a Child with a Nutritional Deficiency

66. 4. Rickets is caused by a lack of sufficient vitamin D in the diet. The vitamin is essential for proper calcium and phosphorus used in the normal development of bones and teeth. Signs of rickets include delayed closure of the fontanels, delayed tooth growth, dental caries, and deformities of the long bones.

Test Taking Strategy—*Analyze to determine what information the question asks for, which is the vitamin deficiency that contributes to the development of rickets. Recall that vitamin D is necessary for the utilization of calcium and a deficiency affects structures that require this mineral. Review the functions of vitamins in normal nutrition if you had difficulty answering this question.*
Cognitive Level—*Applying*
Client Needs Category—*Physiological integrity*
Client Needs Subcategory—*Basic care and comfort*

67. 2, 3, 5. The best dietary sources of calcium are dairy products (including milk, yogurt, and cheese products), soybeans, fortified orange juice, dark green leafy vegetables, sardines, clams, and oysters. Chicken is a good source of protein, and apples have vitamins and antioxidant properties. Broccoli is not a dark green leafy vegetable, and it only has 62 mg of calcium per 1 cup serving.

> *Test Taking Strategy—Analyze to determine what information the question asks for, which is good sources of dietary calcium. Alternative-format "select all that apply" questions require considering each option independently to decide its merit in answering the question. Choose options that identify good dietary sources of calcium. Review normal nutrition and good dietary sources of the mineral calcium if you had difficulty answering this question.*
> **Cognitive Level**—*Applying*
> **Client Needs Category**—*Physiological integrity*
> **Client Needs Subcategory**—*Basic care and comfort*

68. 1, 2, 3, 4. Peanut allergies are more common in children and are the result of direct contact with peanuts, such as ingesting peanuts or products containing peanuts, or indirect contact, such as inhaling peanut dust. The body's immune system mistakenly recognizes peanuts as something harmful. Peanut allergies can be minor or severe and can result in anaphylactic shock and possible death. The signs and symptoms of peanut allergies include hives; itching around the mouth and throat; digestive problems such as nausea, vomiting, diarrhea, and abdominal cramping; and a runny or stuffy nose. Other signs and symptoms include shortness of breath and wheezing, chest tightening, constriction of the airway, and those related to shock, including tachycardia and hypotension.

> *Test Taking Strategy—Analyze to determine what information the question asks for, which is signs and symptoms of an allergic reaction. Alternative-format "select all that apply" questions require considering each option independently to decide its merit in answering the question. Choose options that correlate with manifestations of exposure to an allergen. Review various types of allergic reactions, including ingestants, contactants, and injectants, as well as manifestations that are common among those who have allergies, if you had difficulty answering this question.*
> **Cognitive Level**—*Applying*
> **Client Needs Category**—*Health promotion and maintenance*
> **Client Needs Subcategory**—*None*

69. 1, 2, 3, 4. Foods that contain peanuts or peanut products should be avoided. Some foods containing peanuts are obvious, such as mixed nuts or candy that contains peanuts. Other foods that contain peanuts may be harder to detect; these can include cookies and pastries, ice cream and frozen desserts, energy bars, cereals, and granola.

Additional foods that may contain peanuts are ethnic foods such as Chinese, Thai, Vietnamese, and Mexican. Yogurt and sour cream and cheeseburgers and cola do not contain peanut oil.

> *Test Taking Strategy—Analyze to determine what information the question asks for, which is foods that may contain peanuts. Alternative-format "select all that apply" questions require considering each option independently to decide its merit in answering the question. Choose options that are foods that commonly contain peanuts. Review nutrition and labels on products for ingredients listing peanuts if you had difficulty answering this question.*
> **Cognitive Level**—*Applying*
> **Client Needs Category**—*Health promotion and maintenance*
> **Client Needs Subcategory**—*None*

Nursing Care of a Child with a Musculoskeletal Disability

70. 1. Cerebral palsy is a nonprogressive neuromuscular disorder caused by an injury to the motor-coordinating areas of the brain. Brain surgery cannot help or cure those with this disorder. Physical therapy and other disciplines, such as occupational, speech, and recreational therapy, are often of great benefit to those with cerebral palsy.

> *Test Taking Strategy—Use the process of elimination to select the option that describes correct information about cerebral palsy. Option 4 can be eliminated immediately because cerebral palsy affects motor rather than sensory functions. Options 2 and 3 can be eliminated because they are false statements. Option 1 emerges as the correct answer because it accurately describes cerebral palsy. Review the pathophysiology associated with cerebral palsy and methods for managing the care of a client with this condition if you had difficulty answering this question.*
> **Cognitive Level**—*Applying*
> **Client Needs Category**—*Physiological integrity*
> **Client Needs Subcategory**—*Physiological adaptation*

71. 3. Parents who have children with the same disability are often able to provide emotional support. When these parents meet, they share a common bond and a common burden, and they learn from one another about how to overcome obstacles. Recommending that the child be placed in a long-term care facility, referring the parents to a social welfare agency, or giving them literature to read probably will not help them cope with their problems as effectively as would talking with someone with a similar experience.

> *Test Taking Strategy—Analyze to determine what information the question asks for, which requires*

selecting a method for promoting acceptance of a diagnosis involving a child with special physical needs. Using a network of support (option 3) is better than dealing with a problem in isolation. Review approaches for therapeutically improving coping skills among parents with a child who has a chronic, progressive genetic disorder if you had difficulty answering this question.
Cognitive Level—*Analyzing*
Client Needs Category—*Psychosocial integrity*
Client Needs Subcategory—*None*

Nursing Care of an Adolescent with Appendicitis

72. 3. Absent bowel sounds may be a sign of inflammation and possible obstruction and should be reported immediately. The other findings do not pose as great a threat to the adolescent's health at this time.
   Test Taking Strategy—Note the key word "immediately," which indicates identifying a problem that threatens the safety and well-being of the client. Although all of the options are problematic, the absence of bowel sounds requires immediate attention. Review the complications associated with a ruptured appendix and their manifestations if you had difficulty answering this question.
Cognitive Level—*Analyzing*
Client Needs Category—*Physiological integrity*
Client Needs Subcategory—*Physiological adaptation*

73. 2. Before surgery, the teenager should be given nothing by mouth (NPO) to reduce the risk of aspiration during surgery. Analgesics can mask clinical signs and symptoms needed for a diagnosis; therefore, they should not be given before surgery. Enemas and laxatives should be avoided because they increase peristalsis, which may rupture the appendix. Applying heat to the abdomen is contraindicated because this also may rupture the appendix.
   Test Taking Strategy—Use the process of elimination to select an option that identifies the most appropriate preoperative nursing intervention for a client with appendicitis. Options 3 and 4 are inappropriate and potentially unsafe. Option 1 has merit, but it is not as important as withholding food and fluids to prevent vomiting and aspiration in an anesthetized state. Review interoperative complications and how they can be prevented or minimized if you had difficulty answering this question.
Cognitive Level—*Applying*
Client Needs Category—*Physiological integrity*
Client Needs Subcategory—*Reduction of risk potential*

74. 4. If a total of 1,000 mL is to be given over 8 hours, the nurse needs to divide the amount to be given (1,000 mL) by the total number of hours (8).

$$1{,}000 \text{ mL} \div 8 \text{ hours} = 125 \text{ mL/hour}.$$

   Test Taking Strategy—Note the key information that is necessary for calculating the rate of I.V. fluid administration. These include the volume and number of hours. Review the method for calculating I.V. infusion rates if you had difficulty with this calculation.
Cognitive Level—*Applying*
Client Needs Category—*Physiological integrity*
Client Needs Subcategory—*Pharmacological therapies*

75. 4. Incentive spirometry and deep breathing help prevent respiratory complications that may be experienced by persons having abdominal surgery. Bronchodilators, oxygen, and corticosteroids are used to treat respiratory complications; they are not preventive measures.
   Test Taking Strategy—Use the process of elimination to help select the option that is best for preventing postoperative respiratory complications. Although options 1, 2, and 3 are attractive, they are treatment-related rather than prophylactic. Review postoperative nursing care if you had difficulty answering this question.
Cognitive Level—*Applying*
Client Needs Category—*Physiological integrity*
Client Needs Subcategory—*Reduction of risk potential*

76. 2. Many clients, children and adults alike, are afraid their sutures will pull out if they walk or move too much. The nurse should reassure such clients that the sutures are designed to endure movement and walking. Telling the teenager that walking will not cause discomfort is not true. Although acknowledging the teen's fear is appropriate, the nurse should attempt to respond in a way that helps to resolve the fear. Putting off ambulation is not therapeutic and will not help the client face and resolve fear.
   Test Taking Strategy—Use the process of elimination to guide the selection of an option that represents a therapeutic communication technique. Option 1 is an example of a nontherapeutic communication technique known as giving false reassurance. Option 3 is nontherapeutic because it belittles the client's emotional state. Option 4 is nontherapeutic because it does not provide any method for resolving fears that are real to the client. Option 2 emerges as the correct answer because it provides the client with factual information. Review therapeutic and nontherapeutic communication techniques if you had difficulty answering this question.
Cognitive Level—*Applying*
Client Needs Category—*Psychosocial integrity*
Client Needs Subcategory—*None*

77. **2.** A child with no complications may return to school within 2 weeks of an appendectomy; this generally allows sufficient time for healing and recovery. Limited activities are generally recommended throughout the recovery period.

Test Taking Strategy—Analyze to determine what information the question asks for, which is the usual recovery time after an appendectomy. Recall that a 1- to 2-week recovery period is a conservative estimate for a person whose daily activities are likely to be more energetic than sedentary. Review the postoperative management of a client undergoing an appendectomy if you had difficulty answering this question.
Cognitive Level—Applying
Client Needs Category—Physiological integrity
Client Needs Subcategory—Physiological adaptation

Nursing Care of an Adolescent with Dysmenorrhea

78. **4.** Proper sleep, a well-balanced diet, warm tub baths, application of heat to the abdomen, drinking warm liquids, and moderate exercise are some recommendations the nurse can make to relieve dysmenorrhea (painful menstruation). The other options are not known to relieve menstrual cramps or pain.

Test Taking Strategy—Use the process of elimination to select the option that describes the best measure for relieving dysmenorrhea from among those provided. Options 1, 2, and 3 describe inaccurate and inappropriate nursing measures in relation to relieving menstrual discomfort. Option 4 emerges as the best answer because it includes principles of healthful living and symptomatic treatment. Review dysmenorrhea and methods that are appropriate for its management if you had difficulty answering this question.
Cognitive Level—Applying
Client Needs Category—Physiological integrity
Client Needs Subcategory—Basic care and comfort

79. **2.** During adolescents, peer relationships, more than family, are of a high priority thus the interruption of social functions is of highest priority when considering the effects of dysmenorrhea. Though gym class is a requirement in many schools, many students need to refrain from gym class activities due to illness or injury. The adolescent may return to gym class once dysmenorrhea has subsided. Discussing the symptoms and following up on a treatment plan for the effects of dysmenorrhea typically can be addressed with phone consultation.

Test Taking Strategy—Use the process of elimination to select the option identified as most impacted by the effects of dysmenorrhea. Consider the developmental level of the client when evaluating each option. Note that all options have merit but peers and social
functions are a high priority for the adolescent. Review age appropriate considerations of illness if you had difficulty answering this question.
Cognitive Level—Analyzing
Client Needs Category—Health promotion and maintenance
Client Needs Subcategory—None

80. **3.** The client should take tetracycline hydrochloride (Panmycin) when the stomach is empty and wait 1 hour before eating after taking the drug. The other options are appropriate when taking this medication.

Test Taking Strategy—Analyze to determine what information the question asks for, which is evidence of incorrect understanding of instructions on medication use. Recall that absorption of antibiotics in the tetracycline family is reduced when taken with milk, food, antacids, or mineral supplements containing calcium. Drinking a full glass of water when taking a tetracycline or any other medication promotes pharmacokinetic processes. Review drug information about tetracycline and its administration if you had difficulty answering this question.
Cognitive Level—Applying
Client Needs Category—Physiological integrity
Client Needs Subcategory—Pharmacological therapies

Nursing Care of an Adolescent Who Is Engaging in Risk-taking Behaviors

81. **2.** Methamphetamines, which are central nervous system (CNS) stimulants, can lead to addiction. Their use depletes stores of adrenaline and contributes to the repeated use of the drug to restore pleasure, stimulation, and a sense of well-being. Those who abuse amphetamines may also be involved with the abuse of other substances. It is untrue to state that methamphetamines are tried by "most" adolescents and cause no harm. Methamphetamines are most commonly snorted, injected, swallowed, or smoked, all of which are harmful.

Test Taking Strategy—Use the process of elimination to select an option that provides accurate information about the abuse of methamphetamine. Option 1 can be eliminated because methamphetamines are often a component in harmful polydrug abuse. Option 3 is incorrect because methamphetamines are CNS stimulants, not depressants. Option 4 can be eliminated because methamphetamines are self-administered by a variety of routes. Review drug information about abused CNS drugs if you had difficulty answering this question.
Cognitive Level—Applying
Client Needs Category—Health promotion and maintenance
Client Needs Subcategory—None

82. 4. Signs of methamphetamine abuse include those associated with central nervous system (CNS) stimulants. They include marked nervousness, restlessness, excitability, talkativeness, excessive perspiration, and violent aggressive behavior. The remaining signs are not characteristic of methamphetamine abuse.

> *Test Taking Strategy—Analyze to determine what information the question asks for, which is a sign of methamphetamine use. Refer to the rationale for a description of effects associated with the use of a CNS stimulant like methamphetamine. Review physiologic effects of nervous system stimulation if you had difficulty answering this question.*
> *Cognitive Level—Applying*
> *Client Needs Category—Physiological integrity*
> *Client Needs Subcategory—Pharmacological therapies*

83. 1. Adolescents normally try to develop self-identity. One way of achieving this is through identifying with peers and mimicking group behaviors. The search for intimate relationships usually occurs between ages 18 and 40. Generally, adults demonstrate integrity, not adolescents. Idealism refers to the pursuit of ideas; it is most likely unrelated to amphetamine abuse.

> *Test Taking Strategy—Analyze to determine what information the question asks for, which is the developmental task associated with adolescence. Recall that adolescence is a time when teenagers are attempting to discover who they are as individuals. Review the developmental tasks of various age groups described by Erikson, especially adolescents, and the terms used to identify respective developmental tasks if you had difficulty answering this question.*
> *Cognitive Level—Applying*
> *Client Needs Category—Health promotion and maintenance*
> *Client Needs Subcategory—None*

84. 3. The successful treatment of substance abuse largely depends on the person's desire to become drug-free. Someone who is forced to enter a drug rehabilitation program probably has less of a chance of remaining drug-free than someone who enters a program willingly. Usually a court order is not necessary for participation in a drug abuse program. Merely discussing the dangers of drug abuse is not likely to change the teenager's pattern of substance abuse.

> *Test Taking Strategy—Use the process of elimination to select an option that identifies an accurate and helpful response to a parental query concerning drug treatment. Option 2 is blatantly incorrect. Option 1 is likely to be ineffective because the child probably already knows the dangers of substance abuse, but is most likely in denial. Option 4 is incorrect because using force does not promote success*

in drug treatment. Review approaches for promoting cooperation as it relates to drug treatment if you had difficulty answering this question.
> *Cognitive Level—Analyzing*
> *Client Needs Category—Psychosocial integrity*
> *Client Needs Subcategory—None*

85. 4. Booster doses of tetanus toxoid are recommended during adolescence and once every 10 years thereafter. Smallpox vaccination is no longer advised because it is believed that the disease has been essentially eradicated. The last polio vaccine is given between ages 4 and 6. The *Haemophilus influenzae* type b (Hib) vaccine schedule is completed at 15 months.

> *Test Taking Strategy—Analyze to determine what information the question asks for, which is the recommended schedule for routine immunizations. Recall that a booster of tetanus toxoid is recommended every 10 years. Review the types of routine immunizations and the age at which their initial dose and boosters are recommended if you had difficulty with this question.*
> *Cognitive Level—Applying*
> *Client Needs Category—Health promotion and maintenance*
> *Client Needs Subcategory—None*

86. 1, 2, 3, 4. Tattooing involves the injection of ink into the skin at about 3,000 times per minute. The most common dangers and complications of tattooing involve an allergic reaction to the ink, skin infections because of unsterilized needles, and the transmission of diseases such as tetanus, hepatitis B or C, human immunodeficiency virus (HIV), and syphilis. Tattooing also may result in chronic skin diseases such as psoriasis and dermatitis. Body tattoos can also cause tumors of the skin, which may be benign or even malignant. Tattooing is not associated with heart and lung conditions nor is it associated with spontaneous abortions in tattooed females.

> *Test Taking Strategy—Analyze to determine what information the question asks for, which is risks of tattoos. Alternative-format "select all that apply" questions require considering each option independently to decide its merit in answering the question. Choose options that identify risks associated with tattooing. Review the process of tattooing and its dangers if you had difficulty answering this question.*
> *Cognitive Level—Applying*
> *Client Needs Category—Health promotion and health maintenance*
> *Client Needs Subcategory—None*

Nursing Care of an Adolescent with a Sexually Transmitted Infection

87. 3. A diagnosis of gonorrhea is confirmed when the microorganism is found in the client's vaginal discharge.

This is usually accomplished by viewing a smear sample under a microscope, although cultures of the discharge may also be taken. Cervical biopsy and blood and urine specimen examinations are not used to confirm a diagnosis of gonorrhea.

Test Taking Strategy—Analyze to determine what information the question asks for, which is the type of specimen used to diagnose gonorrhea in a female client. Recall that the microorganism that causes gonorrhea, Neisseria gonorrheae, survives only on moist surfaces within the body and is found most commonly in the vagina of infected females. Review the methods used to diagnose sexually transmitted infections, specifically gonorrhea, if you had difficulty answering this question.
Cognitive Level—Applying
Client Needs Category—Physiological integrity
Client Needs Subcategory—Reduction of risk potential

88. 4. Gastrointestinal upset is one of the adverse reactions to doxycycline (Vibramycin). Potentially serious adverse reactions should be immediately reported to the physician. This medication does not usually discolor the urine. The medication should be taken with a full glass of water; it can also be taken with food or dairy products.

Test Taking Strategy—Use the process of elimination to select the correct information relating to the administration of doxycycline. Options 1, 2, and 3 are not adverse effects of doxycycline (Vibramycin). Review drug-related information about the teaching that is appropriate for a client prescribed doxycycline if you had difficulty with this question.
Cognitive Level—Applying
Client Needs Category—Physiological integrity
Client Needs Subcategory—Pharmacological therapies

89. 3. One or preferably two follow-up smears or cultures should be taken after therapy is completed for clients who have gonorrhea. If the cultures and smears are negative, the client is considered noninfectious. It is unsafe to assume that a client is no longer infectious based on cessation of vaginal discharge, pain-free menstrual periods, or taking prescribed medication; follow-up studies are essential.

Test Taking Strategy—Analyze to determine what information the question asks for, which is identifying how long gonorrhea remains infectious after treatment. Recall that a negative culture 1 week after completing treatment is an indication that a client who had been diagnosed with gonorrhea is no longer infectious. Review sexually transmitted infections, their transmission, how they are cured, and when they require additional treatment if you had difficulty answering this question.

Cognitive Level—Applying
Client Needs Category—Safe and effective care environment
Client Needs Subcategory—Safety and infection control

90. 2.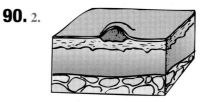

The initial lesions of genital herpes can be described as fluid-filled vesicles, shown in illustration 2. The lesions may become pustules, which in time may become crusted. The other options do not accurately depict genital herpes lesions.

Test Taking Strategy—Use the process of elimination to identify the option that best depicts herpetic lesions. Option 1 can be eliminated because it illustrates a macule, a flat, round, nonpalpable lesion. Option 3 can be eliminated because it illustrates a papule, an elevated, palpable, solid lesion. Option 4 can be eliminated because it illustrates a wheal, an elevated fluid-free lesion with an irregular border. Option 2 emerges as the best answer because the illustration corresponds with a vesicle, a round, elevated lesion that is filled with serum. Review herpes simplex and herpes complex and definitions of the lesions depicted in the options if you had difficulty answering this question.
Cognitive Level—Applying
Client Needs Category—Physiological integrity
Client Needs Subcategory—Physiological adaptation

91. 3. Genital herpes is not associated with sterility; gonorrhea can cause sterility in females. Current studies have identified a close link between genital herpes and prostate cancer in men and cervical cancer in women. Genital herpes also has been closely associated with the occurrence of Hodgkin's disease. Female clients with genital herpes are advised to have Pap tests every 6 months, and male clients are advised to have rectal examinations and prostate-specific antigen (PSA) tests yearly.

Test Taking Strategy—Analyze to determine what information the question asks for, which is evidence that the client has verbalized incorrect information that requires clarification. Review the risks associated with genital herpes if you had difficulty answering this question.
Cognitive Level—Analyzing
Client Needs Category—Health promotion and maintenance
Client Needs Subcategory—None

92. 3. Topical acyclovir (Zovirax) should be applied with a glove or finger cot to prevent spreading the infection. Acyclovir does not provide protection against or prevent recurrence of the disease; however, it does prolong remission and decrease the pain associated with the presence of lesions. Sex partners do not need to be treated with topical acyclovir because it is used to decrease pain and prevent recurrence.

Test Taking Strategy—Use the process of elimination to identify the option that states accurate information. Options 1, 2, and 4 can be eliminated because they are inaccurate. Review the drug treatment of herpes infections, specifically acyclovir, and health teaching about its administration if you had difficulty answering this question.
Cognitive Level—Applying
Client Needs Category—Physiological integrity
Client Needs Subcategory—Pharmacological therapies

93. 4. Sexual contact should be avoided, especially during active disease. The herpes virus can cross the condom membrane; therefore, wearing a condom will not totally ensure protection. Also, douching and taking acyclovir (Zovirax) will not protect against virus transmission.

Test Taking Strategy—Analyze to determine what information the question asks for, which is evidence that the client has verbalized correct information. Option 4 offers the best understanding of herpes virus transmission. Review the methods by which genital herpes is transmitted and methods for interfering with its transmission if you had difficulty answering this question.
Cognitive Level—Evaluating
Client Needs Category—Safe and effective care environment
Client Needs Subcategory—Safety and infection control

94. 3. Malaise, fever, and opportunistic infections are some common symptoms of acquired immunodeficiency syndrome (AIDS). Female clients with AIDS also tend to experience recurrent yeast infections. Other symptoms may include anorexia, weight loss, sore throat, diarrhea, lymph node enlargement, abdominal cramps, thrush, pneumonia, and night sweats. Some people have few or no early symptoms.

Test Taking Strategy—Analyze to determine what information the question asks for, which are the signs and symptoms of an AIDS infection. Recall that signs of any infection are likely to include malaise and fever. Because the human immunodeficiency virus reduces the immune response, an infected person will succumb to infections that healthy individuals are most likely to resist. Review the early and late manifestations of AIDS if you had difficulty answering this question.

Cognitive Level—Understanding
Client Needs Category—Physiological integrity
Client Needs Subcategory—Physiological adaptation

95. 2. Symptoms of acquired immunodeficiency syndrome (AIDS) may appear months or years after the original infection; therefore, the absence of symptoms is no assurance that a sexual partner does not have AIDS. AIDS cannot be cured and the transmission of AIDS cannot be controlled with antiviral drugs. The drugs currently in use may slow disease progression in some people. Telling the adolescent to cease sexual activity is rarely effective.

Test Taking Strategy—Use the process of elimination to help in identifying an accurate statement about AIDS transmission from an asymptomatic person. Review information on the possible time lapse between the initial infection and manifestation of AIDS symptoms if you had difficulty answering this question.
Cognitive Level—Applying
Client Needs Category—Health promotion and maintenance
Client Needs Subcategory—None

96. 1. A high-calorie, bland diet served in small amounts at frequent intervals is best for the adolescent for two reasons. The bland foods will not irritate the lesions in the adolescent's mouth, and the additional calories are needed to prevent weight loss, which is a common finding in adolescents with AIDS. The other diets mentioned may not provide the nutrients needed or may aggravate other problems found in adolescents with AIDS.

Test Taking Strategy—Use the process of elimination to identify the type of diet that is best suited for a client with oral lesions. There are no scientific or therapeutic reasons for the diets identified in options 2, 3, and 4 in relation to managing the care of a client with oral lesions. Review the therapeutic diets listed and indications for their use if you had difficulty answering this question.
Cognitive Level—Applying
Client Needs Category—Physiological integrity
Client Needs Subcategory—Basic care and comfort

97. 4. A ½″ space should be left at the tip of the condom to allow for collection of the ejaculate and to prevent tearing of the condom. Condoms can be damaged by heat and, therefore, should be stored in a cool place. A condom should be applied after the penis is erect. Condoms may or may not be prelubricated. Those that contain a water based lubricant may have the lubricant applied during the manufacturing process or applied at the time of sexual intercourse. A petroleum-based lubricant can degrade the condom material.

Test Taking Strategy—Analyze to determine what information the question asks for, which is accurate information regarding the use of a condom and

maintaining its integrity to prevent pregnancy. Recall that leaving space between the tip of the penis and the end of the condom reduces the potential for altering the integrity of the condom at the time of ejaculation. Review information on how to use a condom if you had difficulty answering this question.
Cognitive Level—*Applying*
Client Needs Category—*Health promotion and maintenance*
Client Needs Subcategory—*None*

98. 1. The client should examine his testicles individually, one at a time, after a warm bath or shower. One testicle is usually slightly larger than the other. Lumps, if detected, are usually found on the sides of the testicles.
Test Taking Strategy—*Analyze to determine what information the question asks for, which is the technique for testicular self-examination and significant findings. Recall that the testes descend when exposed to warmth, making it easier to perform self-examination. Review the procedure for testicular self-examination and signs of testicular cancer if you had difficulty answering this question.*
Cognitive Level—*Applying*
Client Needs Category—*Health promotion and maintenance*
Client Needs Subcategory—*None*

Nursing Care of an Adolescent with Scoliosis

99. 2. Scoliosis, a curvature of the spine that occurs just before puberty, is more common in females and is most often associated with a growth spurt. The cause of most scoliosis is unknown. Children with scoliosis often complain of having difficulty with their clothes fitting properly. Common complaints include an uneven hemline and uneven sleeve length, one shoulder and hip higher than the other, an uneven waist line, and one scapula that is highly pronounced.
Test Taking Strategy—*Analyze to determine what information the question asks for, which is a statement that correlates with a sign of scoliosis. Recall that the spinal curvature of scoliosis disturbs shoulder symmetry. Review scoliosis and its manifestations if you had difficulty answering this question.*
Cognitive Level—*Applying*
Client Needs Category—*Health promotion and maintenance*
Client Needs Subcategory—*None*

100. 1. X-rays are used to confirm a diagnosis of scoliosis. Because the radiation emitted by X-rays carries a risk of causing genetic mutation that may lead to birth defects

in offspring, the nurse should first determine whether there is a possibility that the client is pregnant. The client's allergy status, medication use, and consumption of food are not pertinent to this type of radiologic test.
Test Taking Strategy—*Use the process of elimination to select the option that is most important to ask before performing an X-ray, especially on a female of reproductive age. Recall that exposure to radiation can disrupt cellular structures and function. Review the hazards of radiation exposure on fetal development if you had difficulty answering this question.*
Cognitive Level—*Applying*
Client Needs Category—*Physiological integrity*
Client Needs Subcategory—*Reduction of risk potential*

101. 4. The severity of scoliosis is based on the degree of spinal curvature. Any curvature greater than 20 degrees requires treatment; surgery is indicated if the curvature is 50 degrees or greater. If treatment is not implemented, the curvature will continue to increase. A lateral curvature in the spine causes asymmetry of the thoracic cage with a midline displacement of the sternum, which may affect respiratory function if it becomes pronounced.
Test Taking Strategy—*Use the process of elimination to select the option that identifies the most accurate statement about scoliosis. Option 3 can be eliminated because it describes a significant spinal defect. Recall that the lateral curvature of the spine is more likely to affect organs in the thoracic cavity, making options 2 and 3 incorrect and option 4 the best answer. Review how the severity of scoliosis is determined and the consequence of allowing it to remain untreated if you had difficulty answering this question.*
Cognitive Level—*Analyzing*
Client Needs Category—*Health promotion and maintenance*
Client Needs Subcategory—*None*

102. 1. Curvatures between 20 and 40 degrees usually respond to nonsurgical treatment such as a Milwaukee brace. A Milwaukee brace is a large, cumbersome, full-torso brace that has a bar for the chin and back of the head. The brace is worn an average of 22 to 23 hours per day and should be removed only when the child is taking a bath or swimming. The brace will not cure the curve, but will prevent the progression of the curve. Usually braces are worn for several years until growth is complete. Currently there is an option for an underarm molded brace that is less detectable under clothing. However, this type of brace is not effective in curves of the upper spine, in which case a Milwaukee brace is preferable.
Test Taking Strategy—*Use the process of elimination to identify the option that provides accurate information. Options 2 and 3 can be eliminated because they describe lengthy periods during which the brace is*

not worn. Option 4 can be eliminated because the brace can be removed briefly; for example, while bathing, leaving option 1 as the correct option. Review information about the application of a Milwaukee brace and its use in treating scoliosis if you had difficulty answering this question.
Cognitive Level—*Applying*
Client Needs Category—*Physiological integrity*
Client Needs Subcategory—*Physiological adaptation*

103. **2.** Adolescents are very concerned about appearances and acceptance by their peer group. Because the Milwaukee brace must be worn almost continually, the nurse should discuss ways to help the child find appropriate, stylish attire that hides the brace. This should help the child feel more like peers and ensure better compliance with the treatment plan. The other options are inappropriate.

> *Test Taking Strategy*—*Use the process of elimination to identify the option that is best for promoting compliance in relation to wearing a brace. Options 1, 3, and 4 are not the most therapeutic methods for helping the client adapt and accept wearing the brace and do not foster adolescent socialization. Option 4 is the best answer because it reduces the potential for being identified as being different from peers. Review therapeutic measures for effecting coping, especially in relation to an adolescent whose condition affects self-image, if you had difficulty answering this question.*
Cognitive Level—*Applying*
Client Needs Category—*Health promotion and maintenance*
Client Needs Subcategory—*None*

Dosage Calculations for Children and Adolescents

104. **2.5 mL.**

$$\frac{\text{Desired dose}}{\text{Dose on hand}} \times \text{Total quantity} = X \text{ dose to administer}$$

$$\frac{125 \text{ mg}}{250 \text{ mg}} \times \frac{5 \text{ mL}}{1} = X$$

$$\frac{625}{250} = X$$

$$X = 2.5 \text{ mL}$$

> *Test Taking Strategy*—*Look for key information that facilitates calculating an accurate dosage such as the ordered dose of 125 mg and the supply dose of 250 mg/5 mL. Review the formula for calculating the dosage of oral liquid medication if you had difficulty answering this question.*
Cognitive Level—*Applying*
Client Needs Category—*Physiological integrity*
Client Needs Subcategory—*Pharmacological therapies*

105. **354 mg.**
Begin by converting pounds to kilograms:

$$52 \text{ pounds} \div 2.2 \text{ kg} = 23.6 \text{ kg}$$

Next, use the recommended dose range:

$$15 \text{ mg/kg} \times 23.6 \text{ kg} = 354 \text{ mg}$$

Highest single dose that would be safe: 354 mg

> *Test Taking Strategy*—*Look for key information that facilitates calculating an accurate dosage, such as the weight of the child and the recommended dose based on weight, which is 10 to 15 mg/kg. Review the mathematical process for calculating a dose based on weight if you had difficulty answering this question.*
Cognitive Level—*Applying*
Client Needs Category—*Physiological integrity*
Client Needs Subcategory—*Pharmacological therapies*

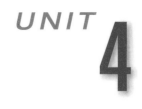

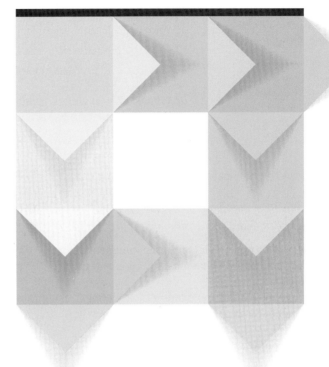

The Nursing Care of Clients with Mental Health Needs

15 The Nursing Care of Infants, Children, and Adolescents with Mental Health Needs

■ Mental Health Needs During Infancy
■ Mental Health Needs During Childhood
■ Mental Health Needs During Adolescence
■ Correct Answers, Rationales, and Test Taking Strategies

Directions: *With a pencil, blacken the space in front of the option you have chosen for your correct answer.*

Mental Health Needs During Infancy

A couple who has been childless for 10 years become parents of a newborn with Down syndrome.

1. To help the parents cope with their disappointment and loss of their "perfect" baby, which nursing action is most appropriate initially?
[ ] **1.** Encourage the parents to verbalize their feelings.
[ ] **2.** Recommend treating the child as a normal newborn.
[ ] **3.** Refer the couple to community resources for assistance.
[ ] **4.** Encourage the parents to consider long-term institutional placement.

When the nurse brings the baby to the mother's room, the father says, "These doctors don't know anything. We're going to consult specialists."

2. Which response by the nurse to the parents is most appropriate at this time?
[ ] **1.** "The physicians here are very well qualified."
[ ] **2.** "This diagnosis is difficult for you to accept."
[ ] **3.** "Why do you feel you need a second opinion?"
[ ] **4.** "It's not as bad as it may seem right now."

The nurse recognizes that the parents are working through the stages of grieving as a result of having a newborn with Down syndrome.

3. The nurse is most correct to support the parents as they move through the grieving process. Place the following stages of the grieving process in the chronologic order in which they will most likely occur. Use all the options.

1. Depression	
2. Anger	
3. Denial	
4. Bargaining	
5. Acceptance	

4. Which of the following information documented by the nurse provides the best evidence that the mother is bonding with her newborn with Down syndrome?
[ ] **1.** The mother smiles and talks to the baby.
[ ] **2.** The mother asks questions about infant care.
[ ] **3.** The mother wants to see visitors who come.
[ ] **4.** The mother feeds and burps the baby.

The nurse notes that the mother appears nervous when the newborn cries during the bath.

5. Which nursing action is most appropriate for the mother at this time?
[ ] **1.** Briefly take over bathing the newborn.
[ ] **2.** Advise the mother to discontinue the bath.
[ ] **3.** Give all future baths in the nursery.
[ ] **4.** Point out the good job being done.

6. As the infant's growth continues, which physical characteristic of Down syndrome is the nurse correct in describing to the parents?
[ ] **1.** Large head and curved index fingers
[ ] **2.** Long fingers and protruding tongue
[ ] **3.** Small head and upward-slanting eyes
[ ] **4.** Simian creases on the soles of the feet

A nurse is assigned to care for several infants in the newborn nursery.

7. Which withdrawal symptom is the nurse most likely to note while observing the newborn of a mother who used heroin during pregnancy?
[ ] **1.** Unresponsiveness
[ ] **2.** Dilated pupils
[ ] **3.** Persistent crying
[ ] **4.** Impaired sucking

8. When caring for a newborn experiencing opioid withdrawal, which nursing intervention should be included in the care plan initially?
[ ] **1.** Reduce environmental stimuli.
[ ] **2.** Touch the newborn frequently.
[ ] **3.** Stroke the newborn's skin gently.
[ ] **4.** Leave the newborn unwrapped.

The mother of the newborn who used heroin during her pregnancy brings the baby to the public health clinic for scheduled immunizations.

9. During the nursing assessment, which of the following suggests that the mother may be continuing to abuse heroin? Select all that apply.
[ ] **1.** The mother states, "I am so tired, I sleep when the baby sleeps."
[ ] **2.** The nurse notes a variety of small ecchymotic areas on the arms and legs of the mother.
[ ] **3.** The mother appears jittery with limited tolerance for the crying of the newborn.
[ ] **4.** The mother has a body odor and the newborn appears unkempt.
[ ] **5.** The mother expresses an inability to afford public transportation to the clinic.
[ ] **6.** The mother states that the father of the child is no longer associated with the family.

10. To ensure optimum mental health of an infant born with a congenital defect such as myelomeningocele, the nurse explains that it is essential for the parents to meet which of the following needs?
[ ] **1.** Autonomy
[ ] **2.** Love
[ ] **3.** Respect
[ ] **4.** Identity

A teenage mother brings her 6-month-old infant to the clinic. She tells the nurse that the baby cries a lot, and she is concerned that the baby is ill.

11. What information is most appropriate for the nurse to collect at this time?
[ ] **1.** The infant's weight and length
[ ] **2.** The infant's breath and heart sounds
[ ] **3.** The infant's head and chest circumference
[ ] **4.** The infant's sucking and grasp reflexes

On examination of the teenager's infant, no signs of illness are identified.

12. What information is most helpful for the nurse to obtain next?
[ ] **1.** The mother's expectations of an infant's behavior
[ ] **2.** How many more children the mother wants to have
[ ] **3.** If the mother plans to finish high school
[ ] **4.** The kinds of toys the mother has for the baby

The mother tells the nurse about being afraid that holding the infant will result in spoiling her baby, so she frequently puts the baby in the crib.

13. Which information given by the nurse to the teenage mother is most appropriate?
[ ] **1.** "Holding the infant fosters a sense of trust."
[ ] **2.** "Grandparents usually spoil babies."
[ ] **3.** "Babies need to be spoiled."
[ ] **4.** "Toddlers are more likely to be spoiled."

14. Which instruction is most important for the nurse to recommend to the teenage mother regarding parenting the infant?
[ ] **1.** "Give the baby a pacifier whenever the baby cries."
[ ] **2.** "Turn on a radio in the room with the baby."
[ ] **3.** "Cuddle and talk to the baby frequently."
[ ] **4.** "Place a brightly colored mobile above the crib."

15. If the teenage mother expresses feeling inexperienced and inadequate in caring for the baby, which referral is best?
[ ] **1.** Project Head Start
[ ] **2.** Planned Parenthood
[ ] **3.** Parent-Teacher Association
[ ] **4.** Parenting classes

16. The nurse is correct in assuming that without adequate nurturing during infancy, the child of the teenage mother is at risk for developing which psychosocial characteristic?
[ ] 1. Inferiority
[ ] 2. Mistrust
[ ] 3. Doubt
[ ] 4. Isolation

The teenage mother returns to the clinic 4 months later. After the nurse and pediatrician assess the infant, a diagnosis of failure to thrive is made.

17. Which assessment findings are most characteristic of a 10-month-old infant with the diagnosis of failure to thrive? Select all that apply.
[ ] 1. The infant cries vigorously when handled.
[ ] 2. The infant fails to achieve developmental milestones.
[ ] 3. The infant appears pale and lethargic.
[ ] 4. The infant eats vigorously when fed.
[ ] 5. The infant has delayed understanding of speech.

The nurse reviews the mother's history to identify factors that may have led to the diagnosis of the infant's failure to thrive.

18. Which of the following risk factors would the nurse expect to note when assessing the mother? Select all that apply.
[ ] 1. The pregnancy was unplanned and unwanted.
[ ] 2. The baby's father abandoned the mother.
[ ] 3. The mother is an adolescent.
[ ] 4. The mother's socioeconomic status is low.
[ ] 5. The mother has a history of alcohol and drug abuse.
[ ] 6. The mother has dropped out of high school.

Mental Health Needs During Childhood

A public health nurse assesses a 2-year-old at the immunization clinic.

19. Which assessment finding is most indicative that the child is developmentally delayed?
[ ] 1. The child is being bottle-fed.
[ ] 2. The child is not toilet-trained.
[ ] 3. The child has no language skills.
[ ] 4. The child cannot draw a picture.

20. Which test finding should the nurse review to more objectively assess the toddler's overall development?
[ ] 1. Denver II Developmental Screening Test
[ ] 2. Scholastic Aptitude Test (SAT)
[ ] 3. Stanford-Binet test
[ ] 4. Wechsler Intelligence Scale for Children test

21. If the mother asks the nurse how to appropriately discipline a child of this age, which response by the nurse is most appropriate?
[ ] 1. "Identify the consequences of unacceptable behavior before it happens."
[ ] 2. "Show disapproval immediately after an unacceptable act."
[ ] 3. "Administer some form of moderate physical punishment."
[ ] 4. "Explain to the toddler why certain behavior is undesirable."

A nursing assistant becomes frustrated by the 2-year-old child's persistent response of "No" whenever the child is asked to do something. The nursing assistant asks the nurse for help.

22. The nurse correctly explains that this is normal behavior for toddlers who are developing which psychosocial characteristic?
[ ] 1. Integrity
[ ] 2. Identity
[ ] 3. Autonomy
[ ] 4. Generativity

23. What is the best suggestion the nurse can give the nursing assistant caring for the 2-year-old child at this time?
[ ] 1. "Let the child choose from two acceptable alternatives."
[ ] 2. "Withhold something the child desires until the child complies."
[ ] 3. "Identify what is expected of the child, rather than ask."
[ ] 4. "Inform the mother if the child continues to be uncooperative."

A 3-year-old child is brought to the emergency department for a sudden, acute episode of an illness with vague symptoms. The child has a history of multiple hospital admissions. The health care team is beginning to suspect Munchausen syndrome by proxy.

24. If this diagnosis is accurate, it is most important for the nurse to assess for which characteristic finding?
[ ] 1. The mother is obsessed with the fear that her child will die.
[ ] 2. The mother is well versed in normal health patterns among children.
[ ] 3. The mother is responsible for creating the child's symptoms.
[ ] 4. The mother is overreacting to minor variations in her child's health.

A 3½-year-old child is scheduled for cardiac surgery. The parents are informed that hospitalization will be prolonged.

25. Which nursing strategy is best to help the child overcome the fear of being in the unfamiliar hospital environment?
[ ] **1.** Bringing a favorite blanket from home
[ ] **2.** Providing age-specific toys while hospitalized
[ ] **3.** Having one or both parents nearby at all times
[ ] **4.** Placing the child in a room with a same-aged child

The parents notice that their child resumed thumb sucking. They explain to the nurse that the child has not done so for more than a year.

26. Which response by the nurse provides the best explanation of the child's behavior?
[ ] **1.** "Thumb sucking is a primitive form of self-stimulation and security."
[ ] **2.** "Thumb sucking is a regressive behavior with a comforting effect."
[ ] **3.** "Thumb sucking substitutes for the missing fluids due to postoperative restriction of fluids."
[ ] **4.** "Thumb sucking satisfies the child's increased need for a familiar touch."

The nurse uses simple, age-appropriate language to explain to the child the purpose and procedure for starting an I.V. infusion.

27. Which additional nursing action is most beneficial for reducing the child's anxiety?
[ ] **1.** Tell the child that the pain will be minimal.
[ ] **2.** Offer the child a reward for good behavior.
[ ] **3.** Let the child handle some of the equipment.
[ ] **4.** Show the child others who have infusing fluids.

28. Which of the following behaviors exhibited by the child demonstrates the most severe reaction to prolonged hospitalization?
[ ] **1.** Clinging to the parents
[ ] **2.** Shaking the crib frantically
[ ] **3.** Thrashing about
[ ] **4.** Ignoring the parents

A parent brings her 2-year-old to the emergency department for treatment of a fractured femur.

29. Which assessment finding would lead the nurse to suspect physical abuse?
[ ] **1.** The child protests when approached by the nurse.
[ ] **2.** The child has patches of missing hair.
[ ] **3.** The child has a fresh bruise on the forehead.
[ ] **4.** The child has an abrasion on the right knee.

30. What information strongly suggests to the nurse that the child's fractured femur is the result of physical abuse?
[ ] **1.** There is evidence of healed fractures.
[ ] **2.** Only the mother witnessed the injury.
[ ] **3.** The child is not fully immunized yet.
[ ] **4.** The child is underweight for height.

After assessing for physical abuse, the nurse suspects that the toddler has also been sexually abused.

31. If the nurse's suspicions are true, which assessment findings require further investigation? Select all that apply.
[ ] **1.** The child demonstrates sexual activity with a doll.
[ ] **2.** The child has a gonorrheal infection.
[ ] **3.** The child is underweight for the corresponding height.
[ ] **4.** The child complains of burning during urination.
[ ] **5.** The child is afraid to be left alone with the suspected parent.
[ ] **6.** The child has trouble sleeping through the night.

32. Which nursing strategy is most appropriate for developing a positive, therapeutic relationship with the abused child at the time of assessment?
[ ] **1.** The nurse should make an effort to have prolonged eye contact with the child.
[ ] **2.** The nurse should maintain a body position at the same level as the child.
[ ] **3.** The nurse should separate the child from the parent during the interview.
[ ] **4.** The nurse should ask the child direct questions about the parent.

33. When the nurse gathers social data from a person suspected of child abuse, which one is most similar to the profile of other child abusers?
[ ] **1.** The person grew up in a divorced household.
[ ] **2.** The person's income is at or below poverty level.
[ ] **3.** The person was the victim of child abuse.
[ ] **4.** The person became a parent after age 25.

34. If the nurse suspects that a child is the victim of abuse, which nursing action is most appropriate to take initially?
[ ] **1.** Refer the parents to Parents Anonymous.
[ ] **2.** Recommend a court appointed legal guardian.
[ ] **3.** Contact a relative to care for the child.
[ ] **4.** Report the facts to child protective services.

35. When interacting with a person suspected of committing child abuse, which attitude on the part of the nurse is most conducive for facilitating a referral to a support group?
[ ] **1.** A friendly attitude
[ ] **2.** An indifferent attitude
[ ] **3.** A sympathetic attitude
[ ] **4.** A nonjudgmental attitude

The parents of a 3-year-old are distressed because their child has been publicly masturbating and ask a nurse for advice.

36. Which nursing suggestion is most helpful for preventing the child from feeling guilty about masturbating?
[ ] **1.** "Interrupt the child casually when masturbation is observed."
[ ] **2.** "Explain to the child that this is an unacceptable practice."
[ ] **3.** "Tell the child that the genitals can be touched only when urinating."
[ ] **4.** "Relate that touching the genitals is something that is done privately."

37. When a nurse observes a 4-year-old with a parent and infant sibling, which is the best evidence that the 4-year-old child is going through the developmental process called identification?
[ ] **1.** The child identifies animals correctly.
[ ] **2.** The child calls the sibling by name.
[ ] **3.** The child pretends to feed a doll.
[ ] **4.** The child accurately points to colors.

A pediatric office nurse prepares a 4-year-old child for his preschool physical examination. The child's mother has also brought her newborn for the first immunization.

38. Which of the mother's remarks is most indicative to the nurse that the preschooler is experiencing anxiety in relation to the new sibling?
[ ] **1.** The child wants to use his father's tools.
[ ] **2.** The child is taking shorter naps in the afternoon.
[ ] **3.** The child cries when toys become broken.
[ ] **4.** The child no longer controls his elimination.

39. The nurse correctly explains that the behavior the preschooler is demonstrating is based on which unmet need?
[ ] **1.** Powerfulness
[ ] **2.** Security
[ ] **3.** Self-confidence
[ ] **4.** Independence

40. Which nursing suggestion is most appropriate to give the preschooler's mother for relieving the 4-year-old child's anxiety?
[ ] **1.** "Give your child some new toys."
[ ] **2.** "Let your child stay up later at night."
[ ] **3.** "Invite the child's grandparents to visit."
[ ] **4.** "Spend more time alone with your child."

The parent of the 4-year-old child asks the nurse what is most helpful in preparing a preschooler for kindergarten.

41. Which nursing suggestion is likely to be most beneficial to the mother?
[ ] **1.** "Give the child simple responsibilities to perform."
[ ] **2.** "Teach the child to print first and last names."
[ ] **3.** "Buy a set of mathematic flash cards that teach addition."
[ ] **4.** "Have the child watch children's daytime television programs."

A mother states that when her 2-year-old child asks for candy at the grocery store and she refuses, the child throws a temper tantrum. She resorts to buying the candy so the child stops kicking and screaming.

42. What is the most appropriate nursing recommendation for eliminating the 2-year-old's tantrums?
[ ] **1.** "Give the child candy before entering the store."
[ ] **2.** "Ignore the child's unacceptable behavior."
[ ] **3.** "Explain to the child that this behavior is childish."
[ ] **4.** "Remind the child of how a big person acts."

The parents of a 3-year-old child with an autism spectrum disorder bring their child to a mental health clinic on a regular basis. Currently, a care conference is planned with the mental health team and the family.

43. When the social worker, who has not had experience with autistic children, asks the nurse to identify signs and symptoms of the disorder, the nurse correctly identifies which finding as most characteristic?
[ ] **1.** Repetitive body movements
[ ] **2.** Intense parental attachment
[ ] **3.** Early sexual development
[ ] **4.** Profound mental retardation

44. When providing care for the 3-year-old autistic child, which behavior is the nurse most likely to note?
[ ] **1.** Constant use of the words "I" and "me"
[ ] **2.** Self-injury without a pain response
[ ] **3.** Flexibility in normal routine
[ ] **4.** Increased interest in others' actions

45. When planning care for an autistic child, which nursing intervention is most appropriate?
[ ] **1.** Providing interactive play activities
[ ] **2.** Applying soft restraints while in bed
[ ] **3.** Using a consistent caregiver
[ ] **4.** Rocking the child as a calming technique

46. If the 3-year-old child is typical of other autistic children, how would the nurse expect the child to respond to its parents?
[ ] **1.** Indifference
[ ] **2.** Friendliness
[ ] **3.** Submissiveness
[ ] **4.** Impatience

47. On the basis of the nurse's knowledge of autistic behavior, which nursing diagnosis is most likely to be a priority at the team conference?
[ ] **1.** Ineffective health maintenance
[ ] **2.** Chronic low self-esteem
[ ] **3.** Risk for activity intolerance
[ ] **4.** Risk for self-directed violence

During the care conference, the parent of the autistic child says that the child helps to get dressed but will not eat independently unless fed by others.

48. Which suggestion by the nurse would be most beneficial for the child's nutrition at this time?
[ ] **1.** "Continue to feed the child until the child tries to pick up food."
[ ] **2.** "Try giving the child finger foods while in the act of dressing."
[ ] **3.** "Leave the food until the child becomes hungry enough to eat it."
[ ] **4.** "Demonstrate how to use a spoon at every meal."

49. If and when the autistic child actually makes an effort to self-feed, which of the following suggestions is most appropriate for the nurse to make?
[ ] **1.** "Note if the self-feeding effort is repeated."
[ ] **2.** "Stop feeding the child thereafter."
[ ] **3.** "Demonstrate approval in some way."
[ ] **4.** "Offer food more frequently during the day."

50. When discussing the home environment with the parents, the nurse should explain that which one of the following is the most appropriate environment for an autistic child?
[ ] **1.** Stimulating, with a variety of sensory experiences
[ ] **2.** Consistent, with a minimum of physical change
[ ] **3.** Flexible, with the freedom to initiate activity
[ ] **4.** Strict, with narrow limits for acceptable behavior

The parents express a desire to leave their autistic child with a responsible person for a few hours occasionally so that they can have relief from the responsibility of constant care and supervision.

51. Which is the most appropriate community resource for the nurse to recommend for respite services?
[ ] **1.** The Office of Family Assistance
[ ] **2.** The American Association on Mental Retardation
[ ] **3.** A local children's day-care facility
[ ] **4.** A home health care agency

The school nurse is conducting a class for parents whose children are about to enter first grade.

52. When describing the characteristic developmental stage of school-age children, which statement by the nurse is most accurate?
[ ] **1.** "School-age children begin developing long-lasting friendships."
[ ] **2.** "School-age children are learning to work beside and with others."
[ ] **3.** "School-age children are preoccupied with finding a purpose in life."
[ ] **4.** "School-age children are striving for independence from others."

The school nurse meets parents and their 7-year-old child to follow up on the child's progress since being diagnosed with attention deficit hyperactivity disorder (ADHD). The child is being treated with methylphenidate hydrochloride (Ritalin).

53. The nurse recognizes that methylphenidate hydrochloride (Ritalin) is classified as which type of drug?
[ ] **1.** Central nervous system depressant
[ ] **2.** Central nervous system stimulant
[ ] **3.** Antidepressant
[ ] **4.** Tranquilizer

54. The nurse advises the parents to look for which change as evidence that methylphenidate hydrochloride (Ritalin) is achieving its desired effect?
[ ] **1.** The child is more alert and active.
[ ] **2.** The child is less easily distracted.
[ ] **3.** The child does not seem fatigued.
[ ] **4.** The child's moods are more stable.

55. When the parents ask about the side effects of taking methylphenidate hydrochloride (Ritalin), the nurse correctly explains that the child may have which common cluster of signs and symptoms?
[ ] **1.** Nausea, vomiting, and diarrhea
[ ] **2.** Fatigue, drowsiness, and dry mouth
[ ] **3.** Insomnia, tachycardia, and anorexia
[ ] **4.** Hypotension, bradycardia, and constipation

56. Which assessment finding best indicates that a child taking methylphenidate hydrochloride (Ritalin) is experiencing an adverse effect?
[ ] **1.** The child has altered elimination patterns.
[ ] **2.** The child develops intolerance to certain foods.
[ ] **3.** The child has an elevated blood pressure.
[ ] **4.** The child has evidence of skin breakdown.

57. The nurse advises the parents of a child taking methylphenidate hydrochloride (Ritalin) that, to avoid potentiating the drug's effects, it is best if their child refrains from consuming which item?

[ ] **1.** Dairy products
[ ] **2.** Cola beverages
[ ] **3.** Processed meats
[ ] **4.** Saturated fats

The school nurse is working with the teacher to assist in providing the best education setting for the child with attention deficit hyperactivity disorder (ADHD).

58. Which of the following nursing interventions is most appropriate to include when preparing a care plan for the child in an educational setting?

[ ] **1.** Work with the teacher to establish clear behavioral expectations for the classroom.
[ ] **2.** Place a chair in the corner of the room as a potential consequence for poor behavior.
[ ] **3.** Allow the child to move about the room as desired provided the behavior is not disruptive.
[ ] **4.** Plan separate learning experiences with more creative assignments and activities.

An 8-year-old child is tentatively diagnosed with leukemia. A bone marrow puncture is part of the diagnostic workup.

59. When providing nursing care, if this child is typical of others the same age with a serious illness, which concept is the most commonly held belief about being ill?

[ ] **1.** Illness is not life-threatening; recovery is assured.
[ ] **2.** Significant others can prevent serious consequences.
[ ] **3.** Discomfort is a punishment for some wrongdoing.
[ ] **4.** Failure to comply with treatment results in parental rejection.

60. To minimize this child's apprehension about the bone marrow puncture, which nursing strategy is most appropriate?

[ ] **1.** Explain the procedure shortly before it is done.
[ ] **2.** Give the information as soon as the test is scheduled.
[ ] **3.** Postpone teaching about the procedure until specific questions are asked.
[ ] **4.** Wait for the physician to explain the procedure to the child and parents.

61. The nurse is aware that whenever preparing a school-age child for a procedure, test, or medical treatment, which is the most important information to convey?

[ ] **1.** When the procedure will take place?
[ ] **2.** Who will perform the procedure?
[ ] **3.** Where the procedure will be performed?
[ ] **4.** What will happen during the procedure?

The child fails to respond to drug therapy for leukemia, and the condition eventually becomes terminal. The parents are unsure of how, or if, they should tell their child about the prognosis.

62. Which rationale offered by the nurse is the best justification for openly discussing the child's prognosis?

[ ] **1.** The child will already have a sense that death is a possibility.
[ ] **2.** Sharing prevents the child from dealing with fears alone.
[ ] **3.** Concealing the truth will be very difficult.
[ ] **4.** Being less than honest is immoral and unethical.

63. Which outcome would the nurse expect to result from providing honest explanations, including discussion about unpleasant experiences, to produce in a seriously ill school-age child?

[ ] **1.** Confidence in caregivers
[ ] **2.** Perseverance in hardship
[ ] **3.** Courage in crises
[ ] **4.** Hope in suffering

A single parent consults the school nurse for help in dealing with an 8-year-old child who has been diagnosed with a learning disability.

64. Which nursing suggestion is most important for preserving the child's self-esteem?

[ ] **1.** Set realistic, achievable goals.
[ ] **2.** Obtain professional tutoring.
[ ] **3.** Help the child with homework.
[ ] **4.** Offer rewards for good grades.

A 9-year-old student is frequently absent from school. When the student attends school, the student talks out of turn, fights with classmates, moves about in the classroom during a lesson, and does not complete the assignments or homework. The student's current grades are inconsistent with past performance. The school nurse plans to speak with the student to determine if there is a health problem that is causing these changes.

65. Which approach is most appropriate when the school nurse speaks with the child?

[ ] **1.** Sit down at the lunch table together.
[ ] **2.** Arrange a meeting in the nurses' office before school.
[ ] **3.** Call the student aside in the hallway between classes.
[ ] **4.** Meet with the student on the playground during recess.

66. If the student reveals all the following information to the nurse, which situation is most likely affecting the recent acting-out behavior?

[ ] **1.** The student's parents are divorcing.
[ ] **2.** The student's favorite pet turtle just died.
[ ] **3.** The student just acquired a paper route.
[ ] **4.** The student is infatuated with a classmate.

The school nurse meets with the teacher to discuss the child's disruptive behavior.

67. Which approach would the nurse recommend for helping the child maintain acceptable behavior in school?
[ ] 1. Send the child to the principal's office when misbehaving.
[ ] 2. Suspend the child until a family conference has been conducted.
[ ] 3. Have the school counselor see the child on a daily basis.
[ ] 4. Consistently enforce reasonable limits for the child's behavior.

A school nurse observes four students who are all approximately 10 years old.

68. Which child in this group is most likely demonstrating behavior commonly associated with first-born children?
[ ] 1. The child who has a low tolerance for frustration
[ ] 2. The child who tends to compromise willingly
[ ] 3. The child who conforms to adult expectations
[ ] 4. The child who is flexible when given choices

A 9-year-old is brought to the emergency department with ketoacidosis secondary to undiagnosed type 1 diabetes mellitus.

69. If the following actions are observed by the nurse as the child improves, which one is the best indication the child is having difficulty accepting the diagnosis?
[ ] 1. The child stays up later than usual watching television.
[ ] 2. The child makes angry remarks to the nurse and parents.
[ ] 3. The child avoids completing homework assignments.
[ ] 4. The child talks on the phone for long periods of time.

70. If the nursing care plan includes the following activities, which one provides the newly diagnosed diabetic child with the most sense of control over the disease?
[ ] 1. Informing the child of laboratory test results
[ ] 2. Providing calorie-controlled dietary instructions
[ ] 3. Supervising self-testing of capillary blood glucose
[ ] 4. Teaching the child the parts of an insulin syringe

The nurse is caring for a 12-year-old who is being seen for Tourette's syndrome.

71. Besides helping the client and family cope with the child's repetitive, purposeless movements, which other problem associated with Tourette's syndrome is essential for the nurse to address?
[ ] 1. Verbal obscenities
[ ] 2. Social withdrawal
[ ] 3. Pathological lying
[ ] 4. Mood swings

72. The symptoms of which other condition that tends to occur concurrently with Tourette's syndrome should the nurse discuss with the parents?
[ ] 1. Schizophrenia
[ ] 2. Attention deficit hyperactivity disorder
[ ] 3. Bipolar disorder
[ ] 4. Obsessive-compulsive disorder

The physician prescribes haloperidol (Haldol) to treat the Tourette's syndrome. The nurse provides the child and parents with information about significant side effects.

73. Besides involuntary tremors, which other side effect should the nurse advise the family to anticipate?
[ ] 1. Muscle spasms
[ ] 2. Muscle weakness
[ ] 3. Muscle atrophy
[ ] 4. Muscle contractures

The parents tell the nurse that they are concerned their child's self-esteem may be jeopardized because of peer ridicule.

74. Which suggestion is most appropriate for the nurse to offer the parents in this situation?
[ ] 1. "Try home-schooling the child."
[ ] 2. "Praise accomplishments as deserved."
[ ] 3. "Avoid discussing peer comments."
[ ] 4. "Show disapproval of negative labels."

Mental Health Needs During Adolescence

A 13-year-old student takes a gun to school and murders a teacher.

75. On the basis of the principles of crisis intervention, when is the best time to provide assistance to those most affected by this incident?
[ ] 1. After the funeral
[ ] 2. Within 6 months
[ ] 3. Immediately
[ ] 4. Six weeks later

76. If the adolescents who witnessed the violence at school are typical of others who experience crises, how are they most likely feeling?
[ ] 1. Helpless
[ ] 2. Depressed
[ ] 3. Angry
[ ] 4. Fortunate

77. When crisis intervention is provided, which nursing action takes priority?
[ ] 1. Explaining the benefits of professional counseling
[ ] 2. Encouraging the survivors to talk about the event
[ ] 3. Reassuring the survivors that they will adapt
[ ] 4. Advising consulting a physician for drug therapy

A 15-year-old girl is being treated in an eating disorders unit for bulimia.

78. When reviewing the assessment data, the nurse would expect to note which characteristic physical finding?
[ ] **1.** Extremely low body weight
[ ] **2.** Erosion of dental enamel
[ ] **3.** Cessation of menstruation
[ ] **4.** Patchy loss of hair

A 17-year-old client is assessed in the emergency department and admitted to the hospital after fainting at school. The client is more than 25% below the normal weight for current height. The teenager is believed to be suffering from anorexia nervosa.

79. During the initial physical examination, the nurse is most likely to detect which finding related to anorexia?
[ ] **1.** Growth of fine body hair
[ ] **2.** Bruises over the upper torso
[ ] **3.** Hyperactive bowel sounds
[ ] **4.** Club-shaped fingertips

80. Which nursing assessment finding differentiates bulimia from anorexia nervosa bulimia in an adolescent with a suspected eating disorder?
[ ] **1.** Body image distortion
[ ] **2.** Purging after meals
[ ] **3.** Decreased self-esteem
[ ] **4.** Binge eating

The nurse reviews the teen's history obtained during admission.

81. Which of the following data best correlate with the profile of a person with anorexia nervosa?
[ ] **1.** The teen is the middle child of three siblings.
[ ] **2.** The teen is a high achiever in school and activities.
[ ] **3.** The teen thinks that classmates are not friendly.
[ ] **4.** The teen experienced many childhood illnesses.

The nursing team meets to plan the anorectic client's care.

82. Which nursing goal is the highest priority at this time?
[ ] **1.** To improve the client's distorted body image
[ ] **2.** To help the client use healthier coping techniques
[ ] **3.** To restore normal nutrition and health
[ ] **4.** To help the client develop assertiveness

The client's parent visits at dinnertime. The parent is overheard to say, "Look at you; you're so thin. Please eat something."

83. Which is most therapeutic for the nurse to say privately to the parent in this situation?
[ ] **1.** "All children know how to frustrate parents."
[ ] **2.** "You need to stop pleading with your child to eat."
[ ] **3.** "You're concerned that your child is starving."
[ ] **4.** "I know how you're feeling; I'm a parent, too."

The mental health technician is frustrated and angry when seeing the anorectic client rearranging the food on the tray but not eating any of it.

84. What is the best guidance the nurse can give the mental health technician caring for the anorectic client?
[ ] **1.** "Blend the food and administer it by tube feeding."
[ ] **2.** "Remind the client that the intake is being recorded."
[ ] **3.** "Review the treatment goals with the client again."
[ ] **4.** "Remove the food without making any comments."

Just before the anorectic client is weighed, the mental health technician tells the nurse that the client drank a full pitcher of water.

85. Which nursing action is most appropriate at this time?
[ ] **1.** Postpone weighing the client until later.
[ ] **2.** Confront the client about what was observed.
[ ] **3.** Say nothing and weigh the client as usual.
[ ] **4.** Subtract 2 lb (0.9 kg) from the client's weight.

A 16-year-old with a cognitive disability is admitted for treatment of a ruptured appendix. The parent reports that the teenager has an intelligence quotient (IQ) in the range of 35 to 50, which approximates that of a 5- to 7-year-old child.

86. If this cognitively disabled client is typical of others of this mental age, what is the nurse most likely to observe?
[ ] **1.** Distress when separated from the mother
[ ] **2.** An exaggerated response to pain
[ ] **3.** Difficulty making his or her needs known
[ ] **4.** Concern over the change in body image

87. If the admitting nurse documents all of the following parental behaviors, which behavior is most likely to suppress this child's ability to reach the maximum potential for development?
[ ] **1.** The parent dresses and undresses the teen.
[ ] **2.** The parent answers all the medical questions.
[ ] **3.** The parent exaggerates the teen's abilities.
[ ] **4.** The parent assumes blame for the teen's condition.

While attempting to help the cognitively disabled adolescent out of bed, the nursing assistant is struck by the teenager.

88. Which nursing statement is the best explanation for the adolescent's behavior?
[ ] **1.** "Aggression is a common behavior manifested by cognitively disabled people."
[ ] **2.** "Aggression is a response that occurs when a person feels threatened."
[ ] **3.** "Aggression is an indication that the client has a poor opinion of the care provided."
[ ] **4.** "Aggression is a common way for adolescents to communicate they are experiencing pain."

89. When the nurse documents the episode during which the client acted out, which wording is best?
[ ] **1.** "Became angry for no reason and an assault occurred."
[ ] **2.** "Hit caregiver unexpectedly even though not provoked."
[ ] **3.** "Struck nursing assistant when being helped from bed."
[ ] **4.** "Attacked nursing assistant without prior warning."

The cognitively disabled client's behavioral outburst is discussed at a team conference.

90. Of the following suggestions, which one would best prevent nursing personnel from becoming injured when providing the adolescent with care?
[ ] **1.** Apply soft wrist restraints before ambulating the client.
[ ] **2.** Ask a parent to care for the client.
[ ] **3.** Explain steps involved in care before touching the client.
[ ] **4.** Medicate the client immediately before ambulation.

A 16-year-old is brought to the emergency department for treatment of a stab wound after a gang-related fight. The teenager is eventually ordered by the court to receive counseling at the community mental health clinic.

91. Which area of the adolescent's social history is most appropriate for the clinic nurse to assess?
[ ] **1.** Peer relationships
[ ] **2.** School performance
[ ] **3.** Church attendance
[ ] **4.** Employment records

92. If the nurse obtains the following data, which factor has the strongest influence on the teenager's development of antisocial behavior?
[ ] **1.** Parental discipline is inconsistent.
[ ] **2.** There are more than three siblings.
[ ] **3.** The family relies on public welfare.
[ ] **4.** Role models do not value education.

93. What information is most important for the nurse to communicate before each group meeting?
[ ] **1.** The date and time of the next meeting
[ ] **2.** The qualifications of the participating therapists
[ ] **3.** That everyone should use first names only
[ ] **4.** That client information is kept confidential

94. If the adolescent demonstrates the following behaviors during group meetings, which is most indicative to the nurse that the client is resisting therapy?
[ ] **1.** The adolescent borrows cigarettes from others.
[ ] **2.** The adolescent laughs inappropriately.
[ ] **3.** The adolescent keeps checking the clock.
[ ] **4.** The adolescent fidgets in the chair.

Family therapy is included in the counseling plan for the adolescent gang member. The client's parent arrives late and is intoxicated.

95. If the adolescent is typical of others who have grown up in an alcoholic family, the nurse would expect to assess for problems in which area?
[ ] **1.** Low self-esteem
[ ] **2.** Managing stress
[ ] **3.** Long-term learning
[ ] **4.** Fear of authority

96. Of the following community resources, which referral is the nurse most likely to suggest for this client?
[ ] **1.** Alcoholics Anonymous
[ ] **2.** Al-Anon
[ ] **3.** Alateen
[ ] **4.** The Substance Abuse Council

97. If the adolescent benefits from therapy that focuses on growing up in an alcoholic household, the nurse is most likely to observe the adolescent developing an ability to do what?
[ ] **1.** Keep promises
[ ] **2.** Trust others
[ ] **3.** Solve problems
[ ] **4.** Honor commitments

A 16-year-old boy has been selected to play on the junior varsity football team. He spends several hours a day in a weight-training facility.

98. When the gym owner asks the teenager if he would like a performance enhancing drug to help increase muscle mass, on what basis is the nurse most accurate in predicting the teen will accept?
[ ] **1.** Several teammates are taking this drug.
[ ] **2.** The team is having a winning season.
[ ] **3.** His parents support his interest in football.
[ ] **4.** He can afford to pay for a substantial supply.

After the adolescent takes the unidentified drug for some time, his weight increases dramatically and his muscles become larger and well-defined.

99. If the unprescribed drug is an anabolic steroid, the nurse is most likely to identify which assessment finding?
[ ] **1.** Enlarged genitalia
[ ] **2.** Bronzed skin
[ ] **3.** Worsened acne
[ ] **4.** Brittle nails

100. Which of the following are behavioral effects of anabolic steroids?
[ ] **1.** Aggression and rage
[ ] **2.** Confusion and doubt
[ ] **3.** Anxiety and depression
[ ] **4.** Paranoia and suicidal ideation

After being suspended from the team for taking anabolic steroids, the teenager tells his parents, "I might as well be dead. My football career is over." The parents call the physician's office asking for help.

101. When the office nurse reviews the current laboratory findings of the client who abuses anabolic steroids, which laboratory test finding is most likely to be abnormal?

[ ] **1.** Thyroid function
[ ] **2.** Liver function
[ ] **3.** Electrolyte panel
[ ] **4.** Blood count

The nurse warns the football player's parents that their son's statements suggest a potential for suicide.

102. Which additional warning signs of suicide should the nurse identify for the parents? Select all that apply.

[ ] **1.** Withdrawal
[ ] **2.** Apathy
[ ] **3.** Angry outbursts
[ ] **4.** Alcohol abuse
[ ] **5.** Delusions
[ ] **6.** Incoherent speech

A 17-year-old has been dating a classmate secretly because the relationship is a constant source of parental conflict. She has also stopped attending church and started smoking cigarettes—something her parents strongly dislike—and she has had sexual intercourse. She has not had a menstrual period for 2 months.

103. When the teenager makes an appointment at a birth control clinic, which nursing attribute is most important to communicate during the initial meeting?

[ ] **1.** Efficiency
[ ] **2.** Intelligence
[ ] **3.** Sympathy
[ ] **4.** Acceptance

104. Which nursing action best conveys an interest in this client and her situation?

[ ] **1.** Making frequent eye contact with her
[ ] **2.** Providing her with free clinic literature
[ ] **3.** Writing down information the client provides
[ ] **4.** Avoiding long pauses between questions

As the adolescent talks with the clinic nurse, she reveals that her parents disapprove of her friends, ideas, and actions.

105. Based on the nurse's knowledge of child development, when adolescents test previously accepted values, which developmental need is being aquired? It is normal for adolescents to test previously accepted values in order to acquire which developmental attribute?

[ ] **1.** Ingenuity
[ ] **2.** Identity
[ ] **3.** Intuition
[ ] **4.** Insight

The receptionist calls the nurse out of the room and tells her that the teenager's mother is on the phone asking why her daughter is being seen.

106. After conferring with the nurse, which response by the receptionist to the mother is most appropriate at this time?

[ ] **1.** "The clinic cannot release that information."
[ ] **2.** "Your daughter will return the phone call shortly."
[ ] **3.** "You may talk to your daughter after her examination."
[ ] **4.** "Your daughter came to the clinic for birth control."

A pregnancy test is performed before a method of birth control is prescribed for the adolescent client. The test result is positive.

107. After receiving the news about her pregnancy, which of the following social data collected by the nurse will be most beneficial to the pregnant adolescent at this time?

[ ] **1.** The teen appears to have a mothering instinct.
[ ] **2.** The teen is making immediate plans for marriage.
[ ] **3.** The teen expects financial support from her boyfriend.
[ ] **4.** The teen has an emotionally supportive family.

A nursing assistant asks the nurse why the pregnant adolescent asked for contraceptive assistance when she probably suspected she was pregnant already.

108. The nurse correctly explains that this client's behavior is an example of which psychological defense mechanism?

[ ] **1.** Displacement
[ ] **2.** Regression
[ ] **3.** Denial
[ ] **4.** Compensation

The parents of an 18-year-old bring their child to a mental health clinic after the child reports hearing voices that say, "You're a bad person."

109. When the parents ask if their child is psychotic, the nurse who is performing the initial interview is most correct in explaining which of the following as a behavior exhibited by psychotic people?

[ ] **1.** They adjust poorly to new situations.
[ ] **2.** They have difficulty in relationships.
[ ] **3.** They cannot differentiate reality from unreality.
[ ] **4.** They feel helpless in resolving problems.

110. When performing a brief check of the client's mental status, which question is most appropriate when the nurse assesses the client's orientation?

[ ] **1.** "What is today's date?"
[ ] **2.** "How did you get here?"
[ ] **3.** "Where were you born?"
[ ] **4.** "Who is the current president?"

As the nurse is documenting in the notes, the hallucinating client asks to read what the nurse is writing.

111. Which nursing action is most appropriate in this situation?
[ ] **1.** Asking the client why he or she is so suspicious
[ ] **2.** Putting the notes away immediately
[ ] **3.** Handing the client the form to read
[ ] **4.** Explaining that it is illegal to read the notes

The 18-year-old client refuses to be admitted to the psychiatric unit of the local hospital.

112. Which nursing explanation regarding involuntary hospital admittance is most accurate?
[ ] **1.** A person cannot be committed involuntarily unless the client is uncooperative at this time.
[ ] **2.** A person cannot be committed involuntarily unless the client poses harm to self or others.
[ ] **3.** A person cannot be committed involuntarily unless the client cancels office appointments.
[ ] **4.** A person cannot be committed involuntarily unless the client refuses to take medications.

The psychiatrist prescribes haloperidol (Haldol), an antipsychotic drug for this client.

113. Which nursing instruction is most appropriate when teaching a client who self-administers haloperidol (Haldol)?
[ ] **1.** "Take the pills on an empty stomach."
[ ] **2.** "Do not skip meals while taking the drug."
[ ] **3.** "Stop taking the drug if sedation occurs."
[ ] **4.** "Rise slowly from a sitting position."

114. Which of the following is the best indication that haloperidol (Haldol) is achieving a therapeutic effect?
[ ] **1.** The client no longer hears voices.
[ ] **2.** The client sleeps more than before.
[ ] **3.** The client thinks of himself or herself as a good person.
[ ] **4.** The client feels more energetic and rested.

Another client is prescribed clozapine (Clozaril), an atypical antipsychotic medication. The client is not feeling well and calls the physician's office for advice.

115. When the client reports the following physical changes to the office nurse, which sign or symptom is considered a serious side effect of clozapine that needs to be reported immediately to the prescribing physician?
[ ] **1.** Frequent diarrhea
[ ] **2.** Severe sore throat
[ ] **3.** Gradual weight loss
[ ] **4.** Ringing of the ears

Correct Answers, Rationales, and Test Taking Strategies

Mental Health Needs During Infancy

1. 1. Verbalizing feelings is an appropriate step toward processing emotional trauma. Emphasizing the newborn's normalcy regardless of the cognitive ability and referring the parents to agencies that provide early intervention would be appropriate eventually, after the parents have had time to react emotionally themselves. It would be inappropriate for the nurse to encourage the parents to seek institutionalization. Any decisions about how to care for their child should be left up to the parents.
> *Test Taking Strategy*—Look at the key words "most appropriate initially," in reference to helping parents cope with disappointment and loss. Although options 2 and 3 are attractive choices, facilitating the parents' verbalization (option 1) is the best initial nursing action. If you had difficulty answering this question, remember that verbalization of feelings helps with the coping process.
Cognitive Level—Applying
Client Needs Category—Psychosocial integrity
Client Needs Subcategory—None

2. 2. Reflecting is an effective communication technique that involves responding to both the feelings and the verbalized content. Reflecting requires empathic responses that facilitate further therapeutic interaction. Defensiveness (option 1) is a nontherapeutic communication technique that implies to the parents that their feelings and actions are unnecessary and foolish. Asking a "why" question (option 3) demands an explanation from the client. This form of communication is nontherapeutic because most clients are not able to verbalize their rationales. Disagreeing (option 4) implies that the parents have no right to feel as they do.
> *Test Taking Strategy*—Analyze to determine what information the question asks for, which is the most appropriate response to the parent's statement. Recall that reflecting is a therapeutic communication technique. Review therapeutic and nontherapeutic communication techniques if you had difficulty answering this question.
Cognitive Level—Applying
Client Needs Category—Psychosocial integrity
Client Needs Subcategory—None

3.

3. Denial

2. Anger

4. Bargaining

1. Depression

5. Acceptance

Grieving is a highly individual experience based on one's coping mechanisms, life experiences, resources, and support system. Although the grieving process encompasses five stages and in many cases follows a progressive course, the parents who are coping with the loss of their "perfect" baby will need to work through the various stages of grief in their own particular order and on their own timeline.

Generally, the first stage of grief involves shock and disbelief, which results in denial. Denial is a coping mechanism that eases the anxiety and pain of the experience. During this stage, the parents ask, "Why me?" and require proof that something is wrong (such as needing to see laboratory values and X-rays). They may request second, third, or fourth opinions; they also may minimize the child's condition, making it seem less serious than it really is.

Anger, the second stage, is commonly directed at others (such as the other spouse, baby, health care provider, or hospital services). The parents may verbalize the unfairness of the situation. They may even express their anger by focusing on inconsequential things such as the light being too bright.

During the bargaining stage (typically, the third stage), the parents try to correct their actions and bargain with God or a higher power. They promise to be a better spouse or parent in an attempt to fix the problem.

Depression, the fourth stage of grieving, is commonly manifested by crying. The parents feel sad and alone and begin planning how to tell their family or friends. Acceptance, the last stage of the grieving process, is characterized by the parents' ability to make plans for their child's future; they may also return to work or their normal routine during this stage.

> *Test Taking Strategy*—Analyze to determine what information the question asks for, which is sequencing the stages of grieving in their usual order of occurrence. Review the stages of grieving, noting the order in which they commonly occur, if you had difficulty answering this question.
> *Cognitive Level*—Remembering
> *Client Needs Category*—Psychosocial integrity
> *Client Needs Subcategory*—None

4. 1. Evidence of bonding includes eye contact, skin contact, touching and stroking, smiling and talking to the infant, and cuddling. Other evidence involves providing basic care, such as changing the baby's diaper and feeding the baby. The other behaviors are normal and appropriate, but they are not the best evidence of bonding.

> *Test Taking Strategy*—Use the process of elimination to help select the option that describes the best evidence of maternal-infant bonding. Options 2 and 3 can be eliminated because they do not reflect any interaction with the infant. Although option 4 may appear attractive, it describes performing tasks rather than a behavior that promotes an emotional bond. Review signs of maternal-infant bonding if you had difficulty answering this question.
> *Cognitive Level*—Applying
> *Client Needs Category*—Psychosocial integrity
> *Client Needs Subcategory*—None

5. 4. Allowing the mother to provide basic care promotes bonding. A mother's self-concept and self-confidence are increased when the nurse offers supportive encouragement. Interfering with parenting skills contributes to parental feelings of insecurity and decreases the mother's confidence.

> *Test Taking Strategy*—Look at the key words "most appropriate" as they refer to a nursing action when a nervous mother bathes a crying infant. Recall that positive reinforcement generally builds self-confidence and the likelihood that the mother will persevere and continue to feel empowered to bathe the infant comfortably in the future. Review outcomes of positive reinforcement if you had difficulty answering this question.
> *Cognitive Level*—Analyzing
> *Client Needs Category*—Psychosocial integrity
> *Client Needs Subcategory*—None

6. 3. A small head, upward-slanting eyes, protruding tongue, curved little finger, round face, flat nose, and simian creases on the palms are characteristic of the physical features of someone with Down syndrome.

> *Test Taking Strategy*—Analyze to determine what information the question asks for, which is a statement that describes a physical manifestation of an infant with Down syndrome. Options 1, 2, and 4 contain incorrect information. Only option 3 includes findings that are all characteristic of Down syndrome. Review the characteristics associated with Down syndrome if you had difficulty answering this question.
> *Cognitive Level*—Remembering
> *Client Needs Category*—Physiological integrity
> *Client Needs Subcategory*—Physiological adaptation

7. 3. Withdrawal from heroin and other abused drugs, whether in a newborn or an adult, is characterized by symptoms somewhat opposite of the drug's action. For example, in heroin withdrawal, newborns are typically hyperactive and irritable, cry constantly, and are unable to be consoled. These particular symptoms place the infant at high risk for child abuse. They are also poor feeders, putting them at risk for failure to thrive.

Test Taking Strategy—Analyze to determine what information the question asks for, which is a sign of an infant's withdrawal from an opiate. Persistent crying (option 3) is the best choice because it describes behavior associated with physiologic stimulation. Review signs of opiate withdrawal in a newborn if you had difficulty answering this question.
Cognitive Level—Applying
Client Needs Category—Psychosocial integrity
Client Needs Subcategory—None

8. 1. Because opioid withdrawal is characterized by central nervous system stimulation, reducing environmental stimuli is a priority when caring for a newborn experiencing its effects. Touching and stroking increase tactile stimuli and are more appropriate when caring for normal newborns. Most infants, including those experiencing withdrawal, are comforted by being wrapped snugly in a blanket.

Test Taking Strategy—Look at the key word "initially" in reference to an appropriate nursing intervention when caring for a newborn during opiate withdrawal. Recall that opiate withdrawal causes central nervous system stimulation. Option 1 is the best choice because it would control stimulating the infant. Review techniques for managing the care of an infant withdrawing from an opiate if you had difficulty answering this question.
Cognitive Level—Analyzing
Client Needs Category—Psychosocial integrity
Client Needs Subcategory—None

9. 2, 3, 4. Heroin is a very addictive narcotic drug. The mother is at high risk for relapse. The nurse should be aware and assess for potential signs of relapse. Having a variety of ecchymotic areas on the arms and legs could indicate that the mother is injecting heroin into the veins. The mother's jitteriness and intolerance of the baby's crying could be indications of withdrawal from a recent use of heroin. Physical withdrawal from opiates is extremely unpleasant. Health problems can result from self-neglect of physical needs. An indication of self-neglect can be the unkempt look of the mother and baby. These considerations are cause for further questioning by the nurse. New mothers are commonly tired as the baby is up frequently at night. It is a good health practice to sleep when the baby sleeps. Neither being unable to afford public transportation nor no longer associating with the baby's father indicates that the mother is abusing heroin.

Test Taking Strategy—Analyze to determine what information the question asks for, which is signs of heroin abuse. Alternative-format "select all that apply" questions require considering each option independently to decide its merit in answering the question. Read the information in the rationale for possible signs of relapse. Review signs of opiate abuse if you had difficulty answering this question.
Cognitive Level—Applying
Client Needs Category—Psychosocial integrity
Client Needs Subcategory—None

10. 2. Meeting an infant's need for love is one of the best foundations for future mental health, regardless of the child's physical or mental status. Love helps the child feel secure and helps the child build self-esteem and trust in others. The needs for autonomy, respect, and identity are also important, but they represent higher-level needs.

Test Taking Strategy—Look at the key word "essential," which indicates a priority. In this case, the question is asking for the most important need to foster when caring for an infant, which is option 2. Review Maslow's hierarchy of needs, which lists the need for love and belonging as having a higher priority than the need for self-esteem or the need for self-actualization, if you had difficulty answering this question.
Cognitive Level—Applying
Client Needs Category—Health promotion and maintenance
Client Needs Subcategory—None

11. 1. Excessive crying is a manifestation of infantile anxiety. Severe anxiety leads to weight loss and stunted, slowed growth, commonly referred to as *failure to thrive*. Failure to thrive can occur from an unsatisfactory relationship with a caregiver. Listening to the heart and breath sounds and measuring the head and chest are appropriate, but they do not readily indicate how this child's growth compares with norms for infants of the same age. Assessing the sucking and grasp reflexes is more appropriate for a newborn infant.

Test Taking Strategy—Look at the key words "most appropriate … at this time" in relation to a nursing assessment that is pertinent for confirming or ruling out an inexperienced mother's concern that her infant's crying indicates illness. Validating that the infant is thriving or not would be reflected in a normal or lower than expected weight, identified in option 1. The other options identify appropriate nursing assessments, but they are not the best nursing assessment initially. Review manifestations of a failure to thrive if you had difficulty answering this question.
Cognitive Level—Analyzing
Client Needs Category—Physiological integrity
Client Needs Subcategory—Physiological adaptation

12. 1. A certain amount of crying is normal for an infant because it is the baby's only means of communicating distress. How a parent reacts to the baby's crying is important. Finding out the parent's expectations helps the nurse determine whether the parent has a realistic perception of the infant's behavior. The other selections do not provide significant additional data needed to analyze the young parent's concern.

Test Taking Strategy—Analyze to determine what information the question asks for, which is a nursing assessment that is indicated after confirming that the infant is not ill. Option 1 is the best choice because, depending on the answer, it helps the nurse clarify normal infant behavior and how to cope with situations that are stressful for the inexperienced mother. Review methods for determining the causes of stress for the mother of an infant if you had difficulty answering this question.
Cognitive Level—Analyzing
Client Needs Category—Health promotion and main-
tenance
Client Needs Subcategory—None

13. 1. "Spoiling a baby" is a commonly used phrase that refers to the notion that frequent holding, cuddling, or immediately responding to an infant's cries ultimately promotes the infant's dependence on the caregiver. Holding the baby promotes the acquisition of trust, a developmental characteristic acquired in infancy. However, neglecting and isolating an infant promotes stress and affects normal development. Infants cannot develop negative effects from being held and touched in an affectionate manner, and they are extremely sensitive to the attitudes and actions of those caring for them. All humans, not just babies or toddlers, need physical and social contact with other humans for adequate nurturing.

Test Taking Strategy—Look at the key words "most appropriate" in reference to nursing information that is accurate and promotes the well-being of the infant. Option 1 clarifies that holding an infant promotes a feeling of safety and security and does not generally spoil an infant. Review measures for promoting growth and development of an infant if you had difficulty answering this question.
Cognitive Level—Applying
Client Needs Category—Health promotion and main-
tenance
Client Needs Subcategory—None

14. 3. Touching and hearing a parent's voice are essential for optimal emotional growth during infancy. Receiving affectionate sensory stimulation helps the infant develop a feeling of trust, the major developmental task during infancy. Inanimate sensory stimulation is appropriate, but physical human interaction is a priority.

Test Taking Strategy—Use the process of elimination to help select the option describing the most important recommendation for parenting from among the options. Recalling Erikson's developmental stage of infancy and the task associated with it leads to selecting option 3, because cuddling and talking to the baby is a means of promoting trust. Options 1, 2, and 4 can be eliminated because they lack any emotional relationship for the infant. Review the developmental tasks associated with the stages of infancy through adolescence if you had difficulty answering this question.
Cognitive Level—Applying
Client Needs Category—Health promotion and main-
tenance
Client Needs Subcategory—None

15. 4. People with expertise in successful child-rearing techniques teach parenting classes. Participants learn by imitating and modeling the behaviors of others in the group. Group members support one another by sharing common experiences. Project Head Start is for preschool children. Planned Parenthood is concerned with family planning. Parent-teacher associations are for parents of school-age children.

Test Taking Strategy—Use the process of elimination to help select the option that identifies an organization that will help an inexperienced mother gain confidence. Read the purposes and missions of the organizations that are identified in the rationale. Review the advantages provided by attending parenting classes if you had difficulty answering this question.
Cognitive Level—Applying
Client Needs Category—Safe and effective care environment
Client Needs Subcategory—Coordinated care

16. 2. Mistrust is the characteristic most likely to develop if infants are not nurtured adequately. Such infants begin to view the world as unsafe and unreliable. The other characteristics—inferiority, doubt, and isolation—are negative attributes acquired at later stages of unfulfilled development.

Test Taking Strategy—Analyze to determine what information the question asks for, which is a negative characteristic acquired during infancy. Recalling Erikson's developmental stage of infancy and possible characteristics that are acquired at that time leads to selecting option 2, because if the infant's need for security is not met, the infant acquires mistrust. Review Erikson's developmental tasks associated with the stages of infancy through adolescence if you had difficulty answering this question.

Cognitive Level—Applying
Client Needs Category—Health promotion and
maintenance
Client Needs Subcategory—None

17. **2, 3, 5.** Failure to thrive is a condition in which the infant falls below the third percentile for weight and length. There are two main reasons why this occurs: organic causes that result from congenital or other physiologic problems, and nonorganic causes that result from poor maternal bonding and lack of parenting skills. Nonorganic causes are regarded as a form of child neglect. In some cases, failure to thrive results from a combination of both causes.

Typical characteristics of an infant who is diagnosed with failure to thrive include a delay in developmental milestones after about the third month and delayed understanding of speech related to the lack of interaction. These infants are typically pale and lethargic. They lack subcutaneous fat, making them thin and wrinkled, often with skin breakdown. They do not cry when handled, but instead stare intensely at people who approach. They are often poor feeders because they lack the strength to eat.

> *Test Taking Strategy—Analyze to determine what information the question asks for, which is signs and symptoms of failure to thrive. Alternative-format "select all that apply" questions require considering each option independently to decide its merit in answering the question. Select options that reflect evidence that the infant's growth and development are behind those associated with a normal infant of similar age. Review growth and development of infants between ages 4 and 6 months if you had difficulty answering this question.*
> *Cognitive Level—Analyzing*
> *Client Needs Category—Health promotion and maintenance*
> *Client Needs Subcategory—None*

18. **1, 2, 3, 4, 5.** Several maternal risk factors—all nonorganic causes—can potentially lead to failure to thrive. Most are associated with an interruption in the maternal attachment process or inadequacy of parenting skills. These risks include an unplanned or unwanted pregnancy, maternal history of teenage pregnancy, alcohol or drug abuse, low socioeconomic status, and a father who is no longer available to provide support. The fact that the mother has dropped out of high school is not necessarily a risk factor for failure to thrive.

> *Test Taking Strategy—Analyze to determine what information the question asks for, which is maternal risk factors for failure to thrive. Alternative-format "select all that apply" questions require considering each option independently to decide its merit in answering the question. Select options that contribute to an infant's failure to thrive. Review psychosocial characteristics of high-risk mothers if you had difficulty answering this question.*

Cognitive Level—Applying
Client Needs Category—Psychosocial integrity
Client Needs Subcategory—None

Mental Health Needs During Childhood

19. **3.** A 2-year-old child typically uses at least single words like "no" and "me" to make ideas understood. Therefore, the absence of language skills would suggest a developmental delay. The other behaviors do not necessarily indicate delayed development. Most children begin drinking from a glass and toilet-training at this stage of development. The ability to draw a picture depends on the development of fine motor skills, which typically begins during the toddler stage with scribbling and is refined as the child grows older and is able to draw simple figures and pictures.

> *Test Taking Strategy—Look at the key words "most indicative" as they relate to identifying an option that describes a delay in expected development of a toddler. Option 3 is most significant because a toddler is generally communicating verbally in some way unless the toddler has a hearing deficit. Review when language skills develop in toddlers if you had difficulty answering this question.*
> *Cognitive Level—Applying*
> *Client Needs Category—Health promotion and maintenance*
> *Client Needs Subcategory—None*

20. **1.** The Denver II Developmental Screening Test measures four major areas of development and can identify developmental delays from infancy through preschool ages. The Scholastic Aptitude Test (SAT) is administered to high school students and is a predictor of academic success. The Stanford-Binet test and the Wechsler Intelligence Scale for Children are IQ (intelligence) tests.

> *Test Taking Strategy—Analyze to determine what information the question asks for, which is a method for objectively determining the toddler's state of development. Recall the purposes of the other diagnostic tests listed, which leads to selecting option 1 as the best answer. Review the purpose for administering the Denver II Developmental Screening Test if you had difficulty answering this question.*
> *Cognitive Level—Remembering*
> *Client Needs Category—Health promotion and maintenance*
> *Client Needs Subcategory—None*

21. **2.** Demonstrating disapproval immediately after unacceptable behavior helps the child associate the undesirable behavior with negative consequences. This approach takes time and consistent reinforcement, but it is the most appropriate form of discipline for a toddler. Toddlers are too young to control their impulses just by identifying potential consequences or receiving explanations for behavioral expectations. Physical punishment tends to teach impressionable youngsters that it is appropriate to be physically violent.

Test Taking Strategy—Look at the key words "most appropriate" as they refer to a method for disciplining a toddler. Recall that a child of this age does not have the capacity to understand logic. Because their actions tend to be impulsive, they are more likely to change their behavior if a parent follows the principle of "cause and effect." In other words, if an unacceptable behavior is immediately followed by a negative consequence, it is more likely to create a learned response. Review the effects of positive and negative reinforcement in relation to learning if you had difficulty answering this question.
Cognitive Level—Analyzing
Client Needs Category—Health promotion and maintenance
Client Needs Subcategory—None

22. 3. To exercise autonomy, toddlers often become defiant and refuse to cooperate with requests, routines, and regulations. At this time, the toddler does not understand the need to abide by rules and requests outside of his or her wants. This often frustrates parents who are trying to guide the toddler. The psychosocial characteristics of integrity, identity, and generativity are acquired at later stages of development.

Test Taking Strategy—Analyze to determine what information the question asks for, which is an accurate explanation for negativity in a toddler. Recall that according to Erikson, toddlers are acquiring autonomy (option 3) at this age, which is evidenced by asserting himself or herself. Review Erikson's developmental tasks associated with early childhood if you had difficulty answering this question.
Cognitive Level—Applying
Client Needs Category—Health promotion and maintenance
Client Needs Subcategory—None

23. 1. To avoid a power struggle, it is best to give the child an opportunity to choose between two acceptable alternatives. Withholding something desirable is not likely to meet with success because a child of this age tends to be quite oppositional when challenged. The child is too young to comprehend abstract explanations. Informing the mother is not likely to change the child's behavior.

Test Taking Strategy—Use the process of elimination to help select the option that identifies the best suggestion for managing the care of a child who is developing autonomy. Option 2 can be eliminated because it uses a power struggle to acquire a toddler's change in behavior. Option 3 can be eliminated because

it exceeds the toddler's cognitive ability. Option 4 can be eliminated because it turns responsibility for managing the toddler's behavior onto the mother rather than the surrogate caregiver, who is the nursing assistant in this case. Option 1 emerges as the best choice because it supports the toddler's autonomy. Review Erikson's developmental tasks associated with early childhood if you had difficulty answering this question.
Cognitive Level—Applying
Client Needs Category—Safe and effective care environment
Client Needs Subcategory—Coordinated care

24. 3. A parent causing physical symptoms in a dependent child is characteristic of Munchausen syndrome by proxy. Consequently, the victim (typically a young child) is subjected to a variety of unnecessary medical procedures. The parent's sole purpose in intentionally producing an illness in a dependent child is to draw attention to the parent for the pain or work associated with caring for an ill child. This condition is considered a form of child abuse and must be reported to the authorities. A parent's fear of the child dying does not automatically make the nurse think of a Munchausen syndrome by proxy diagnosis. Being knowledgeable about developmental norms is important for parents as the child grows. Overreacting to minor health variations is not a characteristic sign of Munchausen syndrome by proxy.

Test Taking Strategy—Use the process of elimination to help select the option that provides the most accurate description of the role of a caregiver with Munchausen syndrome by proxy in relation to the person manifesting physical symptoms. The correct etiology is identified in option 3. Review the psychopathology involved in Munchausen syndrome by proxy if you had difficulty answering this question.
Cognitive Level—Applying
Client Needs Category—Psychosocial integrity
Client Needs Subcategory—None

25. 3. Having one or both parents within sight and touch helps to prevent separation anxiety and provides one of the best coping strategies for dealing with the pain and suffering that the child may experience. The other options listed have secondary therapeutic value.

Test Taking Strategy—Use the process of elimination to help select the option that identifies the best approach for reducing fear in a toddler who must be hospitalized. Although modeling is a method for promoting desired behavior, option 4 does not indicate that the same-aged child is necessarily coping well with his or her fears. Option 2 can be eliminated because toys may distract the child, but they don't reduce fear. Option 1 appears attractive because it represents an item that correlates with a safe and

secure environment, but it is not as beneficial as the presence of a parent, who the child looks to for protection from harm. Review methods for relieving real or imagined fears experienced by a toddler if you had difficulty answering this question.
Cognitive Level—Applying
Client Needs Category—Health promotion and maintenance
Client Needs Subcategory—None

26. 2. Regressive behavior such as thumb sucking is considered a coping mechanism that relieves anxiety. Given the child's circumstances and behavioral observations among others who have experienced stressful situations, this is the most credible explanation among the options listed for the phenomenon.
Test Taking Strategy—Use the process of elimination to help select the option that identifies the best explanation for the resumption of thumb sucking by a toddler. Option 1 can be eliminated because it identifies a reason an infant may have begun sucking the thumb. Option 3 can be eliminated because the toddler's need for fluid should be met through parenteral administration of fluid if oral fluids are restricted. Option 4 may appear attractive, but thumb sucking is not done to meet a need for touch. Option 2 emerges as the best answer because it explains the relationship between resuming a once-abandoned comforting behavior with regression to an earlier age. Review regression as it relates to behavior if you had difficulty answering this question.
Cognitive Level—Applying
Client Needs Category—Psychosocial integrity
Client Needs Subcategory—None

27. 3. Handling equipment whenever possible helps children overcome some of their initial fears. It is important to be honest with children when procedures involve pain. However, the term "minimal" is relative; from the child's perspective, the pain may be more than minimal. Bribing a child by offering a reward is not a therapeutic means of gaining cooperation. Seeing others who have I.V. lines will not necessarily diminish the child's unique feelings and expectations concerning the upcoming procedure.
Test Taking Strategy—Analyze to determine what information the question asks for, which is a beneficial action for reducing a toddler's anxiety in addition to using simple, age-appropriate language. Option 3 can reduce a child's anxiety because children of this age are tactile learners. Handling the equipment may provide some degree of familiarity and reality, which may dispel imagined fears concerning their use. Review learning styles of toddlers if you had difficulty answering this question.
Cognitive Level—Applying
Client Needs Category—Psychosocial integrity
Client Needs Subcategory—None

28. 4. The toddler who is ignoring the parents is practicing a form of detachment, the third stage in typical hospital adjustment. This stage represents the most severe reaction that can occur in a toddler who is hospitalized for a prolonged time. All the remaining options characterize the initial (protest) stage of hospital adjustment. The second (despair) stage is characterized by apathy and withdrawal.
Test Taking Strategy—Look at the key words "most severe reaction" and "to prolonged hospitalization." Children tend to withdraw as an emotional protective mechanism when exposed to a prolonged stressful situation. Review manifestations of impaired adjustment to hospitalization from a toddler's perspective if you had difficulty answering this question.
Cognitive Level—Analyzing
Client Needs Category—Psychosocial integrity
Client Needs Subcategory—None

29. 2. Hair of varying lengths or bald areas may be attributed to pulling on the child's hair during abusive acts. The nurse who finds this during a physical assessment should suspect child abuse. A 2-year-old child is typically very curious and clumsy. It is not unusual to find bruises and abrasions over bony prominences (such as elbows and knees) sustained during falls. However, a bruise over soft tissue such as the abdomen should arouse suspicion. It is also not unusual for a toddler to protest when approached by a health care provider, especially if past experiences with health care providers have been unpleasant.
Test Taking Strategy—Analyze to determine what information the question asks for, which is a finding that suggests the cause of a child's injury is due to abuse rather than accidental trauma. Option 1 can describe a normal response in some children. Options 3 and 4 describe normal physical findings in a toddler. Option 2 is the best answer because such hair loss may be due to abusive hair pulling. Review signs of childhood physical abuse if you had difficulty answering this question.
Cognitive Level—Applying
Client Needs Category—Psychosocial integrity
Client Needs Subcategory—None

30. 1. One classic sign of physical abuse is evidence of scars, bruises, and fractures in varying stages of healing. Being underweight and not fully immunized may raise suspicions of neglect or that the family is financially needy; however, these findings alone do not strongly suggest abuse. Injuries can occur without an adult witness.
Test Taking Strategy—Analyze to determine what information the question asks for, which is a finding that suggests that the cause of a child's injury is abuse. Options 3 and 4 may suggest neglect rather than abuse. Option 2 may be a normal finding. Option 1 is the best answer because it offers a classic sign of

physical abuse. Review signs of childhood physical abuse if you had difficulty answering this question.
Cognitive Level—*Applying*
Client Needs Category—*Psychosocial integrity*
Client Needs Subcategory—*None*

31. **1, 2, 4, 5, 6.** Any sexual activity between a child younger than age 18 years and an adult is classified as sexual abuse. Signs of sexual abuse include demonstrating sexual acts on a doll or other toy, having a sexually transmitted disease (such as gonorrhea), being afraid to be left alone with the perpetrator, and difficulty sleeping (or napping). Other signs of sexual abuse include discussing sexual acts with heightened awareness and vocabulary for the child's age; pregnancy younger than age 15; vaginal or anal tearing; perineal, anal, or vaginal inflammation; symptoms of increased anxiety, such as tics, stuttering, or nail biting; and poor school performance. Burning on urination, especially in young girls, may be a sign of a urinary tract infection; this is not uncommon in toddlers and preschoolers due to poor hygiene and wiping techniques during toileting. However, it does require further investigation because it may be related to a sexually transmitted infection or sexual abuse. Being underweight may be a sign of neglect, not sexual abuse.
Test Taking Strategy—*Analyze to determine what information the question asks for, which is assessment findings suggestive of sexual abuse. Alternative-format "select all that apply" questions require considering each option independently to decide its merit in answering the question. Select all the options that reflect sexual abuse of a toddler. Review signs of childhood sexual abuse if you had difficulty answering this question.*
Cognitive Level—*Applying*
Client Needs Category—*Psychosocial integrity*
Client Needs Subcategory—*None*

32. **2.** The nurse should be positioned at a young child's level, regardless of the reason for interaction, to reduce the child's risk of feeling threatened. Prolonged eye contact tends to heighten anxiety. Victims of child abuse often protect their abusers. Therefore, separating the child from the mother and asking direct questions are not appropriate strategies; they also do not promote a positive nurse–client relationship.
Test Taking Strategy—*Look at the key words "most appropriate" in reference to an approach for developing a positive therapeutic relationship with a child. Recall that positioning oneself at the same level of the client promotes trust and reduces power, authority, and judgment conveyed by a nurse who positions himself or herself higher than the client. Review nonverbal techniques for promoting and*

interfering with therapeutic communication if you had difficulty answering this question.
Cognitive Level—*Analyzing*
Client Needs Category—*Psychosocial integrity*
Client Needs Subcategory—*None*

33. **3.** Commonly, child abusers have been victims of child abuse. Although there are significant stressors for persons raised by a single parent or who are not financially secure, these factors are not uniquely contributory to child abuse. Parents who abuse their children are more often young and immature when the violence begins.
Test Taking Strategy—*Analyze to determine what information the question asks for, which is a characteristic of child abusers. Recall that abuse tends to be perpetuated across generations, making option 3 the best answer. Review factors that contribute to abuse if you had difficulty answering this question.*
Cognitive Level—*Applying*
Client Needs Category—*Psychosocial integrity*
Client Needs Subcategory—*None*

34. **4.** Nurses are among those required by law to report suspected child abuse. Not reporting suspected child abuse is considered a crime. The child protective services agency is responsible for finding a temporary and safe environment such as foster care for the child in future danger. Parents Anonymous is an organization that provides support to those who wish to break the cycle of child abuse. However, the priority at this time is the child's safety.
Test Taking Strategy—*Look at the key words "most appropriate" and "initially," which indicate the need to select an option describing the first nursing action when child abuse is suspected. Recall that nurses, teachers, and others involved in a relationship with a child are legally obligated to report their suspicions of abuse to authorities, as identified in option 4. Proof of abuse is not a requirement for reporting. Review legal aspects related to reporting child abuse if you had difficulty answering this question.*
Cognitive Level—*Analyzing*
Client Needs Category—*Safe and effective care environment*
Client Needs Subcategory—*Coordinated care*

35. **4.** Perpetrators of child abuse, as well as those with other social problems, are more likely to be receptive to seeking help if the nurse conveys a nonjudgmental attitude during the interaction. The other options are not necessarily inappropriate, but they are unlikely to motivate clients toward self-help.
Test Taking Strategy—*Look at the key words "most conducive" as they relate to an attitude that creates a therapeutic relationship with a client who needs*

support for dealing with abuse issues. A nonjudg-mental attitude (option 4) is the best approach to take when encouraging abusers to seek help. Review methods for promoting a therapeutic nurse-client relationship if you had difficulty answering this question.
Cognitive Level—*Applying*
Client Needs Category—*Psychosocial integrity*
Client Needs Subcategory—*None*

36. 4. Giving the child permission to masturbate privately sets limits as to where this is done but does not imply that masturbation is a deviant behavior. Interrupting the practice or providing the child with another alternative may temporarily stop the activity; however, the child would not understand the reason for the diversion. The other choices imply that experiencing pleasure from touching one's body is objectionable.

> *Test Taking Strategy*—*Look at the key words "most helpful" in relation to a method for reducing potential guilt associated with childhood masturbation. Knowing that the behavior is likely to be repeated because it is pleasurable, it is best to provide parameters by which masturbation, a fairly normal activity, can be devoid of judgment as to its morality. Option 1 has merit, but it is not likely to reduce the potential for guilt, making option 4 the best answer. Review suggestions for managing incidences of childhood masturbation if you had difficulty answering this question.*
Cognitive Level—*Applying*
Client Needs Category—*Health promotion and maintenance*
Client Needs Subcategory—*None*

37. 3. Feeding a doll (or changing the doll's diaper or clothes) is most suggestive of the identification process. Identification is behavior that imitates the same-sex parent or other adult. The other behaviors are examples of the child's cognitive development.

> *Test Taking Strategy*—*Look at the key words "best example" as they refer to the process of identification demonstrated in a child's behavior. Imitating the behavior of a parent (option 3) is an example of identification. Review how identification is demonstrated if you had difficulty answering this question.*
Cognitive Level—*Applying*
Client Needs Category—*Health promotion and maintenance*
Client Needs Subcategory—*None*

38. 4. A preschooler who is not accustomed to sharing attention may feel that the new child is taking his or her place. The preschooler may behave like an infant to regain attention or may resort to behavior manifested during an earlier period of development (such as wetting and soiling himself) to feel more secure. It is normal for a 4-year-old child to begin identifying with and imitating the same-sex parent (such as trying to use his father's tools). Preschoolers begin to need less daytime sleep. At this age, crying is a natural emotional response to disappointing events.

> *Test Taking Strategy*—*Analyze to determine what information the question asks for, which is a manifestation of childhood anxiety brought on by the birth of a new sibling. Recall that regression, in this case, can be an attention-getting mechanism as the preschooler perceives a rivalry with the new sibling. This knowledge leads to selecting option 4 as the best answer. Review regression as well as manifestations of sibling rivalry if you had difficulty answering this question.*
Cognitive Level—*Applying*
Client Needs Category—*Health promotion and maintenance*
Client Needs Subcategory—*None*

39. 2. Anxiety occurs when a person perceives a threatening situation. The perceived threat creates a feeling of insecurity. Mental mechanisms (also known as ego defense mechanisms) such as regression are unconsciously or subconsciously used to eliminate or reduce conflict, protect one's self-image, and resolve an emotional dilemma.

> *Test Taking Strategy*—*Analyze to determine what information the question asks for, which is an explanation of the basis for using the ego defense mechanism known as regression. Regression may be used to protect the self in a situation that provokes anxiety and thus insecurity (option 2). Review ego defense mechanisms and the purpose they serve if you had difficulty answering this question.*
Cognitive Level—*Analyzing*
Client Needs Category—*Psychosocial integrity*
Client Needs Subcategory—*None*

40. 4. Anxiety that results from competing for attention is diminished if the parent spends time alone with the child. The other options are appropriate interventions, but they will not necessarily relieve the child's anxiety.

> *Test Taking Strategy*—*Look at the key words "most appropriate" as they refer to advice on a method for relieving a preschooler's anxiety relative to sibling rivalry. Recall that the child is seeking more parental attention, making option 4 the best answer. Review measures for managing sibling rivalry if you had difficulty answering this question.*
Cognitive Level—*Applying*
Client Needs Category—*Health promotion and maintenance*
Client Needs Subcategory—*None*

41. 1. A school-age child must learn to follow directions and carry out a task. Therefore, providing the preschooler with tasks within the level of accomplishment promotes success and a positive feeling about self-competence. Printing the first name may be beneficial, but printing both first and last names is a skill not usually accomplished by 4-year-olds. A preschooler usually has no immediate use for flash cards that teach addition. This skill is typically reserved for 7- to 8-year-old children in first and second grades. Daytime television programs are not necessarily educational.

Test Taking Strategy—Look at the key words "most beneficial" as they refer to a suggestion for preparing a preschooler for kindergarten. Recall that the initial school experience requires sharing with others and following directions from someone other than a parent. This leads to selecting option 1 as the best answer. Review the activities that are appropriate to the level of a 3- to 5-year-old child in preparation for beginning school if you had difficulty answering this question.
Cognitive Level—Analyzing
Client Needs Category—Health promotion and maintenance
Client Needs Subcategory—None

42. 2. Children learn how to manipulate others through certain types of behavior. When a child realizes that a tantrum will not obtain the desired result, the child will most likely discontinue that behavior. Therefore, ignoring the behavior is the best choice. Giving candy beforehand contradicts the principle that candy is not allowed at this time. A young child is more likely to behave based on emotions rather than intellectual logic. Therefore, the preschool child is not likely to accept an explanation about the inappropriateness of the behavior or pleas to act differently.

Test Taking Strategy—Look at the key words "most appropriate" in reference to a technique for eliminating a toddler's temper tantrums. Recall that ignoring undesirable behavior is a form of negative reinforcement that leads to its extinction. Review negative versus positive methods of reinforcing behavior and their outcomes if you had difficulty answering this question.
Cognitive Level—Analyzing
Client Needs Category—Psychosocial integrity
Client Needs Subcategory—None

43. 1. Autism is a psychiatric condition with no known cause. More common among boys, this disorder is characterized by unawareness of external reality, limited or no social interaction, abnormal speech patterns and conversational ability, preoccupation with repetitive behaviors, and a low range of interest in self or others. Autistic children tend to display bizarre body movements. For example,

they rock their bodies, bang their heads, or touch their hands to their faces in peculiar mannerisms. If these movements are interrupted, violent temper tantrums may result. None of the other items describes characteristics of autism.

Test Taking Strategy—Analyze to determine what information the question asks for, which is the most accurate characteristic manifested by a child with autism. Recall that those affected by autism display repetitive, purposeless, and often self-injurious physical mannerisms, making option 1 the best choice. Review manifestations of childhood autism if you had difficulty answering this question.
Cognitive Level—Analyzing
Client Needs Category—Psychosocial integrity
Client Needs Subcategory—None

44. 2. Autistic children are prone to repetitive body movements such as continuous hand clapping. If the behavior is interrupted, they often act impulsively, becoming aggressive causing self-injury. Therefore, they commonly demonstrate insensitivity to pain. Mental retardation is common; diagnosis depends on the clinical presentation and the child's inability to reach developmental milestones. Because of their abnormal speech patterns and inability to communicate effectively, autistic children rarely use the words "I" and "me." Autistic children are also prone to rigid routines, and they show little to no interest in the actions of others.

Test Taking Strategy—Analyze to determine what information the question asks for, which is a behavior commonly manifested by those with childhood autism. Recall that autistic children can be severely self-abusive. Most individuals who do not have autism would cease an action that causes pain, but that is not the case in autism. If you had difficulty answering this question, review the signs and symptoms associated with autism.
Cognitive Level—Applying
Client Needs Category—Psychosocial integrity
Client Needs Subcategory—None

45. 3. A consistent caregiver or primary nurse facilitates development of a trusting relationship. Autistic children have a limited ability to interact with others. Restraints are inappropriate to use on a continual basis because they increase the risk of injury; close supervision is preferred. Rocking is inappropriate because autistic children do not easily tolerate physical contact.

Test Taking Strategy—Look at the key words "most appropriate" as they relate to a planned nursing intervention when caring for a child with autism. Recall that children with autism do not do well with change. Providing consistency, whether with caregivers, the environment, or lifestyle activities, helps promote the child's ability to cope with circum-

stances others may tolerate better. Review nursing interventions for managing the care of a child with autism if you had difficulty answering this question.
Cognitive Level—*Analyzing*
Client Needs Category—*Safe and effective care environment*
Client Needs Subcategory—*Coordinated care*

46. 1. The characteristics of autism are divided into three categories: inability to relate to others, inability to communicate with others, and limited activities and interests. Autistic children tend to show little or no ability to relate to other humans, including their parents. All the remaining examples require interaction with and response to one or more people. This is unrealistic for a child with autism.
Test Taking Strategy—Analyze to determine what information the question asks for, which is the response that is typical of an autistic child to his or her parents. Recall that the term autism implies "unto oneself." Those affected with this disorder tend to lack empathy and the ability to interact with others, which leads to selecting option 1 as the best answer. Review the behavioral characteristics of those affected by autism if you had difficulty answering this question.
Cognitive Level—*Applying*
Client Needs Category—*Health promotion and maintenance*
Client Needs Subcategory—*None*

47. 4. One common behavior among autistic children is a tendency to cause self-harm by head banging, biting, and pulling out hair and fingernails. An autistic child is incapable of, or not responsible for, maintaining his or her own health. Self-esteem is established on the basis of receiving approval or disapproval from others. Because an autistic child is indifferent to the physical presence and opinion of others, low self-esteem is not likely to be a problem. An autistic child's general physical health is unaffected by the mental disorder. Therefore, if the child cannot tolerate activity, it is due to another, unrelated condition.
Test Taking Strategy—Look at the key words "most likely" and "priority," indicating a problem of highest importance when planning the care of a client with autism. Recall that protecting the client from self-injury reflects the first level of Maslow's hierarchy of needs. Although options 1 and 3 also reflect physiologic needs, they are not problems generally experienced by a child with autism. Review the manifestations of autism in relation to the list of nursing diagnoses in the options if you had difficulty answering this question.
Cognitive Level—*Applying*
Client Needs Category—*Safe and effective care environment*
Client Needs Subcategory—*Coordinated care*

48. 1. Children with autism have varying levels of impairment and require full assistance with some or all activities of daily living. When the child demonstrates an attempt at self-feeding, it is appropriate to encourage the child to participate in this aspect of self-care. Learning takes place when a person is ready. Until an autistic child demonstrates some interest, attempts to gain cooperation are likely to be frustrating for the child and the parent.
Test Taking Strategy—Look at the key words "most beneficial" in reference to a suggestion for managing an autistic child's seeming lack of interest in feeding himself or herself. Recall that the child's intake of food is important for health. If and when the child makes an effort to participate, it is important to seize the opportunity to facilitate more involvement in self-feeding. Review motivation in relation to participating in self-care if you had difficulty answering this question.
Cognitive Level—*Analyzing*
Client Needs Category—*Physiological integrity*
Client Needs Subcategory—*Basic care and comfort*

49. 3. Rewards, even in the form of praise, tend to promote repetition of a desired behavior. Noting whether the behavior is repeated is appropriate, but it is not the best technique to use first. It would be unrealistic to expect the child to continue self-feeding after only one attempt. Giving the child more food does not necessarily encourage self-feeding behavior; if it does, obesity is a possible consequence.
Test Taking Strategy—Look at the key words "most appropriate" as they relate to a nursing response to an autistic client's initial efforts at self-feeding. Recall that positive reinforcement potentiates the likelihood that a behavior will be repeated. Praise is a form of positive reinforcement, making option 3 the best choice. Review the outcomes associated with positive and negative forms of reinforcement if you had difficulty answering this question.
Cognitive Level—*Analyzing*
Client Needs Category—*Psychosocial integrity*
Client Needs Subcategory—*None*

50. 2. If an autistic child's possessions, routines, or environment are altered, the child is likely to become upset and combative toward others or self. A stimulating environment creates chaos and distress for an autistic child. A flexible environment with no routines causes anxiety; the child cannot appreciate choices within the flexibility. Limit setting is important, but a rigid, inflexible atmosphere can be distressing.
Test Taking Strategy—Look at the key terms "most appropriate" in reference to the environment best suited for a child with autism. Recall that inconsistency and change are met with acting-out physically

and emotionally, making option 2 the best answer. Review the nursing and home care for managing a client with autism if you had difficulty answering this question.
Cognitive Level—*Analyzing*
Client Needs Category—*Psychosocial integrity*
Client Needs Subcategory—*None*

51. 4. Private home health care agencies employ various levels of health practitioners. An agency of this type selects the surrogate caregiver most appropriate for the type of client and level of care needed. The Office of Family Assistance is a federal agency that administers the Temporary Assistance for Needy Families (TANF) program. TANF is a social welfare program that provides economic assistance to a parent who is unable to financially support the care of one or more children. The American Association on Mental Retardation is concerned with people who are mentally retarded, not mentally ill. Mental retardation usually begins in childhood and is characterized by deficits in intellect and motor and adaptive skills. Autism, however, is a psychiatric (mental) illness with no known cause. Mental illness is a term that describes a broad range of mental and emotional conditions. Most day-care facilities do not provide evening care and might not accept a child with special needs.

 Test Taking Strategy—Analyze to determine what information the question asks for, which is the most appropriate community resource for providing respite care of an autistic child. Recall that a home health care provider offers personnel who provide care; a certified nursing assistant, licensed practical nurse, or registered nurse may provide whatever type of home care is needed (option 4). The other options do not specifically serve this population. Review the types of services provided by the various resources listed in the options if you had difficulty answering this question.
Cognitive Level—*Applying*
Client Needs Category—*Safe and effective care environment*
Client Needs Subcategory—*Coordinated care*

52. 2. Children between the ages of 6 and 11 are acquiring industry, which is characterized by learning to work beside and cooperatively with others. They learn to accept success and defeat, and how to give support to others. The other characteristics are associated with later stages of development.

 Test Taking Strategy—Look at the key words "most accurate" in reference to a characteristic of a school-age child's stage of development. Recall that school-age children are involved in learning, creating, and accomplishing numerous new skills and knowledge, thus developing a sense of industry, which is best identified by the statement in option 2.

Review the activities associated with the development of a person who is school age if you had difficulty answering this question.
Cognitive Level—*Applying*
Client Needs Category—*Health promotion and maintenance*
Client Needs Subcategory—*None*

53. 2. Methylphenidate hydrochloride (Ritalin) is a central nervous system stimulant that acts primarily on the cerebral cortex. The drug decreases hyperactivity and impulsiveness and appears to act in a manner similar to amphetamines. Methylphenidate is effective in 70% to 80% of children.

 Test Taking Strategy—Analyze to determine what information the question asks for, which is the class of drugs to which methylphenidate belongs. Recall that methylphenidate is a central nervous system stimulant that helps those affected by attention deficit hyperactivity disorder (ADHD) to focus on completing a task despite being a stimulant. Review the classification and mechanism of action for methylphenidate if you had difficulty answering this question.
Cognitive Level—*Remembering*
Client Needs Category—*Physiological integrity*
Client Needs Subcategory—*Pharmacological therapies*

54. 2. Some of the chief characteristics of attention deficit hyperactivity disorder (ADHD) include distractibility, difficulty following directions, inability to remain focused on a task, and difficulty sustaining attention. Relief of these symptoms indicates a therapeutic response. Although methylphenidate hydrochloride (Ritalin) is a central nervous system stimulant, it should not cause a child to be more alert, active, or less fatigued than the child was before treatment with the drug. In fact, overstimulation indicates a nontherapeutic or adverse response to the drug. Methylphenidate may cause a child to be less irritable and aggressive, but altering mood is not the primary reason for administering this drug.

 Test Taking Strategy—Analyze to determine what information the question asks for, which is evidence of a therapeutic effect manifested by a child who is receiving methylphenidate to manage symptoms of ADHD. Recall that one of the purposes in prescribing this drug is to reduce distractibility, which will facilitate learning and improve behavior in social and school environments (option 2). Review the desired effects in response to drug therapy with methylphenidate if you had difficulty answering this question.
Cognitive Level—*Analyzing*
Client Needs Category—*Physiological integrity*
Client Needs Subcategory—*Pharmacological therapies*

55. 3. Because methylphenidate hydrochloride (Ritalin) is a central nervous system stimulant, side effects reflect overstimulation, as evidenced by insomnia, tachycardia, and anorexia. Some people experience an intense degree of these symptoms, even with low dosages. The remaining adverse effects are not associated with this particular drug.

> *Test Taking Strategy*—Analyze to determine what information the question asks for, which is the side effects associated with the drug methylphenidate. Recall that methylphenidate is a central nervous system stimulant that could result in the signs and symptoms in option 3. Review the side effects of methylphenidate if you had difficulty answering this question.
> *Cognitive Level*—Remembering
> *Client Needs Category*—Physiological integrity
> *Client Needs Subcategory*—Pharmacological therapies

56. 3. Hypertension is an adverse effect of methylphenidate hydrochloride (Ritalin), which may necessitate switching to a non-stimulating drug such as atomoxetine (Straterra). Food intolerances, altered elimination patterns, and altered skin integrity are not associated with this drug.

> *Test Taking Strategy*—Use the process of elimination to help select the option that identifies the best description of an undesirable side effect associated with methylphenidate. Recall that elevated blood pressure (option 3) is a sign of central nervous system stimulation that has the potential for cardiovascular and cerebrovascular complications. Review the side effects of methylphenidate if you had difficulty answering this question.
> *Cognitive Level*—Applying
> *Client Needs Category*—Physiological integrity
> *Client Needs Subcategory*—Pharmacological therapies

57. 2. Caffeine is present in 75% of all soft drinks. It is an ingredient in all cola products, except those labeled "caffeine-free." Caffeine is a stimulating drug that contributes to overstimulation in a child who is taking methylphenidate hydrochloride (Ritalin).

> *Test Taking Strategy*—Analyze to determine what information the question asks for, which is a dietary product that should be avoided by someone who takes methylphenidate. Recall that methylphenidate is a central nervous system stimulant. Therefore, foods and beverages that also cause physiologic stimulation, such as caffeine (option 2), should be avoided. Review health teaching that is appropriate for those who take or administer methylphenidate if you had difficulty answering this question.
> *Cognitive Level*—Applying
> *Client Needs Category*—Physiological integrity
> *Client Needs Subcategory*—Pharmacological therapies

58. 1. When planning an educational setting care plan, it is most important that the teacher and student have a clear understanding of behavioral expectations. It is essential that the teacher set and maintain consistent limits. Understanding and abiding by the behavioral expectations is a goal for the student. Reminders of consequences such as a chair in the corner of the room are educationally inappropriate and may lower the child's self-esteem. Allowing the child to move about the room is disruptive to others and does not allow the student to focus on the tasks at hand. There is no need to have a separate learning assignment or activity. By understanding the student's needs, the teacher can ensure that the student has the potential to function at the same level as the other students.

> *Test Taking Strategy*—Look at the key words "most appropriate" when applied to a collaborated plan for managing the classroom experiences of a child with ADHD. Whenever there are behavioral problems, regardless of the cause, it is important that everyone involved understands what is and isn't allowed and the consequences if expectations are not met. Option 1 correlates with this principle. Review the purpose for setting limits when there is a potential for behavioral problems if you had difficulty answering this question.
> *Cognitive Level*—Analyzing
> *Client Needs Category*—Safe and effective care environment
> *Client Needs Subcategory*—Coordinated care

59. 3. School-age children tend to view disease and its treatment as a form of punishment, even though they cannot identify the transgression. They have anxiety related to the hospitalization and often perceive parental anxiety. Although school-age children consider adults to be quite powerful, they are aware that serious illnesses have unpredictable outcomes.

> *Test Taking Strategy*—Analyze to determine what information the question asks for, which is a common belief about illness from the perspective of a school-age child. Option 3 correctly describes the belief of many school-age children that illness equates with punishment. Review health beliefs that are common among children if you had difficulty answering this question.
> *Cognitive Level*—Applying
> *Client Needs Category*—Health promotion and maintenance
> *Client Needs Subcategory*—None

60. 1. School-age children tend to fantasize and exaggerate a potentially unpleasant experience. Therefore, it is best to avoid providing information far in advance. However, the child may be totally unprepared if the teaching is postponed until questions are asked or if the nurse assumes that the physician will provide all the information the child needs to know.

> *Test Taking Strategy—Look at the key word "most appropriate" as it relates to a nursing approach for minimizing a child's apprehension before a bone marrow puncture. Recall that the longer a child thinks about the procedure, the greater the chances that the degree of apprehension will increase. Imagined fears tend to overwhelm reality; thus, providing an explanation shortly before the procedure is done (option 1) is the best approach for reducing apprehension. Review principles of teaching clients who are school-age, especially in relation to reducing fear and apprehension, if you had difficulty answering this question.*
> **Cognitive Level**—*Applying*
> **Client Needs Category**—*Psychosocial integrity*
> **Client Needs Subcategory**—*None*

61. **4.** Most children are primarily concerned with how they will be affected by a diagnostic test, procedure, or medical treatment. The nurse must provide honest information and support the child throughout the procedure. The other information is secondary to this.

> *Test Taking Strategy—Look at the key words "most important" in reference to identifying the priority component of information from a child's perspective. Option 4 is the best choice because the items described in the other options are of less importance to a child of this age. Review principles of teaching clients who are school age if you had difficulty answering this question.*
> **Cognitive Level**—*Applying*
> **Client Needs Category**—*Health promotion and maintenance*
> **Client Needs Subcategory**—*None*

62. **2.** Although all the reasons for discussing the prognosis with the dying child are basically true, the best rationale for encouraging open communication is that it facilitates coping and emotional support for both the child and the family while they prepare for the child's inevitable death. Families who have left something unsaid often feel guilt and remorse.

> *Test Taking Strategy—Use the process of elimination to help select an option that accurately describes the best reason for sharing information about a terminal condition with an affected child. Although all the options are credible, dealing with grief and loss are better managed when there is a network of support, as identified in option 2. Review techniques for dealing with grief and loss if you had difficulty answering this question.*
> **Cognitive Level**—*Applying*
> **Client Needs Category**—*Psychosocial integrity*
> **Client Needs Subcategory**—*None*

63. **1.** Providing an ill child with honest explanations about the nature of the condition and upcoming procedures or treatments promotes confidence and trust in caregivers, especially when the reality of the experience is congruent with the teaching. The other characteristics may be acquired, but not as a consequence of an honest nurse–client relationship.

> *Test Taking Strategy—Analyze to determine what information the question asks for, which is the outcome that can be expected from providing honest explanations about potentially unpleasant experiences. Recall, as stated in option 1, that honesty facilitates trust and confidence. Review the impact of honesty on a nurse–client relationship if you had difficulty answering this question.*
> **Cognitive Level**—*Analyzing*
> **Client Needs Category**—*Psychosocial integrity*
> **Client Needs Subcategory**—*None*

64. **1.** Setting achievable goals allows the child the potential for success. Success instills a sense of pride in accomplishment and motivation for improvement. The other suggestions are not inappropriate; however, they are not the best techniques for supporting the child's self-esteem.

> *Test Taking Strategy—Look at the key words "most important" in reference to a method for preserving a child's self-esteem. Recall that self-esteem is a result of one's opinion about self-worth. Mastering tasks and achieving goals (option 1) provides a foundation for building and maintaining positive self-esteem. Review factors that affect self-esteem if you had difficulty answering this question.*
> **Cognitive Level**—*Analyzing*
> **Client Needs Category**—*Health promotion and maintenance*
> **Client Needs Subcategory**—*None*

65. **2.** Privacy is an essential component of a therapeutic environment. Selecting a location where the person cannot be observed or overheard by others facilitates open communication and a therapeutic relationship.

> *Test Taking Strategy—Analyze to determine what information the question asks for, which is the environment that is best for discussing the cause of problematic behavior with a school-age child. Recall that a meeting in the nurse's office is more likely to provide a private and therapeutic environment for discussing serious matters. The lunchroom, hallway, and playground are environments that may trivialize the topic of discussion and make the child an object of ridicule by his or her peers. Review the key principles of privacy and the benefits it offers regarding communication if you had difficulty answering this question.*

Cognitive Level—Analyzing
Client Needs Category—Safe and effective care environment
Client Needs Subcategory—Coordinated care

66. 1. In addition to the death of a parent, divorce is one of the most disruptive events a child can experience. Changes in family structure jeopardize a child's sense of security. Acting out is a behavioral manifestation of conflict. The death of a pet turtle, acquiring a paper route, and an infatuation with a classmate are situations that do not match the manifested behavior. Although these incidences may be stressful to the child, they would not have as intense an emotional impact as parental divorce.
  Test Taking Strategy—Look at the key words "most likely" in reference to the contributing cause of the school-age child's behavior. Of all the options, divorce (option 1) is the greatest stressor. Review childhood stressors and their effect on behavior if you had difficulty answering this question.
Cognitive Level—Applying
Client Needs Category—Psychosocial integrity
Client Needs Subcategory—None

67. 4. Discipline delivered immediately, fairly, and consistently helps a child understand the limits of acceptable and unacceptable behavior. Anxious people need reassurance that someone will enforce limits if they are unable to remain in control. Sending the child to the principal indicates that the teacher is evading personal responsibility for controlling classroom behavior. Suspension isolates the child from any helpful resource and is likely to contribute to continued low academic performance. Sending the child to the counselor on a daily basis is premature and too severe for the behavior manifested at this time. However, the counselor should be informed of the student's behavior and the home situation.
  Test Taking Strategy—Analyze to determine what information the question asks for, which is a method for maintaining acceptable behavior. Option 4 is the best answer because it indicates that there is an established structure that is fairly mediated if a deviation occurs. Knowing the consequences for one's actions tends to limit unacceptable behavior. Review the benefits from setting limits and expectations for behavior if you had difficulty answering this question.
Cognitive Level—Applying
Client Needs Category—Psychosocial integrity
Client Needs Subcategory—None

68. 3. The oldest child in a family tends to be one who conforms to the expectations of adults and who is more affected by criticism, more responsible, and more behaviorally rigid. The youngest child is likely to be less tolerant of frustration and more dependent on others. Middle children are more flexible and independent.

  Test Taking Strategy—Look at the key words "most likely" as they are used in reference to a characteristic behavior commonly manifested by first-born children. Review the rationale for an explanation of how birth order tends to affect behavior. There is sociologic support for identifying a first-born child using the description in option 3. Understand that there are exceptions to any generalization. Review the effects of birth order on attitudes and behavior if you had difficulty answering this question.
Cognitive Level—Applying
Client Needs Category—Health promotion and maintenance
Client Needs Subcategory—None

69. 2. Making angry remarks suggests that this child is demonstrating displacement. Displacement is a psychological defense mechanism in which a person releases feelings onto someone or something else other than the true object of the anger, which in this case is the illness. The other behaviors are more indicative of normal behavior for a child this age, especially one whose usual routine is unstructured due to unusual circumstances.
  Test Taking Strategy—Analyze to determine what information the question asks for, which is the best indication that the child is having difficulty accepting a diagnosis synonymous with lifelong changes. Although all of the options are normal or somewhat negative behaviors, option 2 stands out because it demonstrates a common ego defense mechanism known as displacement. Review ego defense mechanisms and the purposes they serve if you had difficulty answering this question.
Cognitive Level—Applying
Client Needs Category—Health promotion and maintenance
Client Needs Subcategory—None

70. 3. Taking an active role in one's care is the most effective way to acquire a sense of control over a disease. Therefore, actually performing self-testing of blood glucose levels is therapeutic. The other activities are important, but less effective in promoting a sense of control.
  Test Taking Strategy—Analyze to determine what information the question asks for, which is an activity that facilitates a diabetic child's sense of control over a chronic disease. Although all of the options describe activities that are important to living with diabetes mellitus, option 3 is the best answer because the child with diabetes is actually performing a self-care activity rather than being the passive recipient of information. Review the benefits from active participation in self-care if you had difficulty answering this question.
Cognitive Level—Analyzing

Client Needs Category—Health promotion and maintenance
Client Needs Subcategory—None

71. 1. Tourette's syndrome is a genetic disorder that begins manifesting at about age 7. More common among boys, the disorder causes the child to suffer from various tics (rapid, repetitive movements), including vocal tics (repeated use of words or phrases, coughing, barking, snorting, or throat clearing) and motor tics (such as eye movements, neck jerking, facial grimacing, jumping, and touching). Those with Tourette's syndrome tend to utter verbal obscenities or other socially unacceptable words (coprolalia) and make other vocal sounds embarrassing to all concerned. The bizarre activities, which are difficult to control, tend to make the client an object of ridicule or avoidance by those unfamiliar with the condition. If other symptoms in the remaining options occur, they are secondary to the diagnosis or unique to the client.

> *Test Taking Strategy—Use the process of elimination to help select the option that describes a problem unique to clients with Tourette's syndrome that must be addressed to facilitate coping by the family and client. Outbursts of verbal obscenities (option 1) are common among those with this disorder. Addressing this issue helps prepare the client and family for situations in which it occurs. A client with Tourette's syndrome may also have the behaviors identified in options 2, 3, and 4, but they are not commonly associated with the disorder. Review the manifestations of Tourette's syndrome if you had difficulty answering this question.*
> *Cognitive Level—Remembering*
> *Client Needs Category—Psychosocial integrity*
> *Client Needs Subcategory—None*

72. 4. A high percentage of children with Tourette's syndrome also have a varying degree of obsessive-compulsive symptoms such as recurring thoughts, the need to arrange/rearrange objects, or repeatedly complete then undo a task. Medications can help control this behavior if identified. There is no correlation between schizophrenia, attention deficit hyperactivity disorder, or bipolar disorder and Tourette's syndrome.

> *Test Taking Strategy—Analyze to determine what information the question asks for, which is a co-morbid condition of Tourette's syndrome. Although obsessive compulsive symptoms are not manifested by all who have Tourette's syndrome, the incidence is statistically significant enough to include when discussing its symptomatology. Review the manifestations of Tourette's syndrome if you had difficulty answering this question.*
> *Cognitive Level—Remembering*
> *Client Needs Category—Psychosocial integrity*
> *Client Needs Subcategory—None*

73. 1. Antipsychotic drugs such as haloperidol (Haldol) cause a cluster of side effects known as extrapyramidal symptoms. Parkinsonian-like tremors and sudden strong muscle spasms, especially of the neck, are two types of these symptoms. Muscle weakness, muscle atrophy, and muscle contracture are not common side effects.

> *Test Taking Strategy—Analyze to determine what information the question asks for, which is a side effect of the drug haloperidol. Review extrapyramidal symptoms, especially dystonia, that are side effects of antipsychotic medications if you had difficulty answering this question.*
> *Cognitive Level—Remembering*
> *Client Needs Category—Physiological integrity*
> *Client Needs Subcategory—Pharmacological therapies*

74. 2. Self-esteem develops as a consequence of experiencing deserved praise from people the child respects. Positive reinforcement is preferable to focusing on negative behavior. Praise is considered a far healthier approach than sheltering and protecting the child physically or emotionally from peers.

> *Test Taking Strategy—Look at the key words "most appropriate" in reference to a suggested approach for maintaining the self-esteem of a child with Tourette's syndrome, who is subject to potential ridicule by peers. Although options 1, 3, and 4 are methods for either avoiding or countering negative peer remarks, they are not the best methods for promoting self-esteem. Review techniques for building self-esteem if you had difficulty answering this question.*
> *Cognitive Level—Analyzing*
> *Client Needs Category—Health promotion and maintenance*
> *Client Needs Subcategory—None*

Mental Health Needs During Adolescence

75. 3. The best outcomes are obtained when crisis intervention is initiated immediately after the precipitating event. Although crises tend to become resolved even without professional support, the outcomes are less than optimal as time passes.

> *Test Taking Strategy—Use the process of elimination to help select the option that identifies the best time for providing crisis intervention. Crises tend to resolve over time with or without any therapeutic interventions, but not as effectively as if they are dealt with immediately after a significant event. Therefore, option 3 is the best answer. Options 1, 2, and 4 can be eliminated because there is a lapse of time between the event and the identified time frames. Review the principles of crisis intervention if you had difficulty answering this question.*

Cognitive Level—Applying
Client Needs Category—Psychosocial integrity
Client Needs Subcategory—None

76. 1. Most people who experience a crisis have an overwhelming feeling of helplessness. This feeling is a direct consequence of having inadequate coping strategies. The other emotional responses may occur among some individuals, but they are not characteristic of the majority of individuals experiencing crises.

> *Test Taking Strategy—Look at the key words "most likely" that are used in reference to a feeling that is typical when witnessing violence or some other type of psychic trauma. Initially most persons feel helpless (option 1), which is the rationale for providing support when individuals are most vulnerable. Review the impact of a crisis on a person's psychological well-being if you had difficulty answering this question.*

Cognitive Level—Applying
Client Needs Category—Psychosocial integrity
Client Needs Subcategory—None

77. 2. The first step toward resolving a crisis is to have survivors process the event from their perspective. Some individuals require professional counseling, but most do not if crisis intervention is initiated soon after the event. Reassuring survivors that they will adapt may be appropriate, but it is not the most important action to take initially. Drug therapy in the form of minor tranquilizers is usually unnecessary; also, tranquilizing may be detrimental because it tends to interfere with processing the reality of the crisis.

> *Test Taking Strategy—Look at the key word "priority," which requires identifying the most important action to take at this time. Verbalizing the impact the crisis has had (option 2) helps put the event in a more realistic perspective. Review the techniques used in crisis intervention if you had difficulty answering this question.*

Cognitive Level—Analyzing
Client Needs Category—Psychosocial integrity
Client Needs Subcategory—None

78. 2. Bulimia is an eating disorder that is characterized by a preoccupation with food and body weight. Bulimics control their weight by a cycle of purging after eating binges. The disorder is more common among female adolescents and young adults (in their 20s). Most bulimic clients experience a period of depression or guilt after binging on large quantities of high-calorie foods. Because consuming such large amounts causes abdominal distention and pain, the bulimic client typically vomits to lessen the discomfort. Deterioration of dental structures and erosion of tooth enamel results from repeated contact between gastric acid and teeth from self-induced vomiting. Bulimic

clients usually maintain a normal weight. Anorectic clients are more likely to cease menstruating when their body fat is depleted. Loss of hair is also correlated more with the malnutrition of anorexia nervosa.

> *Test Taking Strategy—Analyze to determine what information the question asks for, which is a physical assessment finding common among those who have bulimia. Because bulimia involves binging and purging, dental enamel is prone to deterioration (option 2). Review the signs of bulimia focusing on the effect repeated forced vomiting has on teeth if you had difficulty answering this question.*

Cognitive Level—Remembering
Client Needs Category—Physiological integrity
Client Needs Subcategory—Physiological adaptation

79. 1. Anorexia nervosa is an eating disorder characterized by preoccupation with food, body weight, and extreme weight loss caused by fasting or excessive exercise. Anorexia nervosa usually occurs in young women between ages 13 and 20 and is more common in families who have already had an occurrence of the disorder. Low self-esteem and a distorted body image are major characteristics of the illness. Clients with anorexia nervosa commonly manifest lanugo, a growth of fine downy hair similar to that of newborn infants. It is thought that this occurs to promote or maintain normal body temperature in people who have little or no body fat. Bruises may indicate a vitamin deficiency, but they would not be limited to the upper torso. Generally, bowel sounds are normal in anorectic clients. Clubbing of the fingers is characteristic of conditions causing chronic hypoxia.

> *Test Taking Strategy—Look at the key words "most likely" in reference to a physical finding common to those with anorexia nervosa. Recall that anorectics lose a great deal of subcutaneous and even muscle tissue which interferes with an ability to maintain body temperature. Consequently, there is a fine growth of hair (option 1) that develops as a physiologic mechanism for maintaining near-normal body temperature. Review the signs and symptoms associated with anorexia nervosa if you had difficulty answering this question.*

Cognitive Level—Remembering
Client Needs Category—Physiological integrity
Client Needs Subcategory—Physiological adaptation

80. 4. The distinguishing clinical difference between anorexia nervosa and bulimia is binge eating. Adolescents with bulimia often binge and then purge what they have eaten. Both anorexia nervosa and bulimia have similar symptoms of body image distortion, purging after meals, and decreased self-esteem.

> *Test Taking Strategy—Analyze to determine what information the question asks for, which is an assessment finding that distinguishes between the two eating*

disorders. The key to the answer is the difference in eating patterns. Anorectics are more prone to self-starvation rather than binge eating (option 4). Review the manifestations associated with anorexia nervosa and bulimia if you had difficulty answering this question.
Cognitive Level—*Remembering*
Client Needs Category—*Physiological integrity*
Client Needs Subcategory—*Physiological adaptation*

81. 2. Generally, anorectic clients are characterized as being "perfect" children with above-average scholastic achievement, perhaps due to a fear of failure. They often adhere to a strict program of exercise and are ritualistic in their behaviors. None of the other characteristics listed is unique to clients with anorexia nervosa.
> *Test Taking Strategy*—*Use the process of elimination to help select the option that correlates best with a client who has anorexia nervosa. Recall that individuals with anorexia nervosa are often perfectionist, as described in option 2. They use controlling their food intake as a symbolic way of controlling aspects of their life that may be out of control. Some believe that the family in which the anorectic is a part is dysfunctional. Although the characteristics described in options 1, 3, and 4 are possible, they are not components of the usual cluster of characteristics found in individuals who develop anorexia nervosa. Review the psychosocial factors common among those with anorexia nervosa if you had difficulty answering this question.*
Cognitive Level—*Remembering*
Client Needs Category—*Health promotion and maintenance*
Client Needs Subcategory—*None*

82. 3. Initial treatment of a client with anorexia nervosa focuses on meeting physiological needs. After nutrients, fluids, vitamins, and electrolytes have been administered, attention shifts to the client's psychosocial problems.
> *Test Taking Strategy*—*Look at the key words "highest priority," which in this case applies to the most important goal when managing the care of a client with anorexia. Recall that meeting physiological needs comes before all others according to Maslow's hierarchy of needs. Therefore, option 3 is the best answer. Review the life-threatening consequences of self-starvation if you had difficulty answering this question.*
Cognitive Level—*Analyzing*
Client Needs Category—*Safe and effective care environment*
Client Needs Subcategory—*Coordinated care*

83. 3. Validation is a therapeutic communication technique in which the nurse interprets what is perceived to be

the underlying meaning of the words. If the interpretation is correct, it increases rapport and forms a basis for future collaboration. The techniques of generalizing, giving advice, and responding with a stereotypical statement are examples of nontherapeutic ways of communicating.
> *Test Taking Strategy*—*Look at the key words "most therapeutic" in reference to a response by the nurse to the parent's statement. Option 3 is best from among the listed options because it validates the parent's statement and is an example of therapeutic communication. Review therapeutic and nontherapeutic communication techniques if you had difficulty answering this question.*
Cognitive Level—*Applying*
Client Needs Category—*Psychosocial integrity*
Client Needs Subcategory—*None*

84. 4. Controlling the desire to eat is a nonverbal technique that the anorectic client uses to demonstrate power and control. Getting attention as a result of this behavior reinforces its effectiveness. Consequently, the most appropriate way to handle this situation is to simply remove the food without making any comments. Until a client's malnutrition becomes life-threatening, forced feeding is unethical and inappropriate. Recording intake is not an incentive for eating. The fear of becoming fat in an anorectic client is often greater than a prior commitment to collaborated goals.
> *Test Taking Strategy*—*Use the process of elimination to help select the option that describes the best action to take when an anorectic client arranges rather than eats food. Recall that giving attention to an undesirable behavior is a form of positive reinforcement. Ignoring behavior (option 4) is nonjudgmental. If the client is in a life-threatening state and if the consequences of not eating have been identified clearly to the client, it may become necessary to implement option 1 at some time, but the information in the stem does not address these issues. Options 2 and 3 do not meet the goal of ending the behavior. Review the role reinforcement plays in relation to promoting or extinguishing behavior if you had difficulty answering this question.*
Cognitive Level—*Analyzing*
Client Needs Category—*Safe and effective care environment*
Client Needs Subcategory—*Coordinated care*

85. 2. Confrontation is an effective therapeutic communication technique that allows the nurse to point out differences between an expected behavior and the actual action. Postponing weighing is likely to result in more accurate assessment data. However, this choice of action—as well as saying nothing or subtracting 2 pounds from the client's weight—avoids the greater issue of dealing with the behavior.

Test Taking Strategy—*Look at the key words "most appropriate" as they relate to a nursing response when a client drinks water to falsify the measurement of body weight. Remember that calling attention to an undesirable behavior demonstrates to the client that he or she will be held accountable for the consequences of an observed action. Review the situations in which confrontation, a therapeutic communication technique, are indicated if you had difficulty answering this question.*
Cognitive Level—*Analyzing*
Client Needs Category—*Physiological integrity*
Client Needs Subcategory—*Reduction of risk potential*

86. 1. Separation anxiety is a common response when a cognitively disabled client experiences a change in caretakers in an unfamiliar environment. Pain is a subjective experience; it is erroneous to assume that a client who is cognitively disabled will respond any differently to pain than others with normal intelligence. An adolescent with this cognitive capacity should be able to communicate about basic needs despite the disability. An adolescent with normal cognitive ability is typically concerned about changes in body image; however, such concerns are unlikely for someone at this developmental level.
  Test Taking Strategy—*Analyze to determine what information the question asks for, which is a typical assessment finding in a cognitively disabled client admitted to a hospital. Option 1 is the best answer from among the options provided because it represents a response commonly seen in cognitively disabled clients. Review typical findings in a hospitalized client with an IQ between 35 and 50 if you had difficulty answering this question.*
Cognitive Level—*Applying*
Client Needs Category—*Health promotion and maintenance*
Client Needs Subcategory—*None*

87. 1. Assuming responsibility for skills that can be performed independently, such as dressing and undressing, tends to interfere with the ability to achieve maximum levels of self-care. It is normal for a parent to be the medical historian for nonadult children. Self-blame and exaggerating the child's abilities are indications that the parent is not coping well with the child's condition.
  Test Taking Strategy—*Look at the key words "most likely" in reference to a parental behavior that interferes with the cognitively disabled teen reaching his or her highest potential. Recall that providing too much care stifles a person's independence, making option 1 the best answer. Review methods for promoting the potential of a client with a cognitive disability if you had difficulty answering this question.*

Cognitive Level—*Analyzing*
Client Needs Category—*Health promotion and maintenance*
Client Needs Subcategory—*None*

88. 2. The client's aggressive response is a defensive reaction not unlike that displayed by younger children who perceive themselves to be in threatening situations. Stating that all cognitively disabled people are physically aggressive is an overgeneralization. One incidence of physically lashing out is not sufficient to conclude that the client has a poor opinion of the care provided. Children commonly demonstrate that they are in pain by crying or moaning, not by being aggressive.
  Test Taking Strategy—*Use the process of elimination to help select the option that provides the best explanation for the aggressive act by a cognitively disabled client. Option 1 represents a generalization, option 3 draws a conclusion without proper evidence, and option 4 is an incorrect statement. Option 2 is the best answer because it recognizes the aggressiveness as a defensive reaction. Review the underlying reasons that clients display aggression if you had difficulty answering this question.*
Cognitive Level—*Applying*
Client Needs Category—*Psychosocial integrity*
Client Needs Subcategory—*None*

89. 3. The nurse should take care to document facts, not opinions. Although stating that the nursing assistant was struck while helping the client out of bed requires more elaboration, it is more appropriate than the other choices. Stating that the aggression was a consequence of feeling angry or that the act was spontaneous is inaccurate. The word "attacked" is an emotionally charged term that suggests more violence than actually occurred.
  Test Taking Strategy—*Look at the key words "most appropriate" in reference to documenting an incident involving a client's aggressive action. Recall that documentation should be objective and factual, which supports selecting option 3 as the best answer. Review principles of documentation if you had difficulty answering this question.*
Cognitive Level—*Applying*
Client Needs Category—*Safe and effective care environment*
Client Needs Subcategory—*Coordinated care*

90. 3. To avoid any misperceptions, it is best to offer explanations before physically touching the client. Entering the client's personal space without warning may be interpreted as a threatening act. Restraints are unjustified in this situation. The parent should not be asked to assume total responsibility for caring for the child. Medicating the client with an analgesic is justified if the client experiences pain, but it is best to administer it at least 20 to 30 minutes before an activity.

Test Taking Strategy—*Use the process of elimination to help select the option that provides the best sugges-tion to avoid being struck again by the cognitively disabled client. Options 1 and 2 can be eliminated immediately because using physical or chemical restraints for the benefit of personnel violates the Omnibus Budget Reconciliation Act (OBRA). Option 2 can be eliminated because providing care is the primary responsibility of assigned nursing person-nel. Review how touch may be perceived by an anxious client if you had difficulty answering this question.*
Cognitive Level—*Analyzing*
Client Needs Category—*Safe and effective care envi-ronment*
Client Needs Subcategory—*Coordinated care*

91. 1. The adolescent's attitudes and behavior are influ-enced much more by peers than by school, religion, or employment—although all of these affect the dynamics of each individual.
Test Taking Strategy—*Analyze to determine what information the question asks for, which is the most appropriate data to assess when obtaining a court-ordered client's social history. Recall that during adolescence, teens are influenced more by peers than by any other social factors. Review the psychosocial characteristics of adolescents if you had difficulty answering this question.*
Cognitive Level—*Applying*
Client Needs Category—*Health promotion and maintenance*
Client Needs Subcategory—*None*

92. 1. Inconsistency in setting limits or imposing conse-quences when limits are violated weakens an adolescent's ability to recognize boundaries for behavior. Discipline provides security even if restrictions are not appreciated at the time. Siblings, social status, and role models influence the teen but are not the strongest influence.
Test Taking Strategy—*Analyze to determine what information the question asks for, which is the fac-tor that is most influential in developing antisocial behavior. Recall that individuals who demonstrate antisocial behavior have acquired a very weak or absent superego. The superego can be compared to one's conscience, which is a result of being raised with guidelines about what is right and wrong. Because the primary source for learning right from wrong begins with parental guidance and modeling, inconsistency on the part of parents (option 1) is the best answer from among the options. Review the manner in which a superego forms and how it affects behavior if you had difficulty answering this question.*
Cognitive Level—*Applying*

Client Needs Category—*Psychosocial integrity*
Client Needs Subcategory—*None*

93. 4. Reassuring clients that the information they divulge will remain confidential is perhaps the most important concept to emphasize. Most therapy meetings are scheduled on a day and time that repeats on a regular basis. It is understood that someone who leads a group is qualified to do so. Using first names is common, but indi-cating that this is a practice to follow is less important than stressing confidentiality.
Test Taking Strategy—*Analyze to determine what information the question asks for, which is the most important information to communicate to individu-als who attend group meetings. Recall that personal information must be kept confidential (option 4). Any breach of confidentiality may result in a cessation of communication among members of the group. Lack of free interaction sabotages the therapeutic benefits of group therapy. Review guidelines for partici-pants involved in group therapy if you had difficulty answering this question.*
Cognitive Level—*Applying*
Client Needs Category—*Safe and effective care environment*
Client Needs Subcategory—*Coordinated care*

94. 3. Persistently checking a clock is a nonverbal way of saying that one would rather be someplace else or that the therapy session should be over soon. Such nonverbal behaviors suggest that no value is being obtained from the session. Borrowing cigarettes demonstrates irrespon-sibility. Laughing inappropriately suggests insensitivity. Fidgeting is a sign of anxiety.
Test Taking Strategy—*Analyze to determine what information the question asks for, which is the action that is most indicative of resistance to therapy. Checking the clock (option 3) demonstrates resist-ance to therapy. Review behaviors that demonstrate resistance to therapy such as missing meetings, coming late to meetings, leaving meetings early, and lack of participation at meetings, if you had difficulty answering this question.*
Cognitive Level—*Analyzing*
Client Needs Category—*Psychosocial integrity*
Client Needs Subcategory—*None*

95. 1. Children who have grown up with an alcoholic parent commonly have a problem with low self-esteem. Other dysfunctional attributes include an inability to trust, an extreme need to control, an excessive sense of respon-sibility, and a denial of feelings, which can be carried into adulthood. The other problems may be present in any person exposed to alcoholism, but they are not commonly shared characteristics.

Test Taking Strategy—*Analyze to determine what information the question asks for, which is an outcome from having grown up in an alcoholic family. Alcoholism is a family disease. Recall that life in a family with someone who is an alcoholic is generally filled with disappointments when promises have not been kept, embarrassment by the parent's public intoxication, and lack of physical and emotional attention to needs, which all lead to low self-esteem (option 1). Review the characteristics of children when one or both parents are alcoholics if you had difficulty answering this question.*
Cognitive Level—*Applying*
Client Needs Category—*Psychosocial integrity*
Client Needs Subcategory—*None*

96. 3. All the resources listed are helpful in some way to a person growing up in an alcoholic family. However, the one best suited for an adolescent is Alateen. Alateen focuses on providing support for teenagers in alcoholic families and helping them to see how the alcoholism affects their lives. One of the primary goals is to help break the pattern of alcoholism within the family.

Test Taking Strategy—*Analyze to determine what information the question asks for, which is the agency that is most appropriate for assisting a client with a parent who is an alcoholic. The purpose of Alcoholics Anonymous is to help those who abuse alcohol get and stay sober one day at a time. The purpose of Al-Anon is to help those who live in an alcoholic household understand how the disease affects them personally, making option 2 a choice with some merit. However, Alateen, if it is available in the community, helps adolescents deal with issues that relate to a family member's alcoholism or their own alcohol abuse, making option 3 the best answer. Members who belong to a community's Substance Abuse Council implement strategies to reduce alcoholism and drug abuse within the local area. Review the purpose of the community resources identified in the options if you had difficulty answering this question.*
Cognitive Level—*Remembering*
Client Needs Category—*Safe and effective care environment*
Client Needs Subcategory—*Coordinated care*

97. 2. Learning to trust others is a major sign of accomplishment for children of alcoholic parents. It is often difficult for such children to understand the concept of "normal" trusting relationships because these children have not yet experienced them. Developing the other psychosocial skills listed would be considered positive accomplishments, but they are not commonly identified benefits from therapy aimed at resolving issues from growing up in an alcoholic household.

Test Taking Strategy—*Analyze to determine what information the question asks for, which is the most likely benefit to an adolescent of receiving therapy focused on issues surrounding life with an alcoholic parent. Recall that a child with an alcoholic parent has been disappointed many times by unkept promises and dysfunctional parenting. Consequently, the ability to trust others (option 2) is the best answer. Review the needs of children when one or both parents are alcoholic if you had difficulty answering this question.*
Cognitive Level—*Applying*
Client Needs Category—*Psychosocial integrity*
Client Needs Subcategory—*None*

98. 1. The peer group becomes more influential than parents in determining how adolescents behave. Peer behavior is used as a model for establishing what activities are acceptable or unacceptable. The fact that the team is winning is no more a motivation for taking controlled substances than if the team was losing. Affordability is not necessarily a factor in compromising values.

Test Taking Strategy—*Analyze to determine what information the question asks for, which is the factor that most likely affects an adolescent's willingness to use a nonprescription and perhaps illegal drug. Recall that adolescents are highly influenced by peer behavior and attitudes, making option 1 the best answer. Review peer pressure and how it affects adolescent decision-making if you had difficulty answering this question.*
Cognitive Level—*Applying*
Client Needs Category—*Health promotion and maintenance*
Client Needs Subcategory—*None*

99. 3. Anabolic steroids commonly cause acne in both male and female users, regardless of the age group. Prolonged use of anabolic steroids can lead to hypogonadism in males evidenced by atrophy of the testes. Bronzed skin and brittle nails are unrelated to the use of anabolic steroids.

Test Taking Strategy—*Analyze to determine what information the question asks for, which is an effect of taking an anabolic steroid. Recall that severe acne (option 3), a side effect of anabolic steroids, is not one of the more dangerous or life-threatening effects. Review the side effects of anabolic steroids if you had difficulty answering this question.*
Cognitive Level—*Applying*
Client Needs Category—*Physiological integrity*
Client Needs Subcategory—*Pharmacological therapies*

100. 1. Anabolic steroids are synthetic drugs chemically related to androgens such as testosterone. Androgens and anabolic steroids are associated with aggressive behavior. Severe mental changes, such as uncontrolled rage and personality changes, are common. The other emotional changes are unrelated to steroid use.

Test Taking Strategy—Analyze to determine what information the question asks for, which is behavioral effects associated with anabolic steroids. Recall that males tend to be more aggressive than females, which some attribute to a predominance of testosterone rather than estrogen, making option 1 the best answer. Review the effects of anabolic steroids if you had difficulty answering this question.
Cognitive Level—Remembering
Client Needs Category—Physiological integrity
Client Needs Subcategory—Pharmacological therapies

101. Anabolic steroids have a profound effect on the liver characterized by liver degeneration and dysfunction. Liver enzymes are abnormally elevated. Anabolic steroids do not affect thyroid function, electrolyte levels, or cause atypical blood counts.

Test Taking Strategy—Use the process of elimination to select the option identifying the laboratory test(s) that are most affected by the use of anabolic steroids. Recall that the liver is the organ for metabolizing and detoxifying drugs. Review the pharmacokinetic steps following drug administration which include absorption, distribution, metabolism, and excretion, if you had difficulty answering this question.
Cognitive Level—Remembering
Client Needs Category—Physiological integrity
Client Needs Subcategory—Pharmacological therapies

102. 1, 2, 3, 4. Signs of depression accompany a potential for suicide. Other warning signs include withdrawal from family, friends, and school activities; apathy; angry outbursts or behavior that is out of character; and alcohol or other depressant drug abuse. Delusions and incoherent speech are signs commonly associated with schizophrenia.

Test Taking Strategy—Analyze to determine what information the question asks for, which is warning signs of suicidal ideation. Alternative-format "select all that apply" questions require considering each option independently to decide its merit in answering the question. Select all the options that are signs of suicide. Review signs of a potential for suicide if you had difficulty answering this question.
Cognitive Level—Applying
Client Needs Category—Psychosocial integrity
Client Needs Subcategory—None

103. 4. Acceptance is the basis for developing a therapeutic relationship. An accepting attitude indicates that the client is unique and worthy of respect. Trust develops when a client feels accepted. Empathy, not sympathy, should be demonstrated. The other qualities are desirable but are not as likely to facilitate building trust.

Test Taking Strategy—Analyze to determine what information the question asks for, which is the nursing attribute that is most important when communicating with an adolescent during the initial meeting at a birth control clinic. Recall that a nonjudgmental attitude is best when interacting with a client who is concerned about how his or her actions may be morally or socially perceived. This information supports selecting option 4 as the best answer. Review nursing approaches that promote acceptance in a nurse-client relationship if you had difficulty answering this question.
Cognitive Level—Applying
Client Needs Category—Psychosocial integrity
Client Needs Subcategory—None

104. 1. Eye contact communicates that the nurse is paying attention and considers what the client says to be important. Giving away free literature does not communicate a sincere, personal regard for the client. Writing information is a job-related task. Avoiding pauses could be interpreted as disinterest.

Test Taking Strategy—Use the process of elimination to help select the option that describes the best nursing action for conveying an interest in a client. Option 2 can be eliminated because providing literature is a poor substitute for personal interest. Option 4 can be eliminated because a battery of questions may convey that the nurse's motivation is to end the interaction as soon as possible without concern for the significance to the client. Option 3 can be eliminated because writing information, although it implies what the client says is significant, does not convey interest as much as making eye contact (option 1). Review nursing actions that promote interest during a nurse-client interaction if you had difficulty answering this question.
Cognitive Level—Applying
Client Needs Category—Psychosocial integrity
Client Needs Subcategory—None

105. 2. Teenagers normally go through a period when they reject the standards and ideals of their parents and other adults. By experimenting with new behaviors that are often opposite those of the parents, the adolescent emerges with a unique identity and a lasting set of values. Adolescent rebellion is not likely to facilitate ingenuity, intuition, or insight.

Test Taking Strategy—Analyze to determine what information the question asks for, which is the outcome that results from achieving the developmental tasks during adolescence. Recall that according to Erikson, acquiring identity is an outcome that occurs during adolescence. Review Erikson's stages of development, especially in relation to adolescence, and the attributes that are associated with each stage if you had difficulty answering this question.

Cognitive Level—Remembering
Client Needs Category—Health promotion and maintenance
Client Needs Subcategory—None

106. 1. Client treatment is a confidential matter. Neither the nurse nor other clinic personnel may reveal the client's identity or reason for treatment without the client's consent. All the other actions overtly or covertly divulge a relationship between the clinic and the client; the examples violate the principle of confidentiality.

Test Taking Strategy—Look at the key words "most appropriate" in relation to a parent's request for information about the purpose of the adolescent's visit with the nurse. Recall that health information—even when it involves information on birth control for a minor—is protected by the Health Insurance Portability and Accountability Act (HIPAA). This knowledge leads to selecting option 1 as the best answer. Review the HIPAA legislation and its implications for health care workers if you had difficulty answering this question.
Cognitive Level—Applying
Client Needs Category—Safe and effective care environment
Client Needs Subcategory—Coordinated care

107. 4. One important element in resolving a crisis is the emotional support of significant others. The client's mothering instinct, marriage plans, and financial support are not as beneficial as a family's unconditional love and encouragement.

Test Taking Strategy—Analyze to determine what information the question asks for, which is the attribute that will be most beneficial to an adolescent upon learning about an unplanned pregnancy. Recall that support from significant others (option 4) is most important when dealing with a stressor. Review techniques that are helpful in reducing a stress response if you had difficulty answering this question.
Cognitive Level—Analyzing
Client Needs Category—Psychosocial integrity
Client Needs Subcategory—None

108. 3. Denial is a form of behavior that protects one's consciousness from dealing with a catastrophic situation. Denying a situation keeps anxiety at an acceptable level. Displacement involves discharging angry feelings onto an unrelated person or object. Regression occurs when a person resorts to behavior associated with a younger age. Compensation is characterized by pursuing an activity that ensures success to make up for feeling inadequate.

Test Taking Strategy—Analyze to determine what information the question asks for, which is the ego

defense mechanism that is best exemplified by seeking a method of birth control when a pregnancy possibly already exists. Denial is a psychological defense mechanism that protects the self (ego) from reality. Review ego defense mechanisms and the purpose they serve if you had difficulty answering this question.
Cognitive Level—Remembering
Client Needs Category—Psychosocial integrity
Client Needs Subcategory—None

109. 3. Clients who are psychotic generally have unrealistic and irrational thoughts. Yet these thoughts seem real and logical to the psychotic person. Many people who are mentally healthy experience difficulty in relationships, have problems adjusting to new situations, and feel helpless in resolving some problems.

Test Taking Strategy—Analyze to determine what information the question asks for, which is a behavior manifested by psychotic individuals. Recall that the term psychosis implies the most serious form of mental illness. Clients who are acutely psychotic have difficulty perceiving the reality of their life experiences (option 3). Psychotic individuals need care from mental health practitioners until they are capable of living safely within the community. Review the signs and symptoms associated with psychotic thought processes if you had difficulty answering this question.
Cognitive Level—Applying
Client Needs Category—Psychosocial integrity
Client Needs Subcategory—None

110. 1. Orientation is a person's ability to identify who and where they are, as well as identifying the day, month, and year. Asking how the client arrived is one way to assess the short-term memory. Having the client identify his or her place of birth assesses long-term memory. Asking the client to name the current president assesses the client's knowledge base.

Test Taking Strategy—Look at the key words "most appropriate" in relation to a technique for assessing a client's orientation. Recall that orientation applies to identifying person, place, and time, which is best described in option 1. Review the method for assessing orientation if you had difficulty answering this question.
Cognitive Level—Applying
Client Needs Category—Health promotion and maintenance
Client Needs Subcategory—None

111. 3. According to the American Hospital Association, a client has a fundamental right to review his or her own medical records. Also, the Mental Health Systems Act of 1980 contains a model for the mental health client's bill of rights. It states that a client has the right to access his or her mental health care records except for information provided by third parties and information deemed by a mental health professional to be detrimental to the client's health. Therefore, the nurse should hand the client the notes and allow the client to read them. Asking a "why" question is a nontherapeutic communication technique because it demands an explanation by the client. Putting the notes away is a nonverbal method of denying the client's request; it may also be misinterpreted by the client as an indication that there is something to hide. It is not illegal for clients to read their own medical records.

Test Taking Strategy—Analyze to determine what information the question asks for, which is the most appropriate response to a client's request to read information documented in his or her medical record. Recall that a client has the basic right to access his or her medical records, which is indicated by option 3. However, keep in mind that agencies may have a policy regarding the process that should be followed when a client requests access. This sometimes involves having the client's physician or agency administrator present at the time the medical record is accessed. Agency policy should be reviewed and followed whenever a client makes a similar request. Review the Patient's Bill of Rights, which has become a standard guideline for those providing health care, if you had difficulty answering this question.

Cognitive Level—Applying
Client Needs Category—Safe and effective care environment
Client Needs Subcategory—Coordinated care

112. 2. The most essential criterion for an involuntary commitment is that the client is a clear and present danger to himself or herself or to others. Commitment criteria have been established to protect the client's right to appropriate treatment in the least restrictive setting. There are methods for assessing a client other than involuntary commitment. Neither failure to keep office appointments nor uncooperative behavior is a criterion for involuntary commitment. All competent adults have the right to refuse treatment, which includes not taking medications.

Test Taking Strategy—Analyze to determine what information the question asks for, which is the criterion used to justify an involuntary admission to a mental health facility. Recall that a client has the right to self-determination unless and until the client's actions are dangerous (option 2). Review the legal basis for committing a person involuntarily for mental health treatment if you had difficulty answering this question.

Cognitive Level—Applying
Client Needs Category—Safe and effective care environment
Client Needs Subcategory—Coordinated care

113. 4. Orthostatic hypotension is a side effect commonly associated with traditional antipsychotic drugs such as haloperidol (Haldol). Cautioning a client to rise slowly helps moderate the drop in blood pressure, thereby minimizing the potential for dizziness, fainting, or falling. Taking the medication on an empty stomach or skipping meals does not affect the drug's therapeutic action. This category of drugs is likely to make the client feel drowsy when treatment is initiated. The client should never omit or discontinue taking an antipsychotic drug without first consulting the physician.

Test Taking Strategy—Analyze to determine what information the question asks for, which is the most appropriate teaching for a client taking the drug haloperidol. Recall that taking an antipsychotic medication can cause postural hypotension. To ensure that the client's safety is maintained, it is essential that the nurse include teaching that helps the client avoid injury should loss of consciousness occur. Review the side effects of haloperidol and implications for health teaching if you had difficulty answering this question.

Cognitive Level—Applying
Client Needs Category—Physiological integrity
Client Needs Subcategory—Pharmacological therapies

114. 1. Traditional antipsychotics are most likely to reduce or eliminate psychotic symptoms, such as delusions and hallucinations. They do so by blocking receptors of the neurotransmitter dopamine. Increased drowsiness and sleepiness are undesirable side effects of antipsychotics. It is doubtful that the client will feel more energetic and rested because one of the drug's common side effects is sedation. The drug does not alter the client's self-concept.

Test Taking Strategy—Use the process of elimination to help select the option that identifies the best evidence of haloperidol's therapeutic effect. Recall that psychoses may be accompanied by hallucinations, especially of the auditory type. Consequently, the elimination of this symptom (option 1) is a desired response for a client taking this drug. Option 2 can be eliminated because sedation is an effect that may or may not be desirable. Option 3 can be eliminated because the client's self-concept is not a result of the drug's mechanism of action. Option 4 can be eliminated because it contradicts the usual effects experienced by persons taking this medication. Review the desired outcomes associated with antipsychotic drug therapy if you had difficulty answering this question.

Cognitive Level—Remembering
Client Needs Category—Physiological integrity
Client Needs Subcategory—Pharmacological therapies

115. 2. Antipsychotic drugs can depress the bone marrow's production of blood cells. A severe sore throat suggests that the client does not have sufficient white blood cells (WBCs) to fight off microorganisms. A complete blood count is needed to assess the possibility of this adverse effect. Clozapine (Clozaril) has caused lethal agranulocytosis in 1% to 2% of patients; therefore, a WBC count is performed every week or two for as long as the client receives the drug and for 4 weeks after the drug is stopped. This drug is likely to cause constipation and weight gain. Ringing of the ears (tinnitus) is not associated with clozapine use.

Test Taking Strategy—Look at the key word "immediately" in reference to a symptom suggestive of a serious side effect of clozapine. Recall that suscep- tibility to infection, evidenced by a sore throat, may be related to agranulocytosis, which could have life-threatening consequences. The sore throat identified in option 2 should be reported to the prescriber immediately. Review the unique side effects of clozapine, the importance of monitoring WBC counts on a regular basis, and the significance of abnormal laboratory values to the health of the client if you had difficulty answering this question.

Cognitive Level—Applying
Client Needs Category—Physiological integrity
Client Needs Subcategory—Pharmacological therapies

TEST

16 The Nursing Care of Adult Clients with Mental Health Needs

- Mental Health Needs During Young Adulthood
- Mental Health Needs During Middle Age (35 to 65)
- Mental Health Needs During Late Adulthood (Older than 65)
- Correct Answers, Rationales, and Test Taking Strategies

Directions: *With a pencil, blacken the space in front of the option you have chosen for your correct answer.*

Mental Health Needs During Young Adulthood

A nurse works in a substance abuse clinic where most of the clients are ages 18 to 25.

1. When a 24-year-old with a record of multiple convictions for driving under the influence (DUI) claims not to be an alcoholic, what is the most pertinent assessment question the nurse can ask?
[ ] **1.** "When you drink, do you drink beer or hard liquor?"
[ ] **2.** "Did you begin drinking before or after you were of legal age?"
[ ] **3.** "Do you prefer to drink alcohol rather than soft drinks?"
[ ] **4.** "Are you unable to recall events that occurred while drinking?"

2. What is the most accurate nursing explanation of the first step in recovering from alcoholism?
[ ] **1.** Admitting an inability to control drinking
[ ] **2.** Forming a close support network
[ ] **3.** Relying on some form of religious belief
[ ] **4.** Checking into an inpatient rehabilitation unit

3. Which resource is most appropriate for the nurse to recommend when a client's family asks where they can go for support in coping with an alcoholic family member?
[ ] **1.** Alcoholics Anonymous
[ ] **2.** Recovery Anonymous
[ ] **3.** Al-Anon
[ ] **4.** Synanon

An anonymous caller phones the emergency department and asks the nurse how to tell if someone has been smoking marijuana within the past few hours.

4. The nurse correctly informs the caller that most people have which physical signs after recent marijuana use? Select all that apply.
[ ] **1.** Shivering
[ ] **2.** Inflamed eyes
[ ] **3.** Rapid pulse
[ ] **4.** Restlessness
[ ] **5.** Pinpoint pupils
[ ] **6.** Increased sex drive

5. When asked how long marijuana stays in the body after use, which response by the nurse is most accurate?
[ ] **1.** "It will show up in urine tests 3 to 4 days after use."
[ ] **2.** "Traces may be picked up by sensitive blood tests 8 to 10 weeks later."
[ ] **3.** "Hair analysis can detect marijuana use more than a year before the urine test."
[ ] **4.** "Marijuana leaves the body within 2 hours of smoking it."

6. Which nursing statement regarding the effects of chronic marijuana use is most accurate? Select all that apply.
[ ] **1.** It suppresses motivation.
[ ] **2.** It is physically addicting.
[ ] **3.** It can cause lung cancer.
[ ] **4.** It can suppress respirations.
[ ] **5.** It can affect memory.
[ ] **6.** It suppresses reproductive hormones.

A young couple brings their infant to the emergency department, whereupon, the infant is pronounced dead on arrival. Sudden infant death syndrome (SIDS) is the tentative cause of death.

7. When resuscitation efforts of a young couple's infant son are unsuccessful, which nursing action is most important next?
[ ] **1.** Ask the parents for permission to perform an autopsy.
[ ] **2.** Ask about the possibility of harvesting the infant's organs for transplantation.
[ ] **3.** Check on the parents' choice for the funeral arrangements.
[ ] **4.** Take the parents to a room where they can be with the baby.

8. Which emotional parental response is the nurse most likely to anticipate immediately after the sudden death of their infant?
[ ] **1.** Anger
[ ] **2.** Guilt
[ ] **3.** Fear
[ ] **4.** Depression

9. Which statement is most important for the nurse to convey to the parents after they have been informed of their infant's death?
[ ] **1.** "We did all we could to resuscitate your baby."
[ ] **2.** "The baby would have been brain damaged had he lived."
[ ] **3.** "You did not cause, nor could you have prevented, your baby's death."
[ ] **4.** "Grief support groups are available for situations such as yours."

During a routine clinic visit, the nurse suspects that a 20-year-old is the victim of domestic violence.

10. Which nursing action is most appropriate for determining whether domestic abuse is occurring?
[ ] **1.** Ask directly if domestic abuse is occurring.
[ ] **2.** Arrange a second visit to validate suspicions.
[ ] **3.** Assess the young children for signs of injury.
[ ] **4.** Make inquiries among relatives or neighbors.

11. If the client admits that incidences of domestic abuse are occurring, which nursing intervention is most beneficial?
[ ] **1.** Offering the victim money to leave home
[ ] **2.** Identifying resources for shelter and safety
[ ] **3.** Recommending termination of the abusive relationship
[ ] **4.** Suggesting joint counseling with a therapist or clergyman

12. If a client is typical of other victims who remain in abusive relationships, the nurse is accurate in identifying which of the following as a component of the battered victim's belief system?
[ ] **1.** The potential for danger is not serious.
[ ] **2.** The extended family will provide protection.
[ ] **3.** The victim can prevent the battering.
[ ] **4.** Leaving the batterer is a potential option.

A nurse is a volunteer answering telephone calls on a hotline at a crisis center.

13. When the nurse responds to a call from a 22-year-old rape victim, which instruction is most important before referring the client to the emergency department of the local hospital?
[ ] **1.** "Do not bathe or shower."
[ ] **2.** "Make a sketch of the rapist."
[ ] **3.** "Write down what happened."
[ ] **4.** "Call a 911 operator."

14. When the rape victim arrives at the emergency department, which nursing action is best for relieving the client's anxiety?
[ ] **1.** Determine the victim's last date of menstruation.
[ ] **2.** Collect evidence for criminal prosecution.
[ ] **3.** Assess the extent of the client's injuries.
[ ] **4.** Stay with the client at all times.

15. Which nursing action is the highest priority during the immediate care of a rape victim?
[ ] **1.** Documenting the circumstances of the rape
[ ] **2.** Keeping contact with strangers to a minimum
[ ] **3.** Offering the victim a choice of sedatives
[ ] **4.** Notifying the client's family about the incident

16. What is the best rationale for the nurse to describe emergency department procedures and their purposes to the rape victim before they are implemented?
[ ] **1.** It diminishes feelings of powerlessness.
[ ] **2.** It tends to reduce the client's anxiety.
[ ] **3.** It is a policy of the emergency department.
[ ] **4.** It meets the client's need for teaching.

17. If a rape victim desires medical treatment but objects to having evidence collected for criminal prosecution, which nursing action is most appropriate?
[ ] **1.** Persuading the victim to reconsider the decision
[ ] **2.** Proceeding because it is required
[ ] **3.** Accepting the rape victim's decision
[ ] **4.** Advising the victim to use better judgment

18. What is the most valid reason for the nurse to recommend that the rape victim attend group meetings with others who have been raped?

[ ] **1.** People with similar problems can provide emotional support.

[ ] **2.** Other victims can provide authoritative information about trauma.

[ ] **3.** New friendships can be established with other victims.

[ ] **4.** Self-protective skills can be acquired from others.

19. If the rape victim shares all of the following information during a group session, which nursing findings are most indicative of a severe adjustment reaction? Select all that apply.

[ ] **1.** The victim reports feeling somewhat anxious.

[ ] **2.** The victim describes having sporadic nightmares.

[ ] **3.** The victim has lost weight and eats out of habit.

[ ] **4.** The victim has occasional doubts about self-worth.

[ ] **5.** The victim refuses to have sexual relations.

[ ] **6.** The victim has started to drink wine before bedtime.

A public health nurse must inform a 26-year-old homosexual client that the client has tested positive for human immunodeficiency virus (HIV).

20. Which initial reaction would the nurse expect if the client is typical of others who just received news of this diagnosis?

[ ] **1.** Anger

[ ] **2.** Shock

[ ] **3.** Resentment

[ ] **4.** Depression

21. During a follow-up interview between the nurse and the client, which action by the client is most suggestive of denial about the illness?

[ ] **1.** The client conceals the information from others.

[ ] **2.** The client avoids contact with homosexual friends.

[ ] **3.** The client confronts some former sex partners.

[ ] **4.** The client has intercourse without using condoms.

22. If the nurse identifies all of the following client strengths, which one is most important for coping with this diagnosis?

[ ] **1.** Acceptance by religious leaders

[ ] **2.** A sustained network of support

[ ] **3.** Acquisition of many social acquaintances

[ ] **4.** Sexual tolerance within the community

23. Which statement made by the client diagnosed with human immunodeficiency virus (HIV) would the nurse interpret as the most serious indication of an increased risk for suicide?

[ ] **1.** "I have recurring dreams about dying."

[ ] **2.** "How many people have died from HIV?"

[ ] **3.** "Will I be alert when I'm near death?"

[ ] **4.** "Everyone would be better off without me."

Weeks later, the client with HIV is brought to the hospital by emergency personnel where a diagnosis of attempted suicide is made. The client is admitted and placed on suicide precautions.

24. Which nursing actions are appropriate for preventing self-destructive behavior? Select all that apply.

[ ] **1.** Station a security guard outside the client's room at all times.

[ ] **2.** Remove all cords, wires, and strings in the room.

[ ] **3.** Provide paper dishes and plastic utensils.

[ ] **4.** Assess whether the client has swallowed all medications.

[ ] **5.** Ask a family member to stay with the client during the night.

[ ] **6.** Check in on the client every hour.

The nurse has been working with a bulimic college student to help control the eating disorder.

25. Which recommendation by the nurse is most likely to be effective in helping the client control bulimia?

[ ] **1.** Restrict using the bathroom after meals.

[ ] **2.** Take a daily inventory of food offered at the dormitory.

[ ] **3.** Avoid eating in fast food establishments.

[ ] **4.** Keep a daily calorie count of all foods consumed.

26. If the client has been taking an antidepressant for several weeks, which outcome would be evidence to the nurse of the most desired therapeutic effect?

[ ] **1.** The client is feeling less depressed.

[ ] **2.** The client is eating more nutritiously.

[ ] **3.** The client is having fewer food binges.

[ ] **4.** The client is feeling less suicidal.

At a nurse led group meeting for clients with eating disorders, the client with bulimia tells a very emaciated client, "You're a real loser if you think you've got a weight problem."

27. Which nursing action is most appropriate at this time?

[ ] **1.** Criticize the nature of the client's rude behavior.

[ ] **2.** Support the emaciated client who was targeted by the remark.

[ ] **3.** Invite others in the group to respond to the situation.

[ ] **4.** Embarrass the bulimic client with a similar comment.

An obese 25-year-old with a history of abusing dextroamphetamine (Dexedrine) attends the eating disorder group meeting.

28. Which nursing assessment finding is most suggestive that the obese client is continuing to take dextroamphetamine (Dexedrine)?

[ ] **1.** The client stares blankly into space.

[ ] **2.** The client monopolizes the discussions.

[ ] **3.** The client wears sunglasses indoors.

[ ] **4.** The client slurs words when speaking.

29. Which finding in the client's nursing history strongly suggests lack of achieving the characteristic developmental level expected at this age in the life cycle?
[ ] **1.** The client drifts in and out of relationships.
[ ] **2.** The client worries about financial security.
[ ] **3.** The client questions personal sexual identity.
[ ] **4.** The client hesitates to be assertive.

30. When discussing obesity, which comment is the best indication to the nurse that the client is using the coping mechanism of rationalization to deal with being overweight?
[ ] **1.** "I have many health risks from being obese."
[ ] **2.** "I have real difficulty resisting ice cream."
[ ] **3.** "I know you don't like me because I'm fat."
[ ] **4.** "I can't help being overweight; it's in my genes."

A 27-year-old foreign born client is admitted to the mental health unit with abdominal pain thought to be psychophysiologic in origin. The client is apprehensive and speaks very little English.

31. Which translation method is best when the nurse obtains the client's history?
[ ] **1.** A translation card that includes key words, phrases, and pictures
[ ] **2.** A certified translator who speaks the client's language
[ ] **3.** A hospital housekeeper who speaks the client's language
[ ] **4.** The client's family member who can translate the process

A 30-year-old with a history of substance abuse is admitted to the chemical dependency unit at a local hospital.

32. If the client snorts cocaine on a regular basis, which physical assessment findings will the nurse most likely detect? Select all that apply.
[ ] **1.** Dry, stuffy nose
[ ] **2.** Perforated nasal septum
[ ] **3.** Congested breath sounds
[ ] **4.** Sinus pain under the eyes
[ ] **5.** Elevated blood pressure
[ ] **6.** Inability to sleep

33. If the client's drug screen is positive for cocaine, it is most appropriate for the nurse to advise a staff person to monitor the client closely for which finding?
[ ] **1.** Cardiac arrhythmias
[ ] **2.** Depressed respirations
[ ] **3.** Low heart rate
[ ] **4.** Elevated blood glucose level

While caring for a client who abuses drugs, the client is diagnosed with having Hepatitis B.

34. Which type of precautions should the nurse implement to prevent the transmission of Hepatitis B to others?
[ ] **1.** Standard precautions
[ ] **2.** Contact precautions
[ ] **3.** Airborne precautions
[ ] **4.** Droplet precautions

A young adult who has been diagnosed with schizophrenia is able to function for extended periods of time in the community.

35. During a home visit, which nursing assessment finding is most suggestive that the client is experiencing auditory hallucinations?
[ ] **1.** The client sings a song while walking around the room.
[ ] **2.** The client quickly changes the topic of conversation.
[ ] **3.** The client repeats a sentence over and over again.
[ ] **4.** The client turns an ear as if listening to someone.

36. If a schizophrenic client says, "Wing ding, the world is a ring," which response by the nurse is most therapeutic?
[ ] **1.** "How clever. You've made up a poem."
[ ] **2.** "I don't understand what you mean."
[ ] **3.** "Earth does orbit in a circle."
[ ] **4.** "Tell me more about the world."

37. Which nursing assessment finding is most indicative that the community-based client with schizophrenia needs to be rehospitalized?
[ ] **1.** The client neglects eating, hygiene, and sleep.
[ ] **2.** The client has missed counseling appointments.
[ ] **3.** The client is hesitant about going to work.
[ ] **4.** The client refuses to live with relatives.

38. When caring for a schizophrenic who is receiving risperidone (Risperdal), the nurse is aware that the medication is likely to have which effect on the client?
[ ] **1.** An increased incidence of extrapyramidal symptoms
[ ] **2.** An increased incidence of insomnia and agitation
[ ] **3.** Urine retention from anticholinergic effects
[ ] **4.** Symptoms of anorexia with profound weight loss

39. Before administering medication to the client with schizophrenia, it is essential that the nurse identify the client's name and which additional information?
[ ] **1.** The client's home address
[ ] **2.** The client's insurance carrier
[ ] **3.** The client's date of birth
[ ] **4.** The client's physician name

Mental Health Needs During Middle Age (35 to 65)

A nurse is assigned to care for a 35-year-old client who sustained a severe head injury and brain damage in a motor vehicle accident.

40. During the initial feeding, the client deliberately spits at the nurse. Which action is most appropriate to take first?
[ ] 1. Leave the client's room immediately.
[ ] 2. Indicate that the behavior is unacceptable.
[ ] 3. Act as if the behavior was accidental.
[ ] 4. Stand as far from the bed as possible.

41. If the client's spitting becomes habitual, which intervention is best to include in a care plan to reduce the behavior?
[ ] 1. Establish a significant consequence, such as no television for 30 minutes.
[ ] 2. Wear a face shield or other form of barrier protection when feeding the client.
[ ] 3. Explain how rude it is to spit at other people.
[ ] 4. Identify the health risks associated with spitting.

42. Which nursing action is most appropriate when performing a mental status assessment on this client?
[ ] 1. Ask open-ended questions, such as "How have you been feeling lately?"
[ ] 2. Allow extra time for the client to respond to assessment questions.
[ ] 3. Defer mental status questions to the client's spouse.
[ ] 4. Omit the mental status assessment; the results will be abnormal.

A 42-year-old is assessed in the emergency department to determine the etiology of chest pain.

43. If the client's pain is the result of a panic attack, which findings will the nurse most likely note during the physical assessment? Select all that apply.
[ ] 1. Tachycardia
[ ] 2. Hypotension
[ ] 3. Increased salivation
[ ] 4. Constricted pupils
[ ] 5. Sweating
[ ] 6. Unsteady gait

44. If a diagnosis of panic disorder is accurate, the nurse would correctly assume that the chest pain is related to which cause?
[ ] 1. Unknown cause
[ ] 2. Feigned illness
[ ] 3. Attention-seeking behavior
[ ] 4. Intense fear

45. When interacting with a client experiencing a panic attack, which technique by the nurse is most likely to help reduce the client's anxiety level?
[ ] 1. Stand less than an arm's length away.
[ ] 2. State that everything is going to be okay.
[ ] 3. Instruct the client to take shallow breaths.
[ ] 4. Explain all actions and procedures.

46. Which concept is most important for the nurse to convey to a client during a panic attack?
[ ] 1. The client is safe.
[ ] 2. The client is believed.
[ ] 3. The client is trusted.
[ ] 4. The client is accepted.

47. When the client begins crying and says, "Nurse, I feel like I'm going to die," which response is most therapeutic?
[ ] 1. "Don't cry. It won't help matters right now."
[ ] 2. "You don't want the physician to see you this way."
[ ] 3. "Everyone feels frightened in an emergency."
[ ] 4. "I'll stay with you until you feel better."

The physician prescribes alprazolam (Xanax) to treat the client's panic disorder.

48. What information is most appropriate for the nurse to tell the client about taking alprazolam (Xanax)?
[ ] 1. Avoid consuming alcohol while taking this drug.
[ ] 2. Long-term use will not cause drug dependency.
[ ] 3. This drug can cause insomnia in some people.
[ ] 4. A blood test will be required periodically.

49. The nurse is aware that if the client's panic attacks occur more frequently, the client is likely to develop which common reaction?
[ ] 1. The client will seek out referrals for psychiatric treatment.
[ ] 2. The client will fear venturing from home and will become reclusive.
[ ] 3. The client will take more than the prescribed amount of medication.
[ ] 4. The client will become psychotic and will require psychiatric admission.

The nurse on a mental health unit conducts a group meeting for clients diagnosed with obsessive-compulsive disorder (OCD).

50. Which clients can the nurse most likely expect as members of an obsessive-compulsive disorder (OCD) support group? Select all that apply.
[ ] 1. A 30-year-old who performs handwashing five times per hour
[ ] 2. A 35-year-old who wears gloves when touching a public faucet
[ ] 3. A 40-year-old who is sexually promiscuous
[ ] 4. A 45-year-old who drinks a fifth of whiskey daily
[ ] 5. A 50-year-old who cannot throw anything away
[ ] 6. A 60-year-old who repeatedly checks the locks on locked doors

51. When discussing the care of clients with obsessive-compulsive disorder (OCD) with nursing staff, which treatment options are considered most therapeutic? Select all that apply.
[ ] **1.** Selective serotonin reuptake inhibitors (SSRIs) such as fluvoxamine (Luvox)
[ ] **2.** Electroconvulsive therapy (ECT)
[ ] **3.** Cognitive-behavioral therapy
[ ] **4.** Surgical prefrontal lobotomy
[ ] **5.** Tranquilizers such as diazepam (Valium)
[ ] **6.** A self-help class on the Internet

After having an argument with his spouse on the phone, a client becomes angry and belligerent toward a nursing assistant.

52. The nurse correctly explains to the nursing assistant that the client's behavior is an example of which coping mechanism?
[ ] **1.** Introjection
[ ] **2.** Projection
[ ] **3.** Compensation
[ ] **4.** Displacement

53. Which action is best for the nurse to initially recommend to the nursing assistant to help the angry client maintain self-control?
[ ] **1.** Apply soft restraints and isolate the client.
[ ] **2.** Get the client involved in an activity.
[ ] **3.** Remain calm and appear nonthreatening.
[ ] **4.** Offer to talk to the client's spouse.

54. If the client's anger continues to escalate to potentially violent behavior, which nursing action is most appropriate?
[ ] **1.** Assemble several staff members.
[ ] **2.** Ask the physician to calm the client.
[ ] **3.** Go alone with the client to a private room.
[ ] **4.** Place behavioral restraints within the client's view.

55. If the angry client is out of control and refuses a p.r.n. sedative medication, what is the nurse's most appropriate legal option?
[ ] **1.** The nurse must respect the client's right to refuse the ordered medication.
[ ] **2.** The nurse can administer the medication to protect the safety of self and others.
[ ] **3.** The nurse must get permission from a probate court judge to administer the medication.
[ ] **4.** The nurse should ask the hospital's attorney about the client's right to refuse treatment.

The physician orders four-point behavioral restraints.

56. Once the restraints have been applied, what objective evidence indicates to the nurse that the restraints are too tight? Select all that apply.
[ ] **1.** The client reports being unable to move the right hand.
[ ] **2.** The client's fingers and toes are pale.
[ ] **3.** The client reports having pain.
[ ] **4.** Capillary refill is greater than 6 seconds.
[ ] **5.** There is excoriation around the wrist.
[ ] **6.** The client reports numbness and tingling.

A nurse prepares to teach a 60-year-old client who is highly anxious about a heart catheterization scheduled for tomorrow.

57. Which form of instruction is best when the nurse prepares the anxious client for the procedure?
[ ] **1.** Provide detailed explanations.
[ ] **2.** Use short, simple sentences.
[ ] **3.** Draw elaborate diagrams.
[ ] **4.** Show a teaching DVD.

58. If the nurse documents all of the following information in the database, which finding is probably the most significant source of conflict and anxiety for this client?
[ ] **1.** The client is facing forced retirement.
[ ] **2.** The client has 12 grandchildren.
[ ] **3.** The client is learning to use a computer.
[ ] **4.** The client wants to sell the family home.

A 38-year-old person comes to the clinic to receive information and treatment for a fear of flying.

59. If this client is typical of others with phobias, which coping mechanism is the nurse most correct in suspecting the client has been using to deal with the fear of flying?
[ ] **1.** Suppression
[ ] **2.** Compensation
[ ] **3.** Avoidance
[ ] **4.** Undoing

60. The nurse performs a physical assessment and collects the client's health history. Which assessment findings would the nurse expect to note as the client discusses the phobia related to flying? Select all that apply.
[ ] **1.** Sweating
[ ] **2.** Tachycardia
[ ] **3.** Tremors
[ ] **4.** Shortness of breath
[ ] **5.** Uncontrollable crying
[ ] **6.** Facial tics

The phobic client asks the nurse to explain cognitive therapy, the type of treatment that was recommended by the physician.

61. The nurse accurately explains that cognitive therapy involves which of the following?
[ ] 1. Altering people's irrational beliefs
[ ] 2. Exposing people to things they fear
[ ] 3. Helping people verbalize their feelings
[ ] 4. Rewarding people's altered behaviors

A nurse volunteers to participate in a support group for military personnel with post-traumatic stress disorder (PTSD).

62. When asked to identify the characteristics of post-traumatic stress disorder (PTSD), the nurse correctly responds that most people with this disorder report which findings? Select all that apply.
[ ] 1. Recurring nightmares
[ ] 2. Auditory hallucinations
[ ] 3. Rapidly changing emotions
[ ] 4. Anger that erupts easily
[ ] 5. Ease in being startled
[ ] 6. Trouble concentrating

63. Which therapeutic nursing intervention is most beneficial for a client diagnosed with post-traumatic stress disorder (PTSD)?
[ ] 1. Administering antianxiety medications
[ ] 2. Monitoring the client's physical symptoms
[ ] 3. Encouraging the client to express feelings
[ ] 4. Investigating the client's family interactions

64. When the nurse asks the members of the post-traumatic stress disorder (PTSD) support group to draw pictures of their traumatic experiences, what is the most therapeutic outcome for the activity?
[ ] 1. Each will deal consciously with painful memories.
[ ] 2. The participants will bond emotionally with each other.
[ ] 3. Each person will receive approval from group members.
[ ] 4. The activity will justify participation in the group.

A World War II veteran tells the nurse about feeling startled and fearful whenever attending Fourth of July fireworks displays, and asks for a possible explanation.

65. Which nursing explanation of the client's experiences is most accurate?
[ ] 1. The client was frightened of them as a child.
[ ] 2. The client is fearful of being injured.
[ ] 3. The client associates the event with combat service.
[ ] 4. The client is afraid it will trigger memories.

A 55-year-old has multiple symptoms that do not resemble any specific disorder. The client is anxious and worried because no definite diagnosis has been made.

66. When the anxious client without any specifically diagnosed disorder summons the nurse and reports feeling weak and dizzy, which nursing action is most appropriate at this time?
[ ] 1. Helping the client to relax
[ ] 2. Giving the client something to eat
[ ] 3. Administering oxygen by cannula
[ ] 4. Taking the client's vital signs

The client shares with the nurse about regretting never attending college or having had children.

67. What is the best nursing explanation for the middle aged adult's reminiscences?
[ ] 1. Adults tend to assess their accomplishments at midlife.
[ ] 2. Adults tend to set unreasonable goals at midlife.
[ ] 3. Adults tend to envy others' achievements at midlife.
[ ] 4. Adults tend to question their values at midlife.

One day the undiagnosed client says to the nurse, "Do you think they'll ever be able to find out what's wrong with me?"

68. Which response by the nurse is best in this situation?
[ ] 1. "That is something to discuss with your physician."
[ ] 2. "It sounds like you're feeling discouraged."
[ ] 3. "Let us worry about your lack of progress."
[ ] 4. "You need to practice a little more patience."

After several diagnostic tests, the physician explains to the client that there are no significant findings and diagnoses the condition as hypochondriasis.

69. The nurse reviews the client's medical history, assessing for possible risk factors leading to hypochondriasis. Which of the following reported findings are considered risk factors for this disorder? Select all that apply.
[ ] 1. Family history of hypochondria
[ ] 2. Diagnosed anxiety disorder
[ ] 3. Serious illness as a child
[ ] 4. Witnessed violence in childhood
[ ] 5. Stressful experience with a loved one's illness
[ ] 6. Fear of death or disfigurement

A staff member asks the nurse about the signs and symptoms of hypochondriasis.

70. The nurse is accurate in identifying which of the following signs and symptoms as closely associated with hypochondriasis? Select all that apply.
[ ] **1.** Frequently researching information about specific illnesses and their symptoms
[ ] **2.** Chronic fear that minor symptoms are signs of a serious illness
[ ] **3.** Symptoms that correlate with specific medical diseases are repeatedly reported
[ ] **4.** Interference of the disorder with social life or work
[ ] **5.** Numerous physician visits, sometimes in the same day
[ ] **6.** Obtaining multiple tests for the same symptoms

A client's pastor visits the hospital. On approaching the nurses' station, the pastor tells the nurse that the client has given permission to see the medical record.

71. Which action by the nurse is most appropriate at this time?
[ ] **1.** Telling the pastor to ask the client's physician for permission to access the medical record
[ ] **2.** Asking the pastor to produce evidence of being a certified hospital chaplain
[ ] **3.** Informing the pastor that the medical record is confidential to all but the staff
[ ] **4.** Checking the agency's policy regarding access to medical records with the nursing supervisor

The nursing team holds a conference concerning a 38-year-old who has just been admitted with ulcerative colitis, a psychophysiologic disease.

72. When a nursing assistant asks if *psychophysiologic* means that the client is not really sick, which response by the nurse is most accurate?
[ ] **1.** The client pretends to be sick when needing a rest.
[ ] **2.** The client believes an illness exists, but the tests are all negative.
[ ] **3.** The client would rather be hospitalized than have to work.
[ ] **4.** The client has an illness that is influenced by emotions.

During a team conference, the nurses discuss the care of the client with ulcerative colitis.

73. Which of the following assessments is the highest nursing priority when caring for the client?
[ ] **1.** The number and characteristics of the client's bowel movements
[ ] **2.** How much the client knows about colostomy care?
[ ] **3.** Which coping mechanisms the client uses for handling stress?
[ ] **4.** The types of relationships the client has with peers

The discussion turns to exploring ways to maintain the client's self-esteem while providing rectal hygiene.

74. Which nursing approach is best for managing the client's care?
[ ] **1.** Use a nonjudgmental manner when cleaning the client of stool.
[ ] **2.** Ask the client's spouse to perform hygiene measures.
[ ] **3.** Hold the client responsible for all hygiene.
[ ] **4.** Assign same-gender nurses to care for the client.

The client's spouse confides to the nurse that the client who is recovering from surgery is a chronic alcoholic but has not told the physician.

75. Which finding by the nurse during a postoperative assessment is most indicative of the client's alcoholism?
[ ] **1.** The client's blood pressure is lower than normal.
[ ] **2.** The client's pain is unrelieved with usual dosages of analgesics.
[ ] **3.** The client becomes nauseated after eating.
[ ] **4.** The client's pulse is slow, weak, and irregular.

Approximately 36 hours after admission, the client becomes restless and shouts that the bugs in the room must be exterminated.

76. In this situation, which nursing action is most appropriate?
[ ] **1.** Placing restraints on the client's arms and legs
[ ] **2.** Reassuring the client that the bugs are imaginary
[ ] **3.** Remaining at the client's bedside to reinforce reality
[ ] **4.** Closing the client's door so that others are not alarmed

77. On the basis of the change in the client's condition, which nursing action is most appropriate to perform next?
[ ] **1.** Notify the client's spouse
[ ] **2.** Call the nursing supervisor
[ ] **3.** Inform the physician
[ ] **4.** Document the assessed data

78. While caring for a client who is withdrawing from alcohol, the nurse must assess for what additional complication?
[ ] **1.** Hypothermia
[ ] **2.** Seizures
[ ] **3.** Ascites
[ ] **4.** Jaundice

At the beginning of the next shift, a team member states, "Don't expect me to take care of that good-for-nothing drunk."

79. The nurse counsels the team member privately about the inappropriate remark. What nursing recommendation will be most helpful in understanding and accepting the behavior of clients?
[ ] **1.** Strive to understand one's own behavior
[ ] **2.** Analyze what motivates clients' behavior
[ ] **3.** Become more familiar with abnormal behavior
[ ] **4.** Take courses in behavioral psychology counseling.

A home health nurse is scheduled for daily visits to change the abdominal dressing of a 45-year-old with a history of bipolar disorder.

80. While reviewing the client's psychiatric history, the nurse would expect to note which major characteristic of bipolar disorder?
[ ] **1.** Ritualistic behavior
[ ] **2.** Symbolic aggressiveness
[ ] **3.** Cyclic mood swings
[ ] **4.** Periodic amnesia

The nurse reads that the client is taking lithium carbonate (Lithane) to treat the bipolar disorder and suspects that the client has not been taking the medication as prescribed.

81. When the nurse reviews information about lithium carbonate (Lithane) with the client, which instructions are most important to stress? Select all that apply.
[ ] **1.** Take a high-potency vitamin each morning.
[ ] **2.** Refrain from sexual activity while taking this medication.
[ ] **3.** Notify the physician if urine output increases.
[ ] **4.** Drink 10 to 12 glasses of water per day.
[ ] **5.** Maintain a sufficient salt intake daily.
[ ] **6.** Avoid eating aged cheeses.

82. Which assessment measure is most important for the nurse to monitor to determine whether the client's current dose of lithium carbonate (Lithane) is appropriate?
[ ] **1.** Vital signs
[ ] **2.** Urine volume
[ ] **3.** Drug blood levels
[ ] **4.** Brain wave scans

83. Which findings strongly suggests to the nurse that the client is experiencing an exacerbation of the bipolar disorder? Select all that apply.
[ ] **1.** The client has been spending money extravagantly.
[ ] **2.** The client wants to become a 5-year-old again.
[ ] **3.** The client has been methodically cleaning the house.
[ ] **4.** The client has been staying up late to read.
[ ] **5.** The client demonstrates increased sexual promiscuity.
[ ] **6.** The client has increased anxiety when going outside the house.

Mental Health Needs During Late Adulthood (Older than 65)

A nurse performs a home assessment on a reasonably healthy older adult who chooses to live in a supervised retirement community.

84. If the older adult's sons and daughters are visiting on the day of the scheduled visit, which nursing action is most appropriate before beginning the assessment?
[ ] **1.** Encourage the client's children to offer their comments at any time.
[ ] **2.** Provide a private setting for conducting the assessment.
[ ] **3.** Identify the names and relationships of those present.
[ ] **4.** Offer to share the assessment results with the client's children.

85. Which question by the nurse during the client interview is likely to generate the most information?
[ ] **1.** "Tell me about your family."
[ ] **2.** "Are you currently married?"
[ ] **3.** "Who is your nearest relative?"
[ ] **4.** "Give me a list of your family members."

86. Which question is best for the nurse to ask to assess the client's long-term memory?
[ ] **1.** "What is your current age?"
[ ] **2.** "What is today's date?"
[ ] **3.** "What is your date of birth?"
[ ] **4.** "What occurred last January?"

87. Which action by the nurse can best determine if an older client's inappropriate responses to several questions are due to miscommunication or to impaired cognition?
[ ] **1.** Ask the client to repeat the question before answering it.
[ ] **2.** Ask questions that require only a "yes" or "no" response.
[ ] **3.** Ask the client's next of kin for answers to the questions.
[ ] **4.** Ask questions to which the client is sure to know the answers.

88. Which nursing assessment finding is most atypical of a 65-year-old client?
[ ] **1.** Making errors in copying a line drawing
[ ] **2.** Forgetting the names of longstanding neighbors
[ ] **3.** Recalling information slowly
[ ] **4.** Naming only two of the last three presidents

89. If the client is typical of others of similar age, the nurse can anticipate the client as having which age-related problems? Select all that apply.
[ ] **1.** Dealing with losses
[ ] **2.** Becoming cynical
[ ] **3.** Losing patience
[ ] **4.** Developing hostility
[ ] **5.** Having periods of regret
[ ] **6.** Experiencing episodes of depression

A 68-year-old who is currently being treated for major depression is transferred to a medical unit after an episode of acute abdominal pain.

90. Which of the following nursing assessment data places the client at highest risk for suicide?
[ ] **1.** The client feels hopeless about the future.
[ ] **2.** The client has a plan in mind for suicide.
[ ] **3.** The client states that death would end the misery.
[ ] **4.** The client says the distress is intolerable.

91. If the physician prescribes imipramine hydrochloride (Tofranil) for the client, the nurse should assess for which initial therapeutic drug effect?
[ ] **1.** Absence of suicidal ideation
[ ] **2.** Improved concentration
[ ] **3.** Decreased agitation
[ ] **4.** Regulated mood

92. Which of the following nursing instructions are appropriate to include in the teaching plan of a client who is just beginning treatment with imipramine hydrochloride (Tofranil)? Select all that apply.
[ ] **1.** Avoid eating cheese, chocolate, and pickled foods.
[ ] **2.** Take short naps during the day.
[ ] **3.** Rise from the chair or bed slowly.
[ ] **4.** Expect to wait about 3 weeks before feeling better.
[ ] **5.** Refrain from all sexual activity for 1 month after starting the medication.
[ ] **6.** Use a good sunscreen when outdoors.

93. Which nursing action is especially important when administering medications to a depressed client?
[ ] **1.** Encouraging the client to drink a full glass of water
[ ] **2.** Checking that the client has swallowed all oral medications
[ ] **3.** Giving the medications on an empty stomach before meals
[ ] **4.** Having the client take each medication separately

94. The depressed client undergoes electroconvulsive therapy (ECT). Which of the following outcomes can the nurse most likely expect during the client's immediate recovery period?
[ ] **1.** Brief episodes of absence seizures
[ ] **2.** Sensitivity to light and double vision
[ ] **3.** Short-term memory loss and headaches
[ ] **4.** Periods of unexplained fear and anxiety

The physician prescribes doxepin (Sinequan) to be taken at bedtime for another client with depression.

95. What nursing suggestion is best if the client complains of dizziness on rising after taking doxepin (Sinequan) as prescribed?
[ ] **1.** "Place a cool compress on your forehead."
[ ] **2.** "Get up slowly from a seated position."
[ ] **3.** "Remain in bed with your feet elevated above your heart."
[ ] **4.** "Take some deep breaths before getting out of bed."

A nurse refers a 66-year-old home care client to the mental health clinic for evaluation of a coexisting depressive disorder.

96. If the home health nurse documented all of the following findings, which one is most suggestive that the client is depressed?
[ ] **1.** The client is irritable after grandchildren visit.
[ ] **2.** The client has multiple, unrelated physical complaints.
[ ] **3.** The client takes lengthy naps in the late afternoon.
[ ] **4.** The client cries when talking about a dead spouse.

97. If the nurse notes the following symptoms after the client begins taking duloxetine (Cymbalta), which one is most likely drug-related?
[ ] **1.** Polyuria
[ ] **2.** Diplopia
[ ] **3.** Drooling
[ ] **4.** Insomnia

A nurse who is employed in a long-term care facility observes that a romantic relationship is developing between two residents.

98. Which action is most appropriate if the nurse discovers the oriented older couple having consensual sexual intercourse?
[ ] **1.** Report it to their adult children.
[ ] **2.** Restore a measure of privacy.
[ ] **3.** Suggest they become roommates.
[ ] **4.** Censure their sexual activity.

An older adult client with chronic mental illness is transferred from a long-term state psychiatric hospital to a nursing home for custodial care.

99. If a client with chronic mental illness develops the following symptoms after the physician discontinues haloperidol (Haldol), which symptom is the nurse most likely to attribute to a consequence of the drug therapy?
[ ] **1.** Facial tics
[ ] **2.** Depression
[ ] **3.** Patchy hair loss
[ ] **4.** Daytime lethargy

A client who has had a stroke currently lives in a long-term care facility and struggles to manage activities of daily living.

100. If the client frequently comes to meals with the residue of soap on the face or an unbuttoned shirt, which nursing action is most beneficial to the client's self-esteem?
[ ] **1.** Send the client back to finish.
[ ] **2.** Bathe and dress the client daily.
[ ] **3.** Schedule the client's hygiene activities after meals.
[ ] **4.** Comment on how self-reliant the client is.

A nurse joins a group of older adult clients during reminiscence therapy.

101. Which activity planned by the nurse is most helpful in facilitating reminiscence therapy among older adult clients?
[ ] **1.** Discussing a current event topic
[ ] **2.** Singing popular songs from the 1960s
[ ] **3.** Reading an article from the newspaper
[ ] **4.** Making decorations for a future holiday

102. When one older adult at reminiscence therapy says, "If I had it to do all over again, I wouldn't change a thing," the nurse is most accurate in interpreting this to mean that the client has acquired which developmental characteristic?
[ ] **1.** Trust
[ ] **2.** Integrity
[ ] **3.** Intimacy
[ ] **4.** Autonomy

A group of nurses attends in-service training about documentation issues.

103. The nurses critique a chart entry that says, "States, 'I feel unwanted.' Appears to be confused." Which statement best describes why this entry is unsatisfactory?
[ ] **1.** The nurse who made the entry failed to interpret the significance of feeling unwanted.
[ ] **2.** The nurse who made the entry failed to indicate the importance of the client's statement.
[ ] **3.** The nurse who made the entry failed to substantiate that the client made the quote.
[ ] **4.** The nurse who made the entry failed to describe the evidence of the confused behavior.

The educator conducts in-service training for the nursing staff on cultural considerations related to mental illness, and discusses the barriers to obtaining treatment.

104. When providing care for an Asian client diagnosed with mental illness, which are primary factors in developing a plan of care? Select all that apply.
[ ] **1.** Language
[ ] **2.** Literacy
[ ] **3.** Reticence to report of symptoms
[ ] **4.** Marital status
[ ] **5.** Members of extended family
[ ] **6.** Financial status

A nurse is employed on a special unit for clients with dementia.

105. What is the best nursing action to help reorient a confused client who wanders into other clients' rooms?
[ ] **1.** Place a large sign with the client's name on the door.
[ ] **2.** Keep the room doors on the unit locked at all times.
[ ] **3.** Restrain the client in a wheelchair when unattended.
[ ] **4.** Speak to the client about invading other people's privacy.

A 70-year-old client with dementia removes clothing and walks naked through the halls of a long-term care facility.

106. Which action is most appropriate for the nurse to take first?
[ ] **1.** Remind the client that clothes are required in public.
[ ] **2.** Tell the client to put clothes on again.
[ ] **3.** Explain to the residents that the client is not of sound mind.
[ ] **4.** Take the client to a vacant room nearby.

107. When a nurse orients a newly hired nursing assistant, which of the following instructions is most therapeutic for helping clients with dementia remain oriented?
[ ] **1.** Address all clients using their first name.
[ ] **2.** Ask clients to identify their goals for the day.
[ ] **3.** Assign clients to greet visitors each day.
[ ] **4.** Post large calendars with the current date.

108. During a nursing conference with personnel, which nursing technique is best to stress to the staff for reducing confusion among clients with dementia?
[ ] **1.** Wear an employee name tag when caring for clients.
[ ] **2.** Adhere to a consistent routine of unit activities.
[ ] **3.** Provide diversional activities such as field trips.
[ ] **4.** Distribute a list of the day's scheduled events.

109. What is the best suggestion that the nurse leading the team conference can offer for communicating with clients with dementia?
[ ] **1.** Speak loudly to get the client's attention.
[ ] **2.** Use short sentences when speaking to the client.
[ ] **3.** Use written forms of communication.
[ ] **4.** Allow the client to listen to news programs.

110. When a client with dementia in the nursing facility says, "I want to go home," which response by the nurse is most appropriate?
[ ] **1.** "You are at home."
[ ] **2.** "You are staying here."
[ ] **3.** "You must not like us."
[ ] **4.** "You need to call your family."

The spouse of a client on the dementia unit visits on a daily basis. A nurse who regularly cares for the client notices that the spouse is beginning to show signs of exhaustion and self-neglect.

111. Which nursing intervention is most beneficial for the client's spouse at this time?
[ ] **1.** Suggesting that the spouse make an appointment for a physical examination
[ ] **2.** Discussing modifying the amount of time the spouse devotes to care-giving
[ ] **3.** Reminding the spouse of the scheduled times for visiting clients on the unit
[ ] **4.** Explaining that many staff are available to care for the client

A client who is diagnosed with Alzheimer's disease lives in a long-term care center. The client's daughter visits regularly.

112. One day the client's daughter states to the nurse, "I'm not sure my mom recognizes me." Which response by the nurse is most therapeutic?
[ ] 1. "This is probably the beginning of the end."
[ ] 2. "You're distressed that there isn't an appropriate response to you."
[ ] 3. "Don't worry. The standard of care is being delivered."
[ ] 4. "There will be good days and bad days. Today is a bad day."

113. When the older client with Alzheimer's disease is confused about how to use a fork, which nursing action is best for prolonging the client's ability to maintain self-care?
[ ] 1. Ask the physician to order a liquid diet.
[ ] 2. Position the client to promote mimicking other clients.
[ ] 3. Serve the client first so there is sufficient time to eat.
[ ] 4. Seat the client alone so no one will see any mess that occurs.

The daughter of the client with Alzheimer's disease wants to take the client home for a day.

114. Which nursing assessment is critical for ensuring the client's well-being during the home visit?
[ ] 1. The caregiver's understanding of the symptoms the client manifests
[ ] 2. The caregiver's understanding of when the client must return
[ ] 3. The caregiver's understanding of when to administer medications
[ ] 4. The caregiver's understanding of how to provide hygiene measures

An older adult who is admitted to the hospital is dying of a terminal illness. The client has an advance directive indicating that no heroic measures be used to prolong life.

115. What is the most appropriate nursing action when the terminally ill client's death is imminent?
[ ] 1. Sit quietly and hold the dying client's hand.
[ ] 2. Notify the hospital chaplain of the potential for death.
[ ] 3. Call the funeral home, alerting them of an imminent death.
[ ] 4. Transfer the client to the intensive care unit.

After the death of the terminally ill client, a nursing assistant is extremely distraught.

116. What nursing approach is most beneficial for helping the nursing assistant at this time?
[ ] 1. Sending the nursing assistant home for the rest of the shift
[ ] 2. Terminating the nursing assistant from this type of work
[ ] 3. Allowing the nursing assistant to express feelings
[ ] 4. Asking the nursing assistant to help with postmortem care

Family members of the deceased client are referred to a grief support group.

117. When a new member to the group tells the nursing leader about sensing the presence of the dead spouse in the home, which nursing intervention is most appropriate?
[ ] 1. Recommending more professional counseling
[ ] 2. Assuring the client that it is wishful thinking
[ ] 3. Letting the client be comforted by the experience
[ ] 4. Encouraging the client to stay with relatives

Correct Answers, Rationales, and Test Taking Strategies

Mental Health Needs During Young Adulthood

1. 4. Alcoholism is a chronic, progressive, often fatal disease that has genetic, psychosocial, and environmental elements. It is characterized by alcohol craving, impaired control over drinking, a preoccupation with alcohol, and the use of alcohol despite the consequences (loss of a job, problems with a spouse or significant other, or trouble with the law). Alcoholism is a physical dependency, and abrupt deprivation leads to severe withdrawal symptoms. Alcoholics experience distorted thinking and denial. Although an affirmative answer to all the questions is significant, the most suggestive sign of alcoholism is the occurrence of blackouts. Blackouts are a form of amnesia for actions and events that take place when a person is drinking. Alcoholism is a dependency on alcohol-containing substances; it can occur regardless of the type of alcohol consumed and when the person began drinking. Preferring alcohol over soft drinks is a personal choice; however, choosing to drink alcohol can lead to serious consequences, including the increased risk of developing alcoholism.

> *Test Taking Strategy—Look at the key words "most pertinent" as they refer to an assessment for identifying alcoholism. Option 4 is the best answer from among the options because alcoholics experience blackouts regardless of when they started consuming alcohol. Review the signs and symptoms of alcoholism if you had difficulty answering this question.*
> *Cognitive Level—Analyzing*
> *Client Needs Category—Psychosocial integrity*
> *Client Needs Subcategory—None*

2. 1. Denial is the major barrier to recovery from alcoholism. The first step of Alcoholics Anonymous (AA) and other treatment programs is to admit powerlessness over alcohol. AA does emphasize belief in a higher power, but relying on and participating in an organized religion is not a prerequisite for participation in the treatment program. Forming a close support network is important because the client undergoes many physical, emotional, and lifestyle changes, but this is not the first step to the recovery process. Admission to an inpatient rehabilitation unit is also not a prerequisite to treatment because clients often attend treatment programs after work and on the weekends as outpatients.

> *Test Taking Strategy—Look at the key words "first step" in reference to a sign of recovery for alcoholism. Option 1 is the best answer because accepting responsibility for alcohol dependence must occur before the client can overcome his or her past history. Review the steps in AA's 12-step program,*

> focusing on step one, if you had difficulty answering this question.
> *Cognitive Level—Applying*
> *Client Needs Category—Psychosocial integrity*
> *Client Needs Subcategory—None*

3. 3. Al-Anon is an organization specifically for family members of alcoholics who may or may not be involved in recovery. Alcoholics Anonymous is for recovering alcoholics. Recovery Anonymous is a support group for persons with mental disorders. Synanon is a private organization involved in drug rehabilitation.

> *Test Taking Strategy—Analyze to determine what information the question asks for, which is the organization that offers support for persons who are in a relationship with someone who is alcohol-dependent. Review the purpose of the organizations listed in the options if you had difficulty answering this question.*
> *Cognitive Level—Remembering*
> *Client Needs Category—Safe and effective care environment*
> *Client Needs Subcategory—Coordinated care*

4. 2, 3. Inflammation of the eyes is almost always present after smoking marijuana. Depending on the dose obtained from the drug, the pulse rate can be rapid, causing the user to feel anxious. Other signs include euphoria, drowsiness, light-headedness, and hunger. Shivering accompanies opiate withdrawal, not marijuana use. Restlessness is observed in abrupt alcohol withdrawal or with use of a central nervous system stimulant. Pinpoint pupils are a sign of heroin use, not marijuana use. There is no evidence that marijuana use is related to increased sex drive, although use of marijuana may lead to a reduction of sexual inhibitions. Usually, sexual performance is negatively affected with drugs and alcohol use.

> *Test Taking Strategy—Analyze to determine what information the question asks for, which is the signs and symptoms of marijuana use. Alternative-format "select all that apply" questions require considering each option independently to decide its merit in answering the question. Review signs of marijuana use if you had difficulty answering this question.*
> *Cognitive Level—Applying*
> *Client Needs Category—Psychosocial integrity*
> *Client Needs Subcategory—None*

5. 1. Because urine is easy to obtain and inexpensive to analyze, urine tests are widely used to detect illegal drug use. Marijuana use can be detected in the body 3 to 4 days after use (if urine is used). In fact, most illegal drugs, including cocaine, heroin, amphetamines, barbiturates, and "ecstasy" (MDMA) stay in the body from 3 to 10 days. Samples of blood, hair, tissue, and saliva can also be used to test for illegal drug use, but with greater difficulty.

Hair analysis can detect cocaine that was used more than a year before the urine test. Marijuana is detected by blood tests 3 to 4 weeks after use, not 8 to 10 weeks. Drugs that are used as inhalants (such as glue) leave the body within 2 hours.

Test Taking Strategy—Look at the key words "most accurate" in relation to the length of time during which marijuana use can be detected. Option 1 is the best answer. THC, the main active substance found in marijuana, is generally included in a drug screening test when assessing a suspected substance abuser. Review drug screening for abused substances if you had difficulty answering this question.
Cognitive Level—Remembering
Client Needs Category—Psychosocial integrity
Client Needs Subcategory—None

6. 1, 5, 6. Marijuana is known to produce apathy among those who use it. Consequently, many chronic users become disinterested in school, work, or other social responsibilities. As a result, they fail to reach their potential for success. Chronic use of marijuana affects memory and the ability to learn, similar to the effects associated with chronic alcohol abuse. Chronic marijuana abuse also suppresses hormonal production, causing a decrease in sperm production and inability to ovulate. Marijuana is more likely to be psychologically addicting than physically addicting. The evidence linking marijuana use with lung cancer is inconclusive, but studies do show an increase in the number of colds, bronchitis, and asthma cases among chronic users of marijuana. Breathing may be impaired, but the respiratory center in the brain is not usually suppressed as it is in opiate abuse.

Test Taking Strategy—Analyze to determine what information the question asks for, which is signs of long-term marijuana use. Alternative-format "select all that apply" questions require considering each option independently to decide its merit in answering the question. Choose options that are associated with chronic use of marijuana. Review the consequences of chronic marijuana use if you had difficulty answering this question.
Cognitive Level—Applying
Client Needs Category—Psychosocial integrity
Client Needs Subcategory—None

7. 4. Sudden infant death syndrome (SIDS) is the unexpected, unexplained death of an infant who is typically between age 2 weeks and 1 year old. In most cases, the infant is laid down for a nap or to sleep at night and then, after several hours, is found dead in the crib. Common risk factors include prematurity, low birth weight, and an adolescent or opioid-dependent mother.

Because of the abruptness and finality of the situation, the parents of an infant who died from SIDS have a very difficult time accepting their infant's death. Their most immediate need is to experience the reality of their loss. Facilitating an opportunity to have personal contact with the infant promotes the grieving process. The other nursing actions may be completed at a later time.

Test Taking Strategy—Use the process of elimination to help select the option that is most important to perform first when interacting with the parents of an infant that has not responded to resuscitation efforts. Although all the options are realistic, option 4 is the best answer because it promotes healthy grieving. Review actions that are helpful when grieving a death, especially one that is sudden and unexpected, if you had difficulty answering this question.
Cognitive Level—Analyzing
Client Needs Category—Psychosocial integrity
Client Needs Subcategory—None

8. 2. Most parents feel guilty immediately after the death of a previously healthy infant, as in sudden infant death syndrome (SIDS). They need reassurance that they are in no way to blame for the child's death. Later, the parents may benefit from a professional or support group to help in resolving their anger, fear, and depression.

Test Taking Strategy—Analyze to determine what information the question asks for, which is the emotion most likely to be experienced immediately after the death of a child from SIDS. Option 2 is the best answer because parents feel responsible for protecting children from harm and feel guilty when they erroneously believe they were negligent in some way. Review emotional responses associated with the sudden, unexpected death of a child if you had difficulty answering this question.
Cognitive Level—Applying
Client Needs Category—Psychosocial integrity
Client Needs Subcategory—None

9. 3. It is important to relieve parents of any self-blame after the unexpected death of an infant. Unfortunately, many parents are suspected of child abuse in cases like this. Informing them of the staff's efforts and where grief support may be obtained are appropriate nursing actions, but they are secondary to relieving undeserved guilt. Indicating that the child may have had brain damage is little consolation immediately after the infant's death.

Test Taking Strategy—Use the process of elimination to help select the option that describes the most important statement a nurse can make to parents who have been informed about the death of their child. Option 3 is the best answer because it reinforces that self-blame is not deserved. Options 1 and 4 have merit, but they are not most important initially. Option 2 could be correct; however, the statement is not likely to bring solace to the parents. Review the therapeutic effect of statements offered to grieving parents if you had difficulty answering this question.

Cognitive Level—Analyzing
Client Needs Category—Psychosocial integrity
Client Needs Subcategory—None

10. 1. Domestic abuse is maltreatment by a family member toward someone else living in the household. If the abused individual comes to the emergency department and is treated for trauma (bruising, burns, broken bones, lacerations, or head injuries), the investigation of potential domestic abuse is a priority. Candidly asking if the person is being abused is the most straightforward way to obtain information. Although many victims of abuse protect their abuser, they are not apt to reveal their abuse unless they sense that someone is concerned enough to ask. It is appropriate to assess the children for signs of abuse, but this would be done secondarily. Checking with relatives or friends may damage the nurse-client relationship or jeopardize the victim's safety if the abusive spouse becomes aware of the inquiry. Asking the client to return for a second visit may arouse suspicions in the abuser, which could cause further abuse for the client. The nurse should obtain as much information as possible during the initial visit.

> *Test Taking Strategy—Look at the key words "most appropriate" in reference to the best action for confirming suspicions of domestic abuse. Option 1 is the best approach; however, many victims of abuse are hesitant to reveal how their injuries occurred. Review assessment techniques when managing the care of a client who is the suspected victim of abuse if you had difficulty answering this question.*
> *Cognitive Level—Analyzing*
> *Client Needs Category—Psychosocial integrity*
> *Client Needs Subcategory—None*

11. 2. More than anything else, knowing where there is a safe place to go for help empowers the victim to seek protection when exposed to future violence. Giving out money or personal information such as address or telephone numbers to clients is not professional behavior and is never appropriate. Many women stay in abusive relationships because they think the abuser will change or they feel there is no other alternative. Trying to terminate an abusive relationship may also escalate the frequency or severity of violence. Most male batterers are resistant to change and are unlikely to participate in joint counseling.

> *Test Taking Strategy—Look at the key words "most beneficial" in reference to helping a client who may be the victim of domestic abuse. Option 2 is the correct answer because it offers a means of safety, protection, and support when terminating an abusive relationship. Review interventions for managing situations involving domestic violence if you had difficulty answering this question.*
> *Cognitive Level—Analyzing*
> *Client Needs Category—Psychosocial integrity*
> *Client Needs Subcategory—None*

12. 3. Many victims of family violence believe that, if they behave in an ideal way that is pleasing to the batterer, they can prevent the cycle of abuse. Some persons even blame themselves or believe that they deserve the abuse. Battered individuals feel hopeless and powerless and have a great deal of guilt. Often, abused women have no money and lack the skills and self-esteem to earn it. They need a great deal of support to leave their partners, and extended family members may not be willing to take in the victim because of fear for their own safety. Most victims know that the abuse is serious or even life-threatening, that they may be murdered if they attempt to terminate the relationship, and that their family most likely will be unsupportive.

> *Test Taking Strategy—Analyze to determine what information the question asks for, which is the rationale many victims of domestic abuse use when remaining in a relationship with their abuser. Option 3 is the best answer because abuse victims often erroneously believe they are responsible for the abuse and rationalize that if they avoid contributing behaviors, the abuse will cease or be avoided. Review factors that contribute to long-standing domestic abuse if you had difficulty answering this question.*
> *Cognitive Level—Analyzing*
> *Client Needs Category—Psychosocial integrity*
> *Client Needs Subcategory—None*

13. 1. Rape is forced sexual activity involving intercourse and penetration of an orifice by the penis. It is a deviant behavior and a crime of violence. Sexual assault refers to other forced sex acts (such as oral sex). To preserve possible evidence, a physical examination should be performed before the victim showers or bathes, brushes teeth, douches, changes clothes, or has anything to drink. If there is no report of oral sex, rinsing the mouth and drinking fluids may be permitted. Evidence of pubic hair, semen, skin, and nail samples are some of the data collected from the victim. Although a sketch of the rapist or a written description of the crime may be helpful, rape victims are usually not capable of completing these activities independently. It is inappropriate to recommend calling 911 if the victim is in no immediate danger. However, advising the victim to call a support person is appropriate, but not the most important information to convey.

> *Test Taking Strategy—Analyze to determine what information the question asks for, which is the most important initial instruction to provide a rape victim. Option 1 is the best answer because it facilitates identifying and prosecuting the perpetrator of the crime. Review the process of collecting evidence in crimes involving rape if you had difficulty answering this question.*
> *Cognitive Level—Analyzing*
> *Client Needs Category—Psychosocial integrity*
> *Client Needs Subcategory—None*

14. 4. Assuming that the nurse is female, the most supportive nursing activity is to remain with the rape victim at all times. Such victims of crime suffer a great deal of stress, especially when they must interact with physicians or police officers who are strangers and often men. The other nursing actions are important to the care of rape victims, but they are not as likely to reduce anxiety as the continuous presence of an empathic female nurse.

Test Taking Strategy—Use the process of elimination to help select the best nursing action for relieving a rape victim's anxiety. Option 4 is the best answer because remaining with the rape victim provides emotional support, which tends to reduce anxiety during stressful situations. Review nursing techniques for relieving anxiety if you had difficulty answering this question.
Cognitive Level—*Analyzing*
Client Needs Category—*Psychosocial integrity*
Client Needs Subcategory—*None*

15. 2. Victims of violent crimes are likely to perceive strangers as a threat to their safety. Therefore, a priority for nursing care is to limit the number of client contacts with unfamiliar people, even though the strangers are well-meaning staff. The nurse is responsible for assessing the victim for physical and emotional trauma, whereas the police document the circumstances of the rape. Sedation is generally avoided if at all possible because it interferes with crisis resolution. The nurse must protect the confidentiality of the client. Therefore, notifying the family, unless the client requests it, is not appropriate.

Test Taking Strategy—Look at the key words "highest priority," which implies selecting the most important action from among the options. In this case, option 2 is the best answer, because a rape victim is likely to feel threatened when interacting with anyone with whom she or he has not developed trust. Review therapeutic nursing actions when managing the care of a rape victim if you had difficulty answering this question.
Cognitive Level—*Analyzing*
Client Needs Category—*Psychosocial integrity*
Client Needs Subcategory—*None*

16. 2. Providing explanations helps to reduce anxiety. It is especially important for clients who are trying to manage the stress of a traumatic experience. Giving clients opportunities to make choices is a therapeutic method of diminishing feelings of powerlessness. Although giving information does support standards of care established in the emergency department and meets the client's need for teaching, these are not the primary reasons for explaining care measures to a rape victim.

Test Taking Strategy—Analyze to determine what information the question asks for, which is the rationale for describing procedures and their purposes to a

rape victim. Option 2 is the best answer because knowledge empowers the victim to cope with the unfamiliarity of a rape examination and collection of evidence. Review therapeutic nursing actions when managing the care of a rape victim if you had difficulty answering this question.*
Cognitive Level—*Analyzing*
Client Needs Category—*Psychosocial integrity*
Client Needs Subcategory—*None*

17. 3. Competent adult clients always have the right to make decisions regarding their treatment. Although a nurse may not feel that the decision is in the client's best interests, the client's right to refuse must be respected. Coercion in any form is inappropriate.

Test Taking Strategy—Look at the key words "most appropriate" in reference to a client's refusal to allow collection of evidence involved in a rape. Although the nurse may feel another decision is better, option 3 is the best answer because it respects the client's right to self-determination. Review the right to self-determination and the manner in which it applies to client care if you had difficulty answering this question.
Cognitive Level—*Analyzing*
Client Needs Category—*Safe and effective care environment*
Client Needs Subcategory—*Coordinated care*

18. 1. Although all the options are possible outcomes of the group process, the most desired outcome for a self-help group is that the group members obtain mutual support from one another. Self-help groups allow members to express their feelings openly and honestly. Individual members have been through similar experiences and serve to validate the feelings and experiences of others in the group.

Test Taking Strategy—Look at the key words "most desired outcome" in reference to the goal for participating in a rape support group. Option 1 is the best answer because the rape victim can identify with others who have had a similar experience and may value their comments more so than those of others. Review the purposes for and advantages of participating in support groups if you had difficulty answering this question.
Cognitive Level—*Analyzing*
Client Needs Category—*Psychosocial integrity*
Client Needs Subcategory—*None*

19. 2, 3. Eating out of habit or hardly eating anything is an indication that a rape victim is not recovering readily from the crime. Sleep patterns may also be disturbed. The other behavioral symptoms are more characteristic of normal or mild reactions to the rape trauma and are likely to be relieved with short-term support.

Test Taking Strategy—Analyze to determine what information the question asks for, which is signs of the victim having a severe adjustment reaction. Alternative-format "select all that apply" questions require considering each option independently to decide its merit in answering the question. Choose options that are indicative of a severe adjustment reaction. Review the psychopathology of a severe adjustment reaction if you had difficulty answering this question.
Cognitive Level—Analyzing
Client Needs Category—Psychosocial integrity
Client Needs Subcategory—None

20. 2. Most people are momentarily shocked after receiving bad news. Disbelief or denial typically follows, and the client may believe there have been mistakes in the test results or in the diagnosis. Later, common emotional responses include anger, bargaining, depression, and acceptance—generally in that order.
Test Taking Strategy—Analyze to determine what information the question asks for, which is the most typical reaction when being given life-threatening information. Option 2 is the best answer because it describes a primitive emotional response. The alternative options are intellectual and behavioral responses once the information has been processed. Review Kübler-Ross's stages in dealing with a loss if you had difficulty answering this question.
Cognitive Level—Analyzing
Client Needs Category—Psychosocial integrity
Client Needs Subcategory—None

21. 4. Denial is the failure to acknowledge an unbearable condition or the failure to admit the reality of a situation. It is a protective mechanism. The need to deny may be so overwhelming that it interferes with a person's good judgment to implement safer sex practices and use condoms. Concealing the information and avoiding contact with or confronting others are behaviors more indicative of depression and anger.
Test Taking Strategy—Look at the key words "most suggestive" in relation to evidence of denial. Option 4 is the best answer because the client's action is contrary to believing that he or she may transmit human immunodeficiency virus (HIV) infection to others. Review the ego defense mechanism known as denial and the purposes it serves if you had difficulty answering this question.
Cognitive Level—Analyzing
Client Needs Category—Psychosocial integrity
Client Needs Subcategory—None

22. 2. Having a social network of supportive friends and relatives diminishes a crisis. This promotes subsequent coping. Acceptance by religious leaders, new social

acquaintances, and sexual tolerance do not provide the same quality of emotional support as friends.
Test Taking Strategy—Look at the key words "most important" in reference to identifying a factor that promotes effective coping. Option 2 is the best answer because having support from friends and relatives is better than having to cope with a crisis independently. Review methods for promoting effective coping if you had difficulty answering this question.
Cognitive Level—Analyzing
Client Needs Category—Psychosocial integrity
Client Needs Subcategory—None

23. 4. Some people entertain thoughts of suicide as their only means of relieving others and themselves of the hopelessness of living with a terminal disease. Signs of despair indicate that a client should be closely observed to ensure safety. Dreams may be an indication that the client is fearful of dying. The other remarks are more suggestive of someone seeking information.
Test Taking Strategy—Look at the key words "most serious indication" in relation to a sign of increased risk for suicide. Option 4 is the best answer because it is characteristic of hopelessness and feeling there is no reason that can justify living. Review signs of suicidal ideation if you had difficulty answering this question.
Cognitive Level—Analyzing
Client Needs Category—Psychosocial integrity
Client Needs Subcategory—None

24. 2, 3, 4. The main priority when caring for a suicidal client is safety. The reason for suicidal precautions is to prevent the suicidal client from self-inflicting injuries or achieving death. The most appropriate nursing interventions include removing all cords, wires, and strings located in the room so that the client is unable to use these for hanging or other injuries. Paper plates and plastic utensils are less likely to cause self-inflicted harm than glass plates, glassware, and metal silverware. It is important for the nurse to assess whether the client has swallowed all pills. Some clients, intent on committing suicide, may "cheek" the pills, spit them out after the nurse has left the room, and hoard them for a future suicide attempt. Clients who are suicidal need 1:1 supervision, but this can be achieved by having another nurse or unlicensed staff person watch the client. A security guard is not required. Because 1:1 supervision is needed, checking on the client every hour and asking a family member to stay during the night will not provide the safety that the client requires. Direct supervision must be performed by hospital personnel, not family or friends.
Test Taking Strategy—Analyze to determine what information the question asks for, which is standard suicide precautions. Alternative-format "select all that

apply" questions require considering each option independently to decide its merit in answering the question. Choose options that are standard practices to prevent suicide. Review suicide precautions if you had difficulty answering this question.
Cognitive Level—Applying
Client Needs Category—Psychosocial integrity
Client Needs Subcategory—None

25. 1. Bulimia, also known as *bulimia nervosa,* is an eating disorder in which an individual believes he or she is fat or overweight and attempts to lose weight by self-induced vomiting, excessive exercise, abuse of diuretics or laxatives, and sessions of binging and purging (consuming massive amounts of food and then vomiting). Binging and purging take place privately. Staying out of the bathroom after a meal interferes with the client's opportunities to induce vomiting and use laxatives or enemas to stimulate bowel elimination. Having the client take an inventory of foods offered in the dormitory may precipitate an uncontrollable urge to go on an eating binge. The bulimic's food binges are not isolated to fast food establishments. Recording calories only increases the anxiety that bulimics experience when their eating is out of control.
> *Test Taking Strategy—Look at the key words "most likely" as they relate to a nursing recommendation to help control purging behavior by a bulimic. Option 1 is the best answer because it imposes a restriction that prevents purging while food is still in the stomach. Review methods for managing purging behaviors of persons with bulimia if you had difficulty answering this question.*
> *Cognitive Level—Analyzing*
> *Client Needs Category—Safe and effective care environment*
> *Client Needs Subcategory—Coordinated care*

26. 3. A reduction in binging is the best therapeutic effect for this client because it breaks the binge–purge cycle. The problem with bulimics is not that they do not eat nutritious food, but that they eat too much food. Usually, the food they eat is high in carbohydrates and calories. After eating large amounts of food, bulimics feel guilty and have abdominal discomfort. Purging reduces the guilt and decreases the abdominal pain. Antidepressants work well in controlling the symptoms of bulimics who are not clinically depressed. Usually, bulimics do not display signs of suicide; therefore, the physician would not prescribe antidepressants for reducing suicidal ideation.
> *Test Taking Strategy—Analyze to determine what information the question asks for, which is the most desired effect of antidepressant therapy when used to treat a client with bulimia. Option 3 is the best answer because the goal of therapy is to reduce or eliminate binging, which in turn should reduce or eliminate purging. Review the role of antidepressant*

therapy in managing the cycle of binge-purge behavior in persons with bulimia if you had difficulty answering this question.
> *Cognitive Level—Analyzing*
> *Client Needs Category—Physiological integrity*
> *Client Needs Subcategory—Pharmacological therapies*

27. 3. Peer censure is much more therapeutic than disapproval from the group leader. If the therapist or members of the treatment team react positively or negatively to the individuals involved in the conflict, it is likely to divide the group members and jeopardize group work.
> *Test Taking Strategy—Look at the key words "most appropriate" in reference to interjecting a response to a negative comment by a peer in a group therapy session. Option 4 is the best answer because the nurse who leads the group avoids being the source of censure. Review the role of a leader in group therapy if you had difficulty answering this question.*
> *Cognitive Level—Analyzing*
> *Client Needs Category—Psychosocial integrity*
> *Client Needs Subcategory—None*

28. 2. Being overly talkative is a common sign of use of amphetamines such as dextroamphetamine (Dexedrine). This drug is a stimulant; staring into space and slurring words are side effects typical of depressant types of drugs. Some marijuana users wear sunglasses indoors to disguise their inflamed eyes.
> *Test Taking Strategy—Look at the key words "most suggestive" in relation to current behavior that reflects current amphetamine abuse. Option 2 is the best answer because it correlates with physiologic stimulation. Review the effects associated with central nervous system stimulants, specifically amphetamines, if you had difficulty answering this question.*
> *Cognitive Level—Analyzing*
> *Client Needs Category—Psychosocial integrity*
> *Client Needs Subcategory—None*

29. 1. Young adults who have not acquired the developmental characteristic of intimacy tend to have superficial relationships that are temporary in nature. Worrying about financial security is more common during the middle years of adulthood. A person's sexual identity is established much earlier in life. Assertiveness is more of a unique personality characteristic than one commonly acquired at a particular stage in life.
> *Test Taking Strategy—Analyze to determine what information the question asks for, which is evidence of a failure to achieve intimacy by a young adult. Review Erikson's developmental stages and the results associated with positive and negative outcomes, focusing particularly on the stage of young adulthood, if you had difficulty answering this question.*

Cognitive Level—*Analyzing*
Client Needs Category—*Health promotion and maintenance*
Client Needs Subcategory—*None*

30. 4. Rationalization is a coping mechanism in which a person fails to take responsibility for something by offering some acceptable explanation for it. Indicating health risks from being overweight is an example of intellectualization. The failure to resist ice cream demonstrates that the client has insight into the behavior. Projection is the mechanism of accusing others of one's own feelings that are too painful to acknowledge.

   Test Taking Strategy—*Use the process of elimination to help select the option that best correlates with the ego defense mechanism of rationalization. Option 4 is the best answer because it is a comment in which the client eliminates personal responsibility for obesity by blaming someone or something other than himself or herself. Review the defense mechanism known as rationalization and how it is used to protect the ego (self) if you had difficulty answering this question.*
   Cognitive Level—*Analyzing*
   Client Needs Category—*Psychosocial integrity*
   Client Needs Subcategory—*None*

31. 2. Non–English-speaking clients or those who speak very little English feel more comfortable communicating with and through a certified translator of their own gender. This reduces embarrassment about questions pertaining to genitourinary functions, bowel elimination, reproductive history, and other sensitive issues related to mental health history. Translation cards have key words and phrases in various foreign languages and may be helpful in conveying important words in the foreign language; however, it would be difficult for the nurse to ask all questions included in the admission database using such cards. Having a member of the housekeeping staff translate sensitive history to the nurse is inappropriate. Having a family member translate the information may or may not be a good choice, depending on the nature of the relationship and the level of understanding of medical terminology. Also, the nurse would not be sure that the information is being accurately conveyed.

   Test Taking Strategy—*Analyze to determine what information the question asks for, which is the best method for communicating with a client who speaks English as a second language. Option 2 is the best answer from among the options provided because it involves using a direct objective resource as a translator. Review recommended techniques for communicating with clients with limited ability to understand and respond to spoken English if you had difficulty answering this question.*

Cognitive Level—*Analyzing*
Client Needs Category—*Safe and effective care environment*
Client Needs Subcategory—*Coordinated care*

32. 2, 5, 6. Cocaine is a potent stimulant that can be injected, smoked, or snorted. Snorting occurs when cocaine powder is inhaled through the nose and absorbed into the bloodstream through the nasal tissues. Snorting cocaine on a routine basis may ulcerate, erode, and perforate the nasal mucosa and septum. Because cocaine is a stimulant, the nurse most likely will find an irregular heartbeat that can lead to chest pain. Elevated blood pressure and pulse rate are also common as well as the inability to sleep. Anorexia is also common in frequent users because of the lack of desire to eat. Even with routine use of cocaine, the breath sounds should be clear, not congested. Cocaine users have a runny nose due to the irritation of the drug in the nasal passages; they usually do not have frontal sinus pain.

   Test Taking Strategy—*Analyze to determine what information the question asks for, which is signs of cocaine use. Alternative-format "select all that apply" questions require considering each option independently to decide its merit in answering the question. Choose options that correlate with physical findings associated with use and abuse of cocaine. Review signs of cocaine use and abuse if you had difficulty answering this question.*
   Cognitive Level—*Analyzing*
   Client Needs Category—*Psychosocial integrity*
   Client Needs Subcategory—*None*

33. 1. Cocaine abuse can result in cardiac arrhythmias, chest pain, and death because toxicity may occur anytime and with any dose. Cocaine is a central nervous system stimulant; it increases respirations, heart rate, and blood pressure. The client's blood glucose level may decrease, not elevate, due to calorie use during periods of hyperactivity.

   Test Taking Strategy—*Analyze to determine what information the question asks for, which is the type of assessment finding that is most likely when managing the care of a client who tests positive for cocaine use. Option 1 is the best answer because cardiac symptoms are likely to occur when abusing a central nervous system stimulant. Review consequences associated with the use and abuse of cocaine if you had difficulty answering this question.*
   Cognitive Level—*Analyzing*
   Client Needs Category—*Psychosocial integrity*
   Client Needs Subcategory—*None*

34. 1. Standard precautions that include preventing needlestick and sharps injuries are required to prevent transmission of the hepatitis B virus.

Test Taking Strategy—Use the process of elimination to identify the type of precautions that control a blood borne pathogen like hepatitis B. Recall that contact precautions are used to prevent infectious disease transmission by skin to skin contact or contact with contaminated objects. Airborne precautions are used to block infectious organisms suspended in the air over long distances. Droplet precautions block transmission of pathogens in respiratory secretions within 3 feet of the infected person. The remaining option, standard precautions, is the correct answer. Review transmission based precautions and the manner in which hepatitis B is acquired if you had difficulty answering this question.
Cognitive Level—*Analyzing*
Client Needs Category—*Safe and effective care environment*
Client Needs Subcategory—*Safety and Infection Control*

35. 4. Hallucinations are sensory experiences of which only the client is aware. They may be auditory, visual, olfactory, or tactile. An auditory hallucination involves hearing a voice or sound that no one else perceives. The person rarely volunteers about experiencing altered perceptions. The observant nurse draws inferences based on the client's nonverbal cues.
Test Taking Strategy—Look at the key words "most suggestive" in reference to a manifestation that correlates with experiencing auditory hallucinations. Option 4 is the best answer because it describes behavior that suggests the person is hearing and attending to a voice other than that of the nurse. Review the signs associated with auditory hallucinations if you had difficulty answering this question.
Cognitive Level—*Applying*
Client Needs Category—*Psychosocial integrity*
Client Needs Subcategory—*None*

36. 2. Schizophrenia is a group of mental disorders characterized by a gradual deterioration of mental functioning. As a result of the schizophrenic's disordered thoughts, the client may have difficulty putting thoughts into words. The nurse should never pretend to understand the meaning of a client's illogical statement or twist the words to interpret the statement as something logical.
Test Taking Strategy—Analyze to determine what information the question asks for, which is the most therapeutic response to a client who speaks in rhymes, a phenomenon known as clanging. Option 2 is the best answer because it is never therapeutic to imply that a client's gibberish is understood. Review techniques of therapeutic communication, especially the technique called clarification, if you had difficulty answering this question.

Cognitive Level—*Applying*
Client Needs Category—*Psychosocial integrity*
Client Needs Subcategory—*None*

37. 1. Hospitalization is indicated when a client poses a danger to self or others. In this case, the client is neglecting bodily needs; therefore, hospitalization is warranted. The other options suggest that the client is having problems with socialization skills, but they are not conditions that improve with hospitalization.
Test Taking Strategy—Analyze to determine what information the question asks for, which is the assessment finding that is most indicative of a schizophrenic client's need for rehospitalization. Option 1 is the best answer because society has an obligation to protect a client from self-harm or from harming others. Review the criteria for an involuntary psychiatric admission if you had difficulty answering this question.
Cognitive Level—*Analyzing*
Client Needs Category—*Psychosocial integrity*
Client Needs Subcategory—*None*

38. 2. The most common side effects of risperidone (Risperdal) include insomnia and agitation. Orthostatic hypotension also occurs, with reflex tachycardia. Extrapyramidal symptoms may occur, but to a lesser degree in incidence and severity than those associated with typical antipsychotics. Anticholinergic symptoms such as urine retention are not commonly reported. Weight gain, not loss, may develop.
Test Taking Strategy—Analyze to determine what information the question asks for, which is an effect manifested by a client who is taking the atypical antipsychotic drug risperidone. Because risperidone blocks alpha2-adrenergic receptors in addition to receptors for dopamine type 2 and serotonin type 2, clients may experience signs of hyperactivity such as insomnia and agitation during the early phase of treatment (the first week or two). Review the side effects of atypical antipsychotics, risperidone in particular, if you had difficulty answering this question.
Cognitive Level—*Understanding*
Client Needs Category—*Physiological integrity*
Client Needs Subcategory—*Pharmacological therapies*

39. 3. Besides asking the client's name, a second option is to ask the client to state his or her date of birth.
Test Taking Strategy—Use the process of elimination to select the option with the second identifier before administering a medication or performing a procedure. Recall that the one constant identifying item among the four options is the client's birth date. The remaining options are all subject to change. Review the Joint Commission's National Patient Safety Goals if you had difficulty answering this question.

Cognitive Level—Remembering
Client Needs Category—Safe and effective care environment
Client Needs Subcategory—Safety and infection control

Mental Health Needs During Middle Age (35 to 65)

40. **2.** Regardless of the cause or the client's level of mental functioning, it is important to establish that there are limits for the client's behavior. Leaving the room first is insufficient to correlate the nurse's response and the unacceptable behavior. Ignoring the behavior is more likely to communicate permission to repeat it. The same is true for trying to avoid being a repeat target.

Test Taking Strategy—Look at the key words "most appropriate" in reference to the action a nurse should take first when spat upon by a client with brain damage. Option 2 is the best answer because setting limits and enforcing appropriate consequences are forms of negative reinforcement that may prevent or limit future behavior of a similar nature. Review the outcomes that may result when negative reinforcement is used if you had difficulty answering this question.
Cognitive Level—Analyzing
Client Needs Category—Psychosocial integrity
Client Needs Subcategory—None

41. **1.** One of the best ways to modify behavior is to impose a significant consequence that has been previously communicated to the client. Wearing protective garments will not stop the behavior, although it is appropriate hygienically. It is unrealistic to think that a client with impaired cognition will be persuaded to change behavior as a result of intellectual reasoning.

Test Taking Strategy—Use the process of elimination to help select the option that describes the best approach for reducing a client's inappropriate behavior. Recall that imposing consequences for undesirable behavior (option 1) is a form of negative reinforcement that may reduce or eliminate repeated episodes. Option 2 can be eliminated because it imposes a responsibility on the part of the nurse. Options 3 and 4 can be eliminated because a brain-damaged person may not be able to cognitively understand logic or a form of reprimand. Review the outcomes associated with the use of negative reinforcement if you had difficulty answering this question.
Cognitive Level—Analyzing
Client Needs Category—Safe and effective care environment
Client Needs Subcategory—Coordinated care

42. **2.** To obtain the most valid results from the mental status assessment of a client who is cognitively impaired, it is best to allow extra time for the client to respond to questions. A certain number of open-ended questions are necessary during a mental status examination, regardless of the client's cognitive ability. Omitting the assessment or deferring the entire assessment to someone else violates standards of care.

Test Taking Strategy—Look at the key words "most appropriate" in reference to an option that describes an assessment technique for evaluating the mental status of a client who is cognitively impaired. Recall that a cognitively impaired client may require additional time to process a response to questions. Review the components of a mental status assessment, focusing on modifications that can be implemented for clients with special needs, if you had difficulty answering this question.
Cognitive Level—Applying
Client Needs Category—Health promotion and maintenance
Client Needs Subcategory—None

43. **1, 5, 6.** Panic attacks are one type of anxiety disorder. The physical symptoms are generally a consequence of sympathetic nervous system stimulation, as in the release of adrenaline, which causes an increased heart rate. Other signs and symptoms include palpitations, a bounding heart rate, sweating, unsteady gait, dizziness, shakiness, and feelings of choking. Clients may think that they are having a heart attack or even dying. Sympathetic nervous system stimulation is also associated with hypertension, a dry mouth, and dilated pupils.

Test Taking Strategy—Analyze to determine what information the question asks for, which is the signs and symptoms of a panic attack. Alternative-format "select all that apply" questions require considering each option independently to decide its merit in answering the question. Choose options that reflect sympathetic nervous system stimulation. Review physiologic effects produced by the sympathetic nervous system if you had difficulty answering this question.
Cognitive Level—Applying
Client Needs Category—Psychosocial integrity
Client Needs Subcategory—None

44. **4.** Panic attacks are due to the interplay of biological and physiological factors. A person who begins to experience the symptoms typically fears that the symptoms are life-threatening. The cycle of symptoms followed by fear followed by intensified symptoms creates a vicious circle. To the client experiencing panic attacks, these symptoms are real and usually have a known cause. The client does not feign the attacks or seek attention through them; such attacks are a source of true distress.

Test Taking Strategy—Analyze to determine what information the question asks for, which is the etiology for chest pain experienced by a person during a panic attack. Recall that the person experiencing a panic attack interprets their physical symptoms as life-threatening. The fear of dying (option 4) is the underlying basis for sympathetic nervous system stimulation that constricts arterial blood flow, resulting in chest pain. Review the cause and effects of symptoms associated with a panic attack if you had difficulty answering this question.
Cognitive Level—*Applying*
Client Needs Category—*Psychosocial integrity*
Client Needs Subcategory—*None*

45. 4. Most people experience increased anxiety during situations in which they have no prior experience. To a client who is already anxious, this unfamiliarity adds to the anxiety. Providing explanations and instructions helps to diminish the client's insecurity, thereby decreasing the anxiety. Standing within an arm's length invades a client's personal space and heightens anxiety. Instructing the client to take shallow breaths will not decrease the anxiety and may result in hyperventilation. A more appropriate instruction would be to tell the client to take slow, deep breaths with air going in through the nose and out of the mouth. Telling the client that everything is going to be okay is meaningless reassurance, and this action should be avoided.
Test Taking Strategy—Analyze to determine what information the question asks for, which is a technique for helping to reduce a client's anxiety during a panic attack. Option 4 is the best answer because providing information promotes a sense of security in knowing what to expect. Review techniques for managing anxiety if you had difficulty answering this question.
Cognitive Level—*Analyzing*
Client Needs Category—*Psychosocial integrity*
Client Needs Subcategory—*None*

46. 1. Being reassured about safety helps more than the other actions to reduce the client's feelings of fear and loss of control; feeling safe interrupts the vicious cycle of fear and panic. Being believed, trusted, and accepted are integral to establishing a therapeutic relationship.
Test Taking Strategy—Look at the key words "most important" in reference to the concept that is most therapeutic to convey when interacting with a client during a panic attack. Recall that the client is experiencing intense fear; therefore, conveying a sense of safety is most important. Review nursing interventions when interacting with a person experiencing a panic attack if you had difficulty answering this question.

Cognitive Level—*Analyzing*
Client Needs Category—*Psychosocial integrity*
Client Needs Subcategory—*None*

47. 4. Staying with a frightened client communicates genuine concern, and the presence of a caring person tends to reduce anxiety. The first choice is an example of giving advice, which is a nontherapeutic communication technique. It is inappropriate to try to shame the client with the possibility of physician intervention in response to out-of-control behavior. The third nontherapeutic example is one of generalizing, which disregards this client's right to be considered unique.
Test Taking Strategy—Analyze to determine what information the question asks for, which is the most therapeutic response to the client's statement. Recall that the physical presence of the nurse provides emotional support and reduces fear and anxiety. The other options are examples of nontherapeutic responses. Review techniques of therapeutic and nontherapeutic communication if you had difficulty answering this question.
Cognitive Level—*Analyzing*
Client Needs Category—*Psychosocial integrity*
Client Needs Subcategory—*None*

48. 1. Antianxiety drugs such as alprazolam (Xanax) produce a calming effect. Alcohol consumption with this medication is likely to potentiate the drug's action and endanger the client's safety from profound sedation. Drug dependency is related to this drug's dosage and length of administration. Insomnia is unlikely because the drug causes sedation. Blood levels are not commonly monitored when benzodiazepines such as alprazolam are prescribed.
Test Taking Strategy—Look at the key words "most appropriate" in reference to information about the drug alprazolam. Recall that alprazolam produces sedative effects that could be compounded when taken in combination with other sedative drugs such as alcohol (option 1). Review health teaching that is appropriate for clients taking antianxiety drugs, specifically alprazolam, if you had difficulty answering this question.
Cognitive Level—*Remembering*
Client Needs Category—*Physiological integrity*
Client Needs Subcategory—*Pharmacological therapies*

49. 2. Many clients who experience panic attacks develop agoraphobia, a fear of being in a place or situation where help may be unavailable. Some clients who experience panic attacks seek psychiatric treatment; some take more than the prescribed amount of medication, but these are not characteristic of the majority of individuals with this anxiety disorder. Persons with panic disorder rarely develop psychotic symptoms.

Test Taking Strategy—Analyze to determine what information the question asks for, which is a possible outcome of experiencing repeated panic attacks. Recall that clients tend to associate the place or circumstance under which a panic attack occurs with those attacks and to avoid these in the future. This leads to isolation and a fear of leaving an environment that represents safety and security (option 2). Review the etiology for developing agoraphobia if you had difficulty answering this question.
Cognitive Level—*Applying*
Client Needs Category—*Psychosocial integrity*
Client Needs Subcategory—*None*

50. **1, 2, 5, 6.** Obsessive-compulsive disorder (OCD) is a type of anxiety disorder. Obsessions are irrational thoughts, unwanted ideas, or impulses that occur repeatedly in a person's mind. Obsessions are often intense, frightening, or bizarre and commonly focus on fear of dirt and germs, contamination, and violent or aggressive behavior. Religious thoughts or sexual feelings are also common. Compulsions are the repetitive rituals that individuals perform to lessen anxiety and make them feel temporarily better. Unfortunately, the good feelings do not last, and the cycle begins again. Typical compulsions include excessive washing (particularly of the hands or body), cleaning, checking, counting, arranging, and hoarding. Compulsions commonly occupy a great deal of time, which interferes with work performance and normal lifestyle. Clients with OCD are preoccupied with order, safety, and cleanliness. They are ashamed of their problem and, therefore, try to hide it. Stress and other psychological factors make the problem worse. The disorder usually begins in adolescence or early adulthood. Of the clients listed, those demonstrating OCD tendencies include the client who repeatedly performs handwashing, the client who wears gloves when touching a public faucet, the client who cannot throw anything away, and the client who repeatedly checks and rechecks locked doors. Sexual promiscuity is common among those in a manic phase of bipolar disorder. Drinking a fifth of whiskey every day is indicative of alcoholism.
Test Taking Strategy—Analyze to determine what information the question asks for, which is behaviors common in those with OCD. Alternative-format "select all that apply" questions require considering each option independently to decide its merit in answering the question. Review examples of behaviors that are common among persons with OCD if you had difficulty answering this question.
Cognitive Level—*Remembering*
Client Needs Category—*Psychosocial integrity*
Client Needs Subcategory—*None*

51. **1, 3.** Effective treatment of obsessive-compulsive disorder (OCD) includes the administration of selective serotonin reuptake inhibitors (SSRIs) such as fluvoxamine

(Luvox). Serotonin is thought to be lacking in clients with OCD; SSRIs replace the missing serotonin in the brain. Cognitive-behavioral therapy is also beneficial because it teaches clients how to confront their thoughts and control their rituals. Eventually, anxiety decreases and the clients lessen their preoccupation with thoughts and actions. Electroconvulsive therapy (ECT) is used in some circumstances for clients who have severe depression that is unresponsive to other forms of therapy. Clients with OCD do not need a lobotomy, which involves removal of part of the brain. Tranquilizers are also not used for treatment of this disorder. Clients with OCD need professional help. Self-help classes from the Internet may provide information about the disorder, but most likely will not decrease anxiety enough to break the cycle.
Test Taking Strategy—Analyze to determine what information the question asks for, which is therapeutic actions taken to manage OCD. Alternative-format "select all that apply" questions require considering each option independently to decide its merit in answering the question. Review interventions used to manage OCD if you had difficulty answering this question.
Cognitive Level—*Analyzing*
Client Needs Category—*Safe and effective care environment*
Client Needs Subcategory—*Coordinated care*

52. **4.** Displacement is a coping mechanism in which a person transfers angry feelings for one person onto someone else who is less likely to retaliate with significant consequences. Introjection involves taking on the characteristics of another. Projection is characterized by accusing someone of one's own weaknesses. Compensation is demonstrated by overcoming some inadequacy by excelling at another activity.
Test Taking Strategy—Analyze to determine what information the question asks for, which is the coping mechanism characterized by displays of anger toward an undeserved person or object (option 4). Review the ego defense mechanism known as displacement as well as the other coping mechanisms listed if you had difficulty answering this question.
Cognitive Level—*Remembering*
Client Needs Category—*Psychosocial integrity*
Client Needs Subcategory—*None*

53. **3.** The least restrictive approach should be implemented initially to manage undesirable behaviors. This excludes the application of physical restraints and isolation. By remaining calm, the nurse models the type of behavior that is expected and reduces stimuli that the client may interpret as threatening. The least restrictive approach should be implemented initially which excludes the application of restraints and isolating the client. Physical activity is a way of dissipating anger, but it should not supersede discussing the client's feelings. Although encouraging the client to discuss what triggered the anger would be beneficial, it would be inappropriate to suggest talking to the client's spouse.

> *Test Taking Strategy—Use the process of elimination to help select the option that describes the best initial action the nurse should recommend for helping a client maintain self-control. Recall that anxiety is communicated, and so is calmness. Therefore, option 3 is the best answer. Options 1 and 2 have merit, but they are not the best initial actions. Option 4 is incorrect because it is the client's responsibility to problem-solve by dialoguing with his or her spouse. Review nursing actions that reduce a client's anger and hostility if you had difficulty answering this question.*

Cognitive Level—*Analyzing*
Client Needs Category—*Safe and effective care environment*
Client Needs Subcategory—*Coordinated care*

54. **1.** Gathering staff is a show of force, which is sometimes all that a client needs to realize that it is best to regain self-control. Asking a physician to intervene implies that nurses are unable to effectively manage a disruptive client's behavior. It is unsafe to go anywhere alone with a client who is beyond anger and in danger of losing self-control. Displaying restraints as a means of controlling the client's behavior is an implied threat, which is unethical.

> *Test Taking Strategy—Look at the key words "most appropriate" in reference to managing potentially violent behavior. Recall that the nurse is responsible for ensuring the safety of the client and others. Being confronted by the presence of a team of nursing staff often persuades an individual to avoid any further escalation of potentially dangerous behavior (option 1). Review methods for managing the care of a client who has the potential for becoming violent if you had difficulty answering this question.*

Cognitive Level—*Analyzing*
Client Needs Category—*Psychosocial integrity*
Client Needs Subcategory—*None*

55. **2.** Administering medications against a client's will when the circumstances indicate a danger to the client or others is legally permissible. To avoid liability, documentation must objectively describe the evidence of danger and the lack of success when alternative measures were attempted. In most cases, the nurse should be respectful of the client's right to refuse the medication. However, if the client is demonstrating signs that harm to self or others is possible, the client's rights are waived. The nurse does not need to get permission from a judge to administer the drug, and the hospital attorney does not need to be consulted.

> *Test Taking Strategy—Analyze to determine what information the question asks for, which is the nursing action that is legally sound when an out-of-control*

client refuses sedative medication. Recall that the nurse is obligated to ensure the safety of the client and others (option 2), which justifies overriding the client's objection to medication. Review the legal aspects that apply to administering medication despite its refusal by a client who is out of control if you had difficulty answering this question.

Cognitive Level—*Analyzing*
Client Needs Category—*Safe and effective care environment*
Client Needs Subcategory—*Coordinated care*

56. **2, 4, 5.** Objective data are most important in this case. The nurse must observe for signs of impaired circulation, which include paleness of the fingers and toes and prolonged capillary refill. (Normal capillary refill is about 3 seconds.) In addition, excoriation around the wrist indicates that the restraint is too tight. The excoriation occurs as the client tries to remove the restraints. Usually, if two fingers can be inserted under the restraint, this ensures that circulation and nerve function are not impaired. The nurse must be careful of manipulation by the client regarding subjective data, such as inability to move the hand, numbness, and tingling of the extremities and pain. Judgment regarding these choices is prudent.

> *Test Taking Strategy—Analyze to determine what information the question asks for, which is signs of restraints that are too tight. Alternative-format "select all that apply" questions require considering each option independently to decide its merit in answering the question. Choose options that identify evidence that physical restraints may be causing injury to the client on whom they have been applied. Review assessments and nursing actions that are required when physical restraints are used if you had difficulty answering this question.*

Cognitive Level—*Analyzing*
Client Needs Category—*Physiological integrity*
Client Needs Subcategory—*Reduction of risk potential*

57. **2.** Using short, simple sentences is best when teaching anxious clients who have short attention spans and difficulty concentrating. Detailed explanations or elaborate diagrams would overwhelm an anxious client. DVDs are not as effective as one-on-one instruction in this situation. The nurse needs to periodically assess the client's comprehension and repeat information that is unclear.

> *Test Taking Strategy—Use the process of elimination to determine the form of communication to use when providing information to an anxious client. Recall that anxiety interferes with processing information, especially if it is lengthy and detailed, making option 2 the answer. Review modifications in teaching when providing information to a client who is anxious if you had difficulty answering this question.*

Cognitive Level—Analyzing
Client Needs Category—Psychosocial integrity
Client Needs Subcategory—None

58. 1. Middle-aged adults forced into early retirement are likely to experience a great deal of stress because adults at this stage in life are very concerned with their future financial security. The other events are challenging but probably not major sources of conflict as adults achieve generativity.

Test Taking Strategy—Look at the key words "most significant" in reference to the source of a client's conflict and anxiety. Recall that forced retirement (option 1) is a significant stressor for a client who is 60 years old. Review anxiety-provoking circumstances experienced by older adults if you had difficulty answering this question.
Cognitive Level—Analyzing
Client Needs Category—Psychosocial integrity
Client Needs Subcategory—None

59. 3. Phobic people avoid what they perceive as the cause of their discomfort. Suppression is a coping mechanism in which a person chooses to refrain from thinking about something that is a source of conflict. Compensation is characterized by pursuing an activity that ensures success to make up for feeling inadequate. Undoing is a coping mechanism in which one makes amends for having offended someone.

Test Taking Strategy—Analyze to determine what information the question asks for, which is a coping mechanism that is commonly used to manage fear. Recall that avoiding the source of fear (option 3) is a method of reducing anxiety, although it may not be the most therapeutic approach. Review coping strategies, especially avoidance, if you had difficulty answering this question.
Cognitive Level—Applying
Client Needs Category—Psychosocial integrity
Client Needs Subcategory—None

60. 1, 2, 3, 4. Phobias are a type of anxiety involving persistent, irrational fears. They can be classified as social (public speaking), agoraphobia (fear of crowds or public places), and simple (fear of certain objects or stimuli, such as animals, insects, heights, enclosed spaces, and flying). Common signs and symptoms include sweating, tachycardia and palpitations, tremors, shortness of breath, nausea, and nightmares. The client may manifest such signs and symptoms when coming in contact with the fear or by thinking or discussing the fear. Uncontrollable crying is more indicative of depression, and facial tics are commonly associated with Tourette's syndrome.

Test Taking Strategy—Analyze to determine what information the question asks for, which is signs and symptoms of phobias. Alternative-format "select all that apply" questions require considering each

option independently to decide its merit in answering the question. Because phobic reactions are a result of anxiety, review signs and symptoms of sympathetic nervous system stimulation if you had difficulty answering this question.
Cognitive Level—Applying
Client Needs Category—Psychosocial integrity
Client Needs Subcategory—None

61. 1. Cognitive therapy involves confronting irrational thoughts and behaviors. The expected outcome is that the client will recognize the flaws in thinking and ultimately change the behavior. The remaining options describe desensitization therapy, assertiveness training, and behavioral modification, in that order.

Test Taking Strategy—Analyze to determine what information the question asks for, which is an accurate explanation of cognitive therapy. Review cognitive therapy if you had difficulty answering this question.
Cognitive Level—Applying
Client Needs Category—Health promotion and maintenance
Client Needs Subcategory—None

62. 1, 5, 6. Post-traumatic stress disorder (PTSD) is an anxiety disorder that occurs after exposure to a terrifying situation in which grave life-threatening harm occurred or life was threatened. Traumatic events, including violent personal assaults, natural or human-caused disasters, accidents, or military combat, may trigger PTSD. Clients with PTSD generally reexperience their traumatic events in some way, such as through upsetting dreams, nightmares, or flashbacks. They also are easily startled and have difficulty concentrating. In addition, they avoid people, places, and things that remind them of the event. Some clients have visual hallucinations, but generally not auditory hallucinations. Most have a numbed or blunted emotional response to others with whom they interact.

Test Taking Strategy—Analyze to determine what information the question asks for, which is behavioral signs of PTSD. Alternative-format "select all that apply" questions require considering each option independently to decide its merit in answering the question. Choose options that correlate with the signs and symptoms of PTSD. Review the manifestations of PTSD if you had difficulty answering this question.
Cognitive Level—Analyzing
Client Needs Category—Psychosocial integrity
Client Needs Subcategory—None

63. 3. Clients with post-traumatic stress disorder (PTSD) who are able to recall the precipitating traumatic event use a tremendous amount of energy to control their feelings or suppress the memory of it. Giving clients permission to talk about the traumatic event can be very therapeutic. Many clients with this disorder abuse drugs and alcohol to help numb their consciousness; antianxiety drugs are likely to do the same. Improving damaged relationships is a goal of therapy, but it is not the primary focus of treatment. Monitoring the client's physical symptoms is advisable, but it is not as therapeutic as the use of appropriate communication skills.

Test Taking Strategy—Look at the key words "most beneficial" in reference to a therapeutic nursing intervention when providing care for a client with PTSD. Recall that the underlying cause of PTSD is a traumatic experience after which the client represses feelings. As in all crises, whether in the immediate or distant past, talking about the event is therapeutic. Review therapeutic nursing approaches for managing the care of a client with PTSD if you had difficulty answering this question.
Cognitive Level—Analyzing
Client Needs Category—Psychosocial integrity
Client Needs Subcategory—None

64. 1. Art is used as a therapeutic tool to promote the expression of thoughts or feelings that are too difficult to verbalize.

Test Taking Strategy—Use the process of elimination to help select the option that describes the most therapeutic outcome from drawing a picture depicting the traumatic triggering experience. Recall that clients with PTSD have difficulty verbalizing their thoughts and feelings surrounding the traumatic event. Art can serve as a stimulus for dealing with psychological issues within a safe and supportive environment, as described in option 1. Although the outcomes in the remaining options may occur, none is the most therapeutic outcome underlying the intervention. Review the purposes for art therapy in relation to mental health disorders if you had difficulty answering this question.
Cognitive Level—Analyzing
Client Needs Category—Psychosocial integrity
Client Needs Subcategory—None

65. 3. A stimulus that evokes a physiologic response similar to that of the original traumatic event can trigger intense anxiety. The stimulus of the fireworks is similar to that of gunfire during combat and can reproduce comparable anxiety. If the client had been frightened of fireworks as a child, the client probably would have manifested a continued fear response before the military experience. In this case, the startle response is not associated with a fear of getting injured from the fireworks or a fear of painful memories.

Test Taking Strategy—Analyze to determine what information the question asks for, which is the most accurate explanation for a startle response to a stimulus that seems unrelated to emotional issues. Recall that clients with post-traumatic stress disor-

der (PTSD) tend to repress their thoughts and feelings. Consequently, when exposed to a stimulus that is similar to the traumatic event (option 3), clients may experience emotional distress. Review stimuli that may trigger a reaction in someone who has PTSD if you had difficulty answering this question.
Cognitive Level—Analyzing
Client Needs Category—Psychosocial integrity
Client Needs Subcategory—None

66. 4. Assessment is the first step in the nursing process. Therefore, the nurse should take the client's vital signs before implementing any further action. After completing the assessment and finding the client in no immediate danger, the nurse can gather additional data and implement other nursing interventions.

Test Taking Strategy—Look at the key words "most appropriate at this time" in reference to a nursing response to symptoms experienced by a client with an undiagnosed disorder. Recall that vital signs are one of the basic assessments when caring for any client and should be the initial action taken by the nurse (option 4). Review the purposes for taking vital signs if you had difficulty answering this question.
Cognitive Level—Analyzing
Client Needs Category—Physiological integrity
Client Needs Subcategory—Reduction of risk potential

67. 1. Middle adulthood is characterized as a period of either generativity or stagnation. During this stage in the life cycle, it is common for adults to assess their accomplishments at mid-life. In some cases, those who view themselves as not having accomplished much experience what is known as a midlife crisis. People usually establish goals at an earlier age. Middle-aged people generally do not question their values which were firmly established earlier in adulthood. They may envy others' achievements, but being envious of others is something that happens at all stages of life, not just during middle age.

Test Taking Strategy—Use the process of elimination to help select the option that provides the best nursing explanation for the client's statement about unfulfilled accomplishments. Recall that middle-age is the time during which adults take stock of their accomplishments or lack thereof (option 1). Options 2, 3, and 4 may occur but none are typical of middle-aged adults. Review Erikson's stages of development throughout the life cycle, focusing on middle adulthood in particular, if you had difficulty answering this question.
Cognitive Level—Applying
Client Needs Category—Health promotion and maintenance
Client Needs Subcategory—None

68. **2.** Therapeutic communication requires that the nurse assess hidden meanings within a client's statements or questions, then verbalize the feeling or tone for validation. Deferring discussion to the physician is a form of scapegoating, which conveys to the client that the nurse chooses to remain uninvolved. Telling the client to let the staff worry or to practice more patience is giving advice, which is a nontherapeutic form of communication.

> *Test Taking Strategy*—*Use the process of elimination to help select the option that correlates with a therapeutic response. Option 2 is an example of the therapeutic communication technique known as sharing perceptions. Options 1, 3, and 4 are responses that are nontherapeutic. Review therapeutic and nontherapeutic communication techniques if you had difficulty answering this question.*
> **Cognitive Level**—*Analyzing*
> **Client Needs Category**—*Psychosocial integrity*
> **Client Needs Subcategory**—*None*

69. **1, 2, 3, 4, 5.** Hypochondriasis is a psychological disorder characterized by the belief that real or imagined minor physical symptoms are a sign of serious illness. Even when several doctors assure the person otherwise, a hypochondriac is convinced that he or she has a serious disease. Hypochondriacs are often preoccupied with vague physical complaints, such as fatigue, headaches, nausea, or dizziness. They fear or believe that they have a major disease, despite constant reassurance that they are healthy. Hypochondriacs may even fixate on specific diseases after reading or hearing about them. Risk factors for hypochondria include a family history of hypochondriasis, a diagnosed anxiety disorder, severe illness as a child, witnessed violence in childhood, and stressful experience with a loved one's illness. Fear of death is a common symptom of hypochondriacs, but it is not considered a risk factor.

> *Test Taking Strategy*—*Analyze to determine what information the question asks for, which is risk factors for developing hypochondriasis. Alternative-format "select all that apply" questions require considering each option independently to decide its merit in answering the question. Choose options that correlate with risk factors for hypochondriasis. Review factors that may lead to the development of hypochondriasis if you had difficulty answering this question.*
> **Cognitive Level**—*Applying*
> **Client Needs Category**—*Psychosocial integrity*
> **Client Needs Subcategory**—*None*

70. **1, 2, 4, 5, 6.** Major signs and symptoms of this disorder include becoming knowledgeable about specific illnesses and their symptoms; a chronic fear that minor symptoms are signs of a serious illness; interference with social life, work, or marriage and the loss of income; multiple doctor visits, sometimes several in the same day; and repeated requests for tests for the same symptoms. In many cases, clients go from physician to physician hoping that they will be diagnosed with a physical disease. Client's with hypochondriasis have multiple vague common physical complaints (headache, dizziness, backache, stomach ache) that do not correlate with any particular diagnosis and often change over time.

> *Test Taking Strategy*—*Analyze to determine what information the question asks for, which is signs and symptoms of hypochondriasis that the nurse accurately identifies to a staff member. Alternative-format "select all that apply" questions require considering each option independently to decide its merit in answering the question. Choose options that correlate with the manifestations of hypochondriasis. Review a text that identifies the signs and symptoms of hypochondriasis if you had difficulty answering this question.*
> **Cognitive Level**—*Applying*
> **Client Needs Category**—*Safe and effective care environment*
> **Client Needs Subcategory**—*Coordinated care*

71. **3.** Only hospital employees who are immediately involved in the care of a client may have access to the client's health record. This is a Health Insurance Portability and Accountability Act (HIPAA) regulation designed to protect the client's health information and treatment. Some examples of a client's protected health history include name, address, phone number, age, Social Security number, and insurance or banking account numbers. A signed, written release from the client must be obtained before confidential information is divulged. The nurse must take all necessary measures to safeguard health information in the client's medical record and to maintain confidentiality.

> *Test Taking Strategy*—*Look at the key words "most appropriate" in reference to a request to see the client's medical record. Recall that the HIPAA legislation requires that a client's health information be kept private and confidential. Therefore, the nurse is acting appropriately by refusing to allow the client's pastor access to the medical record (option 3). Review how HIPAA applies to safeguarding health information if you had difficulty answering this question.*
> **Cognitive Level**—*Analyzing*
> **Client Needs Category**—*Safe and effective care environment*
> **Client Needs Subcategory**—*Coordinated care*

72. **4.** A client with ulcerative colitis has an inflamed bowel and experiences severe diarrhea with up to 30 stools per day. Endoscopic examinations and X-rays confirm the presence of pathology; therefore, option 2 is inaccurate. In addition, the client does experience physical symptoms, which makes option 1 incorrect. The exact cause of the disease is unknown, but emotional stress is one of many cofactors. Most clients with psychophysiological diseases would rather work than experience their symptoms.

> *Test Taking Strategy—Analyze to determine what information the question asks for, which is an accurate explanation of the term psychophysiologic. Recall that the mind and body are interrelated during a conference with staff. Consequently, physical disorders can be influenced, as stated in option 4, by a client's emotional status at the time. Review the pattern of exacerbations as they occur in clients with psychophysiological illnesses if you had difficulty answering this question.*
> *Cognitive Level—Applying*
> *Client Needs Category—Safe and effective care environment*
> *Client Needs Subcategory—Coordinated care*

73. **1.** Meeting physiological needs always takes precedence over other needs, including security, love, and belonging. The most important information needed at this time concerns the client's bowel elimination and its impact on fluid status, nutrition, and electrolyte balance.

> *Test Taking Strategy—Use the process of elimination to help select the option that represents the highest assessment priority when caring for a client with ulcerative colitis. Recall that Maslow's hierarchy lists physiological needs as a higher priority than other types of client needs. This principle is reflected in option 1. Review Maslow's hierarchy and how it applies to nursing care if you had difficulty answering this question.*
> *Cognitive Level—Analyzing*
> *Client Needs Category—Safe and effective care environment*
> *Client Needs Subcategory—Coordinated care*

74. **1.** Cleaning stool is never pleasant; however, the nurse can avoid making the client feel responsible for the condition or offensive to others by conveying a nonjudgmental attitude when providing care. Treating the client with dignity will help sustain self-esteem. Having a family member or same-gender nurse clean the stool or making the client responsible for all personal hygiene would not promote self-esteem; in fact, these measures might have the opposite effect.

> *Test Taking Strategy—Use the process of elimination to help select the option that describes the best approach for maintaining a client's self-esteem while providing rectal hygiene. Recall that remaining nonjudgmental, as stated in option 1, avoids projecting negative feelings. Eliminate options 2, 3, and 4 because these measures might lead to a decrease in self-esteem. Review how remaining nonjudgmental enhances the nurse-client relationship if you had difficulty answering this question.*

Cognitive Level—Analyzing
Client Needs Category—Psychosocial integrity
Client Needs Subcategory—None

75. **2.** A consequence of alcohol abuse is a tolerance to all sedative drugs. A need for a higher dosage or more frequent administration can indicate that the client abuses alcohol or some other central nervous system depressant drug. An alcoholic's blood pressure and pulse become abnormally high during withdrawal from alcohol. It is common for postoperative clients to become nauseated after eating.

> *Test Taking Strategy—Look at the key words "most indicative" in reference to an assessment finding that correlates with alcoholism. Recall that chronic abuse of a sedative drug such as alcohol results in cross-tolerance with other drugs in this category. Therefore, option 2 is the best answer because a nonalcoholic client would most likely experience pain relief after administration of a usual dose of an analgesic. Review the phenomenon of cross-tolerance if you had difficulty answering this question.*
> *Cognitive Level—Applying*
> *Client Needs Category—Psychosocial integrity*
> *Client Needs Subcategory—None*

76. **3.** Visual hallucinations occur in advanced withdrawal from alcohol. These are real and terrifying experiences for the alcoholic. To maintain safety and reduce the client's fear and anxiety, it is essential that a nurse remain with the client. Restraints should be used only when all other alternatives for maintaining the safety of the client or others have been exhausted. In the client's mind, the hallucination is real; telling the client that seeing bugs is imaginary is illogical and untrue. Closing the client's door is unsafe and likely to heighten the fear.

> *Test Taking Strategy—Look at the key words "most appropriate" used in reference to the nursing action indicated when a client erroneously believes there are bugs in the room. Recall that it is never therapeutic to desert a client who is distressed. Therefore, option 3 is the best answer. Review how the presence of a supportive person can reduce an anxiety-provoking experience if you had difficulty answering this question.*
> *Cognitive Level—Analyzing*
> *Client Needs Category—Safe and effective care environment*
> *Client Needs Subcategory—Safety and infection control*

77. **3.** It is always best to notify the physician first whenever there is a sudden change in a client's condition. Usually the nursing supervisor is not called unless the client becomes combative or the condition continues to worsen. Alcohol withdrawal is generally treated with one of the minor tranquilizers, such as lorazepam (Ativan), or a central nervous system depressant such as phenobarbital; however, a physician must prescribe these. Notifying the client's spouse may be indicated, but only after the physician has been notified and the client's safety is secured. Documenting the incident is important after the situation is under control.

> *Test Taking Strategy—Look at the key words "most appropriate" used in reference to a nursing action that should be performed next after noting the change in the client's condition. Recall that a significant change in a client's condition requires collaboration between the nurse and the physician. Review the role of collaboration when managing client care if you had difficulty answering this question.*
> *Cognitive Level—Analyzing*
> *Client Needs Category—Physiological integrity*
> *Client Needs Subcategory—Reduction of risk potential*

78. 2. Seizures occur from rebound central nervous system stimulation as the alcohol is metabolized from the client's system. Seizures occur in some clients as early as within the first 24 hours of withdrawal. Of the choices listed, seizures are the most severe. Hyperthermia may occur during alcohol withdrawal. Ascites and jaundice result from liver damage caused by chronic alcohol abuse.

> *Test Taking Strategy—Analyze to determine what information the question asks for, which is a complication that is secondary to alcoholism. Recall that withdrawal from a sedative drug results in stimulating manifestations such as seizures (option 2). Review the signs and symptoms that occur during withdrawal from alcohol if you had difficulty answering this question.*
> *Cognitive Level—Applying*
> *Client Needs Category—Psychosocial integrity*
> *Client Needs Subcategory—None*

79. 1. Staff members are better able to understand client behavior by increasing their own self-awareness. Nurses who are generalists are not academically prepared to analyze a client's motivation or provide psychotherapy. Knowledge of abnormal behavior is important, but it is not the first step in understanding the behavior of others.

> *Test Taking Strategy—Look at the key words "first step" in reference to understanding and accepting negative client behavior. Recall that prejudice is learned. Therefore, understanding the origin of one's own biases helps guard against behaving negatively in relationships with clients. Review how stereotyping affects client care if you had difficulty answering this question.*
> *Cognitive Level—Applying*
> *Client Needs Category—Safe and effective care environment*
> *Client Needs Subcategory—Coordinated care*

80. 3. Bipolar disorder is a serious mental illness characterized by dramatic mood swings. The causes of bipolar disorder are unknown, but there are certain triggers causing the client to have changes in mood. Clients with bipolar disorder, formerly called *manic-depressive disorder,* have cycles in which they display a marked change in mood between mania (abnormal highs) and depression (lows). The disorder is called *bipolar* because of the swings between the opposing poles in mood. Mania often affects thinking, judgment, and social behavior, causing serious problems. Bipolar disorder is a recurring illness that can be treated with long-term medication. The exaggerated mood is followed or preceded by an interval of normal mood.

> *Test Taking Strategy—Analyze to determine what information the question asks for, which is a major characteristic of bipolar disorder. Recall that this disorder is characterized by extreme changes in mood (option 3). Review the manifestations of bipolar disorder if you had difficulty answering this question.*
> *Cognitive Level—Applying*
> *Client Needs Category—Psychosocial integrity*
> *Client Needs Subcategory—None*

81. 4, 5. Lithium carbonate (Lithane) is a mood-stabilizing drug approved for the treatment of mania and for preventing the recurrence of manic-depressive cycles. Clients who take this medication should drink 10 to 12 glasses of water each day and maintain a sufficient salt intake. Sexual activity need not be restricted. Lithium carbonate usually causes polyuria; therefore, notifying the physician about increased urine output is unnecessary. Avoiding aged cheeses or wine is an instruction given to clients who take monoamine oxidase inhibitors (MAOIs), not lithium. Taking a high-potency vitamin is a personal health choice, but it will not affect a therapeutic response to lithium carbonate.

> *Test Taking Strategy—Analyze to determine what information the question asks for, which is client actions to take while receiving lithium. Alternative-format "select all that apply" questions require considering each option independently to decide its merit in answering the question. Choose options that describe health teaching related to the self-administration of lithium carbonate. Review pharmacologic information concerning lithium drug therapy if you had difficulty answering this question.*
> *Cognitive Level—Remembering*
> *Client Needs Category—Physiological integrity*
> *Client Needs Subcategory—Pharmacological therapies*

82. 3. Lithium carbonate (Lithane) has a narrow therapeutic range. Toxic reactions occur when blood levels are higher than 1.5 mEq/L. Common side effects include GI discomfort, nausea, muscle weakness, vertigo, and a dazed feeling. Blood levels are usually drawn throughout therapy, and the lithium dosage is adjusted according to the results.

The client who takes lithium carbonate may develop polyuria, but the volume of urine eliminated is not used to monitor the lithium level. Close monitoring of kidney, cardiovascular, and thyroid functions is important. Neither vital signs nor brain scans are used to evaluate the client's ability to metabolize the lithium dose.

> *Test Taking Strategy—Look at the key words "most important" in reference to determining if the dosage of lithium carbonate is appropriate. Recall that the dosage of lithium is monitored using drug levels in blood specimens (option 3). Review how the absorption, metabolism, and excretion of drugs, lithium carbonate in particular, can be objectively determined by measuring drug levels in blood if you had difficulty answering this question.*
> **Cognitive Level**—*Remembering*
> **Client Needs Category**—*Physiological integrity*
> **Client Needs Subcategory**—*Pharmacological therapies*

83. **1, 5.** Spending money extravagantly and sexual promiscuity are signs that a client with bipolar disorder is having difficulty using good judgment. Wanting to become a 5-year-old again could be interpreted as an example of an altered thought process related to schizophrenia. Methodically cleaning the house could indicate obsessive-compulsive behavior. Staying up late may be a sign of hyperactivity, which often accompanies a manic phase of bipolar disorder, but reading is a sedentary activity that is not characteristic of mania. However, such behavior is not as suggestive of loss of control as the client's spending money extravagantly or sexual promiscuity. Agoraphobia is an anxiety disorder often precipitated by the fear of having no easy means of escape. As a result, sufferers of agoraphobia may avoid public or unfamiliar places.

> *Test Taking Strategy—Analyze to determine what information the question asks for, which is behaviors associated with mania. Alternative-format "select all that apply" questions require considering each option independently to decide its merit in answering the question. Choose options that correlate with behaviors manifested by persons in the manic phase of bipolar disorder. Review the signs of manic behavior if you had difficulty answering this question.*
> **Cognitive Level**—*Applying*
> **Client Needs Category**—*Psychosocial integrity*
> **Client Needs Subcategory**—*None*

Mental Health Needs During Late Adulthood (Older than 65)

84. **2.** Privacy is important whenever the nurse gathers information of a personal nature. Regardless of the environment, clients have the right to expect that what they reveal will be kept private and confidential—even from well-meaning family members. Therefore, asking the

family members to give the client privacy is prudent and advisable.

> *Test Taking Strategy—Look at the key words "most appropriate" in reference to the action that is best before proceeding with the home assessment of an older adult when relatives are present. Recall that clients have a right to privacy, which makes option 2 the best answer. Review the importance of ensuring privacy during a nurse-client interaction if you had difficulty answering this question.*
> **Cognitive Level**—*Applying*
> **Client Needs Category**—*Safe and effective care environment*
> **Client Needs Subcategory**—*Coordinated care*

85. **1.** An indirect leading statement or open-ended question is purposely general and nonspecific. It allows the client to give as much information as desired. Close-ended questions or statements, exemplified in the other three options, elicit facts or sometimes one-word replies.

> *Test Taking Strategy—Analyze to determine what information the question asks for, which is the best communication technique for obtaining information from a client. Recall that open-ended questions (option 1) allow the client to respond in limitless ways. Review the purpose and value of using open-ended questions during nurse-client interactions if you had difficulty answering this question.*
> **Cognitive Level**—*Applying*
> **Client Needs Category**—*Psychosocial integrity*
> **Client Needs Subcategory**—*None*

86. **3.** Asking the client to identify the date of birth is a standard technique for assessing long-term memory. To evaluate the client's response, the nurse should know the answer to the question. Asking the client's current age and today's date helps in the assessment of short-term memory and orientation. Asking what occurred last January is too vague for a valid assessment.

> *Test Taking Strategy—Use the process of elimination to help select the option that describes the best method for assessing long-term memory. Recall that long-term memory involves information about events in the distant past, which is described in option 3. Eliminate options 1 and 2 because these measure short-term memory. Eliminate option 4 because this question is too vague. Review techniques for assessing long-term memory if you had difficulty answering this question.*
> **Cognitive Level**—*Remembering*
> **Client Needs Category**—*Physiological integrity*
> **Client Needs Subcategory**—*Reduction of risk potential*

87. **1.** Asking a client to repeat the question helps to rule out a hearing deficit or possible dementia. A client has a 50% chance of being right when responding only with a "yes" or "no." Asking the next of kin is appropriate if the client is not a reliable historian. Asking questions only the client can answer does not provide comprehensive objective data.

Test Taking Strategy—*Analyze to determine what information the question asks for, which is a method for helping discriminate between miscommunication and impaired cognition when assessing an older client's verbal response. Recall that having a client repeat or paraphrase the question validates that the question has been perceived accurately. Review communication techniques that are useful when assessing clients, especially those who may be experiencing dementia, if you had difficulty answering this question.*
Cognitive Level—*Applying*
Client Needs Category—*Health promotion and maintenance*
Client Needs Subcategory—*None*

88. **2.** Being unable to provide the names of longstanding neighbors is the most significant sign of mental deterioration from among the options provided. In the normal progression of dementia, short-term memory loss is affected followed by long-term memory impairment. The other assessment findings are normal or typical for an adult who is 65 years old.

Test Taking Strategy—*Look at the key words "most atypical" in reference to geriatric assessment data. Recall that significant information from the past tends to be maintained and recalled fairly easily. Therefore, the inability to recall the names of longstanding neighbors (option 2) is suggestive of a change in mental status, which may or may not correlate with the onset of dementia, depending on other findings. Review the signs of dementia if you had difficulty answering this question.*
Cognitive Level—*Applying*
Client Needs Category—*Physiological integrity*
Client Needs Subcategory—*Reduction of risk potential*

89. **1, 6.** Late adulthood is a time when most people deal with multiple losses, including family and friends. These losses may result in depression, which is common in the elderly. Becoming cynical, losing patience, and developing hostility reflect myths about aging that many younger people believe are true. Having periods of regret is not a typical problem for the elderly unless their earlier lives were not what they hoped for.

Test Taking Strategy—*Analyze to determine what information the question asks for, which is normal phenomena of older adulthood. Alternative-format "select all that apply" questions require considering each option independently to decide its merit in answering the question. Choose options that correlate with phenomena that occur during late adulthood. Review the characteristics of older adults*

during that stage in the life cycle if you had difficulty answering this question.
Cognitive Level—*Analyzing*
Client Needs Category—*Health promotion and maintenance*
Client Needs Subcategory—*None*

90. **2.** A plan for suicide indicates that the client has given serious thought to ending life. A client who has developed a suicide plan is much more likely to act on those feelings. The remaining examples are characteristic of passive suicide ideation, which is not associated with as much lethal risk as an active suicide plan.

Test Taking Strategy—*Use the process of elimination to help select the option that describes the highest risk for suicide. Although all of the options have merit, having a plan for how suicide would be accomplished (option 2) represents the highest risk. Review techniques for assessing suicidal ideation in depressed clients if you had difficulty answering this question.*
Cognitive Level—*Applying*
Client Needs Category—*Psychosocial integrity*
Client Needs Subcategory—*None*

91. **3.** Imipramine hydrochloride (Tofranil) is administered for depression. Client manifestations that occur relatively quickly after initiation of the medication include improvement in sleep, appetite, and fewer psychomotor disturbances (agitation and anxiety). Cognitive symptoms of depression, such as low self-esteem, guilt, suicidal ideation, and lack of concentration, tend to improve more slowly. Mood may be the last symptom to improve.

Test Taking Strategy—*Analyze to determine what information the question asks for, which is evidence of an initial therapeutic effect associated with tricyclic antidepressant drug therapy. Recall that there is a lag time in achieving effectiveness when tricyclic antidepressants are administered. Consequently, a decrease in agitation (option 3) is more likely to occur before there is relief of a depressed mood. Review the actions of tricyclic antidepressants and evidence of therapeutic effectiveness if you had difficulty answering this question.*
Cognitive Level—*Analyzing*
Client Needs Category—*Physiological integrity*
Client Needs Subcategory—*Pharmacological therapies*

92. **3, 4.** Imipramine hydrochloride (Tofranil) is a tricyclic antidepressant (TCA) that is used to reduce depression. Nursing instructions should include rising from the chair slowly because this drug has been associated with cardiac problems and electrocardiographic (ECG) changes. Also, as with many older classes of antidepressants, it may take 3 to 4 weeks before the client begins to feel better. Avoiding cheese, chocolate, and pickled foods is related to monoamine oxidase inhibitors (MAOIs), not TCAs.

93. 2. The nurse must check that the depressed client has swallowed all medication. Some clients "cheek" medications, then use them as a method of suicide after accumulating a sufficient quantity. Taking medications with a full glass of water is appropriate for clients who do not have fluid restrictions. Some medications are better absorbed on an empty stomach; some that cause stomach upset are better taken with food. Taking one or all the prescribed drugs at one time is safe as long as the client does not have difficulty swallowing them.

> *Test Taking Strategy—Look at the key words "especially important" in reference to a nursing action that applies to the administration of medication to a depressed client. Recall that depressed clients are potentially suicidal and may hoard medications for a later suicide attempt. The client's act of disguising the fact that medication has been swallowed could facilitate suicide. By checking the client's mouth, including under the tongue and in the buccal cavities, the nurse can determine if the medication has been swallowed. Review the phenomenon known as cheeking as it applies to taking medication if you had difficulty answering this question.*
> *Cognitive Level—Analyzing*
> *Client Needs Category—Safe and effective care environment*
> *Client Needs Subcategory—Safety and infection control*

94. 3. Electroconvulsive therapy (ECT) involves electrically induced seizures in anesthetized clients for a therapeutic effect. ECT is most often used as a treatment for severe major depression that has not responded to other types of treatment and is not a controversial issue in psychiatric circles. After ECT, it is common for clients to experience headaches and temporary retrograde and antegrade memory loss for events nearest in time to the treatment. Proponents of ECT claim that the capacity to remember information eventually returns to the pretreatment level. The effects identified in the other options may occur, but they are not effects associated with ECT.

> *Test Taking Strategy—Look at the key words "most likely" reaction and "immediate" recovery period after ECT. Recall that clients who receive ECT may experience temporary loss of short-term memory and headaches that do not tend to be as severe as those identified in option 3. Review the outcomes associated with the administration of ECT if you had difficulty answering this question.*
> *Cognitive Level—Applying*
> *Client Needs Category—Physiological integrity*
> *Client Needs Subcategory—Reduction of risk potential*

95. 2. Doxepin (Sinequan) and other tricyclic antidepressants may cause orthostatic hypotension, especially in the morning. The nurse should advise rising slowly and dangling the feet over the side of the bed before standing. This helps the client gain balance before walking. Placing a cool compress on the forehead may help the client initially, but orthostatic hypotension is still a concern when the client rises. Advising the client to breathe deeply is used for shortness of breath and hypoventilation, not orthostatic hypotension. Having the client elevate both feet will not decrease dizziness on rising.

> *Test Taking Strategies—Analyze to determine what information the question asks for, which is a nursing suggestion for a client who is most likely experiencing postural hypotension. Ensuring client safety is a priority. Therefore, option 2 is the best answer because it provides time for baroreceptors to stabilize a client's blood pressure. Review methods for managing postural hypotension if you had difficulty answering this question.*
> *Cognitive Level—Analyzing*
> *Client Needs Category—Physiological integrity*
> *Client Needs Subcategory—Pharmacological therapies*

96. 2. Depression in the elderly is often masked under the guise of multiple physical complaints. It is often easier to seek help for physical problems than to verbalize the need for emotional help. Being irritable after a visit from active grandchildren is normal for some older adults. Sleeping a great deal of the time is suggestive of depression, but taking a lengthy nap regularly in the afternoon is not necessarily pathologic. Crying when talking about a dead spouse is normal if the death happened recently. If the crying is brief, it is not interpreted as unresolved grief.

> *Test Taking Strategy—Look at the key words "most suggestive" in reference to a finding that correlates with depressive symptoms in an older adult. Recall that depression can be manifested by both physical and emotional symptoms. Option 2 describes the complaint that many depressed clients present when consulting their primary care provider. Review the signs and symptoms of depression if you had difficulty answering this question.*

Cognitive Level—*Applying*
Client Needs Category—*Psychosocial integrity*
Client Needs Subcategory—*None*

97. 4. Duloxetine (Cymbalta) is classified as a serotonin norepinephrine inhibitor (SNRI) or dual action antidepressant. Drugs in this category tend to cause insomnia, nervousness, blurred vision, sweating, problems with ejaculation, and dry mucous membranes.

  Test Taking Strategy—*Use the process of elimination to help select the option that describes the drug-related symptom that is most likely associated with duloxetine, an SNRI antidepressant. Recall that drugs in this category interfere with the reuptake of norepinephrine and serotonin. Elevated levels of norepinephrine are likely to cause insomnia (option 4). Option 1 can be eliminated because polyuria is more often a side effect of lithium therapy. Option 3 can be eliminated because drooling may occur when taking an atypical antipsychotic medication. Option 2 can be eliminated because it is not commonly associated with any psychotropic medication. Review the side effects of SNRI antidepressants and sertraline in particular if you had difficulty answering this question.*
  Cognitive Level—*Applying*
  Client Needs Category—*Physiological integrity*
  Client Needs Subcategory—*Pharmacological therapies*

98. 2. Providing privacy is appropriate for preserving the sexually active couple's self-esteem. Reporting the clients' sexual behavior to their adult children is inappropriate, as long as the clients are competent and consenting adults. The request to become roommates is better initiated by the residents. Censuring sexuality is inappropriate; even older adults have a need for love and affection.

  Test Taking Strategy—*Look at the key words "most appropriate" in reference to finding older clients in a nursing home having intercourse. Note that the stem indicates that the clients are oriented and thus have the cognitive ability to make decisions. Because sexual intimacy is normal in a romantic relationship and the location of the lovemaking is appropriate, the clients deserve to have their privacy protected. Review the role of the nurse in ensuring privacy if you had difficulty answering this question.*
  Cognitive Level—*Applying*
  Client Needs Category—*Psychosocial integrity*
  Client Needs Subcategory—*None*

99. 1. Involuntary facial movements and tongue and eye movements indicate the development of tardive dyskinesia, a negative consequence of traditional, typical antipsychotic (neuroleptic) drug therapy. The condition is usually irreversible, even after the drug is discontinued. About 20% of those treated with antipsychotic medications in the long-term develop tardive dyskinesia. None of the other assessment findings is linked to antipsychotic drug withdrawal.

  Test Taking Strategy—*Look at the key words "most likely" in reference to a consequence of taking an antipsychotic drug for a prolonged period of time. Recall that tardive dyskinesia, involuntary muscle movements characterized by facial tics (option 1), occurs more often when clients are treated with typical rather than atypical antipsychotic medications. Review potential side effects associated with typical antipsychotic drug therapy if you had difficulty answering this question.*
  Cognitive Level—*Applying*
  Client Needs Category—*Physiological integrity*
  Client Needs Subcategory—*Pharmacological therapies*

100. 4. Self-esteem is promoted by experiencing recognition for accomplishments. Giving genuine praise promotes a positive self-concept. The longer a person can maintain independence, the less likely that physical deterioration will occur. All of the other options communicate an inability to manage self-care satisfactorily.

  Test Taking Strategy—*Look at the key words "most beneficial" in reference to a nursing action that promotes a client's self-esteem. Despite the fact that the client's self-care was imperfect, the client did perform bathing and grooming independently and deserves positive reinforcement for that effort, as indicated by option 4. Review the role of positive reinforcement as a motivation for repeating a desired behavior if you had difficulty answering this question.*
  Cognitive Level—*Applying*
  Client Needs Category—*Psychosocial integrity*
  Client Needs Subcategory—*None*

101. 2. Techniques that may facilitate reminiscing include singing songs from an earlier period and looking at picture albums, old catalogs, movies, and magazines. Discussing current events and reading a recent newspaper article help clients remain oriented to the present. Making holiday decorations is more likely to provide diversional therapy and help clients remain oriented.

  Test Taking Strategy—*Look at the key words "most helpful" in reference to an activity that facilitates reminiscence therapy. Note that reminiscence implies recalling events and experiences from the past, which is characterized by option 2. Review the activities that are generally included in reminiscence therapy if you had difficulty answering this question.*
  Cognitive Level—*Analyzing*
  Client Needs Category—*Psychosocial integrity*
  Client Needs Subcategory—*None*

102. 2. During senescence, it is common for people to review their life experiences. If clients believe that their lives have been satisfying and worthwhile, they acquire integrity. If clients have regrets, they end their lives with a feeling of despair. Trust is acquired during infancy. Intimacy is established during young adulthood. The toddler stage in the life cycle is associated with autonomy.

Test Taking Strategy—*Analyze to determine what information the question asks for, which is the developmental characteristic demonstrated by the client's statement. Recall that integrity is a positive characteristic that develops for some older adults at that stage in the life cycle. Integrity is indicated in option 2 by the client's affirmation that he or she is satisfied with prior life events and relationships. Review Erikson's developmental stages throughout the life cycle and their positive or negative outcomes if you had difficulty answering this question.*

Cognitive Level—*Applying*
Client Needs Category—*Health promotion and maintenance*
Client Needs Subcategory—*None*

103. 4. Words may not mean the same thing to all people. Reporting what was observed is a much more accurate and objective method for documenting behavior, especially in view of the fact that the nurse's notes are part of the permanent record that can be used as admissible evidence in a court of law. None of the other critiques identifies the vague and subjective quality of the nurse's charting.

Test Taking Strategy—*Analyze to determine what information the question asks for, which is the reason the sample documentation is unsatisfactory. Recall that a principle of documentation is that it must be objective rather than subjectively conclude what the nurse has observed. Option 4 offers the best reason this note is unsatisfactory because it supports the lack of objective evidence. Review the principles of documentation if you had difficulty answering this question.*

Cognitive Level—*Applying*
Client Needs Category—*Safe and effective care environment*
Client Needs Subcategory—*Coordinated care*

104. 1, 2, 3. For many clients, regardless of their cultural background, mental illness is an embarrassment and a social stigma. For these reasons, many ethnic and cultural groups are less likely to seek treatment for mental illness. Primary factors that affect developing a plan of care for an Asian client include language, literacy level, and reticence among those who are Asian to report and discuss their physical and mental symptoms with strangers. Marital status, the client's extended family, and financial means are not considered as pertinent as the other options.

Test Taking Strategy—*Analyze to determine what information the question asks for, which primary factors the nurse should consider when planning the nursing care for an Asian client. Alternative-format "select all that apply" questions require considering each*

option independently to decide its merit in answering the question. Choose options that include basic factors for all clients as well as cultural differences. Review factors involved in transcultural care if you had difficulty answering this question.

Cognitive Level—*Analyzing*
Client Needs Category—*Safe and effective care environment*
Client Needs Subcategory—*Coordinated care*

105. 1. Labeling rooms with easily identifiable words or pictures promotes environmental awareness. Sensory cues restore the confused client's ability to reorient. Locking the unit deprives all the clients of a certain amount of freedom and privacy. Physical restraint used unnecessarily is considered battery. A confused client is unable to process information about the consequences of behavior.

Test Taking Strategy—*Use the process of elimination to help select the option that describes the best method for managing a client who wanders. Recall that loss of memory is one of the chief losses experienced by a client with dementia. Providing a cue within the environment, such as described in option 1, may help reorient a client suffering from dementia. Review methods for reorienting clients with dementia if you had difficulty answering this question.*

Cognitive Level—*Analyzing*
Client Needs Category—*Health promotion and maintenance*
Client Needs Subcategory—*None*

106. 4. It is essential that the nurse treat a client with cognitive impairment with dignity. Shielding from public view by taking the client to a vacant room is the most appropriate action for the nurse to take in this situation. It would be inappropriate and a violation of confidentiality to tell others about the client's mental impairment. The other options are better suited for a client with a higher level of cognitive function.

Test Taking Strategy—*Look at the key words "most appropriate" in reference to the first action a nurse should take when a client is naked in a public area. Recall that a client with dementia is not likely to comply with a directive to dress. Nor is the client able to cognitively appreciate the significance of his or her nakedness. Providing an explanation to other clients is also inappropriate and unlikely to solve the situation. Relocating the client to a place out of the view of others (option 4) is the first action the nurse should take. Once in a private place, the nurse can help the client dress appropriately. Review the principles in caring for a client with dementia if you had difficulty answering this question.*

Cognitive Level—*Analyzing*
Client Needs Category—*Psychosocial integrity*
Client Needs Subcategory—*None*

107. 4. Displaying a large calendar with easy-to-read words and numbers in a prominent place is one way to help older clients remain oriented. All of the other options have therapeutic benefits but are not useful in orienting clients to present reality.

> *Test Taking Strategy—Look at the key words "most therapeutic" in reference to a method for helping clients with dementia remain oriented. Recall that orientation involves correctly identifying person, place, and time. A calendar (option 4) would help orient a client, as well as others, to the current day, month, and year (components of time). Review methods for maintaining orientation and reorienting clients with dementia if you had difficulty answering this question.*
> *Cognitive Level—Analyzing*
> *Client Needs Category—Psychosocial integrity*
> *Client Needs Subcategory—None*

108. 2. Consistent repetition in the unit routine helps clients with cognitive impairments stay oriented to activities in which they are expected to participate. Wearing a name tag is a helpful technique, but routinely assigning the same employee to care for the same clients is even better. Altering a set routine of activities with field trips tends to disorient clients, at least temporarily. Clients with dementia are usually incapable of reading and following a written schedule.

> *Test Taking Strategy—Use the process of elimination to help select the option that describes the best technique for reducing confusion experienced by clients with dementia. Recall that inconsistent patterns of activities interfere with the client's ability to process information, but consistent repetitive routines provide some degree of stability and familiarity for the client. Review techniques for reducing confusion in clients with dementia if you had difficulty answering this question.*
> *Cognitive Level—Analyzing*
> *Client Needs Category—Safe and effective care environment*
> *Client Needs Subcategory—Coordinated care*

109. 2. To facilitate attention, concentration, and retention, all verbal communication with a client with late-stage dementia should be brief and simple. Directions are given in understandable language with a minimum of distracting stimuli in the environment. Speaking loudly does not improve memory. Writing down some information may help a client to remember oral instructions, but overall it is not the best recommendation of the choices provided. Listening to a news program helps maintain reality orientation, but it does not promote memory.

> *Test Taking Strategy—Use the process of elimination to help select the option that describes the best method to use when communicating with a client*

with dementia. Recall that a client with dementia has a short attention span and cannot process detailed information, which makes option 2 the best answer. Review techniques for communicating with clients who have altered cognitive function if you had difficulty answering this question.
> *Cognitive Level—Analyzing*
> *Client Needs Category—Psychosocial integrity*
> *Client Needs Subcategory—None*

110. 2. It is best to reinforce that the client is in the appropriate place. Trying to convince a client that this is home may provoke the client or cause further agitation. Treating the request lightly communicates disrespect. Using the family as a scapegoat avoids responsibility for helping the client understand and cope.

> *Test Taking Strategy—Look at the key words "most appropriate" in reference to a nursing response to a dementia client's request to "go home." It is always therapeutic to present reality to a client who has dementia or is otherwise confused due to some other condition. Reality is presented in option 2. Review the value of presenting reality when communicating with a confused or disoriented client if you had difficulty answering this question.*
> *Cognitive Level—Analyzing*
> *Client Needs Category—Psychosocial integrity*
> *Client Needs Subcategory—None*

111. 2. Nurses need to be alert to signs of burnout and exhaustion among family members. A caring staff member encouraging longer periods of separation can relieve the family's potential for feeling guilty. The client's spouse may benefit from a physical examination, but that is not the most therapeutic action in the list of choices. Clients in a long-term health care facility have a right to see visitors at any time within reason. Indicating that the staff is capable of caring for the client's spouse may imply that the spouse is unappreciated or is an inconvenience.

> *Test Taking Strategy—Look at the key words "most beneficial" in reference to helping a client's spouse who shows signs of exhaustion and self-neglect. Recall that visiting less frequently or for shorter periods of time facilitates spending more time for physical and emotional self-care (option 2). Review how respite care is important when caring for a caregiver if you had difficulty answering this question.*
> *Cognitive Level—Analyzing*
> *Client Needs Category—Health promotion and maintenance*
> *Client Needs Subcategory—None*

112. 2. Verbalizing what has been implied is a therapeutic communication technique in which the listener reflects the speaker's expressed thoughts and related feelings.

One of the greatest stressors for family members of clients with Alzheimer's is that those afflicted are physically present but emotionally absent. The remaining responses are clichés. They probably will not encourage the client's daughter to talk more about feelings.

Test Taking Strategy—Look at the key words "most therapeutic" in reference to a nursing response to a statement made by the client's daughter. Option 2, which is the correct answer, is an example of a therapeutic communication technique. Review examples of therapeutic communication techniques if you had difficulty answering this question.
Cognitive Level—Analyzing
Client Needs Category—Psychosocial integrity
Client Needs Subcategory—None

113. **2.** Providing a client with environmental cues relieves confusion. Repetitive reminders help the confused person maintain or relearn how to function. A liquid diet is unappetizing and unnecessary as long as the client can chew, swallow, and digest food naturally. Serving this client early will not eliminate confusion. Seating a client alone deprives the client of any role models to imitate and shows disregard for the client's dignity.

Test Taking Strategy—Use the process of elimination to help select the option that describes the best nursing action for prolonging the ability to self-feed in a client with progressive dementia. Imitation, as identified in option 2, provides visual cues for how to use utensils when eating. Review techniques for managing the care of a client with dementia of the Alzheimer's type if you had difficulty answering this question.
Cognitive Level—Analyzing
Client Needs Category—Health promotion and maintenance
Client Needs Subcategory—None

114. **3.** Drugs are potentially unsafe if not administered correctly. The nurse usually takes the time to explain drug administration verbally in such situations; however, it is also helpful to reinforce verbal instructions with written information. Before the client leaves, the nurse needs to determine that the client's daughter has an accurate understanding of the instructions. The family is most likely already familiar with the other types of information.

Test Taking Strategy—Look at the key words "critical assessment" in reference to a criterion that ensures the client's safety during a home visit. Option 3 is the best answer because errors in administering medications can have dangerous consequences, whereas failing to return the client at the time expected, lack of hygiene measures, and misunderstanding about the client's symptoms are not potentially life-threatening. Review essential information to ascertain when preparing a family member for

a client's home visit if you had difficulty answering this question.
Cognitive Level—Analyzing
Client Needs Category—Safe and effective care environment
Client Needs Subcategory—Safety and infection control

115. **1.** A dying client with an advance directive should not be abandoned even though the client does not want heroic measures taken to extend life. Staying with the client provides comfort and demonstrates caring behaviors while the client dies with dignity. It is premature to call the funeral home. Transferring to the intensive care unit (ICU) is not appropriate because the client's condition does not warrant it. In addition, this would cost the client unneeded expense. Depending on the client's religious preferences, it may or may not be appropriate to notify the hospital chaplain.

Test Taking Strategy—Look at the key words "most appropriate" in reference to providing care to a client whose death is imminent. Recall that it is emotionally and psychologically cruel to leave the client alone when dying. If the nurse cannot remain at the client's bedside, a surrogate should be designated. Review the principles involved in caring for dying clients if you had difficulty answering this question.
Cognitive Level—Analyzing
Client Needs Category—Safe and effective care environment
Client Needs Subcategory—Coordinated care

116. **3.** Expressing feelings to an understanding listener helps facilitate the grieving process. Communication helps people deal openly with their emotions and feelings, which is healthier than suppressing the event's emotional impact. Being sent home or terminated does not help promote grieving. Asking the nursing assistant to perform postmortem care in this emotional state shows a disregard for the traumatic experience.

Test Taking Strategy—Look at the key words "most beneficial" in reference to nursing support for a distraught nursing assistant. Recall that verbalizing thoughts and feelings at the time of a crisis (option 3) is therapeutic for preventing or minimizing ineffective coping, whereas the actions described in the other options are less or even nontherapeutic. Review crisis intervention techniques if you had difficulty answering this question.
Cognitive Level—Analyzing
Client Needs Category—Psychosocial integrity
Client Needs Subcategory—None

117. **3.** Having a paranormal experience, such as sensing a deceased person's presence or seeing or talking to the deceased person, can be comforting. As long as there is no potential for being financially, emotionally, or physically disadvantaged, the nurse should not dispute the bereaved person's experience.

> ***Test Taking Strategy***—*Look at the key words "most appropriate" in reference to a client's paranormal experience. Recall that paranormal experiences are rare, but not uncommon, after the death of a significant other. Implying that the experience is normal and in no way threatening may help the person accept and perhaps value the experience. Review the incidence of paranormal experiences after a death and their significance if you had difficulty answering this question.*
> ***Cognitive Level***—*Analyzing*
> ***Client Needs Category***—*Psychosocial integrity*
> ***Client Needs Subcategory***—*None*

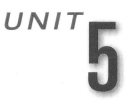

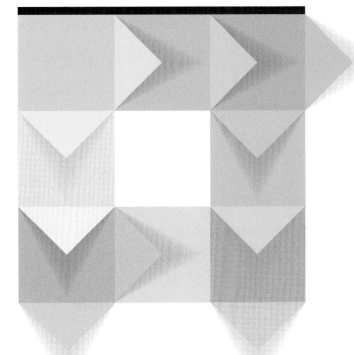

Postreview Tests

Comprehensive Test 1

■ Correct Answers, Rationales, and Test Taking Strategies

Directions: *With a pencil, blacken the space in front of the option you have chosen for your correct answer.*

1. Which assessment findings provide the nurse with the best indications that a client's tracheostomy needs suctioning? Select all that apply.
[ ] **1.** The client's pulse rate is slowed.
[ ] **2.** The client's skin is cool and moist.
[ ] **3.** The client's respirations are noisy.
[ ] **4.** The client is coughing up sputum.
[ ] **5.** The client's pulse oximeter reads 87%.
[ ] **6.** The client's respiratory rate is 32.

2. Before suctioning a client with a tracheostomy, which nursing action should the nurse perform first?
[ ] **1.** Clean the tracheostomy stoma with a sterile, cotton-tipped applicator.
[ ] **2.** Instill 5 mL of saline within the tracheostomy.
[ ] **3.** Administer 100% oxygen for 1 to 2 minutes.
[ ] **4.** Occlude the vent on the catheter for 15 seconds.

3. When changing a sterile abdominal dressing, which nursing actions support the principles of asepsis? Select all that apply.
[ ] **1.** The nurse dons clean gloves to remove the soiled dressing.
[ ] **2.** The nurse places the soiled dressing in a biohazard bag.
[ ] **3.** The nurse performs hand hygiene before donning sterile gloves.
[ ] **4.** The nurse cleans the wound from the outer edge toward the center.
[ ] **5.** The nurse reaches across the sterile field to adjust the wrapper.
[ ] **6.** The nurse touches the client's soiled dressing with sterile gloves.

4. If a client with a conductive hearing loss asks the nurse how a hearing aid improves hearing, which response by the nurse is most appropriate?
[ ] **1.** "A hearing aid amplifies sounds that are present."
[ ] **2.** "A hearing aid makes sounds sharper and clearer."
[ ] **3.** "A hearing aid transmits more distinct, crisp sounds."
[ ] **4.** "A hearing aid eliminates garbled background sounds."

5. The nurse observes a nursing assistant assigned to a client who just returned from having a bronchoscopy. Which action by the nursing assistant would prompt the nurse to intervene?
[ ] **1.** The nursing assistant takes the client's pulse oximeter reading.
[ ] **2.** The nursing assistant offers the client some water.
[ ] **3.** The nursing assistant raises the head of the bed.
[ ] **4.** The nursing assistant takes the client's tympanic temperature.

6. When a client becomes angry and shouts at the nurse because of a dislike for food that was served, which response by the nurse is most appropriate?
[ ] **1.** Say something humorous and promise to call the dietitian.
[ ] **2.** Listen attentively, allowing the client to express opinions.
[ ] **3.** Leave the room, and allow the client a period of privacy.
[ ] **4.** Explain that the diet was ordered by the physician.

7. At the time of a retinal detachment, which symptoms will the client most likely describe to the nurse? Select all that apply.
[ ] **1.** Seeing flashes of light
[ ] **2.** Being unable to see light
[ ] **3.** Feeling discomfort in light
[ ] **4.** Seeing poorly in daylight
[ ] **5.** Having severe eye pain
[ ] **6.** Experiencing wavy vision

8. When the nurse cares for a 3-month-old infant, which medication administration technique is best?
[ ] **1.** Putting the medication in the infant's bottle and giving it during the next feeding
[ ] **2.** Placing the medication in a needleless syringe and administering it orally
[ ] **3.** Giving the medication in a medicine cup while pinching the infant's nose shut
[ ] **4.** Mixing the medication with a small amount of cereal and giving it with a spoon

9. When the nurse cares for a small child in Bryant's traction, which assessment finding is the best indication that the traction is applied properly?

[ ] **1.** The child can sit up without experiencing discomfort.

[ ] **2.** The child can reach the trapeze hanging above the bed.

[ ] **3.** The child's buttocks are raised slightly off the mattress.

[ ] **4.** The child's legs are pulled toward the bottom of the bed.

10. When planning the nursing care for a client in sickle cell crisis, what is the main nursing priority?

[ ] **1.** Administering antibiotics

[ ] **2.** Preventing immobility

[ ] **3.** Relieving discomfort

[ ] **4.** Limiting food and fluids

11. A client newly diagnosed with cancer receives external radiation therapy. Which of the nurse's instructions regarding bathing is most appropriate?

[ ] **1.** Avoid getting the irradiated skin wet.

[ ] **2.** Use body wash instead of bar soap on the irradiated skin.

[ ] **3.** Cover the reddened irradiated area with clear plastic.

[ ] **4.** Use a soft cloth to wash the irradiated skin.

12. If the physician orders "diet as tolerated" for a client the evening of surgery, which diet is most appropriate for the nurse to request initially?

[ ] **1.** Bland diet

[ ] **2.** Soft diet

[ ] **3.** Clear liquid diet

[ ] **4.** Regular diet

13. A pregnant client in the third trimester calls the obstetrician's office and reports to the nurse that she has had a severe headache for the past 2 days. Which nursing action is most appropriate?

[ ] **1.** Ask if the client is having flu or cold symptoms.

[ ] **2.** Advise the client to eliminate coffee and other sources of caffeine.

[ ] **3.** Instruct the client to take two aspirin and lie down for an hour.

[ ] **4.** Request that the client come to the physician's office immediately.

14. Laboratory data for an adult client diagnosed with *Pneumocystis carinii* pneumonia indicate immunosuppression. When the nurse gathers the client's history on admission, what information is most helpful in determining the client's susceptibility to this infection?

[ ] **1.** The client's immunization history

[ ] **2.** The client's family history

[ ] **3.** The client's smoking practices

[ ] **4.** The client's sexual practices

15. Which statement made by the parents of a toddler best suggests to the nurse that the child has cystic fibrosis?

[ ] **1.** "Our child's perspiration is very salty."

[ ] **2.** "Our child vomits immediately after eating."

[ ] **3.** "Our child's stools are soft and bright yellow."

[ ] **4.** "Our child's urine is tea colored."

16. If a client has been taking corticosteroid medication for a prolonged period, which statement to the nurse provides the best indication that the danger related to this medication is understood?

[ ] **1.** "I should never suddenly stop taking my medication."

[ ] **2.** "My reaction time will be slowed while taking this drug."

[ ] **3.** "If I forget to take one dose, I should call the physician."

[ ] **4.** "I shouldn't take this drug for more than 6 months."

17. When monitoring the treatment response of a client with diabetes insipidus, which component of the urinalysis is most important for the nurse to assess?

[ ] **1.** Urine pH

[ ] **2.** Urinary casts

[ ] **3.** Specific gravity

[ ] **4.** Urine bilirubin

18. While visiting a client who takes a prescribed diuretic, how can a home health care nurse best evaluate the drug's effectiveness?

[ ] **1.** Monitor the client's weight.

[ ] **2.** Palpate the client's peripheral pulses.

[ ] **3.** Assess the client's appetite.

[ ] **4.** Elicit the client's reflexes.

19. When applying nitroglycerin ointment to a client's chest, which nursing technique is most appropriate?

[ ] **1.** Squeezing a ribbon of ointment on paper

[ ] **2.** Rubbing the ointment thoroughly into the skin

[ ] **3.** Reapplying the ointment every 4 hours

[ ] **4.** Spreading the ointment directly over the heart area

20. Once parents understand how to open an infant's airway, which instruction regarding rescue breathing is important for the nurse to include when teaching parents of a newborn?

[ ] **1.** "Cover the nose and mouth; blow as much air as is possible."

[ ] **2.** "Cover the nose; blow enough air to make the chest rise 2 inches."

[ ] **3.** "Cover the nose and mouth, blow puffs of air every 3 seconds.

[ ] **4.** "Cover the mouth and pinch the nose closed; blow puffs of air."

21. What are the priorities when planning the nursing care of a 75-year-old hospitalized client who develops pneumonia? Select all that apply.
[ ] **1.** Relieving the cough
[ ] **2.** Maintaining oxygenation
[ ] **3.** Providing nourishment
[ ] **4.** Encouraging independence
[ ] **5.** Administering prescribed antibiotics within 4 hours of admission
[ ] **6.** Obtaining ordered blood cultures within 24 hours of admission

22. When providing nursing care for a client after a sub-total thyroidectomy, which position is best?
[ ] **1.** Supine
[ ] **2.** Semi-Fowler's
[ ] **3.** Lateral
[ ] **4.** Sim's

23. When assessing a client who has attempted suicide by taking an overdose of medication, which question is most important for the nurse to ask initially?
[ ] **1.** "How many pills did you take?"
[ ] **2.** "Why did you take the pills?"
[ ] **3.** "What is the name of the drug?"
[ ] **4.** "Have you attempted suicide in the past?"

24. A 6-year-old child has just had placement of bilateral myringotomy tubes. As the parents prepare for discharge, the nurse correctly includes which instruction in the child's discharge plan?
[ ] **1.** "Instill ear drops in the ears every 4 hours for the first 24 hours."
[ ] **2.** "Speak in a louder voice when talking to the child."
[ ] **3.** "Insert earplugs whenever the child swims or showers."
[ ] **4.** "Irrigate the ears daily with tap water while the tubes are in place."

25. In an adult client, the nurse plans to administer 2 mL of medication I.M. Which technique is most accurate?
[ ] **1.** The nurse adds 2 mL of air to the vial before withdrawing the drug.
[ ] **2.** The nurse withdraws the medication using a tuberculin syringe.
[ ] **3.** The nurse selects the deltoid muscle for injecting the medication.
[ ] **4.** The nurse inserts a $\frac{5}{8}''$ needle into the muscle at a 45-degree angle.

26. Which action by the nurse is most appropriate to assess the neurologic status of a client who has a freshly applied plaster cast to the lower extremity?
[ ] **1.** Asking the client to wiggle the toes
[ ] **2.** Depressing the nail bed to observe the color
[ ] **3.** Feeling the temperature of the toes
[ ] **4.** Palpating the pedal pulses bilaterally

27. The noon blood glucose level of a client with type 1 diabetes mellitus is 250 mg/dL. The physician orders a sliding-scale insulin regimen based on the client's blood glucose level. The order reads, "Give regular insulin using the following scale:"

0 to 140 mg/dL	None
141 to 200 mg/dL	2 units
201 to 250 mg/dL	4 units
251 to 300 mg/dL	6 units
301 to 350 mg/dL	8 units
351 to 400 mg/dL	10 units
Over 400 mg/dL	Notify physician

How many units of insulin should the nurse plan to give?

[ ] **1.** 2 units
[ ] **2.** 4 units
[ ] **3.** 6 units
[ ] **4.** 8 units

28. A homeless person has an enlarged, tender liver, and a hepatitis B infection is suspected. When the nurse obtains all of the following in the client's history, what is the most likely etiologic factor for the disease?
[ ] **1.** The client eats food found in garbage cans.
[ ] **2.** The client drinks a fifth of whiskey per day.
[ ] **3.** The client smokes cigarettes extinguished on the street.
[ ] **4.** The client occasionally shares needles to inject heroin.

29. When the nurse reviews the history of several antepartum clients, which pregnant clients are at greatest risk for developing maternal and fetal complications during pregnancy? Select all that apply.
[ ] **1.** The client who regularly restricts food intake to avoid gaining weight
[ ] **2.** The client who remains sexually active throughout the pregnancy
[ ] **3.** The client who participates regularly in an aerobic exercise program
[ ] **4.** The client who is 36 years old and pregnant for the first time
[ ] **5.** The client who refuses to take her prenatal vitamins due to constipation
[ ] **6.** The client who has a history of a chlamydia infection 3 years ago

30. A physician orders 2 mg/kg of a drug. If the client weighs 88 pounds, how many milligrams of the medication should the nurse administer?

31. A nurse massages the uterus of a postpartum client. Which assessment finding is the best indication that the intended effect of this nursing action has been achieved?
[ ] **1.** Postpartal pain is relieved.
[ ] **2.** The uterus becomes firm.
[ ] **3.** The client passes clots from the vagina.
[ ] **4.** Uterine contractions cease.

32. When a physician orders subcutaneous injections of glulisine (Apidra) insulin, when is the optimum time for the nurse to administer the injection?
[ ] **1.** Between meals
[ ] **2.** At bedtime
[ ] **3.** 15 minutes before a meal
[ ] **4.** 30 minutes after a meal

33. A depressed client tells the nurse, "No one really cares whether I live or die." What is the nurse's most appropriate response?
[ ] **1.** "You're exaggerating! Lots of people care about you."
[ ] **2.** "Talking like that will only make you feel worse."
[ ] **3.** "Tell me why you think no one cares about you."
[ ] **4.** "It sounds like you're feeling ignored or abandoned."

34. Which nursing action is best for determining if a client has a fecal impaction?
[ ] **1.** Auscultating the bowel sounds
[ ] **2.** Measuring the abdominal girth
[ ] **3.** Inserting a finger within the rectum
[ ] **4.** Assessing for diarrhea

35. After a 6-year-old child develops tonsillitis, the nurse instructs the parents to avoid giving the child aspirin or aspirin products. What is the best explanation for the nurse's instruction?
[ ] **1.** Aspirin lowers the temperature and, therefore, can mask a fever.
[ ] **2.** Aspirin can cause symptoms related to Reye's syndrome.
[ ] **3.** Aspirin irritates the stomach and could cause an ulcer.
[ ] **4.** Aspirin reduces inflammation and conceals an infection.

36. What is the best evidence the nurse can use to determine if a postpartum client's Kegel exercises are effective?
[ ] **1.** The client can perform deep-knee bends without back discomfort.
[ ] **2.** The client can touch the toes without abdominal discomfort.
[ ] **3.** The client can do several sit-ups without stopping.
[ ] **4.** The client can stop and restart the flow of urine while voiding.

37. A pregnant client with known human immunodeficiency virus (HIV) infection is admitted to the hospital in active labor. Which method for assessing the fetus is most appropriate for the nurse to perform at this time?
[ ] **1.** Fetal scalp sampling
[ ] **2.** Chorionic villi sampling
[ ] **3.** External fetal monitoring
[ ] **4.** Internal fetal monitoring

38. When a nurse performs a mental status assessment on an adult client with hypothyroidism, which of the following is an expected finding?
[ ] **1.** Quick recall of events
[ ] **2.** Rapid response to questions
[ ] **3.** Bizarre thought processes
[ ] **4.** Impaired cognitive function

39. The nurse is caring for a client who has just been diagnosed with sinus bradycardia. Indicate with an *X* the area on the illustration where the heartbeat's electrical impulse is initiated.

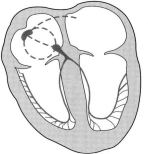

40. When a schizophrenic client claims to see demons in the room, what is the best documentation for the nurse to record?
[ ] **1.** "Experiencing hallucinations"
[ ] **2.** "Frightened by hallucinations"
[ ] **3.** "States, 'Seeing demons in my room'"
[ ] **4.** "Having distorted sensory perceptions"

41. The nurse assists with the delivery of a stillborn infant who is gestationally small with a malformed cranium. To promote the parents' grieving process, which nursing action is most appropriate?
[ ] **1.** Allowing the parents to see and touch their dead infant
[ ] **2.** Covering and shielding the dead infant from parental view
[ ] **3.** Describing the positive characteristics of the dead infant
[ ] **4.** Discharging the mother within 24 hours of delivery

42. Which nursing technique is most accurate for removing an object that completely obstructs the airway of an unconscious adult?

[ ] **1.** Administering abdominal thrusts until the object is dislodged

[ ] **2.** Administering two quick ventilations of air

[ ] **3.** Administering five chest thrusts and a breath

[ ] **4.** Administering 30 chest compressions followed by 2 breaths

43. When the nurse cares for a client with a colostomy, which assessment finding is the best evidence that the client is adjusting to the change in body image?

[ ] **1.** The client wears loose-fitting garments.

[ ] **2.** The client takes a shower each day.

[ ] **3.** The client empties the appliance.

[ ] **4.** The client avoids foods that form gas.

44. After an upper GI X-ray, which of the following is most important for the nurse to monitor?

[ ] **1.** The client's ability to eat

[ ] **2.** The passage of stool

[ ] **3.** The color of the client's urine

[ ] **4.** The client's swallowing ability

45. A 17-year-old unmarried postpartum client is being discharged from the hospital. Which client factor is most indicative to the nurse that the client needs a community-based referral after discharge?

[ ] **1.** The client is a primipara.

[ ] **2.** The client lives alone.

[ ] **3.** The client had a previous spontaneous abortion.

[ ] **4.** The client continues to see the newborn's father.

46. A hospitalized client diagnosed with cancer has a sealed source of radiation inserted into the vagina. Which information is most important to obtain to ensure the safety of the nurse assigned to care for the client?

[ ] **1.** Whether the assigned nurse is sensitive to radiation

[ ] **2.** Whether the assigned nurse is pregnant

[ ] **3.** Whether the assigned nurse has attended the radiation safety inservice

[ ] **4.** Whether the assigned nurse will be reassigned to another unit later in the shift

47. A team conference is scheduled to discuss interventions necessary to resolve the inadequate dietary intake of a client diagnosed with Alzheimer's disease. Which nursing intervention will most likely facilitate an improvement in the client's nutrition?

[ ] **1.** Providing high-calorie finger foods every waking hour

[ ] **2.** Serving foods that are easy to digest

[ ] **3.** Giving the client additional time to eat each meal

[ ] **4.** Asking the client's family for a list of the client's favorite foods

48. Which nursing assessment technique is best for detecting thrombophlebitis in a client's lower extremity?

[ ] **1.** Have the client dorsiflex each foot.

[ ] **2.** Palpate the dorsalis pedis pulses.

[ ] **3.** Observe the client's gait while walking.

[ ] **4.** Compare the color in the client's nailbeds.

49. When the nurse reviews the pattern on an ECG monitor strip, which of the following characteristics are indicative of normal sinus rhythm? Select all that apply.

[ ] **1.** T wave precedes a QRS complex.

[ ] **2.** Heart rate is between 60 and 100 beats/minute.

[ ] **3.** The atrioventricular (AV) node initiates the impulse.

[ ] **4.** Each impulse occurs regularly.

[ ] **5.** Ventricles depolarize and contract.

[ ] **6.** Ventricular rate is slower than the atrial rate.

50. When a hospitalized client diagnosed with Graves' disease is scheduled to undergo a subtotal thyroidectomy, what is the best reason that the nurse omits palpating the thyroid gland?

[ ] **1.** The nurse's action can compress the trachea.

[ ] **2.** The nurse's action can damage the laryngeal nerve.

[ ] **3.** The nurse's action can cause extreme discomfort.

[ ] **4.** The nurse's action can cause thyroid storm.

51. Which statement made by an alcoholic client who takes disulfiram (Antabuse) is the best indication that the nurse should provide further health teaching?

[ ] **1.** "If I miss one dose of the drug, I'll experience nausea, vomiting, and fainting."

[ ] **2.** "I can get very sick if I consume alcohol in any form while taking this drug."

[ ] **3.** "I can have a reaction even 2 weeks after I stop taking this drug."

[ ] **4.** "I shouldn't apply aftershave lotion or cologne to my skin while taking this drug."

52. In preparation for a client's discharge, the nurse discontinues an I.V. line. Which nursing action is essential at this time?

[ ] **1.** Applying pressure to the insertion site for 5 minutes

[ ] **2.** Putting on clean gloves before removing the I.V. line

[ ] **3.** Checking the client's blood glucose level after removal

[ ] **4.** Reporting the amount of blood loss to the physician

53. A few days before having a malignant growth removed from the colon, the client says to the nurse, "I'm scared that I'll have to have a colostomy. What if the surgeon can't get all of the cancer?" Which nursing response is most therapeutic?

[ ] **1.** "There is no need to worry or be afraid. Trust me."

[ ] **2.** "Tell me more specifically about your concerns."

[ ] **3.** "You know as well as I that you have an excellent surgeon."

[ ] **4.** "Try to relax. Worrying will only make matters worse."

54. While assisting a physician, during which component of a physical examination should the nurse provide the physician with a topical anesthetic agent?
[ ] **1.** When testing deep tendon reflexes
[ ] **2.** When removing vaginal secretions
[ ] **3.** When measuring intraocular pressure
[ ] **4.** When examining the tympanic membranes

55. If a client with type 1 (insulin-dependent) diabetes mellitus receives 5 units of NPH insulin every morning at 7 A.M., the nurse should closely monitor the client for signs of hypoglycemia at what time?
[ ] **1.** 3:00 P.M.
[ ] **2.** 12:00 A.M.
[ ] **3.** 7:30 A.M.
[ ] **4.** 10:00 P.M.

56. When a nurse cares for a client with a nasogastric tube immediately after gastric surgery, which of the following is essential to report to the charge nurse or physician?
[ ] **1.** The client reports having a sore throat.
[ ] **2.** The client rates pain at a 5 on the 0 to 10 pain scale.
[ ] **3.** The client reports feeling nauseated.
[ ] **4.** The client has bright red drainage in the tube.

57. The nurse caring for a middle-aged adult would expect which characteristic behavior indicating the developmental task of generativity?
[ ] **1.** The client expresses fear of having further serious illnesses.
[ ] **2.** The client wishes to know the purpose of the medications.
[ ] **3.** The client wants to write a personal memoir of childhood.
[ ] **4.** The client desires to learn more about using a computer.

58. Which culturally sensitive nursing technique is best for determining whether a male Jewish client follows religious orthodox customs?
[ ] **1.** Ask if the client speaks the Hebrew language.
[ ] **2.** Inquire about the client's dietary preferences.
[ ] **3.** Question whether the client wears a yarmulke.
[ ] **4.** Assess whether the client has been circumcised.

59. Which nursing action is most appropriate when a chest tube is inadvertently pulled from its insertion site?
[ ] **1.** Quickly covering the opening to keep out air
[ ] **2.** Reinserting the displaced chest tube
[ ] **3.** Checking the client's breath sounds
[ ] **4.** Telling the client to hold his or her breath

60. When developing the care plan of a client who has a nasogastric (NG) tube for gastric decompression, which nursing order should be revised?
[ ] **1.** Encourage liberal oral fluid intake every hour.
[ ] **2.** Use normal saline when irrigating the NG tube.
[ ] **3.** Offer throat lozenges every 4 hours, as needed, for discomfort.
[ ] **4.** Provide oral hygiene every 4 hours during the day and as needed.

61. If the nurse is giving an enema to an adult client, how far should the enema tip be inserted into the anal canal?
[ ] **1.** 1″ to 2″ (2.5 to 5 cm)
[ ] **2.** 3″ to 4″ (7.5 to 10 cm)
[ ] **3.** 5″ to 8″ (15 to 20 cm)
[ ] **4.** 9″ to 10″ (22.5 to 25 cm)

62. Which technique should the nurse plan to use when giving perineal care to an uncircumcised male client?
[ ] **1.** Use a separate wash cloth to clean the anal area.
[ ] **2.** Retract the foreskin; then wash the glans penis.
[ ] **3.** Wash the scrotum prior to washing the penis.
[ ] **4.** Clean the penis with normal saline solution.

63. An adult comes to the clinic with recurring back pain. Which information is most important for the nurse to obtain before developing a teaching plan?
[ ] **1.** The client's age
[ ] **2.** The client's occupation
[ ] **3.** The client's gait
[ ] **4.** The client's medications

64. Which advice is most appropriate for the nurse to give to a person whose friend has been raped?
[ ] **1.** Always act happy and enthusiastic around the victim.
[ ] **2.** Prevent the victim from avoiding people.
[ ] **3.** Encourage the victim to talk about the traumatic experience.
[ ] **4.** Suggest frequent vacations or pleasurable activities.

65. A client from the Far East is visiting in the United States and becomes ill, requiring hospitalization. The nurse observes the client's spouse placing a knife beneath the client's pillow to "cut" the pain. Neither the client nor the spouse speaks English. Which nursing action is most appropriate at this time?
[ ] **1.** Explain through a translator that analgesic drugs will be administered to control pain.
[ ] **2.** Explain through a translator that sharp objects pose a safety hazard to the client and others.
[ ] **3.** Explain through a translator that a form must be signed relieving the agency of responsibility.
[ ] **4.** Explain through a translator that the staff will leave the knife in place as long as desired.

66. Which nursing assessment finding provides the best indication that a client with nephrotic syndrome (acute glomerulonephritis) has experienced a therapeutic effect from corticosteroid therapy?
[ ] 1. Increase in body weight
[ ] 2. Increase in muscle mass
[ ] 3. Increase in urine output
[ ] 4. Increase in blood pressure

67. During the night, a client is startled and continues to worry about an alarm that sounded from the electronic I.V. infusion pump. Which nursing intervention is most appropriate to relieve the client's anxiety at this time?
[ ] 1. Infuse the solution by gravity.
[ ] 2. Explain why the alarm sounded.
[ ] 3. Give a prescribed tranquilizer.
[ ] 4. Stay until the client's sleep is restored.

68. An adolescent single parent tells the nurse about being frustrated because of sleeplessness since the baby was born 3 months ago. Which nursing response is most appropriate?
[ ] 1. Explain that this is normal, and suggest asking a family member or friend for occasional relief.
[ ] 2. Explain that parenting is a big responsibility and suggest that the client reconsider adoption.
[ ] 3. Explain that frustration usually precedes abusive behavior and must be reported.
[ ] 4. Explain that sleeplessness is temporary, and encourage the client to be patient until the situation improves.

69. A home health nurse visits a postpartum client with a breast abscess. The client has purulent drainage from one breast and is receiving antibiotic therapy. Which information is most appropriate for the nurse to give the client to help prevent the spread of the infectious microorganisms elsewhere?
[ ] 1. "Take your antibiotics until the drainage is gone."
[ ] 2. "Keep your breasts supported in a tight bra."
[ ] 3. "Shower daily and wash your hands frequently."
[ ] 4. "Apply warm compresses at least four times a day."

70. A postoperative client asks the nurse why performing leg exercises is important. The best explanation is that leg movement that involves contracting and relaxing leg muscles helps to prevent which condition?
[ ] 1. Loss of muscle strength
[ ] 2. Formation of blood clots
[ ] 3. Swelling of the extremities
[ ] 4. Development of varicose veins

71. If a child with asthma receives aminophylline (Truphylline) by I.V. infusion, which side effect is the nurse most likely to observe?
[ ] 1. Bradycardia
[ ] 2. Drowsiness
[ ] 3. Restlessness
[ ] 4. Hypotension

72. A resident of a long-term care facility is depressed. As the nurse explores probable reasons for the client's depression, which of the following are most likely to be the causative factors? Select all that apply.
[ ] 1. History of previous depression
[ ] 2. Overstimulation
[ ] 3. Loss of independence
[ ] 4. Chronic illnesses
[ ] 5. Reminders of death and dying
[ ] 6. Food and drug interactions

73. Which prescribed antibiotic should the nurse question before administering it to a child younger than age 8?
[ ] 1. Cefazolin (Kefzol)
[ ] 2. Amoxicillin (Amoxil)
[ ] 3. Tetracycline hydrochloride (Tetracyn)
[ ] 4. Gentamicin (Garamycin)

74. Which response is most appropriate when an older client with Alzheimer's disease in a long-term care facility says, "I must leave so I can be home when my children return from school?"
[ ] 1. "Nonsense! Your children are adults with their own children."
[ ] 2. "I'm sure a neighbor will take care of them for a while."
[ ] 3. "I'll call the school and tell them to expect you later."
[ ] 4. "You're in a nursing home. I'm your nurse."

75. A nurse conducts a "Healthy Heart" class for community leaders and informs them that they should chew an aspirin if they feel they are having chest pain. What is the best rationale for this instruction?
[ ] 1. Aspirin is administered for its analgesic action.
[ ] 2. Aspirin is administered for its antipyretic action.
[ ] 3. Aspirin is administered for its antiinflammatory action.
[ ] 4. Aspirin is administered for its antiplatelet action.

76. What is the best location for the nurse to assess for a pulse when performing cardiopulmonary resuscitation on an infant?
[ ] 1. Over the radial artery
[ ] 2. Over the femoral artery
[ ] 3. Over the brachial artery
[ ] 4. Over the carotid artery

77. If the nurse finds a client who has fallen out of the hospital bed, which nursing action is best to perform initially?
[ ] 1. Reporting the accident to the client's family
[ ] 2. Helping the person back to bed or a chair
[ ] 3. Placing an alarm device on the bed.
[ ] 4. Checking the client's physical condition

78. Following the delivery of an infant, what is the best indication to the nurse that a healthy parental-newborn attachment is developing?
[ ] 1. The parents observe the care of the newborn.
[ ] 2. The parents are happy with the newborn's gender.
[ ] 3. The parents watch and listen to the newborn.
[ ] 4. The parents touch and talk to the newborn.

79. In which client would a nurse expect bleeding between menstrual periods an indication of a serious problem that requires further evaluation?
[ ] **1.** A client taking oral contraceptives
[ ] **2.** A client on hormone replacement therapy
[ ] **3.** A client who is perimenopausal
[ ] **4.** An adolescent who recently began menstruating

80. The nursing team in a long-term care facility evaluates the effectiveness of interventions used to improve a confused client's orientation. Which client action provides the best evidence of progress in accomplishing the goal?
[ ] **1.** The client walks with others to the dining room.
[ ] **2.** The client dresses without difficulty.
[ ] **3.** The client locates the bathroom without assistance.
[ ] **4.** The client talks to family on the telephone.

81. Which nursing instruction is correct when teaching a client with asthma how to use a dry powder inhaler?
[ ] **1.** "Inhale the medication slowly over 10 seconds."
[ ] **2.** "Hold your breath for 10 seconds before exhaling."
[ ] **3.** "Swallow any oral drug residue quickly."
[ ] **4.** "Cough immediately after inhaling the dry powder."

82. Which nursing assessment finding is the best indication that a 2-year-old has symptoms related to otitis media?
[ ] **1.** The child has a runny nose.
[ ] **2.** The child is irritable.
[ ] **3.** The child swallows frequently.
[ ] **4.** The child tugs at an ear.

83. If all of the following drugs are prescribed on an "as needed" (prn) basis, which one is most appropriate for the nurse to administer to a client with Ménière's disease during an acute attack?
[ ] **1.** Acetaminophen (Tylenol)
[ ] **2.** Meclizine (Antivert)
[ ] **3.** Meperidine (Demerol)
[ ] **4.** Triazolam (Halcion)

84. After a thyroidectomy, for which electrolyte imbalance is it most appropriate for the nurse to monitor to detect?
[ ] **1.** Hypokalemia
[ ] **2.** Hyponatremia
[ ] **3.** Hypomagnesemia
[ ] **4.** Hypocalcemia

85. Which nursing action is best for preventing skin breakdown when a client with jaundice complains of severe itching?
[ ] **1.** Bathing the client with very warm water
[ ] **2.** Dusting the client's body with cornstarch
[ ] **3.** Trimming the client's fingernails
[ ] **4.** Using hypoallergenic bed linens

86. A new client has arrived at the gynecologist's office for an annual examination and Papanicolaou test. Before the physical examination, the nurse is conducting a reproductive and sexual assessment. Place the nursing actions in the order they would be completed by the nurse, beginning with the first action and ending with the last. Use all the options.

1. Ask the client to use the bathroom to urinate.	
2. Introduce yourself and explain the sequence of events.	
3. Help the client into the stirrups for the physical examination.	
4. Focus on general questions related to sexual health and reproduction.	
5. Have the client change into a hospital gown and offer a sheet to cover her lap.	
6. Take vital signs and obtain information about the client's last menstrual period.	

87. A client with hyperparathyroidism is prone to hypercalcemia. Which nursing interventions are most appropriate to include in this client's care plan? Select all that apply.
[ ] **1.** Monitor the client's cardiac rhythm.
[ ] **2.** Provide a high fluid intake.
[ ] **3.** Observe for signs of muscle spasms.
[ ] **4.** Take hourly vital signs.
[ ] **5.** Assess the client for low blood sugar.
[ ] **6.** Evaluate the client's joints for dysfunction.

88. Which nursing assessment findings best suggest that a client has an abdominal aortic aneurysm? Select all that apply.
[ ] **1.** A pulsating mass felt when palpating the client's abdomen
[ ] **2.** An extra heart sound heard during chest auscultation
[ ] **3.** Uneven chest movements noted when observing respirations
[ ] **4.** A hollow sound heard when percussing the abdomen
[ ] **5.** A report of lower back pain by the client
[ ] **6.** A finding of cool and cyanotic extremities

89. If a known substance abuser presents to the emergency department with tachycardia and chest pain, what is the most appropriate question for the nurse to ask?
[ ] **1.** "When did you last use heroin?"
[ ] **2.** "When did you last use cocaine?"
[ ] **3.** "When did you last use barbiturates?"
[ ] **4.** "When did you last use marijuana?"

90. From among the following options, which nursing assessment finding provides the best evidence that a client remains adequately oxygenated while a tracheostomy is suctioned?
[ ] **1.** The heart rate stays within 88 to 92 beats/minute.
[ ] **2.** The client's pulse is bounding.
[ ] **3.** The client remains alert during suctioning.
[ ] **4.** The client's capillary refill remains stable at 5 seconds.

91. A friend shares with a nurse about being engaged to be married. The nurse knows that the friend's fiancé has tested positive for human immunodeficiency virus (HIV). What is the nurse legally obligated to do?
[ ] **1.** Inform the friend of the fiancé's HIV infectious status.
[ ] **2.** Recommend that the friend be tested for HIV antibodies.
[ ] **3.** Advise the friend to postpone the marriage indefinitely.
[ ] **4.** Safeguard information in the fiancé's health history.

92. During the first stage of a client's labor, the nurse finds that the fetal heart rate decreases during a contraction and returns to normal at the end of the contraction. Which nursing action is most appropriate in response to the assessment finding?
[ ] **1.** No action is indicated at this time.
[ ] **2.** Notify the physician immediately.
[ ] **3.** Place the client in a supine position.
[ ] **4.** Elevate the head of the client's bed.

93. Which comment made by a client who is taking aspirin is most likely related to an adverse effect of drug therapy?
[ ] **1.** "My thoughts are racing."
[ ] **2.** "I'm urinating a lot."
[ ] **3.** "I've developed diarrhea."
[ ] **4.** "I hear buzzing in my ears."

94. Which statement provides the best indication that a client understands the nurse's teaching about alprazolam (Xanax), a newly prescribed medication?
[ ] **1.** "I should not drink alcohol while taking this drug."
[ ] **2.** "I will need to continue taking this drug for life."
[ ] **3.** "I might have some insomnia."
[ ] **4.** "I will need a blood test periodically."

95. A 78-year-old client arrives at the hospital and is suspected of having pneumonia. Which laboratory tests should the nurse monitor that will confirm the initial diagnosis?
[ ] **1.** Complete blood count (CBC) and chest X-ray
[ ] **2.** Hemoglobin and hematocrit
[ ] **3.** Pulmonary function tests and lung biopsy
[ ] **4.** Electrolytes and lung computed tomography scan

96. The nurse instructs the parents of a toddler about caring for their child's plaster leg cast. Which instruction is most accurate regarding the drying of the child's cast?
[ ] **1.** Increase the temperature of the room.
[ ] **2.** Turn the child every 1 to 2 hours.
[ ] **3.** Fan the wet cast with folded newspaper.
[ ] **4.** Take the child outside in the sun during the day.

97. Which statement made by a primigravid client at 38 weeks' gestation the best indication to the nurse that lightening has occurred?
[ ] **1.** "I don't have to urinate as frequently now."
[ ] **2.** "My backaches are relieved."
[ ] **3.** "I can breathe so much easier now."
[ ] **4.** "I've noticed slight contractions lately."

98. The nurse assesses for a pulse on an elderly unresponsive client and finds it weak and thready. In the absence of breathing, which of the following provides the best evidence that rescue breathing by the nurse is being performed appropriately?
[ ] **1.** The chest rises when air is forced in.
[ ] **2.** The pupils of both eyes are dilated.
[ ] **3.** A carotid pulse is palpated at the neck.
[ ] **4.** The nurse forms a seal over the victim's nose.

99. After having a rectal tube in place for 20 minutes, a client's abdominal distention remains unrelieved. What is the most appropriate nursing action at this time?
[ ] **1.** Rotate the tube several times within the rectum.
[ ] **2.** Insert the rectal tube farther into the rectum.
[ ] **3.** Remove the tube, and reinsert it in 2 to 3 hours.
[ ] **4.** Replace the tube with one of larger diameter.

100. A client begins taking phenytoin (Dilantin) for seizures, and the nurse provides instructions regarding the medication and its side effects. Which nursing instruction is most accurate?
[ ] **1.** "Drink generous amounts of fluid."
[ ] **2.** "Weigh yourself daily."
[ ] **3.** "Gradually taper the dosage."
[ ] **4.** "Perform regular oral hygiene."

101. When the nurse performs cardiopulmonary resuscitation on a 6-month-old infant, which cardiac compression technique is correct?
[ ] **1.** The nurse interlocks fingers of both hands.
[ ] **2.** The nurse uses two fingers of one hand.
[ ] **3.** The nurse uses the heel of one hand.
[ ] **4.** The nurse uses the palm of one hand

102. The nurse teaches a client the signs and symptoms of a myocardial infarction (MI), what is the most correct explanation for the etiology of the chest pain?
[ ] **1.** Ischemia of the heart muscle
[ ] **2.** Damage to the coronary arteries
[ ] **3.** Impending circulatory collapse
[ ] **4.** Left ventricular muscle fatigue

103. A hospitalized client in heart failure receives furosemide (Lasix) twice per day. As the nurse monitors the client's laboratory test values, which one should be reported to the physician immediately?
[ ] **1.** Potassium: 3.0 mEq/L
[ ] **2.** Sodium: 137 mEq/L
[ ] **3.** Calcium: 9.1 mg/dL
[ ] **4.** Chloride: 102 mEq/L

104. When caring for the newborn of a mother who has heavily consumed alcohol throughout the pregnancy, which nursing assessment finding is most likely to be observed in the newborn?
[ ] **1.** Lethargy
[ ] **2.** Irritability
[ ] **3.** Flaccidity
[ ] **4.** Jaundice

105. The nurse administers a minor tranquilizer to an anxious client and evaluates its effectiveness 30 minutes later. Which nursing assessment technique provides the best indication of the drug's effectiveness?
[ ] **1.** Assessing the client's facial expressions
[ ] **2.** Asking the client to rate the anxiety from 0 to 10
[ ] **3.** Observing the length of time a client sleeps
[ ] **4.** Monitoring the client's interactions with others

106. A client is 1 day postoperative after a below-the-knee amputation. As the nurse changes the dressing for the first time, the client says, "I just can't look at it!" Which comment by the nurse is most appropriate at this time?
[ ] **1.** "Just look away until you feel ready."
[ ] **2.** "Maybe you should consider getting counseling."
[ ] **3.** "If it were me, I'd be curious to see how it looks."
[ ] **4.** "Come on! It doesn't look that bad."

107. For a client with a lower respiratory tract infection, when is the best time for the nurse to perform postural drainage?
[ ] **1.** When the client has an empty stomach
[ ] **2.** When the client is short of breath
[ ] **3.** When the client experiences coughing
[ ] **4.** When the respiratory therapist orders it

108. Which nursing assessment finding provides the earliest indication that a client is hypoxic?
[ ] **1.** The client is cyanotic.
[ ] **2.** The client is disoriented.
[ ] **3.** The client is restless.
[ ] **4.** The client is hypotensive.

109. A 75-year-old client has a perineal prostatectomy for cancer of the prostate. After surgery, which nursing action is essential to include in the client's care plan?
[ ] **1.** Instruct the client to perform Valsalva's maneuver during defecation.
[ ] **2.** Place the client in high Fowler's position immediately after surgery.
[ ] **3.** Administer laxatives to promote bowel elimination.
[ ] **4.** Provide perineal care after each bowel movement.

110. A nurse notices that a coworker has left the computer screen on while still logged into the system. The nurse leaves the screen as it is and tries to locate the coworker. A visitor is observed reading the computer screen. Who is responsible for this Health Insurance Portability and Accountability Act (HIPAA) violation? Select all that apply.
[ ] **1.** The nurse who found the screen
[ ] **2.** The nurse's coworker who left the screen
[ ] **3.** The visitor who was reading the screen
[ ] **4.** The institution where the coworker works
[ ] **5.** The client's primary care physician
[ ] **6.** The manager of the department

111. A client diagnosed with a GI bleed has received an order for a blood transfusion. Place the nursing actions in the order in which they are performed, beginning with the first and ending with the last action. Use all options.

1. Monitor vital signs at 15-minute to hourly intervals during the infusion.	
2. Assist the registered nurse (RN) in gathering supplies to start an I.V. line using an 18-gauge needle.	
3. Identify the client with a licensed coworker at the bedside.	
4. Assist the registered nurse (RN) in obtaining informed consent for the blood transfusion.	
5. Assist the registered nurse (RN) in infusing the blood within 4 hours.	
6. Dispose of the blood bag and tubing in a biohazard container.	

112. When the nurse obtains the health history of a client diagnosed with an inguinal hernia, what information is most likely a contributing factor for the problem?
[ ] **1.** The client had an umbilical hernia as a child.
[ ] **2.** The client does not get much physical activity.
[ ] **3.** The client lifts heavy mailbags as a postal worker.
[ ] **4.** The client has been underweight most of his or her adult life.

113. The physician orders an immune assay enzyme test to confirm a diagnosis of acute bronchiolitis secondary to respiratory syncytial virus (RSV) infection for a 12-month-old child. Which type of specimen is most appropriate for the nurse to collect?
[ ] **1.** Throat swab
[ ] **2.** Nasal secretions
[ ] **3.** Sputum specimen
[ ] **4.** Blood specimen

114. An obstetric nurse is discharging a mother and newborn. While escorting the family to the car, which of the following nursing observations demonstrate correct car seat placement? Select all that apply.
[ ] **1.** The car seat is facing the rear in the passenger's front seat.
[ ] **2.** The base of the seat is tethered to a hook on the floor.
[ ] **3.** A parent is seated beside the car seat.
[ ] **4.** The car seat is facing forward in the back seat.
[ ] **5.** The car seat is placed between the parents in the front seat.
[ ] **6.** The car seat is facing the rear in the back seat.

115. The nurse finds a client with diabetes weak, perspiring, and shaking. If all of the following assessment findings are present after the nurse gives the client three 15 g glucose tablets, which one provides the best indication that the nurse has managed the client's symptoms successfully?
[ ] **1.** The client feels much better.
[ ] **2.** The client's skin is warm.
[ ] **3.** The client's blood glucose level is 80 mg/dL.
[ ] **4.** The client's blood pressure is 122/78.

116. When obtaining the health history of a female with thrombophlebitis, the nurse should ask if the client routinely takes which medication?
[ ] **1.** Iron supplement
[ ] **2.** Oral contraceptive
[ ] **3.** Nasal decongestant
[ ] **4.** Stomach antacid

117. After the physician's explanation of the risks and benefits of a transurethral resection of the prostate (TURP), which statement offers the best indication to the nurse that the client understands the effect this surgery will have on sexual function?
[ ] **1.** "I won't ejaculate normally anymore."
[ ] **2.** "I won't have orgasms anymore."
[ ] **3.** "I won't have erections anymore."
[ ] **4.** "I won't desire to have sex anymore."

118. If a postoperative client received an overdose of heparin, which antidote can the nurse anticipate the physician will order?
[ ] **1.** Protamine sulfate
[ ] **2.** Naloxone hydrochloride (Narcan)
[ ] **3.** Vitamin K
[ ] **4.** Calcium gluconate

119. A non–English-speaking Hispanic client is admitted to the hospital to rule out myocardial infarction. What information should the nurse obtain when performing a cultural assessment? Select all that apply.
[ ] **1.** The client's food preferences
[ ] **2.** When the client's last bowel movement occurred
[ ] **3.** The client's primary language
[ ] **4.** Whether the client can tell time
[ ] **5.** The client's religion
[ ] **6.** Whether the client is in pain

120. When a nurse is unable to log on to the computer to document care for a client, what action by the nurse is most appropriate in this circumstance?
[ ] **1.** Forego documentation because access has been denied.
[ ] **2.** Ask for a coworker's ID and password to complete documentation.
[ ] **3.** Call technical support, notifying them of the situation.
[ ] **4.** Find an unattended computer that is on to complete documentation.

121. Which nursing intervention is most appropriate for meeting the needs of an infant with congenital heart disease?
[ ] **1.** Respond quickly to the infant's crying.
[ ] **2.** Place the infant in the prone position.
[ ] **3.** Avoid holding and cuddling the infant.
[ ] **4.** Use a firm, small-hole nipple for feedings.

122. When instructing a postoperative client about the use of enoxaparin (Lovenox), which statement should the nurse include about the drug's therapeutic action?
[ ] **1.** "It promotes wound-tissue healing."
[ ] **2.** "It breaks up clots that have formed."
[ ] **3.** "It decreases postoperative bleeding."
[ ] **4.** "It reduces formation of blood clots."

123. The physician orders enoxaparin (Lovenox). To prevent bruising, which actions by the nurse are most appropriate when administering the drug that is supplied in a prefilled syringe? Select all that apply.
[ ] **1.** Instruct the client to avoid rubbing the injection site for 1 hour.
[ ] **2.** Waste extra medication by holding the syringe and needle pointed toward the floor.
[ ] **3.** Expel the air bubble before giving the medication.
[ ] **4.** Flick the drop of medication off the tip of the needle before injecting.
[ ] **5.** Inject the medication using a 10-degree angle into the client's thigh.
[ ] **6.** Apply firm direct pressure to the site afterwards for 5 minutes.

124. When a child is referred to the school nurse for frequent brief staring episodes accompanied by unresponsiveness, which type of seizure disorder can the nurse most likely expect that the child is experiencing?
[ ] **1.** Myoclonic
[ ] **2.** Absence
[ ] **3.** Partial
[ ] **4.** Clonic

125. After attending an inservice program on the Emergency Medical Treatment and Active Labor Act (EMTALA), a nurse is correct in identifying that the law applies to which of the following clients? Select all that apply.
[ ] **1.** A client who is brought to the hospital after a suicide attempt
[ ] **2.** A client who has been physically abused by a spouse
[ ] **3.** A client who is shot by police while holding a hostage
[ ] **4.** A client who is in preterm labor about to deliver
[ ] **5.** A client who is transferred from the hospital back to the nursing home
[ ] **6.** A client who has no insurance and is unable to pay for treatment

126. Which action by the nurse will best prevent a newborn from experiencing heat loss secondary to evaporation?
[ ] **1.** Wrapping the infant in warmed blankets
[ ] **2.** Thoroughly drying the child after bathing
[ ] **3.** Positioning the crib away from outside windows
[ ] **4.** Positioning the crib away from air conditioning vents in the nursery

127. When caring for a 30-year-old pregnant client who has been diagnosed with gestational diabetes, which statement is the best indication to the nurse that the client understands the disorder?
[ ] **1.** "The disorder was present during my childhood."
[ ] **2.** "The disorder is controlled with oral hypoglycemics."
[ ] **3.** "The disorder will probably go away after I deliver."
[ ] **4.** "The disorder may cause me to have a small baby."

128. Which assessment finding would the nurse expect in a 7-month-old infant admitted to the hospital with a tentative diagnosis of bacterial meningitis?
[ ] **1.** Decreased white blood cell count
[ ] **2.** Bulging fontanel
[ ] **3.** Low-pitched cry
[ ] **4.** Increased glucose in cerebrospinal fluid

129. During a conference on seizure disorders at a parent-teacher association (PTA) meeting, the school nurse is correct in identifying which condition as the most common etiological risk factor?
[ ] **1.** Head trauma that results in long-term brain changes
[ ] **2.** Illegal drug use that results in unconsciousness
[ ] **3.** A sequela of a neurological disorder like meningitis.
[ ] **4.** Recent spinal cord damage from a sports accident

130. While assisting with a health screening clinic at a local preschool, the nurse would expect to observe which developmental characteristic among the 6-year-old participants?
[ ] **1.** The children are usually very reserved.
[ ] **2.** The children tend to enjoy pretend play.
[ ] **3.** The children tend to show little or no reaction to criticism.
[ ] **4.** The children almost always finish tasks they have started.

Correct Answers, Rationales, and Test Taking Strategies

1. **3, 5, 6.** Typical signs that a tracheostomy needs suctioning include noisy respirations, dyspnea, and increased respiratory and pulse rates. The pulse oximeter measures the oxygenation in the tissues. Because the airway (and therefore oxygenation) is affected, the client's pulse oximeter readings will be decreased. Auscultation of the chest helps most to determine when to suction a tracheostomy.

> *Test Taking Strategy—Analyze to determine what information the question asks for, which is assessment findings that indicate a need to suction a tracheostomy tube. Alternative-format "select all that apply" questions require considering each option independently to decide its merit in answering the question. Review the indications for suctioning, which include signs of hypoxia and adventitious lung sounds, if you had difficulty answering this question.*
> *Cognitive Level—Analyzing*
> *Client Needs Category—Physiological integrity*
> *Client Needs Subcategory—Physiological adaptation*

2. **3.** Before suctioning, the nurse gives the client oxygen to prevent hypoxemia and hypoxia while removing air and debris from the upper airway. After inserting the catheter, the nurse positions the tip at the desired level, usually 6″ to 10″ (15 to 25 cm), occludes the vent, and twists the catheter to remove it. Afterward, the client is reoxygenated a second time. Usually, cleaning the tracheostomy stoma is done last after the sterile procedure is completed, following the general principal of "clean to dirty." Instilling saline into a tracheostomy tube is no longer recommended.

> *Test Taking Strategy—Look for the key word "first," indicating a priority. Recall that airway and breathing as well as Maslow's hierarchy of needs call for meeting physiological needs before all others. Preserving adequate oxygenation is the most important nursing action. Review the procedure for suctioning natural and artificial airways if you had difficulty answering this question.*
> *Cognitive Level—Analyzing*
> *Client Needs Category—Physiological integrity*
> *Client Needs Subcategory—Reduction of risk potential*

3. **1, 2, 3.** It is appropriate to use clean gloves to remove a soiled dressing, to place the soiled dressing in a container that acts as a barrier against transmitting microorganisms that may be present, and to perform hand washing before donning sterile gloves. The most appropriate aseptic technique for cleaning wounds is to work in such a way that debris and microorganisms are carried away from the impaired skin. Therefore, wounds should always be cleaned starting at the wound itself and working outward. Reaching across the sterile field and touching the soiled dressing with sterile gloves will compromise sterility.

> *Test Taking Strategy—Analyze to determine what information the question asks for, which is the correct steps to take to ensure aseptic wound care. Alternative-format "select all that apply" questions require considering each option independently to decide its merit in answering the question. Choose those actions that support the principles of medical and surgical asepsis thereby controlling the transfer of pathogens to the nurse, other agency personnel, and the client. Review principles of asepsis if you had difficulty answering this question.*
> *Cognitive Level—Analyzing*
> *Client Needs Category—Safe and effective care environment*
> *Client Needs Subcategory—Safety and infection control*

4. **1.** A hearing aid amplifies sound waves transmitted by air and bone conduction. Hearing aids do not improve the quality of the sounds by making them crisper, sharper, or less garbled.

> *Test Taking Strategy—Use the process of elimination to select an option that describes an accurate response to the client as it relates to the use of a hearing aid. Recall that most hearing aids worn by clients with a conductive hearing loss do not filter sounds; they only increase the volume of sounds to the wearer. Options 2, 3, and 4 are inaccurate statements, Review the use of hearing aids if you had difficulty answering this question.*
> *Cognitive Level—Analyzing*
> *Client Needs Category—Physiological integrity*
> *Client Needs Subcategory—Basic care and comfort*

5. **2.** Food and fluids are withheld temporarily after a bronchoscopy until the gag reflex returns. If the gag reflex is absent, aspiration may occur. Taking vital signs, the pulse oximeter reading, and tympanic temperature are appropriate measures that provide a baseline for further care. Raising the head of the bed is a safe action.

> *Test Taking Strategy—Analyze to determine what information the question asks for, which is an action that could be unsafe in a client who has just undergone a bronchoscopy. Providing oral fluids (option 2) to a client who may be unable to clear his or her airway is an unsafe action. Review implications for care in relation to a client who has had topical anesthesia in the airway if you had difficulty answering this question.*
> *Cognitive Level—Analyzing*
> *Client Needs Category—Safe and effective care environment*
> *Client Needs Subcategory—Coordinated care*

6. **2.** It is therapeutic to allow an angry person to express feelings within social limits. By remaining neutral, the nurse demonstrates acceptance of the client as an individual and acts as a role model in helping the client regain control. Using humor, leaving the client, or providing an explanation may add to the angry feelings; the client may interpret these actions to mean that the circumstances leading to anger are unimportant.

> *Test Taking Strategy—Use the process of elimination to select an option that identifies a therapeutic response involving an angry client. Option 1 can be immediately eliminated because it is nontherapeutic to be frivolous when confronted by a client's anger. Option 3 can be eliminated because deserting a client who is angry is not therapeutic. Option 4 may have merit, but it is not likely to decrease the client's anger. Option 2 then emerges as a therapeutic response because it allows the client to express himself or herself. Review therapeutic approaches when dealing with a client who is angry if you had difficulty answering this question.*
> *Cognitive Level—Analyzing*
> *Client Needs Category—Psychosocial integrity*
> *Client Needs Subcategory—None*

7. **1, 6.** Retinal detachment occurs when the retina's rods and cones separate from the choroid layer. A detached retina is a serious problem, often seen in middle-aged and elderly clients, that requires immediate attention. Most clients with a retinal detachment describe seeing flashes of light or wavy or watery vision. Only the most profoundly blind cannot see light. Photophobia, or feeling discomfort in light, is associated with many primary and secondary disorders; however, those with retinal detachment do not generally experience it. The client with a retinal detachment generally retains vision in a large portion of the retina. The visual defect is evident only in the area of the tear or separation of the sensory layer from the pigmented layer. Therefore, in the intact retina, vision during daylight is unchanged. Clients experiencing retinal tears and detachment usually have no eye pain.

> *Test Taking Strategy—Analyze to determine what information the question asks for, which is symptoms of retinal detachment. Alternative-format "select all that apply" questions require considering each option independently to decide its merit in answering the question. Select options that correlate with the symptoms experienced by a client experiencing a retinal detachment. Review the signs and symptoms of retinal detachment if you had difficulty answering this question.*
> *Cognitive Level—Analyzing*
> *Client Needs Category—Physiological integrity*
> *Client Needs Subcategory—Physiological adaptation*

8. **2.** Giving an infant medication using a needleless syringe or dropper helps reduce the incidence of choking, coughing, and vomiting. The medication should be placed between the cheek and gum and administered slowly as the infant swallows. Calibrated nipples may also be used to administer medication to infants. Medications are not routinely given in an infant's bottle because the infant may not finish the bottle and may not get the prescribed amount of medication. Pinching a child's nose is not recommended because this action increases the chance of aspiration. Solid (not liquid) forms of medication may be crushed and mixed with jelly, cereal, pudding, or applesauce. However, solid foods should not be given to infants younger than age 4 or 5 months old because they still possess the extrusion reflex; the food will be spat out and not swallowed.

> *Test Taking Strategy—Use the process of elimination to select the option that accurately describes how to administer medication to an infant. Option 1 can be eliminated because it does not ensure that the infant will receive the full amount of the drug unless the entire contents of the formula are consumed. Eliminate options 3 and 4 because they are potentially unsafe. Option 2 emerges as the correct choice. Review techniques for administering liquid medication to an infant if you had difficulty answering this question.*
> *Cognitive Level—Applying*
> *Client Needs Category—Physiological integrity*
> *Client Needs Subcategory—Pharmacological therapies*

9. **3.** When a child is in Bryant's traction, the buttocks just clear the mattress. The ropes that lead to pulleys above the bed keep the child's legs at a 90-degree angle to the trunk. The child should not sit up or use a trapeze. The legs are pulled toward the ceiling.

> *Test Taking Strategy—Use the process of elimination to select an option that describes the best indication that Bryant's traction is functioning appropriately. Option 1 can be eliminated because the client is lying supine with the legs elevated and, therefore, should not sit up. Option 2 can be eliminated because the client has no need to use a trapeze. Option 4 can be eliminated because it describes an undesirable position for a client in this type of traction. Review how Bryant's traction is applied if you had difficulty answering this question.*
> *Cognitive Level—Applying*
> *Client Needs Category—Physiological integrity*
> *Client Needs Subcategory—Basic care and comfort*

10. **3.** Red blood cells are formed in the bone marrow found in long bones and in the sternum. In sickle cell anemia, a genetic disorder affecting the hemoglobin on red blood cells causes them to appear like a sickle or crescent instead of being round. Consequently, the malformed red blood cells cannot move easily through blood vessels. During sickle cell crisis, the red blood cells clump together and obstruct the arteries, causing the client severe pain, especially in the chest, joints, and abdomen. Consequently, the priority nursing goal is to relieve the client's discomfort and pain. Analgesics are routinely administered and adjusted according to the client's response. Activity is usually limited during sickle cell crisis to prevent hypoxia. Antibiotics are not administered for clients with this disorder. Fluids are necessary to prevent dehydration, which can exacerbate the problem.

> *Test Taking Strategy*—*Look for the key words "main priority" in relation to the care of a client in sickle cell crisis. Recall that a client in sickle cell crisis experiences severe joint pain. Relieving pain therefore has the highest priority. Review the signs and symptoms of a client experiencing sickle cell crisis if you had difficulty answering this question.*
> *Cognitive Level*—*Applying*
> *Client Needs Category*—*Physiological integrity*
> *Client Needs Subcategory*—*Physiological adaptation*

11. 4. To avoid additional injury to radiated skin, the client is instructed to use gentle washing with warm water and a soft cloth. Water will not harm the skin, but harsh soaps, lotions, alcohol-based cosmetics, and rubbing the skin should be avoided. It is the client's choice which type of cleanser to use. Regardless of whether the client chooses body wash or bar soap, it should be mild and nonabrasive to avoid injury to the skin. Covering the reddened area with clear plastic will not serve any therapeutic purpose, and the tape used to hold the plastic may cause further skin breakdown.

> *Test Taking Strategy*—*Use the process of elimination to select an option that accurately describes instructions for bathing when a client is receiving external radiation therapy. Options 1, 2, and 3 can be eliminated because they are inaccurate instructions. Review nursing care of the skin as it relates to radiation therapy if you had difficulty answering this question.*
> *Cognitive Level*—*Applying*
> *Client Needs Category*—*Physiological integrity*
> *Client Needs Subcategory*—*Basic care and comfort*

12. 3. A clear liquid diet is generally offered initially after surgery. This diet moistens the mouth, provides fluid and some energy-supplying calories, and stimulates peristalsis. It is also the least likely diet to contribute to nausea or vomiting. If tolerated well, the client can progress to a full liquid, soft, or regular diet.

> *Test Taking Strategy*—*Analyze to determine what information the question asks for, which is a diet that is safe initially for a client in the early stage of recovering from anesthesia. Because nausea and vomiting can be precipitated in the presence of solid food in the diet, option 3 is the best answer. Review types of diets and their indications if you had difficulty answering this question.*
> *Cognitive Level*—*Analyzing*
> *Client Needs Category*—*Physiological integrity*
> *Client Needs Subcategory*—*Basic care and comfort*

13. 4. Any pregnant client in the third trimester with a persistent, severe headache needs to be promptly examined by a physician. A persistent headache may be insignificant, but it is also a sign of pregnancy-induced hypertension (PIH), formerly known as *toxemia* or *eclampsia*. The other suggestions may be appropriate after the client has been medically assessed.

> *Test Taking Strategy*—*Use the process of elimination to identify the best action to take in response to a client who may be developing PIH. Options 1, 2, and 3 can be eliminated because they overlook the seriousness of the situation. Review the signs and symptoms of PIH if you had difficulty answering this question.*
> *Cognitive Level*—*Analyzing*
> *Client Needs Category*—*Physiological integrity*
> *Client Needs Subcategory*—*Reduction of risk potential*

14. 4. Acquired immunodeficiency syndrome (AIDS) is suspected when individuals succumb to opportunistic infections such as *Pneumocystis carinii* pneumonia. Because sexual transmission is the most common mode of acquiring human immunodeficiency virus (HIV), assessing a client's sexual practices is important. If the client does not report any high-risk sexual practices, the nurse may assess the possibility of I.V. drug use or a history of having received blood or blood products. A client's immunization history, family history, and smoking practices are not likely to provide etiologic information about this opportunistic infection.

> *Test Taking Strategy*—*Use the process of elimination to identify an option that describes a risk factor associated with the acquisition of AIDS. Options 1, 2, and 3 can be eliminated because they are inconsequential to acquiring AIDS. Option 4 emerges as the correct answer. Review the risk factors associated with contracting AIDS if you had difficulty answering this question.*
> *Cognitive Level*—*Applying*
> *Client Needs Category*—*Health promotion and maintenance*
> *Client Needs Subcategory*—*None*

15. 1. Cystic fibrosis is a hereditary disease that affects the mucus glands of the lungs, liver, pancreas, and intestines. It is usually diagnosed in early childhood. Thick mucus production, as well as an immunocompromised condition, results in frequent lung infections. Diminished secretion of pancreatic enzymes causes poor growth, fatty diarrhea, and deficiency of fat-soluble vitamins. Parents of children with cystic fibrosis commonly report that the child's perspiration tastes very salty. This is attributed to the fact that children with cystic fibrosis lose large amounts of salt in their perspiration. Vomiting immediately after eating is not a usual sign of cystic fibrosis, but it is associated with pyloric stenosis. Soft, bright yellow stools are characteristic of a breast-fed infant. In cystic fibrosis, the stools are large, foamy, and foul-smelling. Tea-colored urine is a symptom of acute glomerulonephritis, a kidney disease, not cystic fibrosis.

Test Taking Strategy—*Use the process of elimination to select an option that best describes a finding that suggests a child has cystic fibrosis. Option 2 can be eliminated because it suggests a GI obstruction. Option 3 can be eliminated because it describes a potentially normal finding. Option 4 can be eliminated because it is more likely associated with a disorder involving some other organs, such as the liver, gallbladder, or kidneys. Review the signs and symptoms of cystic fibrosis if you had difficulty answering this question.*
Cognitive Level—*Applying*
Client Needs Category—*Physiological integrity*
Client Needs Subcategory—*Physiological adaptation*

16. 1. For the person who takes corticosteroids for a prolonged time, abruptly discontinuing the medication can cause life-threatening consequences. Acute adrenal insufficiency (also known as *addisonian crisis* or *adrenal crisis*) can occur, leading to possible death due to fluid volume depletion, hypotension, and shock. Taking a steroid medication does not interfere with a person's reaction time. A missed dose does not warrant consulting the physician. Although prolonged corticosteroid therapy causes many side effects, individuals may take the medication for long periods of time.
Test Taking Strategy—*Use the process of elimination to identify an accurate understanding about corticosteroid therapy. Option 2 can be eliminated because steroids do not cause sedation. Option 4 can be eliminated because safe steroid therapy may be required for longer than 6 months. Option 3 has some merit because it describes an interruption in the schedule of medication administration, but it is not as significant as abruptly discontinuing self-administration (option 4). Review the implications of corticosteroid therapy if you had difficulty answering this question.*
Cognitive Level—*Applying*
Client Needs Category—*Physiological integrity*
Client Needs Subcategory—*Pharmacological therapies*

17. 3. Diabetes insipidus is characterized by excessive urine production and elimination as a result of alterations in antidiuretic hormone. The specific gravity, which measures the concentration of the urine, is an indication of the ratio of water to dissolved substances. In diabetes insipidus, the specific gravity is 1.002, little more than water. As the client improves, the specific gravity is expected to increase as less water is excreted in the urine.
Test Taking Strategy—*Look at the key words "most important," which suggests a priority. Although there are many reasons for monitoring urinary pH, urinary casts, and bilirubin, because diabetes insipidus results in excretion of large volumes of fluid, monitoring the specific gravity of urine provides an indication of the magnitude of the pathophysiology of diabetes insipidus or its response to treatment. Review the function of antidiuretic hormone and how it is affected by diabetes insipidus if you had difficulty answering this question.*

Cognitive Level—*Applying*
Client Needs Category—*Physiological integrity*
Client Needs Subcategory—*Reduction of risk potential*

18. 1. Weighing the client daily to weekly is an appropriate way of monitoring the effectiveness and compliance of a client who takes a diuretic at home. Other valuable assessments include measuring the client's blood pressure, listening to breath sounds, and inspecting the skin and lower extremities for signs of edema. Pulse rate, appetite, and reflexes are not affected by diuretics.
Test Taking Strategy—*Use the process of elimination to identify the best method for evaluating a therapeutic response to diuretic therapy. Options 3 and 4 may be eliminated because diuretics do not suppress the appetite nor do they diminish or increase reflexes. Although option 2 has some merit because it suggests palpation, the focus of the palpation would be to detect the presence and severity of peripheral edema. Option 1 emerges as the best answer. Review nursing assessments that are pertinent when caring for a client receiving a diuretic if you had difficulty answering this question.*
Cognitive Level—*Applying*
Client Needs Category—*Physiological integrity*
Client Needs Subcategory—*Pharmacological therapies*

19. 1. Nitroglycerin is a medication used to dilate coronary arteries. To apply topical nitroglycerin ointment, the nurse squeezes a ribbon of the drug onto calibrated application paper. The paper is then placed on the client's chest, back, or arms, but not directly over the heart area. Applying the ointment over the heart may interfere with the assessment of heart sounds or obtaining an apical pulse rate. The paper is covered with plastic wrap and taped to hold it in place. The drug should not be rubbed into the client's skin. The nurse must avoid coming into direct skin contact with the ointment while measuring or applying it; such contact can result in absorption of the medication into the nurse's skin, causing a severe headache. The nurse must follow the physician's orders regarding reapplication of the ointment. Usually, nitroglycerin ointment is left on longer than 4 hours.
Test Taking Strategy—*Use the process of elimination to identify the option that accurately describes the technique for applying nitroglycerin ointment. Option 2 can be eliminated because the drug is absorbed without being rubbed into the skin. Option 4 can be eliminated because the ointment is generally applied to the arms, upper chest, or back rather than over the heart. Option 3 has merit, but the frequency of application may vary among prescribers. Review the technique for applying nitroglycerin ointment if you had difficulty answering this question.*
Cognitive Level—*Remembering*
Client Needs Category—*Physiological integrity*
Client Needs Subcategory—*Pharmacological therapies*

20. 3. Rescue breathing is performed when the infant has a pulse but is not breathing. After sealing both the nose and mouth with the rescuer's mouth, the infant is given controlled, gentle breaths (described as puffs of air) from the rescuer. The volume is just enough to make the chest rise lasting 1 second and repeated every 3 seconds for 2 minutes and reassessing for a pulse every 2 minutes to determine if compressions are required.

> *Test Taking Strategy—Analyze to determine what information the question asks for, which is the manner in which rescue breathing is administered to an infant. Recall that the volume of air that is administered must be comparable to the infant's lung capacity and that it is unlikely that a rescuer could pinch an infant's nose when performing rescue breathing. The infant's chest should rise, but a rise of 2 inches is excessive. Review the technique for administering rescue breathing to an infant if you had difficulty answering this question.*

Cognitive Level—Remembering
Client Needs Category—Physiological integrity
Client Needs Subcategory—Physiological adaptation

21. 2, 5, 6. Maintaining and improving oxygenation is a priority goal when planning the nursing care of a client with an acute respiratory tract infection. Airway and breathing are always a priority for every client. The Joint Commission has established quality indicators regarding care of clients who are diagnosed with pneumonia. These quality indicators require that pneumonia clients be given antibiotics within 4 hours of admission and that blood cultures be obtained within 24 hours of admission, preferably before administration of the antibiotics. If blood cultures are not easily obtained before giving antibiotics, the antibiotics are still given. In some circumstances, such as when the client's airways contain moist secretions, it is important to promote rather than relieve coughing. Nourishment is important in the care of any client with an infection, but impaired breathing is more life-threatening than a brief reduction in caloric intake. Eventually, the client can begin assuming self-care; however, during the acute phase of illness, the nurse should promote rest and offer assistance to reduce the client's oxygen requirements.

> *Test Taking Strategy—Analyze to determine what information the question asks for, which is the priority actions to take in the case of a client with pneumonia. Alternative-format "select all that apply" questions require considering each option independently to decide its merit in answering the question. Review the nursing activities for managing a client with pneumonia if you had difficulty answering this question.*

Cognitive Level—Analyzing
Client Needs Category—Safe and effective care environment
Client Needs Subcategory—Coordinated care

22. 2. A client with a subtotal thyroidectomy has a neck incision. Therefore, elevating the head, as in semi-Fowler's position, tends to relieve edema and decrease the potential for airway obstruction. Controlling edema will help the client talk and feel more comfortable; however, these are secondary benefits.

> *Test Taking Strategy—Use the process of elimination to select the option that describes the position that is best for a client who has had a subtotal thyroidectomy. Recall that a horizontal neck incision is used to remove the thyroid gland. The location of the incision has the potential for compromising ventilation. Elevating the head facilitates breathing and reduces swelling and related pain at the incision site leading to option 2. A supine, lateral, and Sim's positions, therefore, can be eliminated. Review the nursing management of a client who has undergone a thyroidectomy in relation to preventing or minimizing complications if you had difficulty answering this question.*

Cognitive Level—Applying
Client Needs Category—Physiological integrity
Client Needs Subcategory—Reduction of risk potential

23. 3. Determining what drug has been taken is essential in determining the potential effects and the treatment needed. Although determining the approximate number of pills and when they were taken will help to assess the potential lethality of the overdose, this information is not as critical initially. While the client's life is threatened, discussing the reason for the overdose is not a priority. Asking about previous suicide attempts is not important initially but will be a necessary question once the client is stabilized.

> *Test Taking Strategy—Use the process of elimination to select an option that describes the most important data when assessing a client who has overdosed. Options 2 and 4 are not facts that relate to the immediate status of the client. Option 1 has merit, but the client may not be able to provide an accurate answer. Option 3 emerges as the best answer. Review data collection in cases of overdose if you had difficulty answering this question.*

Cognitive Level—Analyzing
Client Needs Category—Physiological integrity
Client Needs Subcategory—Reduction of risk potential

24. 3. Myringotomy tubes are small tubes that are surgically placed into the child's eardrum to help drain the fluid out of the middle ear to reduce the risk of ear infections. The tubes may be made of plastic, metal, or Teflon. Earplugs are used as a barrier against water entering the tubes used to equalize pressure within the middle ear. The introduction of water from such activities as swimming or showering can cause suppurative (pus-producing) otitis media. The child's hearing should improve as pressure within the middle ear is relieved. Instilling ear drops or water for irrigation is contraindicated for the same reasons that water from swimming and showering is prohibited from entering the ears.

Test Taking Strategy—Use the process of elimination to select the option that provides correct information for parental management of a child with bilateral myringotomy tubes. Options 1 and 4 can be eliminated because they are unsafe. Option 2 is incorrect because hearing is improved. Option 3 is the best choice from among the options. Review the care of a client with myringotomy tubes if you had difficulty answering this question.
Cognitive Level—*Applying*
Client Needs Category—*Health promotion and maintenance*
Client Needs Subcategory—*None*

25. **1.** Adding a volume of air equal to the amount of drug to be withdrawn from a vial increases the pressure within the vial and facilitates filling the syringe. A tuberculin syringe holds a maximum volume of 1 mL; therefore, it will not accommodate the 2-mL volume of medication needed in this situation. The deltoid muscle is not used when the volume of the medication exceeds 1 mL. It is appropriate to select a 1½″ to 2″ (3.8 to 5 cm) needle to reach the depth where muscle is located. The needle is inserted at a 90-degree angle when administering an I.M. injection.

Test Taking Strategy—Use the process of elimination to select the option that accurately describes the technique for administering an intramuscular (I.M.) injection. Option 2 can be immediately eliminated because its capacity is 1 mL. Although the deltoid muscle (option 3) can be used for an I.M. injection, the 2-mL volume contradicts its selection as an injection site. Option 4 has some merit depending on the size of the client, but the question stem does not provide that information. Option 1 remains as the best answer. Review the technique for administering an I.M. injection if you had difficulty answering this question.
Cognitive Level—*Understanding*
Client Needs Category—*Physiological integrity*
Client Needs Subcategory—*Pharmacological therapies*

26. **1.** Observing whether a client can move the fingers or toes of a casted extremity is the best method for assessing neurologic function because muscles cannot move unless the nervous system is intact. Monitoring capillary refill, feeling the skin temperature, and palpating the pedal pulses are appropriate techniques for assessing a client's vascular status.

Test Taking Strategy—Use the process of elimination to select the option that accurately describes a technique for performing a neurologic assessment. Options 2, 3, and 4 are incorrect because the purpose of the described assessment techniques is to determine if circulation is adequate or impaired. Option 1 is the best answer. Review the methods for assessing an extremity after the application of a cast and the significance of the assessment findings if you had difficulty answering this question.

Cognitive Level—*Understanding*
Client Needs Category—*Physiological integrity*
Client Needs Subcategory—*Reduction of risk potential*

27. **2.** A sliding scale is a type of insulin regimen used to regulate blood glucose levels throughout the day. The amount of insulin to administer is based on the client's capillary blood glucose measurement. In this case, because the blood glucose level is 250 mg/dL, the nurse should plan to give 4 units of insulin.

Test Taking Strategy—Analyze to determine what information the question asks for, which is the administration of the proper dose of insulin, according to a client's blood sugar level. Review the use of a sliding scale when administering insulin if you had difficulty answering this question.
Cognitive Level—*Applying*
Client Needs Category—*Physiological integrity*
Client Needs Subcategory—*Pharmacological therapies*

28. **4.** Hepatitis B is a serious form of liver inflammation/disease caused by infection with the hepatitis B virus (HBV). Hepatitis B can be acute or chronic. Some people may be asymptomatic but carry HBV in their blood and pass the infection on to others. HBV enters the bloodstream through breaks in the skin or mucous membranes and is transmitted by infected blood, serum, semen, vaginal fluid, and sharing of contaminated needles. Viruses depend on living cells to grow and reproduce. Therefore, it is extremely unlikely that the virus could be transmitted by smoking cigarettes long since extinguished. Hepatitis A is associated with eating unsanitary, contaminated food. Hepatitis B is not caused by drinking alcohol.

Test Taking Strategy—Use the process of elimination to select the option that best correlates with a risk factor for the acquisition of hepatitis B. Option 3 can be immediately eliminated because it does not describe a transmission factor for hepatitis B. Option 1 may appear attractive because it could be a source for transmitting hepatitis, but not hepatitis B. Option 2 can cause alcoholic hepatitis, a precursor of cirrhosis, but this is not an infectious type of hepatitis. Review the methods of transmitting hepatitis B if you had difficulty answering this question.
Cognitive Level—*Applying*
Client Needs Category—*Physiological integrity*
Client Needs Subcategory—*Physiological adaptation*

29. **1, 4.** Reasonable weight gain is expected during pregnancy. Poor nutrition due to poverty or lack of knowledge is a leading contributor to high-risk pregnancies. To ensure the health of both the mother and her fetus, it is important for the mother to eat a variety of foods. Many physicians do not restrict sexual activity during pregnancy unless complications, such as uterine bleeding or placenta previa, are evident or the membranes rupture. A certain amount of regular exercise is preferable to sporadic activity. The type and amount of exercise depends on the health, habits, and obstetric history of each client. Pregnancy beyond age 35 is considered a risk factor due to potential chromosomal abnormalities. Refusal to take prenatal vitamins does not necessarily pose a risk for the client or her baby, but the client needs to be instructed about the benefits of vitamins. Having a history of a chlamydia infection (a sexually transmitted infection) several years ago does not put the client or fetus at risk during this pregnancy.

> *Test Taking Strategy*—*Analyze to determine what information the question asks for, which is risk factors for pregnancy complications. Alternative-format "select all that apply" questions require considering each option independently to decide its merit in answering the question. Review prenatal risk factors if you had difficulty answering this question.*
> *Cognitive Level*—*Applying*
> *Client Needs Category*—*Physiological integrity*
> *Client Needs Subcategory*—*Reduction of risk potential*

30. **80 mg.**

There are 2.2 pounds per kilogram; therefore, 88 pounds divided by 2.2 equals 40 kg. Because the client should receive 2 mg for every kilogram, the nurse multiplies $2 \times 40 = 80$ mg. Using the ratio-and-proportion method, the dosage is calculated as follows:

Step 1 (known ratio to unknown ratio):

$$\frac{2 \text{ mg}}{1 \text{ kg}} = \frac{X \text{ mg}}{40 \text{ kg}}$$

Step 2 (cross-multiply and solve for X):

$$1\,X = 80$$
$$X = 80 \text{ mg}$$

> *Test Taking Strategy*—*Analyze to determine what information the question asks for, which involves pediatric dosage calculation. Review the steps involved in calculating dosages if you had difficulty answering this question.*
> *Cognitive Level*—*Applying*
> *Client Needs Category*—*Physiological integrity*
> *Client Needs Subcategory*—*Pharmacological therapies*

31. **2.** Massaging the uterus causes the myometrium to contract and become firm, occluding the blood vessels and thereby controlling postpartum bleeding. This is more accurate than expressing clots from the vagina. The client may experience pain when the uterus is massaged. The discomfort is due to uterine contraction, which intensifies (not ceases) as the uterus is massaged.

> *Test Taking Strategy*—*Use the process of elimination to identify the option that identifies the expected outcome from uterine massage. Option 1 can be eliminated immediately because massaging the*

uterus is not performed for the purposed of relieving pain. Option 3 may appear attractive because clots may be expelled as a consequence of uterine massage, but that is not its purpose. Option 4 can be eliminated because that is not an expected consequence of uterine massage. Once unlikely options are eliminated, option 2 remains as the best answer. Review the purpose for massaging the uterus after delivery of an infant and its expected result if you had difficulty answering this question.
> *Cognitive Level*—*Evaluating*
> *Client Needs Category*—*Physiological integrity*
> *Client Needs Subcategory*—*Reduction of risk potential*

32. **3.** Glulisine (Apidra) is a rapid-acting insulin used to reduce a client's blood sugar prior to consuming a meal. Because it is rapid-acting, it should be administered within 15 minutes before or within 20 minutes after starting a meal. It is not appropriate to administer glulisine after the completion of a meal or between meals. Glargine (Lantus) insulin is administered at bedtime.

> *Test Taking Strategy*—*Analyze to determine what information the question asks for, which is the optimum time to administer glulisine (Apidra) insulin. Recall that rapid-acting insulins, like glulisine (Apidra), aspart (Novolog), and lispro (Humalog) begin lowering blood sugar within 15 minutes of administration. To avoid hypoglycemia, the client should have food available soon after the injection is given. Review types of insulin and their time of onset if you had difficulty answering this question.*
> *Cognitive Level*—*Applying*
> *Client Needs Category*—*Physiological integrity*
> *Client Needs Subcategory*—*Pharmacological therapies*

33. **4.** Paraphrasing the content of the client's statement is a therapeutic communication technique that helps the client know that the message was heard and how it was interpreted. This technique will likely encourage the client to continue verbalizing. Classifying the statement as an exaggeration is belittling. Telling the client that talking will contribute to sadness is an indirect way of saying that this line of communication should cease. Demanding an explanation by asking "why" is also a block to therapeutic communication because it requires that the client justify a rationale for the statement and puts the client on the defensive.

> *Test Taking Strategy*—*Use the process of elimination to identify the most therapeutic communication technique for responding to the client's statement. Options 1, 2, and 3 can be eliminated because they all contain nontherapeutic elements. Review therapeutic and nontherapeutic communication techniques if you had difficulty answering this question.*
> *Cognitive Level*—*Analyzing*
> *Client Needs Category*—*Psychosocial integrity*
> *Client Needs Subcategory*—*None*

34. 3. The only reliable method for confirming the presence of hard, dry stool within the rectum is digital examination. Auscultating bowel sounds and measuring abdominal girth are appropriate physical assessment techniques, but they do not aid in determining whether the client has a fecal impaction. Assessing for diarrhea is always important in relation to fluid and electrolyte imbalances, but it may not be an indication of fecal impaction. Leaking stool, but not diarrhea, may be associated with a fecal impaction because the stool above the impaction may be seeking a path for elimination. It is important to differentiate which is the case.

Test Taking Strategy—Use the process of elimination to help select the assessment that is best for identifying the presence of a fecal impaction. Options 1, 2, and 4 have merit because they relate to assessments of GI function, but they are not as conclusive as a digital examination (option 3). Review the assessment of bowel elimination as it relates to a fecal impaction if you had difficulty answering this question.
Cognitive Level—*Analyzing*
Client Needs Category—*Physiological integrity*
Client Needs Subcategory—*Basic care and comfort*

35. 2. Aspirin can cause Reye's syndrome in children. Reye's syndrome is a potentially fatal disease that causes damage to the brain, liver, and kidneys. It is associated with aspirin consumption by children age 8 years or younger. The disease causes the brain to swell and the liver to become fatty, enlarged, and firm. The kidneys also change appearance. Severe brain damage or death may result if early detection is not made. To reduce the potential for developing this disorder, salicylates are avoided.

Test Taking Strategy—Use the process of elimination to identify an accurate rationale for avoiding the administration of aspirin to a child. Options 1, 3, and 4 have some aspirin does relieve a fever and reduce inflammation. Gastric irritation is a side effect of aspirin use, but it is unlikely that aspirin would be given to a child in a quantity or frequency for this to occur when managing most childhood ailments. Option 2 emerges as the best answer. Review the correlation of aspirin as a risk factor for Reye's syndrome if you had difficulty answering this question.
Cognitive Level—*Applying*
Client Needs Category—*Physiological integrity*
Client Needs Subcategory—*Pharmacological therapies*

36. 4. If the pubococcygeal muscles are being contracted and relaxed properly during the performance of Kegel exercises, the client should be able to stop and restart the flow of urine during voiding. Kegel exercises are performed to prevent or relieve stress incontinence; they are ineffective in relieving back pain, improving abdominal tone, or performing sit-ups.

Test Taking Strategy—Use the process of elimination to identify the option that best describes the expected effect when Kegel exercises are performed. Options 1, 2, and 3 can be eliminated because the pubococcygeal muscles do not innervate actions such as deep-knee bends, touching the toes, or performing sit-ups. Review the purpose for performing Kegel exercises if you had difficulty answering this question.
Cognitive Level—*Evaluating*
Client Needs Category—*Health promotion and maintenance*
Client Needs Subcategory—*None*

37. 3. External fetal monitoring minimizes the risk of exposing the fetus to the mother's human immunodeficiency virus (HIV)-infected blood. Fetal scalp blood sampling and internal fetal monitoring are invasive techniques that would increase the fetus's risk of exposure to HIV. Chorionic villi sampling is a prenatal test that can detect genetic abnormalities such as Down syndrome.

Test Taking Strategy—Note the key words "most appropriate" and "HIV infection." Although all of the options are methods for fetal assessment, the best answer is option 3 because it is most conducive for preventing blood-borne viral transmission to the unborn fetus. Review techniques of fetal assessment and their risk for transmitting blood-borne infections if you had difficulty answering this question.
Cognitive Level—*Analyzing*
Client Needs Category—*Safe and effective care environment*
Client Needs Subcategory—*Safety and infection control*

38. 4. Persons with hypothyroidism (myxedema) are most likely to demonstrate a general slowing of thought processes. Although persons with hypothyroidism are slow in responding, their thought processes are usually based in reality. Quick recall of events, rapid verbal responses, and bizarre thinking are uncharacteristic of clients with this disorder.

Test Taking Strategy—Analyze to determine what information the question asks for, which is the expected outcome when performing a mental status assessment of a client with hypothyroidism. Hypothyroidism contributes to diminished cognitive function, making option 4 the best answer. Review the signs and symptoms of hypothyroidism if you had difficulty answering this question.
Cognitive Level—*Applying*
Client Needs Category—*Physiological integrity*
Client Needs Subcategory—*Physiological adaptation*

39.

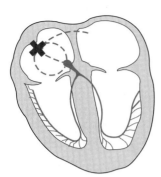

In a sinus rhythm, the sinoatrial (SA) node initiates the electrical impulses. The SA node is located in the upper part of the right atrium.

> *Test Taking Strategy—Analyze to determine what information the question asks for, which is the location of the natural pacemaker. Review the physiology of cardiac electrical conduction and locations of the structures in the conduction pathway if you had difficulty answering this question.*
> ***Cognitive Level****—Remembering*
> ***Client Needs Category****—Physiological integrity*
> ***Client Needs Subcategory****—Physiological adaptation*

40. **3.** Charting must be as clear and objective as possible. Quoting the client is always appropriate. Interpreting or labeling what the nurse suspects is occurring is not the best form of documentation.

> *Test Taking Strategy—Use the process of elimination to select the best documentation of the nurse's interaction with the client who is most likely experiencing a hallucination. Recall that documentation should be objective rather than a subjective nursing interpretation. Review do's and don'ts of documentation if you had difficulty answering this question.*
> ***Cognitive Level****—Applying*
> ***Client Needs Category****—Safe and effective care environment*
> ***Client Needs Subcategory****—Coordinated care*

41. **1.** Having direct contact with a stillborn infant tends to initiate healthy grieving. Although providing a verbal description that focuses on the infant's attributes is therapeutic, it is not as personal as seeing and touching the infant. Preventing any interaction between the parents and infant interferes with the grief process. Many postpartum clients are discharged within 24 to 48 hours of delivery; this would have no bearing on resolving the grief of a perinatal loss.

> *Test Taking Strategy—Use the process of elimination to select an option that describes an appropriate nursing measure for coping with the delivery of a stillborn infant. Option 2 can be eliminated immediately because it interferes with grieving a loss. Option 3 can be eliminated because a verbal description of the infant is not considered effective for resolving the*

exaggerated images the parents may have. Option 4 can be eliminated because an early discharge interferes with verbalizing thoughts and feelings that may help in the process of grieving. Option 1, then, becomes the best answer to the question. Review nursing measures for resolving the perinatal death of an infant if you had difficulty answering this question.
> ***Cognitive Level****—Analyzing*
> ***Client Needs Category****—Psychosocial integrity*
> ***Client Needs Subcategory****—None*

42. **1.** To remove an object from the airway of an unconscious, nonpregnant adult, the rescuer administers forceful thrusts upward from the abdomen. If the adult is conscious, abdominal thrusts are repeated until the object is dislodged or the victim becomes unconscious. If the client is unconscious, the rescuer should gently assist the client to the floor, look inside the mouth, and attempt to ventilate using two breaths. Resuscitation efforts and chest compressions should begin if there is no pulse. Ventilating the client is ineffective as long as the airway is obstructed; however, attempts at ventilation should be made until emergency medical assistance can arrive.

> *Test Taking Strategy—Use the process of elimination to help select the option that accurately describes the technique for performing the abdominal thrust maneuver. Options 2 and 4 can be eliminated because they describe actions involving the performance of cardiopulmonary resuscitation (CPR). Option 3 can be eliminated because it inaccurately identifies the ratio of chest compressions to breaths in the event that CPR is required. Review the technique for relieving an obstruction in the airway of an adult if you had difficulty answering this question.*
> ***Cognitive Level****—Analyzing*
> ***Client Needs Category****—Physiological integrity*
> ***Client Needs Subcategory****—Physiological adaptation*

43. **3.** Performing self-care indicates that a client has progressed from denial and anger to a stage of acceptance. Wearing loose-fitting garments can be viewed as an attempt to hide the change in body image. Although showering daily and avoiding gas-forming foods are appropriate, they may only be an indication that the client is self-conscious about possible fecal odor.

> *Test Taking Strategy—Note the key words "best evidence." Select the most accurate description among the options demonstrating that a client with a colostomy is coping with a change in body image. Review Kübler-Ross's stages of grieving, focusing on "acceptance," if you had difficulty answering this question.*
> ***Cognitive Level****—Evaluating*
> ***Client Needs Category****—Psychosocial integrity*
> ***Client Needs Subcategory****—None*

44. **2.** After any GI procedure that uses barium as a contrast medium, the nurse should monitor the client's bowel elimination. Retained barium can cause constipation and even bowel obstruction. A laxative or some other method of promoting the passage of the stool is needed if elimination is delayed. The stool color appears white or chalky as barium is eliminated. Assessing the color of the client's urine and the ability to swallow and eat are unrelated to the consequences of the radiographic procedure.

Test Taking Strategy—Note the key words "most important," which indicate a priority. Because the retention of barium administered as contrast medium during an upper GI X-ray may be life-threatening, it represents the highest priority for assessment. Review the nursing management of a client undergoing an upper GI X-ray if you had difficulty answering this question.
Cognitive Level—Analyzing
Client Needs Category—Physiological integrity
Client Needs Subcategory—Reduction of risk potential

45. **2.** An adolescent mother who lives alone is most likely in need of financial assistance and the emotional support that various organizations, including a teen parenting group, can provide. The client's primipara status and previous spontaneous abortion are unrelated to her ability to care for herself and her newborn. The fact that the client continues to see the newborn's father is no guarantee that he will provide the level and type of support this young mother needs.

Test Taking Strategy—Use the process of elimination to identify an option that accurately describes the need for a referral for an adolescent after delivery of an infant. Although option 1 has merit, it can be eliminated because it does not necessarily mean that the adolescent does not have a person to consult regarding care of the infant. Options 3 and 4 are not as significant in relation to a need for support and help in caring for the newborn as option 2, which suggests that the client is isolated and does not have access to a network for immediate support. Review the potential emotional and financial needs of a teenage mother after discharge if you had difficulty answering this question.
Cognitive Level—Analyzing
Client Needs Category—Safe and effective care environment
Client Needs Subcategory—Coordinated care

46. **2.** The care of clients with radioactive implants is best assigned to nonpregnant nurses because acute or chronic exposure to ionizing radiation can cause gene mutation and birth defects. All nurses—male and female, pregnant and nonpregnant—are at risk for radiation if precautions of time, distance, and shielding are not followed. Whether the nurse has attended the radiation safety inservice or is being reassigned to another unit later in the shift are topics that the charge nurse may need to know; however, they are not as important as the staff nurse's pregnancy status.

Test Taking Strategy—Look at the key words "most important," which suggest a priority; in this case, ensuring safety. Because exposure to radiation can affect rapidly growing cells, which includes the fetus

of a pregnant nurse, it is the most important priority to consider when assigning this client's care. Review the hazards of exposure to internal sources of radiation if you had difficulty answering this question.
Cognitive Level—Analyzing
Client Needs Category—Safe and effective care environment
Client Needs Subcategory—Safety and infection control

47. **1.** High-calorie finger foods are best for clients with Alzheimer's disease, who find it almost impossible to sit or stand in one location for more than a few minutes. The problem is not the quantity or variety of food, the time available for eating, the client's personal preferences, or digestibility of food; rather, the underlying problem for these clients is their limited attention span and ability to concentrate on any physical task.

Test Taking Strategy—Use the process of elimination to help select the option that accurately identifies a method for facilitating a desired outcome. Option 2 can be eliminated because serving easily digestible food does not necessarily resolve an inadequate intake. Option 3 can be eliminated because the problem does not involve insufficient time to eat. Option 4 has some merit, but it is not as likely to address the problem as much as providing high-calorie food at frequent intervals. Review dietary measures for meeting the nutritional needs of clients if you had difficulty answering this question.
Cognitive Level—Analyzing
Client Needs Category—Health promotion and maintenance
Client Needs Subcategory—None

48. **1.** To detect the presence of thrombophlebitis, the nurse has the client dorsiflex each foot separately and notes if the client experiences calf pain. The presence of calf pain is considered a positive Homans' sign and needs to be reported immediately. Although palpating the pedal pulse to assess the client's distal arterial blood flow comparing the color in the client's nailbeds and observing for evidence of guarding while walking can provide supportive evidence of thrombophlebitis, these are not the primary assessment techniques for detecting the disorder. Comparing the color in the client's nailbeds helps assess if circulation is bilaterally comparable, but monitoring the temperature of the unaffected leg offers no useful comparative value in this situation.

Test Taking Strategy—Use the process of elimination to select the option that accurately describes the assessment technique for identifying thrombophlebitis in a lower limb. Options 2 and 4 have merit because they reflect techniques for identifying compromised circulation, but they are not the best technique for identifying a sign that suggests that the client has thrombophlebitis. An impaired gait, as suggested in option 3, may be related to pain associated with thrombophlebitis, but it is vague and nonspecific. Review Homans' sign and how it is elicited if you had difficulty answering this question.

Cognitive Level—Analyzing
Client Needs Category—Physiological integrity
Client Needs Subcategory—Reduction of risk potential

49. **2, 4, 5.** A normal heart rate is between 60 and 100 beats/ minute. Each impulse occurs regularly, producing a regular heart rate. The ventricles depolarize and contract to pump blood through the system. The atrioventricular (AV) node is the gatekeeper, sending impulses to the ventricles. The sinoatrial (SA) node initiates the impulse. P waves, which are the impulses from the SA node, precede the ventricular repolarization of the QRS complex. Ventricular rates, which are slower than atrial rates, are indicative of heart blocks.

Test Taking Strategy—Analyze to determine what information the question asks for, which is options that correlate with signs of normal sinus rhythm. Alternative-format "select all that apply" questions require considering each option independently to decide its merit in answering the question. Review the waveforms in normal cardiac conduction and the findings that accompany normal sinus rhythm if you had difficulty answering this question.
Cognitive Level—Applying
Client Needs Category—Physiological integrity
Client Needs Subcategory—Physiological adaptation

50. **4.** If the thyroid gland is manipulated preoperatively or during its surgical removal, any preoperative palpation increases the client's risk of developing thyroid crisis or storm, a life-threatening condition. An enlarged thyroid gland can compress the trachea, but that is not the basis for omitting palpation of the gland. The laryngeal nerve may be damaged during surgical removal of the thyroid gland, but palpating the thyroid preoperatively would not contribute to nerve damage. The client may experience minor discomfort if the gland is palpated, but discomfort is not a basis for omitting glandular palpation.

Test Taking Strategy—Analyze to determine what information the question asks for, which is the rationale for omitting the palpation of the thyroid gland in a client with Graves' disease. Review the pathophysiology of Graves' disease and the effect of high levels of the hormone thyroxine if you had difficulty answering this question.
Cognitive Level—Applying
Client Needs Category—Physiological integrity
Client Needs Subcategory—Reduction of risk potential

51. **1.** Missing a dose of disulfiram (Antabuse) will not cause a drug reaction. The reaction occurs when the client ingests alcohol or applies it to the skin. To ensure that a reaction does not occur, the client must abstain from alcohol for at least 2 weeks or more after discontinuing the drug.

Test Taking Strategy—Use the process of elimination to help select the option that describes an indication of ineffective learning in relation to the self-administration of disulfiram. Options 2, 3, and 4

can be eliminated because they are accurate statements. Option 1 emerges as an example of incorrect information because missing a dose is not likely to cause a drug reaction. Review the actions and precautions that relate to disulfiram if you had difficulty answering this question.
Cognitive Level—Evaluating
Client Needs Category—Physiological integrity
Client Needs Subcategory—Pharmacological therapies

52. **2.** Standard precautions are followed for every client, regardless of the potential for direct contact with blood, such as when removing an I.V. device from its site. Normally, blood glucose levels are not checked after the I.V. solution is discontinued, unless the solution contained large amounts of dextrose, such as in total parenteral nutrition. Blood loss should be minimal or nonexistent when the I.V. line is discontinued. Usually direct pressure is not needed for a prolonged period of time unless the client is receiving anticoagulant therapy.

Test Taking Strategy—Note the key term "essential," which indicates a priority nursing action. Options 3 and 4 can be immediately eliminated because they are unrelated to discontinuing an I.V. line. Option 1 has some merit because applying pressure is a method for controlling bleeding; however, applying pressure for 5 minutes is generally needed when discontinuing an arterial (not venous) line. Option 2 then becomes the most obvious correct answer. Review the nursing actions involved in discontinuing an I.V. infusion if you had difficulty answering this question.
Cognitive Level—Analyzing
Client Needs Category—Safe and effective care environment
Client Needs Subcategory—Safety and infection control

53. **2.** When a client verbalizes or manifests symptoms of anxiety, it is best for the nurse to help the client express any concerns. Belittling fears by saying "There is no need for fear," using a reassuring cliché such as "trust me" or "you have an excellent surgeon," and giving advice such as "try to relax" are all nontherapeutic ways of communicating.

Test Taking Strategy—Use the process of elimination to help select the option that demonstrates a therapeutic communication technique. Options 1, 3, and 4 are examples of nontherapeutic communication techniques, leaving Option 2 as the best answer. Review therapeutic and nontherapeutic communication techniques if you had difficulty answering this question.
Cognitive Level—Analzying
Client Needs Category—Psychosocial integrity
Client Needs Subcategory—None

54. **3.** Topical anesthesia is needed when a tonometer is used to measure the pressure within a client's eyes. The anesthetic, prepared in liquid eyedrop form, makes it possible to apply the tonometer to the cornea without the client feeling as if something is touching the eye. The other assessment procedures include using a reflex hammer, a vaginal speculum, and an otoscope—none of which requires the application of a topical anesthetic.

> *Test Taking Strategy—Look at the key word "essential," which indicates a priority nursing action. Options 1, 2, and 4 do not create discomfort during the course of assessment. Review methods for performing the assessments listed if you had difficulty answering this question.*
> *Cognitive Level—Analyzing*
> *Client Needs Category—Physiological integrity*
> *Client Needs Subcategory—Reduction of risk potential*

55. **1.** NPH is an intermediate-acting type of insulin. The onset of action is 1 to 3 hours, and the peak effect occurs in 6 to 12 hours. Hypoglycemia can occur at the expected onset and again when the insulin level peaks. In this case, the NPH insulin should peak sometime between 1 P.M. and 7 P.M., during which time the nurse should assess for hypoglycemia. Therefore, checking the client's glucose level at 3:00 P.M. would be appropriate. Because the client has breakfast at 7:00 A.M. and eating raises blood glucose levels, the nurse will not detect hypoglycemia at 7:30 A.M. Checking the glucose level at 10:00 P.M. or 12:00 A.M. is well beyond the time for peak action to occur.

> *Test Taking Strategy—Analyze to determine what information the question asks for, which is the most likely time for hypoglycemia to develop after early-morning administration of intermediate-acting insulin. Review the onset, peak, and duration of intermediate-acting insulin if you had difficulty answering this question.*
> *Cognitive Level—Applying*
> *Client Needs Category—Physiological integrity*
> *Client Needs Subcategory—Pharmacological therapies*

56. **4.** Bright red drainage indicates that the client is bleeding internally. Bright red drainage suggests arterial bleeding which is more serious than dark red blood which suggests venous bleeding. Preventing life-threatening consequences depends on prompt collaboration with the physician. The nurse can use comfort measures to relieve a sore throat, which is not a life-threatening condition. Nausea is common after surgery or if the gastric tube is obstructed. Depending on further assessment, the nurse may administer a prescribed antiemetic or solve the reason the gastric tube may not be draining properly. On the pain scale of 0 to 10, a rating of 5 indicates moderate pain that the nurse could reduce by administering a prescribed analgesic without consulting the physician.

> *Test Taking Strategy—Look for the key term "essential," which indicates a priority assessment finding to report. The appearance of bright red drainage is*

more indicative of a threat to the client's physical well-being than the findings described in options 1, 2, and 3. Review the signs associated with arterial bleeding if you had difficulty answering this question.*
> *Cognitive Level—Analyzing*
> *Client Needs Category—Physiological integrity*
> *Client Needs Subcategory—Reduction of risk potential*

57. **3.** Eric Erikson describes generativity as a concern for leaving something of worth to society. Adults older than age 40 typically seek to identify a positive contribution for which they will be most remembered. For some, their legacy is having been a good parent, an upstanding citizen, or a community volunteer; for others, more tangible activities, such as writing or painting, are their legacy.

> *Test Taking Strategy—Analyze to determine what information the question asks for, which is an example of generativity. Review the developmental stage of middle adulthood if you had difficulty answering this question.*
> *Cognitive Level—Understanding*
> *Client Needs Category—Health promotion and maintenance*
> *Client Needs Subcategory—None*

58. **2.** Asking about dietary practices is the most direct method among the options provided for determining if the client follows an orthodox Jewish lifestyle. Hebrew is commonly spoken by individuals who have emigrated from Israel. Reform, conservative, and orthodox Jewish men may wear a yarmulke, or skullcap, especially on the Sabbath or when attending synagogue. Many Christian men, as well as Jews, are circumcised.

> *Test Taking Strategy—Analyze to determine what information the question asks for, which is the practices associated with orthodox Judaism. Review the cultural beliefs and actions expected of persons who practice orthodox Judaism if you had difficulty answering this question.*
> *Cognitive Level—Analyzing*
> *Client Needs Category—Psychosocial integrity*
> *Client Needs Subcategory—None*

59. **1.** To reduce the potential for recollapsing the lung, air is prevented from entering the opening from which a chest tube has been pulled. When the tube comes out, its sterility is compromised. If the tube is to be replaced, a new, sterile tube must be used. Holding the breath may help temporarily, but the client cannot sustain this effort. Breath sounds should be assessed, but only after the chest tube has been reinserted.

> *Test Taking Strategy—Look at the key words "most appropriate," which suggests a priority nursing action. Select the option that identifies the best nursing response after removal of a chest tube from its insertion within the pleural space of a client. Review the nursing management of a client with a closed*

chest drainage system if you had difficulty answering this question.
Cognitive Level—*Analyzing*
Client Needs Category—*Physiological integrity*
Client Needs Subcategory—*Reduction of risk potential*

60. 1. Fluids are restricted to a few ice chips or small sips of water. Because the nasogastric (NG) tube is connected to suction, providing oral fluids liberally would deplete electrolytes as the gastric contents are suctioned into the suction canister. The nurse must follow the physician's written order or the facility's standards for care when irrigating an NG tube. Normal saline is the solution of choice because if plain water or distilled water is used, it would deplete electrolytes as they diffuse into the watery solution. Relieving throat discomfort and providing oral hygiene are appropriate nursing care measures.

> **Test Taking Strategy**—*Analyze to determine what information the question asks for, which is an unsafe action when managing the care of a client with an NG tube. Review the consequences of providing plain water to a client whose NG tube is connected to suction if you had difficulty answering this question.*

Cognitive Level—*Analyzing*
Client Needs Category—*Safe and effective care environment*
Client Needs Subcategory—*Coordinated care*

61. 2. The tip of the enema tubing is inserted approximately 3″ to 4″ (7.5 to 10 cm) when giving an enema to an adult client. This allows the tube to enter the anal canal and pass the internal sphincter, where the solution is instilled. Introducing the tube farther may injure mucous membranes. Introducing it a shorter distance places the solution in the rectum and causes the client to expel the enema before it can be effective.

> **Test Taking Strategy**—*Analyze to determine what information the question asks for, which is the appropriate distance to insert an enema tubing tip. Review the procedure for administering an enema to an adult if you had difficulty answering this question.*

Cognitive Level—*Remembering*
Client Needs Category—*Safe and effective care environment*
Client Needs Subcategory—*Safety and infection control*

62. 2. Retracting the foreskin is necessary to remove secretions and prevent infection. The foreskin is replaced after the area is cleaned. The anal area is washed after the penis and scrotum are cleaned; a separate wash cloth is unnecessary. Usually the penis is cleaned before the scrotum. The penis is washed with plain or soapy water; normal saline solution is unnecessary for this procedure.

> **Test Taking Strategy**—*Analyze to determine what information the question asks for, which is appropriate actions to take when performing perineal care of an uncircumcised male. Review the importance of*

retracting and replacing the foreskin of an uncircumcised male if you had difficulty answering this question.
Cognitive Level—*Analyzing*
Client Needs Category—*Physiological integrity*
Client Needs Subcategory—*Reduction of risk potential*

63. 2. Knowing a client's occupation and the type of work performed provides valuable information about whether or not to include principles of body mechanics in a teaching plan for a client with recurrent back pain. The client's age and energy level affect the strategies selected for providing the health teaching. Observing the client's gait is more medically diagnostic because if one limb is shorter than the other, it may suggest an alteration in the alignment of spinal vertebrae. Assessing the client's medications may prove helpful when developing a care plan, especially if the medications are used to treat musculoskeletal problems. However, knowledge of medications the client is taking is not as helpful as exploring the occupation of the client and the type of work performed.

> **Test Taking Strategy**—*Look at the key words "most important," which suggests a priority. Because low back pain is generally associated with the use of poor body mechanics and lifting objects incorrectly, determining the client's occupation is the most important data to obtain from among the options provided.*

Cognitive Level—*Analyzing*
Client Needs Category—*Physiological integrity*
Client Needs Subcategory—*Reduction of risk potential*

64. 3. Talking and dealing with an anxiety-provoking experience is healthier than avoiding or suppressing it. Failing to deal with the terror of an event can also lead to post-traumatic stress disorder. Most victims can detect insincerity when others pretend to be happy in their presence. Although interacting with others who have experienced a similar traumatic event is therapeutic, socializing for the sake of socializing is not. Taking vacations and participating in pleasurable activities are forms of stress management, but they serve as distractions and delay processing the impact of a traumatic event.

> **Test Taking Strategy**—*Use the process of elimination to help in selecting an option that describes a therapeutic action when interacting with a client who has been raped. Option 1 can be immediately eliminated because it is not compatible or empathetic with the trauma the client has experienced. Option 2 can be eliminated because it is not readily accomplished nor is it realistic. Option 4 can be eliminated because it interferes with experiencing the reality of the situation. Option 3 emerges as the correct option because it promotes verbalization about the feelings of the traumatized client.*

Cognitive Level—*Analyzing*
Client Needs Category—*Psychosocial integrity*
Client Needs Subcategory—*None*

65. 4. As long as a health belief has no detrimental effect, it is best to integrate it in the care plan. Rejecting an otherwise neutral cultural practice interferes with a therapeutic nurse-client relationship. However, the nurse must be mindful of the client's need for safety and the safety needs of the other clients and staff.

> *Test Taking Strategy—Use the process of elimination to select the option that is culturally appropriate. Option 1 implies that the spouse's action is not as important as an approach used by practitioners of Western medicine. Option 2 can be eliminated because it implies that the spouse's action jeopardizes the safety of others. Option 3 can be eliminated because it suggests that tolerating the spouse's action comes with relief from responsibility. Option 4 emerges as the correct answer because it respects the client and spouse's cultural belief when it does not compromise the health and safety of the client or others. Review nursing actions that support transcultural care if you had difficulty answering this question.*

> **Cognitive Level**—*Analyzing*
> **Client Needs Category**—*Psychosocial integrity*
> **Client Needs Subcategory**—*None*

66. 3. Corticosteroid therapy reduces the immunologic injury to the nephrons. As the nephrons recover, the client's urine output increases. Weight gain is a nontherapeutic effect of steroids due to altered glucose metabolism and sodium retention. Long-term and short-term high-dose therapies with corticosteroids are likely to create muscle weakness and atrophy. Blood pressure decreases from previously hypertensive levels as renal function improves.

> *Test Taking Strategy—Use the process of elimination to help select an option that describes a positive outcome associated with corticosteroid therapy. Option 1 can be eliminated because weight gain is undesirable. Option 2 can be eliminated because it is associated with anabolic steroids, such as analogues of testosterone. Option 4 can be eliminated because treatment of nephrotic syndrome and its related fluid retention should reduce blood pressure rather than raise it. Option 3 emerges as the best choice. Review the rationale for managing nephrotic syndrome with corticosteroid therapy and its expected outcomes if you had difficulty answering this question.*

> **Cognitive Level**—*Evaluating*
> **Client Needs Category**—*Physiological integrity*
> **Client Needs Subcategory**—*Pharmacological therapies*

67. 2. One of the best techniques for reducing a hospitalized client's anxiety is to explain procedures before performing them and offer instructions about any equipment involved in the client's care. Many hospitalized clients exaggerate the significance of common procedures and equipment and sometimes overreact to unaccustomed sights and sounds. In this case, the nurse should explain why the alarm sounded to help calm the client. Switching the infusion to gravity flow without explaining why is unlikely to relieve the client's anxiety. A tranquilizer or hypnotic medication should not be given until the results of other nursing interventions have been evaluated. Staying until the client falls asleep may be time-consuming and will keep the nurse from other nursing duties.

> *Test Taking Strategy—Use the process of elimination to help select an option that describes the best nursing intervention for relieving anxiety. Option 1 has some merit, because it eliminates the potential for an alarm from an electronic infusion device. Option 3 appears to be a good answer because administering a tranquilizer relieves the symptoms of anxiety, but it does not help relieve the real or imagined fear that precipitated the anxiety. Although staying with a client is supportive (option 4), it is not realistic if it involves a great deal of time because it could interfere with the performance of other responsibilities required of the nurse. Option 2 emerges as the best answer because it provides the client with factual information. Having knowledge provides power because it allows processing information realistically. Review methods for relieving anxiety if you had difficulty answering this question.*

> **Cognitive Level**—*Analyzing*
> **Client Needs Category**—*Psychosocial integrity*
> **Client Needs Subcategory**—*None*

68. 1. It is not unusual for any new parent to feel frustrated and overwhelmed by parenting demands. Explaining to the adolescent that this is normal and suggesting coping methods and occasional respite from family or friends are appropriate nursing measures in this case. Suggesting that the client place the newborn for adoption is extreme, given the circumstances. The information as presented does not warrant reporting the situation to child protective services. Telling the parent to be patient does not help deal with the situation at hand.

> *Test Taking Strategy—Use the process of elimination to help identify the option that is most supportive for helping a frustrated young mother with a newborn. Eliminate option 2 immediately because suggesting adoption is severe and unjustified. Option 3 can be eliminated because a threat interferes with a therapeutic nurse–client relationship. Option 4 may be appealing because it poses the promise that the client's frustration will eventually be relieved by being patient. Option 1 emerges as the best answer because it provides a solution to the client's sleep deprivation. Review methods for promoting a therapeutic nurse–client relationship if you had difficulty answering this question.*

> **Cognitive Level**—*Analyzing*
> **Client Needs Category**—*Psychosocial integrity*
> **Client Needs Subcategory**—*None*

69. 3. Cleaning with soap and water is one of the best methods for reducing transmission of microorganisms. Supporting the breasts and applying warm compresses provide comfort but have no effect on preventing the transmission of microorganisms elsewhere. The entire course of antibiotics should be taken, not just until symptoms subside.

Test Taking Strategy—Use the process of elimination to help identify the option that supports a principle of asepsis. Options 2 and 4 can be immediately eliminated because they do not interfere with disease transmission. Option 1 has merit because it treats the client's infection, but if the client stops taking the antibiotic before completing the full course, it will encourage resistant organisms. Washing with soap and water (option 3) is a proven method of preventing disease transmission, and therefore is the correct answer. Review principles of asepsis especially as they apply to wound care if you had difficulty answering this question.
Cognitive Level—*Applying*
Client Needs Category—*Safe and effective care environment*
Client Needs Subcategory—*Safety and infection control*

70. 2. The main reason for performing leg exercises is to promote venous circulation, thereby preventing the formation of blood clots. Leg exercises are generally used as an alternative when ambulation and activity are less than adequate. Exercise helps to maintain muscle strength, reduces dependent edema, and relieves blood congestion in varicose veins. However, these are secondary benefits of leg exercises.

Test Taking Strategy—Use the process of elimination to help select an option that describes an evidenced-based reason for performing leg exercises postoperatively. Option 1 looks attractive because exercise does build muscle tone, but that is not the potential problem among postoperative clients. Option 3 also has merit because muscle contraction promotes drainage of fluid into lymphatic vessels, but most postoperative clients do not have edema in the extremities. Although activity promotes venous circulation and can relieve swelling of the legs in clients who have varicose veins (option 4), this is not the reason leg exercises are considered a standard of care for postoperative clients. Option 2 emerges as the best answer. Review the purpose for performing leg exercises in the postoperative period if you had difficulty answering this question.
Cognitive Level—*Applying*
Client Needs Category—*Physiological integrity*
Client Needs Subcategory—*Reduction of risk potential*

71. 3. Aminophylline (Truphylline), a bronchodilator, is most likely to produce stimulating effects, such as restlessness, insomnia, irritability, tachycardia, and hypertension. It is sometimes difficult to differentiate between the effects of the drug therapy and the manifestations of hypoxia.

Breath sounds and respiratory effort are monitored frequently along with vital signs. Drug blood levels are monitored to evaluate a person's ability to metabolize the drug; dosages are adjusted based on the response. Bradycardia, drowsiness, and hypotension are all opposite to the stimulating effects associated with aminophylline.

Test Taking Strategy—Analyze to determine what information the question asks for, which is a side effect of I.V. aminophylline. I.V. aminophylline produces sympathetic nervous system stimulation, which is evidenced by restlessness (option 3). Review the side effects of sympathomimetic drugs and aminophylline in particular if you had difficulty answering this question.
Cognitive Level—*Remembering*
Client Needs Category—*Physiological integrity*
Client Needs Subcategory—*Pharmacological therapies*

72. 1, 3, 4, 5. Depression is fairly common among residents in long-term care facilities. A decline in the ability to care for personal activities of daily living, loss of personal independence, and continual reminders of death and dying are typically associated with nursing home placement and subsequent depression. In addition, some residents of long-term care facilities have had earlier episodes of depression or mental illness; many suffer from chronic illnesses or pain that limits their mental and physical functioning. Inactivity rather than overstimulation is associated with depression among residents. Food and drug interactions are usually not associated with depression.

Test Taking Strategy—Analyze to determine what information the question asks for, which is causative factors for depression in residents of long-term care facilities. Alternative-format "select all that apply" questions require considering each option independently to decide its merit in answering the question. Review stressors experienced uniquely by older adults and their potential for contributing to depression if you had difficulty answering this question.
Cognitive Level—*Applying*
Client Needs Category—*Psychosocial integrity*
Client Needs Subcategory—*None*

73. 3. Tetracycline hydrochloride (Tetracon) is not recommended for children younger than age 8 unless its use is absolutely necessary. This family of antibiotics causes permanent yellow, gray, or brown tooth discoloration. Penicillins, cephalosporins, and aminoglycosides will not discolor a child's teeth.

Test Taking Strategy—Analyze to determine what information the question asks for, which is a potential risk associated with the administration of an antibiotic when given to a client who is younger than age 8 years. Review the listed antibiotics for potential adverse effects if you had difficulty answering this question.
Cognitive Level—*Remembering*
Client Needs Category—*Physiological integrity*
Client Needs Subcategory—*Pharmacological therapies*

74. 4. It is best to first promote reality orientation when any client with dementia becomes confused. Disagreeing may agitate the client, interfering with the effectiveness of any provided therapy. Collaborating in the delusion by offering to call the school or indicating that a neighbor will care for the children contributes to the altered thought processes.

> *Test Taking Strategy—Use the process of elimination to help select the option that describes a therapeutic communication technique. Options 1, 2, and 3 can be eliminated because they are not therapeutic. Option 4 emerges as the best answer because it helps orient the client to the "here and now." Review therapeutic and nontherapeutic communication techniques if you had difficulty answering this question.*
> *Cognitive Level—Applying*
> *Client Needs Category—Psychosocial integrity*
> *Client Needs Subcategory—None*

75. 4. Aspirin is used during the acute stages of a myocardial infarction (MI) primarily for its antiplatelet action. This action helps restore blood flow through the arteries. Chewing an aspirin is recommended because it has more rapid effects than swallowing it whole. Aspirin also has analgesic, anti-inflammatory, and antipyretic actions, but none of these is the reason for its administration during a possible MI.

> *Test Taking Strategy—Use the process of elimination to help select an option that describes an evidence-based rationale for using aspirin at the time of a life-threatening cardiac event. Although options 1 and 2 and 3 are accurate, there is no correlation between these actions and its use during a cardiac event. Option 4 is the best answer because aspirin interferes with platelet aggregation. Review the effect of aspirin in relation to the clotting mechanism if you had difficulty answering this question.*
> *Cognitive Level—Applying*
> *Client Needs Category—Physiological integrity*
> *Client Needs Subcategory—Pharmacological therapies*

76. 3. The brachial artery is used to assess for a pulse during cardiopulmonary resuscitation (CPR) of an infant. The rationale is that an infant's neck is short and fat, which makes assessing the carotid pulse difficult. Also, the airway of an infant is short, soft, and compliant, so palpating for a carotid pulse may close or occlude the infant's airway. The radial and femoral arteries are not routinely used when assessing a client of any age during CPR. The femoral artery may be used, but this requires taking off the clothes and diaper which will cost valuable time.

> *Test Taking Strategy—Analyze to determine what information the question asks for, which is the location for assessing a pulse on an infant during CPR. Recall the anatomic differences of infants compared with others. Review guidelines for performing CPR*

on an infant if you had difficulty answering the question.
> *Cognitive Level—Understanding*
> *Client Needs Category—Physiological integrity*
> *Client Needs Subcategory—Physiological adaptation*

77. 4. The nurse's initial action is to assess the client's physical condition before attempting any change in the client's position. After examining the client, the nurse should solicit adequate help to move the client to a safer, more comfortable place, usually the bed or chair. It is appropriate to place a bed alarm device after the client is assessed. It is always important to keep the family informed as to the client's condition (within Health Insurance Portability and Accountability Act [HIPAA] regulations), but this should not take priority over assessing the client for injury. After all the data are collected and the nurse provides comfort and reassurance to the client, the accident should be reported to the unit manager, risk manager, and physician. A written description of the accident and its outcome is recorded and kept on file in the risk management office.

> *Test Taking Strategy—Look at the key word "initially" in reference to a nursing action after finding a client who has fallen from the bed. Recall that assessment is the first step in the nursing process. Review the steps in the nursing process and the policy and legalities concerning sharing information with the family if you had difficulty answering this question.*
> *Cognitive Level—Analyzing*
> *Client Needs Category—Safe and effective care environment*
> *Client Needs Subcategory—Safety and infection control*

78. 4. The best evidence of healthy parent–newborn attachment is that the parents hold, touch, and talk to their newborn child. Physical contact tends to stimulate the beginning of parental love and protectiveness. It communicates comfort and security to the infant. Being pleased with the baby's gender is a positive sign, but it is not as indicative of the future relationship between parents and an infant. Observing others caring for the infant or watching from a distance is not as effective as eye-to-eye and direct skin contact in promoting bonding.

> *Test Taking Strategy—Use the process of elimination to help select the option that identifies the best description of healthy parent-newborn attachment. All of the options describe positive behaviors, but option 4 indicates physical and verbal interaction, which has a higher level of promoting attachment than the others. Review evidence of attachment between parents and newborn infants if you had difficulty answering this question.*
> *Cognitive Level—Evaluating*
> *Client Needs Category—Health promotion and maintenance*
> *Client Needs Subcategory—None*

79. 2. Metrorrhagia, vaginal bleeding between regular menstrual periods, is significant in a woman who is receiving hormonal replacement therapy because it may signal cancer, tumors of the uterus, or other gynecologic problems that require further evaluation. Bleeding between menstrual periods by a woman taking oral contraceptives is not usually serious. Dysfunctional irregular bleeding may also occur in individuals at the opposite ends of the reproductive lifespan, such as adolescents and perimenopausal women, and usually is not as much of a concern.

> *Test Taking Strategy—Analyze to determine what information the question asks for, which is identifying the client for whom gynecologic bleeding is most pathologic. Options 1, 3, and 4 describe blood loss that can be explained physiologically. Review the significance of abnormal gynecologic bleeding and its relationship to pathologic conditions if you had difficulty answering this question.*

Cognitive Level—Applying
Client Needs Category—Physiological integrity
Client Needs Subcategory—Physiological adaptation

80. 3. A sign that a client is oriented is the ability to find the appropriate room without assistance. Walking with others is not evidence that the client can independently find the dining room. The ability to dress is evidence that the client is able to perform activities of daily living but does not reflect improvement in orientation. Talking on the telephone indicates that the client has retained the ability to communicate verbally.

> *Test Taking Strategy—Use the process of elimination to help select the option that describes the best evidence that a client's orientation has been restored. The tasks in options 2 and 4 do not require orientation to perform. Option 1 may seem attractive, but walking with others does not require orientation on the part of the client. Option 3 emerges as the best answer because it indicates the client has used a level of cognitive thinking for finding a specific location within the environment. Review how to assess orientation if you had difficulty answering this question.*

Cognitive Level—Evaluating
Client Needs Category—Psychosocial integrity
Client Needs Subcategory—None

81. 2. It is best to hold inhaled medication in the lungs for 10 seconds or longer to maximally disperse the inhaled drug throughout the lungs. Because distribution of the powder depends on the efficacy of the inhalation, clients are taught to take a rapid, deep breath when inhaling to deliver the dry powder to the lungs. Swallowing the medication fails to distribute the drug to the appropriate location for absorption. Coughing causes the medication to be confined to the upper airways.

> *Test Taking Strategy—Analyze to determine what information the question asks for, which is to identify a correct instruction when teaching a client how to use a dry powder inhaler. Options 1, 3, and 4 describe incorrect instructions in relation to using a dry powder inhaler because they would either result in inadequately inhaling the dry powder or facilitating its anatomic dispersal. Review the technique for using a dry powder inhaler if you had difficulty answering this question.*

Cognitive Level—Understanding
Client Needs Category—Physiological integrity
Client Needs Subcategory—Pharmacological therapies

82. 4. A young child may not be able to verbally indicate the location of discomfort. Pulling at the infected ear is a common indication of a middle ear infection. Irritability, a runny nose, and swallowing frequently can be signs of many problems; however, they are not specific to an otitis media infection.

> *Test Taking Strategy—Use the process of elimination to help select the option that accurately describes a nonverbal assessment finding that correlates with a middle ear infection. Options 1 and 2 appear attractive because they may accompany a middle ear infection, but they can also be associated with other conditions. Option 3 may indicate the accumulation of pharyngeal secretions, but not necessarily a middle ear infection. Option 4 emerges as the correct choice. Review signs of a middle ear infection, especially in relation to a toddler, if you had difficulty answering this question.*

Cognitive Level—Applying
Client Needs Category—Physiological integrity
Client Needs Subcategory—Physiological adaptation

83. 2. Ménière's disease is a disease of the inner ear that results in episodes of dizziness (vertigo), ringing in the ears (tinnitus), and hearing loss. It has no known cause, and the frequency and severity of the attacks vary. Several types of medications may be used during an acute attack. Some include central nervous system depressants, such as diazepam (Valium) or lorazepam (Ativan). Meclizine (Antivert) is an antivertigo-antiemetic drug that is commonly prescribed for motion sickness and vertigo due to vestibular disease. Acetaminophen (Tylenol) has antipyretic and analgesic actions and is not usually used for Ménière's disease. Meperidine (Demerol), an opioid analgesic, is also not used for this disease. Triazolam (Halcion), a benzodiazepine, is commonly prescribed for sleep, not vertigo and tinnitus.

> *Test Taking Strategy—Use the process of elimination to help select the option that identifies a medication used to relieve a symptom experienced during an acute attack of Ménière's disease, which likely includes nausea and dizziness. Options 1, 3, and 4 are drugs used to manage symptoms other than*

those associated with an acute attack of Ménière's disease. Review the symptoms experienced by a person with Ménière's disease as well as the action of meclizine if you had difficulty answering this question.
Cognitive Level—*Remembering*
Client Needs Category—*Physiological integrity*
Client Needs Subcategory—*Pharmacological therapies*

84. 4. Calcium is chiefly regulated in the blood by parathyroid hormone and calcitonin (a hormone released by the thyroid). After a thyroidectomy, clients are monitored for hypocalcemia because it is possible that the parathyroid glands may have been accidentally removed. Hypocalcemia is manifested by tingling and numbness of the extremities and mouth and muscle contractions of the fingers and hands. The other choices are not related to a thyroidectomy.
Test Taking Strategy—*Use the process of elimination to help select the option that accurately identifies the electrolyte imbalance that may occur as a complication after a thyroidectomy. Options 1, 2, and 3, which identify low potassium, sodium, and magnesium, in that order, are not electrolyte imbalances that commonly occur after removing the thyroid. Option 4 identifies an electrolyte imbalance that is a potential complication of thyroidectomy and for which the nurse should monitor the client. Review the nursing care of a client undergoing a thyroidectomy if you had difficulty answering this question.*
Cognitive Level—*Analyzing*
Client Needs Category—*Physiological integrity*
Client Needs Subcategory—*Physiological adaptation*

85. 3. The fingernails are cut short to maintain skin integrity. Some health care professionals also recommend that the client wear cotton gloves to prevent opening the skin in case scratching cannot be controlled. Warm water accentuates the itching sensation. Dry cornstarch absorbs perspiration but does not relieve itching. Because jaundice is not related to an allergic reaction, using special hypoallergenic linens is inappropriate.
Test Taking Strategy—*Use the process of elimination to help select the option that identifies the best intervention to prevent or limit impairment of skin integrity secondary to itching. Option 1 can be eliminated immediately because bathing with very hot water may intensify itching. Options 2 and 4 may appear as attractive options, but their implementation is useful for reasons other than limiting trauma to the skin. Review methods for preventing or reducing skin impairment secondary to itching if you had difficulty answering this question.*
Cognitive Level—*Evaluating*
Client Needs Category—*Physiological integrity*
Client Needs Subcategory—*Basic care and comfort*

86.

| 2. Introduce yourself and explain the sequence of events. |
| 1. Ask the client to use the bathroom to urinate. |
| 4. Focus on general questions related to sexual health and reproduction. |
| 6. Take vital signs and obtain information about the client's last menstrual period. |
| 5. Have the client change into a hospital gown and offer a sheet to cover her lap. |
| 3. Help the client into the stirrups for the physical examination. |

Completing a reproductive history and physical examination can be stressful for the client. To ease the client's anxiety and build a trusting relationship, the nurse should begin with an introduction (2) and explain the sequence of events. Next, the nurse should allow the client to use the bathroom (1), especially if the bathroom is in the hall. Next, the nurse begins collecting the client history, focusing first on general questions about sexual health and reproduction before addressing more detailed concerns (4). Then the nurse should take a set of vital signs for baseline and ask the client about her last menstrual period (6). Next, the nurse should step out of the examination room and allow the client to change into a hospital gown (5). Lastly, just before the physician arrives for the physical examination, the nurse helps the client into the stirrups (3).
Test Taking Strategy—*Look at the key words "nursing actions" and "first to last," and organize the appropriate sequence during a reproductive and sexual nursing assessment. Review how a reproductive assessment and pelvic examination is performed if you had difficulty answering this question.*
Cognitive Level—*Remembering*
Client Needs Category—*Health promotion and maintenance*
Client Needs Subcategory—*None*

87. 1, 2, 6. A client with hyperparathyroidism is prone to forming kidney stones. Therefore, keeping the urine dilute and promoting frequent urinary elimination by providing a high fluid intake help reduce the potential for stone formation. Hypercalcemia also increases the risk of cardiac arrhythmias and calcification around the surfaces of articular joints. Taking vital signs hourly is extreme unless the client begins to become symptomatic for arrhythmias. Muscle spasms are common in clients with hypocalcemia, not hypercalcemia. Low blood sugar is not associated with hyperparathyroidism.

Test Taking Strategy—Analyze to determine what information the question asks for, which is signs of hypercalcemia. Alternative-format "select all that apply" questions require considering each option independently to decide its merit in answering the question. Review evidence of the signs of hypercalcemia and methods for monitoring their manifestation if you had difficulty answering this question.
Cognitive Level—*Applying*
Client Needs Category—*Physiological integrity*
Client Needs Subcategory—*Physiological adaptation*

88. 1, 5, 6. An aneurysm is the ballooning or dilation of a blood vessel as a result of a weakness in the vessel wall. The aorta is commonly affected by high blood pressure. Smoking and age are other factors related to an abdominal aortic aneurysm. When the descending aorta develops an aneurysm, an examiner may feel a pulsating abdominal mass. Other signs and symptoms include mild midabdominal or back pain, peripheral emboli, and cool, cyanotic extremities. Extra heart sounds are associated with disorders of the conduction system or heart failure, not abdominal aortic aneurysms. Uneven chest movements are more often a sign of a pneumothorax or flail chest. Hollow sounds are normal assessment findings when percussing most areas of the abdomen.
Test Taking Strategy—Analyze to determine what information the question asks for, which is signs of an abdominal aortic aneurysm. Alternative-format "select all that apply" questions require considering each option independently to decide its merit in answering the question. Review the signs of an abdominal aortic aneurysm, including signs of its rupture, if you had difficulty answering this question.
Cognitive Level—*Applying*
Client Needs Category—*Physiological integrity*
Client Needs Subcategory—*Physiological adaptation*

89. 2. Cocaine is a central nervous system stimulant that increases blood pressure and heart rate and causes cardiac arrhythmias. Any or all of these cardiovascular effects can result in chest pain, tachycardia, or palpitations in an otherwise young, healthy person. Opioids, including heroin; barbiturates; and marijuana are central nervous system depressants that are more likely to cause bradycardia and hypotension.
Test Taking Strategy—Use the process of elimination to help select the option that identifies the abused substance most associated with the client's presenting symptoms. Options 1, 3, and 4 can be eliminated because they are central nervous system depressants. Option 2, because it is a central nervous system stimulant, emerges as the correct answer. Review the substances listed and evidence of their abuse if you had difficulty answering this question.
Cognitive Level—*Applying*
Client Needs Category—*Physiological integrity*
Client Needs Subcategory—*Pharmacological therapies*

90. 1. If a pulse oximeter is not used, a heart rate that remains within 60 to 100 beats/minute is within normal limits, indicating that the client is adequately oxygenated and not suffering from hypoxia. Tachycardia, bounding pulses, and arrhythmias are warning signs of oxygen deprivation. Noting the client's alertness is not the best method for evaluating the client's oxygenation status during suctioning. Normal capillary refill is about 3 seconds, not 5.
Test Taking Strategy—Use the process of elimination to help select the option that identifies the best evidence of adequate oxygenation. Option 4 can be immediately eliminated because it describes abnormal assessment data. Option 2 can be eliminated because a full pulse rather than a bounding pulse is considered normal. Although option 3 appears to have some merit, it does not indicate adequate oxygenation as well as option 1. Review assessment findings that indicate adequate oxygenation if you had difficulty answering this question.
Cognitive Level—*Evaluating*
Client Needs Category—*Physiological integrity*
Client Needs Subcategory—*Physiological adaptation*

91. 4. The nurse has an ethical and legal responsibility to protect the confidentiality of the person who is human immunodeficiency virus (HIV) positive. When persons test positive for HIV, they are provided counseling and education concerning measures for preventing its transmission. Legally, HIV-infected persons are required to divulge their infectious status to any and all potential sex partners. When safe sex practices and blood and body fluid precautions are followed, it is possible to prevent transmission of HIV from an infected person to a noninfected person. All of the remaining options are inappropriate.
Test Taking Strategy—Look at the key words "legally obligated." Select an option that describes compliance with the Health Insurance Portability and Accountability Act (HIPAA) of 1996, which protects a client's health information. Review HIPAA legislation and its implications for health care workers if you had difficulty answering this question.
Cognitive Level—*Analyzing*
Client Needs Category—*Safe and effective care environment*
Client Needs Subcategory—*Coordinated care*

92. 1. Early decelerations are usually benign and require no intervention. However, the nurse should continue to monitor the client to detect the presence of late decelerations, a more serious condition that requires intervention. If late decelerations occur, the nurse should turn the client to a side-lying position, elevate the legs, and notify the physician.
Test Taking Strategy—Use the process of elimination to help select the most appropriate nursing action based on the assessment finding. Because the described assessment finding is normal, option 1 is the best answer. Options 2, 3, and 4 would be

appropriate depending on the significance of an abnormal finding. Review normal and abnormal characteristics of fetal heart rate during active labor if you had difficulty answering this question.
Cognitive Level—*Analyzing*
Client Needs Category—*Health promotion and maintenance*
Client Needs Subcategory—*None*

93. 4. Buzzing, or tinnitus (ringing in the ears), is a common adverse effect experienced by individuals who take large, frequent doses of aspirin. GI upset and prolonged bleeding are other adverse effects associated with aspirin. Racing thoughts, polyuria, and diarrhea are not associated with aspirin use.

Test Taking Strategy—*Analyze the information about which the question asks, which is a statement that reflects an effect associated with aspirin. Option 1 can be immediately eliminated because aspirin does not affect cognitive ability. Although aspirin can cause gastric irritation, its use is not likely to cause diarrhea or increased urination. Option 4 emerges as the best answer. Review the effects and adverse effects of aspirin if you had difficulty answering this question.*
Cognitive Level—*Applying*
Client Needs Category—*Physiological integrity*
Client Needs Subcategory—*Pharmacological therapies*

94. 1. The combination of alcohol and a minor tranquilizer can cause central nervous system and respiratory depression. Many people have died accidentally or purposely when these two drugs are mixed. Generally, minor tranquilizers are given in low doses for short periods of time while an individual develops other effective coping techniques. Benzodiazepines such as alprazolam (Xanax) cause drowsiness rather than insomnia. Blood tests are generally unnecessary to monitor the effectiveness of benzodiazepine drug therapy.

Test Taking Strategy—*Use the process of elimination to help select an option that reflects accurate client learning in relation to prescribed alprazolam. Options 2, 3, and 4 are all incorrect statements that have no relationship to alprazolam. Option 1 emerges as the best answer because use of alcohol can potentiate the drug's sedative effect. Review the action of alprazolam and implications for health teaching if you had difficulty answering this question.*
Cognitive Level—*Evaluating*
Client Needs Category—*Physiological integrity*
Client Needs Subcategory—*Pharmacological therapies*

95. 1. The most common diagnostic tests for pneumonia are a complete blood count (CBC) (with white blood cell count) and a chest X-ray. Other diagnostic and laboratory tests used to establish a diagnosis include a sputum culture and Gram stain, arterial blood gas studies, pulse oximetry, blood cultures, and a bronchoscopy. Pulmonary function tests, hemoglobin and hematocrit, electrolyte levels, and

lung computed tomography scan are not used to diagnose pneumonia but may be used to diagnose other pulmonary disorders.

Test Taking Strategy—*Use the process of elimination to select the option that confirms or rules out pneumonia. Because pneumonia is a respiratory infection, it is most likely that the client will have an elevated white blood cell count and density in areas of the lungs where inflammation has occurred; these findings could be identified by the tests in option 1. Review the laboratory and diagnostic tests listed and their related purposes if you had difficulty answering this question.*
Cognitive Level—*Applying*
Client Needs Category—*Physiological integrity*
Client Needs Subcategory—*Reduction of risk potential*

96. 2. Frequently turning a client with a wet plaster cast helps to dry the complete circumference of the cast. The room would need to be heated to an uncomfortably high temperature to have a significant effect on drying the cast. Manually fanning the cast is tedious and time consuming. It would be impractical to take a client outside in the sun to dry a plaster cast.

Test Taking Strategy—*Use the process of elimination to help select the most accurate instruction as it relates to drying a plaster cast. Option 1 can be eliminated because a plaster cast produces heat as a chemical reaction, which in combination with heating the environment may elevate the toddler's temperature to an unsafe level. Option 3 can be eliminated because it is too inefficient. Option 4 can be eliminated because it is not a recommended method for drying a cast, and exposure to the sun may dry the cast surface before it dries the area next to the skin. Option 2 emerges as the best answer. Review the care of a client with a freshly applied plaster cast if you had difficulty answering the question.*
Cognitive Level—*Applying*
Client Needs Category—*Physiological integrity*
Client Needs Subcategory—*Basic care and comfort*

97. 3. When a pregnant client says that breathing is eased, it is an indication that lightening has occurred. This means that the fetus has settled into the pelvic inlet. Laypersons often remark that the baby has "dropped." Multipara clients may not experience this phenomenon until just before or during true labor. Urination generally increases with lightening because of the pressure exerted by the fetus on the bladder. Lightening may increase the incidence of backaches due to the descent of the fetus and relaxation of the pelvic joints before delivery. Braxton Hicks contractions are irregular, weak uterine contractions. When these contractions become more noticeable, they indicate impending labor.

Test Taking Strategy—*Use the process of elimination to help select an option that describes evidence of lightening during pregnancy. Options 1, 2, and 4 can be eliminated because they are unrelated or contradictory*

to the physical signs associated with lightening. Option 3 emerges as the best answer. Review the phenomenon known as lightening and its physiologic effects if you had difficulty answering this question.
Cognitive Level—*Applying*
Client Needs Category—*Health promotion and maintenance*
Client Needs Subcategory—*None*

98. 1. Seeing the chest rise is the best evidence that rescue breathing is being performed appropriately. A rising chest indicates that the airway is open and no air is leaking from the victim's nose or mouth. It also indicates that the rescuer is administering a sufficient volume of air. Dilated pupils are a sign that the brain is not receiving adequate oxygenation. A pulse indicates that cardiac compressions are unnecessary. The rescuer needs to seal or cover both the nose and the mouth.
Test Taking Strategy—*Use the process of elimination to help select the option that describes the best evidence of successfully oxygenating an unconscious client using rescue breathing. Option 2 can be immediately eliminated because dilated pupils are an indication of brain damage. Option 3 can be eliminated because the presence of a pulse is a positive sign of heart contraction and circulation of blood. Option 4 can be eliminated because it does not describe a correct technique when resuscitating a victim. Option 1 emerges as the best answer. Review the technique for performing rescue breathing and indications of its effectiveness if you had difficulty answering this question.*
Cognitive Level—*Evaluating*
Client Needs Category—*Physiological integrity*
Client Needs Subcategory—*Physiological adaptation*

99. 3. If a rectal tube has not brought relief after about 20 minutes, it is best to remove the tube temporarily and reinsert it a few hours later to allow the gas to travel farther down the large intestine. Rotating a rectal tube or replacing the tube with a larger one does not increase its effectiveness. If a rectal tube is already inserted correctly beyond the internal rectal sphincter, inserting it farther will not improve the potential for relieving abdominal distention.
Test Taking Strategy—*Use the process of elimination to select an option that describes the best action after having left a rectal tube in place for 20 minutes. Option 1 can be eliminated because if intestinal gas is in the area of the rectal tube, it would travel through the opening and external lumen. Although option 2 looks attractive, it can be potentially unsafe. Option 4 can be eliminated because replacing the current tube with a larger size does not ensure effectiveness. Option 3 emerges as the best answer because it may take additional time for peristalsis to move the intestinal gas toward the rectum. Review the use of a rectal tube for reducing abdominal distention if you had difficulty answering this question.*
Cognitive Level—*Analyzing*
Client Needs Category—*Physiological integrity*
Client Needs Subcategory—*Basic care and comfort*

100. 4. One of the side effects of phenytoin (Dilantin) is gingival hyperplasia. Therefore, attention to good oral hygiene is required. Phenytoin does not require additional fluid intake. Weight gain rarely occurs when taking this medication; therefore, daily weights are not necessary. To adequately control seizures, the client must take the prescribed dosage daily. It must never be tapered without a physician's order.
Test Taking Strategy—*Use the process of elimination to help select an option that accurately describes appropriate teaching of a client who has been prescribed phenytoin. Options 1 and 2 can be eliminated because this drug does not affect fluid retention or fluid loss. Option 3 can be eliminated because the client should remain compliant with the dosing instruction. Knowledge that phenytoin can cause gingival hyperplasia leads to selecting option 4 as the best answer. Review the side effects of phenytoin and implications for teaching if you had difficulty answering this question.*
Cognitive Level—*Applying*
Client Needs Category—*Physiological integrity*
Client Needs Subcategory—*Pharmacological therapies*

101. 2. Because of the disproportionate size of an adult's hand compared with an infant's heart and chest, the rescuer uses just two fingers to perform the chest compressions on an infant who is 1 year old or younger. The rate of compressions for an infant is 100 per minute. The heel of one hand may be used on children between ages 1 and 8. The interlocked fingers of both hands are used when performing chest compressions on individuals older than age 8. The palms of the hands are not used during chest compressions regardless of the victim's age.
Test Taking Strategy—*Use the process of elimination to help select the option that accurately describes the recommended method for administering chest compressions on an infant. Options 1 and 3 identify how to administer chest compressions on older victims; option 4 is incorrect regardless of the victim's age. Review the guidelines for administering chest compressions if you had difficulty answering this question.*
Cognitive Level—*Remembering*
Client Needs Category—*Physiological integrity*
Client Needs Subcategory—*Physiological adaptation*

102. 1. A myocardial infarction (MI) results from inadequate blood circulation to the heart muscle, resulting in poor myocardial oxygenation. Diminished oxygenation leads to ischemia or angina pain. Pain that accompanies an MI is not caused by damage to the arteries, impending circulatory collapse, or left ventricular muscle fatigue.
Test Taking Strategy—*Use the process of elimination to help select the option that accurately identifies the etiology of angina. Option 2 can be eliminated because damage to the myocardium is a consequence of inadequate oxygenation rather than the*

cause of ischemic pain. Options 3 and 4 can be eliminated because they describe consequences resulting from dysfunctional heart function and cardiac rhythm. Option 1 emerges as the best answer. Review the etiology of angina if you had difficulty answering this question.
Cognitive Level—*Understanding*
Client Needs Category—*Physiological integrity*
Client Needs Subcategory—*Physiological adaptation*

103. 1. Potassium levels are normally between 3.5 mEq/L and 5.0 mEq/L. Because the potassium level is less than 3.5 mEq/L, it is considered hypokalemia. Furosemide (Lasix) is a diuretic that depletes potassium. Therefore, the nurse should monitor the client's potassium daily. All of the other laboratory test values listed are within normal limits.
Test Taking Strategy—*Look at the key words "reported immediately," which indicates a priority nursing action. There is a narrow physiologic range of potassium in the blood; it is the only laboratory value that is abnormal in this list, which indicates that option 1 is the correct answer. Review normal values of serum electrolytes and the significance of abnormal blood levels of potassium if you had difficulty answering this question.*
Cognitive Level—*Analyzing*
Client Needs Category—*Physiological integrity*
Client Needs Subcategory—*Reduction of risk potential*

104. 2. Infants who are born with fetal alcohol syndrome tend to be extremely irritable at birth. As they mature, they may develop disorders characterized by hyperactivity. Lethargy, flaccidity, and jaundice are not exhibited by infants with fetal alcohol syndrome.
Test Taking Strategy—*Use the process of elimination to help select the option that best describes a finding associated with a newborn experiencing alcohol withdrawal. Because alcohol, a central nervous system depressant, blocks stimulating neurotransmitters while it is present in the blood, alcohol withdrawal is accompanied by physiologic stimulation. Options 1 and 2 can be eliminated because they reflect central nervous system depression. Option 4 can be eliminated because jaundice can be either a common newborn physiologic finding associated with high bilirubin in the blood or a consequence of liver damage that generally accompanies chronic alcohol abuse. Option 2 emerges as the best answer. Review the effects of alcohol withdrawal in a newborn infant if you had difficulty answering this question.*
Cognitive Level—*Applying*
Client Needs Category—*Psychosocial integrity*
Client Needs Subcategory—*None*

105. 2. One of the best ways to quantify the client's subjective response to a medication is to use some form of rating scale. The heart rate and blood pressure may be lowered with antianxiety medication, but that does not help evaluate the client's perception. The other assessment techniques are too vague to be significant.
Test Taking Strategy—*Use the process of elimination to help select an option that best describes the effectiveness of a minor tranquilizer. Option 1 can be eliminated because the data elicited are subjective. Option 3 appears attractive because it describes a calming effect. Option 4 may appear attractive, but it does not specifically describe the client's behavior during social interactions. Option 2 emerges as the best answer because it requires a more quantitative assessment, similar to the method used when performing a pain assessment. Review methods for assessing anxiety if you had difficulty answering this question.*
Cognitive Level—*Evaluating*
Client Needs Category—*Physiological integrity*
Client Needs Subcategory—*Pharmacological therapies*

106. 1. Although it is therapeutic to involve a client with a change in body image during care, acceptance of the change in body image cannot be rushed. Therefore, it is best for the nurse to accept the client's behavior and choice without judgment. This shows respect for the individual's unique effort to cope. In the early postoperative period, it is premature to suggest that the client needs professional counseling to adjust. How the nurse would deal with the same circumstance is immaterial. Saying that the stump does not look that bad is an evaluative statement based on the nurse's experience.
Test Taking Strategy—*Look at the key words "most appropriate." Select an option that reflects empathy when interacting with a client experiencing a change in body image. Options 2, 3, and 4 are judgmental and lack empathy. Review the meaning of empathy and how it applies to a nurse–client relationship if you had difficulty answering this question.*
Cognitive Level—*Analyzing*
Client Needs Category—*Psychosocial integrity*
Client Needs Subcategory—*None*

107. 1. Postural drainage is performed before eating or after consumed food has left the stomach. Done on a full stomach, the positioning, coughing, or expectorating may cause the person to feel nauseated and vomit. Vomiting may result in aspiration. Postural drainage is performed according to a scheduled routine to mobilize secretions, not just when an individual feels short of breath or is actively coughing. Although the respiratory therapist is consulted when planning postural drainage, this is not the deciding factor as to when it takes place.
Test Taking Strategy—*Use the process of elimination to select an option that accurately describes the optimum time for performing postural drainage.*

Although options 2 and 3 may appear attractive, shortness of breath and coughing should not limit the performance of postural drainage. Option 4 can be eliminated because postural drainage can be initiated independently by a nurse. It does not depend exclusively on a directive from a respiratory therapist, although the intervention could be a result of their mutual collaboration when caring for a client with a respiratory problem. Review the technique for performing postural drainage and when it is best performed if you had difficulty answering this question.
Cognitive Level—*Analyzing*
Client Needs Category—*Physiological integrity*
Client Needs Subcategory—*Reduction of risk potential*

108. 3. The earliest signs of hypoxia are manifested by behavioral changes, such as restlessness, apprehension, anxiety, decreased judgment, and drowsiness. As hypoxia progresses, the nurse typically observes dyspnea, tachypnea, and tachycardia. The client's blood pressure may become elevated due to anxiety. Cyanosis is one of the last signs the nurse is likely to observe in a client who is hypoxic.

> *Test Taking Strategy—Look at the key words "earliest indication." Select the option that is manifested in the beginning stage of hypoxia. Options 1, 2, and 4 are late signs. Review assessment findings associated with hypoxia, focusing on those that appear early and those that appear later, if you had difficulty answering this question.*
> **Cognitive Level**—*Applying*
> **Client Needs Category**—*Physiological integrity*
> **Client Needs Subcategory**—*Physiological adaptation*

109. 4. Maintaining cleanliness is of highest priority after a perineal prostatectomy because the client is at high risk for wound infection from organisms present in stool. Straining during defecation is contraindicated; therefore, performing Valsalva's maneuver (bearing down against a closed glottis) is inappropriate. A high Fowler's position can contribute to discomfort in the perineal incisional area. Laxatives are generally too harsh for prophylactically maintaining comfortable stool elimination.

> *Test Taking Strategy—Look at the key word "essential," which indicates a priority. The location of the surgical incision increases the potential for an infection that may have life-threatening consequences. Therefore, option 4 is the best answer. Options 1, 2, and 3 describe unsafe or inappropriate nursing actions. Review nursing care of a client undergoing a perineal prostatectomy if you had difficulty answering this question.*
> **Cognitive Level**—*Analyzing*
> **Client Needs Category**—*Safe and effective care environment*
> **Client Needs Subcategory**—*Safety and infection control*

110. 1, 2, 4, 6. HIPAA is an acronym for the Health Insurance Portability and Accountability Act of 1996, which provides guidelines to protect a client's health information. In this case, there were four responsible parties: the nurse that found the violation but did not correct it, the nurse's coworker who left the terminal unattended while still logged on, the manager of the unit who has 24-hour accountability for the employees of the department and, ultimately, the facility where both nurses work. In this case, the visitor is not responsible for the violation because HIPAA regulations only pertain to health care providers. Fortunately, the physician is not involved in this situation.

> *Test Taking Strategy—Analyze to determine what information the question asks for, which is responsible parties in the case of a violation of HIPAA guidelines. Alternative-format "select all that apply" questions require considering each option independently to decide its merit in answering the question. Review HIPAA legislation and the implications for health care workers if you had difficulty answering this question.*
> **Cognitive Level**—*Applying*
> **Client Needs Category**—*Safe and effective care environment*
> **Client Needs Subcategory**—*Coordinated care*

111.

4. Assist the registered nurse (RN) in obtaining informed consent for the blood transfusion.
2. Assist the registered nurse (RN) in gathering supplies to start an I.V. line using an 18-gauge needle.
3. Identify the client with a licensed coworker at the bedside.
1. Monitor vital signs at 15-minute to hourly intervals during the infusion.
5. Assist the registered nurse (RN) in infusing the blood within 4 hours.
6. Dispose of the blood bag and tubing in a biohazard container.

Before the transfusion, the client must sign an informed consent that provides the risks and benefits of the transfusion (4). After the informed consent is obtained, blood for type and crossmatch should be drawn, and the blood requisition should be completed and sent to the blood bank. Before the transfusion, an 18-gauge or 20-gauge I.V. line must be started with normal saline solution infusing (2). Once the blood is ready for transfusion and is present on the unit, the client must be identified at the bedside by two licensed nurses. These two nurses will also compare the information on the blood bag with that of the printed blood bank requisition and compare it to the client's arm bracelet (3). Vital signs must be taken at the beginning of the transfusion for baseline, after 15 minutes, and then according to facility policy (1). To prevent bacterial growth, blood must be infused within 4 hours of being started (5). After the blood has been infused, the blood bag and tubing should be disposed into a biohazard container (6).

Test Taking Strategy—Analyze to determine what information the question asks for, which is the proper sequence for nursing actions when assisting with a blood transfusion. Review the procedures for administering a unit of blood if you had difficulty answering this question.
Cognitive Level—Understanding
Client Needs Category—Safe and effective care environment
Client Needs Subcategory—Safety and infection control

112. **3.** The most common cause of a hernia is performing an activity that increases intra-abdominal pressure, such as lifting heavy objects. Increasing intra-abdominal pressure causes the intestine to protrude through areas in the abdominal musculature that are structurally weak. There is no correlation between having an umbilical hernia as a child and having an inguinal hernia as an adult. Inactivity plays a role in weakening abdominal muscles; however, in this situation, the client's hernia is most likely due to heavy lifting. Being underweight is not a factor related to inguinal hernias.

Test Taking Strategy—Use the process of elimination to help select the option that best identifies an etiology for developing an inguinal hernia. Option 1 can be eliminated because having had an umbilical hernia does not increase the risk for acquiring an inguinal hernia, neither does option 4, which suggests a relationship between low body weight and the development of a hernia. Option 2 may be an attractive choice, but it is not as significant as option 3 which is the correct answer. Review the etiologies associated with developing an inguinal hernia if you had difficulty answering this question.
Cognitive Level—Applying
Client Needs Category—Physiological integrity
Client Needs Subcategory—Physiological adaptation

113. **2.** Respiratory syncytial virus (RSV) is highly contagious and is spread by droplet contamination. It is associated with lower respiratory tract infections (bronchiolitis and pneumonia) in children younger than age 2. Hospitalization is usually required with RSV, and the main goal is to assist the child to breathe. An immune assay enzyme test to confirm RSV infection requires a specimen of nasal secretions. Throat swabs, sputum specimens, and blood specimens are not used to perform this particular diagnostic test.

Test Taking Strategy—Look at the key words "most appropriate" and "specimen." Knowing the type of secretions that most likely harbor RSV leads to selecting option 2 as the best answer. Review RSV, its mode of transmission, and tests to confirm the diagnosis if you had difficulty answering this question.
Cognitive Level—Analyzing
Client Needs Category—Physiological integrity
Client Needs Subcategory—Reduction of risk potential

114. **2, 6.** The car seat for a newborn should be tethered to a stationary area of the car, such as a hook on the floor. Correct car seat placement includes placing the seat in the rear seat and in a rear-facing position. Even though it is helpful to have the mother seated beside the car seat, this is not required.

Test Taking Strategy—Analyze to determine what information the question asks for, which is appropriate use of an infant car seat. Alternative-format "select all that apply" questions require considering each option independently to decide its merit in answering the question. Review the use of a car seat for ensuring the safety of an infant if you had difficulty answering this question.
Cognitive Level—Understanding
Client Needs Category—Safe and effective care environment
Client Needs Subcategory—Safety and infection control

115. **3.** The described symptoms are typical of a hypoglycemic reaction. Therefore, a normal non-fasting blood glucose level between 80 and 110 mg/dL is the best evidence that hypoglycemia has been corrected. The blood pressure is generally within normal limits or increased during hypoglycemia because of anxiety and adrenaline secretion. Assessing the blood pressure or skin temperature is not as valuable in determining the client's response to the nursing intervention. (Clients who perspire during a hypoglycemic reaction usually have skin that is cool and moist; the return to a warm temperature may be an indicator of other things, not just response to treatment.) Objective data such as a blood glucose levels are more accurate than having the client verbalize feeling better.

Test Taking Strategy—Use the process of elimination to help select the option that describes the best evidence of having successfully relieved an episode of hypoglycemia. Although options 1, 2, and 4 indicate that the client is stable, option 3 is the best objective evidence that the blood sugar is within a normal range. Review the signs and symptoms of hypoglycemia if you had difficulty answering this question.
Cognitive Level—Evaluating
Client Needs Category—Physiological integrity
Client Needs Subcategory—Physiological adaptation

116. 2. Oral contraceptives containing estrogen place individuals taking them at risk for thromboembolic disease. The risk of blood clot formation is from 3 to 11 times higher with this form of birth control than with other birth control measures. A history of blood clots is generally a contraindication to taking oral contraceptives. Iron supplements, nasal decongestants, and antacids do not promote the formation of blood clots.

> *Test Taking Strategy—Analyze to determine what information the question asks for, which is information in the client's history that correlates with the development of a thrombus. Knowing that there is a correlation between contraceptives containing estrogen and thrombus formation leads to selecting option 2 as the best answer. There is a greater increase in risk for thrombi if the client also smokes. Review the drug categories listed, noting especially the risks associated with contraceptives containing estrogen, if you had difficulty answering this question.*
> *Cognitive Level—Analyzing*
> *Client Needs Category—Physiological integrity*
> *Client Needs Subcategory—Pharmacological therapies*

117. 1. After a transurethral resection of the prostate (TURP), men experience retrograde ejaculation. That is, ejaculation is dry during orgasm. Semen is deposited within the bladder. The first voiding after intercourse is likely to appear cloudy because it contains the seminal fluid and sperm. Because of this change in physiology, men can expect to be unable to impregnate a sexual partner. Despite retrograde ejaculation, after a TURP men experience orgasms, achieve erections during sexual excitement, and maintain normal libidos.

> *Test Taking Strategy—Look at the key terms "best indication" and "understanding sexual function," and assess the options as they relate to a client's understanding of the effects of TURP. Option 1 is the best answer because it represents the likelihood of experiencing retrograde ejaculation. Options 2, 3, and 4 do not describe consequences of having a TURP. Review the sexual outcome after a TURP if you had difficulty answering this question.*
> *Cognitive Level—Evaluating*
> *Client Needs Category—Health promotion and maintenance*
> *Client Needs Subcategory—None*

118. 1. Heparin is an anticoagulant. The antidote for an overdose of heparin is protamine sulfate. Naloxone hydrochloride (Narcan) is used for respiratory depression and opioid overdoses. Vitamin K is the antidote for warfarin (Coumadin) overdose. Calcium gluconate is given to treat tetany or as the antidote for magnesium overdose when magnesium levels are toxic in pregnancy induced hypertension (PIH).

> *Test Taking Strategy—Analyze to determine what information the question asks for, which is the antidote to use for managing an overdose of heparin.*

Option 1 is the correct answer. Option 2 is used for managing an overdose of a sedative drug like a narcotic. Option 3 is used to manage an overdose of an anticoagulant like warfarin. Option 4 is used to manage tetany or hypermagesemia. Review the use of heparin and how an overdose is managed if you had difficulty answering this question.
Cognitive Level—Remembering
Client Needs Category—Physiological integrity
Client Needs Subcategory—Pharmacological therapies

119. 1, 3, 5. Cultural information can be invaluable when providing care for clients who are of a different culture, ethnicity, or religion. Therefore, performing a comprehensive cultural assessment will improve the client's care. Assessment of the client's food preferences is important because eating is important to recovery. Food preferences and diet may also be the cause of the disorder. The client's primary language and ability to speak and understand treatment goals and discharge instructions are important for the nurse to assess. Assessing language also provides information about whether an interpreter might be needed during the hospitalization. The client's religion is important to assess because of its possible prevalence in the client's daily life and current health practices and beliefs. Bodily functions, such as bowel movements, urination, and menstruation, are sensitive topics that most clients from a different culture are reluctant to discuss with the nurse during the initial admission assessment. Breast and penis or scrotal diseases as well as reproductive disorders are also topics that may be embarrassing for the client to discuss (especially if the client's language skills are inadequate or the client's understanding of the language is limited).

Asking the client to tell time is an inappropriate question. What the nurse really needs to know is the significance of time to the client because attitudes about time vary culturally. In some cultures, such as in the United States, life is scheduled around a strict time frame; being "on time" is a value. However, in some cultures time is less important. Personal interactions, human contacts, and official business are more highly valued.

Asking the client about pain is not part of the cultural assessment. What the nurse really needs to know is how the client expresses pain based on cultural, ethnic, and religious beliefs and values.

> *Test Taking Strategy—Analyze to determine what information the question asks for, which is the components of the cultural assessment. Alternative-format "select all that apply" questions require considering each option independently to decide its merit in answering the question. Review the components of a culturally based assessment if you had difficulty answering this question.*
> *Cognitive Level—Analyzing*
> *Client Needs Category—Psychosocial integrity*
> *Client Needs Subcategory—None*

120. 3. Although computer documentation is by data entry rather than on paper, computerized charting is still considered a legal medical record and can be subpoenaed in court. A nurse's ID and password are secure and private and should never be shared under any circumstance. The nurse should call technical support, explain that access has been denied, and have technical support assist with regranting access to the password and ID. Forgoing documentation is not appropriate because if an action was not documented, it was not done. Computers should never be left on and unattended, and the nurse should never attempt to use one that is. In addition, the nurse should never use or ask to use anyone else's password or ID to gain access to the computer. These actions are grounds for disciplinary action in most institutions.

Test Taking Strategy—Look at the key word "most appropriate," and select an option that reflects compliance with the principles of documentation requiring that each entry be made by the person who records the information. Therefore, obtaining assistance from technical support (option 3) is the best answer for this question. Review guidelines for documentation whether it is written or entered on a computer if you had difficulty answering this question.

Cognitive Level—Analyzing
Client Needs Category—Safe and effective care environment
Client Needs Subcategory—Coordinated care

121. 1. Measures should be taken to minimize crying because excessive crying increases oxygen demand, which increases cardiac workload. The infant should be placed in semi-Fowler's position. Holding is encouraged to decrease the infant's anxiety and cardiac workload. The infant is fed using a soft nipple with a large hole to decrease the effort required to suck.

Test Taking Strategy—Look at the key words "most appropriate" in relation to the needs of an infant with a congenital heart condition. Recognizing that crying can affect oxygenation, which is impaired due to cardiovascular pathology, leads to selecting option 1 as the best answer. Option 2 does not promote oxygenation. Option 3 is appropriate for meeting the emotional needs of the infant and minimizing distress, but it is not as specific as option 1. Option 4 would require energy, which increases the need for oxygen. Review nursing care of a client with a congenital heart condition if you had difficulty answering this question.

Cognitive Level—Analyzing
Client Needs Category—Physiological integrity
Client Needs Subcategory—Reduction of risk potential

122. 4. Enoxaparin (Lovenox) is a subcutaneously administered anticoagulant that reduces the risk of developing deep vein thrombosis and pulmonary emboli after surgical procedures when the client cannot ambulate as usual. There is no indication that enoxaparin has any effect on tissue healing or limiting bleeding, and it does not break up clots that have formed.

Test Taking Strategy—Analyze to determine what information the question asks for, which is the desired action of enoxaparin. Knowing that enoxaparin is an anticoagulant leads to selecting option 4 as the best answer. Option 2 may look attractive, but heparin and its derivatives do not lyse clots that already exist; they only prevent clots from forming. Review the action of enoxaparin if you had difficulty answering this question.

Cognitive Level—Understanding
Client Needs Category—Physiological integrity
Client Needs Subcategory—Pharmacological therapies

123. 1, 2, 4. Enoxaparin (Lovenox) is an anticoagulant that, when prepackaged, contains a nitrogen bubble that must be left intact in the syringe (not expelled before giving). Its purpose is to propel the medication deeper into the tissue, thereby minimizing bruising. Bruising is also minimized if the medication is not allowed to run down the sides of the needle, as would happen if the needle was pointed up toward the ceiling. Bruising will also be minimized if the nurse flicks the drop of Lovenox from the tip of the needle before injecting it. In addition, the client should be instructed to avoid rubbing the site for at least an hour after administration. Firm direct pressure to the injection site will cause bruising. Direct pressure should only be done when prolonged bleeding occurs, but should not be evident with subcutaneous injections. Enoxaparin is given at a 90-degree angle, usually into the abdomen, where faster absorption of the medication is possible.

Test Taking Strategy—Analyze to determine what information the question asks for, which is nursing actions when administering enoxaparin. Alternative-format "select all that apply" questions require considering each option independently to decide its merit in answering the question. Review the technique for injecting a low molecular weight heparin if you had difficulty answering this question.

Cognitive Level—Analyzing
Client Needs Category—Physiological integrity
Client Needs Subcategory—Pharmacological therapies

124. 2. Absence seizures occur most frequently in childhood and adolescence. They involve a lapse of consciousness for 5 to 10 seconds with a blank facial expression and often include frequent repetitive movements. Afterward, the child typically resumes normal activity as if there had never been any seizure activity. Myoclonic and clonic seizures involve motor function disturbances. Partial seizures are common types of seizures that do not result in loss of consciousness, but they are not the most common type for this age-group.

Test Taking Strategy—Analyze to determine what information the question asks for, which is a type of seizure characterized by blinking and brief episodes of inattentiveness. This leads to selection option 2 as the best answer. Review the manifestations of seizures listed if you had difficulty answering this question.
Cognitive Level—Applying
Client Needs Category—Physiological integrity
Client Needs Subcategory—Physiological adaptation

125. 1, 2, 3, 4, 6. The Emergency Medical Treatment and Active Labor Act (EMTALA) requires hospitals and ambulance services to provide care to anyone who requires emergency medical treatment regardless of that person's ability to pay. EMTALA applies when an individual with a medical emergency comes to the emergency department. It does not pertain to clients who are classified as inpatients. An emergency medical condition is when a client has acute symptoms of sufficient severity that absence of immediate medical attention could jeopardize the client's health, impair body function, result in dysfunction to an organ, or cause pain. The types of clients that warrant emergent medical treatment include clients with psychiatric disturbances; clients who have a history of substance abuse or sexual, physical, and mental abuse; clients who are a threat to themselves or others; and clients who demonstrate aggressive or violent behavior, attempted suicide, depression, or the inability to perceive danger. Other circumstances that constitute emergent medical conditions involve pregnant women who are in labor. EMTALA pertains when there is not adequate time to transfer to another hospital or the transfer poses a threat to the woman or her unborn child. If a client has an emergent medical condition, the hospital must stabilize the client within the capability of the hospital before transferring to another institution or discharging.
Test Taking Strategy—Analyze the information about which the question asks, which is the clients covered by EMTALA. Alternative-format "select all that apply" questions require considering each option independently to decide its merit in answering the question. Review the EMTALA and its implication for health care workers and the clients who require emergency care if you had difficulty answering this question.
Cognitive Level—Applying
Client Needs Category—Safe and effective care environment
Client Needs Subcategory—Coordinated care

126. 2. Removing moisture from the infant's body will prevent heat loss by evaporation, which occurs when a liquid is converted to a vapor. Wrapping an infant in a warmed blanket prevents heat loss by conduction, which occurs if the infant's skin comes into direct contact with a cold surface or object. Positioning the crib away from outside windows on cold days prevents heat loss by radiation,

which occurs if the infant is placed near cold objects. Positioning the crib away from air conditioning vents prevents heat loss by convection, which occurs if the infant comes into contact with cold moving air.
Test Taking Strategy—Use the process of elimination to help select the option that describes the best method for preventing evaporative heat loss in an infant. Options 1, 3, and 4 can be eliminated because they describe ways of preventing heat loss by means other than evaporation. Review methods by which heat loss occurs if you had difficulty answering this question.
Cognitive Level—Analyzing
Client Needs Category—Health promotion and maintenance
Client Needs Subcategory—None

127. 3. Gestational diabetes usually does not persist after delivery of the baby. Some women who have had gestational diabetes develop type 2 (non–insulin-dependent) diabetes mellitus, but this is not usually the case. Gestational diabetes is present only during pregnancy; therefore, it could not be present in the client's childhood. Oral hypoglycemics are not given during pregnancy because they may harm the fetus. Women who have diabetes during pregnancy are more prone to having large-for-gestational age babies.
Test Taking Strategy—Analyze to determine what information the question asks for, which is a statement that reflects an accurate understanding of gestational diabetes. Option 3 is inaccurate. Options 1, 2, and 4 are all inaccurate statements. Review gestational diabetes and its relation to health if you had difficulty answering this question.
Cognitive Level—Evaluating
Client Needs Category—Physiological integrity
Client Needs Subcategory—Physiological adaptation

128. 2. One of the manifestations of bacterial meningitis is a bulging fontanel, which occurs secondary to increased intracranial pressure. The white blood cell count may be elevated with any type of bacterial infection. The infant will usually have a high-pitched, not a low-pitched, cry. The glucose level in cerebrospinal fluid is decreased, not increased, in bacterial meningitis.
Test Taking Strategy—Analyze to determine what information the question asks for, which is a diagnostic finding that correlates with bacterial meningitis in an infant. Knowing that an inflammation of the meninges is accompanied by swelling of localized tissue and that the fontanels are not fused at this age leads to the selection of option 2 as the best answer. Options 1, 3, and 4 all describe findings that are not associated with bacterial meningitis affecting a 7-month-old infant. Review the age at which fontanels fuse as well as the pathophysiology that correlates with bacterial meningitis, especially as it affects an infant, if you had difficulty answering this question.

Cognitive Level—Applying
Client Needs Category—Physiological integrity
Client Needs Subcategory—Physiological adaptation

129. 1. Head trauma resulting in long-term brain changes increases the risk of seizure disorder by approximately 50%. No correlation is noted between drug use and seizure disorder. Seizures may accompany meningitis especially when there is a high fever, but there is only a 4% to 10% possibility that a seizure disorder would follow recovery from meningitis. A seizure is not related to spinal cord trauma.

> *Test Taking Strategy—Look at the key words "most common risk factor" and "seizure disorder." Select the option that shows an accurate relationship between these key words, which is option 1. Options 2, 3, and 4 do not accurately identify risk factors for a seizure disorder. Review risk factors associated with a seizure disorder if you had difficulty answering this question.*

Cognitive Level—Applying
Client Needs Category—Health promotion and maintenance
Client Needs Subcategory—None

130. 2. Children at this age are magical thinkers and enjoy pretend play. As they grow older and begin interacting more with other children, their interest in pretend play decreases. Six-year-old children commonly are very busy, boisterous, and bossy; are sensitive to criticism; and usually have short attention spans, demonstrated by beginning one or more tasks but rarely completing them.

> *Test Taking Strategy—Analyze to determine what information the question asks for, which is a developmental characteristic of a school-age child. Option 2 correctly describes a characteristic of a school-age child. The remaining options are not characteristics of young school-age children. Review the developmental characteristics of school-age children if you had difficulty answering this question.*

Cognitive Level—Applying
Client Needs Category—Health promotion and maintenance
Client Needs Subcategory—None

Comprehensive Test 2

Directions: With a pencil, blacken the space in front of the option you have chosen for your correct answer.

1. A client comes to the clinic complaining of epigastric pain. The client reportedly takes several nonprescription over-the-counter medications on a regular basis. Which drug identified by the nurse is most likely related to the client's current complaint?
[ ] **1.** Milk of magnesia, which the client takes for constipation
[ ] **2.** Aspirin, which the client takes for arthritis
[ ] **3.** Nyquil (combination medication containing acetaminophen, dextromethorphan, doxylamine, and pseudoephedrine), which the client takes to fall asleep
[ ] **4.** Benadryl (diphenhydramine), which the client takes for allergy symptoms

2. A client who is 3 months' pregnant complains to the nurse of feeling tired. Which nursing advice is best to give this client?
[ ] **1.** "Do most of your work just after lunch."
[ ] **2.** "Increase your prenatal vitamins to two."
[ ] **3.** "Sleep later in the morning."
[ ] **4.** "Rest whenever you feel tired."

3. A pregnant client comes to the prenatal clinic for a routine visit. As the nurse is completing a nutritional analysis, it is determined that the client needs additional iron. Which food is best for the nurse to include in a diet plan for this pregnant client who needs additional iron?
[ ] **1.** Potatoes
[ ] **2.** Legumes
[ ] **3.** Oranges
[ ] **4.** Cheese

4. An unconscious adult is brought to the emergency department and is suspected of overdosing on heroin. Which initial medication would the nurse have on hand ready for physician's orders?
[ ] **1.** Methadone hydrochloride (Dolophine)
[ ] **2.** Succinylcholine chloride (Anectine)
[ ] **3.** Naloxone hydrochloride (Narcan)
[ ] **4.** Pancuronium bromide (Pavulon)

5. The postpartum nurse is reviewing the physician's orders for a bisacodyl (Dulcolax) suppository. If the nurse is caring for the following postpartum clients, for which client would the nurse need the physician's orders clarified?
[ ] **1.** A client who has hemorrhoids
[ ] **2.** A client who is breast-feeding
[ ] **3.** A client who has a third-degree perineal tear
[ ] **4.** A client who had a vacuum extraction delivery

6. A client with abdominal pain has been diagnosed with gallstones. When the client asks about treatment to remove the gallstones with extracorporeal lithotripsy. What is the best explanation of this method of treatment that the nurse can provide?
[ ] **1.** "Extracorporeal lithotripsy dissolves gallstones with strong chemicals."
[ ] **2.** "Extracorporeal lithotripsy pulverizes gallstones with shock waves."
[ ] **3.** "Extracorporeal lithotripsy removes gallstones with a special endoscope."
[ ] **4.** "Extracorporeal lithotripsy removes gallstones by binding them to a sticky resin."

7. A client who is 4 months' pregnant states that she lives on a limited income and has a problem purchasing enough meat to supply sufficient protein for her diet. Which food can the nurse recommend to supplement the client's meat source?
[ ] **1.** Broccoli
[ ] **2.** Cauliflower
[ ] **3.** Fortified cereal
[ ] **4.** Dried beans

8. When teaching a postmenopausal client about breast self-examination, which instruction by the nurse is most accurate?
[ ] **1.** "Examine your breasts on awakening."
[ ] **2.** "Examine your breasts on the first day of the month."
[ ] **3.** "Examine your breasts after you finish your shower."
[ ] **4.** "Examine your breasts before your mammogram."

9. The urine of a client who is 6 months' pregnant tests positive for albumin. The nurse correctly assumes that the client is probably developing which complication of pregnancy?

[ ] **1.** Preeclampsia
[ ] **2.** Liver impairment
[ ] **3.** Amniotic embolism
[ ] **4.** Gestational diabetes

10. A 10-year-old child is admitted to the hospital with endocarditis secondary to rheumatic fever. Which assessment finding in the child's medical history is most consistent with this condition?

[ ] **1.** The child had a congenital heart defect at birth.
[ ] **2.** The child had a recent untreated streptococcal infection.
[ ] **3.** The child has consistently had clubbing of the fingers.
[ ] **4.** The child failed to receive proper immunizations for measles.

11. A pregnant client is admitted to the labor and delivery area with vaginal bleeding. The physician's routine admission orders include the administration of an enema. Which action by the nurse is most appropriate?

[ ] **1.** Administer the enema as ordered.
[ ] **2.** Withhold the enema at this time.
[ ] **3.** Give the enema if the client reports constipation.
[ ] **4.** Substitute a laxative for the cleansing enema.

12. A client had a hysterectomy 10 hours ago. The nurse assesses the client and finds that her blood pressure has fallen abruptly. Which action by the nurse is most appropriate at this time?

[ ] **1.** Continue to monitor the blood pressure every 15 minutes.
[ ] **2.** Document the information on the client's chart.
[ ] **3.** Inform the surgeon about the client's condition.
[ ] **4.** Change the client to a Fowler's position.

13. A postoperative client who just had a transurethral prostatectomy asks why he must drink so much water. Which response by the nurse is most accurate?

[ ] **1.** "It helps keep the catheter unobstructed."
[ ] **2.** "It promotes excretion of toxic wastes."
[ ] **3.** "It helps increase your bladder capacity."
[ ] **4.** "It promotes postoperative bladder retraining."

14. The physician performs a vaginal examination on a client in labor and states that the client is completely effaced and fully dilated. At this time, the nurse correctly plans to meet the needs of the client who is entering which stage of labor?

[ ] **1.** First
[ ] **2.** Second
[ ] **3.** Third
[ ] **4.** Fourth

15. When a female client requires urinary catheterization, where should the nurse insert the catheter? Indicate the correct location on the diagram with an X.

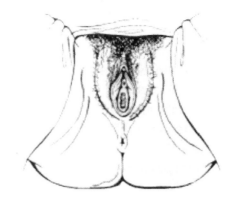

16. A resident of a long-term care facility has a history of repeated falls after attempting to get up from the wheelchair. Which instruction to the nursing team is most appropriate to prevent further client falls?

[ ] **1.** "Use a sheet to tie the client to the wheelchair."
[ ] **2.** "Keep the client within view at all times."
[ ] **3.** "Assess client needs on a frequent basis."
[ ] **4.** "Let me know if she needs to be sedated."

17. The nurse is assessing for side effects from the administration of a dose of penicillin (Bicillin). Which assessment finding best justifies withholding the next I.M. administration of penicillin until consulting the prescribing physician?

[ ] **1.** The client states that the injection sites are painful.
[ ] **2.** The client shows the nurse a red, itchy rash.
[ ] **3.** The client's body temperature is 100°F (37.8°C).
[ ] **4.** The client complains of a sore mouth.

18. The admitting nurse documents a client's dietary information. Which information is most likely to contribute to the client's complaint of constipation?

[ ] **1.** The client eats five daily servings of fresh vegetables.
[ ] **2.** The client eats breakfast cereal with skim milk daily.
[ ] **3.** The client drinks four glasses of liquids per day.
[ ] **4.** The client substitutes grains and beans for meat.

19. The nurse is assigned six clients during the afternoon shift on a medical-surgical unit. After receiving report on the following clients, arrange the clients in the most appropriate order of nursing assessment.

1. A young adult who has been given discharge instructions but is awaiting a ride
2. A new postoperative client being transferred by the nursing assistant into a bed
3. An elderly client admitted with unstable angina who reports sternal chest pain
4. An adult who is awaiting transport to the operating room for surgery in 1 hour
5. A client with an afternoon blood sugar reading of 285 mg/dL
6. A client with history of gallstones reporting abdominal pain of 7 out of 10

20. A postoperative client asks the nurse to explain the purpose of the abdominal Penrose drain. Which statement by the nurse best explains the reason for using a Penrose drain?

[ ] **1.** "A Penrose drain decreases scar tissue formation."
[ ] **2.** "A Penrose drain helps fluid escape from the surgical area."
[ ] **3.** "A Penrose drain provides a means for irrigating the wound."
[ ] **4.** "A Penrose drain releases accumulating intestinal gas."

21. During a home health visit, the nurse asks the parents of a 7-year-old to describe how they give the child's medication through a gastrostomy tube. Which response by the parents indicates the need for additional teaching?

[ ] **1.** "We crush the medication finely and mix it with 30 mL of warm water."
[ ] **2.** "Before giving the medication, we flush the tube with 50 mL of water."
[ ] **3.** "We mix the medication into the bag of tube-feeding formula before instilling it."
[ ] **4.** "We flush the tube with 50 mL of water after administering the medication."

22. The nurse recognizes that a safe pediatric dose of oral cephalexin (Keflex) is 25 mg/kg/day in four equally divided doses. What is the safe single dose in milligrams for a child weighing 44 pounds?

23. A physician orders postural drainage for a client with pneumonia. Which nursing action best facilitates a therapeutic outcome for the client?

[ ] **1.** Placing the client in a supine position
[ ] **2.** Encouraging the client to cough deeply
[ ] **3.** Having the client breathe through the mouth
[ ] **4.** Instructing the client to breathe slowly

24. A 75-year-old client comes to the diabetic clinic for a scheduled visit. Which assessment finding indicates that the client with diabetes requires additional teaching regarding foot care?

[ ] **1.** The client has placed lamb's wool between the toes.
[ ] **2.** The client trims calluses with a nail clipper.
[ ] **3.** The client's toenails are short and cut straight across.
[ ] **4.** The client wears white nonelastic foot socks.

25. When preparing a client for insertion of a nasogastric (NG) tube, how should the nurse position the client's neck to facilitate introducing the tube into the nostril?

[ ] **1.** Flexed
[ ] **2.** Extended
[ ] **3.** Rotated to the left
[ ] **4.** Hyperextended

26. When providing discharge instructions to a client receiving warfarin sodium (Coumadin), the nurse teaches the importance of regular monitoring for which laboratory value?

[ ] **1.** Platelet levels in the blood
[ ] **2.** Partial thromboplastin time (PTT)
[ ] **3.** Circulating blood volume
[ ] **4.** International Normalized Ratio (INR)

27. A previously healthy client comes to the emergency department complaining of severe nausea and vomiting hours after eating in a restaurant. Which assessment question best determines if a food-borne pathogen is the cause of the client's symptoms?

[ ] **1.** "What foods did you eat?"
[ ] **2.** "Did you take something for your nausea?"
[ ] **3.** "Did your food look spoiled?"
[ ] **4.** "Have you ever had food poisoning?"

28. If the care plan of a client receiving internal radiation therapy includes all the following nursing interventions, which intervention requires revision because it is unsafe?

[ ] **1.** Maintain a radiation symbol on the outside wall or door to the client's room.
[ ] **2.** Inform all non-nursing personnel that the client is receiving radiation therapy.
[ ] **3.** Wear a radiation-monitoring badge when providing care to the client.
[ ] **4.** Assign the same personnel to consistently care for the client.

29. Which question is essential for the nurse to ask before a client undergoes an intravenous pyelogram (IVP)?

[ ] **1.** "Are you afraid of needles?"
[ ] **2.** "Have you ever had X-rays taken?"
[ ] **3.** "Do you have any allergies to seafood?"
[ ] **4.** "Have you experienced fear of confined places?"

30. Which diversional activity is best to include in the care plan of a client with recent loss of vision?

[ ] **1.** Listening to a radio or audiotapes
[ ] **2.** Talking with other clients on the unit
[ ] **3.** Listening to television
[ ] **4.** Reading books set in Braille

31. An 8-year-old child is brought to the emergency department after falling from a swing. Which assessment finding provides the nurse with the best evidence that the child has a compound fracture?

[ ] **1.** Complaint of pain at the injury site
[ ] **2.** Abnormal mobility of the injured extremity
[ ] **3.** Grinding sensation over the injury site
[ ] **4.** Bone protruding at the injury site

32. If a client is to receive 1,000 mL of dextrose 5% in normal saline solution over an 8-hour period, the nurse correctly sets the infusion pump to administer which hourly volume?

[ ] **1.** 50 mL
[ ] **2.** 100 mL
[ ] **3.** 125 mL
[ ] **4.** 150 mL

33. Which laboratory test result, if elevated, is most indicative to the nurse that a child has rheumatic fever?

[ ] **1.** Antinuclear antibody test
[ ] **2.** Antistreptolysin O titer
[ ] **3.** Heterophile antibody titer
[ ] **4.** Fluorescent antibody test

34. A 350-pound (159-kg) client with diabetes is hospitalized. The nurse plans to give the client's morning insulin in the abdomen. Which needle angle is most appropriate?

[ ] **1.** 15 degrees
[ ] **2.** 30 degrees
[ ] **3.** 45 degrees
[ ] **4.** 90 degrees

35. When planning discharge instructions for a client who has had a prostatectomy, which information is most appropriate for the nurse to include?

[ ] **1.** Avoid eating foods containing roughage.
[ ] **2.** Avoid heavy lifting and strenuous exercise.
[ ] **3.** Use an enema if constipation occurs.
[ ] **4.** Limit fluid intake to eight glasses per day.

36. When caring for a client with expressive (motor) aphasia, which nursing intervention specifically addressing the expressive (motor) aphasia is best to include in the care plan of this client?

[ ] **1.** Use a louder than normal voice when communicating with the client.
[ ] **2.** Write questions and directions for the client to read.
[ ] **3.** Speak in short sentences to promote understanding.
[ ] **4.** Give the client time to respond to questions.

37. A chest tube was placed in a client with a hemothorax 4 hours ago and was connected to a closed water-seal drainage system. When the oncoming shift nurse assesses the system, which assessment finding should be reported immediately?

[ ] **1.** Approximately 2 cm of water is in the water-seal chamber.
[ ] **2.** The water-seal chamber is bubbling continuously.
[ ] **3.** Dark, bloody drainage is in the collection chamber.
[ ] **4.** Diminished breath sounds are heard in the lung with the hemothorax.

38. A client has returned to the nursing unit after a cardiac catheterization. When assessing the client's femoral pulse, where should the nurse's fingers be placed?

[ ] **1.** Behind the knee
[ ] **2.** On the dorsum of the foot
[ ] **3.** Into the inguinal area
[ ] **4.** Over the lower tibia

39. Which nursing assessment finding is the best indication that a pregnant client is in the transition phase of labor?

[ ] **1.** The client states that she feels a gush of water coming from her vagina.
[ ] **2.** The client states that she feels as if she needs to have a bowel movement.
[ ] **3.** The client tells her coach not to touch her but also asks not to be left alone.
[ ] **4.** The client asks for blankets and tells the nurse that she cannot stop shivering.

40. The nurse asks a postpartum client to explain how she performs Kegel exercises. Which description provides the best evidence that she is performing Kegel exercises correctly?

[ ] **1.** "I tighten, and then alternately relax, my perineal muscles."

[ ] **2.** "I lie supine and alternately raise and lower my legs."

[ ] **3.** "I tighten my abdominal muscles for 45 seconds for a total of 10 repetitions."

[ ] **4.** "I roll from side to back to side four to six times an hour."

41. The nurse is administering specific allergens for a client's allergy testing from a multiple-dose vial. Which nursing action demonstrates the correct technique for withdrawing a parenteral drug from a multiple-dose vial?

[ ] **1.** Withdrawing the entire volume in a syringe, then discarding the unneeded portion

[ ] **2.** Injecting 1 mL more of air than the amount of the drug to be withdrawn

[ ] **3.** Refrigerating the medication vial for 10 minutes before withdrawing the drug

[ ] **4.** Injecting the same volume of air into the vial as liquid that will be removed

42. A home care nurse is instructing a family member on administering an injection. When the family member demonstrates the injection technique for the nurse, which technique is potentially unsafe?

[ ] **1.** The family member wears clean gloves when administering the injection.

[ ] **2.** The family member discards the empty syringe in a biohazard container.

[ ] **3.** The family member recaps the needle securely before discarding the syringe.

[ ] **4.** The family member uses an alcohol swab to disinfect the injection site.

43. When caring for a child with hemophilia, which assessment finding should the nurse immediately report to the physician?

[ ] **1.** The child is experiencing anorexia.

[ ] **2.** The child has discomfort from joint pain.

[ ] **3.** The child's mood is somewhat depressed.

[ ] **4.** The child has developed nasal congestion.

44. A client arrives in the emergency department with symptoms of a fever, muscle rigidity, elevated or labile blood pressure, and confusion. A diagnosis of neuroleptic malignant syndrome (NMS) is made. Which of the following evidence supports this diagnosis?

[ ] **1.** The client was prescribed an antipsychotic medication 2 weeks ago.

[ ] **2.** A magnetic resonance imaging (MRI) scan revealed a past bleed in the occipital lobe of the brain.

[ ] **3.** The white blood cell count was documented on the laboratory report as 6,100 cells/mcg.

[ ] **4.** The family reports the client has had an increase in stress at work.

45. When an unlicensed nursing assistant provides care for a 10-month-old infant, which observation indicates to the nurse that the technician requires additional teaching?

[ ] **1.** The room temperature is set at 75°F (23.8°C) during the infant's bath.

[ ] **2.** For oral hygiene, the infant's teeth are swabbed with wet gauze.

[ ] **3.** Before bathing, the water temperature is checked with an elbow.

[ ] **4.** The infant's chest is sprinkled with baby powder after the bath.

46. In the emergency department, the nurse notes multiple needle punctures on a client's arms. The nurse correctly suspects that the client is abusing which category of drugs?

[ ] **1.** Opiates

[ ] **2.** Barbiturates

[ ] **3.** Amphetamines

[ ] **4.** Hallucinogens

47. An older adult client is comatose and on life support. The family asks that life-support measures be discontinued. Which method is best for determining whether it is appropriate to carry out the family's request?

[ ] **1.** Considering the cost of continued life-support measures

[ ] **2.** Checking if the client's insurance covers life-support measures

[ ] **3.** Validating that all immediate relatives are in total agreement

[ ] **4.** Examining the specifications in the client's advance directive

48. When a client ingests a toxic substance either intentionally or accidentally, which initial information is most important for the nurse to obtain?

[ ] **1.** The client's age

[ ] **2.** Who found the client

[ ] **3.** The substance involved

[ ] **4.** The client's medical history

49. A nursing assistant voices concern for personal safety when assigned to care for a client with acquired immunodeficiency syndrome (AIDS). Which information from the nurse is best for allaying the nursing assistant's fears?

[ ] **1.** The life expectancy for AIDS clients is longer than in previous years.

[ ] **2.** AIDS is commonly transmitted by contact with blood and body fluids.

[ ] **3.** Standard precautions can prevent human immunodeficiency virus (HIV) transmission.

[ ] **4.** If infected, workers' compensation will cover the cost of care.

50. Immediately after a pregnant client's membranes rupture, which nursing action is a priority?
[ ] **1.** Monitoring the fetal heart rate
[ ] **2.** Beginning antibiotic administration
[ ] **3.** Putting a waterproof pad beneath the client
[ ] **4.** Placing the client in Trendelenburg's position

51. An elderly client presents to the physician's office with symptoms of a respiratory infection. Based on the nurse's knowledge, which of the following risk factors increases the client's susceptibility to pneumonia? Select all that apply.
[ ] **1.** Sudden weight gain
[ ] **2.** Smoking and alcohol intake
[ ] **3.** Anemia and hyperactive gag reflex
[ ] **4.** Dehydration
[ ] **5.** Decreased force of cough
[ ] **6.** Deteriorating cilia in the respiratory tract

52. In which of the following positions is it best for the nurse to place the client with suspected heart failure?
[ ] **1.** Semi-sitting (low Fowler's)
[ ] **2.** Left side-lying (Sims')
[ ] **3.** Sitting upright (high Fowler's)
[ ] **4.** Lying supine with the head lowered (Trendelenburg's)

53. When the client with a slow-bleeding cerebral aneurysm asks for assistance to the toilet for a bowel movement, which nursing response is most appropriate?
[ ] **1.** Comply with the client's request.
[ ] **2.** Obtain a bedside commode.
[ ] **3.** Place the client on a bedpan.
[ ] **4.** Remove the stool digitally administering a suppository.

54. If the nurse collects all of the following data when performing a newborn's initial assessment, which assessment finding is most important to report?
[ ] **1.** Blue hands and feet
[ ] **2.** Flaccid muscle tone
[ ] **3.** Heart rate over 100 beats/minute
[ ] **4.** Loud, vigorous cry

55. A maintenance worker in a health agency comes to a nurse after receiving a minor finger burn. Which first-aid measure is correct in this situation?
[ ] **1.** Apply petroleum jelly to the burn.
[ ] **2.** Cover the burn with nonallergenic tape.
[ ] **3.** Immerse the burned area in cool water.
[ ] **4.** Place the burned area in warm water.

56. Which nursing assessment finding provides the best evidence that a client with acute angle-closure glaucoma is responding to drug therapy?
[ ] **1.** Swelling of the eyelids is decreased.
[ ] **2.** Redness of the sclera is reduced.
[ ] **3.** Eye pain is reduced or eliminated.
[ ] **4.** Peripheral vision is diminished.

57. Which nursing action is most correct before instilling eardrops in a client's ear?
[ ] **1.** Warm the medication to room temperature.
[ ] **2.** Refrigerate the medication for 30 minutes.
[ ] **3.** Clean the outer surface of the dropper.
[ ] **4.** Fill the dropper with no more than 1 mL of medication.

58. Which teratogenic effect is most likely to occur among the fetuses of pregnant women who chronically consume alcohol?
[ ] **1.** Mental retardation
[ ] **2.** Congenital cataracts
[ ] **3.** Seizure disorders
[ ] **4.** Missing limbs

59. Which initial nursing response is best if a child confides information that indicates sexual abuse?
[ ] **1.** Persuade the child to provide details.
[ ] **2.** Examine the child for genital injuries.
[ ] **3.** Let the child know he or she is believed.
[ ] **4.** Look for signs of sexually transmitted infections.

60. The nurse assesses a client with chronic alcoholism who has been drinking up to the time of admission. During which time frame after admission is the nurse most likely to observe initial signs of alcohol withdrawal in this client?
[ ] **1.** 1 to 2 hours
[ ] **2.** 4 to 6 hours
[ ] **3.** 12 to 72 hours
[ ] **4.** 3 to 7 days

61. When caring for a client who has been burned around the face and neck, which assessment finding should the nurse immediately report to the physician?
[ ] **1.** Fluid overload
[ ] **2.** Signs of hemorrhage
[ ] **3.** Signs of infection
[ ] **4.** Respiratory distress

62. The nurse is completing a care plan for an immobile client. Which nursing measure for preventing contractures is best to include in the care plan?
[ ] **1.** Encourage the client to perform isometric exercises.
[ ] **2.** Help the client to perform range-of-motion (ROM) exercises.
[ ] **3.** Elevate the client's extremities on pillows.
[ ] **4.** Use a pressure-relieving mattress.

63. When assessing a client with severe burns, which assessment finding provides the best evidence that the wound is infected?
[ ] **1.** The wound has a foul odor.
[ ] **2.** The eschar is black.
[ ] **3.** The leukocyte count is 5,000/mm^3.
[ ] **4.** The heart rate is increased.

64. A 6-year-old child is recovering from acute non-infectious gastroenteritis. The physician provides orders to advance the child's diet to solid food. Which food choice is best for the nurse to offer the child initially?
[ ] **1.** Vanilla pudding
[ ] **2.** Chicken broth
[ ] **3.** Oatmeal and milk
[ ] **4.** Unsweetened applesauce

65. The nurse is working for a mental health group home facility. In planning therapeutic activities for the population, which activity is most appropriate for a client with generalized anxiety disorder?
[ ] **1.** Playing cards
[ ] **2.** Assembling models
[ ] **3.** Using a treadmill
[ ] **4.** Painting pictures

66. A client who takes furosemide (Lasix) for heart failure comes to the clinic for a routine visit. The client's laboratory report reveals a potassium level of 3.1 mEq/L. Which question elicits the best information to assess whether the client is demonstrating signs and symptoms of hypokalemia?
[ ] **1.** "Have you been having leg cramps or muscle weakness?"
[ ] **2.** "Have you noticed a slowing of your heart rate?"
[ ] **3.** "Have you had a rapid weight gain lately?"
[ ] **4.** "Have you noticed if your speech has become slurred?"

67. When a client with type 1 diabetes comes to the clinic for a routine visit, which question should the nurse plan to ask in relation to possible complications?
[ ] **1.** "When did you have your vision checked?"
[ ] **2.** "What's the color of your urine?"
[ ] **3.** "What's your usual blood pressure?"
[ ] **4.** "Have you had any heart palpitations?"

68. When collecting data from the parent of a child who is suspected of having rheumatic fever, the nurse demonstrates an accurate understanding of the etiology by asking if the child has recently had which condition?
[ ] **1.** Chickenpox
[ ] **2.** Sore throat
[ ] **3.** Influenza
[ ] **4.** Roseola

69. Which assessment finding would the nurse expect to find in a child who has rheumatic fever?
[ ] **1.** Urticaria
[ ] **2.** Hypothermia
[ ] **3.** Hypotension
[ ] **4.** Arthralgia

70. A primigravid client at 42 weeks' gestation is having a nonstress test. Which finding provides the best evidence of an unfavorable response to the test?
[ ] **1.** Fetal heart rate accelerations are at least 15 beats/minute above baseline.
[ ] **2.** Fetal movement is detected within 20 minutes of beginning the nonstress test.
[ ] **3.** More than two fetal heartbeat accelerations occur during a 20-minute to 30-minute period.
[ ] **4.** Each fetal heart rate acceleration lasts less than 15 seconds.

71. The radiologist uses a red marker to identify a cancerous area on the client's skin in preparation for radiation treatments. Which action is essential to this client's nursing care?
[ ] **1.** Removing the red marks using acetone after each treatment
[ ] **2.** Washing the skin with mild soap and tepid water when bathing
[ ] **3.** Keeping the irradiated skin exposed to air at all times
[ ] **4.** Rubbing lotion into the irradiated area after each treatment

72. A client with an ulcer has been taking aluminum hydroxide gel (Amphojel) for 3 days. Which symptom reported to the nurse is most likely a side effect of the antacid?
[ ] **1.** Constipation
[ ] **2.** Flatus
[ ] **3.** Dry mouth
[ ] **4.** Dyspepsia

73. A nursing assistant is assigned to care for a 5-year-old child with acute lymphoblastic leukemia. Which of the nursing assistant's actions indicates that additional teaching is needed?
[ ] **1.** The nursing assistant performs oral care using a sponge-type brush.
[ ] **2.** The nursing assistant assesses the child's temperature rectally.
[ ] **3.** The nursing assistant maintains protective isolation precautions.
[ ] **4.** The nursing assistant places a sheepskin under the bony prominences.

74. The physician prescribes pantoprazole (Protonix) for a client with peptic ulcer disease. When the client asks the nurse to explain the medication's action, which description is most correct?
[ ] **1.** "Pantoprazole makes gastric secretions more acidic."
[ ] **2.** "Pantoprazole covers the ulcer with a protective barrier."
[ ] **3.** "Pantoprazole inhibits gastric acid production."
[ ] **4.** "Pantoprazole blocks histamine receptors in the stomach."

75. Which volume of solution is most appropriate when irrigating a client's colostomy?
[ ] **1.** 50 to 100 mL
[ ] **2.** 100 to 150 mL
[ ] **3.** 250 to 500 mL
[ ] **4.** 500 to 1,000 mL

76. As the nurse gathers data from the medical record of an adolescent tentatively diagnosed with type 1 diabetes mellitus, the nurse would expect to note which history finding?
[ ] **1.** A sudden onset of symptoms
[ ] **2.** A Progressive weight gain
[ ] **3.** Treatment with oral hypoglycemic agents
[ ] **4.** A marked decrease in urine output

77. A client has hemiparalysis from a recent stroke. Which technique should the nurse avoid when changing the client's position in bed?
[ ] **1.** Logrolling the client from side to side
[ ] **2.** Sliding the client to move up in bed
[ ] **3.** Lifting the client using a mechanical lift
[ ] **4.** Having the client use an overhead trapeze

78. When administering eyedrops, in which anatomic location should the nurse apply the drops?
[ ] **1.** Inner canthus
[ ] **2.** Outer canthus
[ ] **3.** Upper conjunctival sac
[ ] **4.** Lower conjunctival sac

79. Which laboratory test would the nurse expect the physician to order to determine the infectious status of a 6-month-old infant whose mother tests positive for human immunodeficiency virus (HIV) infection?
[ ] **1.** Enzyme-linked immunosorbent assay (ELISA)
[ ] **2.** Polymerase chain reaction (PCR) test
[ ] **3.** Western blot blood test
[ ] **4.** Rapid plasma reagin (RPR)

80. Which nursing assessment technique is most appropriate to determine whether a 25-year-old substance abuser's unresponsiveness is related to a heroin overdose?
[ ] **1.** Checking the size of the client's pupils
[ ] **2.** Measuring the client's blood pressure
[ ] **3.** Observing the client's response to pain
[ ] **4.** Smelling the odor of the client's breath

81. The nurse is caring for a pregnant client who is in labor and receiving epidural anesthesia. Which position should the nurse avoid when repositioning this client?
[ ] **1.** Supine
[ ] **2.** Semi-Fowler's
[ ] **3.** Right side-lying
[ ] **4.** Left side-lying

82. The nursing team develops a teaching plan for a 10-year-old client with newly diagnosed diabetes who also has attention deficit hyperactivity disorder (ADHD). Which teaching strategy is most appropriate?
[ ] **1.** Providing individualized teaching in a quiet environment
[ ] **2.** Planning group teaching with other children with ADHD
[ ] **3.** Administering consequences for inappropriate behavior
[ ] **4.** Varying the method of instruction for each session

83. A client whose spouse died 1 month earlier tells a nurse about a plan to sell their home and move in with a daughter and son-in-law. Which nursing response is most appropriate?
[ ] **1.** Encourage the client to move on with her life.
[ ] **2.** Congratulate the client on making a hard decision.
[ ] **3.** Caution the client to postpone making major changes.
[ ] **4.** Suggest the client look into renting an apartment.

84. Which nursing action is most therapeutic for helping an older adult resolve grief associated with the death of a spouse?
[ ] **1.** Recommend taking a cruise with other senior citizens
[ ] **2.** Inform the client that grieving takes about 6 months
[ ] **3.** Allow the client to verbalize feelings about the loss
[ ] **4.** Refer the client to an accountant for financial advice

85. At a routine home health visit, the nurse observes that an elderly client has several arm and leg bruises. The nurse reviews the client's history, which reveals that the client moved in with an adult child 1 month ago. Which assessment finding best indicates that the older adult is a victim of elder abuse?
[ ] **1.** The client sleeps on a couch in the living room.
[ ] **2.** There are conflicting explanations for the injury.
[ ] **3.** The home requires extensive cleaning.
[ ] **4.** The client has lost weight in the past month.

86. Which of the following nursing orders is appropriate for the practical nurse to add to the care plan of a client who has just undergone a modified mastectomy?
[ ] **1.** Keep the arm on the operative side at the level of the heart.
[ ] **2.** Avoid taking blood pressures using the arm on the operative side.
[ ] **3.** Encourage abduction exercises of the arm on the operative side.
[ ] **4.** Empty the wound drainage container every 24 hours.

87. Which information regarding estrogen deficiency is most appropriate for the nurse to include in the discharge teaching of a client who has had her ovaries removed?
[ ] **1.** Hot flashes and a feeling of warmth are common.
[ ] **2.** Menstrual periods are accompanied by heavy flow.
[ ] **3.** Leg cramps may occur during sleep and inactivity.
[ ] **4.** Orgasms may be absent or reduced in the future.

88. The adult children of an older parent consult the nurse about relocating their aging parent from their home to a long-term care facility. Which nursing suggestion is most therapeutic for facilitating the parent's transition to the long-term care facility?
[ ] **1.** Identify the costs and services of several facilities.
[ ] **2.** Involve the parent in planning the relocation.
[ ] **3.** Consult the parent's physician about the planned move.
[ ] **4.** Label all the client's belongings with the client's name.

89. When planning the nursing care of a client who has undergone an abdominal hysterectomy, which nursing measure is most helpful for preventing postoperative complications and facilitating an early discharge?
[ ] **1.** Reestablishing oral fluids and nutrition
[ ] **2.** Promoting ambulation and movement
[ ] **3.** Maintaining accurate intake and output
[ ] **4.** Exploring feelings about altered image

90. When a nurse discusses hospice care with the family of a terminally ill client, which statement is most accurate?
[ ] **1.** "Hospice nurses give better care than hospital nurses."
[ ] **2.** "Hospice nurses give around-the-clock care at home."
[ ] **3.** "Hospice nurses empower personal end-of-life decisions."
[ ] **4.** "Hospice nurses help extend predicted life expectancy."

91. The school nurse is supervising a group of children in the classroom. Which characteristic behavior would the nurse expect to note when observing an 8-year-old child with attention deficit hyperactivity disorder (ADHD)?
[ ] **1.** The child has difficulty understanding instructions.
[ ] **2.** The child is uninterested in the surroundings.
[ ] **3.** The child refuses to play with others.
[ ] **4.** The child often fidgets and squirms.

92. The newborn infant of a diabetic mother is admitted to the nursery. Which nursing intervention is most important to perform initially when providing care for this infant?
[ ] **1.** Check the newborn's blood glucose level.
[ ] **2.** Perform a gestational age assessment.
[ ] **3.** Assess for signs of neurologic deficits.
[ ] **4.** Begin phototherapy immediately.

93. The goal for the initial treatment of a client with newly diagnosed myasthenia gravis is to determine an effective maintenance dose of pyridostigmine (Mestinon). Which nursing assessment finding is the best evidence that the medication is achieving a therapeutic effect?
[ ] **1.** Dilated pupils
[ ] **2.** Increased muscle strength
[ ] **3.** Regular heart rhythm
[ ] **4.** Improve bowel elimination

94. A 17-year-old client is seen in the dermatology clinic for treatment of acne. Which nursing instruction is essential when teaching about how to avoid secondary infections and scarring?
[ ] **1.** Avoid wearing cosmetics.
[ ] **2.** Apply a drying agent nightly.
[ ] **3.** Avoid squeezing blackheads.
[ ] **4.** Scrub with a mild face soap.

95. A client has undergone an inguinal hernia repair and is preparing for discharge. Which instruction by the nurse is most appropriate?
[ ] **1.** Avoid forceful coughing.
[ ] **2.** Empty the bladder often.
[ ] **3.** Sleep on the operated side.
[ ] **4.** Limit early ambulation.

96. A client requires gastric decompression. Immediately after a Salem sump tube is inserted, which nursing action is correct?
[ ] **1.** The nurse checks the tube for proper placement.
[ ] **2.** The nurse connects the tube to mechanical suction.
[ ] **3.** The nurse irrigates the tube to keep it patent.
[ ] **4.** The nurse offers the client sips of ice water.

97. A client takes ibuprofen (Motrin) for discomfort associated with osteoarthritis. The best evidence that the client understands the hazards of taking this nonsteroidal anti-inflammatory drug (NSAID) is the ability to identify which common side effect?
[ ] **1.** Double vision
[ ] **2.** Transient dizziness
[ ] **3.** Irregular pulse
[ ] **4.** Upset stomach

98. An employee of a chemical plant comes to the emergency department for treatment of severe chemical burns. Which is the most appropriate emergency nursing treatment for this type of burn?
[ ] **1.** Irrigate the area with large amounts of water
[ ] **2.** Cover the burn with a sterile dressing
[ ] **3.** Apply a thick layer of petroleum jelly to the area
[ ] **4.** Rub the burned skin with crushed ice

99. The nurse is assigned a client with significant dementia and limited communication. The client has a moist cough. The nurse can best determine if oropharyngeal suctioning is necessary based on which assessment finding?
[ ] **1.** Type of cough
[ ] **2.** Sputum color
[ ] **3.** Ability to raise sputum
[ ] **4.** Respiratory rate

100. The family of a 78-year-old client brings the client to the hospital after falling, striking the head, and briefly losing consciousness. Which instruction is most important for the nurse to convey to the family before discharging the client from the emergency department?
[ ] **1.** Give the client extra fluids for the next 72 hours.
[ ] **2.** Keep the client flat in bed for the next several days.
[ ] **3.** Notify the physician if the client is difficult to arouse.
[ ] **4.** Check the client's eyes, ears, and nose for signs of bleeding.

101. A 12-year-old client is brought to the physician's office for evaluation of a fractured right arm. Which nursing assessment finding is the best indication that there is an infection under a client's cast?
[ ] **1.** There is a long crack in the cast
[ ] **2.** There is a foul odor coming from the cast
[ ] **3.** There is on the cast surface
[ ] **4.** There is an indentation in the cast

102. To avoid the potential for Reye's syndrome, it is best for the nurse to recommend that parents avoid administering which drug to their young children?
[ ] **1.** Acetaminophen (Tylenol)
[ ] **2.** Ibuprofen (Advil)
[ ] **3.** Aspirin (Anacin)
[ ] **4.** Naproxen (Naprosyn)

103. When preparing to withdraw a medication from an ampule, which technique should the nurse use?
[ ] **1.** Allow the ampule to stand undisturbed for a minute after shaking it.
[ ] **2.** Tap the ampule stem with a fingernail a few times.
[ ] **3.** Hold the ampule upside down, then quickly invert it.
[ ] **4.** Roll the ampule gently between the palms of the hands.

104. Which nursing observation is the best evidence that a client's traction is maintained correctly?
[ ] **1.** The client's legs are parallel to the bed.
[ ] **2.** The client states that comfort is not compromised.
[ ] **3.** The counterweights are hanging free of the floor.
[ ] **4.** The client's feet are resting against the footboard.

105. Which cluster of nursing assessment findings is the best indication that a client is developing pulmonary edema?
[ ] **1.** Bradycardia, transient confusion, mild anxiety
[ ] **2.** Orthopnea, sudden dyspnea, elevated blood pressure
[ ] **3.** Tachycardia, decreased respiratory rate, weak pulse
[ ] **4.** Flushed face, hypotension, thick tenacious sputum

106. A 5-year-old child is scheduled to have a cardiac catheterization at 8 A.M. Which of the following provides the best evidence to the nurse that the child has been appropriately prepared for the procedure?
[ ] **1.** The child's chest has been cleansed with an antiseptic solution.
[ ] **2.** The parents state that the child has had nothing by mouth since 6 A.M.
[ ] **3.** The child has been shown pictures of the cardiac catheterization laboratory.
[ ] **4.** The parents state that the child will be unconscious during the procedure.

107. Which is the first step the nurse should take when planning a bladder retraining program for an incontinent client?
[ ] **1.** Determine the client's voiding patterns.
[ ] **2.** Limit the client's oral fluid intake.
[ ] **3.** Develop a regular schedule for urination.
[ ] **4.** Requisition a portable bedside commode.

108. Which observation by the nurse offers the best evidence that a paraplegic client understands the correct way to empty the bladder using Crede's maneuver?
[ ] **1.** The client inserts a straight catheter into the urethra using clean technique.
[ ] **2.** The client takes several deep breaths from the diaphragm before trying to void.
[ ] **3.** The client exhales slowly and steadily while tensing the abdominal muscles.
[ ] **4.** The client applies light pressure over the bladder area with the dominant hand.

109. The care plan for a 7-year-old child with partial-thickness burns indicates that the client should be placed in the prone position for 2 hours each shift. If the nursing assistant carries out the care plan correctly, the nurse will observe that the child is positioned in what manner?
[ ] **1.** On the back
[ ] **2.** On the side
[ ] **3.** On the abdomen
[ ] **4.** In a sitting position

110. The nurse assesses a newborn infant who has just been admitted to the nursery from the delivery room. Which nursing assessment finding is the best indication that the infant is experiencing respiratory distress?
[ ] **1.** An abdominal breathing pattern
[ ] **2.** A respiratory rate of 40 breaths/minute
[ ] **3.** An irregular breathing pattern
[ ] **4.** Grunting sounds on expiration

111. A client who has advanced cancer is taking a chemotherapy drug. Which effect is the client most likely to report to the nurse as a consequence of the drug therapy?
[ ] **1.** Hair loss
[ ] **2.** Abdominal distention
[ ] **3.** Deepening of the voice
[ ] **4.** Significant weight loss

112. A surgical client experiences abdominal incisional discomfort when coughing postoperatively. Which nursing intervention is most appropriate for reducing the client's discomfort?
[ ] **1.** Provide client instruction to flex both knees while coughing.
[ ] **2.** Have the client lie supine with back support before trying to cough.
[ ] **3.** Teach to apply light pressure to the incision with a pillow while coughing.
[ ] **4.** Administer an analgesic soon after coughing.

113. A liquid nutritional supplement is ordered for an older adult who is not eating adequately. When is the best time for the nurse to provide the supplement?
[ ] **1.** Just before the noon meal
[ ] **2.** At the noon meal with other food
[ ] **3.** Immediately after eating lunch
[ ] **4.** Between breakfast and lunch

114. Which nursing intervention is most appropriate for preventing urine and stool from soiling the hip-spica cast of an 18-month-old child?
[ ] **1.** Insert cotton wadding between the cast and the skin in the perineal area.
[ ] **2.** Cover the edges of the cast around the perineum with a waterproof material.
[ ] **3.** Offer the bedpan at more frequent intervals.
[ ] **4.** Place plastic pants over the perineal area.

115. A nurse assists the physician for a lumbar puncture. Which of the following is the most appropriate client position for this procedure?
[ ] **1.** The client is in the prone position with the head turned to the side.
[ ] **2.** The client is in the recumbent position with the feet slightly elevated.
[ ] **3.** The client is in the supine position with the head of the bed elevated 45 degrees.
[ ] **4.** The client is in the side-lying position with the knees drawn up and back flexed.

116. A nurse and a nursing assistant are transferring an adult client from the bed to a wheelchair. Which nursing intervention is best for ensuring the client's safety during the transfer?
[ ] **1.** Putting slippers on the client's feet
[ ] **2.** Locking the wheels on the wheelchair
[ ] **3.** Raising the upper side rails on the bed
[ ] **4.** Showing the client how to use the trapeze

117. The nursing team is caring for clients on a medical-surgical unit when the fire alarm sounds. Which nurse on the team acts most appropriately to contain a fire?
[ ] **1.** The nurse who closes all the inside doors
[ ] **2.** The nurse who returns to the nurses' station
[ ] **3.** The nurse who searches for signs of smoke
[ ] **4.** The nurse who stays with an immobile client

118. If the physician orders the irrigation of a client's urinary catheter but does not specify the type of solution to use, which solution would be the nurse's first choice?
[ ] **1.** Distilled water
[ ] **2.** Warm tap water
[ ] **3.** Sterile normal saline solution
[ ] **4.** Diluted hydrogen peroxide

119. If a client has obstructive jaundice, which assessment finding is the nurse most likely to observe?
[ ] **1.** Urine that is very dark brown
[ ] **2.** Saliva that is tan and thick
[ ] **3.** Stool that is green and watery
[ ] **4.** Skin that is pale and quite dry

120. After observing a brown discoloration on the washcloth while bathing an African American child, a nursing assistant reports a suspicion that the child's hygiene has been neglected. Which statement by the nurse provides the best explanation for the discoloration noted by the nursing assistant?
[ ] **1.** "African Americans bathe less to avoid dry skin."
[ ] **2.** "This is a normal finding from shedding skin cells."
[ ] **3.** "Soap removes melanin from epidermal tissue."
[ ] **4.** "The skin of African Americans tends to retain oil."

121. When a nurse performs a mental status examination on an older adult, the previously cooperative client becomes silent when asked to spell "world" backwards. Which response by the nurse is most appropriate at this time?
[ ] **1.** Discontinue assessing the client.
[ ] **2.** Go on to another mental assessment.
[ ] **3.** Assume the client has early signs of dementia.
[ ] **4.** Presume the client is functionally illiterate.

122. Which goal is most appropriate when the nurse manages the care of an older adult client who has osteoporosis?
[ ] **1.** The client will consume more dairy products.
[ ] **2.** The client will acquire increased bone density.
[ ] **3.** The client will ambulate without falling.
[ ] **4.** The client will be restrained in a wheelchair.

123. Which nursing assessment finding is most likely associated with the long-term effects of diabetes mellitus?
[ ] **1.** Diminished vision
[ ] **2.** Frequent indigestion
[ ] **3.** Urine retention
[ ] **4.** Tremors at rest

124. A 5-year-old child is being discharged after undergoing a tonsillectomy and adenoidectomy. When preparing discharge instructions for the parents, which information is most appropriate for the nurse to include?
[ ] **1.** "Children commonly will have a great deal of pain for the first 7 days."
[ ] **2.** "Your child will have difficulty swallowing for about 3 weeks."
[ ] **3.** "Your child may expectorate bright red blood for about 1 week."
[ ] **4.** "A transient earache for about 1 to 3 days is a common complaint."

125. The nurse teaches a client how to change the ostomy appliance in preparation for discharge home. Which suggestion is most helpful for ensuring that the appliance remains attached?
[ ] **1.** Empty the collection bag frequently.
[ ] **2.** Limit fluid intake throughout the day.
[ ] **3.** Change the appliance each morning.
[ ] **4.** Avoid eating gas-forming vegetables.

126. Which nursing assessment finding is considered abnormal when performing a gestational age assessment on a full-term infant?
[ ] **1.** Lanugo covers the shoulders, back, and forehead
[ ] **2.** The infant exhibits a strong Moro reflex
[ ] **3.** There are anterior transverse creases on the soles of the feet
[ ] **4.** The infant assumes a fully flexed posture

127. The emergency department physician prescribes alteplase (Activase), a thrombolytic drug, after a client's myocardial infarction. Which statement about the therapeutic action of this medication should the nurse explain to the client?
[ ] **1.** The medication lowers the client's anxiety level.
[ ] **2.** The medication lowers the systolic blood pressure.
[ ] **3.** The medication prevents the risk of arrhythmias.
[ ] **4.** The medication dissolves any clots in the circulation.

128. The nurse is developing a care plan for the residents of an assisted living facility. Which of the following physiological changes are characteristic of aging? Select all that apply.
[ ] **1.** Cardiac output declines.
[ ] **2.** The gag reflex is weaker.
[ ] **3.** Renal blood flow decreases.
[ ] **4.** Gastric motility increases.
[ ] **5.** Serum albumin level decreases.
[ ] **6.** The amount of body water increases.

129. The nurse is caring for a client who requires a venipuncture for I.V. therapy. After checking the physician's orders and explaining the procedure to the client and assembling all of the equipment, the nurse performs all of the following actions in order of priority. Indicate the correct order in which the procedure is performed. Use all the options.

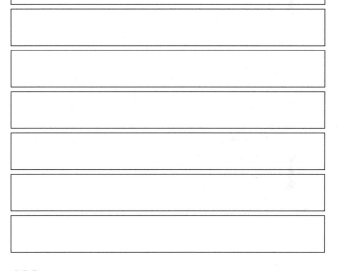

1. Clean the venipuncture site thoroughly.

2. Withdraw the needle and connect the tubing.

3. Apply a tourniquet and palpate veins.

4. Hold the skin taut, and pierce the skin, entering the vein.

5. Note the blood in the chamber, and release the tourniquet.

6. Wash your hands and then put on gloves.

130. Which of the following nursing interventions is most helpful in preventing loneliness in a new resident of a long-term care facility?
[ ] **1.** Initiate reminiscence therapy weekly.
[ ] **2.** Provide group activities.
[ ] **3.** Provide individual visits.
[ ] **4.** Allow the resident to watch television.

131. A nurse in an acute care setting is a member of the ethical care practices committee. Which of the following topics would the nurse expect to be considered by the committee as an ethical concern?
[ ] **1.** A 15-year-old mother who decides to place her baby for adoption
[ ] **2.** A client who refuses to take the prescribed medications
[ ] **3.** An elder who reports being physically abused
[ ] **4.** A nurse who witnesses another nurse taking a client's medication

Correct Answers, Rationales, and Test Taking Strategies

1. 2. Aspirin is used as an anti-inflammatory, analgesic, antipyretic, and antiplatelet agent. It is a known gastric irritant. It should be taken with a full glass of water, food, or milk. Enteric-coated or buffered forms of aspirin help prevent gastric irritation and reduce the risk of bleeding. None of the other medications is associated with gastric irritation.

> *Test Taking Strategy—Look at the key words "most likely related" and "epigastric pain." Review the drugs listed to identify a drug that could cause this side effect, which is aspirin (option 2), and the side effects of the drugs listed if you had difficulty answering this question.*

Cognitive Level—*Applying*
Client Needs Category—*Physiological integrity*
Client Needs Subcategory—*Pharmacological therapies*

2. 4. Getting additional rest is the best choice among the options for restoring energy during the demands of pregnancy. Although it is beneficial to modify the work routine to take advantage of times of peak energy, early morning is usually more of a prime energy time than midafternoon. It is inadvisable to take more than the prescribed dose of a medication, including vitamins. Daytime napping is appropriate, even if the naps are short and frequent.

> *Test Taking Strategy—Use the process of elimination to select the option that describes the best advice for managing fatigue experienced by a woman in the first trimester of pregnancy. Option 2 can be eliminated because it is never wise to take excessive doses of vitamins containing fat-soluble vitamins, which are stored rather than excreted in urine. Options 1 and 3 may not be realistic depending on the client's lifestyle and work-related responsibilities, which the stem does not identify. Option 4 emerges as the best answer. Review the problems associated with early pregnancy and nursing measures for their management if you had difficulty answering this question.*

Cognitive Level—*Applying*
Client Needs Category—*Physiological integrity*
Client Needs Subcategory—*Basic care and comfort*

3. 2. Good sources of iron include liver, lean meats, legumes, dried fruits, leafy green vegetables, whole grain, and fortified cereals. Potatoes, oranges, and cheese are not good sources of iron. However, citrus fruits in the diet help with iron absorption.

> *Test Taking Strategy—Use the process of elimination to select the option with the best example of a food source of iron. Option 1 can be eliminated because potatoes are a source of potassium, not iron.*

Option 3 can be eliminated because oranges are a source of ascorbic acid (vitamin C). Option 4 can be eliminated because cheese is a good source of calcium. Review food sources of iron in a nutritional text if you had difficulty answering this question.

Cognitive Level—*Analyzing*
Client Needs Category—*Physiological integrity*
Client Needs Subcategory—*Basic care and comfort*

4. 3. Heroin is an opioid derived from morphine. Naloxone hydrochloride (Narcan) is an opioid antagonist that reverses the effects of opioids. Methadone hydrochloride (Dolophine) is an opiate-like drug used for detoxification and for clients in treatment programs for opioid abstinence. Both succinylcholine chloride (Anectine) and pancuronium bromide (Pavulon) are powerful neuromuscular junction blocking agents used as adjuncts to anesthetics.

> *Test Taking Strategy—Analyze to determine what information the question asks for, which is an antidote used to manage an overdose involving heroin. Option 3 is the best answer from among the choices provided. Review the uses of the drugs listed if you had difficulty answering this question.*

Cognitive Level—*Applying*
Client Needs Category—*Physiological integrity*
Client Needs Subcategory—*Pharmacological therapies*

5. 3. Laxative use is contraindicated for postpartum clients with a third-degree or fourth-degree laceration because this type of laceration extends into the rectal sphincter. Instead of a laxative, a stool softener is usually prescribed. To avoid constipation, clients are encouraged to increase fluid intake and ambulate. Hemorrhoids and a vacuum extraction are not reasons for omitting laxatives or enemas. Consideration is given to ordering bisacodyl (Dulcolax) suppositories to breast-feeding women because small amounts of metabolites are excreted in breast milk. However, bisacodyl suppositories are still used during pregnancy and lactation.

> *Test Taking Strategy—Analyze to determine what information the question asks for, which is the client for which a bisacodyl (Dulcolax) suppository is unsafe. Because bisacodyl is a harsh laxative, it has the potential to further injure a postpartum client with a third-degree tear (option 3) during the expulsion of stool. Option 2 has merit, but because the prescribed medication is in a suppository form, it is less likely to produce sufficient systemic effects that would affect a nursing infant. Review the classifications of laxatives verses stool softeners if you had difficulty answering this question.*

Cognitive Level—*Analyzing*
Client Needs Category—*Physiological integrity*
Client Needs Subcategory—*Pharmacological therapies*

6. 2. Persons with only a few gallstones and mild symptoms experience relief by the application of shock waves (lithotripsy) that pulverize the stones. The smaller stones then move into the intestinal tract and are excreted in the stool.

> *Test Taking Strategy—Analyze to determine what information the question asks for, which is how lithotripsy eliminates stones in the gallbladder. Knowing the mechanism by which lithotripsy is administered leads to the selection of option 2. Review information on lithotripsy, which is also used to pulverize kidney stones, if you had difficulty answering this question.*
> **Cognitive Level**—*Understanding*
> **Client Needs Category**—*Physiological integrity*
> **Client Needs Subcategory**—*Reduction of risk potential*

7. 4. Dried beans, rice, peanut butter, peanuts, and whole grains are examples of plant proteins that are cheaper than animal proteins, such as meat, chicken, fish, and dairy products. Plant proteins taken in a sufficient amount or combined with a small amount of meat can satisfy the protein needs of a pregnant woman. Broccoli and cauliflower are vegetables that add significant sources of fiber and vitamins to the diet. Fortified cereal includes vitamins and minerals such as folic acid, B vitamins, and iron, depending on the cereal.

> *Test Taking Strategy—Analyze to determine what information the question asks for, which is an alternative source of dietary protein. Dried beans (option 4) are the best source of protein from among the options provided. Review food sources of dietary protein if you had difficulty answering this question.*
> **Cognitive Level**—*Understanding*
> **Client Needs Category**—*Physiological integrity*
> **Client Needs Subcategory**—*Basic care and comfort*

8. 2. Postmenopausal women generally pick an arbitrary date, such as the first day of the month, and perform breast self-examination (BSE) on that date each month. If the client is still menstruating, the best time to examine the breasts is 2 to 3 days after a period, when the breasts are not tender. The time of day is not pertinent. It is better to examine the breasts during a shower, when the client's fingers can easily glide over the breast tissue. Breasts should be examined monthly rather than once a year.

> *Test Taking Strategy—Use the process of elimination to select the option that describes accurate information about performing a BSE by a postmenopausal client. Option 2 is the only accurate instruction. Review information about the technique for performing BSE, especially when the client is no longer menstruating, if you had difficulty answering this question.*
> **Cognitive Level**—*Analyzing*
> **Client Needs Category**—*Health promotion and maintenance*
> **Client Needs Subcategory**—*None*

9. 1. The presence of albumin in the urine is one of the primary signs of preeclampsia, which is also referred to as *toxemia of pregnancy* and *pregnancy-induced hypertension*. Other warning signs include hypertension, severe headache, excessive swelling of the hands and feet, double vision, and nausea and vomiting. The excretion of albumin in the urine is not a sign of liver impairment, amniotic embolism, or gestational diabetes.

> *Test Taking Strategy—Analyze to determine what information the question asks for, which is the significance of finding albumin in a pregnant client's urine. Recall that albumin is a protein that should not be present in urine. When a pregnant client develops albuminuria, it could be an indication of preeclampsia (option 1). Review albuminuria and its significance, especially as it relates to a pregnant client, if you had difficulty answering this question.*
> **Cognitive Level**—*Applying*
> **Client Needs Category**—*Physiological integrity*
> **Client Needs Subcategory**—*Reduction of risk potential*

10. 2. Endocarditis is an infection or inflammation of heart valves. There is an association between infections with group A hemolytic streptococci and the development of rheumatic fever complicated by endocarditis. To prevent rheumatic heart disease and endocarditis, the American Heart Association recommends that children with streptococcal infections receive antibiotic therapy during their acute illness for at least 10 full days. Poverty and lack of health insurance often deter parents from seeking medical treatment for ill children. Endocarditis is not generally associated with birth defects, clubbing of the fingers, or failure to receive immunizations for the usual childhood infectious diseases.

> *Test Taking Strategy—Look at the key words "most consistent with" and "rheumatic fever." Recall that endocarditis, a sequela of rheumatic fever, is linked to a prior streptococcal infection (option 2). Review the factors that contribute to rheumatic fever and endocarditis if you had difficulty answering this question.*
> **Cognitive Level**—*Applying*
> **Client Needs Category**—*Physiological integrity*
> **Client Needs Subcategory**—*Physiological adaptation*

11. 2. Not all clients admitted to the obstetric department are given an enema, but some physicians include an enema as part of their routine admission orders. It is appropriate to withhold an enema for clients who are experiencing vaginal bleeding and to collaborate with the physician. Enemas given during labor are not used for constipation but to evacuate stool to prevent contamination of the sterile field during delivery or to stimulate uterine contractions. The nurse should consult the physician before substituting a laxative for an enema.

Test Taking Strategy—*Look at the key words "most appropriate," "pregnant client," and "administration of an enema." Recall that when an obstetric client has vaginal bleeding, an enema may be contraindicated. Review care of a client in the antepartum period if you had difficulty answering this question.*
Cognitive Level—*Analyzing*
Client Needs Category—*Physiological integrity*
Client Needs Subcategory—*Reduction of risk potential*

12. 3. The nurse's ultimate responsibility is for the client's safety. A change in vital signs is a sign of systemic complications, such as hemorrhage and shock, and should be reported immediately. After notifying the charge nurse and physician, the nurse should then take frequent vital signs to provide a baseline for further treatment. Documenting the information, which is necessary, does not help the client improve. Fowler's position may lower, not raise, the blood pressure.

Test Taking Strategy—*Look at the key information in the stem, which relates that the blood pressure has fallen abruptly in a client in an early postoperative period and asks for the "most appropriate" nursing action. The blood pressure should have stabilized by this time postoperatively. An abrupt fall in blood pressure is an indication of bleeding or hemorrhage. Processing this information leads to selecting option 3 as the best answer. Review signs of hypovolemic shock and postoperative nursing care if you had difficulty answering this question.*
Cognitive Level—*Analyzing*
Client Needs Category—*Physiological integrity*
Client Needs Subcategory—*Reduction of risk potential*

13. 1. A large oral intake keeps the urine dilute and less likely to obstruct a urinary catheter with blood clots and tissue debris. A large fluid volume does promote the excretion of toxic wastes, but that is not the best answer in this situation. The bladder capacity of a prostatectomy client is unaffected by the surgery. Specific exercises are used to promote bladder retraining.

Test Taking Strategy—*Look at the key words "most accurate response" to a question about the reason for increasing oral fluid intake posed by a client who has undergone a transurethral resection of the prostate (TURP). Recall that there is a great deal of tissue and blood loss associated with a procedure that is performed through the urethra. Consequently, it is imperative to consume a high volume of fluid to keep the catheter patent. Review the postoperative nursing care of a client who has undergone a TURP if you had difficulty answering this question.*
Cognitive Level—*Analyzing*
Client Needs Category—*Physiological integrity*
Client Needs Subcategory—*Reduction of risk potential*

14. 2. The second stage of labor begins when the cervix is completely effaced and fully dilated; this stage of labor ends with delivery of the neonate. During the first stage of labor, the client has regular contractions that serve to dilate and thin the cervix. During the third stage of labor, the placenta is delivered. During the fourth stage of labor, the mother is monitored closely for complications such as hemorrhage.

Test Taking Strategy—*Analyze to determine what information the question asks for, which is the stage of labor that correlates with complete effacement and full dilation. These data correspond with option 2. Review the stages of labor and their characteristics if you had difficulty answering this question.*
Cognitive Level—*Understanding*
Client Needs Category—*Physiological integrity*
Client Needs Subcategory—*Reduction of risk potential*

15.

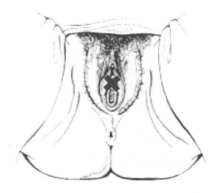

The nurse inserts the urinary catheter in the urinary meatus, which lies just above the vaginal opening and below the clitoris.

Test Taking Strategy—*Analyze to determine what information the question asks for, which is the location of the urinary meatus. Review illustrations of the female anatomy, especially the location of the urinary meatus in relation to the clitoris, vagina, and rectum, if you had difficulty answering this question.*
Cognitive Level—*Understanding*
Client Needs Category—*Physiological integrity*
Client Needs Subcategory—*Reduction of risk potential*

16. 3. The first instruction to the nursing team in preventing falls is to assess why the client is trying to get out of the chair. Regular assessment of the client's needs and then follow-up action is the best course of action. A medical order is required before a restrictive restraint is applied. Tying a person in a chair with a sheet is ineffective for preventing falls because the client can slip under the sheet and onto the floor. Keeping a client within sight at all times is impractical. Sedation, a form of chemical restraint, should be the last means of keeping the client safe.

Test Taking Strategy—Look at the key terms "most appropriate" and "prevent." Recall that assessment is the first step in the nursing process, which makes option 3 the best answer. Options 1, 2, and 4 can be eliminated because they are impractical and violate the client's rights. Review the steps in the nursing process if you had difficulty answering this question.
Cognitive Level—*Analyzing*
Client Needs Category—*Safe and effective care environment*
Client Needs Subcategory—*Coordinated care*

17. 2. The presence of a rash is highly suggestive of an allergic reaction, which is common among individuals who are sensitive to penicillins. Before administering subsequent doses, the nurse needs to withhold the dose and notify the physician. The nurse uses alternative I.M. injection sites and rotates each injection site when a site becomes painful. A body temperature of 100°F (37.8°C) indicates that the client is responding to the infecting pathogen and would not be an indication to withhold the antibiotic. A sore mouth can be the result of a superinfection caused by yeast or fungus as a result of frequent or multiple antibiotic use. A sore mouth does not warrant withholding the medication; however, it does require further investigation.

Test Taking Strategy—Look for the key words "best justifies withholding" in relation to identifying an undesirable effect of penicillin. Options 1 and 3 are not reasons for withholding the medication. Although the sore mouth (option 4) is not normal, it probably is not specific to penicillin, and is not usually a basis for withdrawing an antibiotic. Consequently, option 2, which may be a sign of an allergic response, is the best answer. Review the side effects that are common among clients who receive antibiotics if you had difficulty answering this question.
Cognitive Level—*Analyzing*
Client Needs Category—*Physiological integrity*
Client Needs Subcategory—*Pharmacological therapies*

18. 3. Four glasses of fluid per day is an inadequate volume of liquid to ensure moist stool. A healthy daily fluid intake includes 1,200 to 1,500 mL of water and beverages, along with an additional 700 to 1,000 mL of water from food sources. Eating five servings of vegetables, eating cereal with skim milk, and substituting plant protein sources for meat are healthy dietary choices, and would not contribute to constipation. Increasing dietary fiber promotes regular elimination of moist, bulky stools.

Test Taking Strategy—Use the process of elimination to identify the food source that contributes most to constipation. Options 1 and 4 can be eliminated immediately because they promote bowel elimination. Option 2 may or may not promote elimination, depending on whether the cereal is high in fiber; the fact that it is eaten with skim milk would not contribute to constipation. Option 3 emerges as the best choice because

it is less than the recommended daily amount. Inadequate fluid intake contributes to constipation. Review common causes of constipation and its management if you had difficulty answering this question.
Cognitive Level—*Applying*
Client Needs Category—*Physiological integrity*
Client Needs Subcategory—*Basic care and comfort*

19.

1. A young adult who has been given discharge instructions but is awaiting a ride
2. A new postoperative client being transferred by the nursing assistant into a bed
3. An elderly client admitted with unstable angina who reports sternal chest pain
4. An adult who is awaiting transport to the operating room for surgery in 1 hour
5. A client with an afternoon blood sugar reading of 285 mg/dL
6. A client with history of gallstones reporting abdominal pain of 7 out of 10

The nurse must prioritize the nursing assessments after the report to include those clients needing immediate attention due to unstable status first, followed by those clients with needs that are not as pressing. In this situation, the nurse's first priority is the client with unstable angina who is experiencing sternal chest pain. The nurse should recognize this condition as a potential emergency requiring immediate medication and physician notification depending on the assessment findings. The nurse would then complete a nursing assessment of the client returning from surgery. The period immediately after surgery is a crucial time to have postoperative complications. The nurse is responsible for documenting the client's condition on return to the medical-surgical unit. Although abdominal pain is not unusual for the client with gallstones, a pain level of 7 out of 10 requires the administration of pain medication. A nursing assessment is completed before pain medication administration to assess the characteristics of the pain. The client with an elevated blood sugar reading would be assessed next. A thorough assessment of any signs and symptoms of hyperglycemia would be completed and, typically, insulin would be given. Although a blood sugar of 285 mg/dL is elevated and requires nursing action, it is not at an emergency level. The nurse would then assess the client scheduled for surgery in 1 hour. Assessing the preoperative status and making certain that the preoperative protocols are followed is the nurse's responsibility. The last priority is the client who is discharged and awaiting a ride home. The client remains the responsibility of the nurse until the client has been documented to have left the building.

Test Taking Strategy—Analyze to determine what information the question asks for, which is the highest priority to lowest priority of clients for a nursing assessment. Determine which clients are less stable than others. Review Maslow's hierarchy of needs if you had difficulty answering this question.
Cognitive Level—*Analyzing*
Client Needs Category—*Safe and effective care environment*
Client Needs Subcategory—*Coordinated care*

20. 2. A Penrose and other types of open drains are placed within an operative site to help drainage escape from a surgical wound. Drains in a wound do not decrease scar formation. A drain is not used to irrigate a wound. A drain may remove air if it is in the area of a wound, but it is not used to release intestinal gas. Nasogastric and nasointestinal tubes are used to remove air and secretions from the stomach or intestine.

Test Taking Strategy—Use the process of elimination to help select the option that provides the most accurate reason for an open drain such as a Penrose drain. Option 3 can be eliminated immediately because wounds are not irrigated through a Penrose drain. Option 4 can be eliminated because the distal end of the drain is in tissue, not the lumen of an intestine. Option 1 has some merit because the wound heals more effectively if fluid and debris are removed, but it is not the best answer. Option 2 emerges as the most accurate explanation. Review the purpose of open wound drains if you had difficulty answering this question.
Cognitive Level—*Understanding*
Client Needs Category—*Physiological integrity*
Client Needs Subcategory—*Physiological adaptation*

21. 3. Medications should never be mixed with the total volume of tube-feeding formula because if the total volume is not ingested, the child will not receive the full amount of medication. Medications should be given separately from the formula. The procedures described in the remaining options are safe and appropriate.

Test Taking Strategy—Analyze the information about which the question asks, which in this case reflects an inaccurate technique for administering medication through a gastrostomy tube. Options 1, 2, and 4 are accurate statements; option 3 is incorrect. Review how to administer medications through a gastrostomy tube if you had difficulty answering this question.
Cognitive Level—*Analyzing*
Client Needs Category—*Physiological integrity*
Client Needs Subcategory—*Pharmacological therapies*

22. 125 mg.
To solve the calculation, first use the approximate equivalent of 2.2 pounds = 1 kg to find the child's weight in kg:

$$\frac{44 \text{ lb}}{2.2} = 20 \text{ kg}$$

Next, calculate the total daily dose for this child by multiplying the dose by the child's weight in kg:

$$25 \text{ mg} \times 20 \text{ kg/day} = 500 \text{ mg/day}$$

To find the safe amount given in a single dose, divide by 4 (the total number of doses given in 1 day):

$$\frac{500 \text{ mg}}{4} = 125 \text{ mg/dose}$$

Test Taking Strategy—Analyze to determine what information the question asks for, which involves calculating a single dose of medication based on the weight of the client. Review the mathematical process for calculating pediatric dosages if you had difficulty answering this question.
Cognitive Level—*Applying*
Client Needs Category—*Physiological integrity*
Client Needs Subcategory—*Pharmacological therapies*

23. 2. Coughing increases intrathoracic pressure, which facilitates raising and expelling secretions from the airways. The client's body position during postural drainage depends on which lobe(s) of the lung needs draining. Lying supine does not encourage drainage from the lungs because it does not capitalize on using gravity. Breathing through the mouth is not related to postural drainage and elimination of secretions. Breathing slowly may increase tidal volume, but it does not promote elimination of pulmonary secretions.

Test Taking Strategy—Use the process of elimination to help select the "best" option for promoting a therapeutic outcome when performing postural drainage. Option 1 can be immediately eliminated because a supine position does not support the gravitational movement of lung secretions. Option 4 can be eliminated because an optimum result from postural drainage is unrelated to breathing slowly. Option 3 may look somewhat like an attractive answer, but coughing (option 2) is best for loosening and raising retained pulmonary secretions. Review the technique for performing postural drainage if you had difficulty answering this question.

Cognitive Level—*Analyzing*
Client Needs Category—*Physiological integrity*
Client Needs Subcategory—*Physiological adaptation*

24. 2. Because of the changes in circulation in the lower extremities related to the disease process, it is important for the client with diabetes to observe good foot care. Further teaching is needed in this case because the client is at risk for cuts, injury, and infection by trimming calluses with a tool like a nail clipper that has a sharp cutting surface. Using lambs wool to prevent pressure among adjacent toes and having toenails that are short and straight are appropriate when practicing good foot care. Nonelastic white foot socks are appropriate to avoid interfering with blood circulating to the lower extremities. Wearing white socks can help diabetics detect draining lesions better than those that are dark colors. Other instructions regarding diabetic foot care include avoiding going barefoot; wearing well-fitting shoes; washing, drying, and covering injuries with sterile gauze; applying lotion to the feet daily; and keeping the feet clean and dry and nails short. In addition, the client should carefully examine the feet daily for blisters, cuts, and redness.

Test Taking Strategy—*Analyze to determine what information the question asks for, which is an assessment finding regarding diabetic foot care that requires additional teaching. Options 1, 3, and 4 are accurate, but option 2 represents a risk for vascular and wound-healing complications for a diabetic client. Review diabetic foot care if you had difficulty answering this question.*

Cognitive Level—*Applying*
Client Needs Category—*Physiological integrity*
Client Needs Subcategory—*Reduction in risk potential*

25. 4. When introducing a nasogastric (NG) tube into a nostril, it is best to have the client sit upright with the neck hyperextended. This position helps the nurse to guide and direct the tip of the tube toward the pharynx. After the tube is in the oropharynx, the nurse instructs the client to flex the neck and lower the chin to the chest. Then, the nurse advances the tube into the stomach. Neck flexion, extension, and rotation of the neck do not facilitate insertion or advancement of an NG tube.

Test Taking Strategy—*Analyze to determine what information the question asks for, which is the correct position of the neck before inserting an NG tube into a client's nostril. Hyperextension (option 4) is the recommended position at this point during*

tube insertion. Review the technique for inserting an NG tube and the positions described in the options if you had difficulty answering this question.

Cognitive Level—*Analyzing*
Client Needs Category—*Physiological integrity*
Client Needs Subcategory—*Reduction of risk potential*

26. 4. The International Normalized Ratio (INR) is the laboratory test used to assess the effectiveness of warfarin sodium (Coumadin) therapy. Blood levels are obtained on a regular basis to assess the blood's coagulation status. Warfarin sodium works by interfering with the formation of vitamin K–dependent clotting factors in the liver. Platelet levels are unaffected by warfarin sodium. Partial prothrombin time (PTT) is used to assess the effectiveness of heparin, not warfarin, therapy. The circulating blood volume remains unchanged with warfarin sodium.

Test Taking Strategy—*Analyze to determine what information the question asks for, which is the laboratory test used to monitor clients receiving warfarin (Coumadin). Option 1 may seem to have merit because platelets, also known as thrombocytes, are involved in blood clotting, but that is not the substance affected by warfarin. Option 2 may appear to have merit, but PTT is used to monitor clients receiving heparin. Review how the effect of warfarin is monitored to determine the dosage and ensure the safety of the client if you had difficulty answering this question.*

Cognitive Level—*Analyzing*
Client Needs Category—*Physiological integrity*
Client Needs Subcategory—*Pharmacological therapies*

27. 1. Identifying the foods ingested is important in assessing the potential source of the gastroenteritis. Foods of an animal source are primarily involved in outbreaks of food-borne gastroenteritis. Common foods include milk, eggs, and meat such as poultry. The pathogens tend to grow and reproduce when the food is not refrigerated properly or is undercooked. Recently, tomatoes, spinach, and lettuce have been documented as sources of *Escherichia coli* outbreaks due to possible improper handling of the food. The appearance, flavor, and odor of contaminated food may be unaffected. Whether a client has previously had a food-borne infection does not necessarily reflect a diagnostic relationship to the present symptoms. Taking something for nausea does not help determine the cause of the problem.

Test Taking Strategy—*Use the process of elimination to select the option that represents the best assessment for determining if a food source is related to the client's symptoms. Option 2 can be eliminated because it focuses on the client's self-treatment. Option 4 can be eliminated because a prior incident of food poisoning does not necessarily provide critical information about the client's current health problem.*

Option 3 may look like it has merit, but food-borne pathogens do not always cause food to look or taste tainted. Option 1 emerges as the best answer. Review common causes of food-borne gastroenteritis and information that may indicate the etiology of gastroenteritis if you had difficulty answering this question.
Cognitive Level—*Applying*
Client Needs Category—*Safe and effective care environment*
Client Needs Subcategory—*Safety and infection control*

28. 4. Care of a client receiving internal radiation therapy is best rotated among all nonpregnant members of the nursing team because rotating care minimizes the time any one individual is exposed to radiation. It is safe and appropriate to warn personnel and visitors of a potential hazard, both verbally and using universal symbols. Radiation badges measure the amount of radiation exposure to the caregiver; therefore, each person involved in the client's care wears a different badge.

Test Taking Strategy—*Analyze to determine what information the question asks for, which is an unsafe intervention involving the care of a client receiving internal radiation therapy. Options 1, 2, and 3 all describe methods for ensuring the safety of persons who may have reason to be in contact with the client. Option 4 describes a potentially unsafe practice. Review the risks involved in caring for a client receiving internal radiation and precautions that are appropriate in the client's care if you had difficulty answering this question.*
Cognitive Level—*Applying*
Client Needs Category—*Safe and effective care environment*
Client Needs Subcategory—*Coordinated care*

29. 3. An intravenous pyelogram (IVP) is used to evaluate the structures of the urinary system and to assess renal function. An iodine-based dye injected intravenously is commonly used. After injection, the dye passes into the kidneys. X-rays are taken about 30 minutes later. A history of allergies is most important, especially if the client has a history of an allergy to iodine or seafood (which contains iodine). Allergic reactions vary from mild flushing and itching to anaphylactic shock. Delayed response to the dye can occur 2 to 6 hours after the test. If the client is allergic to iodine, the physician is notified before the client has the IVP. Urine output is monitored after the test. The other choices are not essential for the nurse to ask before the IVP.

Test Taking Strategy—*Look at the key word "essential," which indicates a priority. The question that is most important to ask is option 3, because the client may have a cross-sensitivity to the contrast medium used during an IVP if the client is allergic to seafood. Review the process involved in an IVP and potential hazards for a client on whom this test is performed if you had difficulty answering this question.*

Cognitive Level—*Analyzing*
Client Needs Category—*Safe and effective care environment*
Client Needs Subcategory—*Safety and infection control*

30. 1. Of the four options, listening to a radio or audiotapes is the most appropriate diversional activity for a client with a recent loss of vision. The newly blind client may not be ready to interact with others as a means of diversion. Listening to television may create anxiety because the client can only hear, not see, what is happening. Reading books set in Braille requires special education and time to practice the technique.

Test Taking Strategy—*Use the process of elimination to select the best diversional activity for a client who recently became blind. Option 4 can be immediately eliminated because it takes a long time to learn Braille. Option 3 can be eliminated because the media of television is designed primarily for sighted individuals. Option 2 may appear to have merit because it does provide diversion, but it is not the best answer. Option 1 emerges as the best answer. Review nursing care of a client with impaired vision, focusing on techniques for providing appropriate diversional activities if you had difficulty answering this question.*
Cognitive Level—*Analyzing*
Client Needs Category—*Physiological integrity*
Client Needs Subcategory—*Basic care and comfort*

31. 4. A compound fracture is one in which the bone pierces the skin and the bone is exposed. Pain, impaired mobility, and crepitation (grinding sensation) can be present in closed fractures as well; therefore, these findings do not provide the best evidence of a compound fracture.

Test Taking Strategy—*Use the process of elimination to select an option that provides the best description of a compound fracture. Options 1, 2, and 3 are signs and symptoms of any type of fracture, whether simple or compound. Option 4 emerges as the best answer because it is unique to compound fractures. Review the types of fractures and their complications if you had difficulty answering this question.*
Cognitive Level—*Applying*
Client Needs Category—*Physiological integrity*
Client Needs Subcategory—*Physiological adaptation*

32. 3. To determine the number of milliliters of an I.V. solution to infuse in 1 hour, the total quantity (in this example, 1,000 mL) is divided by the total hours of infusion (in this example, 8 hours). Therefore, the hourly volume is 125 mL.

Test Taking Strategy—*Analyze to determine what information the question asks for, which involves a calculation that yields the appropriate hourly volume of I.V. fluid based on the physician's order. Review the mathematical process for calculating I.V. infusion rates if you had difficulty answering this question.*

Cognitive Level—*Applying*
Client Needs Category—*Physiological integrity*
Client Needs Subcategory—*Pharmacological therapies*

33. 2. An antistreptolysin O test is useful in the diagnosis of rheumatic fever. This test detects antibodies to the enzymes of the streptococcus group A, which is thought to cause rheumatic fever, glomerulonephritis, bacterial endocarditis, scarlet fever, and other related conditions. The antinuclear antibody test is used to diagnose lupus erythematosus. The heterophile antibody titer is performed to determine if a person has infectious mononucleosis. The fluorescent antibody test is used to diagnose syphilis.

   Test Taking Strategy—*Look at the key words "most indicative" in relation to the laboratory test for confirming or ruling out a diagnosis of rheumatic fever. Option 2 is the correct answer; the other tests are associated with disorders other than rheumatic fever. Review diagnostic tests used when a client is suspected of having rheumatic fever if you had difficulty answering this question.*
   Cognitive Level—*Applying*
   Client Needs Category—*Physiological integrity*
   Client Needs Subcategory—*Physiological adaptation*

34. 4. Because the client is overweight, inserting the needle at a 90-degree angle is the most appropriate technique. Using a ⅝″ needle rather than a ½″ needle will allow the insulin to reach the subcutaneous tissue. A 15-degree angle is used for intradermal injections, such as in tuberculosis tests. A 30-degree angle is not used with subcutaneous injections. If the client were of normal weight, a 45-degree angle for the injection would be appropriate.

   Test Taking Strategy—*Look at the key words "most appropriate" and the information about the client's weight as they relate to the angle in which insulin is injected within the abdomen. Option 4 identifies the appropriate angle for reaching the subcutaneous depth in a client with excessive abdominal adipose tissue. Review techniques for administering a subcutaneous injection within the abdomen, especially when a client is obese, if you had difficulty answering this question.*
   Cognitive Level—*Analyzing*
   Client Needs Category—*Physiological integrity*
   Client Needs Subcategory—*Pharmacological therapies*

35. 2. Discharge teaching for a client who has undergone a prostatectomy includes the warning to avoid heavy lifting and strenuous exercise until the physician permits these activities. Constipation is avoided by eating foods high in roughage; enemas are also avoided. A liberal fluid intake is encouraged.

   Test Taking Strategy—*Look at the key words "most appropriate" in relation to discharge instructions after a prostatectomy. Option 2 is the best answer for ensuring that the client does not experience a* postoperative complication during the recovery period. Review postoperative instructions for a prostatectomy if you had difficulty answering this question.
   Cognitive Level—*Analyzing*
   Client Needs Category—*Physiological integrity*
   Client Needs Subcategory—*Reduction of risk potential*

36. 4. A client with expressive aphasia hears normally and understands verbal communication but has an impaired ability to provide a clear verbal response. Communication is improved in many instances if the nurse gives the client time to use motions or signs, write an answer (if able), or try to speak. Even though the speech of a client with expressive aphasia is greatly impaired, some affected people can be understood if the listener is patient. It is incorrect to assume that a client with aphasia is also intellectually compromised.

   Test Taking Strategy—*Use the process of elimination to select the option that is best when interacting with a client who has motor aphasia. Options 1 and 3 can be immediately eliminated because hearing and processing information are not problematic for a client with motor aphasia. Option 2 may appear attractive, but it is the client who may respond by writing because he or she is speech impaired. Option 4 emerges as the best answer. Review the differences between expressive and receptive aphasia if you had difficulty answering this question.*
   Cognitive Level—*Analyzing*
   Client Needs Category—*Physiological integrity*
   Client Needs Subcategory—*Basic care and comfort*

37. 2. Continuous bubbling is abnormal in the water-seal chamber but is normal in the suction-control chamber. Continuous bubbling in the water-seal chamber generally indicates an air leak in the tubing between the client and the water-seal chamber. The source of the air leak needs to be determined, or the therapeutic benefit of the water-seal drainage system will be compromised. The water seal is being maintained by the 2 cm of water. Bloody drainage is normal and a sign that the blood is being evacuated from the thorax. Breath sounds are usually diminished in clients with a hemothorax.

   Test Taking Strategy—*Look at the key word "immediately," which identifies a priority. Options 1, 3, and 4 describe normal or expected assessment findings. Option 2 is an indication that there is an air leak, which must be managed as soon as possible. Review nursing care of a client with closed water-seal chest drainage if you had difficulty answering this question.*
   Cognitive Level—*Analyzing*
   Client Needs Category—*Physiological integrity*
   Client Needs Subcategory—*Physiological adaptation*

38. 3. After cardiac catheterization, the nurse needs to assess the femoral pulse, which is located in the client's groin. The popliteal pulse is felt behind the knee. The pedal pulse is felt on the dorsum of the foot. The posterior tibial pulse is felt in the lower leg.

Test Taking Strategy—Analyze to determine what information the question asks for, which is the appropriate location of the fingers when assessing the femoral pulse. Knowing that the femoral pulse is located in the groin area, option 3 is the best answer. Review the names and locations of peripheral pulses if you had difficulty answering this question.
Cognitive Level—*Applying*
Client Needs Category—*Physiological integrity*
Client Needs Subcategory—*Reduction of risk potential*

39. 3. During the transition phase of active labor, the client may not tolerate touch but fears being left alone. Other signs of transition include nausea and vomiting, trembling of the lower extremities, irritability, and fear of losing control. Rupture of the membranes may occur spontaneously or artificially at any point during labor. The urge to push (the same feeling as the urge to have a bowel movement) occurs during the second stage of labor. Shivering is a normal response that may occur after delivery, during the fourth stage of labor.

Test Taking Strategy—Use the process of elimination to help select the option that correctly describes the transition phase of active labor. Options 1, 2, and 4 are observed in other stages of labor. Review the stages of labor and their characteristics if you had difficulty answering this question.
Cognitive Level—*Applying*
Client Needs Category—*Health promotion and maintenance*
Client Needs Subcategory—*None*

40. 1. Kegel exercises involve tightening and relaxing the pelvic floor muscles. The exercises are performed 4 or more times per day and from 5 to 20 times each session. Performed consistently, Kegel exercises prevent or relieve stress incontinence, shorten the second stage of labor, promote healing of perineal and rectal incisions, and increase the potential for sexual orgasm.

Test Taking Strategy—Use the process of elimination to help select the option that accurately describes the technique for performing Kegel exercises. Options 2 and 4 can be eliminated because Kegel exercises do not involve leg raising or rolling from side to side. Option 3 may look attractive, but Kegel exercises are not performed to strengthen abdominal muscles. Because Kegel exercises increase the tone of perineal muscles to prevent or relieve stress incontinence, option 1 emerges as the correct answer. Review the purpose and technique for performing Kegel exercises if you had difficulty answering this question.

Cognitive Level—*Applying*
Client Needs Category—*Health promotion and maintenance*
Client Needs Subcategory—*None*

41. 4. The correct procedure is to instill a volume of air equal to the volume that will be removed. Instilling air increases the pressure within the vial and facilitates removal of the drug. Omitting air instillation creates a vacuum in the vial when the drug is withdrawn. Injecting more air than the amount of the drug withdrawn creates excessive pressure in the vial, which may force the plunger out of the syringe. It is generally unnecessary to refrigerate a drug before withdrawing it from a vial unless the manufacturer recommends refrigeration.

Test Taking Strategy—Use the process of elimination to help select the option that identifies the correct technique for withdrawing a parenteral medication from a multidose vial. Option 1 is incorrect because only a portion of the medication is needed. Option 3 can be eliminated because refrigerating the vial for 10 minutes is not a standard practice. After eliminating these two choices, you are left with two options that both suggest injecting air into the vial; after analyzing these, eliminate option 2 because instilling 1 mL more of air than the amount of volume to withdraw is excessive. Option 4 emerges as the correct answer. Review the technique for withdrawing medication from a multidose vial if you had difficulty answering this question.
Cognitive Level—*Analyzing*
Client Needs Category—*Physiological integrity*
Client Needs Subcategory—*Pharmacological therapies*

42. 3. Recapping needles is a potentially hazardous action that can lead to needle-stick injuries and possible transmission of blood-borne pathogens. Wearing gloves, depositing sharp items in a biohazard container, and swabbing the site are safe and appropriate actions.

Test Taking Strategy—Analyze to determine what information the question asks for, which is an unsafe practice when administering an injection. Option 3 is unsafe because it increases the risk for acquiring a blood-borne pathogen if a puncture occurs. If capping a needle is desired, it can be done by "scooping" the needle cover before administering the medication to protect the fingers and hand of the person administering the injection, but recapping is never done after the injection is given. Review measures for avoiding injuries from sharp equipment such as needles attached to syringes if you had difficulty answering this question.
Cognitive Level—*Evaluating*
Client Needs Category—*Physiological integrity*
Client Needs Subcategory—*Pharmacological therapies*

43. 2. Mild to severe joint pain indicates bleeding into the joint, which can lead to joint deformities or destruction. Hemophiliacs with symptoms suggestive of bleeding need immediate medical attention. There is no direct connection between hemophilia and anorexia or nasal congestion. Depression may develop as a consequence of coping with a chronic illness. Depression indicates a need for additional nursing assessment for suicidal ideation and continued close observation.

Test Taking Strategy—Look at the key word "immediately," which indicates a priority. Joint pain (option 2) is the assessment finding most suggestive of a serious complication in a client with hemophilia. Review the potential complications that place a client with hemophilia at risk if you had difficulty answering this question.
Cognitive Level—Analyzing
Client Needs Category—Physiological integrity
Client Needs Subcategory—Reduction of risk potential

44. 1. Neuroleptic malignant syndrome (NMS) is a life-threatening condition characterized by fever, muscle rigidity, autonomic instability, and cognitive changes such as delirium. The most common cause of the condition is antipsychotic medication use. Generally the higher the client dosage, the more common the occurrence of the condition. Rapid and large changes in dosage can also trigger the condition. Having a past bleed on a magnetic resonance imaging (MRI) scan, having a low white blood cell count, or experiencing stress at work are not contributing factors in the development of NMS.

Test Taking Strategy—Analyze to determine what information the question asks for, which is a factor associated with the development of NMS. Knowing that antipsychotic drugs are also referred to as neuroleptics should lead to the selection of option 1 as the best answer. Review the side effects associated with antipsychotic medications if you had difficulty answering this question.
Cognitive Level—Applying
Client Needs Category—Physiological integrity
Client Needs Subcategory—Physiological adaptation

45. 4. The use of body powder on an infant is not recommended because of the risk for pneumonitis secondary to aspiration of the talc. A room temperature between 72°F and 75°F (22.2°C and 23.9°C) is appropriate. Wiping the teeth with gauze is appropriate oral care for an infant; as an alternative, having the infant drink water cleans the mouth. It is also appropriate to use the elbow to assess the bath water temperature because the elbow is sensitive to temperature variations.

Test Taking Strategy—Analyze to determine what information the question asks for, which involves identifying a practice performed by an unlicensed nursing assistant that needs changing. Option 4 is potentially unsafe and needs to be eliminated. Review the haz-ards associated with using baby powder on an infant if you had difficulty answering this question.
Cognitive Level—Analyzing
Client Needs Category—Safe and effective care environment
Client Needs Subcategory—Coordinated care

46. 1. Two abused drugs that may be injected into a vein are cocaine and heroin. Heroin is an opiate. Opiates are any drug containing or derived from opium. Cocaine is a stimulant; it is purified from the leaves of the cocoa plant. Cocaine is also commonly snorted through the nose or inhaled by smoking. Heroin is injected directly into a vein or under the skin, a technique known as "skin-popping." Barbiturates, amphetamines, and hallucinogens are more commonly self-administered by the oral route.

Test Taking Strategy—Analyze to determine what information the question asks for, which is a category of drugs among the options that are commonly injected intravenously. Heroin and some other opiate derivatives can be parenterally self-administered; drugs in the other categories are not. Review signs of opiate abuse if you had difficulty answering this question.
Cognitive Level—Applying
Client Needs Category—Physiological integrity
Client Needs Subcategory—Pharmacological therapies

47. 4. An advance directive is a legal document that describes how a client wishes to be treated or not treated should the client at some future time be unable to make this decision independently. The client may also select a spokesperson, such as the physician or a spouse, to act as a proxy regarding using or withholding medical treatment. Financial cost or insurance is not considered a priority in arriving at an ethical decision. It is unnecessary for all the client's relatives to agree or disagree on discontinuing life support.

Test Taking Strategy—Analyze to determine what information the question asks for, which is a legal basis that guides the nurse when faced with a request to cease life support. Ensuring that there is an advance directive (option 4) indicating the client's choice as to whether life support is desired or not is the first step. In addition, the physician should document that the client's condition is hopeless for recovery before the nurse follows a medical order for discontinuing life support. Review advance directives and their purpose if you had difficulty answering this question.
Cognitive Level—Analyzing
Client Needs Category—Safe and effective care environment
Client Needs Subcategory—Coordinated care

48. 3. Correct treatment of poison ingestion and the possible administration of an antidote depend on identification of the specific substance ingested. The client's age, who discovered the client, and the client's medical history are relevant but of lesser importance than identifying the substance.

Test Taking Strategy—Look at the key words "most important" in relation to obtaining assessment data about a toxic substance. Option 3 is the best choice from among the four options because identifying the substance may or may not have life-threatening consequences, or at the very least, can provide guidance on the treatment approach that is appropriate. Review information pertinent to assessing the client who ingests a toxic substance if you had difficulty answering this question.
Cognitive Level—*Analyzing*
Client Needs Category—*Physiological integrity*
Client Needs Subcategory—*Physiological adaptation*

49. 3. Reinforcing the fact that standard precautions can block the transmission of the virus from the client to the health care worker is the best information among the choices. Being told the sources of transmission is not as reassuring as reiterating how the transmission is blocked. Although many infected people are living longer, that information is not likely to give peace of mind. Health care workers who are occupationally infected with HIV may not qualify for workers' compensation benefits because it is difficult to prove that a specific incident resulted in infection.

Test Taking Strategy—Use the process of elimination to help select the option that is better than the others for allying a fear of contracting acquired immunodeficiency syndrome (AIDS). Option 1 can be eliminated because even knowing that life expectancy for an infected person has been somewhat increased, it does not compare to that of an uninfected person. Option 4 can be eliminated because the client's chief concern about AIDS is the potential for an early death rather than the need for financial assistance with the cost of care. Option 2 has some merit, but it is not as good an answer as option 3, which reinforces that Standard Precautions can prevent the transmission of human immunodeficiency virus. Review standard precautions and the modes of HIV transmission if you had difficulty answering this question.
Cognitive Level—*Analyzing*
Client Needs Category—*Safe and effective care environment*
Client Needs Subcategory—*Safety and infection control*

50. 1. Immediately after the membranes have ruptured, the nurse monitors the fetal heart rate to detect fetal distress. Natural or artificial rupture of the membranes may result in prolapse of the umbilical cord, which is followed by compression of the cord and interference with fetal oxygenation. Antibiotics are not routinely given when the amniotic membranes rupture. The physician may decide to place the client on antibiotics if the membranes have been ruptured for an extended time. Applying pads does not take priority over assessing for fetal distress. In the event of a prolapsed cord, the client is placed in Trendelenburg's position to assist with relieving umbilical cord compression.

Test Taking Strategy—Look at the key word "priority," which indicates that an immediate action is required. Knowing that the umbilical cord can be compressed once the fetus is no longer buoyed by the amniotic fluid should lead to selecting option 1. Review the nursing action that is indicated after the rupture of membranes if you had difficulty answering this question.
Cognitive Level—*Analyzing*
Client Needs Category—*Physiological integrity*
Client Needs Subcategory—*Reduction of risk potential*

51. 2, 5, 6. Pneumonia occurs most commonly in clients who are in a weak, immunosuppressed state; have chronic disorders, such as acquired immunodeficiency syndrome (AIDS), diabetes, cardiac or pulmonary disorders, cirrhosis, cancer, or renal failure; are malnourished, smokers, or alcoholics; or have been exposed to toxic airborne substances. Other risk factors for pneumonia include immobility and recent general endotracheal intubation or surgery. Risk factors for pneumonia also occur from the aging process, such as having a decreased force of cough, reduced number of alveoli, weakened respiratory muscles, deteriorating cilia, and air trapping in the respiratory system. Sudden weight gain, anemia, and dehydration are not considered risk factors for pneumonia. Aspiration pneumonia can occur if the client has a hypoactive, not a hyperactive, gag reflex.

Test Taking Strategy—Analyze to determine what information the question asks for, which is risk factors for pneumonia. Alternative-format "select all that apply" questions require considering each option independently to decide its merit in answering the question. Review risk factors for developing pneumonia if you had difficulty answering this question.
Cognitive Level—*Applying*
Client Needs Category—*Physiological integrity*
Client Needs Subcategory—*Physiological adaptation*

52. 3. Sitting upright with the feet and legs elevated reduces the myocardial workload. This position also allows for maximum expansion of the thoracic cavity. Low Fowler's position is used if the client cannot tolerate the upright position. Neither lying on the side nor lying with the head lowered would be advisable.

Test Taking Strategy—Look at the key word "best" in relation to a therapeutic position for a client in heart failure. Recall that a high Fowler's position (option 3) lowers the diaphragm and reduces compression of the heart and lungs. Review the rationale for placing a client in high Fowler's position if you had difficulty answering this question.
Cognitive Level—*Applying*
Client Needs Category—*Physiological integrity*
Client Needs Subcategory—*Physiological adaptation*

53. 3. Clients with slow-bleeding cerebral aneurysms are kept quiet to prevent additional or heavy bleeding. Until the physician indicates that it is safe for the client to increase activity, it is best for the nurse to position the client on a bedpan rather than on a bedside commode. Digital removal of stool is appropriate if the client has an impaction. Clients such as this one, who must avoid straining when defecating, are generally given a daily stool softener to facilitate ease of elimination.

Test Taking Strategy—Look at the key words "most appropriate" in relation to a nursing response to a request for ambulatory assistance from a client with a bleeding cerebral aneurysm. Ensuring the client's safety and reducing the potential for a complication should guide to selecting option 3 as the best answer. Review the effects of activity on a bleeding cerebral aneurysm if you had difficulty answering this question.
Cognitive Level—Analyzing
Client Needs Category—Physiological integrity
Client Needs Subcategory—Reduction of risk potential

54. 2. Flaccid muscle tone in a newborn must be reported immediately. A healthy newborn is generally active and displays kicking of the feet and flexion of the arms. The hands and feet may appear blue (acrocyanosis) for a short time after delivery while the rest of the body is pink. As the newborn's respirations improve and the baby is warmed, skin color tends to become pink overall. It is normal for a healthy newborn to have a pulse rate over 100 beats/minute and a loud, vigorous cry.

Test Taking Strategy—Look at the key words "most important," which suggest a priority. Option 2 describes a pathophysiological assessment finding that should be reported immediately. The remaining options are considered normal for a newborn infant. Review normal and abnormal assessment findings of a newborn if you had difficulty answering this question.
Cognitive Level—Analyzing
Client Needs Category—Physiological integrity
Client Needs Subcategory—Physiological adaptation

55. 3. Minor burns over a small area are treated first by immersing the affected part in cool water. Cool compresses may also be applied. Ointments or salves are not applied to minor burns. Normally, a dressing is unnecessary for minor burns. However, when a dressing is necessary, sterile gauze is applied over the area and anchored with nonallergenic tape above and below the burn site.

Test Taking Strategy—Analyze to determine what information the question asks for, which is the appropriate action to take when caring for a minor burn involving a finger. Recall that the depth and extent of a burn, as well as its discomfort, can be reduced by stopping the burning process. This leads to selecting

option 3 as the best answer from among the options. Review first-aid measures for minor burns if you had difficulty answering this question.
Cognitive Level—Analyzing
Client Needs Category—Physiological integrity
Client Needs Subcategory—Physiological adaptation

56. 3. Glaucoma is an eye disorder characterized by increased pressure in the eye. There are three types of glaucoma: closed-angle (acute), open-angle (chronic), and congenital. Closed-angle glaucoma is characterized by acute pain. Therefore, a therapeutic response after the treatment of closed-angle glaucoma is a reduction or elimination of pain within the eye. Swollen eyelids are not a manifestation of closed-angle glaucoma. The conjunctiva, not the sclera, is red during an acute attack of closed-angle glaucoma. Loss of peripheral vision is a pathologic consequence of untreated or ineffectively treated glaucoma.

Test Taking Strategy—Look at the key words "best evidence" in relation to a positive response to drug therapy for a client with acute angle-closure glaucoma. Recalling that a client with this disorder experiences pain during an acute episode leads to the conclusion that its reduction or absence is a sign of a therapeutic response. Review the signs and symptoms associated with acute angle-closure glaucoma if you had difficulty answering this question.
Cognitive Level—Applying
Client Needs Category—Physiological integrity
Client Needs Subcategory—Pharmacological therapies

57. 1. Liquid and ointment otic (ear) preparations are warmed to room temperature if they have been stored in a cool or cold area. Instilling cold medication into the ear is uncomfortable. Unless the dropper is grossly covered with debris or wax, it is unnecessary to clean it routinely. There are no general limitations on the maximum volume instilled within the ear. The anatomic size of the client's ear canal and the prescribed dose of medication are guidelines for the amount of drug administered.

Test Taking Strategy—Use the process of elimination to help select the option that accurately identifies an action that is appropriate before instilling eardrops. Option 2 can be eliminated because refrigerated or cold eardrops may precipitate dizziness when instilled. Option 3 can be eliminated because it is unlikely to cause any major consequences if there is contact between the ear and the dropper. Option 4 can be eliminated because only drops of medication are instilled regardless of how much volume is contained in the dropper. Review the technique for instilling eardrops if you had difficulty answering this question.
Cognitive Level—Analyzing
Client Needs Category—Physiological integrity
Client Needs Subcategory—Pharmacological therapies

58. 1. Fetal alcohol syndrome may result as a consequence of a mother who chronically consumes alcohol during pregnancy. The syndrome leads to mental and physical retardation or structural anomalies involving the head, eyes (widely set), ears, and heart. As children with this syndrome get older, some develop attention deficit hyperactivity disorder. Cataracts, seizures, and missing limbs are not closely associated with fetal alcohol syndrome.

> *Test Taking Strategy—Analyze to determine what information the question asks for, which is the potential effect on a fetus as a result of chronic maternal alcohol consumption. Knowing that fetal alcohol syndrome, which is accompanied by mental retardation, is a potential consequence of maternal alcohol consumption leads to selecting option 1 as the best answer. Review the manifestations of fetal alcohol syndrome if you had difficulty answering this question.*
> **Cognitive Level**—*Applying*
> **Client Needs Category**—*Physiological integrity*
> **Client Needs Subcategory**—*Pharmacological therapies*

59. 3. When the subject involves sexual abuse, the best initial response is to assume a child is telling the truth. After that, nursing actions such as those in the alternative options are appropriate.

> *Test Taking Strategy—Use the process of elimination to help select the option that identifies the best initial response to being informed by a child about sexual abuse. Option 1 can be eliminated immediately because the details surrounding the abuse are not necessary. Options 2 and 3 are actions that may be required later by someone trained in forensics and care of a sexually abused person. Option 3 remains as the best answer because it provides a mechanism for building trust and the potential for helping stop any future abuse. Review measures that are appropriate when there is a revelation of any kind of abuse by a child if you had difficulty answering this question.*
> **Cognitive Level**—*Analyzing*
> **Client Needs Category**—*Psychosocial integrity*
> **Client Needs Subcategory**—*None*

60. 2. The nurse may begin to observe withdrawal symptoms from alcohol as early as 4 to 6 hours after the last drink, especially in clients who have a pattern of consuming large amounts of alcohol on a regular basis. Further signs of alcohol withdrawal may continue for 12 to 72 hours. Initially, clients have a progressive elevation in their vital signs, tremors, and diaphoresis. If withdrawal is uncontrolled, seizures and hallucinations may also occur.

> *Test Taking Strategy—Look at the key words "most likely time frame" in relation to initial signs of alcohol withdrawal. Signs of withdrawal occur soon after the last drink in someone who chronically consumes alcohol. Alcoholics often resume drinking on awakening to reduce or eliminate withdrawal symptoms after having consumed alcohol at bedtime.*

> *This information leads to choosing option 2 as the best answer. Review the manifestations of alcohol withdrawal and the expected time for these to occur if you had difficulty answering this question.*
> **Cognitive Level**—*Understanding*
> **Client Needs Category**—*Psychosocial integrity*
> **Client Needs Subcategory**—*None*

61. 4. Burns around the face and neck may compromise breathing as a consequence of inhaling heated air and debris or the swelling of burned tissue. Initially, the burned client will have a fluid volume deficit related to fluid shifts. Hemorrhage does not commonly occur with burns unless there has been an additional injury, such as a wound or fracture. Signs of infection are not evident initially but may occur several days after the injury.

> *Test Taking Strategy—Look at the key word "immediately," which suggests a priority. Recall that any compromise in the airway and breathing can be life-threatening. This leads to selecting option 4 as the best answer. Review the nursing care of a client with burns involving the face and neck if you had difficulty answering this question.*
> **Cognitive Level**—*Analyzing*
> **Client Needs Category**—*Physiological integrity*
> **Client Needs Subcategory**—*Physiological adaptation*

62. 2. Frequent range-of-motion (ROM) exercises, along with regularly changing a client's position, help to prevent contractures. Isometric exercises maintain muscle tone but do not prevent contractures. Elevating extremities on pillows promotes venous circulation and decreases edema but does not necessarily prevent contractures. Pressure-relieving devices maintain capillary blood flow, which is necessary for maintaining tissue integrity, not preventing contractures.

> *Test Taking Strategy—Use the process of elimination to help select the option that is best for preventing contractures. Options 3 and 4 can be eliminated because they are better suited for maintaining skin integrity. Option 1 may seem correct, but isometric exercises tend to improve or maintain muscle size and tone. Option 2 emerges as the best answer because it involves keeping joints flexible. Review the purpose for ROM exercises and measures for preventing contractures if you had difficulty answering this question.*
> **Cognitive Level**—*Analyzing*
> **Client Needs Category**—*Physiological integrity*
> **Client Needs Subcategory**—*Basic care and comfort*

63. 1. A foul wound odor indicates an infection. The odor of infection is different from the odor associated with burn exudate. Eschar normally turns black after a time. A white blood cell (WBC) count of 5,000/mm³ is normal and, therefore, not an indicator of infection. Tachycardia might occur if an infection is present, but there are other physiological explanations for a rapid heart rate.

Test Taking Strategy—Use the process of elimination to help select the option that describes a finding that correlates with the presence of infection in a burn wound. Option 2 can be eliminated because eschar is an expected finding in a severe burn. Option 2 can be eliminated because it is a normal finding; an elevated WBC count would be more likely. Option 4 has merit, because a client is likely to be tachycardic if a systemic response to an infection has developed, but option 1 is the best answer because it indicates that once-healthy tissue is being damaged by pathogenic organisms. Review the signs of localized infection in a burn wound if you had difficulty answering this question.
Cognitive Level—*Applying*
Client Needs Category—*Physiological integrity*
Client Needs Subcategory—*Physiological adaptation*

64. 4. For a client recovering from gastroenteritis, nonirritating solid foods are added to the diet first. Foods such as bananas, rice, applesauce, toast (BRAT), tea, and yogurt (BRATTY) are provided initially. Milk products are among the last foods reintroduced to the diet because milk and milk products can be hard to digest. However, yogurt helps to recolonize the bowel with beneficial bacteria. Vanilla pudding contains milk, and milk is usually added to oatmeal or cereal. Salty broths such as chicken broth are also avoided. Furthermore, chicken broth is not a solid food.
Test Taking Strategy—Analyze to determine what information the question asks for, which is identifying a food that is provided when eating is initially resumed in the course of managing gastroenteritis. Options 1 and 3 can be eliminated because they contain dairy products. Option 2 can be eliminated because it is a clear liquid rather than a solid food. Review the progression of foods that are appropriate for a client recovering from gastroenteritis if you had difficulty answering this question.
Cognitive Level—*Analyzing*
Client Needs Category—*Physiological integrity*
Client Needs Subcategory—*Basic care and comfort*

65. 3. Large muscle activities that release nervous energy such as using a treadmill are best for clients with generalized anxiety disorder. Playing cards, assembling models, and painting are too sedentary.
Test Taking Strategy—Look at the key words "most appropriate" in relation to selecting an activity that is therapeutic for a client with generalized anxiety. Recall that symptoms of anxiety are a result of sympathetic nervous system stimulation. An activity that depletes accumulated energy, as in option 3, is the best answer. Review measures for reducing or eliminating anxiety if you had difficulty answering this question.
Cognitive Level—*Analyzing*
Client Needs Category—*Psychosocial integrity*
Client Needs Subcategory—*None*

66. 1. Normal potassium levels are between 3.5 and 5.0 mEq/L. A value lower than 3.5 mEq/L indicates hypokalemia. Signs of hypokalemia include muscle weakness, leg cramping, shallow respirations, shortness of breath, irregular rapid heart rate, electrocardiographic (ECG) changes, confusion, depression, lethargy, and GI symptoms. Rapid weight gain is a sign of hypernatremia (elevated sodium level). Slurred speech is a sign of hypophosphatemia (low phosphate level).
Test Taking Strategy—Analyze to determine what information the question asks for, which is a means for validating hypokalemia, which is option 1. Options 3 and 4 are associated with electrolyte imbalances other than hypokalemia. Review the signs and symptoms of hypokalemia if you had difficulty answering this question.
Cognitive Level—*Analyzing*
Client Needs Category—*Physiological integrity*
Client Needs Subcategory—*Physiological adaptation*

67. 1. Diabetes commonly causes altered blood flow to the retina, resulting in a condition known as diabetic retinopathy. Such changes can lead to poor vision and possible blindness. Consequently, clients with diabetes should have their vision checked at least once per year and should be instructed to notify their physician if sudden vision changes occur. Cataracts related to the increased levels of blood glucose may also occur in clients with diabetes. Diabetes is associated with polyuria, but the color of the urine is not typically noted when evaluating for signs and symptoms of diabetes. Neither elevated blood pressure nor heart palpitations are complications of diabetes. Other complications of diabetes include periodontal disease and changes in the circulation of the lower extremities that can result in ulcerations, increased infections, gangrene, and amputations. In addition, changes in the peripheral nerves can cause weakness and pain as well as impaired GI, genitourinary, and vasomotor functioning.
Test Taking Strategy—Analyze to determine what information the question asks for, which is a query that could elicit information relating to a complication of diabetes mellitus. Recall that one complication of diabetes is retinopathy, which leads to selecting option 1. Diabetics should have a yearly eye examination by an ophthalmologist. Review the complications of diabetes mellitus if you had difficulty answering this question.
Cognitive Level—*Analyzing*
Client Needs Category—*Health promotion and maintenance*
Client Needs Subcategory—*None*

68. 2. Rheumatic fever may follow a streptococcal infection. Therefore, a history of a recent sore throat, which may have been due to *Streptococcus* microorganisms, is pertinent to the diagnosis. Viral infections, such as influenza, chickenpox, and roseola, are not known to be associated with rheumatic fever.

> *Test Taking Strategy—Analyze to determine what information the question asks for, which is identifying a factor that may contribute to the etiology of rheumatic fever. Recall that a pharyngitis caused by a streptococcal infection can precede rheumatic fever, making option 2 the correct answer. Review the causes of rheumatic fever if you had difficulty answering this question.*
> **Cognitive Level**—Applying
> **Client Needs Category**—Health promotion and maintenance
> **Client Needs Subcategory**—None

69. 4. Joint pain and tenderness (arthralgia) involving one or more joints is noted when assessing a client with rheumatic fever. Urticaria, hypothermia, and hypotension are not typically associated with rheumatic fever.

> *Test Taking Strategy—Analyze to determine what information the question asks for, which is a sign or symptom that relates to rheumatic fever. Recall that migratory joint pain accompanies rheumatic fever. Therefore, option 4 is the best answer. Review the manifestations of rheumatic fever if you had difficulty answering this question.*
> **Cognitive Level**—Applying
> **Client Needs Category**—Physiological integrity
> **Client Needs Subcategory**—Physiological adaptation

70. 4. When performing a nonstress test, each incident of heart rate acceleration must last for at least 15 seconds. For a nonstress test to be considered favorable, there must also be at least two fetal heart rate accelerations of at least 15 beats/minute within a 20-minute to 30-minute time frame. Fetal movement must be present.

> *Test Taking Strategy—Use the process of elimination to help select the option that best correlates with evidence of an unfavorable response during a nonstress test. Options 1, 2, and 3 all report findings that are considered favorable fetal responses to a nonstress test. Option 4 is the correct choice because accelerations lasting less than 15 seconds are an unfavorable response. Review the process by which a nonstress test is performed on a pregnant female and indications of normal and abnormal responses if you had difficulty answering this question.*
> **Cognitive Level**—Evaluating
> **Client Needs Category**—Health promotion and maintenance
> **Client Needs Subcategory**—None

71. 2. Because mechanical friction further traumatizes skin affected by radiation, the client's skin should be cleaned with mild soap and tepid water and then patted dry. Vigorous rubbing over the area could cause skin dam-

age. The marks are never removed because they are meant to remain on the skin throughout radiation therapy. The irradiated skin is protected from direct sunlight. Clothing that covers the area of treatment must fit loosely.

> *Test Taking Strategy—Look at the key word "essential," which indicates a priority. Recall that radiation affects normal skin as well as the cancerous tumor. To avoid further trauma to healthy tissue, option 2 is the correct answer. Review the nursing care of a client undergoing radiation therapy if you had difficulty answering this question.*
> **Cognitive Level**—Analyzing
> **Client Needs Category**—Physiological integrity
> **Client Needs Subcategory**—Physiological adaptation

72. 1. Constipation is a side effect of antacids containing aluminum and calcium. Antacids containing magnesium cause a laxative effect. An antacid should relieve dyspepsia. Flatus and a dry mouth can occur for a number of reasons, but they are not generally a side effect of an antacid.

> *Test Taking Strategy—Look at the key words "most likely" in relation to a side effect of an antacid containing aluminum hydroxide. Recall that aluminum hydroxide produces its effects in the GI tract, making option 1 the correct answer. Review the effect antacids have on bowel elimination if you had difficulty answering this question.*
> **Cognitive Level**—Understanding
> **Client Needs Category**—Physiological integrity
> **Client Needs Subcategory**—Pharmacological therapies

73. 2. Temperature assessment by the rectal route is avoided when a child has leukemia because of the danger of causing injury and bleeding. A sponge or gauze is appropriate to use for mouth care to prevent gums from bleeding. Children with leukemia are maintained in protective isolation because of their compromised immune status. A sheepskin is placed under bony prominences for comfort.

> *Test Taking Strategy—Analyze to determine what information the question asks for, which is an evaluation of the nursing assistant's actions. Examine the options to identify an action that is being performed incorrectly or unsafely. Recall that a client with leukemia is prone to bleeding because platelet levels are generally decreased. This leads to selecting option 2, which could cause injury. Review the nursing care of a client with leukemia if you had difficulty answering this question.*
> **Cognitive Level**—Evaluating
> **Client Needs Category**—Safe and effective care environment
> **Client Needs Subcategory**—Coordinated care

74. 3. Pantoprazole (Protonix) is a proton pump inhibitor that inhibits the production of gastric secretions, making the gastric contents less acidic. Some antiulcer medications, such as sucralfate (Carafate), form a protective coating similar to mucus at the ulcer site. This layer shields the irritated tissue from further irritation by hydrochloric acid and pepsin. Antacids neutralize gastric secretions, raising their pH. Histamine antagonists reduce gastric acid production by blocking histamine-2 receptors.

Test Taking Strategy—Use the process of elimination to help select the option that correctly identifies the rationale for using pantoprazole in ulcer therapy. Option 1 can be immediately eliminated because increasing gastric acidity is undesirable. Options 2 and 4 have merit because ulcers can be treated with medications that produce these effects. However, because pantoprazole is a proton pump inhibitor, option 3 is the best explanation of its action. Review the mechanism of action of the different classes of medications used to treat ulcers if you had difficulty answering this question.

Cognitive Level—Understanding
Client Needs Category—Physiological integrity
Client Needs Subcategory—Pharmacological therapies

75. 4. The volume used to irrigate a colostomy is the same as the volume used to administer a cleansing enema. Commonly, the volume for a cleansing enema and colostomy irrigation is between 500 and 1,000 mL.

Test Taking Strategy—Use the process of elimination to help select the option that identifies a standard volume used for a cleansing enema administered to an adult. Options 1, 2, and 3 are lower than the usual amount. Option 4 emerges as the best answer. Review the process of irrigating a colostomy if you had difficulty answering this question.

Cognitive Level—Understanding
Client Needs Category—Physiological integrity
Client Needs Subcategory—Basic care and comfort

76. 1. The main difference between type 1 and type 2 diabetes is the sudden onset of symptoms. Type 2 diabetic patients usually have gradual onset of symptoms. The signs and symptoms include polydipsia, polyuria (not a decrease in urine output), polyphagia, nocturia, and weight loss (not weight gain). The onset of diabetic symptoms in children is often associated with ketoacidosis, which is a life-threatening condition. Insulin, not oral hypoglycemic agents, is used to treat adolescent clients with type 1 diabetes.

Test Taking Strategy—Analyze to determine what information the question asks for, which is a characteristic associated with type 1 diabetes mellitus. Type 1 diabetes mellitus is marked by a sudden onset (option 1). Review the signs and symptoms of type 1 diabetes mellitus and their differences in relation to

type 2 diabetes if you had difficulty answering this question.

Cognitive Level—Applying
Client Needs Category—Physiological integrity
Client Needs Subcategory—Physiological adaptation

77. 2. Sliding a client up in bed causes friction, which can injure the skin, predisposing it to breakdown and pressure ulcers. It is better to logroll the client or use a mechanical lift or a trapeze to change positions. When rolling a client, the nurse must maintain the correct anatomic position, keeping the limbs supported. A mechanical lift is particularly useful if the client is large or difficult to move. The lift moves and holds the client when moving in or out of bed. By holding onto the trapeze, the client can assist the nurse in turning and repositioning.

Test Taking Strategy—Analyze to determine what information the question asks for, which is an incorrect or unsafe positioning technique when caring for a client who is paralyzed on one side of his or her body. Recall that friction, which can be produced by sliding a client in bed, can impair the integrity of the skin. This knowledge leads to selecting option 2 as the answer. Review techniques for preventing skin impairment when changing the position of a client who has compromised mobility if you had difficulty answering this question.

Cognitive Level—Analyzing
Client Needs Category—Physiological integrity
Client Needs Subcategory—Basic care and comfort

78. 4. Eyedrops are instilled into the lower conjunctival sac. Before instilling eyedrops, the nurse should first ask the client to look up, then pull the lower lid margin downward by exerting pressure over the bony prominence of the cheek.

Test Taking Strategy—Analyze to determine what information the question asks for, which is the preferred anatomic location for administering eyedrops. Recall that the goal is to instill the medication into a pocket of tissue and avoid the distribution of eye medication into the lacrimal duct located in the inner canthus. This knowledge leads to selecting option 3 as the correct answer. Review the technique for administering liquid eye medication if you had difficulty answering this question.

Cognitive Level—Understanding
Client Needs Category—Physiological integrity
Client Needs Subcategory—Pharmacological therapies

79. 2. A polymerase chain reaction (PCR) test is a more reliable test than the enzyme-linked immunosorbent assay (ELISA) or Western blot test for determining the human immunodeficiency virus (HIV) status of infants and young children. The Western blot test and the ELISA both evaluate the presence of IgG antibodies that can cross the placenta and give a false-positive result if the mother is HIV positive. The PCR test detects HIV, not antibodies, and is therefore more reliable. The rapid plasma reagin (RPR) test is a serologic test used to detect syphilis.

> *Test Taking Strategy—Analyze to determine what information the question asks for, which is the diagnostic test that confirms or rules out HIV infection in an infant. Option 4 can be eliminated because it does not test for HIV. Recall that the preferred test is different in an exposed infant than in an adult. This leads to selecting option 2 as the correct answer. Review the different types of diagnostic tests used for HIV, focusing on the test that is best used for infants and children, if you had difficulty answering this question.*

Cognitive Level—*Applying*
Client Needs Category—*Physiological integrity*
Client Needs Subcategory—*Physiological adaptation*

80. 1. Heroin, like morphine, causes the pupils to constrict. Although a person with a heroin overdose might be hypotensive, this finding is not as significant as finding pinpoint pupils. There may be multiple reasons why the client does not respond to pain. Heroin does not produce a characteristic breath odor as occurs with alcohol consumption or medical conditions such as diabetic ketoacidosis.

> *Test Taking Strategy—Look at the key words "most appropriate" in relation to an assessment technique that relates to a heroin overdose. Recall that the pupils of those who abuse heroin are generally pinpoint in size. Although the other options are general assessments that are indicated when initially caring for an unconscious client, the outcome of option 1 contributes to confirming or ruling out an opiate overdose as the cause of the client's unresponsiveness. Review signs and symptoms of an opiate overdose if you had difficulty answering this question.*

Cognitive Level—*Analyzing*
Client Needs Category—*Psychosocial integrity*
Client Needs Subcategory—*None*

81. 1. The supine position is contraindicated for a client receiving epidural anesthesia because it causes vena cava compression and results in maternal hypotension. Hypotension reduces placental perfusion and fetal oxygenation. Semi-Fowler's and right or left side-lying positions do not compress the vena cava and are, therefore, more appropriate.

> *Test Taking Strategy—Analyze to determine what information the question asks for, which is an incorrect or unsafe position for a client who is receiving epidural anesthesia. Based on the potential for the risks identified, option 1 is the correct answer. Review the safe positions for a client receiving epidural anesthesia if you had difficulty answering this question.*

Cognitive Level—*Analyzing*
Client Needs Category—*Physiological integrity*
Client Needs Subcategory—*Reduction of risk potential*

82. 1. The child who has attention deficit hyperactivity disorder (ADHD) requires an environment free of distractions to facilitate processing information. Group teaching creates a greater potential for distraction. Rewarding desirable behavior is considered more therapeutic for effecting change than administering punishment. Having a consistent routine also proves to be more effective than varying the routine.

> *Test Taking Strategy—Look at the key words "most appropriate" in relation to a teaching method that is best for a child with a short attention span and who is easily distracted. These factors support choosing option 1 as the answer. Review the characteristics of ADHD, focusing on techniques for promoting learning, if you had difficulty answering this question.*

Cognitive Level—*Analyzing*
Client Needs Category—*Psychosocial integrity*
Client Needs Subcategory—*None*

83. 3. After the death of a spouse, it is important to eventually develop a new identity, learn new life skills, engage in new activities, and establish new relationships. Until the acute grief is resolved, however, it is important to delay making major changes. Rushing into decisions too soon often leads to regrets later. Suggesting that the client look into renting an apartment or congratulating the client's decision is inappropriate and nontherapeutic.

> *Test Taking Strategy—Look at the key words "most appropriate" as they relate to a nursing response to a client who is making major lifestyle changes while still recovering from a significant loss. Option 3 is the best answer because the client may not be able to fully evaluate the consequences of decisions made at this time. Review the process of dealing with significant losses and their physical, psychological, and emotional effects if you had difficulty answering this question.*

Cognitive Level—*Analyzing*
Client Needs Category—*Psychosocial integrity*
Client Needs Subcategory—*None*

84. 3. Verbalization allows the bereaved to express emotions connected with grief. Many people need to continue processing their grief over and over again, and they may not receive that opportunity from others who feel inadequate to deal with the emotional pain. Grieving is unique to each person, but it may take several years to resolve the loss of a significant person. Giving advice is nontherapeutic; clients may fear losing the nurse's support if they do not take the advice. Recommending a cruise with other senior citizens or referring the client to an accountant for financial advice is unlikely to resolve the client's grief.

> *Test Taking Strategy—Look at the key words "most therapeutic" as they relate to helping a person cope during the process of grieving. Recall that it is always therapeutic to engage a person with emotional issues to dialogue about the personal*

effects of the loss. Supporting this principle leads to selecting option 3 as the best answer. Review principles of therapeutic communication, especially in relation to resolving grief, if you had difficulty answering this question.
Cognitive Level—*Analyzing*
Client Needs Category—*Psychosocial integrity*
Client Needs Subcategory—*None*

85. 2. Home health care nurses must guard against making assumptions when their clients' environments do not reflect their own values and standards. In this case, although there are obvious health hazards in the home environment, such as its lack of cleanliness, the most suspicious finding suggesting elder abuse is the conflicting explanations about the cause of the client's injuries. Although a private bedroom is more desirable than sleeping on a couch, this may be the only option at this time. The cause of the client's weight loss should be investigated, but it is not necessarily the most suspicious finding indicating elder abuse because it may have a medical cause.

> *Test Taking Strategy—Analyze to determine what information the question asks for, which is an assessment finding that supports the hypothesis that the client's trauma is due to abuse. Recall when assessing a victim of abuse, regardless of age, that there are often variations in the explanations for how the injuries occurred. The inconsistency tends to confirm the suspicion that the real reason is being concealed. Review signs of abuse, focusing on elder abuse, if you had difficulty answering this question.*
Cognitive Level—*Evaluating*
Client Needs Category—*Psychosocial integrity*
Client Needs Subcategory—*None*

86. 2. Procedures that can affect the circulation in the affected arm, such as taking a blood pressure, giving injections, instilling I.V. solutions, and having laboratory blood draws, must be avoided to decrease the potential for ineffective tissue perfusion. The affected arm should be elevated above the heart. The arm on the operative side Abduction exercises of the arm on the operative side are temporarily restricted. The wound drainage container should be emptied at least once a shift or more often as the volume accumulates.

> *Test Taking Strategy—Use the process of elimination to determine which nursing order is appropriate to add to a care plan of a client in the early postoperative period following a mastectomy. Recall that clients who have had a breast removed are at risk for compromised circulation of blood and lymph in the arm on the operative side. Review the postoperative care following a mastectomy if you had difficulty answering this question.*
Cognitive Level—*Analyzing*
Client Needs Category—*Physiological integrity*
Client Needs Subcategory—*Reduction of risk potential*

87. 1. Symptoms similar to menopause such as hot flashes tend to occur when the ovaries are surgically removed. If there are no contraindications, estrogen replacement therapy can relieve many of the uncomfortable symptoms. Menstrual periods cease when the ovaries are removed. Leg cramps are unrelated to the oophorectomy but are important to report to the physician if they occur. Orgasms are unaffected by removal of the ovaries.

> *Test Taking Strategy—Look at the key words "most appropriate" as they relate to discharge teaching for a client who is predisposed to estrogen deficiency secondary to having the ovaries removed. Recall that when estrogen levels fall during the perimenopausal period, which is no different hormonally than when the ovaries are removed, clients experience physiologic phenomena such as hot flashes and sweating (option 1). Review the physiologic manifestations associated with menopause if you had difficulty answering this question.*
Cognitive Level—*Analyzing*
Client Needs Category—*Physiological integrity*
Client Needs Subcategory—*Physiological adaptation*

88. 2. Involving the older adult in planning the transition to the long-term care facility reduces feelings of powerlessness. Feeling that one is part of the solution is better than feeling that one is part of the problem. Obtaining factual information, consulting the physician, and reinforcing positive expected outcomes are helpful but futile if the client feels a loss of control. Labeling the client's clothes is a task that is helpful but does not aid in the client's psychosocial transition.

> *Test Taking Strategy—Look at the key words "most therapeutic" in relation to transitioning an older adult to a care facility. Recall that older adults have been accustomed to making their own decisions. To promote acceptance and ownership of a change, it is important to include the person most affected in the decision-making process, which leads to selecting option 2. Review methods for being a change-agent if you had difficulty answering this question.*
Cognitive Level—*Analyzing*
Client Needs Category—*Psychosocial integrity*
Client Needs Subcategory—*None*

89. 2. Ambulation and movement help in preventing thrombi and hypostatic pneumonia. Early ambulation also promotes resumption of peristalsis, which facilitates oral nutrition. Although nutrition and fluids are important, the client's needs can be met temporarily with parenteral therapy. Intake and output are measures for assessing and evaluating whether fluid replacement and output are adequate. The client's emotional adjustment demands the nurse's attention, but physical recovery is primary to the discharge goals.

> *Test Taking Strategy—Look at the key words "most helpful" as they relate to preventing a postoperative complication. Although all of the options are components of appropriate postoperative nursing care,*

option 2, if not addressed, may lead to interference in the client's recovery and extension of the client's hospitalization. Review postoperative nursing care and measures to avoid complications if you had difficulty answering this question.
Cognitive Level—*Analyzing*
Client Needs Category—*Physiological integrity*
Client Needs Subcategory—*Reduction of risk potential*

90. 3. Hospice nurses are dedicated to facilitating the personal preferences of dying clients and managing how they wish to live and die. Secondarily, they are committed to supporting family members, who tend to be the primary caregivers. Calling hospice nurses "better" nurses is too subjective a statement. Hospice nurses have the same basic education and technical skills as hospital nurses. Hospice nurses make frequent or daily visits to the home, depending on the client needs, but do not provide around-the-clock care. Although some dying clients live longer than expected, that is not an expected outcome of hospice care.
Test Taking Strategy—*Use the process of elimination to select a statement that identifies the role hospice care when a client is terminally ill. This leads to selecting option 3 as the best answer. Review the mission of hospice care if you had difficulty answering this question.*
Cognitive Level—*Analyzing*
Client Needs Category—*Psychosocial integrity*
Client Needs Subcategory—*None*

91. 4. The child with attention deficit hyperactivity disorder (ADHD) has such characteristic symptoms as difficulty concentrating, disruptive behavior, failing to complete tasks, constantly moving and fidgeting, and acting in a loud and noisy manner. The child understands but does not follow directions well because of being easily distracted. Lack of interest in surroundings and refusal to play with others are not characteristic of this disorder.
Test Taking Strategy—*Analyze to determine what information the question asks for, which is a behavior manifested by a child with ADHD. Recall that the child suffers from hyperactivity, as the title of the disorder suggests, which leads to selecting option 4 as the answer. Review the characteristics of a person diagnosed with ADHD if you had difficulty answering this question.*
Cognitive Level—*Applying*
Client Needs Category—*Psychosocial integrity*
Client Needs Subcategory—*None*

92. 1. Infants of diabetic mothers are commonly hypoglycemic at birth or shortly thereafter; therefore, the first nursing action is to assess the blood glucose level. If hypoglycemia is not detected and treated with either oral or I.V. glucose, the infant may develop severe, irreversible central nervous system damage and may die. Infants of diabetic mothers are often large for their gestational age, but this assessment does not take priority over determining

whether the infant is hypoglycemic. The infant of the diabetic mother is also at risk for respiratory distress and hyperbilirubinemia. However, before receiving oxygen or phototherapy, the infant should be evaluated to determine if there is a need for treatment.
Test Taking Strategy—*Look at the key words "most important" and "initially," which suggest the need to select the priority from among the options. Recall that the infant's blood glucose level, which was elevated in utero, will quickly decrease when it is separated from the source of maternal glucose. Hypoglycemia has the potential for being life-threatening. Therefore, option 1 is the answer. Review care of a newborn infant born to a diabetic mother if you had difficulty answering this question.*
Cognitive Level—*Analyzing*
Client Needs Category—*Physiological integrity*
Client Needs Subcategory—*Reduction of risk potential*

93. 2. Pyridostigmine (Mestinon) is a drug commonly used to treat myasthenia gravis. It belongs to a group of cholinergic drugs that promote skeletal muscle contraction. Therefore, the goal of drug therapy is to obtain optimal muscle strength. Signs that the drug levels are nontherapeutic (too low) include signs of the disease itself, such as rapid fatigability, drooping eyelids, and difficulty breathing. The other options are unrelated to myasthenia gravis.
Test Taking Strategy—*Use the process of elimination to help select the therapeutic effect associated with the administration of pyridostigmine. Options 1, 3, and 4 can be eliminated because they describe functions that are controlled by other than skeletal muscles. Review the action and therapeutic use of pyridostigmine if you had difficulty answering this question.*
Cognitive Level—*Understanding*
Client Needs Category—*Physiological integrity*
Client Needs Subcategory—*Pharmacological therapies*

94. 3. Squeezing blackheads and pimples can cause spread of infection and scarring of the skin. A client with acne can wear cosmetics but should avoid those that are oil based. Makeup should be removed nightly with mild soap. Drying agents reduce skin oil that tends to accumulate on the skin surface and occlude hair follicles.
Test Taking Strategy—*Look at the key word "essential" as it applies to a priority for teaching a client with acne how to avoid secondary infections and scarring. Although cleanliness and reducing oily secretions from the face help reduce the lesions, the hands are sources of organisms that may enter lesions as they are traumatically manipulated (option 3). Review the importance of handwashing as a medically aseptic technique if you had difficulty answering this question.*
Cognitive Level—*Analyzing*
Client Needs Category—*Physiological integrity*
Client Needs Subcategory—*Basic care and comfort*

95. 1. To avoid undue strain and tension on the repaired muscle, clients who have undergone a hernia repair must avoid any activity that increases intra-abdominal pressure. Coughing, heavy lifting, sneezing, and straining to have a bowel movement can lead to an incisional hernia until the repaired area has healed. There is no reason for emptying the bladder any more frequently than to maintain comfort. There are no restrictions on turning. Ambulation is not limited unless the client develops a surgical complication.

> *Test Taking Strategy—Look at the key words "most appropriate" as they relate to discharge instructions for a client after repair of an inguinal hernia. Recall that coughing increases intra-abdominal pressure, creating internal force on the incision. Because it is weak at this time, not having healed completely, the tissue is susceptible to developing another hernia. Review the postoperative nursing management of a client after repair of a hernia if you had difficulty answering this question.*
>
> **Cognitive Level**—*Analyzing*
> **Client Needs Category**—*Physiological integrity*
> **Client Needs Subcategory**—*Reduction of risk potential*

96. 1. After inserting the tube, the nurse should check for placement of the tube in the stomach by aspirating stomach contents and injecting air into the stomach while auscultating with a stethoscope. (An X-ray may be ordered to verify placement.) If the client turns blue, has difficulty speaking, or begins to cough or wheeze, the tube is removed immediately because it is either in the client's trachea or is occluding the airway. Suction is applied after tube placement has been verified. Irrigation is usually performed when there are large clots or tissue debris occluding the tubing. Irrigation is not done unless tube placement has been verified. Although the client is not allowed to drink or eat, the nurse may offer small sips of water or ice chips sparingly after the tube is connected to suction.

> *Test Taking Strategy—Look at the key word "immediately" as it relates to a nursing action after inserting a Salem sump tube. Recall that a nasogastric tube has the potential for entering the airway. Thus checking its placement (option 1) is the priority action. Review the sequence of nursing actions when inserting a nasogastric tube if you had difficulty answering this question.*
>
> **Cognitive Level**—*Analyzing*
> **Client Needs Category**—*Physiological integrity*
> **Client Needs Subcategory**—*Reduction of risk potential*

97. 4. The most common adverse reactions to nonsteroidal anti-inflammatory drugs (NSAIDs) include nausea, vomiting, abdominal discomfort, diarrhea, constipation, and gastric or duodenal ulcers. Double vision, transient dizziness, and irregular pulse are not common side effects of NSAIDs.

> *Test Taking Strategy—Analyze to determine what information the question asks for, which is correct information the client identifies as common side effect of NSAID therapy. Recall that NSAIDs should be taken with food because when taken on an empty stomach, they cause gastric irritation, which can possibly lead to ulcer formation and gastric bleeding. Review the side effects of NSAIDs and methods for reducing their development if you had difficulty answering this question.*
>
> **Cognitive Level**—*Evaluating*
> **Client Needs Category**—*Physiological integrity*
> **Client Needs Subcategory**—*Pharmacological therapies*

98. 1. Emergency treatment of a chemical burn is directed at diluting and removing the substance as rapidly as possible by flushing the skin with large quantities of water. Applying a sterile dressing may cause tissue to adhere to the skin and pull tissue from the burn area. Specific dressings for burns will be applied after dilution and removal of the chemical from the skin. Applying a thick layer of petroleum jelly is not appropriate in the emergency department; specific burn ointments are commonly used. Rubbing the skin intensifies the burn injury.

> *Test Taking Strategy—Look at the key words "most appropriate" as they relate to the emergency nursing care of a chemical burn. Recall that reducing and eliminating contact between the corrosive substance and the skin will minimize the injury and is the first action the nurse should take (option 1). Review first-aid measures when responding to an incident involving a chemical burn if you had difficulty answering this question.*
>
> **Cognitive Level**—*Analyzing*
> **Client Needs Category**—*Physiological integrity*
> **Client Needs Subcategory**—*Physiological adaptation*

99. 3. Oropharyngeal suctioning is performed when the client is unable to cough and raise sputum. Other indications of the need for suctioning include dyspnea, cyanosis, and moist breath sounds. Identifying the type of cough, sputum characteristics, and respiratory rate are important assessments, but they are not criteria for determining the necessity for suctioning a client.

> *Test Taking Strategy—Analyze to determine what information the question asks for, which is the best evidence of a need for oropharyngeal suctioning. Recall that coughing and expectoration are the usual means by which accumulated pulmonary secretions are cleared from the airway. Therefore, if a client cannot perform either or both of these actions, the nurse must clear the airway for the client with suction. Review indications for suctioning the airway if you had difficulty answering this question.*
>
> **Cognitive Level**—*Applying*
> **Client Needs Category**—*Physiological integrity*
> **Client Needs Subcategory**—*Physiological adaptation*

100. 3. A change in the client's level of consciousness is a clinical indication of intracranial bleeding. If drowsiness or sleepiness occurs and the client cannot be easily aroused, the physician should be notified. Drinking extra fluids or keeping the client in bed is usually unnecessary. Although it is important to observe for signs of bleeding, the most dangerous bleeding occurs within the skull.

> *Test Taking Strategy—Look at the key words "most important" as they relate to discharge instructions provided to the family of an older adult who experienced trauma secondary to a fall. Recall that head trauma, identified in the stem, can cause slow bleeding within the cranium, a life-threatening consequence. The increased intracranial pressure can lead to altered consciousness. Therefore, option 3 is the priority information to convey at the time of discharge. Review the signs and symptoms of a closed head injury and complications such as a subdural bleed if you had difficulty answering this question.*
> **Cognitive Level**—*Analyzing*
> **Client Needs Category**—*Physiological integrity*
> **Client Needs Subcategory**—*Reduction of risk potential*

101. 2. The presence of a foul or unusual odor from within a cast indicates an infection. A crack or indentation in the cast does not indicate infection but compromises the integrity of the cast. Blood on the cast surface indicates bleeding beneath the cast.

> *Test Taking Strategy—Use the process of elimination to help select the option that best describes the possibility that an infection exists beneath the cast. Recall that purulent drainage is accompanied by a foul odor, which leads to selecting option 1 as the answer. Review signs and symptoms of an infection related to fractures and casting if you had difficulty answering this question.*
> **Cognitive Level**—*Applying*
> **Client Needs Category**—*Physiological integrity*
> **Client Needs Subcategory**—*Physiological adaptation*

102. 3. The primary concern associated with the use of aspirin to treat a fever in children is Reye's syndrome. The American Academy of Pediatrics recommends that aspirin and combination products containing aspirin not be taken by anyone younger than 19 years during an illness accompanied by a fever. Acetaminophen (Tylenol) is safe for the relief of minor symptoms, such as fever and headache. Ibuprofen (Nuprin) and naproxen (Naprosyn) are effective in relieving pain.

> *Test Taking Strategy—Analyze to determine what information the question asks for, which is a drug that is associated with the development of Reye's syndrome. Knowledge of this relationship leads to selecting option 3. Review the factors that contribute to the development of Reye's syndrome if you had difficulty answering this question.*
> **Cognitive Level**—*Understanding*
> **Client Needs Category**—*Physiological integrity*
> **Client Needs Subcategory**—*Pharmacological therapies*

103. 2. The best technique for bringing medication to the base of an ampule is to tap the stem several times with a fingernail. Allowing the ampule to stand, flipping the ampule back and forth, or rolling the ampule does not bring the medication trapped in the ampule stem into the base of the container.

> *Test Taking Strategy—Analyze to determine what information the question asks for, which is an appropriate nursing action when withdrawing medication from an ampule. Recall that medication sometimes collects above the narrow neck of the glass ampule. Tapping the stem tends to facilitate moving the trapped medication into the lower portion of the ampule. Review the technique for withdrawing parenteral medication from an ampule if you had difficulty answering this question.*
> **Cognitive Level**—*Analyzing*
> **Client Needs Category**—*Physiological integrity*
> **Client Needs Subcategory**—*Pharmacological therapies*

104. 3. One of the necessary criteria for maintaining the effectiveness of traction is that the weights must hang free of the floor. The legs may or may not be parallel to the bed, depending on the type of traction applied. Although comfort is a desirable outcome of traction, it is not an indication of the traction's effectiveness. If the feet resist the pull of traction by resting on the footboard, the traction's efficiency is reduced.

> *Test Taking Strategy—Use the process of elimination to help select the option that describes the best evidence that traction is able to function correctly. Option 1 can be eliminated because it is not a principle that can be applied to all types of traction. Option 2 may appear attractive, but comfort is not necessarily an indication of correctly applied traction. Option 4 can be eliminated because it describes a factor that interferes with the function of traction. Option 3 emerges as the correct answer. Review the nursing care of a client in traction if you had difficulty answering this question.*
> **Cognitive Level**—*Evaluating*
> **Client Needs Category**—*Physiological integrity*
> **Client Needs Subcategory**—*Basic care and comfort*

105. 2. The symptoms of pulmonary edema include orthopnea (sitting up to improve breathing), sudden dyspnea, pink frothy sputum, cyanosis, bounding pulse, elevated blood pressure, severe apprehension, and moist or gurgling respirations.

> *Test Taking Strategy—Analyze the information about which the question asks which is the best indication that a client is developing pulmonary edema. Recall that pulmonary edema is accompanied by respiratory distress as the client has more and more difficulty maintaining adequate exchange of gases at the alveolar-capillary membranes. Option 2 is most descriptive of the manifestations associated with this*

pathophysiology. Review the signs and symptoms exhibited by a client developing pulmonary edema if you had difficulty answering this question.
Cognitive Level—*Applying*
Client Needs Category—*Physiological integrity*
Client Needs Subcategory—*Physiological adaptation*

106. 3. If an actual visit to the cardiac catheterization laboratory cannot be arranged, showing the child pictures of the laboratory and equipment will facilitate the teaching process. The site of catheter insertion is the femoral artery or an antecubital vessel; therefore, the chest would not be cleaned with an antiseptic. The child should have nothing by mouth for at least 4 hours before the procedure. For this procedure, the child will be lightly sedated but not unconscious.

Test Taking Strategy—Analyze to determine what information the question asks for, which is evidence that a child has been prepared appropriately for a cardiac catheterization. Recall that a 5-year-old will be best prepared by using pictures (option 3). Options 1, 2, and 4 are not accurate statements. Review teaching strategies appropriate for a school-age child if you had difficulty answering this question.
Cognitive Level—*Evaluating*
Client Needs Category—*Health promotion and maintenance*
Client Needs Subcategory—*None*

107. 1. The initial step in planning a bladder retraining program is determining the client's voiding pattern. Knowing the voiding pattern helps the nurse develop an individualized voiding schedule. Limiting fluid intake is not recommended; the client needs an adequate fluid intake to keep the urine dilute and prevent a fluid deficit. Requisitioning a commode, if appropriate for the client, is done after collecting data about the voiding pattern.

Test Taking Strategy—Analyze to determine what information the question asks for, which is the first step to take when planning bladder retraining. Recall that assessment is the first step in the nursing process, which leads to selection of option 1. Review the components of bladder retraining if you had difficulty answering this question.
Cognitive Level—*Analyzing*
Client Needs Category—*Physiological integrity*
Client Needs Subcategory—*Basic care and comfort*

108. 4. The client performs Crede's maneuver by positioning the hands on the abdomen and applying light pressure over the bladder to initiate voiding. Voiding is achieved without the use of a catheter. The maneuver does not require any special breathing techniques.

Test Taking Strategy—Analyze to determine what information the question asks for, which is the correct method for performing Crede's maneuver. Recall that Crede's maneuver is a technique for facilitating urination by applying manual pressure over the

bladder (option 4). Review the purpose and manner in which Crede's maneuver is performed if you had difficulty answering this question.
Cognitive Level—*Evaluating*
Client Needs Category—*Physiological integrity*
Client Needs Subcategory—*Basic care and comfort*

109. 3. The prone position is one in which the client is placed on the abdomen. If a supine position is indicated, the client is placed on the back. A side-lying position is a lateral position. A sitting position is referred to as Fowler's position.

Test Taking Strategy—Analyze to determine what information the question asks for, which is the body position that correlates with being prone. Recall that a prone position is one in which a person is face down (option 3). Review body positions, focusing on the prone position, if you had difficulty answering this question.
Cognitive Level—*Evaluating*
Client Needs Category—*Physiological integrity*
Client Needs Subcategory—*Basic care and comfort*

110. 4. Grunting on expiration is a signal of respiratory distress, indicating that effort is needed to move air out of the lungs. Newborn infants normally have a respiratory rate between 30 and 60 breaths/minute. In addition, they normally breathe abdominally and have an irregular breathing pattern.

Test Taking Strategy—Use the process of elimination to help select the option that identifies a characteristic of respiratory distress manifested by a newborn. Options 1, 2, and 3 may appear attractive, but they all describe normal breathing characteristics in a newborn infant. Review normal and abnormal characteristics of respiration in newborns if you had difficulty answering this question.
Cognitive Level—*Applying*
Client Needs Category—*Physiological integrity*
Client Needs Subcategory—*Physiological adaptation*

111. 1. Chemotherapeutic drugs are given to cure cancers, decrease tumor size, or prevent or treat metastases. The side effects of these drugs vary, depending on the length of treatment and the specific drug used. Common side effects of chemotherapy include anorexia, nausea and vomiting, diarrhea, soreness or ulcerations of the mouth, loss of hair (baldness), bone marrow depression, and the inability to fight infection. Voice changes and abdominal distention are not usually associated with chemotherapeutic drugs. Weight loss usually results from the cancer itself, although weight loss can occur due to anorexia, nausea, vomiting, and diarrhea.

Test Taking Strategy—Look at the key words "most likely" as they relate to a consequence of cancer chemotherapy. Recall that drugs used to treat cancer target fast-growing and reproducing cells, which include the hair, GI mucosa, blood cells, and fetal tissue. This leads to selecting option 1 as the best

answer from among the options provided. Review common side effects of drugs used to treat cancer if you had difficulty answering this question.
Cognitive Level—*Applying*
Client Needs Category—*Physiological integrity*
Client Needs Subcategory—*Pharmacological therapies*

112. 3. Placing a pillow on the abdomen and applying firm, light pressure reduces strain on the incision, which reduces discomfort. Flexing the knees or lying supine are not as likely to promote comfort as applying pressure. It is more advantageous to administer an analgesic shortly before, rather than after, a client coughs or performs other activities that cause discomfort.

> *Test Taking Strategy*—*Look at the key words "most appropriate" in relation to a nursing intervention to minimize incisional discomfort caused by coughing after surgery. Recall that placing pressure over the incision limits movement that triggers pain receptors in the traumatized tissue. Review the techniques that reduce incisional pain if you had difficulty answering this question.*

Cognitive Level—*Analyzing*
Client Needs Category—*Physiological integrity*
Client Needs Subcategory—*Basic care and comfort*

113. 4. Liquid nutritional supplements are best offered between meals so that the supplement is not substituted for the meal. If the supplement is given before a meal, the client may not eat an adequate amount of food. If it is given with or soon after a meal, the client may be too full to consume the entire volume.

> *Test Taking Strategy*—*Use the process of elimination to help select the option that corresponds with the best time for offering a nutritional supplement. Recall that the term "supplement" implies "in addition to"; in this case, in addition to a meal. This leads to the selection of option 4 as the best answer. Review methods for increasing the dietary intake of a client with imbalanced nutrition if you had difficulty answering this question.*

Cognitive Level—*Analyzing*
Client Needs Category—*Physiological integrity*
Client Needs Subcategory—*Basic care and comfort*

114. 2. Covering the edges of the cast with waterproof material such as plastic helps prevent soiling the cast. Cotton wadding should not be inserted unless ordered by the physician. Offering the bedpan at more frequent intervals does not necessarily prevent soiling of the cast, especially if the child is not toilet trained (which is usual for an 18-month-old child). Plastic pants are contraindicated because they hold moisture and contribute to the disintegration of the cast.

> *Test Taking Strategy*—*Look at the key words "most appropriate" in reference to a recommended intervention for preventing a hip-spica cast from being*

soiled by urine or feces. The desired technique is one that acts as a barrier to these substances (option 2). Review the nursing care of a client in a hip-spica cast if you had difficulty answering this question.*
Cognitive Level—*Analyzing*
Client Needs Category—*Physiological integrity*
Client Needs Subcategory—*Basic care and comfort*

115. 4. When a lumbar puncture is performed, the client is placed either in a side-lying position, with the knees drawn up and the back flexed, or in a sitting position, with the back flexed. Both of these positions increase the space between the vertebrae to facilitate insertion of the needle within the lumbar interspaces with minimal trauma. Neither the prone position nor the recumbent position is appropriate for increasing the vertebral space. Sitting in the supine position with the head of the bed at a 45-degree angle will not allow access to the vertebral space needed for the procedure.

> *Test Taking Strategy*—*Analyze to determine what information the question asks for, which is the correct position that facilitates performing a lumbar puncture. Because the physician must have access to the spine and the space between the vertebrae to insert the needle, option 4 is the best answer. Review positioning options when assisting with a lumbar puncture if you had difficulty answering this question.*

Cognitive Level—*Analyzing*
Client Needs Category—*Physiological integrity*
Client Needs Subcategory—*Reduction of risk potential*

116. 2. Locking the wheels ensures that the wheelchair remains in place during the transfer. Although wearing slippers provides warmth and some protection for the client's feet, doing so is not as important as locking the wheels. Raised side rails and a trapeze can help the client change positions, but they are not the best safety measures during a transfer.

> *Test Taking Strategy*—*Use the process of elimination to help select the option that describes the safest method for transferring a client from a bed to a wheelchair. Although slippers (option 1) are preferred over bare feet, unless they have nonskid soles, they do not necessarily contribute to the client's safe transfer. Option 3 appears attractive because the client can use the upper side rails for support, but it is not the best answer. Option 4 can be eliminated because a trapeze is not used during a transfer. Option 2 is the best remaining answer. Review the technique for assisting an uncompromised client from bed to a wheelchair if you had difficulty answering this question.*

Cognitive Level—*Analyzing*
Client Needs Category—*Physiological integrity*
Client Needs Subcategory—*Basic care and comfort*

117. 1. Closing doors helps keep the fire confined to its location of origin and slows or prevents its spread into other areas. It is important to assemble with others at the nurses' station to await instructions, but this activity is appropriate only after the environment is secured. Searching for smoke takes valuable time better spent closing doors. Staying with an immobile client is admirable, but nurses have a responsibility to ensure the protection of all clients, not just one who may be difficult to evacuate.

Test Taking Strategy—Analyze to determine what information the question asks for, which is an action that contains a fire. Recall that one of the methods used to prevent or limit the spread of a fire is closing open doors (option 1). Doing so first ensures the safety of clients and personnel on the nursing unit. Review a fire plan to identify appropriate actions to take if you had difficulty answering this question.
Cognitive Level—*Evaluating*
Client Needs Category—*Safe and effective care environment*
Client Needs Subcategory—*Safety and infection control*

118. 3. Unless the physician orders otherwise, the standard for care is to use sterile normal saline solution when irrigating an indwelling catheter because the urinary tract is considered sterile. Normal saline solution is an isotonic solution that will not damage cells. It is incorrect to use an unsterile solution of distilled water or tap water. Hydrogen peroxide is not commonly used when irrigating urinary catheters.

Test Taking Strategy—Analyze to determine what information the question asks for, which is an appropriate solution for irrigating an indwelling catheter. Recall that a sterile solution is a necessity to avoid introducing pathogens into the lumen of the catheter and ultimately into the bladder. Option 3 is the only choice that identifies this type of solution. Review the technique for irrigating an indwelling catheter if you had difficulty answering this question.
Cognitive Level—*Analyzing*
Client Needs Category—*Physiological integrity*
Client Needs Subcategory—*Reduction of risk potential*

119. 1. A client with obstructive jaundice characteristically has dark brown urine. The change in color is due to the excretion of bilirubin through the kidneys rather than through the intestinal tract. In addition to dark brown urine, clay-colored stools are evident. The other physical assessments have no relationship to obstructive jaundice.

Test Taking Strategy—Look at the key words "most likely" as they refer to an assessment finding unique to a client with obstructive jaundice. Dark brown urine is seen in clients with this disorder (option 1). Review the signs and symptoms associated with obstructive jaundice if you had difficulty answering this question.
Cognitive Level—*Applying*
Client Needs Category—*Physiological integrity*
Client Needs Subcategory—*Physiological adaptation*

120. 2. Everyone sheds dead skin cells during bathing. In African American clients, the dead skin cells are more obvious because the cells retain their dark pigmentation. This finding is commonly misinterpreted as a disregard for hygiene. Soap cannot physically or chemically remove pigmentation.

Test Taking Strategy—Use the process of elimination to help select the option that best explains the brown discoloration on a washcloth when bathing a client of color. Recall that melanin is the skin pigment found in higher amounts in African Americans. The statements in options 1 and 4 can be eliminated because they are not scientifically accurate. Option 3 can be eliminated because soap removes dirt, debris, and epidermal cells, but not necessarily melanin. Review the cultural differences associated with African Americans and the related transcultural care if you had difficulty answering this question.
Cognitive Level—*Applying*
Client Needs Category—*Safe effective care environment*
Client Needs Subcategory—*Coordinated care*

121. 2. After allowing sufficient time for a response, moving on to another area of assessment shows respect for the client; however, the nurse must document the lack of response in the client's assessment. Failure to respond to one area of assessment does not justify discontinuing further efforts to assess mental status. With only limited data, it is inaccurate to assume that a client who does not respond is demented or illiterate.

Test Taking Strategy—Look at the key word "most appropriate" in reference to an appropriate response to a cooperative client's silence when assessing a component of a mental status examination. Showing respect for a client is a principle that is important in all nurse–client interactions. Therefore, by moving on, the nurse avoids embarrassing the client or contributing to the client's frustration. Option 2 is the appropriate action to take from among the choices provided. Review characteristics of a therapeutic nurse–client relationship if you had difficulty answering this question.
Cognitive Level—*Analyzing*
Client Needs Category—*Psychosocial integrity*
Client Needs Subcategory—*None*

122. 3. Preventing falls is a major goal when caring for clients with osteoporosis. Even a minor fall can result in a fracture. Consuming dairy products is a healthy behavior, but it is not likely to reverse longstanding osteoporosis. Increasing bone density is a goal of medical therapy. Having osteoporosis does not justify restraining a client in a wheelchair.

Test Taking Strategy—Look at the key words "most appropriate" as they refer to a goal when caring for a client with osteoporosis. Recall that osteoporosis weakens the density of bones. Preventing a

fall (option 3) is the best answer because it identifies a realistic short-term goal that relates to safety. Options 1 and 2 have merit, but the identified goals cannot be achieved in a short period of time. Option 4 is totally inappropriate. Review the differences between short-term and long-term goals if you had difficulty answering this question.
Cognitive Level—*Analyzing*
Client Needs Category—*Safe and effective care environment*
Client Needs Subcategory—*Coordinated care*

123. 1. Clients with diabetes mellitus are prone to developing visual changes that may result in blindness. Other major diabetic complications include renal failure, coronary artery disease, increased susceptibility to infection, changes in circulation, and peripheral nerve damage. Indigestion, urine retention, and tremors are significant problems, but they are not commonly associated with diabetes mellitus.
> *Test Taking Strategy*—*Analyze to determine what information the question asks for, which is an assessment finding that correlates with a complication experienced by persons who have had diabetes for an extended period. Recall that retinopathy is a complication of diabetes mellitus that is manifested by diminished vision (option 1). Review the complications of diabetes mellitus and their manifestations if you had difficulty answering this question.*
> **Cognitive Level**—*Applying*
> **Client Needs Category**—*Physiological integrity*
> **Client Needs Subcategory**—*Physiological adaptation*

124. 4. A transient earache for 1 to 3 days is common after a tonsillectomy and adenoidectomy. The discomfort is due to pain referred from the throat to the ear. When giving discharge instructions, the nurse should advise parents of the possibility of earache. Severe pain for the first 7 days after surgery, difficulty swallowing for 3 weeks, and expectorating bright red blood are not normal and should be brought to the physician's attention.
> *Test Taking Strategy*—*Look at the key words "most appropriate" in reference to discharge instructions for parents of a child who has undergone a tonsillectomy and adenoidectomy. Recall that a mutual nerve innervates the throat and ears, and so trauma to the throat secondary to removing the tonsils may be experienced as an earache, making option 4 the best answer. Parents need to know that the symptom is temporary and is not an indication of a complication. Review the discharge instructions after a child's tonsillectomy and adenoidectomy if you had difficulty answering this question.*
> **Cognitive Level**—*Analyzing*
> **Client Needs Category**—*Physiological integrity*
> **Client Needs Subcategory**—*Reduction of risk potential*

125. 1. Emptying the collection bag decreases the weight and pull on the skin to which the appliance is attached. Fluids are not restricted; restricting fluids concentrates the urine and increases the risk of dehydration, skin irritation, and infection. To avoid skin impairment, an appliance is generally not changed on a daily basis; however, a loose or uncomfortable appliance must be changed. It is unlikely that avoiding gas-forming foods would have any effect on appliance attachment.
> *Test Taking Strategy*—*Analyze to determine what information the question asks for, which is a suggestion for ensuring attachment between an ostomy appliance and the peristomal skin. Recall that the larger the volume of stool contained within an appliance, the greater the stress on the adhesive holding the appliance in place. This should lead to selecting option 1 as the best answer. Review health teaching related to managing an ostomy appliance if you had difficulty answering this question.*
> **Cognitive Level**—*Analyzing*
> **Client Needs Category**—*Physiological integrity*
> **Client Needs Subcategory**—*Physiological adaptation*

126. 3. The full-term infant usually has plantar creases over the entire surface of the soles of the feet. The presence of anterior transverse creases is associated with prematurity. Lanugo over the shoulders, back, and forehead is a normal finding in the full-term newborn. A strong Moro reflex and a fully flexed posture are also characteristic of the full-term newborn.
> *Test Taking Strategy*—*Analyze to determine what information the question asks for, which is an abnormal finding during the assessment of a full-term infant. Option 3 describes an abnormal finding. Review normal assessment findings of newborn full-term infants if you had difficulty answering this question.*
> **Cognitive Level**—*Applying*
> **Client Needs Category**—*Health promotion and maintenance*
> **Client Needs Subcategory**—*None*

127. 4. Alteplase (Activase) converts plasminogen to plasmin, which is then able to degrade the fibrin present in clots. The therapeutic action is to dissolve clots, restoring blood flow. The medication does not lower anxiety or systolic blood pressure, nor does it prevent arrhythmias.
> *Test Taking Strategy*—*Analyze to determine what information the question asks for, which is an explanation of the therapeutic action of alteplase. Recall that alteplase is a thrombolytic agent, the action described in option 4. Review the action of thrombolytic agents and the mechanism by which they achieve their desired effect if you had difficulty answering this question.*
> **Cognitive Level**—*Understanding*
> **Client Needs Category**—*Physiological integrity*
> **Client Needs Subcategory**—*Pharmacological therapies*

128. 1, 2, 3, 5. When developing a care plan for older adults, it is important for nurses to recognize the wide variety of physiologic changes that occur with aging and how such changes impact daily life. For example, the efficiency and contractile strength of the heart diminish with aging, resulting in decreased cardiac output. The risk for aspiration increases due to a weaker gag reflex and a delay (not increase) in gastric emptying. Renal blood flow and glomerular filtration rate decrease by 50% between ages 20 and 90. Serum albumin levels also decrease, resulting in less availability of albumin for binding with drugs. Older adults have less body water, causing drier mucous membranes.

Test Taking Strategy—Analyze to determine what information the question asks for, which is characteristic changes associated with aging. Alternative-format "select all that apply" questions require considering each option independently to decide its merit in answering the question. Select options that correlate with physiologic changes among older adults. Review physiological differences between individuals who make up the gerontologic population and adults in younger age groups if you had difficulty answering this question.
Cognitive Level—Applying
Client Needs Category—Physiological integrity
Client Needs Subcategory—Physiological adaptation

129.

6. Wash your hands and then put on gloves.
3. Apply a tourniquet and palpate veins.
1. Clean the venipuncture site thoroughly.
4. Hold the skin taut, and pierce the skin, entering the vein.
5. Note the blood in the chamber, and release the tourniquet.
2. Withdraw the needle and connect the tubing.

Before any procedure, the nurse needs to review the physician's order for accuracy, and then assemble the needed equipment on a convenient space close to the client. Next, the nurse must wash the hands and put on gloves before touching the client. Assessing the vein status thoroughly is essential to ensuring a successful puncture on the initial attempt. After selecting an appropriate vein, the nurse cleans the venipuncture site by wiping thoroughly and allows the site to dry. Holding the skin taut, the nurse pierces the skin with the needle, watching for a blood return in the catheter chamber. After noting the blood return, the nurse releases the tourniquet, withdraws the needle, and attaches the I.V. tubing. Lastly, the nurse documents the site of the I.V. line, the size of the catheter, the date and time, and that the I.V. line is infusing without difficulty.

Test Taking Strategy—Look at the key words "order in which the actions are performed," which requires identifying a sequence from start to finish. In this case, list the steps when performing a venipuncture in the correct order. Review the steps in starting an I.V. infusion if you had difficulty answering this question.
Cognitive Level—Analyzing
Client Needs Category—Physiological integrity
Client Needs Subcategory—Reduction of risk potential

130. 3. An individual visit with a new resident of a long-term care facility is most beneficial in helping the resident adjust to the new environment and decrease loneliness. Reminiscence therapy is beneficial to promote memory but must be done more frequently than weekly to aid in loneliness. Group activities are important ways to promote socialization; however, individuals can be lonely in a group. Watching television does not aid in decreasing loneliness.

Test Taking Strategy—Look at the key words "most helpful" in reference to preventing loneliness experienced by a client who has just been transitioned to a long-term care facility. Recall that preserving and continuing relationships with others that are significant to the client reduce feelings of loneliness, as suggested in option 3. Review methods for meeting the emotional needs of older clients who are living separate from family and friends by choice or necessity if you had difficulty answering this question.
Cognitive Level—Analyzing
Client Needs Category—Psychosocial integrity
Client Needs Subcategory—None

131. 4. An ethical dilemma occurs when there is a conflict in values and a distinction between right and wrong. Nurses are accountable for reporting the unethical practices of other nurses. Taking a client's medications is unethical. It is not an ethical dilemma to place a baby for adoption. A client has the right to refuse medications. Elder abuse is a criminal matter that involves law-enforcement agencies. Nurses are accountable for documentation and referral.

Test Taking Strategy—Analyze the information about which the question asks, which is the type of concerns referred to an ethical practices committee. Read the rationale to help recall the realm into which the options fall. Option 4 describes an ethical concern that may result in the loss of the nurse's license depending on the seriousness of the incident, its validation, and the decision of the committee. Review the mission of ethics committees if you had difficulty answering this question.
Cognitive Level—Understanding
Client Need Category—Safe and effective care environment
Client Needs Subcategory—Coordinated care